HEALTH SYSTEMS PERFORMANCE ASSESSMENT

DEBATES, METHODS AND EMPIRICISM

HEALTH SYSTEMS PERFORMANCE ASSESSMENT

DEBATES, METHODS AND EMPIRICISM

Edited by

Christopher J.L. Murray and David B. Evans

World Health Organization
Geneva

WHO Library Cataloguing-in-Publication Data

Health systems performance assessment : debates, methods and empiricism / edited by
Christopher J.L. Murray, David B. Evans.

    1. Health care evaluation mechanisms 2. Outcome assessment (Health care)
    3. Health care surveys — methods 4. Quality of health care 5. Empirical research
    I. Murray, Christopher J.L. II. Evans, David B.

    ISBN 92 4 156245 5   (NLM classification: W 84.1)

Design and production: Digital Design Group, Newton, MA USA
Printed in Canada by Webcom, Ltd.
Cover: **Sheet Discussing Cosmology and the Light of the Sun and Moon from *Codex Leicester*
by Leonardo da Vinci.** Image credit: Seth Joel/Corbis. Image is courtesy of Corbis at URL: http:
//www.corbis.com.

Table of Contents

PART IV: METHODS AND EMPIRICISM

INPUTS

FINANCING

PROVISION AND COVERAGE

RESOURCE GENERATION

STEWARDSHIP

POPULATION HEALTH

LIST OF TABLES

LIST OF FIGURES

LIST OF BOXES

Foreword

High quality scientific evidence is increasingly available to help the providers of health care make decisions about what types of investigations to order for an individual patient, and how to treat any health problems that are identified. "Evidence-based medicine" has been facilitated by the availability of results from different types of clinical trials, epidemiological studies, and meta-analyses which allow the results of many small studies to be combined in a way that reduces the uncertainty about the overall effect of clinical interventions.

This evidence is critical to the way that the World Health Organization fulfils part of its mandate, the part linked to setting standards and providing technical advice on clinical issues. To illustrate, WHO recently developed a set of internal "guidelines for guidelines" that specify the steps that should be taken to ensure any clinical guidelines released or endorsed by WHO are based on the best available scientific evidence (URL: http://www.who.int/health-systems-performance/).

While clinical guidance is one important part of WHO's mandate, the Organization also receives continual requests from countries to provide advice on how best to organize and manage health systems. It is critical that this advice be based on rigorous scientific evidence, but when I took office in 1998, it became clear that there was little systematic evidence on what makes health systems perform well and what makes them perform badly. One reason was that there were few clear statements of what health systems were supposed to achieve, so the case-studies that existed measured outcomes and goal attainment in a variety of ways. Another was that it is clearly much more difficult to base evidence in this area on the same types of trials that are typically used to show evidence of clinical effectiveness. It is rarely possible, for example, to randomize parts of a country into experimental groups to assess the impact of different types of health system reforms.

Policy advice on health system development has, until recently, been based on case-studies and, sometimes, ideology. Case-studies can be useful, just as case-reports provide valuable information to clinicians. On the other hand, evidence-based clinical medicine cannot exist without epidemiological studies, which operate on the premise that, although all individuals are different in many ways, there is much to be learned from what they have in common. This is also important in the area of health systems performance. All systems and cultures are different in many ways, but there is a great deal of knowledge to be gained from the experiences of groups of countries taken together, learning from common experience.

This volume reports on five years of work to strengthen the scientific evidence-base on health systems performance. It began with the development of a framework that clearly specifies a parsimonious set of key goals to which health systems contribute, a framework widely discussed with experts, policy-makers and the governing bodies of WHO. After a series of consultations on specific components, the first set of figures on goal attainment and health system efficiency was published in *The World Health Report 2000* for all 191 countries that were then Members of the Organization.

That report generated an enormous amount of interest and debate among policy-makers and the scientific community, and it was decided that WHO should report on the performance of the health systems of its Member States at regular intervals. To facilitate this, a further series of consultations was held, and I established an independent Scientific Peer Review Group to review the techniques proposed by the Secretariat for future rounds of performance assessment. I am delighted to introduce this volume, which traces the history of this work, openly reports the debates and criticisms, and describes the methods proposed for future rounds of performance assessment after the peer review and consultation process.

This is not the end of the work. Science advances over time with open debate. I am sure the techniques and methods will develop further over the next decades, but I am also sure that the area of health systems performance assessment is now moving in the right direction. The movement towards basing health policy development and advice on rigorous scientific evidence has begun.

Gro Harlem Brundtland
Director-General
World Health Organization

LIST OF ACRONYMS

AFRO	WHO Regional Office for Africa	EPHF	Essential Public Health Functions
AMRO	WHO Regional Office for the Americas	EURO	WHO Regional Office for Europe
APNHAN	Asia Pacific National Health Accounts Network	FFC	Fairness in Financial Contribution
BNE	Basic Need Expenditure	GCC	Gulf Co-operation Council
BOD	Burden of Disease	GIS	Geographic Information System
CARICOM	Caribbean Community	GPE	WHO Global Programme on Evidence for Health Policy
CEA	Cost-Effectiveness Analysis	HALE	Healthy Life Expectancy
CES	Conference of European Statisticians	HDI	Human Development Index
DALE	Disability-Adjusted Life Expectancy	HFC	Household Financial Contribution
DALYs	Disability-Adjusted Life Years	HIPC	Heavily Indebted Poor Countries
DEA	Data Envelopment Analysis	HIS	Health Information System
DFID	Department for International Development, UK	HOPIT	Hierarchical Ordered Probit
DHS	Demographic and Health Surveys	HPCM	Hierarchical Partial Credit Model
DIF	Differential Item Functioning	HSPA	Health Systems Performance Assessment
DRD	Deputy Regional Director	ICD	International Classification of Diseases
DTP3	Diphtheria-Tetanus-Pertussis Vaccine (Three Doses of)	ICF	International Classification of Functioning, Disability and Health
EC	European Commission, European Communities	ICIDH	International Classification of Impairments, Disabilities and Handicaps
ECE	Economic Commission for Europe	II	Inequality Index
ECLAC	Economic Commission for Latin America and the Caribbean	ILO	International Labour Organization
EHSPI	Enhancing Health Systems Performance Initiative of WHO	IMF	International Monetary Fund
EIP	WHO Evidence and Information for Policy Cluster	IMR	Infant Mortality Rate
		JPRM	Joint Programme Review Mission
EMRO	WHO Regional Office for the Eastern Mediterranean	LE	Life Expectancy
		MMR	Maternal Mortality Ratio

NGO	Non-Governmental Organization
NHA	National Health Accounts
OECD	Organisation for Economic Co-operation and Development
ONUSIDA/ SIDALAC	UNAIDS/AIDS Program of the Economic Commission for Latin America in Spanish
PAHO	Pan American Health Organization
PHC	Primary Health Care
PPP	Purchasing Power Parity
REVES	International Network on Health Expectancy (French: Réseau sur l'Espérance de Vie En Santé)
ROC	Receiver Operating Characteristic
SEARO	WHO Regional Office for South-East Asia
SMPH	Summary Measures of Population Health
SPRG	Scientific Peer Review Group
UC	Universal Coverage

U5-MR	Under-Five Mortality Rate
UNDP	United Nations Development Programme
UNICEF	United Nations Children's Fund
USAID	U.S. Agency for International Development
WB	World Bank
WHA	World Health Assembly
WHO	World Health Organization
WHO-CHOICE	WHO CHOosing Interventions that are Cost-Effective Initiative
WHOCC	WHO Collaborating Centres
WHR	World Health Report
WHS	World Health Survey
WPRO	WHO Regional Office for the Western Pacific
WR	WHO Representative
YLD	Years Lived with Disability
YLL	Years of Life Lost

List of Affiliations

The affiliation for all authors except those specified below is:
Evidence and Information for Policy Cluster (EIP)
World Health Organization
Avenue Appia 20
CH-1211 Geneva 27
Switzerland

Affiliations of Non-EIP Authors

Dr Omar B. Ahmad
School of Public Health
University of Ghana
P.O. Box LG13
Legon, Accra
Ghana

Dr Rob M.P.M. Baltussen
Institute for Medical Technology
    Assessment (iMTA)
Erasmus University Rotterdam
P.O. Box 1738, Room L3-121
3000 DR Rotterdam
Netherlands

Ms Lydia Bendib
Officer for Surveillance of Risk
    Factors Related to NCDs
Noncommunicable Diseases and
    Mental Health Cluster
World Health Organization
Avenue Appia 20
CH-1211 Geneva 27
Switzerland

Prof. Gouke J. Bonsel
Public Health Methods Unit
Dpt. Social Medicine, Room J3-
    304
Amsterdam Medical Centre
P.O. Box 22660
1100 DD Amsterdam
Netherlands

Dr Yang Cao
Department of Health Statistics
Faculty of Health Services
Second Military Medical
    University
Shanghai 200433
People's Republic of China

Mr Charles Darby
Social Science Administrator
Agency for Healthcare Research
    and Quality
540 Gaither Road
Rockville, Maryland 20850
United States of America

Dr Philip Davies
Deputy Secretary
Health and Ageing
Mail Drop Point 84
GPO Box 9848
ACT 2601, Canberra
Australia

Dr Julio Frenk
Minister of Health
Secretaria de Salud
Lieja 7
06696 Mexico, D.F.
Mexico

Dr Michel Guillot
Center for Demography and
    Ecology
University of Wisconsin-Madison
1180 Observatory Drive
Madison, WI 53706
United States of America

Dr Piya Hanvoravongchai
Researcher
International Health Policy
    Program, Thailand (IHPP)
Ministry of Public Health
Bangkok
Thailand

Dr Gary King
David Florence Professor of
    Government
Center for Basic Research in the
    Social Sciences
34 Kirkland Street, Room 2
Harvard University
Cambridge, MA 02138
United States of America

Dr Bao Liu
Department of Health Economics
School of Public Health
Fudan University
138 Yi Xue Yuan Road
Shanghai 200032
People's Republic of China

Dr Alan D. Lopez
Head, School of Population
    Health
Professor of Medical Statistics
    and Population Health
The University of Queensland
Herston Road
Herston Qld 4006
Australia

Dr Amala de Silva
Department of Economics
University of Colombo
Colombo
Sri Lanka

Ms Maria Villanueva
Social Scientist
Behavioural Risk Factor
    Surveillance Group
Department of Noncommunicable
    Disease Prevention and Health
    Promotion
Noncommunicable Diseases and
    Mental Health Cluster
World Health Organization
Avenue Appia 20
CH-1211 Geneva 27
Switzerland

Mr Riadh Zeramdini
Department of Econometric and
    Economic Policy (DEEP)
Ecole des Hautes Etudes
    Commerciales (HEC)
CH-1015 Lausanne
Switzerland

ACKNOWLEDGEMENTS

Putting together a book of this size and scope is a long, complex, and challenging undertaking. Stanislava Nikolova was the managing editor and played the lead role in keeping authors on track, editing their prose, liaising with printers and layout experts, editing text and proofs, and generally ensuring that the book was completed. Without her untiring, cheerful, and competent work, this book could never have been completed, and the editors and authors owe her an enormous debt of gratitude.

Emmanuela Gakidou's fine eye was key to the design of the cover and her motivational and organizational skills were invaluable in keeping the process on track. In addition, Emmanuela and Margaret Hogan kindly diverted time from other projects to proofread long and complicated texts. Sandrine Bijotat-Combe, Gabriella Covino, Sonia Enna, Sue Piccolo, Margaret Squadrani, and Marie-Claude von Rulach provided diverse and important inputs—from arranging consultation meetings, to preparing the report of the Scientific Peer Review Group, to typing printing contracts. Marc Kaufman and his team guided the production process in a competent, professional, and patient manner. The inputs of all of these people are gratefully acknowledged.

A large part of the initial encouragement and intellectual stimulation for the World Health Organization's work on health systems performance assessment originated with Julio Frenk, who played a key role in developing the framework that is the basis of this volume. This intellectual and organizational debt is acknowledged with thanks. We are also grateful to the authors of the chapters for their intellectual input and hard work over a number of years. Their willingness to revise drafts on numerous occasions and to accept many suggested changes was important to the successful completion of the process. Many people in addition to the authors contributed to the preparation of the different chapters, and they are gratefully acknowledged in the individual chapters. Finally, Professor Sudhir Anand as Chair, and the members of WHO's Scientific Peer Review Group (SPRG) on health systems performance assessment, stimulated the authors to make important improvements and modifications to the methods and empirical work, reflected in this volume. The opinions expressed in the text remain, of course, those of the authors.

Parts of the work presented in this volume have been supported by a number of funders. We would like to particularly note the support over a number of years of the United Kingdom Department for International Development. The United States Agency for Healthcare Research and Quality (AHRQ) seconded Charles Darby to work with WHO on the development of the concept and measurement of responsiveness which served as an important impetus to that work. Research on the development of anchoring vignettes, the household survey instruments for health state description and valuation, National Health Accounts and catastrophic health payments were supported by grants from the National Institute on Aging (P01-AG17625).

CJLM
DBE

Part I

INTRODUCTION

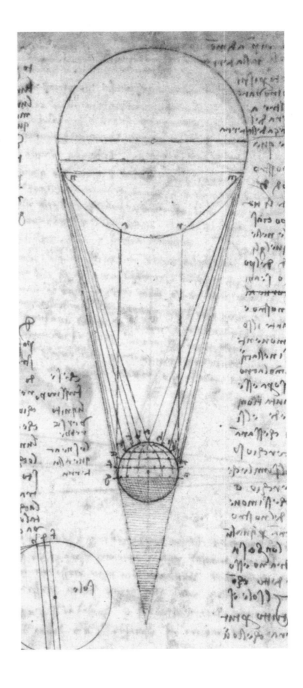

Chapter 1

Health Systems Performance Assessment: Goals, Framework and Overview

Christopher J.L. Murray, David B. Evans

Introduction

Over the last five years, WHO has undertaken a major effort to establish a common conceptual framework for health systems performance assessment, to foster the further development of tools to measure its components, and to work with countries in applying these tools to measure and then to improve health systems performance. The first milestone in this work, the publication of *The World Health Report 2000 (1)*, has generated considerable media attention, controversy in some countries, and debate in academic journals. The interest and discourse on alternative approaches to measuring health systems performance stimulated by the *Report* has, through a broad process of engagement, led to an important evolution of the WHO framework and methods for health systems performance assessment.

This volume brings together in one place the substance of many of these key debates and reports, methodological advances, and new empiricism reflecting the evolution of the WHO approach since the year 2000. Specifically, the volume presents many differing regional and technical perspectives on key issues, major new methodological developments, and a quantum increase in the empirical basis for cross-country performance assessment. It also gives the full report of the Scientific Peer Review Group's exhaustive assessment of these new approaches.

In this chapter, the primary motivation of WHO's work on health systems performance and its specific objectives are outlined. A brief history of this work, including some of the key debates and resolutions in the Executive Board of WHO and the establishment and report of a Scientific Peer Review Group (SPRG), provides important contextual information. The final

framework for health systems performance assessment that has emerged from the consultative and review process is then presented in some detail. This is followed by a concise overview of the different parts of the book, highlighting areas which contain new methods and empiricism, as well as the way the recommendations of the SPRG have influenced the development of the work. The chapter concludes with a few reflections on the overall process.

Goals and Objectives for WHO's Work on Health Systems Performance Assessment

Decision-makers in low-, middle- and high-income countries are faced with five common problems as they struggle to make appropriate choices to improve the performance of their health systems. These problems, and the potential of WHO to contribute to addressing them, provide the motivation for the work on health systems performance that has developed in the Organization since July 1998.

First, national and international discourse on the often complicated issue of health system design or reform is hampered by the lack of clarity about the nature of the fundamental or intrinsic goals for health systems. National debates on health policy frequently have focused on short-run objectives or instrumental goals such as cost containment, expanding public infrastructure, reducing waiting times or introducing user fees. Policy dialogue can often lose sight of the primary goal of the health system, improving population health. WHO, by fostering a common framework and language for health systems analysis, can help various national actors identify end-goals and the means to achieve them. Given WHO's historical emphasis on equity, a health system's framework can highlight the critical importance of this challenge. Embedding this emphasis on equity in the formulation of the goals and the analytical framework for health systems is justified not only by WHO's commitments reflected in strategies such as Health For All, but also by the evidence that populations in most countries give high priority to issues of equity (2). The fact that sometimes equity seems to fall off national health policy agendas reinforces the necessity of articulating its importance among the end-goals of a health system, in a coherent framework of inputs, processes, outputs and outcomes.

Second, often if a decision-maker has sought advice on an issue of the design or reform of a health system, the answer has depended substantially on which consultant or expert is asked. A question on how to finance a health system may elicit answers ranging from the imposition of public sector user fees, to the expansion of social insurance or the creation of medical savings accounts. The diversity of responses to the same question in the same context is in contrast to the convergence of answers from different clinicians on the appropriate management of acute myocardial infarction. This marked difference between health systems and clinical advice reflects the comparative development of the evidence-base for the two areas. Decades of activity by the evidence-based medicine movement and the widespread use of randomized clinical trials to explore the efficacy of interventions has led to greater consistency of clinical approaches to solving similar problems. In contrast, the evidence-base on how to improve the performance of health systems is still lacking.

When health system reforms have the potential to affect millions, why is the evidence-base relatively weak, leaving room for ideology and personal opinion to be among the main inputs into health policy debates? Part of the reason must be that the experimental designs to evaluate health system policies more rigorously are difficult to organize both technically and politically. Part of the reason may be that sufficient research resources have not been invested in the systematic evaluation of policy. In addition, we believe that the absence of a common framework for analysing health systems has impeded progress. When nearly every study uses a somewhat different approach to defining inputs, processes, outputs and outcomes, and a different set of measurement methods, it is difficult to build a global knowledge base. A key goal, there-

fore, for WHO's work on health systems performance, is to contribute over a period of decades to a stronger global evidence base on what works and what does not for health systems. This long-term vision will be greatly facilitated by the development and adoption of a common framework and measurement methods.

Third, in many countries, health systems are fragmented and actors consider only pieces of the puzzle at one time. Decision-makers may feel accountable only for the resources and activity in their direct day-to-day managerial control. The Government, however, in its role as steward of the entire health system, must assume responsibility for the totality of the health system and its contribution to key social goals such as improved health. It is important to create an accountability framework that encourages decision-makers to consider the big picture. A culture of accountability for outcomes means that the media, legislature, executive and civil society all recognize that their actions should be judged by their impact on outcomes. A culture that keeps the focus and energy of society on outcomes, including equity, can have a profound influence on policy in the medium and long terms. Accountability for outcomes requires an accepted framework for the end-goals of health systems, affordable metrics of these outcomes, and transparency. Through its work on health systems performance assessment, WHO is committed to providing countries with a coherent set of tools that can be employed to foster outcomes accountability.

Fourth, in many countries and in international debates, attention has been focused on delivering certain proven technologies to improve health, such as immunization for children or DOTS for tuberculosis.[1] Using the most cost-effective technologies to improve health or reduce health inequalities is an important dimension of health policy. Making sure that new technologies or new strategies to deliver these technologies are rapidly incorporated into health systems is also a high priority. Unfortunately, health system issues such as building human resource capacity, the organization of health service provision, or the development of financing methods that do not exclude the poor, often fail to capture the same policy attention as technology choice. One important goal for WHO's work on health systems performance is to encourage a balanced view of the importance of health system platforms for delivering the right technologies to the right people. A common framework and set of measurement methods, as presented in this volume, can help provide such a balanced context for policy debate.

Finally, the complexity of health system issues and the use of specialized technical language have often limited wide participation in national policy debate. Reflecting WHO's constitutional commitment to providing health information to the general public, one final goal for the development of the WHO framework for health systems performance assessment has been to empower civil society and the general public to become active participants in the formulation of national health policies.

Bearing these broad strategic goals in mind, the specific objectives for WHO's work on health systems performance have been fourfold. The first is to develop a framework for describing, analysing, and ultimately improving the performance of health systems, which is flexible enough to be useful for both developing and developed countries. The second is to develop effective and affordable tools that can be used by national decision-makers to provide timely and relevant information on the performance of their systems. This information can inform strategic decision-making and programme management, and allow progress towards national targets to be monitored and policies to be evaluated. Objective three is to develop tools for national decision-makers in a manner that maximizes the potential for shared learning across countries. In this way, national efforts to monitor performance will contribute to a growing global evidence base on what works and what does not. The final objective is to undertake periodic assessments of the performance of the health systems in the 192 WHO Member States and report this information to national policy-makers and the world public health community.

These specific objectives have only been partially achieved. The work in this volume presents the framework, a number of important tools to monitor performance, and widespread experience with some of these tools. There is not yet a great deal of information available on the range of national experiences using these tools, but the information base is growing. Mexico, Indonesia, Iran, and Uganda, for example, have now had considerable experience applying the framework and associated measurement tools. Some tools, such as measurement methods for assessing the availability of human resources or provider quality, are still being actively developed. To fully achieve the goals and objectives of WHO's work on health systems performance will require long-term efforts. The present volume is an important milestone in this work, but it is only one step on a long road.

THE WORLD HEALTH REPORT 2000, CONSULTATIVE PROCESS ON HEALTH SYSTEMS PERFORMANCE ASSESSMENT AND THE WAY AHEAD

Since July 1998, the Organization has been active in building the evidence base on what makes health systems work. One reason that the Evidence and Information for Policy Cluster (EIP) was created in WHO was to coordinate this work. EIP has formulated a common framework for health systems performance assessment, developed and refined indicators, proposed and tested measurement tools, and assisted countries as requested in their application and interpretation for policy purposes.

WHO's efforts have built on several decades of work on the measurement and analysis of health systems undertaken in a number of related fields. As reflected in more detail in the relevant chapters dealing with health system functions, there has been substantial and important work on the overall challenge of assessing performance through structure, process and outcome. The proposed indicators and measurement strategies for the social goals to which health systems contribute have benefited from the extensive literature on measuring individual and population health, social inequalities in health, equity in health finance, and patient satisfaction. The work presented in this book continues this rich tradition.

The WHO approach has also involved extensive consultation with the research and policy communities, governments and the Governing Bodies of WHO. The conceptual framework was first published in early 2000 and was presented and discussed in the Executive Board and World Health Assembly (3). It was then peer reviewed and published in the international scientific literature (4). The framework, indicators and measurements were presented in substantial detail in *The World Health Report 2000* (1). The report reflected not only the work to develop a consistent framework for analysis that could be used in a standard way in all countries, but also the development of new and innovative tools for measuring key outcomes and inputs to health systems. It involved a huge empirical effort to measure health system attainment and efficiency in all 191 countries that were then members of the Organization.[2]

To make this work more useful to policy-makers, estimates of the uncertainty intervals around key outcomes were reported side by side with the estimates of goal attainment for each country. This is the first time, to our knowledge, that an international agency has reported the uncertainty around the figures it publishes. The techniques used to develop the report have been published in technical discussion papers that were made available on the internet after the release of *The World Health Report 2000*, and many components have been peer reviewed and published (5–20).

The publication of *The World Health Report 2000* with its country rankings attracted a huge amount of media attention as well as subsequent interest and debate involving governments, donor agencies, NGOs, and the scientific community (21–35). It also led to a considerable number of requests from Member States of the Organization for information and technical assistance on how to apply the tools in their settings, in a number of cases for the purposes of subnational performance assessment. Because of the great interest in the topic and its evident importance to governments, the Director-General decided to report on the health systems performance of the countries that are members of WHO on a regular basis, a decision endorsed by the Executive Board of the Organization. It took note "with satisfaction of the measures proposed by the Director-General to help Member States contribute to the WHO assessment of their health system performance regularly, namely…to compile a report on the performance of Member States' health systems every two years."[3]

To ensure that the methods continued to develop, strengthened by broad consultation with Member States and the scientific community, a wide range of activities were undertaken. Six regional consultations were held with representatives of governments and the academic community from countries in all regions of WHO. Technical consultations on different aspects of health systems performance under way since 2000 were broadened to include a range of topics raised at the regional consultations. More than 170 technical experts and health policy-makers from over 69 countries participated in the regional and technical consultations. The reports of all consultations are included in their entirety in this volume, the regional consultations in Part II and the technical consultations in Part III. The Director-General also established a Scientific Peer Review Group (SPRG) to review the framework and methods proposed by the Secretariat for the next round of analysis. In addition, all the reports of the regional and technical consultations, plus the available scientific literature, were provided to the SPRG for its consideration. The complete report of the SPRG is included in this volume.

In response to the input from the consultations and the wider debate, WHO continued to develop the methodologies. It also sought new sources of data which included the establishment of the WHO Multi-country Survey Study on Health and Responsiveness 2000–2001, designed to pilot new approaches to measuring health, responsiveness, and household financial contributions to the health system from representative population surveys. Sixty-three countries participated. Drawing on this work, the consultations and the wider debate, the Secretariat proposed a modified framework to the SPRG and a mode of analysis for the second round of performance assessment.[4]

At the same time, an Advisory Board was established to inform the Director-General on the process surrounding the peer review. It consisted of three members of the Executive Board and three from the Advisory Committee on Health Research (ACHR), chaired by Professor M. Fathalla from Egypt who was also the chair of the ACHR. It met twice, finally reporting that "the review process had been comprehensive, objective, transparent and informative."

The SPRG was chaired by Professor Sudhir Anand from the University of Oxford. It comprised 13 independent experts, at least two from each of the six WHO Regions, with a balance between technical experts and users of evidence about health systems performance. It had three meetings between November 2001 and May 2002. Members reviewed documentation from the consultations and the Secretariat, and considered external submissions. They were also provided with copies of all published debates about the methods and results, as well as with any unpublished documents that were available.[5] Members of the SPRG had access to relevant WHO staff and all associated documentation. They chose to work interactively with WHO, often suggesting new ways of undertaking various components of the work that were then tested by WHO and the results reported back to the SPRG. The chair of the SPRG also visited Brazil to meet with government and academic critics. Brazil was selected because it was the country where criticism of *The World Health Report 2000* had perhaps been the strongest.

The review identified several issues that were strategic rather than scientific in nature. These strategic issues included: the importance of ongoing scientific input into the exercise of health systems performance assessment; whether health system indicators should be published alphabetically or ranked; whether an overall composite measure of health system goal attainment should be published; the importance of strengthening national capacity to monitor health systems performance; and the need for an explicit data audit trail for published figures. In January 2003, the Director-General made proposals to the Executive Board on each of these strategic issues, reproduced in the annex of this chapter. Based on the discussions at the Executive Board, the Director-General proposed that for the next round of performance assessment, a composite measure of attainment would not be published, but that development work on composites would continue with the possibility that they would be included in future rounds. The proposals were accepted by the Executive Board.

Subsequent chapters of this book report the approaches to performance assessment emerging from the consultations and the peer review process. Science is, of course, never static, and the methods and applications will continue to develop over time through experience in applying the methods at the national and subnational levels, and through interactions with governments and the scientific community. These refinements will, we hope, be reflected in future editions of this volume.

A FRAMEWORK FOR HEALTH SYSTEMS PERFORMANCE ASSESSMENT

In this section, the final framework emerging from the consultations and the peer review process is presented briefly, as it is important to understanding the way the components, described in subsequent chapters, fit together. Some of the key debates about the components are highlighted in the next section of this

chapter, which outlines the organization of the book, and considerably more detail is found in the chapters that report on the deliberations of the SPRG and the regional and technical consultations.

DEFINITION OF THE HEALTH SYSTEM

The health system could be defined in a number of ways. The narrowest draws the boundaries tightly around the activities under the direct control of the Ministry of Health, which are often a relatively limited set of personal curative services. It is depicted as the smallest circle in Figure 1.1 and would exclude activities such as the marketing of insecticide impregnated mosquito nets or taxes designed to reduce the use of tobacco or alcohol products.

The second definition corresponds to the second smallest circle in Figure 1.1 and is more inclusive. The system comprises personal medical and non-personal health services, but not intersectoral actions designed specifically to improve health. The type of intersectoral actions in which WHO has long been engaged, such as water and sanitation programmes, would not be included. Stewards of the health system would have no incentive to advocate for the introduction of anti-smoking legislation if they took responsibility only for this narrow set of health actions.

The third definition includes all actors, institutions and resources that undertake health actions—where the primary intent of a health action is to improve health. It is broader than personal medical and non-personal health services. It incorporates selected intersectoral actions in which the stewards of the health system take

Figure 1.1   Boundaries of the health system

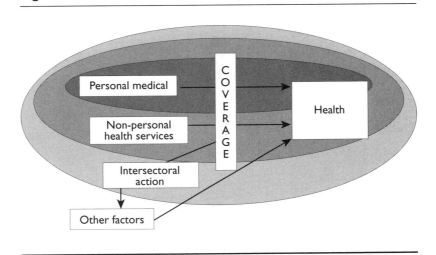

responsibility to advocate for health improvements in areas outside their direct control, such as legislation to reduce fatalities from traffic accidents. This is shown by the largest circle in Figure 1.1.

The final option would be to define the health system as including all actions that might contribute to improving health. It would comprise every box in Figure 1.1 because all areas of human endeavour, e.g. agriculture, education, tourism, can influence health status. There would no longer be any operational distinction between the health system and any other system, and it would not be possible to assess the performance of the health system separately.

The definition proposed by WHO after the consultations and endorsed by the SPRG, is the third option. Its use would encourage governments, as stewards of the health system, to focus on a definable set of actions whose primary intent is to improve health. Ministries of health would take responsibility for personal and non-personal interventions, but also for encouraging a limited set of intersectoral actions designed specifically to improve health.

GOALS

To be outcome-focused, it is necessary to define a set of goals and to measure progress towards achieving them. The health system contributes towards many outcomes that are socially desirable, including improving health, educational attainment, and individual incomes. A set of criteria is needed to determine which goals are intrinsically valued and which of those should be measured routinely.

Two criteria were used to define a goal as intrinsically valued.

■ It is possible to raise the level of attainment of the goal while holding the level of all other intrinsic goals constant—i.e. an intrinsic goal must be at least partially independent of all other goals. Partial independence does not mean completely independent, only that it is possible for the goal to vary independently from the other intrinsic goals.

■ Raising the level of attainment of an intrinsic goal is always desirable—more is always better than less. If the levels of attainment of other intrinsic goals are kept constant and raising the level of attainment of a given goal is not necessarily desirable, it is an instrumental and not an intrinsic goal.

An instrumental goal is desirable because it contributes to the attainment of an intrinsic goal. More

is not necessarily better than less, holding attainment of the intrinsic goals constant.

To warrant measuring attainment of an intrinsic goal regularly, two additional criteria apply. The health system must be able to make a large enough contribution to the goal to justify the expense of measuring it regularly, and it must be feasible to measure the goal's impact on the health system on a regular basis.

It is universally accepted that the defining goal of health systems, the reason why they exist, is to improve health. There are two components to this intrinsic goal. The system should seek not only to improve the average *level of population health*, but also to reduce *health inequalities* in the population.

When individuals interact with the health system, it influences their well-being through improvements in health, but their well-being is also affected by other aspects of these interactions, related to the way they are treated and the environment in which they are treated. This is defined as health system responsiveness, the second intrinsic goal. Again, concern lies not just with increasing the average *level of responsiveness*, but also with reducing *inequalities in responsiveness* within the population.

The third intrinsic goal is the *fairness in financial contribution* to the health system. After a considerable debate, a fair system was defined as one in which household contributions to finance the health system represent an equal sacrifice. Equal sacrifice means that no household would become impoverished or pay an excessive share of its income to finance the health system. It also means that poor households should contribute a smaller share of their incomes to the system than rich households.

There are, therefore, three intrinsic goals and five components in the final framework (Table 1.1). Each intrinsic goal meets the criteria established above. More health (or more responsiveness and more fairness in financial contribution) is always better than less, holding attainment on the other goals constant. Even though improved responsiveness can encourage

Table 1.1   Intrinsic goals to which the health system contributes

	Level	Distribution
Health	✓	✓
Responsiveness	✓	✓
Financial contribution		✓
	Quality	Equity

people to seek care, thereby improving health, it is possible to increase responsiveness by providing better amenities, for example, with no impact on health outcomes. The three goals are partially separable, and the impact of the system is sufficiently large to warrant measuring them regularly.

It is recognized that educational attainment and income-earning potential might meet the criteria of an intrinsic goal, but it is not practical to routinely measure and report the contribution of the health system to those goals. It might, however, be useful to undertake this type of exercise from time to time, as illustrated in the report of the Commission on Macroeconomics and Health which shows the impact of health on economic growth and income (36). The commission's work was valuable in focusing the attention of the international community on the role of health in economic development.

HEALTH SYSTEM FUNCTIONS

Four basic functions contribute to determining the observed levels of goal attainment: financing, service provision, resource generation, and stewardship. This is illustrated in Figure 1.2.

Health system financing is the process by which revenues are collected, accumulated in fund pools, and allocated to specific health actions. It includes revenue collection, fund pooling, and purchasing. Service provision refers to the way inputs are combined to allow the delivery of a series of interventions or health actions. These comprise personal health services—preventive, diagnostic, therapeutic, or rehabilitative—and non-personal services such as

mass health education, legislation, and the provision of basic sanitation facilities.

Health systems also include institutions that produce inputs—particularly human resources, physical resources such as facilities and equipment, and knowledge—to the functions of service provision and financing. Education and research centres, construction firms, and an array of organizations producing technologies such as pharmaceutical products, devices and equipment fulfil these roles. Strategies for resource generation, the third function, can be critical to allowing the health system to perform to its potential or restricting its ability to do so.

Stewardship is a neglected function in many health systems, extending beyond the conventional notion of regulation. It involves setting, implementing and monitoring the rules of the game for the health system; assuring a level playing field among all actors in the system (particularly purchasers, providers and patients); and identifying strategic directions for the health system as a whole (37).

Although these functions were defined in the original framework, and *The World Health Report 2000* summarized the available evidence relating them to goal attainment and efficiency, WHO has now begun to formulate indicators of how well they are being performed so that they can be measured regularly alongside the measurement of key outcomes. For example, the effective coverage of key interventions is an important indicator of the service provision function, and mediates the way inputs are transformed into the outcomes that people value. This is reflected in Figure 1.1. Information on the way the four functions

Figure 1.2   From functions to outcomes

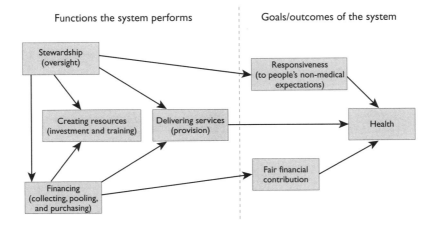

are being performed will be a direct entry point to the development of policies designed to improve performance and will give policy-makers the opportunity to "drill down" to identify the areas responsible for their observed levels of intrinsic goal attainment.

INPUTS

The ability to produce desirable outcomes and the ability to perform key functions appropriately depend on the inputs available to the system. National Health Accounts provide important information on the money value of all resources used by the system. It is also useful to have information on individual components if possible—in particular the availability of human and physical resources of different types. Low levels of goal attainment could be due to inadequate resources or to inappropriate combinations of the available resources. Information on the quantities of inputs and how they are combined is as important to the development of policy as information on health system functions and end-goal attainment.

ATTAINMENT AND EFFICIENCY

Efficiency relates the levels of goal attainment to the inputs used to achieve them. The vertical axis in Figure 1.3 depicts goal attainment, while the horizontal axis shows the quantity of inputs used by the system. M is the maximum achievable outcome for the inputs, taking into account non-health system determinants. L is the minimum possible level of goal attainment in the absence of inputs, necessary because health would not be zero in the absence of the system—e.g. the entire population would not die if the health system failed to exist.[6] Efficiency is defined as the ratio of attainment (above the minimum) to the maximum possible attainment (also above the minimum), i.e. what proportion of the potential health system contribution to goal attainment is actually achieved for the observed level of resources. At point A, it is $e/(e + f)$.

Efficiency measures the extent to which the resources used by the health system achieve the goals that people value. It is not an intrinsic goal because it is not valued for its own sake. It is simply a way of ensuring that the resources available to the system are combined to produce the maximum possible benefit to society—e.g. it is instrumental to achieving the goals important to people.

Efficiency had been called "performance" in *The World Health Report 2000*. The SPRG accepted the recommendation of a number of regional consultations that the term "performance" should be redefined to include the entire range of activities from measuring goal attainment, to the efficiency of input use, to the way the system is functioning. Efficiency would then be used in the narrower sense to capture how well inputs are utilized and combined to produce the outcomes people desire.

Efficiency could be measured in terms of attainment on a single goal or in terms of a composite indicator of attainment. *The World Health Report 2000* reported efficiency in terms of health alone, and in terms of a weighted sum of attainment on the three intrinsic goals. As shown earlier, the SPRG felt that the question of whether to report composite attainment in future rounds of performance assessment was a strategic rather than a scientific issue, and the Director-General has decided that it will not be included in the second round.

This framework determines the organization of the remainder of the book, particularly Part IV. Part IV, described below, begins with the inputs to the health system, before considering recent developments relating to the functions and intrinsic goals. Composite attainment and efficiency are then examined before focusing on key methodological questions relating to data availability and analysis. It concludes by addressing the issue of how best to ensure the policy relevance of health systems performance assessment.

ORGANIZATION OF THE BOOK

This volume is organized into five parts. The first is this chapter which introduces the health systems performance assessment framework and its evolution from July 1998 to June 2003. The second contains the

Figure 1.3   Defining health system efficiency

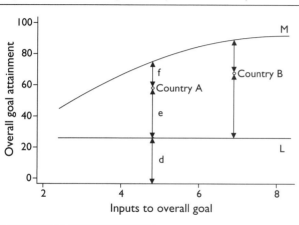

reports of the six consultations held in each of WHO's Regions. These consultations involved broad participation of national experts and decision-makers. The third part comprises the reports of the technical consultations on specific topics related to health systems performance assessment. In a number of cases, the technical consultations were organized in response to ideas and suggestions that emerged from the regional consultations. As noted above, the full report of the SPRG is found in Part V.

The bulk of the book is in Part IV, covering the methods and empiricism relating to different components of the health systems performance assessment framework. Some of this work was prepared for presentation to the SPRG, and incorporates reflections on the debates since the publication of *The World Health Report 2000*. Other chapters report the results of more recent work in response to the final recommendations of the peer review. The tools and methods presented in Part IV provide the basis of future rounds of health systems performance assessment.

Part IV begins with two chapters, 16 and 17, on methods for quantifying the *inputs* to health systems and then using this information for policy purposes. The work WHO has undertaken to develop National Health Accounts for all its Member States is described. This detailed and painstaking exercise has resulted in the production of unprecedented information on total and per capita health expenditures with a breakdown into private, public, and external. The tables routinely reported by WHO in its annual *World Health Report* also provide information on expenditures channelled through private and social insurance mechanisms.

The SPRG emphasized the importance of continuing this work and expanding the breakdown of health expenditure to give more detail, on functions and beneficiaries for example. It also encouraged the Organization to move towards quantifying the levels of physical capital and human resources available to each Member State. Efforts to move in this direction are reported in the chapter on the resource allocation function, described subsequently.

The World Health Report 2000 did not attempt to define or measure indicators of how the four functions of health systems were being performed. The need to develop a series of "process" indicators for the functions was a strong recommendation of the SPRG, the technical and regional consultations, and the wider debate. This would provide timely information to policy-makers about which parts of their systems are working as desired, and which parts are not.

In addition, the SPRG underlined that it was important not only to develop indicators, but also to provide guidance to countries about how the financing function affects goal attainment and efficiency. The work undertaken in WHO to define indicators for this function is described in Chapter 18, while the development of health financing policies based on the best available evidence is the focus of Chapter 19. The goal is to provide countries with information on what types of financing systems are associated with high levels of health systems performance.

The service provision and coverage function is particularly important for countries seeking to understand the reasons for their measured levels of health systems performance. From the regional consultations and the broader global debate, it became clear that information on the delivery of key interventions to people who needed them would supplement information on inputs, functions, and outcomes such as health, responsiveness, and fairness in financial contribution. Coverage of key interventions can be thought of as a health system output that mediates the way the health system contributes to achieving the goal of improving population health.

Coverage is defined in Chapter 20 as the probability that an individual who needs an intervention will obtain it. The idea is familiar in the fields of immunization or tuberculosis control where coverage figures are routinely reported, but it can be generalized to all types of interventions. The technical consultation on conceptualizing and measuring coverage also showed that it can be transformed from an *ex post* measure of the percentage of a population which received an intervention to an *ex ante* construct of the probability that a person who needs an intervention will receive it (38). Chapter 20 then incorporates the quality of an intervention by defining effective coverage as the probability that a person needing the intervention obtains the potential health gain achievable from it—effective coverage is contingent firstly on receiving the intervention in a timely manner, and secondly on receiving it at a level of quality necessary to assure the potential gain in health. Chapter 21 broadens the discussion of service provision to define a variety of additional indicators of how this function is being performed.

The effective coverage concept is applied to the assessment of diphtheria-tetanus-pertussis (DTP3) and measles vaccination in Chapter 22. This work not only illustrates the approach, but also provides important evidence on the limitations of health service delivery registries as a tool for monitoring coverage.

Inequalities in effective coverage are illustrated using DTP3 and measles vaccination in Chapter 23.

As effective coverage is the means through which health systems can influence population health, the possibility of disaggregating gaps into those due to the physical unavailability of technologies, lack of financial access, lack of physical access, and problems with cultural acceptability and provider quality would be valuable to policy-makers. This type of information would show the areas in which action is necessary to improve coverage. The conceptual framework for this is presented in Chapter 20, and work to develop an approach to measuring these gaps in practice is continuing.

The resource generation function is critical if countries are to successfully scale-up interventions to meet the Millennium Development Goals now that more resources are becoming available for health from external or domestic sources. Shortages of human resources are particularly important because they cannot be overcome in the short term except, perhaps, through migration. The role of out-migration in exacerbating such shortages in poor countries is particularly important for analysis. Proposals to measure and report indicators of the resource generation function are presented in Chapter 24.

The SPRG welcomed the emphasis that WHO placed on the stewardship function in *The World Health Report 2000*, something which had been neglected in many debates about health systems performance and the role of government. Since the measurement of stewardship poses significant conceptual and technical challenges, it encouraged WHO to continue work on developing indicators for this function which would be useful for policy purposes. Proposals are found in Chapter 25.

With the discussion of inputs and functions, Part IV then moves to recent methodological developments relating to the measurement of the five key health system outcomes and associated empirical work. The level of population health is described in nine chapters covering all the components required for producing the final summary measure of population health, healthy life expectancy (HALE). This set of chapters begins with a presentation of key concepts (Chapters 26 and 27), followed by a description of the methods for measuring mortality with an empirical analysis of how mortality varies across WHO Member States (Chapters 28 and 29). Next are three chapters on non-fatal health outcomes (Chapters 30–32), including a review of the health state valuations that allow fatal and non-fatal outcomes to be combined into one summary measure of population health. The SPRG welcomed the effort made by WHO, reported in Chapter 32, to improve health state valuation methods. It also endorsed the proposal to use valuations derived from the forthcoming World Health Survey as a basis for calculating levels of population health in the future.

A summary measure of population health (SMPH), healthy life expectancy, is described in Chapter 33, building on the inputs of the preceding chapters, and variations in HALE across the world are reported as well. The SPRG affirmed the value of reporting and comparing health levels over time and across countries using a SMPH, and it argued that the use of a SMPH complements, rather than competes with, information on each component part. That being said, WHO will continue to make information on the components of HALE—fatal and non-fatal outcomes and the health state valuations used to combine them—available to countries. This is the reason for dedicating nine chapters of this volume to population health, reporting on each of the components of HALE as well as on the overall SMPH.

The concept and measurement of health inequality generated some of the most contentious debates subsequent to the publication of *The World Health Report 2000*, largely relating to three issues (39–44). The first was that WHO chose to report total inequality in health outcomes rather than inequality between social groups. Total inequality measures allow the identification of both between-group and within-group inequalities. Within a population, people in the tails of the distribution, i.e. those with the lowest levels of health, can be identified so analysts and policy-makers are able to determine if these people have any common characteristics and how their health can be improved. Total inequality is clearly a function of the between-group inequality (regardless of how groups are defined) and the within-group inequality; it provides the context to interpret differences between groups.

The second issue for health inequality was that information on health outcomes for adults was not available at the individual level. Therefore, the indicator was based on inequality in child survival using data from the Demographic and Health Surveys (DHS). Data were imputed for countries in which there had been no DHS survey based on the observed relationship between inequality and other variables from the DHS data.

Thirdly, there was a debate about whether the total inequality in health outcomes was of interest to policy-makers, or whether they were concerned only with those parts of inequality thought to be unfair or directly under their control. During the technical consultation on health inequalities, it was debated whether voluntary or genetic risks should be excluded from the assessment of total variation. For example, variations in health linked to the first cannot be considered to be unfair, while many of those linked to the second cannot be reduced as yet by health actions.

The SPRG recommended that the total health inequality or "pure health inequality" approach be developed further at both a methodological and an empirical level, while acknowledging that measuring inequality between socioeconomic groups is important to policy-makers. Ideally, an indicator of inequality in HALE is desirable, but this requires further development of methods to measure inequality in adult health expectancies, possibly using small-area data.

The major conceptual issues and debates involved in measuring and comparing health inequalities across countries are covered in Chapter 34, while the three subsequent chapters focus, respectively, on between-group versus within-group variation, determinants of inequality in child survival using the results of surveys in 39 countries, and the methods proposed for measuring inequality in the risk of adult mortality in subsequent rounds of analysis.

Five chapters cover fairness in household financial contribution. *The World Health Report 2000* proposed a definition of fairness in which the sacrifice created by financial contributions to the health system should be equal across households, independent of their health status or their utilization of health services. This "equal sacrifice" principle was operationalized as an equal share of each household's capacity to pay. The motivation for this definition was that the goal of the health system was not to redistribute income, but to ensure that the financial burden of paying for the system was distributed across households in a fair manner.

Considerable debate ensued from the publication of the index of fairness in household financial contribution in *The World Health Report 2000*. One of the main concerns was that the fairness concept espoused by WHO did not take into account the income redistributive effect of health payments. Chapter 38 reports the observed distribution of household financial contributions in the 59 countries for which reliable data were available at the end of 2002, and explores the impact of those contributions in the space of household financial burden and income. It shows that concerns with the impact of health payments on income

distribution are different from the concerns which the financial burden payments place on households. Both approaches offer useful information to policy-makers: concern with the income space shows how many households are pushed into poverty as a result of health payments, for example, while concern with the burden space identifies the extent to which payments are fairly distributed across households. For this reason the SPRG endorsed WHO's proposal to report indicators of the impact of financial contributions in both the burden and income spaces.

Definitional, empirical, and technical challenges involved in determining the fairness in household financial contribution using survey data supplemented by information from other sources are the focus of Chapter 39. It draws extensively on the debate, consultations, and deliberations of the SPRG, and highlights areas in which further development is necessary. Chapter 40 reports updated estimates of the fairness in financial contribution for an expanded set of countries, using the modified methods emerging from the debates over the past two years, while observed levels of unfairness are disaggregated into their horizontal and vertical components in Chapter 41. This chapter suggests that horizontal inequality—where households with similar means contribute different proportions of their capacities to pay to the health system—is a more pervasive form of inequality than vertical inequality linked to the regressivity of payments.

The final chapter on fairness in financial contribution (Chapter 42) focuses on ways to identify households that face financial catastrophe because of health payments. Surprisingly, some households face financial catastrophe not only in poor countries where out-of-pocket payments form a high proportion of health expenditure, but also in wealthy European countries with forms of social health insurance. A focus on this indicator allows policy-makers to concentrate their efforts on the set of people most at risk because of the way the health system is financed.

Responsiveness was a new concept introduced in *The World Health Report 2000*. The regional consultations had generally agreed that people expected more from their health systems than simply the production of health, and that the quality of basic amenities provided by the system and its client orientation influenced well-being. However, there was less agreement about the appropriate domains of responsiveness, the weights for these domains, and the method of measurement. Some observers believed that the patient satisfaction surveys undertaken in a number of European countries captured the concept of responsiveness (*45*).

As a result of these debates, responsiveness is formally defined in Chapter 43 along with the rationale for choosing a particular set of domains. A criticism of the original method used to measure responsiveness was that it allowed a system which excluded many users but was very responsive to the few people it served to appear more responsive overall than a system that served everyone, but could not afford to be equally responsive to each person. This was considered to be counterintuitive, so a way of incorporating excluded non-users into the analysis was developed and is reported in the chapter. A case is also made that responsiveness differs importantly from patient satisfaction—responsiveness measures what actually happens when individuals come in contact with the health system, not whether their encounter with it meets their expectations as clients (*46*).

Many commentators had criticized *The World Health Report 2000* for measuring responsiveness using key informants (*21;27;45*). Accordingly, WHO embarked on a Multi-country Survey Study (MCSS) in 2000–2001, designed partly to pilot a questionnaire that could be used to obtain information on patient experiences from representative household surveys. It was fielded in 63 countries. The psychometric properties of the responsiveness questions are reported in Chapter 44, which also describes how the questions were modified for subsequent inclusion in the World Health Survey that went to the field in over 70 countries in 2002.

The MCSS also allowed another common criticism of *The World Health Report 2000* to be tested. It had been widely suggested that the weights of the different domains of responsiveness would vary across cultures, and that some cultures might even give a zero weight to particular domains. Chapter 45 shows that this did not happen in the countries included in the MCSS—no domain was ever valued at zero. Although there was some variation in domain weights across settings, the variation was certainly less than suggested by some critics. Overall levels of responsiveness for the countries included in the Multi-country Survey Study are reported in Chapter 46, while Chapter 47 describes the observed extent of inequality in responsiveness across individuals within each participating country.

The World Health Report 2000 combined country scores on each of the five outcomes into a composite attainment score partly for the purposes of estimating health system efficiency. As mentioned earlier, the SPRG argued that the question of whether to continue to report a composite attainment score for each country in the future was essentially a policy or strategic decision for WHO rather than a technical one, although it raised a number of technical questions that would need to be addressed if WHO chose to do so. The SPRG acknowledged the usefulness of measuring health system efficiency, which could be estimated either in terms of composite attainment or for each outcome separately. Again, it raised a number of technical problems related to the measurement of efficiency that have yet to be resolved.

No additional estimates of overall attainment or efficiency have been made since the publication of *The World Health Report 2000*. Chapter 48 explores a key question raised repeatedly in discussion of the original work, that the weights used to combine attainment on each of the five outcome indicators would vary across countries because of differing country priorities. There is, indeed, some variation in the weights derived from household surveys, but it is not very large. Chapter 49 shows that even relatively large changes in weights would have had little impact on the country attainment ranks produced by the original work. The two chapters suggest that should WHO decide to report overall attainment in the future, an option would be to estimate two alternatives—one using the average weight across countries and one using the countries' own weights.

Some of the key questions that remain to be answered when measuring health system efficiency are considered in Chapters 50–52. One important technical question is how to treat the fact that there is often a considerable lag between introducing an intervention and its impact on outcomes such as improving population health, something that is difficult to incorporate into a traditional efficiency analysis in the absence of a long time series of data on inputs used and the outcomes that are obtained. One possible method of dealing with some of these questions, using multiple indicator models, is proposed in Chapter 52.

Some of the strongest and most widespread criticisms of *The World Health Report 2000* related to data quality and availability (*29;31;33*). One important concern was that in the absence of primary data, many estimates reported for fairness in financial contribution, responsiveness, health inequalities, non-fatal health outcomes, death rates, and life tables had been based on covariates. Another source of criticism was that the data sources and assumptions made in the analyses were not adequately documented (*33*).

The SPRG recommended that WHO make particular efforts to obtain as much primary data as possible and to explain the assumptions and extrapolations used in the treatment of missing data for the next round of health systems performance assessment. It endorsed the World Health Survey as a means of increasing the availability of primary data and recommended that WHO ensure that it is implemented at the earliest possible stage in countries with the least developed health information systems.

The SPRG also emphasized the importance of ensuring that any data collected and reported as part of the health systems performance assessment exercise are comparable across countries. It welcomed WHO's work to develop innovative approaches to enhancing the cross-population comparability of data using vignettes and measured tests, and made a number of technical suggestions and recommendations on how this work could progress in the future.

Key *measurement challenges* form the focus of Chapters 53–58. Recent work on cross-country comparability is reported in Chapters 53 and 55. Where self-reported items are used to measure health status, responsiveness, or other constructs, problems of comparability can emerge because individuals use response categories in different ways. The anchoring vignette approach with its associated compound hierarchical ordered probit (CHOPIT) statistical model provides one strategy for enhancing comparability of survey data. A systematic difference in the use of response categories across individuals or groups in the vignettes can be captured and used to adjust the responses on the individual's own experience to make it comparable with the responses of others. The anchoring vignette approach has been incorporated into the World Health Survey.

Chapter 54 discusses the role of evidence in four important areas: strategic decision-making, programme implementation or management, monitoring of outcomes or achievements, and evaluation of what works and what does not in health systems. It argues that the time-frame for these uses differs, ranging from the immediate for strategic decision-making to the long-term for building an evidence base to evaluate alternative strategies in order to improve health systems performance. In addition, the requirements for strength of evidence vary for the four uses. The chapter discusses the nature of evidence for each of the uses and the inter-relationships between them, finally proposing a consistent approach to generating and disseminating evidence for all four uses. This is built on five guiding principles: validity, reliability, comparability, consultation, and explicit audit trail. The potential of these principles to help clarify debates on the nature of evidence, differences between country data and estimates, and mechanisms to ensure independent monitoring are described.

Given the importance of understanding the contribution of poverty to the observed total inequality in health, responsiveness, and coverage, special emphasis has been given to developing valid, reliable and low-cost methods to identify households with low levels of permanent income. Chapter 56 provides a validation study of this approach in a low-, middle- and high-income country. This approach and the analytical model, a version of a hierarchical ordered probit model for dichotomous variables (DIHOPIT), have also been used in the design of the World Health Survey.

Chapters 57 and 58 focus on efforts to increase the availability of primary data using the WHO Multi-country Survey Study on Health and Responsiveness 2000–2001 and the World Health Survey (WHS) which went into the field in 2002. The MCSS has provided the empirical basis for many of the developments presented in this volume. Experience with the MCSS instrument and the 12-country WHS pilot study have also provided a rich empirical basis for the finalization of the WHS instrument. The WHS will be completed in 72 countries during 2003.

The objective of health systems performance assessment is not measurement for its own sake. It requires measurement—of inputs to the health system, of the way functions are performed, and of outcomes. It requires regular measurement. It requires the use of consistent methods and tools in this measurement. But this measurement is only useful to the extent that it provides the information policy-makers need to improve the performance of their health systems and, through it, the well-being of ordinary people. Without this, health systems performance assessment would become an academic exercise rather than a policy tool. For this reason, the last two chapters of Part IV, Chapters 59 and 60, focus on ways to increase the policy relevance of health systems performance assessment, while each of the chapters including empirical work also centres on the policy use of the information presented.

REFLECTIONS

WHO's first attempt to assess the performance of the world's health systems in *The World Health Report 2000* generated enormous interest, debate, and in many cases, a policy response. Health system issues have assumed more importance in a number of countries and internationally as a result. Certain neglected topics such as the burden of catastrophic health payments, especially in low- and middle-income countries, have become important policy issues—Iran and Mexico have enacted legislation, one of the primary purposes of which is to address fairness in financial contribution. In some cases, the speed of policy response has been impressive. Relevant, valid, reliable, and timely information on health systems performance can make a real difference if it is made available to the broad array of actors in a country.

The evolution of thinking and work on health systems performance assessment reflected in this volume reaffirms the primary goals presented at the beginning of this chapter. The WHO framework helps focus attention on outcomes, particularly inequalities in health, responsiveness, and financial contributions. At the same time, the framework holds the potential to help decision-makers identify opportunities for improving health systems performance by increasing coverage of effective interventions through modulating financing, resource generation, service provision, and stewardship. Widespread and repeated application of the framework at the national and subnational level will inevitably lead to an expanded evidence base that can be used to share knowledge and experience on what works and what does not.

Improving our collective understanding of the determinants of health systems performance is a long-term endeavour. The science of measuring performance and its causes will evolve steadily. Even a limited set of comparable data on inputs, functions, outputs, and outcomes of health systems will stimulate new hypotheses and further research. We hope that the work represented in this volume will be a catalyst for increased global attention to the challenge of improving health systems performance.

NOTES

1   DOTS is directly observed treatment, short course (see URL: http:// www.who.int/gtb/dots/whatisdots.htm).

2   Since that time, Timor Leste has joined WHO as its 192nd member.

3   The full text of Resolution EB107.R8 of 19 January 2001 can be found at URL: http:// www.who.int/gb.

4   The proposal is available at URL: http://www.who.int/ health-systems-performance/.

5   These are also listed at URL: http://www.who.int/health-systems-performance/.

6   Inputs, particularly health expenditure, are likely to be positively correlated with most non-health system determinants of goal attainment such as education and housing. Therefore, the minimum possible across countries would be seen to rise with increases in inputs due to this correlation.

REFERENCES

(1)   World Health Organization. *The World Health Report 2000. Health Systems: Improving Performance.* Geneva, World Health Organization, 2000.

(2)   Gakidou E, Murray CJL, Evans DB. Quality and equity: preferences for health system outcomes. In: Murray CJL, Evans DB, eds. *Health systems performance assessment: debates, methods and empiricism.* Geneva, World Health Organization, 2003.

(3)   World Health Organization. *Health system performance assessment. Report by the Secretariat.* Executive Board, 107th Session (Geneva, 15–23 January 2001), Document EB107/9. Geneva, World Health Organization, 2001.

(4)   Murray CJL, Frenk J. A framework for assessing the performance of health systems. *Bulletin of the World Health Organization,* 2000, 78(6):717–731.

(5)   Kawabata K. A new look at health systems. *Bulletin of the World Health Organization,* 2000, 78(6):716.

(6)   Murray CJL et al. Modified logit life table system: principles, empirical validation, and application. *Population Studies,* 2003, 57:1–18.

(7)   Mathers CD et al. Global patterns of health expectancy in the year 2000. In: Robine JM et al., eds. *Determining health expectancies.* Chichester, John Wiley & Sons, 2003:335–358.

(8)   Mathers CD et al. Healthy life expectancy in 191 countries, 1999. *The Lancet,* 2001, 357:1685–1691.

(9)   Mathers CD et al. Global patterns of healthy life expectancy for older women. *Journal of Women & Aging,* 2002, 14:99–117.

(10) Mathers CD et al. Healthy life expectancy: comparison of OECD countries in 2001. *Australian and New Zealand Journal of Public Health,* 2003, 27 (forthcoming).

(11) Mathers CD, Salomon JA, Murray CJL. Infant mortality is not an adequate summary measure of population health. *Journal of Epidemiology and Community Health,* 2003, 57(5):319.

(12) Murray CJL et al., eds. *Summary measures of population health: concepts, ethics, measurement and applications.* Geneva, World Health Organization, 2002.

(13) Murray CJL et al. *World mortality in 2000: life tables*

for 191 countries. Geneva, World Health Organization, 2002.

(14) Murray CJL, Gakidou E, Frenk J. Health inequalities and social group differences: what should we measure? *Bulletin of the World Health Organization*, 1999, 77: 537–543.

(15) Salomon JA, Murray CJL. The epidemiologic transition revisited: compositional models for causes of death by age and sex. *Population and Development Review*, 2002, 28:205–228.

(16) Salomon JA, Murray CJL. A multi-method approach to measuring health state valuations. *Health Economics* (forthcoming).

(17) Evans DB et al. Comparative efficiency of national health systems: cross national econometric analysis. *British Medical Journal*, 2001, 323:307–310.

(18) Evans DB et al. Measuring quality: from the system to the provider. *International Journal for Quality in Health Care*, 2001, 13:439–446.

(19) Xu K et al. Understanding household catastrophic health expenditures: a multi-country analysis. *The Lancet*, 2003 (forthcoming).

(20) Gakidou E, King G. Measuring total health inequality: adding individual variation to group-level differences. *International Journal for Equity in Health*, 2002, 1.

(21) Almeida C et al. Methodological concerns and recommendations on policy consequences of the World Health Report 2000. *The Lancet*, 2001, 357:1692–1697.

(22) Department for International Development (DFID) UHSRC. *World Health Report 2000: Summary and comments (Draft: 10 July 2000)*. London, Department for International Development, 2000. URL: http://www.dfid.gov.uk/

(23) Hurst J. Performance measurement and improvement in OECD health systems: overview of issues and challenges. In: Organisation for Economic Co-operation and Development, ed. *Measuring up: improving health system performance in OECD countries*. Paris, Organisation for Economic Co-operation and Development, 2002.

(24) McKee M. Measuring the efficiency of health systems. The world health report sets the agenda, but there's still a long way to go. *British Medical Journal*, 2001, 323: 295–296.

(25) Murray CJL et al. Science or marketing at WHO? A response to Williams. *Health Economics*, 2001, 10(4): 277-282.

(26) Navarro V. Assessment of the World Health Report 2000. *The Lancet*, 2000, 356:1598–1601.

(27) Navarro V. World Health Report 2000: responses to Murray and Frenk. *The Lancet*, 2001, 357:1701–1702.

(28) Ollila E, Koivusalo M. Values, ideologies and evidence-based recommendations—The World Health Report 2000: WHO's health policy drifting off course. In: Häkkinen U, Ollila E, eds. *The World Health Report 2000: what does it tell us about health systems? Analyses by Finnish experts*. Helsinki, National Research and Development Center for Welfare and Health (STAKES), 2000.

(29) Oswaldo Cruz Foundation, Ministry of Health, Brazil. *Report of the Workshop "Health Systems Performance: The World Health Report 2000"*. Rio de Janeiro, 14–15 December 2000. URL: http://www.who.int/health-systems-performance/docs/articles/oswaldocruz_report.pdf

(30) Travassos C, Buss PM. The controversial World Health Organization report. *Cadernos de Saúde Pública*, 2000, 16:890–891.

(31) Uga AD et al. Considerations on methodology used in the World Health Organization 2000 Report. *Cadernos de Saúde Pública*, 2001, 17:705–712.

(32) Wibulpolprasert S, Tangcharoensathien V. Health systems performance—what's next? *Bulletin of the World Health Organization*, 2001, 79:489.

(33) Williams A. Science or marketing at WHO? A commentary on 'World Health 2000'. *Health Economics*, 2001, 10(2):93–100.

(34) Williams A. Science or marketing at WHO? Rejoinder from Alan Williams. *Health Economics*, 2001, 10(4): 283–285.

(35) Ministry of Health, Viet Nam. *Comments and suggestions of Viet Nam Ministry of Health/Health Policy Unit as regards the World Health Report 2000*. Hanoi, Viet Nam, 2001.

(36) WHO Commission on Macroeconomics and Health. *Macroeconomics and health: investing in health for economic development. Report of the Commission on Macroeconomics and Health: Executive Summary*. Geneva, World Health Organization, 2001.

(37) Saltman RB, Ferroussier-Davis O. The concept of stewardship in health policy. *Bulletin of the World Health Organization*, 2000, 78:732–739.

(38) World Health Organization. Technical consultation on effective coverage in health systems. In: Murray CJL, Evans DB, eds. *Health systems performance assessment: debates, methods and empiricism*. Geneva, World Health Organization, 2003.

(39) Braveman P, Starfield B, Geiger HJ. World Health Report 2000: how it removes equity from the agenda for public health monitoring and policy. *British Medical Journal*, 2001, 323:678–681.

(40) Houweling TA, Kunst AE, Mackenbach JP. World Health Report 2000: inequality index and socioeco-

nomic inequalities in mortality. *The Lancet*, 2001, 357: 1671–1672.

(41) Leon DA, Walt G, Gilson L. Recent advances: international perspectives on health inequalities and policy. *British Medical Journal*, 2001, 322:591–594.

(42) Szwarcwald CL. On the World Health Organization's measurement of health inequalities. *Journal of Epidemiology and Community Health*, 2002, 56:177–182.

(43) Wolfson M, Rowe G. On measuring inequalities in health. *Bulletin of the World Health Organization*, 2001, 79: 553–560.

(44) Murray CJL, Gakidou E, Frenk J. Response to P. Braveman et al. *Bulletin of the World Health Organization*, 2000, 78(2):234–235.

(45) Blendon RJ, Kim M, Benson JM. The public versus the World Health Organization on health system performance. *Health Affairs*, 2001, 20(3):10–20.

(46) Murray CJL, Kawabata K, Valentine N. People's experience versus people's expectations. *Health Affairs*, 2001, 20(3):21–24.

ANNEX 1.1
WHO's Proposed Responses to the Strategic Issues Identified by the Scientific Peer Review Group

Assessment of Health Systems' Performance
(Extract from document EB111/6)

Action on Strategic Issues

Scientific input. In order to ensure continued scientific input and peer review of the approaches and methods for health systems' performance assessment, the Director-General is establishing five advisory groups consisting of internationally renowned experts from all WHO regions, to advise on the scientific content of the work. The groups will cover: (a) measurement of population and individual health; (b) health and health system inequalities; (c) coverage of interventions and responsiveness; (d) statistical methods relating to issues such as cross-population comparability, projections and health system efficiency; and (e) the four key functions of health systems.

Rankings. In the regional consultations and Board discussions, the question of rankings has raised considerable debate. There are several options. As in *The world health report 2000*, functions and outcomes tables could be presented for each indicator of health system inputs, with each Member State ranked from 1 to 192. Alternatively, for each indicator, separate tables could be presented by region with countries ranked within regions. Another option is to present tables alphabetically with countries assigned into several groups (e.g. from A to E) on the basis of attainment according to each indicator. After careful consideration of these options, the last approach is proposed.

Composite attainment. A composite measure of health system outcomes is an important starting point in the assessment of health system efficiency. In the regional and technical consultations, efficiency was identified as an important dimension of health systems' performance. For these reasons, it is proposed to report a composite of health system outcomes in addition to each outcome individually. The weighting would be the average of the weights derived from representative population surveys that provided answers to questions on the importance of the five outcomes.

Capacity for national reporting. National capacity for data collection and analysis needs strengthening for both the performance of health systems and for health-related Millennium Development Goal indicators. The country cooperation strategy has proved valuable for identifying needs as perceived by Member States. Capacity-building has been introduced, with, for instance, training workshops for country teams on relevant topics. WHO has also begun to work directly with country teams to adapt performance assessment tools to their settings and to analyse the results in a way that is directly relevant for policy use at the national level. This work includes surveys focusing on health, responsiveness and coverage, analysis of burden of disease and assessment of the tools for choosing interventions that are cost-effective.

Consultation with Member States and explicit data audit trails. In view of the recommendations of the consultations and the Scientific Peer Review Group, information published by WHO will adhere to the following principles. First, figures for indicators should be based on methods that produce valid, reliable and comparable results. Secondly, all figures reported by WHO should have undergone a cycle of consultation with the relevant Member State; this will ensure that the best available evidence has been used and that appropriate steps have been taken to respond to situations in which data have limitations. Thirdly, there should be an explicit data audit trail for each figure published; this would make available the primary data source, where possible, and all the analytical steps undertaken to yield a given figure. The scientific advisory group on statistical methods created by the Director-General would have an important role to play in reviewing estimation methods used in deriving figures and ensuring that the methods produce valid, reliable and comparable figures.

Part II

REGIONAL PERSPECTIVES ON PERFORMANCE ASSESSMENT

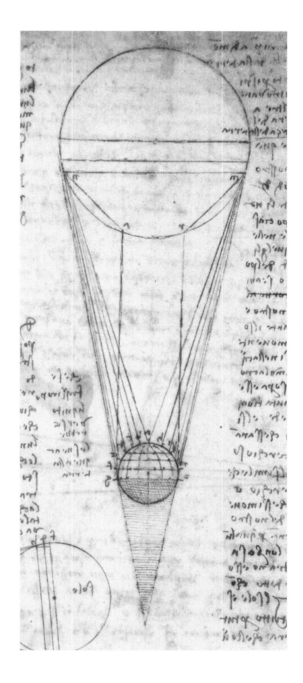

Chapter 2

AFRICAN REGIONAL CONSULTATION ON HEALTH SYSTEMS PERFORMANCE ASSESSMENT[1]

WHO REGIONAL OFFICE FOR AFRICA

MEASURING HEALTH

Agreement has been reached on the fact that the current health indicators no longer define health adequately and that there is a need for a summary measure that captures the multidimensionality of health, i.e. HALE. This regional consultation has identified a number of concerns that would accompany the introduction of such a measure and has formulated recommendations on how to address them.

CONCERNS

The principal concerns are as follows: with HALE adopted and widely used, what would happen to other indicators of health status (IMR, U5-MR, MMR, Adult MR, etc.)? How useful is HALE at the district level for programmes, for decision-makers and for other actors? How sensitive is it to change over a short period of time (i.e. an interval of two years)? What is its added advantage? No less important, do too many confusing and competing concepts (DALE, DALY, HALE, etc.) exist already?

RECOMMENDATIONS

After the adoption of the new summary measure, the concept HALE, a package should be defined to explain it in a very simple manner. Appropriate training for all has to be provided. Policy-makers need to fully understand it. Finally, both the new measure and the old ones (IMR, MMR, U5.MR, etc.) have to continue being used.

DATA REQUIREMENTS

Data are available, but the main concerns expressed at this regional consultation are the weakness of health information systems, the weakness of vital registration systems, the insufficient use of the available data and of alternative sources of data, and the lack of capacity in general. For the gradual solving of the above-mentioned concerns, it was recommended that the WHO/HQ share and update the inventory of data sources and surveys; the national health information systems be strengthened; the minimal indicators for health systems performance assessment be agreed upon; the new summary measure be relevant at the operational district level and easily understood by all; ICHDI be institutionalised and training undertaken.

MEASURING FAIR FINANCING

CONCERNS

The regional consultation pointed out several concerns associated with the ability to measure fair financing. First, the composite index emphasizes what goes in, not what comes out. Second, the formula does not take account of "non-formal" health care. It also does not include indirect costs such as transport, loss of income, time, etc. The formula itself is appropriate, but data are not yet available to support it. In addition, fairness in financial contribution index focuses on the proportion of spending on health of total income, but misses the importance of threshold financing of systems. Finally, the fairness in financing index does not consider issues of transparency.

RECOMMENDATIONS

The consultation underlined the need for advocating for a minimal financing level (threshold) and transparency, as well as for defining the cost of minimum health.

MEASURING RESPONSIVENESS

The participants in the regional consultation agreed on the appropriateness of the seven dimensions of responsiveness. However, the following concerns and additions were raised.

CONCERNS

Responsiveness is a subjective measure. A number of its seven dimensions are not relevant under some conditions in the African Region, i.e. confidentiality, choice of provider, prompt attention. Moreover, in addition to being client-oriented, the responsive measure should also focus on epidemiological changes, equity and the public health function.

RECOMMENDATIONS

WHO's progressive work should be directed towards improving the responsiveness goal and measures to reflect the Region's perspective. The measurement of responsiveness should extend to traditional medicine, the private sector and other related sectors such as water and sanitation. The quality of care, social acceptability of the system and its capacity to deal with emergency situations form an additional dimension of responsiveness to be considered.

METHODOLOGICAL ISSUES

With respect to the methodology used to measure responsiveness, the concerns discussed included the complexity of the construct and instruments; the perception of responsiveness as subject to demographic variation and health outcomes; the literacy level as a possible confounding factor in household surveys; the fact that several data sources exist to address responsiveness, especially from surveys. As a response to these methodological concerns, it was suggested that a triangulation of data collection method for measuring responsiveness should be adopted, assuring continuity of data collection and assessment even at the district level. In addition, methods for measuring responsiveness in private and traditional sectors need to be developed and simplified to allow countries to undertake the process of assessment by themselves. Finally, the ongoing review and development of methods and tools has to continue.

PROCESS OF IMPLEMENTATION

The consultation's recommendations regarding the implementation of the measurement of responsiveness were: the establishment of a multidisciplinary body to control the process; the linking of the process with ongoing research activities (e.g. the Demographic and Health Surveys) for cost-effectiveness; the adaptation of the instrument and the obtainment of baseline data from country-wide interventions like EBM, HIV/AIDS, through RC and RPM discussions, countries' dialogue, and support of WHO; the use of assessment outcome as a tool for influencing policy decisions on health; the building of skills capacity in a country in order for the country to take charge of the processes of data gathering and analysis.

HEALTH FUNCTION: GENERATION OF RESOURCES

CONCERNS

The issues of maintenance are especially critical in the African Region. In the face of its countries' reality, the adaptation of technology coming from other regions is difficult. The regional integration of health facilities needs to be strengthened through the promotion of centres of excellence. At the same time, reinforcing the adequacy of the training programme would present the challenge of reforming the Region's educational systems. Lastly, the role of the Ministry of Health is significant for human resource development.

RECOMMENDATIONS

The goal of WHO is to strengthen the African countries' capacity for strategic planning in the domain of health human resources development. The countries for their part need to build human resources through the promotion of regional integration, a culture of maintenance and the allocation of appropriate resources for its implementation.

FINANCING FUNCTION

CONCERNS

Revenue Collection

- Governments should look at their policies relating to revenue collection and the retention of revenue collected by the health sector. It is only when such revenue is retained, rather than lost to the pool of governmental funds, that its effect in terms of improving performance can be assessed.

- Donors have to operate within the government's revenue collection and pooling policy. Otherwise it will be difficult to trace donor funds or ensure that such funds are available to improve performance.

- It is necessary for countries to build capacity in the areas of revenue collection, pooling and purchasing to make for ease of implementation of the sub-functions of revenue collection, pooling and purchasing.

- Funds have to be managed effectively when collected, pooled or used for purchases. Supervision and feedback on the utilization of funds are crucial.

- There is a need to consider revenue collection within the ambit of poverty, i.e. what is being collected from who? Does collection policy address issues of equity? This also applies to pooling. Those who are poor should not be excluded from pools and should be able to benefit from them as well.

- Pooling systems, especially insurance, must be re-evaluated. This is given the likelihood of insurance to avoid a high-risk group such as HIV/AIDS patients (considered against the background of the scourge of HIV/AIDS in Africa).

- The ethical issues relating to purchasing should be estimated. What types of services are purchased?

Financing Arrangements

- A public/private mix for revenue collection, funds pooling and purchasing should exist.

- The levels of involvement of the various tiers of government in the three sub-functions of revenue collection, pooling and purchasing should be monitored.

- The number, size and coverage of pools should be evaluated.

- An allocation mechanism has to be used for purchasing, in order to decide personal health services versus non-personal health services, geographical spread of provision of services, etc.

RECOMMENDATIONS

- The index of fair financial contribution for the sub-function of revenue collection, funds pooling and purchasing has to be assessed.

- The prepayment issue should be reviewed as it relates to pooling. This is particularly due to the government tax revenue that is viewed as a form of prepayment.

- Transparency and accountability should be considered in the three sub-functions of revenue collection, pooling and purchasing.

- Further development is requested in response to the need of having a composite index for each of the sub-functions in relation to performance.

- WHO should review countries' experiences in the area of health financing and provide them with relevant orientation to improve their financing systems.

- WHO is expected to assist countries with orientation to fix a minimum threshold of funding the health sector. What is the minimum expenditure?

- The cost of revenue collection should be considered *vis-à-vis* what is collected.

- Countries are requested to pay more attention to the quality issues in the case of purchases.
  How do we ensure that the quality desired is purchased and paid for?

- Audits should be considered for financing. Budgeting systems should also be thought of because there is often a difference between what is budgeted and what is actually released to the health sector.

FUNCTION OF SERVICE PROVISION

CONCERNS

The current definition of private sector does not include traditional medicine. The present collaboration mechanism with the private sector has failed to provide accurate and timely data from them. The investigation of service provision should go beyond the consideration of services under the direct responsibility of the Ministries of Health. Multiple data sources (SIG, surveys within and outside of health sectors) should be used.

RECOMMENDATIONS

Countries should strengthen the mechanisms of collaboration with their private sectors, including traditional medicine, in order to obtain the data required for the process of health systems performance assessment. They should also reinforce their information systems and define appropriate tools and methods to evaluate the private sector. The exploration of the provision of services should exceed the traditional services under the responsibility and guidance of the Ministry of Health.

STEWARDSHIP FUNCTION

CONCERNS

It was recognized that stewardship plays a major role in health systems. As a function it needs further investigation as well as the development of a set of tools and methods suitable for its assessment. The domain of existing information, policies and regulations should be considered the main building indicator for the assessment of the stewardship function.

RECOMMENDATIONS

Special attention needs to be paid to the assessment of the stewardship function through the development of indicators, tools and surveys. This assessment should be undertaken by the individual countries with the support of WHO.

IMPROVING EVIDENCE

CONCERNS

- The countries' health information systems need to be strengthened.

- The capacity for data warehousing has to be developed.

- Surveys must be linked with national health information systems.

- Ownership and the local capacity are to be cultivated by working with local institutions and staff (statisticians, epidemiologists, demographers, data specialists).

- The existing capacity and its needs have to be established, and gaps have to be addressed.

- Key health systems performance indicators should be incorporated into routine national health information systems.

- Under WHO's leadership, measures, approaches and methodologies for health systems performance assessment are to be harmonized with the ongoing efforts of other agencies.

- Research in various countries has to be promoted and supported.

- All efforts should be directed towards sustainability, capacity building, institutionalization and shift from the project approach.

- The countries' bureaucracy has to be involved in the process.

- The assessment and use of elements of the composite index is very important in guiding improvements in health systems performance.

- Whereas global comparisons are significant, there is an urgent need for country and regional reports, which will afterwards form part of *The World Health Report*.

- People working on the countries' data systems should be targeted for the upcoming course in Johannesburg, 10–22 October 2001.

RECOMMENDATIONS

Collaboration with research and management institutions, schools of public health and other agencies must be promoted in order to provide quality support to countries and to contribute to the evidence generation in the WHO Survey Programme. Health survey aspects need to be integrated in various ongoing surveys, e.g. Demographic and Health Surveys, to ensure sustainability. Routine methods and survey data should be incorporated into national health information systems. A number of specialists in the area of evidence are necessary to provide technical support to countries. A regional database should be established with indicators to monitor and assess health outcomes and to develop capacity for linking of data sets (creating data warehouses).

NOTES

1 Harare, Zimbabwe, 18–20 July 2001

Chapter 3

AMERICAN REGIONAL CONSULTATION ON HEALTH SYSTEMS PERFORMANCE ASSESSMENT[1]

WHO REGIONAL OFFICE FOR THE AMERICAS

INTRODUCTION

The Regional Consultation of the Americas on Health Systems Performance Assessment called together 70 experts and political decision-makers from 19 Member States. Also present were staff members of the Pan American Health Organization/Regional Office for the Americas of the World Health Organization (PAHO/ AMRO), the Cluster of Evidence and Information for Policy of the World Health Organization (WHO/ HQ), the U.S. Agency for International Development (USAID), the World Bank, the World Bank Institute, the *Convenio Hipólito Unanue* and the Caribbean Community (CARICOM), as well as observers from the WHO Regional Office for Europe and WHO Regional Office for the Western Pacific.

The objectives of the consultation were:

- To discuss different conceptual and methodological approaches to assess the performance of health systems.

- To take stock of different country and regional experiences in the Americas related to health systems performance assessment.

- To identify the critical issues for furthering the conceptual and methodological development of a framework for measuring the performance of health systems that could be applied by countries on a regular basis and informed to WHO periodically.

- To discuss the linkage between health systems performance assessment practices and health systems policy and managerial decision-making processes.

- To define an agenda of international technical cooperation in support of countries' efforts to measure the performance of health systems.

The participants received a document entitled *Critical Issues Health Systems Performance Assessment* as reference material. Both the agenda of the meeting and the document were prepared jointly by the Evidence and Information for Policy Cluster (EIP cluster) from WHO headquarters and by the Division of Health Systems and Services Development of PAHO/WHO. During the plenary sessions of the first two mornings, the programme permitted experts with various perspectives to examine methodological and conceptual matters related to *The World Health Report 2000*, as well as the broader topic of measurement of health systems performance. The presentations were followed by open discussions, which reflected the various viewpoints of the experts and participants.

There was a concerted effort to orient the debate towards the future and to contribute to the development of a clear definition of a performance assessment framework and sound data that are useful to countries. The Director of PAHO/WHO, Dr George Alleyne, set the tone by inviting a respectful, constructive and open debate that would help move the process forward. The first two morning sessions covered the topics of: a) Conceptual Basis and Scope of Health Systems Performance Assessment, and b) Furthering the Framework for Health Systems Performance Assessment Used in *The World Health Report 2000*: Gaps Identified and Challenges Ahead. Discussion panels followed presentations by Dr Christopher J.L. Murray and Dr Daniel Lopez-Acuña.

During the first two afternoons, the participants were divided into four groups in order to respond to a series of discussion questions (see Annex 3.1). The first two days ended with a presentation by a Rapporteur on the main issues discussed in each group. The third day included presentations of country experiences. The afternoon session was focused on linking performance assessment to political and managerial decision-making. The final session included a summary of the principal discussions of the working groups. The Director of PAHO/AMRO, Dr Alleyne, closed the meeting.

This report summarizes the principal issues that were raised during the consultation, including discussions at both the plenary sessions and the working groups. The document is organized into two sections. In the first, the principal lessons learned from *The World Health Report 2000* health systems performance assessment framework are summarized. In the second section, recommendations to review the WHO conceptual framework and the indicators used to evaluate the performance of health systems are formulated.

Health Systems Performance Assessment Framework: Lessons Learned

General Observations

- Definitions of the health system, its boundaries, and its objectives vary from country to country and are related to different societal values. In many countries, these definitions are part of legal frameworks (constitutions, health laws and others). Therefore, there are important limits to countries' comparisons in terms of the performance of their health systems when the systems are defined in so many different ways.

- Health systems performance assessment has to be linked to political and managerial decision-making on the health system and not be viewed as an academic exercise. Many participants shared the opinion that a gap exists between *The World Health Report 2000* and its use by those responsible for the political decisions in the health sector. It was suggested that this gap might be partly due to the fact that the indicators included in the report did not allow policy-makers to directly assess what steps they could take to improve performance in the short term.

- Some participants were of the opinion that both at the national and international levels, the criteria for assessing the performance of health systems, as well as the indicators used, should be established by consensus. This extensive consultation should lead to a transparent framework, data collection and criteria for analysis. Otherwise the polemics

on the criteria and the indicators tend to cloud the results of the assessment and its possible use by policy-makers and other interested actors.

- The equating of "performance" with "efficiency" as in *The World Health Report 2000* was considered to be too narrow. It was suggested that performance should be defined as "the set of activities and programmes carried out in order to achieve objectives and goals that have been previously established." Consequently, performance assessment should be seen as "the quantitative and qualitative appraisal that shows the degree of achievement of the objectives and the goals." It was decided that efficiency is one among several possible dimensions of the performance of health systems. Accordingly, the revision of the conceptual framework should stem from a careful review of the dimensions of performance, particularly intermediate goals and indicators that mediate between inputs and outcomes, to which the system contributes.

Objectives and Results of Health Systems

- Improving health is the ultimate goal to which societies expect their health systems to contribute. Depending on the perspective one takes, responsiveness and fair financing may be considered final goals of the health systems, but not the ultimate goal, or may rather be perceived as attributes of the health system or intermediate goals.

- The delivery of personal services, non-personal services and intersectoral actions are only one way of improving the health of the population. Factors linked to political and socioeconomic conditions, environment, genetics, and individual and collective behaviour have a powerful influence on health. It is necessary to advance knowledge of how these factors interact, how they influence the health status of individuals and populations, and therefore how they contribute to the attainment of the ultimate goal of the health system over and above the performance of the system itself.

- The "time factor" makes the previous analysis even more complex and significantly influences the analysis of performance. Poor health status may be the result of decisions made fifteen years ago and its influence on the present situation may not always be easy to establish.

- All of the above emphasizes the importance of paying particular attention to the functions and intermediate objectives of health systems (what health systems are actually doing and what they could do better) and not just focusing performance assessment on some distant final objectives (what "should be done").

THE BOUNDARIES OF THE HEALTH SYSTEM AND THE DEFINITION OF RESPONSIBILITY AND ACCOUNTABILITY

■ There was considerable discussion about the relationship between the boundaries of the health system and the accountability of government for its performance. A number of participants argued that each country defined its own system differently and expected the government to be responsible in different ways. Therefore it was not possible to define a common framework for health systems performance assessment. Simultaneously, other participants argued that international comparisons with a common framework were useful even if individual countries would want to modify the framework for their own internal purposes.

■ Related to the variation in legal definitions, which can be imprecise or outdated, but also to the identification of actors and the flow of financial and non-financial resources of the system, most definitions tend to minimize the importance of the subsystems of self-care and informal care. The initiative to prepare National Health Accounts, currently in progress in numerous countries, can help to fine tune the definition.

■ In most countries, those responsible for health policy tend to be accountable for actions linked to the delivery of personal and non-personal health services.

■ Greater variability among countries exists in the policies where the health system is only one among various sectors involved. Those responsible for health policy often try to take the lead in intersectoral actions with strong impact on the health of populations, but they do not always achieve it. Thus, the accountability for the effects of these policies is often not clear.

■ Finally, there are situations (for example, war and peace, social violence, etc.) and policies (for example, economic policy), which strongly influence health status. They are outside of the health system's immediate realm of responsibility. At most, those responsible for the health system can

develop a certain advocacy role, but it is the entire government (or even the society at large) that is responsible. Again, there was no general agreement about how broadly or narrowly to define the system and the areas of accountability of policy-makers.

COMPARABILITY AMONG THE HEALTH SYSTEMS OF COUNTRIES

■ Unlike the comparison of the performance of the health system of a country with itself over time, the comparability of the performance of health systems between countries was viewed as something desirable, but difficult to carry out for technical and political reasons.

■ In order for it to serve as a stimulus for the formulation of health policies in countries, the terms of comparison (the conceptual framework, the variables that operate it and the indicators of measurement) should be subject to consensus among those to be compared.

■ The three dimensions of evaluation utilized in *The World Health Report 2000* were discussed. In the first place, it was considered that the use of DALE to measure the ultimate final goal of health does not directly include dimensions of positive health nor of the quality of life related to health. It was suggested that its role as the only indicator used for assessing the attainment of the ultimate goal of health be reviewed.

Secondly, it was discussed that the current concept of "responsiveness" encompasses some dimensions of quality of care, but deals only with the demand side. It does not take into account, for example, the technical quality of the supply side. It does not include direct measures of the degree of response to health-seeking behaviours of the population or of user satisfaction, nor does it consider cultural variability among countries and within the same country.

Thirdly, the concept and measure of "fair financing" were evaluated. It was decided that these concentrate exclusively on one side of the problem, the share of household expenditures devoted to health. They do not take into account the effect of public expenditure in public health and personal care. They do not permit the assessment of how progressive or regressive the financing of the health system is, and consequently do not refer to the full spectrum of financial protection with respect to health. Finally, it was considered that from an ethical perspective, the concept is debatable since it assumes that fair financing is the same as pure proportional financing.

■ It was suggested that other instruments and already existing measures should be examined. These can serve as secondary sources and/or support measures to revise the framework of analysis of performance of health systems and to refine the underlying concepts. The challenge consists precisely in being able to integrate data from various sources in a way that generates relevant knowledge for decision-making that is capable of improving the performance of health systems.

■ The usefulness of a single composite index in constructing a scale of attainment for classifying the performance of the health systems of countries, as was employed in *The World Health Report 2000*, was widely discussed. The opinions included criticisms of the usefulness of the composite index to feed policy design, implementation and evaluation, of the methodology used for its calculation, and of the appropriateness of its publication when the calculations are based on estimates and projections rather than on actual data. Some participants shared the view that summary indexes may be utilized politically for ensuring that attention is gained for the health system.

The aggregate index of performance, and the scale of attainment that ranks countries according to the index, raises questions such as: who does the ranking and what is the ranking for? Both can detract from the substance of the debate: to compare in order to improve.

It was also pointed out that policy-makers need to be able to identify the contributions of the different components of the health system. For example, they need to have the capacity to separate the contribution of personal services, non-personal services and intersectoral actions to the performance of the system and to the ultimate final goal of health. This would help them decide if they should allocate resources in a different manner, commensurate to the type of contribution identified in the performance assessment exercises.

Recommendations for Furthering the Conceptual Framework and the Indicators Utilized by WHO to Assess Health Systems Performance

Introduction

During the meeting an opinion was expressed that health systems performance assessment should include a broad range of activities instead of equating the term performance with efficiency. This will allow the users of performance assessment to consider whether progress is being made with regard to specific goals and whether the appropriate activities are being undertaken to promote the achievement of these goals.

The value of this would be in identifying the problem areas requiring special attention, as well as the best practices, which can serve as models. Thus, performance assessment could also be a tool for regulation and resource allocation.

It was proposed by PAHO/AMRO that performance assessment could be compared to a "dashboard," equipped with multiple gauges that make possible the scrutiny of different dimensions of the performance of health systems. This could allow for assessing the degree of attainment of the intermediate goals and the different ways in which the functions of the systems operate.

The Multiple Dimensions of Health Systems Performance

■ Multiple measures can be related to actions for which national agencies could be held responsible. These measures should be pragmatic and connected with policy and managerial decision-making in the health sector. They should rely on the identification of indicators of performance measurement for the different dimensions of the health system: resources, functions, intermediate goals and final goals.

■ The suggestions on how to evaluate the intermediate goals included:
  a) Access—if patients receive the services needed in the right place and at the right time.
  b) Relevance—if the provision of the service is relevant to the needs and if it is based on an established standard.
  c) Continuity—how the services are related among themselves, including coordination, integration and conduction.

d) Sustainability—capacity of systems to provide infrastructure, such as work force, establishments and equipment, in addition to being innovative and responsive to the needs that can arise.

e) Efficiency—technical efficiency or the capacity to achieve better results at the lowest cost.

f) Competence—providers with knowledge and aptitudes that are appropriate for the care they provide.

g) Acceptability—how efficient are the health systems with regard to the expectations of the citizens.

■ It was considered important to define procedures to measure the performance of the function of the steering role of health authorities, taking into account the roles assumed in the majority of the countries at the central, intermediate and local levels of government.

■ It was noted that performance measurement of the essential public health functions, as currently being done in the Region of the Americas, illustrates the potential of a tool for assessing the institutional capacities of the health authority. It measures one specific domain within the stewardship/steering role function of the health system. It may be used for continuous improvement of public health practice and for reorienting resource allocation into public health actions. It does it through a participatory and transparent process within each country, in which 11 essential public health functions are measured. The results do not include a global indicator and they are not oriented towards the construction of a summary measure that compares countries.

Rethinking Health Systems Performance Assessment

■ As part of rethinking and improving health systems performance assessment, it was considered appropriate to advance a framework that takes into account four dimensions: the inputs and/or resources, the functions, the results or intermediate objectives, and the final objectives of the system.

■ Health systems performance assessment also has to be linked to both the definition of the desired change contained in health sector reform agendas and to the actual possibility of implementing changes.

■ At present, there are some national experiences designed to assess the performance of the health systems in several countries of the Region of the Americas, which should be taken into account and analysed.

■ Performance assessment efforts should incorporate the different areas of analysis (national, intermediate, local) and the different functions of the systems. They should also consider several potential recipients (political decision-makers, the public and other interested actors).

Constructing Relevant Indicators

■ The indicators should be grouped in relation to the previously selected dimensions. A careful definition of terms is required. Some indicators can be used to evaluate more than one dimension.

■ A careful balance should be established between information that is available and communicated periodically by countries and information that is desired, but still unavailable. A process for strengthening data collection, and for estimating the costs and the time required for making data readily available should be defined. It is necessary to find an equilibrium between all the possible factors that could influence the results, the capacity of the system to produce timely information and the capacity of the administrators to analyse and process the information.

■ These indicators should be adaptable to changes in policy and administrative decisions both in the short and in the medium run. The data and methodologies for calculations should be transparent and reproducible.

■ The implications of the inclusion of the health systems performance assessment indicators in routine health information systems requires a careful evaluation by experts of the Member States. A central objective of this consultation is to determine the minimum set of indicators that should be monitored routinely, the relationships between quantitative and qualitative indicators, central and complementary indicators, and the relationships between indicators collected regularly and the conducting of periodic surveys.

WHO Technical Support to Countries for Health Systems Performance Assessment

■ WHO should further develop its capacity to provide technical support in performance assessment of health systems. This implies continuous discussions between the Organization and the Member States.

■ Improving the common understanding of the relationships between state of health and health systems is a long-term process. In addition to documenting the results of that relationship, future reports should emphasize the process that leads to the development of the framework, the measures and the indicators. The formulation of global indicators also implies long-term research efforts that should involve those who are responsible for health policies, researchers and other interested actors. WHO should use its leadership in order to make this process a more inclusive one.

■ WHO should re-examine the methodology of the health systems performance assessment in close collaboration with countries and with its own experts in different clusters and regions. The Organization should play a critical role in the development of standards; in bringing together experts in order to compare and contrast different approaches used in countries; in building consensus on the best ways to ensure comparability between countries with regard to health status, health expenditure, health systems organization and other relevant dimensions of the systems.

■ WHO should support countries' efforts in order to develop capacities to:
   a) Dialogue on national health policies.
   b) Evaluate the resources, functions, intermediate objectives and final objectives of health systems,

as well as the degree of achievement of desired changes.
   c) Examine the ability of current health information systems to generate the necessary data.
   d) Undertake the measurement of performance at national and subnational levels.
   e) Develop appropriate policy responses.

■ WHO should make better use of its collaborating centers, other national institutions, as well as strengthen the exchange of information among its different units and regional offices.

Further Steps

■ The results of the consultation will be considered in the work undertaken in this area in the Region of the Americas. They will be transmitted to World Health Organization headquarters to be incorporated into the recommendations made by other regions to the formulation, which will be presented to the Executive Board in January 2002.

■ PAHO/AMRO will organize a work group that, before the end of September, will begin an in-depth analysis of the subject matter and expand the recommendations made in the consultation.

■ The result of both discussions will be presented to a special session, to be scheduled during the Directive Council Meeting, which will take place during the last week of September 2001. The objective of this session will be to inform the delegations of all the Member Countries and to hold a forum for debate that will also be conveyed to WHO headquarters.

Notes

1 Washington, DC, USA, 8–10 May 2001

ANNEX 3.1
GUIDELINES FOR WORKING GROUP

8 MAY 2001

Discussion Session One

1. Which goals and primary outcomes of the health system should be considered when we assess its performance?

2. Where should we establish the boundaries of the health system? Who formulates that definition and how comparable are performance measurements when the definitions of health systems vary?

3. How do the goals of the current WHO framework align with Member States' goals?

4. Should health policy-makers and stewards of the health system be equally accountable for what they are directly responsible (personal and non-personal services), for what they are only partially responsible (intersectoral action) and for what they are not directly responsible?

5. Which other instruments/measures pertaining to other constituent parts of human development that have an influence on health should be developed?

6. What is the comparability of the measures of responsiveness and financial fairness among countries?

9 MAY 2001

Discussion Session Two

1. What are we referring to when we discuss health systems performance? What does it encompass?

2. Is performance assessment of the health system best served by the calculation of a single combined index subject to weights given to each variable, or by a series of indicators that can provide information on the different domains of health system performance (resources, functions, intermediate goals and final goals)? How can they be more directly linked to action?

3. What are the key indicators of functions and intermediate goals that should be developed to assess the performance of health systems so they provide meaningful information for their improvement?

4. How do WHO data sources and methodologies improve the Member States' abilities to move from data to action and to actually impact policies and programmes?

5. What research and development are needed to support the performance measurement of intermediate goals and health system functions?

Chapter 4

Eastern Mediterranean Regional Consultation on Health Systems Performance Assessment[1]

WHO Regional Office for the Eastern Mediterranean

Session One: Opening Addresses

The Regional Consultation on Health Systems Performance Assessment was convened by the WHO Eastern Mediterranean Regional Office in Ain Saadeh, Lebanon on 9 July 2001. In his address to the meeting, the Regional Director, HE Dr Husein Gezairy, welcomed the participants and thanked the Government of Lebanon for hosting the meeting of experts and scientists from WHO headquarters and the Region (refer to the list of attendance in Annex 4.1).

Dr Gezairy stated that the main objective of the regional consultation was to review critically the WHO conceptual framework on health systems, with respect to scientific foundations, methodologies and tools used to measure health system performance and to suggest potential refinements. The consultation was also invited to recommend measures to improve system assessment through better data gathering and processing, capacity building and other means to insure the reliability of information, the transparency of the process and the ownership of performance measurement exercise by countries and the WHO Regional Office. "It is hoped that the discussions would assist in the preparation of a regional strategy on health system development aimed at improving health system performance."

Dr Albert Jokhadar, speaking on behalf of HE Mr Soleiman Frangieh, Minister of Public Health of the Republic of Lebanon, welcomed the participants. He declared that the health care system of Lebanon suffers from a lot of problems in spite of its expanded resources (12% of the GDP) and its potential strengths. Dr Jokhadar noted that civil disturbances were not the only reason for the problems facing the health care system. "The liberal economy permits the unrestrained acquisition of expensive medical equip-

ment, the establishment of health facilities anywhere investors choose, and the variable quality of manpower, from the very best to the less capable. There have been several attempts at reforms, to no avail as of now. We hope that the proposed reforms of Minister Frangieh will fare better. This is likely to be an arduous and long undertaking, which will require the support of all concerned, nationally and internationally."

The meeting then elected by acclamation Dr Gharama Al Raee (Yemen) as Chairman and Dr Nabil Kronfol as Rapporteur.

Session Two: Regional Response to the Health Systems Performance Exercise

Improving the Performance of Health Systems: Building on *The World Health Report 2000* (Dr David B. Evans)

Dr David B. Evans, Director of the Global Programme on Evidence for Health Policy (GPE) at WHO headquarters, made a presentation titled *Improving the Performance of Health Systems: Building on The World Health Report 2000*. Dr Evans indicated that health system performance assessment has three objectives: to monitor and evaluate the attainment of critical outcomes and the efficiency of a health system in a way that allows comparison over time and across systems; to build an evidence-base on the relationship between the design of the health system and its performance; and to empower the public with information relevant to well-being.

Dr Evans defined the key concept of a "health action" as any activity whose primary intention is to improve health. This concept has set the boundaries of health systems in the framework. The social goals to which the health system contributes were defined as good health, responsiveness and fairness in financial contribution. The level and distribution across the population were important to assure quality, equity, and efficiency.

Dr Evans proceeded with the measurement indices for the framework. He introduced healthy life expectancy (HALE), previously termed DALE (disability-adjusted life expectancy) in the report. HALE is based on life expectancy, includes non-fatal health outcomes, and is calculated using data from epidemiology and health studies such as child mortality surveys. The health system should seek to improve the level of population health, but also to reduce inequalities in health outcomes.

The second goal of health systems, the responsiveness element, was measured in the *The World Health Report 2000* through the survey of key informants. This index focuses on measuring what happens when system and person interact. It addresses the legitimate levels of expectations of the population and is different from patient satisfaction. It includes two main components: respect for the individual and the orientation of the system to the users' expectations. These have the following components: dignity, confidentiality, autonomy, prompt attention to needs, access to social support networks, quality of basic amenities and relative choice of provider(s). Again, health policy-makers should be concerned with improving the level of responsiveness and with reducing inequalities in it.

The third goal, fairness in financial contribution, highlights the fact that some ways of financing health are more fair than others, given that the two other goals are held constant. Most people would agree that catastrophic payments are unfair. Dr Evans introduced the concepts of horizontal equity (when similar groups contribute the same shares of income) and vertical equity (when the rich pay a higher percentage of the income than the less privileged). A fair financial contribution would mean that all households pay the same proportion of their non-subsistence income on health.

The framework proposes two summary measurements: attainment, defined as the achievement of goals singly and in a composite manner, and performance, which is attainment related to resources available and other non-health system inputs to the production of health system outcomes (efficiency). Separate efficiency is calculated for health and for the composite goal.

Dr Evans underlined four functions of health systems: the financing role through revenue collection,

fund pooling and purchasing of services; the provision of health services, both personal and non-personal; resource generation; and stewardship. According to him, the main purpose is to evaluate the system, not to compare across Member States.

The conceptual issues that have been debated since the release of the *The World Health Report 2000* are:

- Narrow (direct control by health authorities) versus broad accountability (the stewardship role of the health authority).

- The issue of causal attribution: multiple factors contribute to socially valued outcomes, including the health system. Multivariate analysis was used to measure the impact of each contributor.

- The mediating factors or intermediate goals: WHO has started an initiative to measure coverage with critical interventions along with efforts to develop measures of performance of the different functions of health systems.

- Performance and time: economic studies of efficiency measure output compared to the maximum that would be possible. For health systems, important time lags exist between actions and outcomes, and the definition of the maximum depends on the time over which the stewards of the system should be held accountable.

- Universal weights for key outcomes: how much does the weight for key outcomes vary across populations and individuals and how could comparisons be made?

The debate on the methodologies proposed in the *The World Health Report 2000* centered on the measurement of HALE (DALE), the challenges for measuring non-fatal health outcomes, the core domains of health and the need to enhance cross-population comparability. New life tables were constructed for 191 countries and were sent to respective Member States for discussion. More than 70 countries are currently involved in the WHO Multi-country Survey Study on Health and Responsiveness. DHS surveys are available from 65 countries, with vital registration data from more than 30 countries, to review the measurement of health inequality. Sample population surveys, the gold standard, are being conducted to measure responsiveness and to compare the results with the responses from key informants used in the first version of the framework. New data collection is ongoing in 70 countries to assess fairness in financial contribution.

Finally, efficiency assessment is being improved by an update of National Health Accounts and estimation of the production function. A second stage analysis would explore the factors that may explain differences in efficiency across different health systems. The evaluation will take place every two years, taking into consideration the suggestions of the Member States and their inputs into the assessment.

Response of Dr Abdul Aziz Saleh (DRD)

Dr Abdul Aziz Saleh, Deputy Regional Director WHO/EMRO, introduced the Region's response. "We see this initiative as an activity to improve the national health systems in the Member States. This should be complementary to the previous activities undertaken. These efforts should leave an impact, not a mere document. The initiative ought to have been at the country level first and should have been based on national capabilities. The challenge of this meeting will be to marry this model with the capabilities of the national staff in the Member States."

The interest of the Member States was shifted to the rankings. The best rank (out of seven) was chosen and used for public opinion. Little debate was generated at the country level on the technical merits of the framework.

The Deputy Regional Director commented on the fact that the report was anchored on data while the validity of these data could be challenged. He underlined the need to strengthen national information systems in order to calculate the recommended indices, as well as to simplify the measurement tools so they can be used by the Member States. In addition, he suggested that in-country comparisons between different regions ought to be made. Dr Saleh ended his speech with the conviction that the objective of this consultation is to develop health systems at the national level along with national expertise. In this manner the framework would be useful beyond its academic merits.

The Regional Position (Dr Belgacem Sabri)

The regional response was presented by Dr Belgacem Sabri, Director of Health Systems and Community Development at WHO/EMRO. Dr Sabri began his presentation by stating that a healthy debate was generated by the release of *The World Health Report 2000*. In his opinion, the latter proposed a technically sound framework for health systems since it delineated appropriately the boundaries of health systems, clari-

fied their goals and functions, and recommended tools for the measurement of their performance.

Dr Sabri also mentioned the reservations expressed regarding the data used in *The World Health Report 2000*, in particular their accuracy, timeliness and extrapolations from limited data. He pointed out that since there was limited involvement of the Regional Office and the Member States in this exercise, a concern should be raised about the ownership of the framework and hence its sustainability. Therefore, it would be necessary to further refine the framework by enriching the concept, filling in the gaps, adapting the tools, investing in capacity building and strengthening health systems.

EMRO was invited to contribute to this framework as early as the Harare meeting. Information was disseminated to WHO staff and discussions were held at the Regional Consultative Committee and at the Regional Committee. The need to involve the Regional Office and the Member States in order to promote the ownership of the framework was stressed, together with the need to further improve data sources and to link this exercise with the strengthening of health systems. Briefing was carried out in several countries of the Region, namely Iran, Morocco, Syria and Tunisia. Previously there had been a close interaction with the countries to discuss the framework and a positive collaboration with HQ to organize briefings, technical discussions, background papers and joint visits to several countries. The Regional Committee recommended that a regional strategy for mapping health systems functions be outlined so that their performance and the collection of evidence to support the framework be improved.

Dr Sabri talked about the importance of supporting the limited capabilities at the Regional Office and at the country level in order to prepare for the adoption of the framework. Since the data for performance assessment was scarce, it was necessary to build the capacity to promote the analytical tools in health systems whether for the burden of disease (BOD) studies or National Health Accounts (NHA), cost analysis and cost-effectiveness (CEA). A network of professionals, as well as national and regional educational institutions, ought to be involved in the process as well.

Dr Sabri's presentation also informed the participants in the consultation that EMRO had promoted the use of household surveys to measure fairness in financial contribution (Syria). Plans had been made to include the responsiveness questionnaire in national population based surveys. At the same time, it had been attempted to assess national health information systems with a special focus on epidemiological intelligence, and to bridge with national statistical departments in Iran, Lebanon, Syria and Tunisia. Partnerships with geo-political groupings such as the League of Arab States, ESCWA, ECA, AGFUND and researchers in academic institutions had been promoted as well. "To support these and other activities, extra-budgetary resources are needed. The Regional Office capabilities for the development of normative activities, for technical coop-eration and for the establishment of the regional observa-tory on health systems must be reinforced," insisted Dr Sabri. Similarly, the Member States ought to be sup-ported in conducting studies such as National Health Accounts, population based surveys, national obser-vatories, burden of disease and cost-effectiveness studies. The decentralization of health systems, based on pri-mary health care principles, the autonomy of hospitals, the referral system, the development of human resources and national information systems ought to be supported.

Eight countries are involved in the initiative to enhance performance assessment: Jordan, Morocco, Iran, Lebanon, Oman, Pakistan, Syria and Tunisia. The initiative, which will be extended to other coun-tries, includes capacity building through training on analytical tools, development of a network of experts, and mapping of health systems functions with the identification of tools to measure improvement.

Dr Sabri concluded with the expectation that this consultation would submit concrete proposals to improve the framework (contents, tools and owner-ship), as well as support arrangements to strengthen capacity building in analytical tools. The outline of a regional strategy to promote the use of the frame-work and to reinforce health systems performance was indicated. The tools and methods for data and performance measures should be mastered.

DISCUSSION

Participants engaged in a discussion of the regional position paper and the framework proposed by HQ. A concern was expressed that primary health care, which has been the linchpin for 24 years, seemed to have been forgotten rather than built upon. The intersectoral col-laboration, the managerial process, and quality issues had also been marginalized in the framework. There was little to document the progress achieved by coun-tries; rather an emphasis had been placed on economic criteria such as GDP. It was decided that the frame-work ought to be used to strengthen capacity at the national level; it should be a means to this end, not an

end by itself. The importance of the framework was that it drew attention to the assessment of performance of health systems, "it got us focused." Yet it did not give answers as to why some countries are doing well and how they achieved this.

Dr Habib Latiri, WHO Representative in Lebanon, described the progress achieved by WHO in the coun-try through the conduct of several studies and sur-veys, very much in concert with those proposed in the framework and requested by WHO/HQ. There was support of the involvement by WHO representatives in this consultation. However, concerns were raised as to the sustainability of this effort if resources were not made available, given the needs of the Regional Office and the Member States. On a different note, some participants expressed the opinion that this framework, though valid academically, fell short in practice. It was suggested that more use ought to be made of time-tested classical indicators. Another con-cern was that decision-making at WHO was moving away from the realm of physicians towards that of economists. A similar process has not occurred in most Member States and this could present some difficulty in espousing the framework.

Dr Gezairy moved the discussion to another level: what about the future? What are the possibilities of making information available in a timely manner in the future? Will this exercise strengthen national health care systems? How can capacity be built? What resources will be made available? Is it better to aban-don the current indicators or to continue to use them in addition to those proposed in the framework?

Dr Evans responded to these comments by stress-ing that the goal of this consultation was precisely to convey information to the Member States and to build cooperation. Although the framework is "academic" and based on research, a lot could be obtained from currently available data. Dr Saleh and Dr Sabri re-emphasized that the objective of the consultation was to look towards the future.

SESSION THREE: ASSESSMENT OF HEALTH SYSTEMS PERFORMANCE

PART ONE

Measuring Health and Health Inequalities (Dr Alan D. Lopez)

Dr Alan D. Lopez, Coordinator of the Epidemiology and Burden of Disease team at WHO/HQ discussed issues related to the measurement of health and health inequalities. He emphasized first the importance of using the healthy life expectancy instead of simple life expectancy since the goal of health care is to improve health, not merely to prolong life. Also, the measurement of pure inequality, together with inequality among social classes, in health are important for health policy.

Dr Lopez stated that the following inputs required for these measurements were used: population and mortality by age and sex, distribution of the population in varying levels of health and incidence, prevalence and duration of illnesses. The data sources were, and continue to be, vital registration records, sample registration records or survey and census data. Vital registration remains the gold standard for cause of death.

To measure health, life tables were constructed for 191 countries. Good sources of data were available for 72 countries, representing 24% of the world population (1.4 billion). Incomplete data were available for 50 countries, representing 58% of the world population. In this group, the under-registration of mortality required adjustment using demographic techniques, matching with other surveys such as the DHS for child mortality under age of 5 years. For the third group of countries with some vital registration records and other surveys but inadequate time-series, tables were constructed using supplementation from other surveys and estimates of adult mortality. This group consisted of 13 countries (3% of world population), and included South Africa, Tanzania and Jordan. Finally, in 56 countries (15% of population) no direct information on adult mortality was available. A new WHO model life table system based on child mortality levels was used to estimate life tables, including estimates of uncertainty.

As far as cause of death data are concerned, vital registration remains the best source (one third of deaths worldwide); the other option is verbal autopsy.

To calculate DALE, disability prevalence could be obtained from burden of disease studies and from health or disability surveys with adjustment. There is a need to obtain prevalence of health states by severity, along with preference weights, to value time spent in poor health.

The measurement of inequalities in health across individuals in a population implies that health is a critical component of well-being and that equality in health is desirable. Group inequalities are different across social classes, education groups, income levels and geographical areas. The choice of a measure of inequality is a normative choice. How much weight ought to be given to the tails or to the spread

of inequality? Should we compare people to the mean or to all other individuals in the population? Two measures were proposed: individual-mean differences and interindividual differences. The next step is to measure inequality in DALE. To this end, individual records from census or surveys need to be linked to death registries. In addition, information on covariates (income, education, place of residence, age, etc.) ought to be obtained. This would require linking health surveys or census records to death registries or a random sample from the census followed by a household survey.

Summarizing Reflections on Health Status and Health Inequalities

Dr Adnan Hyder from Johns Hopkins University and WHO Temporary Advisor commented that several researchers had critiqued the measurement of health status and health inequalities. Some argue that DALE and DALYs have not been accepted universally, that many countries lack valid data and that the disability weights are uncertain. Others question the value of ranking countries. As for health inequality, a comparison of the WHO index with socioeconomic inequalities in 15 developed and 43 developing countries has revealed that the index does not correspond to the size of the socioeconomic inequalities in mortality. Therefore, it should not be interpreted as a reflection of the socioeconomic inequalities in health, nor should it be used to replace them. Equity in health is defined differently in different societies: some countries have equity goals, others do not. How to achieve equity in an efficient manner remains to be answered.

Dr Hyder reflected that several of these critiques are being addressed by WHO, while others need to be evaluated at the regional and country levels. The following part of Dr Hyder's presentation consisted of a summary of the burden of disease study he had conducted for Pakistan. This study was implemented using the existing data in the country and revealed important insights into its disease profile, such as the prevalence of injuries and cardiovascular diseases.

Dr Lopez indicated that some developing countries like Pakistan were able to conduct burden studies that highlighted disease patterns previously underestimated by policy-makers. "Many countries have far more data than they think they have. A rigorous analysis of these data is required." He added that innovative ways to collect data exist and that with constant monitoring, the exercise would not be a burden but an opportunity to revise and develop a country's HIS (a goal underscored by Dr Saleh). The use of DALE need not and should not replace the other indicators. Dr Lopez made this final comment: "You manage what you measure and you invest in what you manage. Do not make the best the enemy of the good."

SESSION FOUR: ASSESSMENT OF HEALTH SYSTEMS PERFORMANCE

PART TWO

Measuring Fairness in Financial Contribution

Dr Evans indicated that the construction of fairness in financial contribution (FFC) is conditional on a society's efforts to redistribute income. The concern for fairness in financial contribution reflects three factors: horizontal equity, catastrophic expenditure and progressivism. Catastrophic payments are unfair if financial systems are organized in a way that households may have to pay a catastrophic share of non-subsistence effective income (capacity to pay, defined as > 50%) to improve or protect their health. Horizontal inequity is so defined when similar groups are contributing very different shares of their capacity to pay towards the health system. This is also considered an unfair financial contribution. Vertical inequity is the concern that the rich pay a larger share of their income to the health system than the poor (or we say rich pay more than poor), even after taking into account the society's efforts to redistribute income. Fairness in financial contribution is perfectly fair if all households pay the same proportion of their non-subsistence effective income on health.

In response to the debates, new primary data has been obtained from 70 countries (constituting 94 data points over time). The new survey data are being analysed in six countries in the EMR region in addition to Pakistan, which had a household survey that contributed new data to *The World Health Report 2000*.

Dr Evans clarified that the construction of the fairness in financing index was also a subject of debate. Two options were predominant: to use the actual food expenditure or the basic need expenditure (BNE) as the denominator. The BNE was calculated by the United Nations in 1985 as a minimum of 1 dollar per person per day. This measurement could be adjusted for inflation and household size, as well as using UN food purchasing power parity PPP instead of the overall PPP. There is evidence that food expenditures do not rise as fast as income, hence progressivism is built into the index.

Preliminary results reveal a quasi-linear relationship between the percentage of expenditures on catastrophic illness and FFC in most countries. This might become the reason to adopt the percentage of expenditures on catastrophic illness as the index since people understand it more readily. However the question is whether 50% is the appropriate cut-off point.

As it was explained in the presentation, the data requirements to construct FFC are the private out-of-pocket health expenditures obtained from household income and expenditures surveys, all levels of government taxation, payments to health insurance by households and employers, and other types of payment and insurance.

Dr Hussein Salehi (Iran) commented on the presentation and raised several issues:

■ The index reported in *The World Health Report 2000* is a composite index, which is supposed to measure overall performance and efficiency of every health system in a comparable manner. It is important to note at the very beginning that the concept of efficiency is somewhat different from the concept of allocative, technical or pareto efficiency as used in economic theory.

■ The index is very sensitive to the weight of each of its five components and although we can learn a lot from each component, there is less confidence in the use of the overall index to evaluate performance and to justify interventions.

■ The index does not include the amount different countries spend on health. For example, Iran spends 6% of its GDP on health, Lebanon 12%. Both variations and hidden expenditures exist. Also, there are many oil producing countries in the EMR. Part of their governments' budgets are financed through oil revenues, which will affect the fairness in financing index in an unfavourable way.

■ The issue of subsidies (multiple exchange rates) is not addressed properly in the methodology of fairness in financial contribution.

■ Inflation rates have been recognized by WHO as an issue, but exactly at what level one should start making adjustments is not known.

■ Should the ranking of countries determine the need for change in the health care system?

■ The household expenditure survey is not generally balanced for technical reasons. The samples taken from rural and urban areas are not proportional to the population. A standard way to solve this problem should be introduced. Differences also exist in household surveys between rural and urban areas. The rural households pay far less on house rent and therefore their percentage expenditures on health may appear higher.

- The ownership of household surveys is usually the central statistics agency or the Ministry of Planning, not the Ministry of Health.

- The age structure of the population in the EMR includes higher proportions of children and elderly, both of which are groups that spend more on health care.

- In the informal sector, few people pay the correct amount of taxes.

- Manuals are needed to assist in the measurement of the indices used in the framework. However, who is to support the financing of such studies? International organizations provide the needed funds at present, but what about the sustainability of these efforts?

- Social security may mean different things in different countries and systems.

- Technical assistance is required to calculate the index.

Dr Zineddine Idriss (Morocco) was asked to comment on the presentation. His remarks were:

- The index is not compulsory for countries and like the Human Development Index, it could be calculated by the international organizations concerned. Moreover, similar efforts may not be supported by national governments since they divert funds from more needed programmes in health. Governments ought to support the attempts of international organizations and furnish them with the available information, along with their analysis of the situation.

- The ranking is but an indicator.

- In Morocco, there are problems with equity in the financing of health services. The interest the government had in the NHA study was to find out the percentage of households experiencing catastrophic payments for health care.

- The expenditures of households (the denominator) may yield doubtful results.

Dr Robert Kasparian (Lebanon) was third to comment on the presentation. He gave an overview of the financing of health services in Lebanon, indicating the difficulties faced in the household surveys regarding the data on income and health expenditures, as well as the measures taken to improve the validity of the information collected. Dr Kasparian focused on the following issues:

- The framework does not address the problems related to the accessibility of health services.

- Countries that have no elaborate tax-based income will find it difficult to determine income and expenditures.

- The definition of households in the GCC countries is blurred. Many leave their families behind (expatriate workers) and the size of the household and its expenditures may be misleading.

- The incompleteness of data may lead to misplacement in the ranking of countries. If Pakistan, 64th in rank, spends little on health care, the index should be backed up by other indicators.

- Is fairness in financial contribution an intrinsic goal of health systems?

Dr Sabri stressed the importance of developing guidelines. He pointed out that the current information might not be user friendly, but this is being examined at present. In addition, household surveys are important instruments and although they are owned by official agencies other than the health authorities, efforts should be made to negotiate the use of raw data and to provide those responsible for the surveys with the questions and the information needed. In so doing, the health authorities would assist in the design of the survey. Furthermore, household surveys are expensive and the necessary resources must be found to assure their sustainability.

Dr Saleh added that the index is complex and needs to be simplified. Dr Gezairy asked how the weights within the framework were assigned and whether a model should be proposed first to see if it will work. Dr Mechbal indicated that most countries have surveys, but the problem exists in the fact that health authorities have little input in the design of these surveys. Efforts ought to be expanded to capture this information and other data from international and regional agencies. Mr Azzam was of the opinion that the manuals used in surveys and national health accounts have to be standardized. Dr Al Raee raised the issue that the participants might be forgetting that the primary goal of health systems is to provide health care to the population, not to undertake costly surveys. Finally, these indices were promoted by the World Bank and other economic institutions.

Dr Evans responded to these comments in this manner:

- The weights were tested in studies performed in many countries, and these proved that the assignment of health a 50% weight in the score is in line with their findings.

- The index is not a description of the financing system of health care. It is only an index much like life expectancy. The country may decide what to do with its findings and it can detect progress over time as well.

- The index of fairness in financial contribution is not an indicator of efficiency. It does not indicate waste or overuse.

- The framework can only be sustained if the country feels that it owns it.

- The fundamental goal of health systems is good health. The responses to surveys in various countries will decide whether fairness is an intrinsic goal, but so far the surveys have demonstrated that people value it highly. Many countries did not know much about the other goals highlighted in *The World Health Report 2000,* since they were accustomed to measuring health indices.

- The guidelines will be distributed once they have been tested in the field.

SESSION FIVE: ASSESSMENT OF HEALTH SYSTEMS PERFORMANCE

PART THREE

Measuring Responsiveness (Dr Somnath Chatterji)

Dr Chatterji's presentation began with the statement that measuring responsiveness is the subject of a multi-country survey study designed to test indices for cross-country comparison. The survey instrument consists of several modules on health, responsiveness and financing. The health module is based on a review of existing assessment instruments, taking into consideration criteria such as culturally sensitive tests, reliability of the instrument and cross-population comparability. In order to improve on cross-country comparability, vignettes and performance tests were designed and are being field tested.

Self-reported health data in surveys may yield responses that vary by country and by population subgroups. Norms, expectations and other determinants are the underlying causes for the difficulties in cross-country comparisons. Efforts are being made to develop a common survey instrument that has cross-cultural comparability possibilities, is both reliable and valid, and can be calibrated. The instrument is conducted through interviews lasting about 75–90 minutes. Postal surveys may also be used although they have a far lower response yield (46% versus 95%). A compressed brief interview form is also being tested with a yield of 65%. Quality control includes a re-test of 10% and a random check of 10% as well. A minimum of 5 000 adult responses is required. To shorten the interview time, some of the modules could be used, rather than all.

The experience of Egypt in this effort was described by Dr Samy Gadalla. Egypt participated in the earlier stages, namely the key informant survey, the household survey, the postal survey and the multimethod valuation exercise. In the last key informant survey of April 2001, 350 responses were elicited. Respondents were pleased with this new concept of responsiveness. Dr Gadalla underlined the need for training, coordination, ranking and calibration of vignettes (which are culturally sensitive). Instead of the Likert's scale, a 0–1 range was deemed preferable.

Dr Farid Aboul Hassanin (Iran) commented on the experience of Iran. The responsiveness survey was carried out for the first time. It was a resource-consuming instrument based on interviews. Dr Aboul Hassanin expressed a concern about the sustainability and the continuity of these efforts. According to him, the interviews are long and have to be adjusted when the respondents are old or illiterate. The interviews could be structured into two parts: health alone and then responsiveness. It is necessary for technical competence to be developed in order to strengthen confidence, ownership and thus advocacy. Political support and commitment are also essential. "We are lagging behind the WHO headquarters on many issues related to the framework. The concept keeps on changing, which leads to some frustration". The significance of the collaboration with universities was noted as well.

Dr Noureddine Achour (Tunisia) made these remarks: Are the techniques used complementary or alternates? In other words, is the postal survey a different option from interviews? How are the respondents chosen in the mail survey? The issue of illiteracy of some respondents, as well as the differences in value systems, must be tested to ensure the validity of the information. Dr Achour questioned the inclusion of responsiveness as an important criterion in health systems assessment. Its introduction in some developing countries may diminish the interest of respondents to medical issues, such as the availability of medications, and re-orient the discussion to hotel services such as food and cleanliness. Dr Achour's concern was that responsiveness might be more beneficial to developed societies rather than to those in mutation or transition. The latter are likely to have other priorities.

In the general discussion that followed, Dr Tawfic Khoja expressed the opinion that little attention is paid to the GCC countries, presumably because they are wealthy. At the same time, developing capacity is needed in these countries to undertake the assessment. Dr Dolly Bassili reported that in Lebanon, the interview took about three hours to complete instead of 90 minutes because the translation itself was not easy. This might lead to a low response rate and delays. A lot of comments included the issue of cultural comparability. Dr Rafic Baddoura (Lebanon) wanted to know how the seven items of "responsiveness" were selected and whether they could be deleted or modified since some of the items could be considered closer to health than others. The responses could be affected by the health status of the respondent (for example, responses of older population and children). Dr Raouf Ben Ammar (Morocco) warned that there is a gap on the conceptual front between WHO headquarters and the Region; between what is done by HQ and what is to be expected. "We want to work with HQ to have this initiative succeed. We must expand efforts to close the gap through training and openness of HQ to inputs from other cultures. Resources are needed to test the model in different cultures." Dr Ibrahim Abdel Rahim (WR Oman) indicated that a shorter version of the questionnaire may be more useful, and that one may broaden the concept of responsiveness to include other elements.

Dr Chatterji thanked the participants for their contribution and insisted upon the fact that the process of measuring responsiveness is a work in progress. It is also not just an effort of WHO headquarters, but has involved partnerships with many international experts and collaborating centres. A specific consultation on responsiveness with representatives from all regions is going to take place in Geneva in September. Dr Chatterji further clarified that currently the interview is long because it contains several modules, while later only some of them will be chosen. He ended his presentation with the view that the participants need to

work together in order to obtain applicable and valid results.

Session Six: Furthering the WHO Framework on Health Systems Performance Assessment

Health Systems Performance: Assessing and Improving Functions (Dr Abdelhay Mechbal)

Dr Abdelhay Mechbal, WHO/EMRO Regional Advisor, Research, Policy and Cooperation, opened the sixth session of the Regional Consultation with the work done to further the WHO framework. He indicated that the following issues need to be addressed: tools to evaluate health systems functions have to be developed; the delivery and stewardship functions need to focus on the attainment of intermediate goals, such as accessibility and effective coverage; health systems performance measurement has to be turned into a tool for planners and managers at the national and subnational levels; and countries must be assisted in understanding the impact of their policies and interventions on the population in most need, as well as in analysing and monitoring the performance of health care providers.

Dr Mechbal mentioned some of the recent international developments since the release of *The World Health Report 2000*:

- The focus on scaling up of health systems to improve the health outcomes of the poor is an effort supported by the United Nations, the European Community and the G8 countries. There is growing support to increase funding for interventions that successfully address the major communicable diseases, such as malaria, tuberculosis, and HIV/AIDS. Funds are also needed to improve the capacity of health systems. This necessitates an adjustment of the health systems functions to deliver successfully and increase these services.

- The goal of "health financing" has also received attention. WHO's policy has been to support evidence-based policy recommendations on revenue collection, pooling of funds and purchasing of services. A WHO policy monograph on alternative health financing arrangements is being produced in collaboration with the regional offices and leading experts in the field. Universal financial protection is the underlying theme, that is, protection of households from catastrophic financial contributions. In the policy monograph, WHO will focus on methods to collect revenues with an emphasis on prepayment mechanisms. In its discussion of approaches to pooling revenues, it will analyse issues regarding the number and size of pools and population coverage. Finally, the purchasing of interventions section will include discussion of what to buy, whom to buy for, how to purchase, the preferred provider payment mechanism and the contractual relationships appertaining.

Recently, the Regional Office has supported the Member States in the area of health financing. The future role of social health insurance in the Gulf Cooperation Council countries was discussed at a meeting in Abu Dhabi. Work on contracting for services is on its way in the African Region. There is a need to develop, strengthen and maintain information databases and to make these available for researchers and scientists. To this end, the National Health Accounts initiative has been launched in collaboration with country institutions. A National Health Accounts Producer's Guide for low- and middle-income countries is being prepared. In addition, plans are being made to increase country and regional capacity to update and use this information for policy analysis.

■ Stewardship was highlighted as an important goal of health systems in the proposed framework. The components of stewardship need to be clarified, in particular the formulation of health policy, regulation and intelligence. This will require defining a vision of health systems and their directions, setting fair rules for the provision of services, assessing performance and sharing information. Development of national skills in policy analysis and strategic planning is of importance. WHO may also assist the Member States in the design of legislation in certain critical areas such as the private delivery of health care. WHO supports activities like the monitoring and evaluation of systems performance, monitoring expenditures and developing health system profiles. These activities will connect the health systems performance assessment model with managerial practices and decision-making processes at the local, regional and national levels. They will also enable the identification of key health systems requirements that determine the effective provision of health interventions.

■ Access to effective interventions has been an important concern for the Organization before

and since the release of the framework. The goal is to strengthen the capacities of health systems to produce the maximum possible health gain for poor and vulnerable populations through the investment of scarce resources in critical interventions and to ensure the fair distribution of benefits from such investments. WHO is striving to produce a parsimonious set of indicators, instruments and methods to obtain valid, reliable and comparable coverage figures for different health interventions. Another objective is a framework for the analysis of health systems functions and their impact on the provision of critical interventions. This ought to provide an action-oriented decision tool for policy-makers and managers. Effective coverage is defined in this context as the proportion of the population that receives effective health services out of the target population that needs these services. To achieve these objectives on effective coverage, several major tasks are involved. First comes the need to identify interventions that produce significant health gain, particularly among the poor. Cost-effective interventions must be decided on. The most appropriate coverage indicators and tools for collecting data on coverage must be selected. The measurement of coverage must be tested and piloted. Finally, a tool that will help incorporate data on effective coverage into the planning and management of services must be developed.

In all of these developments, work will be carried out in consultation with the Member States and in close collaboration with other programs at HQ, Regional Offices, country offices, other international organizations and research institutions.

■ Another intermediate goal, which needs to be pursued to strengthen the capacity of health systems to produce maximum possible health gain, is that of the improved performance of the providers, whether these are hospitals, clinics or practitioners. To help achieve this intermediate goal, WHO will strive to develop a parsimonious set of indicators to monitor quality, responsiveness and efficiency, as well as instruments and methods to obtain the most valid, reliable and comparable data. This will provide an action-oriented decision tool for policy-makers and managers at the subnational and national levels. It will also assist in the translation of evidence into policies and strategies for effective coverage. To assess the performance and quality of providers, WHO will use the same analytical approach as used in the framework for the national system. The key challenge will be to take into account the risk profile of the client population. WHO plans to develop and test the methods for assessing providers in the next two years.

ENRICHING THE WHO FRAMEWORK: A REGIONAL CONTRIBUTION (DR NABIL KRONFOL)

Dr Nabil Kronfol, Temporary Advisor to WHO/EMR, discussed the proposed framework and suggested additions as part of the EMR's contribution to this worldwide effort.

> "In the Eastern Mediterranean Region, in depth discussions took place at the Regional Office and at the Regional and Consultative Committee meetings about the new conceptual framework used to define health systems and to measure their performance. A consensus was reached on the need to enrich the technically sound framework while efforts should be made to better clarify the tools and methods applied to measure system performance and to supply these tools to the Regional Office and the countries. The latter should make use of the framework to develop and strengthen health systems and to improve their performance in order to achieve the goals of health for all through primary health care,"

remarked Dr Kronfol.

> "Very few would doubt the importance of assessing performance of any human activity or the evaluation of any human system. It is therefore imperative to start this discussion paper by praising the efforts expanded by the WHO and the authors of this report. They have proposed a framework for the assessment of health systems that is serious, innovative and remarkable as to its intellectual vision and quantitative methods. Moreover, this is not merely a model for health care systems, but for health systems in general and even for the very concept of health. The strengths of the logic that permeates the framework and the advanced quantitative models used for the measurement of the indicators can not be underestimated. It is therefore appropriate to begin this discussion paper by adopting the overall framework as an important initial effort to performance assessment,"

added Dr Kronfol.

Many opinions and suggestions have been put forward to complement this effort. This is to be expected given the far-reaching impact that the framework has had and will have for years to come. It is indeed not only to be expected, but also encouraged, in order to

have the framework "owned" by the Member States and the WHO Regions. It would be regrettable if the intellectual power that has been expended would not ultimately lead to a universal adoption of and support for the framework as the one framework for the assessment of the performance of health systems worldwide. It is with this strong, favourable disposition towards the proposed framework that the forthcoming comments are introduced for discussion.

It has not been easy to assess the performance of health systems. Efforts to that effect have been made over the past three decades and are a testimony to the importance of this goal as well as to its complexity. This and other considerations have prompted the development of the framework discussed today.

Dr Kronfol then reviewed the functions, goals, boundaries and monitoring tools proposed by *The World Health Report 2000*. According to him, the intrinsic goals of health systems are well outlined in the report.

The framework proposes indicators for the following three goals and their components.

The level of health is measured using disability-adjusted life expectancy or DALE. The importance and relevance of this indicator for the measurement of "good health" is undoubted. However, this is a summary indicator adjusted to a 0–1 scale for a specified number and range of conditions. It includes an adjustment for years spent in poor health. (Incidentally, this adjustment deducts about 6–7 years from the life expectancy or some 10% of an individual's life span. This is an important finding, which policy-makers should consider in order to reduce years spent in disability). Policy-makers are unlikely to have issues with this summary indicator of health status. However, intermediate indicators are needed to uncover specific causes of morbidity and mortality that impact on the value of DALE. In addition, indicators for the non-health components that impact on the health of individuals and communities ought to be defined. This may also serve to identify actions directly under the control of health agencies versus other equally important actions under the responsibility of non-health sectors, such as indices for the environment, nutrition, education and others. This effort would also serve to provide measurement tools for the advocacy role and the stewardship function of health agencies.

Countries or regions may have the same overall value for DALE, yet have varying causes and different intermediate indicators. We argue that intermediate indicators are useful and ought to be included in the assessment of performance as "diagnostic" indicators. The calculation of such indicators would facilitate the evaluation of health programmes and would draw attention to the risks that threaten good health in a particular community or country. WHO should take into consideration the need to strengthen national capabilities in mastering the burden of disease tool through training and provision of technical expertise. Training and research institutions, as well as the WHO collaborating centres, should be used in capacity building.

The goal of responsiveness to the legitimate non-health needs of the population is an important feature in the assessment of health systems. To quantify this goal, key informants were used to estimate the level and distribution, as well as the extent of differences between population subgroups. Further efforts are needed to refine this measurement and the criteria for this quantification. Debate has centred again on this important goal. The seven elements of the observance of human rights, those being dignity, privacy, autonomy, choice of providers, prompt attention to needs, quality of basic amenities, and access to social support, bring up the issues of accessibility and utilization of health facilities and resources. The questionnaire used to capture responsiveness through population-based surveys could be reviewed for the sake of incorporating social and cultural peculiarities.

The interaction of the individual with the system forms the basis of the goal of responsiveness. Yet these same elements are at the core of the concepts of accessibility and utilization.

Accessibility is hindered by social, cultural, financial, geographical and financial factors. Without smooth and easy accessibility, the use of services provided is seriously hampered. Without utilization of services, whether personal or non-personal, the achievement of good health may be curtailed. One may even question the relevance of the provision of medical services (noted correctly as an important function of health systems within the framework) if individuals and communities fail to take advantage of it.

In their paper, Murray and Frenk recognize the importance of access to care, but they argue that it is "an instrumental goal whose attainment will raise the level of health, responsiveness and fairness in financing." They further note that "if we hold the level and distribution of the three goals constant and change the level of access, this would not be intrinsically valued. Improved access to care is desirable insofar as it improves health, reduces health inequalities and

enhances responsiveness." One could argue, however, that although accessibility and utilization are not goals of the health care system, they remain at the very core of health system performance and at the centre of the interaction of individuals and communities with the health care system. They ought to be measured as additional and independent components of health systems performance. Hypothetically, if communities were to refrain from accessing or utilizing the health services, what quantitative measures would be adopted for responsiveness? If people fail to take advantage of services, the seven components of responsiveness cannot be measured, nor would fairness in financing be relevant. The framework would thus fail to measure two of its three goals. It should also be noted that the measurement of accessibility and utilization serves to highlight the factors impeding the benefit of individuals from health programs, and thus can be considered diagnostic indicators.

One model of health care systems describes the interaction between providers and users as the essence of the process of these systems. In this model, clients or users with a health need are considered the inputs to the system. Users with a modified need are the outputs. Facilities and resources are described as the structural (or internal) elements and components of any health care system. The other sectors of the economy and country (environment, education, etc.) are the external environment. The process of transformation of health needs hinges on the provider-user interaction. This process is indeed the result of accessibility in all its elements. Utilization is the result of this accessibility. In this model, the outcomes are "good health" (measured by morbidity and mortality indicators), responsiveness (measured by satisfaction, compliance, etc.) and financing (cost and affordability).

Dr Kronfol maintained, "The intent of this interjection is certainly not to replace the framework by that model. We have already indicated our acceptance of the framework and our commitment to its use and adoption as the new framework for assessing performance. The purpose of this comparison is to indicate that accessibility and utilization are indeed important elements of health care systems, which ought to be included in the assessment of performance." One option could be to secure access for all to the various components of primary health care as indicated in the Alma Ata consideration.

Moreover, the inclusion of accessibility and utilization within the framework serves to integrate the past efforts of the Organization with the present framework and the future adoption of it. It may not be prudent to disregard or discard decades of efforts by the Organization to promote the notions of access and utilization through its well-known programme, Global Strategy for Health for All, through primary health care and the associated indicators of achievement. The integration of these indicators into the proposed framework serves to facilitate its understanding and adoption at present. It will maintain a desired continuity without undermining the essence of the framework or its future potential as the criterion for assessment.

In the background paper for the Regional Consultation of AMRO/PAHO, the scope of performance assessment was discussed and "it was suggested that it might be considered as a broad menu of activities. This would allow HSPA to cover consideration of whether progress is being made toward specified goals and whether appropriate activities are being undertaken to promote the achievements of these goals. The value of this would be to identify problem areas that may require special attention and best practices that can serve as a model." Similar comments were expressed in the SEARO paper.

In any case, there is a need to monitor the efficiency of health care systems at both national and subnational levels, using production and coverage indicators. These indicators should be constructed in view of the contribution of the intermediate goals to the intrinsic goals.

Measurements of accessibility and utilization could be developed using the proposed "tracer" method for a specified number of services and interventions. A set of cost-effective strategies is currently being proposed and evaluated as the minimum basic package that ought to be made available to individuals and communities. A suggestion for this package may consist of integrating some or all the programmes of primary health care within this set of minimum interventions and health services. Indicators for these activities and programmes have benefited from the test of time and from their universal use over the past two decades. This pre-test minimizes the impact of social, cultural and economical differences across and within countries.

If this amendment meets resistance or the proposed framework of HSPA cannot accommodate these concerns, a composite overall index of performance may be suggested. This would maintain the proposed HSPA as is, but would give it a weight of perhaps 75–80%

of the overall indicator of performance. The remaining 20–25% would then be allocated to the agreed upon measures of accessibility and utilization. This arrangement provides the needed flexibility to underscore the importance of interim goals and strategies, as well as a certain weight for diagnostic indicators of health systems.

Several comments were made as to the validity of the indicators introduced in the framework, i.e. the numbers used for measurement. The authors noted that some indicators were estimates. There is no doubt that the calculation of these indicators would be refined in the new version.

In its efforts to assist this process, WHO/EMRO will establish an observatory for the health care systems of the Member States in the Region. In addition to its functions, the observatory will supply updated and validated information on these health systems. This information will provide the indicators for the forthcoming *World Health Reports*. In fact, the framework for assessing performance may be adopted by the observatory as one component of the template for the analysis of health systems in the Region.

ENHANCING HEALTH SYSTEM PERFORMANCE INITIATIVE (DR PHYLLIDA TRAVIS)

Dr Phyllida Travis, Scientist at WHO/HQ, described the current activities undertaken as part of the Enhancing Health System Performance Initiative. The initiative encompasses work with a variety of countries (21 countries so far) to use the health systems performance assessment framework as a tool for the analysis of their health systems, as a method to inform their health policies and as a means to improve performance.

The initial emphasis has been on assessment of performance (the "diagnostic phase"). Self-assessment of goals has been undertaken by countries with WHO support. They use the common framework, but a flexible set of activities is involved. Seminars have been held to discuss the preliminary findings. More recently, there has been a shift from assessment towards other activities: the joint investigation of the underlying reasons for poor performance; the application of the approach at subnational levels; and the provision of technical advice on specific issues, such as regular monitoring of performance and financing policies.

A variety of strategies have been employed to encourage discussion and use of findings within countries: obtaining a high level of MOH support and attention from the start; encouraging greater breadth of analysis so that decision-makers can understand the trade-offs in achievements across the multiple goals of health systems; obtaining quick results so that early feedback can be provided; minimizing labour and costs by using routine data whenever possible; involving national partners in method development; and promoting links with other global activities and agencies.

These strategies inevitably create some challenges. High level of MOH support generates high expectations. The demands for technical support are stretching the available resources within WHO. The quality of available data and the continuing development of methods can create some uncertainty for national investigators.

The future directions of this initiative consist of several components: a greater amount of joint analytical work on the functions of health systems; better documentation and dissemination of findings, perhaps the preparation of short country-specific briefs; and fostering country interaction through inter-country and inter-regional seminars, and the development of regional networks. All of these will require an increased policy and system support from different departments and levels in WHO.

REGIONAL INITIATIVES TO STRENGTHEN HEALTH SYSTEM PERFORMANCE (DR BELGACEM SABRI)

Dr Belgacem Sabri, Director of Health Systems and Community Development at WHO/EMRO, described the regional initiatives to strengthen health system performance. He indicated that "since Alma Ata in 1978, countries have started to monitor and evaluate the policies of health for all and the appertaining strategies. This exercise has included several indicators: of input, process, output, coverage, outcome and quality of life. These efforts are carried out jointly by the Member States and WHO, both contributing to assess coverage by preventive programs, the environment, access and outcomes.

The inclusion of other health determinants helped to stress intersectoral linkages and the principle of community empowerment. In some WHO regions, targets were set and countries were assessed in relation to these targets. The findings from these evaluation and monitoring efforts were used to improve the performance of health systems.

The focus during that period was on services and outcome indicators. However, the framework was cumbersome and not focused, as it was not meant to assess the performance of health systems. The access

to the components of primary health care and the boundaries of health systems were not defined well; the resources devoted or shifted to PHC were not clearly captured. The merit of the new WHO framework is the clarification of the boundaries of health systems, their goals and their functions. The functions and goals will determine the efforts needed to improve performance through more focused interventions. However, some analytical work is expected from WHO in the assessment of the various functions and in identifying ways and means to improve them.

Some of the regional initiatives in this respect have included strengthening of information and support to health legislation; capacity building including the reinforcement of analytical capability of policy and decision-makers; and institutional development.

To accomplish these efforts, the capabilities at the Regional Office must be strengthened. It is planned that an observatory function be developed. This will be the repository of information on health systems in the Region. It will support the assessment and forecasting of needs. It will also undertake the monitoring and evaluation of health sector reforms and health system performance.

Models for health system functions (normative work) have to be developed. This underscores the importance of joint efforts between HQ and the regions. Research institutions ought to be involved and supported financially in this effort. Additional resources must be mobilized through an increase in the regular budget allocations (JPRM) and in the provision of extra-budgetary funds from WHO headquarters.

The regional consultation took note of the recent developments to further the WHO framework on health systems performance assessment. There was general agreement that this framework is a valid document, which needs to be endorsed, albeit with some refinement. It was equally stressed that the goals of health for all are still valid, as are the programmes of primary health care.

In his summary, Dr Evans indicated that the initiative to develop this framework had come originally from the Member States, which needed support to evaluate and perhaps restructure their health systems. Mistakes may have occurred in the process, but an attempt is being made to correct them. Finally, Dr Evans underlined the fact that this is a WHO initiative, not one imposed or suggested by other organizations.

The plenary adjourned at this time.

Later in the evening on Tuesday, 10 July 2001, the expert group meetings were held to discuss the methodological issues related to burden of disease, financing and responsiveness elements.

Session Seven: Recommendations

The regional consultation met on Wednesday morning for three hours in two groups. The purpose of the exercise was to prepare recommendations that were to be reviewed by the entire group following this exercise. The first group was coordinated by Dr Nabil Kronfol; the second, by Dr Sameen Siddiqui (Pakistan).

Although the two groups submitted their recommendations separately, there was close similarity between them. That is why the recommendations are grouped together here. They focus on:

- The ownership of tools and methods by countries and EMRO.
- The enrichment of the framework.
- The strengthening of information support to the performance exercise.
- Mapping of health system functions.
- Improvement of health systems performance.

The Ownership of Tools and Methods by Countries and EMRO

- The regional consultative group endorses the WHO framework and supports its adoption and implementation. The framework is a technically sound one for health systems: it delineates the boundaries, clarifies the goals and the functions, and proposes tools to measure health systems. It needs to be enriched as suggested herewith, in particular as far as the accuracy, timeliness, extrapolations of the limited data available and its ownership by the Member States and the Regional Offices. The group welcomes the openness of WHO to discuss the framework and appreciates the invitation of the EM Regional Office to that effect.

- It is necessary to plan the contribution of the Eastern Mediterranean Region to the further development of the framework. To that effect, funds ought to be committed from HQ (primarily from extra-budgetary resources). It is recommended that this contribution be guided by the Division of Health Systems and Community Development to include *inter alia* the establishment of a regional observatory for health systems and national focal points

to follow up on the process and findings of health systems assessment.

- This activity will involve capacity building (detailed below) in the Member States and the Regional Office. A regional forum may be called periodically to share and discuss the process and studies. National focal points and health authorities ought to find ways to link with national statistical departments and relevant ministries, such as the Ministry of Planning. Cooperation with research centres and academic institutions is highly recommended. The Regional Office is invited to develop partnerships with geopolitical groups to support this initiative (The League of Arab States, the Conference of the Arab Ministers of Health, the Health Ministers of the GCC countries, AGFUND, ESCWA, etc.).

- The Regional Office and the Member States ought to monitor the utilization of the framework in the Region and recommend changes, additions and modifications as these evolve during the application and testing of the framework. All of the above measures would develop the sense of "ownership" of the framework and its tools by the Region and the Member States.

- It is recommended that measures be taken to improve the process of system assessment through better data gathering and processing, capacity building and other means to insure the reliability of the information, the transparency of the process and the ownership of the performance measurement exercise by the Member States and WHO Regional Office. This will assist in the preparation of a regional strategy on health systems development aimed at improving health systems performance.

- Accessibility and utilization remain at the very core of health systems performance and at the centre of interaction between individuals and communities. It is recommended that accessibility and utilization be measured as additional components of health systems assessment. Indicators of accessibility and utilization serve as "diagnostic" indicators to recognize impeding factors. Moreover, the inclusion of accessibility and utilization would serve to integrate the past efforts of WHO with the present framework. This will maintain a desired continuity without undermining the essence of the framework.

Enrichment of the Framework

- It is important to focus on the functions of health systems and to develop their indicators. Why only these three functions and not others? Research is recommended to validate the proposed framework. How do functions vary within the Region, by country? Stewardship is critical and requires a lot of attention. What does it mean? How can it be described?

- The efficiency of health care systems has to be monitored at both the national and the subnational levels, using production and coverage indicators. The latter should be constructed in view of the contribution of the intermediate goals to the intrinsic goals of health systems.

- The initiative to enhance health systems performance must be supported. It purports to work with a variety of countries to use the framework to analyse their health systems, inform health policies and improve performance. Periodic reports on this initiative ought to be released and circulated for the benefit of the Member States.

- The framework has been proposed by health professionals and economists. It is advised that additional researchers from other disciplines (anthropology, sociology, education) be invited to review the functions and contribute to their further development.

- Health systems should secure a minimum of interventions (such as PHC components, essential PH functions) to be referred to as a package of essential clinical care. This set of cost-effective interventions could integrate some or all the programs of PHC, along with indicators that need to be tested and used after validation. Efforts to assess the coverage of effective interventions are being made.

- The weights of the index ought perhaps to be adjusted in light of the responses from all WHO regions including Europe. Some of the elements need to be validated. The available tools must be simplified. Alternative methodologies must be searched for and validity must be checked. Is the composite index valid to measure health systems? What techniques have been validated and what are experimental?

- As far as financing is concerned, the overall level of financing is not included. The components of the index need more attention and ought to be more explicit. Efforts should be expanded to promote the use of household surveys to measure fairness in financial contribution. The framework should also focus on the distribution of resources and cross-subsidy as a mechanism of social solidarity.

- With reference to responsiveness, the issues of cultural sensitivity and quality of care must be further explored and highlighted. The responsiveness questionnaire has to be translated into the local language and incorporated into national population-based surveys. The factors related to access and health components should be disentangled as they highly impact user satisfaction. Questionnaires need to be adapted to regional and country priorities and to be made culture-sensitive. They need to be validated, as do the proposed vignettes.

- Regarding health inequality, "inequity" must be addressed as traditionally defined, with differentials in access, coverage and utilization.

- Intermediate indicators are useful and must be included in the performance of assessment, possibly as "diagnostic" indicators. Intermediate goals are also needed, especially relating to coverage, access and utilization.

- The currently ongoing application of the framework to facility level is a welcome addition.

- It is recommended that success stories on the various functions drawn from an array of countries be prepared and circulated as illustrations. This is especially relevant to the elements of responsiveness and fairness in financing.

- The technical papers and reports have to be made available in the official languages of the Organization in order to involve the scientists and researchers from non-English speaking countries into this worldwide process of health systems performance assessment.

- It is recommended that manuals prepared for study, such as NHA, BOD, and CEA, be made user-friendly. This will facilitate the integration of these important tools into the information systems of countries.

The Strengthening of Information Support to the Performance Exercise

- It is recommended that national information systems be strengthened through the use of ICD-10, the collection of vital statistics, the promotion of health systems research and the use of data available from surveys and studies undertaken by other organizations.

■ Access to information, reports and data needs to be improved. A regional observatory of health systems is recommended to review data, generate relevant information and serve as the liaison with in-country units.

■ The development of capacity is critical to enhance understanding and ownership, and to undertake burden of disease studies, cost effectiveness analysis and national health accounts. Technical support to the Member States is needed and ought to be provided in a more unified manner. Further information on social insurance and health financing schemes is of significance.

■ Indicators for the different levels of care across national and subnational levels ought to be included or added to the framework as "diagnostic" indicators.

■ The framework has to be integrated within national health information systems. To that effect, systems must be evaluated as to the level of decentralization and capability in epidemiological intelligence. The focus is not to improve the information system, but the health system, and then to assess the needs for information. How will this information be used by policy-makers for action and decision?

■ A transparent mechanism to estimate data when not available ought to be described.

■ It is strongly recommended that performance assessment be discussed with the national authorities before the release of the next *World Health Report* to the media. The information used in the assessment ought to be shared with the national authority.

Mapping of Health System Functions

■ It is recommended that efforts be made to support the mapping of health systems' functions through the assessment of existing national and regional capabilities for analytical work, the evaluation of health system functions and plans to strengthen these functions.

■ A concern exists that the framework would bypass the current system.

■ Another concern is that the current framework cannot be used on a continuous basis as proposed.

In the first place, the recommended studies are time-consuming and require extensive resources in manpower and funds. To date the latter have been external funds. The health authorities of some countries may find it difficult to justify expenditures on such studies instead of allocating the meagre resources available to the provision of medical services.

Improvement of Health Systems Performance

■ Policy-makers have to be educated in order to understand what these indicators mean. The correlation between HSPA and health sector reform efforts ought to be clarified.

■ There is an intersection of elements of PHC with HSPA. Which are the complementary parts? How does the improvement of the health system contribute to overall development? This is an important issue for policy-makers in the Region.

■ It is recommended that the data and information obtained from the performance assessment exercise be used in the preparation of the biennium.

■ Support to health system development is of critical importance. The health authorities must be strengthened to develop capacity in policy development, strategic thinking, coordination of functions, institution of national health accounts, promotion of national observatories for health systems and support to priority setting through BOD studies, CEA and other surveys.

■ The decentralization of health systems based on PHC principles must be pursued and activated. This includes support to hospital autonomy, improving access to PHC programmes and adapting PHC to new challenges.

■ The development of human resources must be maintained, in particular to develop capabilities in policy analysis and formulation, strategic planning and management, economics, epidemiology and leadership.

Summary

■ Develop tools to evaluate health systems functions.

■ Focus on the attainment of intermediate goals. The development of intermediate indicators (function-specific) is important as well.

- Make health systems performance measurement a tool for planners and managers at the national and subnational levels. This will entail education and information for policy-makers.

- Assist countries in understanding the impact of their policies and interventions on the population in most need.

- Assist countries in the analysis and monitoring of the performance of health care providers. Increase the country and regional capacity to update, maintain and use information for policy analysis. Information ought to be readily available.

- Stewardship and its components ought to be better defined in terms of health policy formulation, regulation and intelligence. This will require defining a vision and a direction for health systems, setting fair rules for regulation and cooperation in intelligence-gathering and sharing of information.

- Identification of key health systems requirements that determine the effective provision of health interventions. These include the strengthening of the capacities of health systems to produce the maximum possible gain for poor and vulnerable populations from the investment of scarce resources in critical interventions and to ensure fair distribution of benefits from such investments.

- Identify cost-effective interventions that would produce significant health gain, particularly among the poor. Select the most appropriate coverage indicators and tools for collecting coverage data. Pilot these measurements and develop a tool that will help incorporate data on effective coverage into the planning and management of health services.

- Define explicitly the intersection with primary health care.

- Capacity development in the EMRO.

- Assessment of information by country for the application of HSPA.

- Comprehensive approach and institutionalization of HSPA.

NOTES

1 Ain Saadeh, Lebanon, 9–11 July 2001

Dr Gamal Al Sayad
Epidemiology Specialist
Minister of Health
P.O. Box 12
Bahrain

Dr Lamia AL Tahou
Head of Planning & Programme
  Department
C/o Ministry of Health
Manama

Dr Hassan Salah
Cairo
Egypt

Dr Sami Gadallah
36. El Sheikh Ahmed El Sawy str.
Nasr City
Cairo
Egypt

Dr Farid Aboul Hassanin
DG of Primary Health Care
  Programme
C/o WR
Iran

Dr Hussein Salahi
Health Economist
C/o WR
Iran

Dr Mohsen Naghavi
Epidemiologist and Head of BOD
  Team
C/o WR
Iran

H.E. Mr Sleiman Franjieh
Minister of Public Health
Beirut
Lebanon

Mr Marwan Hamada
Minister of Displaced
C/o WR
Lebanon

Dr Walid Ammar
C/o WR
Lebanon

Dr Dolly Bassili
C/o WR
Lebanon

Dr Adnan Mrowa
C/o WR
Lebanon

Mr Robert Kasparian
C/o WR
Lebanon

Dr Abla El Sebai
C/o WR
Lebanon

Dr Hala Nawfal
C/o WR
Lebanon

Dr Maral Tutelian
C/o WR
Lebanon

Dr Iman Nwaihid
C/o WR
Lebanon

Dr Rafik Baddoura
C/o WR
Lebanon

Dr Abdu Jurios
C/o WR
Lebanon

Dr Zineddine M. Idriss
C/o WR
Morocco

Dr Abderrahmane Zahi
C/o WR
Morocco

Dr Ali Jaafar
Director General
Ministry of Health
Muscat
Oman

Dr Sameen Siddiqui
C/o WR
Pakistan

Ms Wafa Salloum
C/o WR
Syria

Dr Mohmoud Dashash
C/o WR
Syria

Dr Suleiman Mashkouk
C/o WR
Syria

Dr Tawfik Ahmed Khoja
Executive Director for Gulf
  Cooperation Council States
Saudi Arabia

Dr Mazen Khadra
C/o WR
Syria

Dr Kamil Al Mirghani
Professor in Community
  Medicines
C/o WR
Sudan

Dr Noureddine Achour
C/o MOH
Tunisia

Dr Mohamed Hsairi
C/o MOH
Tunisia

Mr Gharama Al Raee
C/o WR
Yemen

WHO Secretariat

Dr Hussein A. Gezairy
Regional Director
WHO/EMRO

Dr Abdel Aziz Saleh
Deputy Regional Director
WHO/EMRO

Dr Belgacem Sabri
Director, Health Systems and
Community Development
WHO/EMRO

Dr David B. Evans
Evidence and Information
   for Policy
WHO/HQ

Dr Habib Latiri
WR/Lebanon
WHO/Beirut

Dr Raouf Ben Ammar
WR/Morocco
WHO/Rabat

Dr Ibrahim Abdel Rahim
WR/Oman
WHO/Muscat

Dr Abdullah S. Assa'edi
WR/Syria
WHO/Damascus

Dr Christopher J.L. Murray
Executive Director
Evidence and Information for
   Policy
WHO/HQ

Dr Alan D. Lopez
Evidence and Information for
   Policy
WHO/HQ

Dr Somnath Chatterji
Evidence and Information for
   Policy
WHO/HQ

Dr Phyllida Travis
Evidence and Information for
   Policy
WHO/HQ

Dr Abdelhay Mechbal
Regional Adviser, Research
Policy and Cooperation
WHO/EMRO

Dr El Fatih EL Sammani
Regional Adviser, Emerging
   Diseases
WHO/EMRO

Dr Amina Al Ghamry
Temporary Adviser
WHO/EMRO

Dr Nabil Kronfol
Temporary Adviser
WHO/EMRO

Dr A. Hyder Adnan
Temporary Adviser
WHO/EMRO

Dr Alissar Radi
Medical Officer
WHO/Lebanon

Mrs Ferial Khalil
DHS/Senior Secretary
WHO/EMRO

Ms Ghada Ragab
DHS/Secretary
WHO/EMRO

Chapter 5

EUROPEAN REGIONAL CONSULTATION ON HEALTH SYSTEMS PERFORMANCE ASSESSMENT[1]

WHO REGIONAL OFFICE FOR EUROPE

INTRODUCTION

The launch of *The World Health Report 2000* and its framework for health systems performance assessment (HSPA) has prompted vigorous discussion at the technical and professional levels globally and across the European Region. In response to the debate among the Member States and the academic and policy-making communities, the Director-General of the World Health Organization put in place a far-reaching consultation process.

The Regional Consultation of the European Region on HSPA took place on 3–4 September 2001. Forty-two experts from 22 Member States participated. Ten staff members from the WHO Regional Office for Europe and the Cluster of Evidence and Information for Health Policy of the World Health Organization, Geneva were involved. The meeting brought together representatives of ministries of health, research institutes and international organizations, including the OECD and the World Bank.

The Consultation was targeted at technical experts in the field and senior policy-makers. It was intended to build on the very substantial work carried out in the area since the publication of *The World Health Report 2000* and to be mindful of ongoing developments in response to the feedback already received. In particular, the Consultation was planned to follow the contributions of other regions, academics, practitioners and the WHO headquarters team around: refining data (touching on survey instruments and disability, responsiveness work and vignettes, absolute poverty, subsistence and national health accounts); clarifying terminology (separating efficiency, performance and attainment); broadening concepts (addressing inequality, stewardship, intermediate goals amenable to change, mediating factors

and coverage) and developing tools (training, manuals, assessment methods and the Enhancing Health Systems Development Initiative).

It was also explicitly decided that the meeting should not focus primarily on detailed methodological aspects, but should address how applicable *The World Health Report 2000* is in supporting countries. Discussion then would go beyond the issues of measurement and diagnosis to concentrate on improving performance.

The meeting was designed to highlight progress with HSPA methodology and to set out the options for addressing the remaining issues before working through the practical policy implications. Time was set aside to consider what a particular country ranking meant in terms of performance failures and successes, and to identify the implications for improving health system functions like resource generation, financing, provision or stewardship. It was also anticipated that the meeting would address the cost and effectiveness of alternative strategies for improving these functions.

The objectives of the meeting were therefore to:

- Review the key methodological aspects of the HSPA with a focus on recent progress, identify the remaining issues and gaps, and consider complementary measures to strengthen the framework.

- Present the results of the most recent HSPA work in the European Region and ascertain some of the methodological and policy implications of the developments.

- Discuss the linkage between health systems performance results and health systems policy and managerial processes, with a particular emphasis on explaining performance and improving the functions of the health system.

■ Provide recommendations for the next steps in strengthening the methodology and improving the applicability of the HSPA to health system development in the Member States.

The meeting was structured to address these objectives and was divided into three core sessions, which led participants through a purposeful series of discussions on: measuring health systems performance: methodological issues and developments; explaining performance: linking health system functions with performance; and improving performance: policy implications.

Every session was introduced by a presentation from WHO headquarters on current thinking and developments, with a second paper from an invited expert setting out complementary views and approaches. These were followed by a panel discussion, in which each of three discussants brought country experience to bear on the issues, and then by a plenary.

The meeting was underpinned by detailed preparations, among which was the specially commissioned paper by Prof. Martin McKee. Prof. McKee summarized the debate around *The World Health Report 2000* and raised a series of questions, which facilitated discussion at the consultation. In addition, the document capturing the developments in thinking as the Regional Consultations progressed was updated. A comprehensive selection of background papers and resources was made available to the participants and posted on the web site constructed for this purpose. These papers together with reports from all presentations are available at http://www.observatory.dk/20010815_1.htm.

The present report is structured in accordance with the conceptual approach to the meeting outlined above. It is acknowledged that the boundaries between the core sessions are at best permeable and that there is inevitably an overlap between themes. Nonetheless, the focus on measuring, explaining and improving performance in sequence was invaluable in shaping the thinking. It moved the meeting from reviewing the technical dimensions of measurement, through a consideration of how different broad dimensions of health system functioning contribute to overall performance, to a more detailed look at the kind of working (or not) interventions, the evidence on their role in the functions and performance of the system itself, and what policy-makers and WHO can do to support implementation.

The remainder of the report is divided into three sections, which follow the logic of the consultation, with a concluding section that sets out the conclu-

sions and recommendations made. The report seeks to record the width and depth of the debate and to capture its richness. It cannot, however, hope to include every element of the discussion. It will highlight those areas that the participants felt were particularly important or in need of further development or which contained clear lessons to be learned.

MEASURING HEALTH SYSTEMS PERFORMANCE: METHODOLOGICAL ISSUES AND DEVELOPMENTS

RATIONALE

The session was to focus on the conceptual and methodological debates around the construction of the HSPA framework, the indicators employed and the composite index, with particular attention to recent developments. The key areas addressed within the session were:

■ The boundaries of the health system.

■ The scope, coherence and timing of performance measures.

■ The choice and measurement of goals (health, responsiveness and fairness of financing) and alternative measures.

■ The methodology of measuring health (levels and distribution), responsiveness (levels and distribution) and fairness in financing.

■ Estimating overall health systems performance.

■ Building and using a composite index and ranking.

■ Data collection, availability, quality, validity and sustainability.

PRESENTATIONS

Peter Smith chaired the session. Prof. Martin McKee summarized the debate around *The World Health Report 2000*, touched on values, face validity, choice and coherence and raised key questions for the consultation. Dr Christopher J.L. Murray then addressed the debates around HSPA and some of the issues in the literature. He also presented the new methodological developments as reflected in the HSPA background paper, and discussed the preliminary results from the current HSPA exercise. Dr Murray noted the construction of new life tables, adjustments in the approach to responsiveness, and the new surveys used to measure fairness in financing.

Three parallel question and answer sessions on healthy life expectancy (Dr Colin D. Mathers), responsiveness (Ms Nicole B. Valentine and Dr Bedirhan Üstün) and fairness in financial contribution (Dr Christopher J.L. Murray and Dr Abdelhay Mechbal) at the end of the day, addressed specific issues regarding data collection, and developing and using indicators in countries.

DISCUSSION

The discussants Dr Erik Nord, Dr Bruce Rosen, and Dr Markus Schneider raised a wide range of issues, including data quality and face validity, the value of ranking countries globally versus subregional comparisons, the need to link measurements to actions, the politics of ranking and of marketing the report, trend analysis in a changing methodological environment, non-accountable differences and the separation in time of interventions and outcomes. The plenary discussion was also wide-ranging. The main conclusions are outlined below.

SCOPE, COHERENCE AND TIMING OF PERFORMANCE MEASURES

There was an agreement on the need for clarity about the scope of performance measures and their coherence across the whole performance measurement framework. The highlighted points included:

- The need to establish a link between health systems action and health outcome, and in particular to address the complicating factor of the time frame in which health outcomes can be measured. Further work is necessary to address the coherence of the time period of health actions and when performance gains can be identified and related to it.

- It is important for accountability to choose broad, as opposed to narrow, health system boundaries and of ensuring long-term rather than short-term measures of performance.

- The definition of health system boundaries implied by life expectancy was broad, while the approach to measure responsiveness and fairness in financing was narrower, focusing mostly on personal health services, which tended to introduce incongruity between the dimensions of health systems performance.

- The scope to adjust indicators for responsiveness in the public health domain to make the boundaries more congruent, for example, reflecting public access to information and support in smoking cessation, to supplement the current focus on responsiveness of personal health services.

- The possibility of revising fairness in financial contribution to include a redistributive element between population groups and thus to "match" the population approach implied by life expectancy measures and perhaps reflect time lag and expenditure.

- The desirability of incorporating a measure of country-specific appropriateness of interventions into work on coverage in order to ensure that the position of the most vulnerable populations will be reflected, regardless of the size of the groups or their isolation.

DATA COLLECTION, AVAILABILITY, QUALITY AND SUSTAINABILITY

There were significant problems associated with population data, particularly given the lack of census data or information on disability and health state preferences. A number of participants argued that the treatment of ignorance as uncertainty tended to undermine the confidence in *The World Health Report 2000*. The meeting decided that:

- More details on methodology, data sources and assumptions needed to be published to achieve real transparency. Particular efforts to explain the treatment of missing data and to signpost extrapolation and assumptions would create greater confidence.

- Thought should be given to the impact of data collection exercises on countries. It would be worth exploring options to integrate country data collection into the measurement processes; taking steps to ensure the new World Health Survey and other new instruments do not compete with or undermine existing country work; and "stretching" the two-year cycle to allow for the fact that collecting timely data on financing and responsiveness may be overly burdensome for countries.

- The next report should address the problems of establishing a denominator in countries in conflict, with displaced populations and/or large migrant worker populations and/or excluded minority groups.

Notwithstanding these points, the meeting welcomed the scientific peer review and the current developments led by WHO headquarters to enhance the methodology through a series of consultations.

ESTIMATING OVERALL HEALTH SYSTEMS ATTAINMENT AND PERFORMANCE

The meeting covered building and using a composite index of attainment and performance ranking overlapping issues as separate. There was a consensus that aggregate measures can be very useful, but that they create a number of dilemmas regarding:

■ Meaning and communicating meaning. It is not clear what policy-makers understand by the different health outcome and fairness in financing measures. It was agreed that more specific and detailed information should be transmitted to policy-makers, particularly through disaggregated measures and intermediate indicators, which would help explain the results of the composite indices and signpost the way forward for policy-making.

■ Values and the value judgements implicit in the measures, with their inherently political implications. It was pointed out that values are not universal and that policy-makers with different value systems operating in essentially political environments would extract different messages from the report. The meeting believed that the values in the report should be made more explicit.

■ Country specificity and whether different weights should be used in different countries to reflect the range of country contexts.

RANKING PERFORMANCE

The meeting went on to discuss ranking of performance. It became clear that the issues around the construction of the overall health systems attainment index are further complicated when this index is adjusted to produce an overarching performance measure, which includes the notion of what the maximum goal achievement would be given financial and human capital constraints (using a frontier production approach). Although the exercise had been successful in attracting attention and giving rise to the whole consultation idea, the use of ranking in further HSPA exercises should be reassessed. Certainly the concerns raised above were compounded with questions on the advisability of comparing countries in this way and the alternatives available. The meeting wanted to see

any ranking carried out and made as useful as possible through the use of transparent and comprehensible measures, and through any or a combination of the following:

■ A middle way, ranking countries in line with individual indicators (that are simplified and fully explained) and without using an overall performance index.

■ Grouping countries by region (subregion), socioeconomic status or health care system "type" and ranking only within these groups, using the overall attainment index rather than the performance measure in order to make the exercise as meaningful and useful to policy-makers as possible.

■ Introducing bench-marking initiatives, which would concentrate on providing useable information on performance to policy-makers.

■ Focusing on aberrant results and outliers that would illustrate extremes of performance rather than overall ranking.

The participants were concerned about the use of the report to address change over time. Comparisons over a number of years were desirable and valuable for decision-makers. However, the main preoccupation was that the next report would give rise to comparisons of performance with the first report and to inferences about trends, despite the fact that the two would be based on quite different data sets and methodologies. Finally, a number of participants voiced concerns that the impact of the next report would be undermined if it was seen to pursue a strategy (of ranking and a composite index) without taking on board the suggestions made.

EXPLAINING PERFORMANCE: LINKING HEALTH SYSTEMS FUNCTIONS WITH PERFORMANCE

RATIONALE

The session was planned to balance the fact that much of the broad debate around the HSPA framework had focused on measurement of the broad health system goals and the composite index. The intention was to look inside the "black box" of global health systems performance to address what policy-makers need to know about individual functions like service provision, resource generation or stewardship, if they are to oppose poor efficiency, performance and ranking.

In particular, it was to consider how policy-makers might understand the bench-marks of the best performers and learn from them, while using the HSPA exercise to decide which functions to reform in order to improve performance. Issues addressed included: analysing, measuring and monitoring the performance of individual health system functions; using instrumental or intermediate goals and mediating factors, such as coverage; and assessing causal attribution.

PRESENTATIONS

Dr Mikko Viennonen chaired the session. Mr Orvill B. Adams outlined current work and recent developments in WHO headquarters on health systems functions assessment. He identified intermediate goals that were relatively amenable to short-term change as a key tool in developing strategies for change. He also focused on the provision of services (particularly, the coverage of critical interventions) and the approaches to measuring stewardship. Mr Jeremy Hurst then outlined the approach of the OECD to performance measurement and highlighted some of the experiences of OECD countries, touching on key actors, levers for change and the boundaries between professional roles and policy/management.

DISCUSSION

Dr Elena Varavikova, Dr Reinhard Busse and Dr Juha Teperi raised a number of questions as to how policy-makers were to use a report that at times compounded differences with policy choices. They emphasized the need to address the ultimate goal of achieving improved health systems, to signpost areas for policy-making action and to make pragmatic lessons more accessible. The suggested options included: the provision of analytical descriptions of health system status and reforms to allow policy-makers to identify the steps that enhance performance; the use of avoidable deaths as a more relevant marker for policy-makers, working with countries to select usable "problem indicators;" and the separate reporting of subnational and regional data to facilitate action at an appropriate level (of particular importance in countries of the size and with the variations of the Russian Federation). The plenary discussion amplified these themes. The main conclusions are outlined below.

FROM OVERALL HEALTH SYSTEMS PERFORMANCE TO UNDERSTANDING INDIVIDUAL FUNCTIONS

The report was welcomed for asserting the importance of health systems in health and in terms of national policy responses and expenditure. However, the meeting decided that there were still "conceptual and methodological gaps" in the way the measures of overall health systems performance reflected the performance of individual functions. In addition, more work was necessary on the assessment of individual functions in order to understand how they contribute to the "global" level of health systems performance. Another issue was the significant opportunity cost associated with further work on the "global" approach to measuring overall health systems performance relative to the measurement of individual functions. The value of further investment is fast approaching its ceiling.

The meeting suggested that rather than elaborating on measures of overall performance, which would not advance understanding of individual functions, there should be a more determined focus on intermediate indicators and mediating factors.

USING INTERMEDIATE INDICATORS OR MEDIATING FACTORS

The meeting acknowledged the value of the work done on intermediate measures and, in particular, the advances in the areas of coverage and stewardship. Presenters and discussants provided a number of useful suggestions and illustrations, and there was a clear consensus about the need to continue and expand current efforts to assess mediating factors and develop intermediate indicators. The consultation also recognized the country concerns that work on functions needed to feed into decision-making. The following were considered necessary:

- Thought needs to be given to the choice of indicators to ensure that these appropriately link with system performance and health outcome evidence.

- Process and outcome ought to be reflected upon.

- A systematic qualification and classification of health care system characteristics would support efforts to address functions and intermediate indicators.

- Further consideration of how intermediate goals might cut across functions is important.

- Work on coverage needs to look not just at the access to a number of key interventions, but also at a framework of understanding which includes risk factors.

- Disability-adjusted life expectancy needs to distinguish between people with lower life expectancy and those who are sicker.

- Applicability in both high- and low-spending countries needs to be addressed either through the choice of "all-purpose" indicators or through the establishment of tailored indicator sets.

COMPLEMENTARY AND QUALITATIVE POLICY ANALYSIS MEASURES

Several participants expressed the opinion that the work to date was overly skewed towards quantitative dimensions of analysis. The meeting called for:

- The development of complementary and qualitative measures.

- The use of a conceptual framework mapping health systems functions as a diagnostic tool to explain the relationship between the various functions, between functions and performance, and to highlight policy implications. The Health Systems in Transition profiles, currently ongoing in the European Region were cited as a good example of such tool.

- An analysis of core issues, which would combine a systematic examination of individual functions with in-depth consideration of country case-studies.

- Additional case-study work, country policy reviews and studies of the implementation of change.

IMPROVING PERFORMANCE: POLICY IMPLICATIONS

RATIONALE

This session focused on the "ultimate goal" of the HSPA initiative: improving health systems performance. The premise was that poor performance is the upshot of "failing" functions and that these can be addressed by appropriate interventions where there is the political will and the managerial capacity to select and implement appropriate strategies. The discussion was intended to cover how countries can judge the likely impact of available interventions and, specifically, how they can best understand the evidence

of their effectiveness and the obstacles to implementation. Issues addressed included:

- Securing evidence about the health system interventions that do or do not work.

- The prerequisites for implementation of interventions, including managerial and political capacity.

- National efforts towards and capacities for performance assessment and improvement.

- The importance of communications with policymakers.

- The role of WHO's technical support.

PRESENTATIONS

Prof. Tom van der Grinten chaired the session. Dr Abdelhay Mechbal discussed recent developments in WHO headquarters on the linkage between HSPA and policy-making. He highlighted the work of WHO's Enhancing Health Systems Performance Initiative (EHPI) to support countries in improving performance, the introduction of new measures and the efforts to extend consultation and ownership. Mr Joe Kutzin then provided a country perspective, reporting on the issues involved in implementing and using the HSPA to improve health systems performance in Kyrgyzstan. He addressed the need to understand the planning and the step-by-step implementation process of national policy development and the importance of political support, technical capacity and information systems in achieving change.

DISCUSSION

Dr Pavel Brezovsky, Dr Isabel de la Mata and Dr Andrzej Rys led a discussion that tackled directly the political implications of the HSPA initiative and explored the impact on politicians of doing well or badly. The importance of persuading politicians of the case for health, of outlining explicit solutions to the problems identified and of engaging with the public through effective communication, was underlined. An animated plenary discussion developed these themes. The main conclusions are outlined below.

DEVELOPING AND OBTAINING EVIDENCE ON POLICY INTERVENTIONS

The meeting expressed a commitment to providing policy-makers with the evidence base needed for them to take appropriate and effective action. These were considered crucial:

- A renewed focus on secondary research that would build on existing evidence and expertise in support to link key health interventions to health systems strategies.

- The delivery of case-studies, qualitative analyses and synthesized materials setting out the implications of the evidence available.

- More detailed work on the context in which implementation takes place.

- Action-oriented tools to support politicians and managers in translating evidence into enhanced performance.

- The work of the European Observatory on health care systems was mentioned by several participants as an example of how to carry out these evidence functions in support of policy-makers.

ANALYSING THE PROCESS OF IMPLEMENTATION OF INTERVENTIONS

It was agreed that political capacity and managerial skills were crucial in allowing countries to act on performance-related evidence. The participants stressed that:

- The very particular circumstances within countries would be enormously influential in determining how a given process would take place.

- Full consideration should be given to individual country circumstances, the socioeconomic and political context, national capacities and skills.

- The report needed to tap into the political concerns of policy-makers more explicitly.

WORKING MORE EFFECTIVELY TO SUPPORT COUNTRIES

It was suggested that countries be fully involved as partners at all stages of the process. In particular, it was hoped that:

- A review of the Member States' perceived needs and the management information they seek would help identify the most appropriate indicators.

- More use would be made of data already collected in countries.

- More focus could be put on working transparently with countries and experts as full partners.

COMMUNICATING THE RESULTS

The meeting went on to address the importance of communication. The process of working with countries is not only scientific, but also political and needs to be handled with care. The Member States and the academic community need to be involved throughout and the results have to be discussed with the Member States before being released.

- A marketing strategy should be developed to ensure that the next report delivers clear messages that politicians and the public can understand (providing simple explanations of complex issues).

- Consideration should be given to how terms and concepts translate and to the tone in which recommendations and conclusions are presented to countries.

- The presentation of findings should be reviewed in light of the fact that "weariness" can set in and that reporting counter-intuitive findings undermines the impact on national policy-makers, as well as the report's effectiveness in prompting action.

- A more comprehensive and transparent technical annex should be provided clarifying all the data and methodological issues.

WHO SUPPORT

It was acknowledged that the EHSPI was a positive undertaking and a useful way forward. However, the consultation decided that it needed to be strengthened and that:

- While capacity building on measurement was valuable, it was not sufficient as an approach to supporting countries.

- Further attention should be given to the diagnosis of failing functions.

- Particular efforts should be made to collect and draw lessons from the available evidence on alternative interventions.

- Summaries of all consultations (regional and technical) should be published together with information on responses and methodological advances.

- The credibility and sustainability of the exercise would ultimately depend on the degree to which WHO managed to achieve transparency and partnership.

Conclusions

In essence, the consultation stated that the HSPA exercise had significant potential and that for it to be truly effective, it needed to bridge the gaps between measuring at a global level, the individual functions and the interventions that result in change. It also has to address directly the issues of methodology and transparency. Work was planned to continue on the key methodological aspects discussed over the course of the consultation and in particular, on the congruence of measures, intermediate indicators and the composite indices. Ultimately, work must adapt to national circumstances, capturing within-country differences, as well as common aspects across borders, using national data available and drawing on the full breadth of analytical and qualitative tools to deal with country challenges.

The participants suggested that the very considerable achievements of *The World Health Report 2000* should be built on in line with the understanding arrived at. A coherent evaluation process, which would address the report's impact and influence in countries, should be put in place. The evaluation should include an examination of how the report was received, how the ways it was communicated affected uptake by decision-makers and how the experience so far is likely to affect the sustainability of the process. The evaluation should also consider the opportunity cost of the whole exercise (including the resource consumption by both WHO and the Member States) and set it against other approaches to analysing health systems in order to establish whether the approach is the most effective use of limited resources.

HSPA was agreed to be a key milestone in health systems performance work and to have enhanced the debate. It was evaluated as positive and necessary. The meeting looked forward to the changes in content and process, which it believed would deliver significant improvements in terms of relevance, usefulness in countries and sustainability.

Summary of Recommendations

Key and fundamental shifts that the participants wanted to see included:

- Greater coherence of performance measures.
- More detail and transparency on data collection, availability and methodology.

- The problems of developing composite indicators and the values underpinning the process made much clearer and a more detailed sensitivity analysis carried out.

- Global ranking downplayed in favour of more meaningful comparisons.

- Further work on the overall measure of performance (rather than on evaluating individual functions) reassessed in light of the opportunity costs involved and possible diminishing returns on investment.

- Continued and strengthened work on intermediate indicators development.

- The inclusion of more qualitative and descriptive policy analysis and a stronger role for evidence on the workings of health systems.

- A clear focus on obtaining and assessing evidence on individual interventions that achieve change with use of secondary research and thematic analysis.

- More evidence on the national context, political capacities and skills in a country as a key factor in successful (or unsuccessful) implementation of change.

- A real country presence, building sustainable and enduring relationships with national counterparts, drawing on data already collected in countries and on their understanding of issues.

- Clear and effective communication (keeping countries informed in advance, involving them, developing and applying an appropriate marketing strategy). More strategic approaches to marketing and dissemination.

- A stronger EHSPI going beyond capacity building in measurement to work on assessing functions and obtaining evidence on interventions and implementing change.

- A comprehensive evaluation, including attention to opportunity cost.

Notes

1 Copenhagen, Denmark, 3–4 September 2001

3 SEPTEMBER 2001

| 8:00–8:30 | Registration |

Introductory Session

| 8:30–8:45 | Opening Address [Dr Marc Danzon] |
| 8:45–9:00 | Background, Objectives and Structure of the Regional Consultation [Dr Josep Figueras] |

Session One
Measuring Health Systems Performance: Methodological Issues and Developments

9:00–9:30	*The World Health Report 2000*: Advancing the Methodological Debate [Professor Martin McKee]
9:30–10:30	Health Systems Performance Assessment: Building on *The World Health Report 2000* [Dr Christopher J.L. Murray]
10:30–11:00	Coffee Break
11:00–11:30	Panel Discussion
11:30–12:30	Plenary Discussion
12:30–14:00	Lunch
14:00–15:00	Plenary Discussion (continued)
15:00–15:30	Coffee Break

Session Two
Explaining Performance: Linking Health Systems Functions with Performance

| 15:30–16:00 | Assessing Health Systems Functions: Recent Developments [Mr Orvill B. Adams] |
| 16:00–16:30 | OECD Approach to Performance Measurement and Improvement [Mr Jeremy Hurst] |

16:30–17:00	Plenary Discussion
17:00–18:00	Parallel Methodological Question–Answer Sessions 1. Healthy Life Expectancy 2. Responsiveness 3. Fairness in Financial Contribution
18:00	Reception

4 SEPTEMBER 2001

Session Two (continued)
Explaining Performance: Linking Health Systems Functions with Performance

9:00–9:30	Panel Discussion
9:30–10:30	Plenary Discussion
10:30–11:00	Coffee Break

Session Three
Improving Performance: Policy Implications

11:00–11:30	Working with Countries to Improve Performance: Recent Developments [Dr Abdelhay Mechbal]
11:30–12:00	Improving Performance: A Country Perspective [Mr Joe Kutzin]
12:00–12:30	Panel Discussion
12:30–14:00	Lunch
14:00–15:30	Plenary Discussion
15:30–15:45	Coffee Break

Closing Session

15:45–16:15	Summary of the Regional Consultation
16:15–16:45	Plenary Discussion
16:45–17:00	Closing Address [Dr Marc Danzon]

LIST OF PARTICIPANTS

Temporary Advisers

Dr P.D. Amudjev
Deputy Director
National Centre of Health
  Informatics
15 D. Nesterov Str.
1431 Sofia
Bulgaria

Professor Sudhir Anand
St. Catherine's College
Oxford OX1 3 UJ
United Kingdom

Dr Rifat A. Atun
DFID Resource Centre for Health
  Systems
27 Old Street
London EC1V 9HL
United Kingdom

Mr Gabi Bin-Nun
Deputy Director General
Health Economics and Health
  Insurance
Ministry of Health
2 Ben Tabei Street
P.O. Box 1176
Jerusalem 91010
Israel

Mr Nick Boyd
Branch Head
International & Industry Division
(International & Constitutional
  Branch)
Department of Health
Room 539, Richmond House
79 Whitehall
London SW1A 2NS
United Kingdom

Dr Pavel Brezovsky
Director
Department of Health Care
Ministry of Health
P.O. Box 81 - Palackého nàm 4
CS-128 01 Prague 2
Czech Republic

Dr Reinhard Busse
Head of the Madrid Hub
European Observatory on Health
  Care Systems
Escuela Nacional de Sanidad (ENS)
C/Sinesio Delgado 8
E-28029 Madrid
Spain

Dr Jan Bultman
Principal Health Specialist
Europe and Central Asia Region
World Bank
1818 H Street, NW
Washington, D.C. 20433
USA

Dr I. de la Mata
Deputy Director of Health
  Planning
Ministry of Health
Paseo del Prado 18–20
E-28071 Madrid
Spain

Dr Antonio Duran-Moreno
Tecnicas de Salud
Avda. Republica Argentina
18 Entresuelo
E-41011 Sevilla
Spain

Mr Alfred Ehrenclou
Ministry of Health and Social
  Affairs
P.O. Box 8011
N-0030 Oslo
Norway

Dr Jens R. Eskerud
Adviser
Department of Hospital Policy
Ministry of Health and Social
  Affairs
PO Box 8011 Dep
0030 Oslo
Norway

Prof. Pedro Ferreira
School of Economics
University of Coimbra
Centro de Estudos e Investigaçao
  em Saude
Av. Dias da Silva 165
3004-512 Coimbra
Portugal

Mr Sophus Garfield
8.division
Ministry of Health
6 Holbergsgade
1057 Copenhagen K
Denmark

Dr Alessandro Ghirardini
Senior Officer
Health Planning Department
Piazzale dell'industria 20
I-00144 Rome
Italy

Dr George Gotsadze
Curatio International Foundation
80 Abeshidze Str., P.O. Box 56
Tbilisi 380079
Georgia

Dr Michel Grignon
Credes
1, rue Paul Cézanne
F 75008 Paris
France

Mr Jeremy W. Hurst
Head of Health Policy Unit
Social Policy Division
Directorate for Educ. Empl. Lab.
  & S. Aff
O.E.C.D.
2 rue André-Pascal
F-75775 Paris Cedex 16
France

Dr Danguole Jankauskiene
Social Medicine Centre
Medical Faculty of Vilnius
  University
Seskines 24
2010 Vilnius
Lithuania

Mr Jesper Soeholt Joergensen
8. division
Ministry of Health
6, Holbergsgade
1057 Copenhagen K
Denmark

Dr Adam Kozierkiewicz
Director, National Centre for
  Health Information Systems
38/40 –Dluga Street
00-238 Warsaw
Poland

Dr Pieter G. N. Kramers
Deputy Head
Department of Public Health
  Forecasting
National Institute of Public
  Health and the Environment
  (RIVM)
Antonie van Leeuwenhoeklaan
  9-POB 1
NL-3720 BA Bilthoven
Netherlands

Prof. Allan Krasnik
Danish Association of Social and
  Administrative Medicine
Institute of Public Health
PANUM Institute, Univ. of
  Copenhagen
Blegdamsvej 3
DK-2200 Copenhagen N
Denmark

Prof. Maksut Kulzhanov
Rector
Kazakhstan School of Public
  Health
19a Utepov Str.
Almaty 480060
Kazakhstan

Dr S. Mariotti
Laboratory of Epidemiology and
  Biostatistics
Istituto Superiore di Sanita
Viale Regina Elena 299
I-00161 Roma-Nomentano
Italy

Dr Vlasta Mazankova
Director
Institute of Health Information
  and Statistics of the Czech
  Republic
Palackého nam 4, P.O. Box 60
CS-128 01 Prague 2
Czech Republic

Prof. Martin McKee
Head
WHO Collaborating Centre for
  Health of Societies in Transition
Research Director
European Observatory on Health
  Care Systems
London School of Hygiene and
  Tropical Medicine
Keppel Street
GB-London WC1E 7HT
United Kingdom

Dr Eric Nord
SAHT Folkehelsa
P.O. Box 4404 Nydalen
N-0403 Oslo
Norway

Dr Ferenc Oberfrank
Permanent Secretary of State
OEP foigazgato
Vaci ut 73/A
H-1139 Budapest
Hungary

Dr Bruce Rosen
Director
Program for Health Policy
  Research
Brookdale Institute
POB 13087
Jerusalem 91130
Israel

Dr Andrzej Rys
Under-Secretary of State
Ministry of Health
Ul. Miodowa 15
00-952 Warsaw
Poland

Mme A.M. Sacre-Bastin
Conseiller f.f. – Attaché Santé
Ministère des Affaires sociales
  de la Santé publique et de
  l'Environnement
Cité administrative de l'Etat
Quartier Esplanade 3
B-1010 Bruxelles
Belgium

Dr Markus Schneider
Direktor
Beratungsgesellschaft für
Angewandte Systemforschung
  BASYS
Reisingerstrasse 25
D-86159 Augsburg 1
Germany

Dr Jorge Simoes
Health Economicst
Health Advisor to the President
  of POR
Presidencia da Republica
Palacio de Belem
11349-022 Lisbon
Portugal

Prof. Aris Sissouras
General Director
Hellenic Healthy Cities Network
National Institute for Social
  Research
(EKKE)
14–18, Mesogeion Avenue
GR-11527 Athens
Greece

Prof. Peter C. Smith
Economics and Related Studies
Heslington
University of York
York YO10 5DD
United Kingdom

Dr Juha Teperi
Director
Dept. of Research on Health and
    Social Services
STAKES
Siltasaarenkatu 18, P.O.Box 220
00531 Helsinki
Finland

Mrs Anne-Sofie Trosdahl Oraug
Senior Adviser
Ministry of Health and Social
    Affairs
Postboks 8011
N-0030 Oslo
Norway

Prof. Tom van der Grinten
Department of Health Policy and
    Management
Erasmus University
PO Box 1738
NL-3000 DR Rotterdam
Netherlands

Dr Elena Varavikova
Monitoring of Health Losses Unit
Room 323
Central Research Institute of
    Information and Organization
    of Public Health
Dobrolubova 11
127254 Moscow
Russian Federation

WHO Secretariat

Mr Orvill B. Adams
Evidence and Information for
    Policy
WHO/HQ

Ms Jennifer Cain
Research Officer
European Observatory on Health
    Care Systems
Division of Information, Evidence
    and Communication
WHO/EURO

Dr Yves Charpak
Senior Policy Adviser to the
    Regional Director
WHO/EURO

Mr Philip Davies
Evidence and Information
    for Policy
WHO/HQ

Dr Marc Danzon
Regional Director
WHO/EURO

Dr Anca Dumitrescu
Director
Division of Information, Evidence
    and Communication
WHO/EURO

Ms Ainna Fawcett-Henesy
Regional Adviser
Health Systems
Division of Country Support
WHO/EURO

Dr Josep Figueras
Regional Adviser
Head of the Secretariat and
    Research Director
European Observatory on Health
    Care Systems
Division of Information, Evidence
    and Communication
WHO/EURO

Dr Milagros Garcia-Barbero
Head
WHO European Office for
    Integrated Health Care Services
Barcelona
Spain

Dr Josep Goicoechea Utrillo
Director
Division of Country Support
WHO/EURO

Dr Elke Jakubowski
Research Officer
European Observatory on Health
    Care Systems
Division of Information, Evidence
    and Communication
WHO/EURO

Mr Joe Kutzin
Senior Resident Advisor, MANAS
    Project
Division of Country Support

Dr Itziar Larizgoitia
Evidence and Information for
    Policy
WHO/HQ

Ms Suszy Lessof
Project Manager
European Observatory on Health
    Care Systems
Division of Information, Evidence
    and Communication
WHO/EURO

Dr Abdelhay Mechbal
Evidence and Information for
    Policy
WHO/HQ

Dr Christopher J.L. Murray
Executive Director
Evidence and Information for
    Policy
WHO/HQ

Ms Carolyn Murphy
Division of Administration and
    Management Support
WHO/EURO

Dr Remis Prokhorskas
Statistician, Health Information
    Unit
Division of Information, Evidence
    and Communication
WHO/EURO

Dr T. Bedirhan Üstün
Evidence and Information
    for Policy
WHO/HQ

Ms Nicole B. Valentine
Evidence and Information for
  Policy
WHO/HQ

Dr Mikko Vienonen
Special Rep. of the Director-
  General
World Health Organization Office
for the Russian Federation
28 Ostozhenka ulitsa
119034 Moscow
Russian Federation

Mr Ib Vinther-Jørgensen
Regional Adviser
Informatics Support
Division of Administration and
  Management Support
WHO/EURO

Chapter 6

SOUTH-EAST ASIAN REGIONAL CONSULTATION ON HEALTH SYSTEMS PERFORMANCE ASSESSMENT[1]

WHO REGIONAL OFFICE FOR SOUTH-EAST ASIA

INAUGURAL SESSION

The WHO Regional Office for South-East Asia (SEARO), in collaboration with the EIP Cluster of WHO headquarters, organized a regional consultation and a technical workshop on health systems performance assessment, at SEARO, New Delhi, India from 18 to 21 June 2001. The agenda and programme of work are provided in Annex 6.1. A total of 53 national participants, high-level health officials at policy and programme levels, senior public health and social scientists, and other technical experts from countries of the Region attended the meeting. In addition, there were nine staff members from the WHO country offices, as well as seven staff members from WHO headquarters and SEARO.

Dr S. P. Agarwal (India) was elected Chairperson, Dr K. C. S. Dalpatadu (Sri Lanka) as Vice Chairperson, Dr Soewarta Kosen (Indonesia) and Dr Than Tun Sein (Myanmar) as Rapporteurs.

Inaugurating the consultation, Dr Uton Muchtar Rafei, Regional Director, welcomed the participants and thanked WHO headquarters for providing both technical and financial support. He mentioned that over the past few years, WHO had focused its attention on identifying the reasons for the wide variation in health status of the Member Countries and the ways and means to bridge the gaps among them. WHO developed a framework for health systems performance assessment and the results of its work were reflected in *The World Health Report 2000*. This succeeded in generating widespread interest among governments, international agencies and other development institutions to improve understanding on assessment and improvement of health systems performance.

Most of the Member Countries in SEAR were at the lower end of the ranking scale. This situation prompted a serious concern in these countries that have been trying hard to improve their performance on all fronts. The Regional Director, in consultation with the Ministers of Health of the Region, organized a meeting of the High Level Task Force, attended by senior health officials from all Member States of the Region at SEARO in mid-July 2000.

The Task Force reviewed *The World Health Report 2000*, particularly the concepts, principles and methods used and the results obtained, and recommended that WHO should develop simple and practical mechanisms to measure responsiveness, using appropriate culture-specific parameters. It also suggested that there should be a continuous, two-way dialogue on data verification among the countries, the regional offices and WHO headquarters with all possible sources within the Organization and with other UN agencies, especially for the preparation of future *World Health Reports*. The subject was further debated at the 16th meeting of Health Ministers held in Kathmandu in August 2000, and at the 53rd session of the WHO Regional Committee held in New Delhi in September 2000.

The World Health Report 2000 raised considerable interest and discussion, some positive and some negative. The Director-General, in her report on health systems performance assessment to the 107th session of the WHO Executive Board in January 2001, indicated that WHO would establish a peer review group and a technical consultation process. These will review the framework and methodology of health systems performance assessment and will produce the WHO reports on assessment of health systems performance every two years after consultation with the Member States.

The Executive Board requested that the Director General undertake a series of actions: a) to initiate a scientific peer review of health systems performance methodology as part of the technical consultation process, including updating on methodology and new data sources relevant to the performance assessment of health systems; b) to ensure that WHO consults with the Member Countries and shares the results and recommendations of the scientific peer review; c) to develop a multiyear plan for further research and development of the framework and its relevant indicators to assess the effectiveness and efficiency of health systems as part of the technical consultation process; d) to report to the Member Countries on the impact of health systems performance reports on their policies and practices. After a thorough debate, the Executive Board endorsed this initiative of the Director General. The next WHO report on the assessment of health systems performance will be available by October 2002.

The Regional Director informed that SEARO had strengthened its efforts to build the capacity of the Member Countries to better assess their health systems performance through a global programme—Enhancing Health Systems Performance Initiative (EHSPI). WHO initially identified four countries from the South-East Asia Region: India, Indonesia, Myanmar and Thailand, as pilot countries for this global initiative, for field-testing the tools and techniques for assessing health system performance (based on concept, methodologies and tools developed by WHO). After starting the implementation of the EHSPI activities in late 2000 and early 2001, Nepal and Sri Lanka showed interest and joined the programme.

The progress of the implementation of the global initiative on health systems performance assessment was reviewed and discussed at the Sixth Meeting of Health Secretaries held at Yangon, Myanmar, in February 2001. Keeping in view the importance of the topic and in order to have better in-depth knowledge and experience on health systems performance assessment in the countries of the Region, a regional consultation and a technical workshop on health systems performance assessment were organized jointly by the WHO Regional Office and headquarters.

The main objectives of the regional consultative meeting and the technical workshop were:

■ To listen to and reflect on the widest possible range of views and ideas on health systems performance assessment, to be carried out by WHO for reporting to the Member States every two years.

■ To identify gaps in the process of data collection, analysis and reporting, with the idea to improve the completeness and quality of the available data on key outcomes related to health systems.

REGIONAL CONSULTATION

HEALTH SYSTEMS PERFORMANCE ASSESSMENT

Dr David B. Evans, Director (GPE), WHO/HQ, presented an overview of the development on health systems performance assessment (HSPA) both within WHO and at country levels since the launch of *The World Health Report 2000*, as well as the main elements of the framework and related concepts of HSPA. He explained that the objectives of HSPA are: to build an evidence-base on the relationship between the design of the health system and its performance, thus empowering policy-makers for evidence-based decision-making, and to monitor and evaluate the attainment of critical outcomes and the efficiency of the health system in a way that allows comparison over time and across systems. In his presentation, the following issues were addressed at length: the WHO framework, boundaries of the health system and the measurement methods used in *The World Health Report 2000*; indicators to measure the level and distribution of health, the level and distribution of responsiveness, the distribution of fairness in financial contribution and the measurement of health system efficiency; conceptual and methodological debates, which have emerged since the launching of the report; recent developments, gaps and additional challenges as regards furthering the framework for health systems performance assessment; linking HSPA to policy-making and managerial decision-making.

Dr David Evans elaborated on methods for measuring population health using a summary measurement—healthy life expectancy (HALE, previously DALE), and of carrying on a further analysis by measuring health inequality, health responsiveness and fairness in financial contribution. The basic concept and methods used for measurement of attainment of a healthy state and overall health systems performance were discussed. The attainment of a healthy state is the achievement of health goals, as a single or composite attainment, similar to the human development index. The performance assessment (the efficiency measurement) is the attainment related to resources available and other non-health system inputs to the health system outcomes. In addition, Dr Evans cited examples to demonstrate how functions of the health system have been considered in the assessment process.

The conceptual debates, especially on boundaries, accountability, causality, timing, socially desirable goals, weights assigned, scope of performance, practical policy links and intermediate indictors were explained in detail. Regarding boundaries and accountability, an appropriate definition of the health system would depend on the concept of accountability. The stewards of the health system should ensure that health outcomes are the highest possible for personal and non-personal services and advocacy for intersectoral action. It is also important to consider if a broad definition is appropriate or not. On causality, there was still a dispute about whether it was necessary to measure only those indicators that the Ministry of Health could influence and which are known to change the final outcomes, such as number of children fully immunized, or whether one should measure final outcomes and drill down to causal factors.

It was also revealed that there were two viewpoints on the definition of the maximum level of possible goal attainment. One was to use the maximum level for the resources (health system and non-health system) available to the Ministry of Health in the present year. The second one suggested to use the maximum level for resources available if appropriate policies were followed then and in the past. However, these two viewpoints are intrinsically linked to accountability and boundaries.

Regarding goals and weights, it could be argued whether the goals of health, responsiveness and fairness in financial contribution (FFC) capture all the possible goals or not. It can be queried whether "caring" and "community participation" could be included in the responsiveness component.

The relationship between economic growth and health in both directions is well known. In this context, one needs to consider whether health can contribute enough to make it worthwhile to measure it routinely. *The World Health Report 2000* used 50% weights on health, 25% on responsiveness and 25% on fair financing. It is important to reconsider whether the weights assigned are appropriate or not. The usefulness can vary from country to country, depending on their requirement.

In *The World Health Report 2000*, the performance of health systems was considered similar to their efficiency. In health, performance assessment is the review of a range of activities to improve health outcomes. Efficiency is included as one component. The framework in the report was criticized by a few because

it measured inputs against the final outcomes. Some argued that key factors or indicators that influenced the final outcomes should be identified. It is also crucial to have stronger links between the functions and the final outcomes of the health system.

With reference to the methodological debates, there were challenges for measuring non-fatal health outcomes, such as on core domains of health, differential item functioning, linking individual data on health state with condition-specific epidemiology, and comparing time spent in different health states with time lost due to premature mortality. These issues could be sorted out and discussed further in the regional consultations to be held in all WHO regions and in different WHO forums.

Standardized survey instruments are needed to measure the critical domains of health and their valuation. In addition to reliability and within-population validity, cross-population comparability is extremely important. It has to be enhanced through framing reliable and valid questions to be used in all populations. WHO is developing strategies to refine the cross-population comparability through the use of item response theory, hierarchical ordered probit (HOPIT) and compound HOPIT (CHOPIT), calibration tests, vignettes and comparable subgroups. Future efforts of WHO to measure responsiveness would include a component of facility-based observation. Another challenge to be faced is that the poor often rate the same services as more responsive than the rich.

Debates continued on technical issues, such as formulae and data collection for measuring fairness in financial contribution, operations options for subsistence expenditure, estimating efficiencies, and composition of stewardship, such as defining the vision and direction of the health system (health policy formulations), setting fair rules of the game (regulations), assessing performance and sharing information (intelligence).

Following the presentation, the participants discussed and expressed their opinion and observations as follows:

- The components of stewardship should cover various aspects, such as policy formulation, legislation, regulation, partnership through national and international collaboration and evidence-based policy making. Restructuring of the Ministries of Health and the health systems is inherently linked to stewardship in health.

- WHO should strike a balance between diagnostic activities related to health systems and actions to be taken to improve it; comprehensive versus selective assessment to be taken; and generation of evidence-based information *vis-à-vis* building capacity at the country level. There must be a good balance between academic methodology development and practical policy orientation. Practical aspects must be seriously considered in order to accord proper attention to the relevant technical areas.

■ Tools for measuring effective stewardship should be developed, especially in countries with decentralized setting. Health systems performance assessment is to be used as an effective tool not only at the central level. It also needs to be applied for subnational HSPA, which can provide detailed information for policy at the peripheral levels of the health system.

■ As the components of the health system include private hospitals and clinics, as well as the health services provided by NGOs, it is important that WHO considers the role played by these institutions in the assessment of health systems performance.

■ Effective coverage, like proportion of the population who received coverage of a health intervention, is also an important area to be considered in conducting HSPA. To select a parsimonious set of coverage indicators to best represent health systems performance is not an easy task. However, WHO should attempt to venture into this area so that health systems functions can be assessed appropriately.

■ The ranking of countries according to their health systems performance causes great concern to national authorities due to several reasons ranging from political sensitivity to technical soundness of the methodology. In this respect, ranking countries by groups using appropriate categorization criteria may be one option for consideration. Instead of observing the ranks, countries should see which particular variable is causing its rank to fall, so that proper action can be taken to improve the situation.

■ Countries need to have a consensus on a national framework for health systems performance assessment, especially to be carried out at the subnational level. There is an urgent need to develop a minimal and essential dataset, a priority disease pattern, and a review of the existing health information system and survey capacities at the country level.

MEASURING HEALTH SYSTEMS PERFORMANCE

This section focuses on technical comments on the concept, methods, data requirement and uses of healthy life expectancy, health inequality, responsiveness, and fairness in financial contribution.

Dr Prasanta Mahapatra (India) summarized the concept and use of healthy life expectancy. He briefly described the summary measures of population health, the properties of healthy life expectancy, the data required for computing it, the disability prevalence estimates, the construction of abridged life tables and disability-adjusted life tables. He stated that the age- and sex-specific death rates, which are essential for calculating the life-years lost (YLL) component of the disability-adjusted life expectancy (DALE), are often available in the countries from the vital registration system and are in some cases incomplete. It is the morbidity and disability data that are difficult to obtain. It is necessary to strengthen the data collection systems (including vital registration) on incidence and prevalence of morbidity and disability in the SEAR countries.

Dr Soewarta Kosen (Indonesia) touched upon the summary measures of population health (SMPH), the minimal criteria of SMPH for measuring performance, the disability-adjusted life expectancy (DALE), the calculation of health life expectancy, the potential problems, the defining and measuring of health states and desirable properties to evaluate SMPH.

He emphasized that SMPH should reflect changes in incidence, prevalence, health state severity and mortality, and it should be possible to communicate the results to the public, media, and decision-makers. He also indicated that potential problems of SMPH are cross-population comparability and unavailability of data, such as for constructing population life tables, prevalence of individuals in different health states of interest (non-fatal health outcomes) and severity weights or preferences for time spent in those health states. He concluded by saying that DALE is the most appropriate tool for measuring the level of population health and there is a need to develop a standard disability or health status instrument that incorporates severity levels, which should be cross-culturally valid. It was also suggested to develop methodologies to address cultural and non-health related factors.

Following the presentation, the following observations and remarks were made:

■ Summary measures of population health (SMPH) could be used with appropriate standardization methods for comparison of the health situation of countries with diverse data-generating systems. However, reliability and availability of data required for SMPH are important issues, to which all Member Countries should give prior importance.

- Systematic review of national health information systems in the countries is essential so that necessary reform measures could be made to generate reliable and valid data required for computing SMPH. In this aspect, capacity building for the health professionals working in the national health information systems is *sine qua non*.

Dr Viroj Tangcharoensathien (Thailand) and Dr U Than Tun Sein (Myanmar) described various aspects related to health inequalities. Dr Viroj highlighted that equity indicators are very data demanding and it is also difficult to construct a full set of indicators. Dimensions of equity should include health, health outcome, access, responsiveness, finance and population groups across which disparities might be monitored.

With respect to responsiveness indicators, he elaborated that two distinctions of responsiveness must be made, i.e. satisfaction and acceptability (depends on the expectations), and patient experiences (describing the objective and the characteristics of health service delivery). He mentioned the possibility of adapting the efficiency indicators used for OECD countries. The latter had proposed to use low-level efficiency indicators in the performance framework, such as unit costs. There are no current efforts to produce composite, high-level indicators of efficiency in the OECD countries.

In order to overcome the deficiencies in the area of equity indicators, Dr Tangcharoensathien suggested two possible actions. The first is to achieve consensus on the national framework of performance assessment and to revisit the existing databases, surveys and relevant reports to facilitate generating data for performance assessment. The second set of possible actions is to start with modest and tangible pieces, such as hospital performance (efficiency, quality, access), responsiveness (action-oriented, patient rights, participatory, publicity and civil society involvement) and rapid improvement of overall performance defining measurement tools, non-health sector determinants on health, social inequalities in the context of health, political dimensions of inequality, and stagnation of financing reforms in developing countries, user fees, prepayment of social insurance. As an example, he said that Thailand used 22 performance indicators for hospital accreditation.

Dr U Than Tun Sein made observations on the health inequality concept, measurement methods, data requirements and their uses. He mentioned that equity issues relating to health and health care were placed high on the policy agenda because certain groups of people faced heavier burden of illness and greater exposure to health hazards. They also had less access to health services. Health services for the poor have varying quality. In other words, because of inequity, there are socially disadvantaged groups and areas. He highlighted different perspectives on equity, such as equity in health and in health care. In his opinion, not all inequalities are unjust, but all inequities are the product of unjust inequalities. He also pointed out that inequities cannot be measured directly, while inequalities can. WHO's framework for measuring inequality is used to measure it across the Member Countries.

Dr U Than Tun Sein continued with the significance of detailed work to develop measurement methodologies to monitor health and health care inequalities at distinct levels within individual countries. He described the different dimensions of inequality, emphasizing the need for further improvements in the vital registration system as part of the national routine health information systems. Most countries would not be able to afford to conduct large-scale surveys on a regular basis.

He proposed that serious consideration be given to turning the existing health management information systems into equity relevant information systems. Development of a sentinel area is an important domain to be considered. Specific criteria are needed to select sentinel areas. Data collection procedures in sentinel areas should be under special scrutiny, otherwise it may be of less value for comparison between different countries. Sentinel areas data collection systems may not provide national averages. It is useful for monitoring inequalities between different parts of a country. National health information is crucial for practical action and for promoting the consciousness on equity issues of the decision-makers.

He concluded that one should not sway away from the fundamental purpose of improving the unjust and unfair status in the health of the socially disadvantaged that constitute the majority in many parts of the world. Discrepancies in the quality of data and measurement techniques used between different countries should be kept to the minimum possible. The possibility of creating health equity monitoring sentinel sites over different parts of a country should be considered.

The following observations and comments were made after the presentation:

■ The dimension of equity is so wide that it is impossible to include every domain in it. However, health outcomes in various perspectives, accessibility and responsiveness aspects should be included in conducting the HSPA.

■ WHO's inequality measurement has focused on a wide range of fatal and non-fatal health outcomes. In order to make it more effective, routine data generation, collection and analysis of national health information systems must be able to supply reliable and valid data. It is impossible and too costly to carry out surveys all the time.

■ The concept of equity in health must produce full coverage with equal opportunity to access, utilization and quality of health services, as well as the identification and correction of avoidable unjust and unnecessary factors that impair the health of the population.

■ From policy and social consideration perspectives, culturally and scientifically acceptable indicators for differing social positions should be incorporated in developing the measurement methods for health inequality.

Dr Agus Suwandono (Indonesia) and Dr Amala de Silva (Sri Lanka) made presentations on their experience with responsiveness. Dr Agus Suwandono pointed out that given the importance of learning more about how to measure and improve responsiveness in the SEAR, it is critical to have close collaboration among the Member Countries. He described in detail the responsiveness concept to analyse the performance of the health system. According to him, this concept is a breakthrough: an improved concept of using epidemiology and quantitative measurements, added to qualitative and other social measurements to be applied in the public health field. This concept gives the opportunity to the elements and domains of respect and client orientation of health care to contribute towards the measurement of the health systems performance. If this concept, already applied with its related methods in the developed countries, can be modified to take into account various social and cultural issues, religious beliefs and other ground realities prevailing in these countries, it will be more appropriate for application in developing countries.

Dr Suwandono stated that the concept of health responsiveness mostly reflected the curative part of the overall health system. It concentrated on the overall health system without delineating clinical, public and private health services. It did not take into account the preventive, promotive and rehabilitative aspects of a health system, and it still regarded the public, indigenous and private sectors, which in most developing countries were different entities, as one integral part of the system. The concept looked into the responsiveness of providers to the community needs and demands in health services. It did not reflect the responsiveness of health providers to the needs of the programmes, which actually could be measured by coverage indicators. In some developing countries such as Indonesia, with the integration of health and social welfare programmes, the concept of health responsiveness should also be adjusted by social welfare indicators.

Various methods of measuring responsiveness had been carried out in Indonesia. All of them were complementary to each other in terms of purpose of survey, sampling, data collection methods and domains. Each method had its own advantages and disadvantages.

Household surveys are very expensive and a lot of effort is required to obtain proper sampling frame, sampling method, questionnaire design and overall survey preparation, such as training of data collectors, transportation, data collection, validation and management.

The mail survey seems to be a very practical way to receive the health responsiveness data. However, there are some disadvantages of this method, especially in the developing countries. It is very difficult to obtain a good response rate, to control the validity of the data and to construct appropriate sampling frame. Some questionnaires have been filled in by the same person after colluding with the post office personnel.

The new approach of a snowball method for a key informant survey is very difficult to be carried out in Indonesia, due to the unwillingness of the respondents to pass it on to other potential respondents.

According to WHO, the ideal tool to implement measurement would be free of error and would faithfully reproduce either what happens or the perception of what happens. Unfortunately, no error-free device exists. Therefore, the possible tools to be used in this health responsiveness measurement are to be based on the results of people's observations and reports. The WHO strategy is to measure the consumers' reports and ratings of the experience with their care, rather than their satisfaction.

According to WHO, the rating items require the respondent to evaluate the experience in the context of the sub-elements of responsiveness. A respondent's level of expectation is likely to play some role in the formulation of an answer. However, the rating items are distinct from satisfaction items in that they do not ask the respondent to say how satisfied he or she is.

The WHO strategy employs an approach that will combine cognitive and field-testing. These two techniques used jointly provide the best evidence on the reliability and validity of the instruments, as well as guidance on how to revise them for future use. Every angle of data collection in a health responsiveness survey is carefully taken into account in order to obtain valid and reliable data. However, based on the Indonesia experiences, several problems have been observed.

It required a lot of time for items to be asked and for tests and exercises to be carried out. The average amount of time needed to complete one questionnaire was 3.5 hours (between 3–4 hours). The respondents became tired and bored. Most of them felt tired after 60 minutes of the interview and the exercise and were reluctant to continue.

Rating and scoring, which can be classified as subjective measurements, were influenced significantly by the respondents' cultural background, religious group and the local value system.

Some visualization was rejected by the respondents because it was very difficult to visualize things that they had not experienced. There was an understanding that similar situations would never really happen to them in the future. In some cases when a respondent was asked to visualize a condition of schizophrenia, severe depression or paraplegia, he or she refused to do so, due to supernatural or religious reasons.

Operational definitions of some terminology in responsiveness need to be described in a clear manner, for example, home visit. Moreover, some measurement methods, such as ranking and the thermometer scale are redundant.

In several questions related to health status, three or more aspects of a condition are asked, making it difficult for the respondent to imagine the situation (for example: run, heavy sport, etc.).

The WHO strategy for the responsiveness survey presents an integrated approach for collecting and using data for measuring and improving responsiveness. The strategy is built on a strong research base and is drawing on stakeholders to provide input and guidance. The most serious problem is the validation of the respondent's answers to the questions asked by the data collector, based on the available health responsiveness questionnaires and exercises.

Dr Amala de Silva (Sri Lanka) elaborated on the issue of choosing the domains of responsiveness: How were they chosen, are there only eight items, how are they defined, and are they equally important? She also stressed the importance of the elements of responsiveness and noted that the household survey results currently suggest that prompt attention and dignity are considered the most important elements, while autonomy and social support networks during care are the least important. One may need to see whether ranking is related to country, gender, or income levels, and whether the importance of ranking changes over time. Dr Amala de Silva was of the opinion that access to social support networks during care should also consider the following issues: visits from relatives and friends, provision of food and other consumables by family and friends, and opportunity for carrying out religious and cultural practices.

The participants made the following observations and comments on the presentation:

- The concept of health responsiveness has provided new insight as a public health indicator for measurement of non-health outcomes. The latter are generally related to various cultural issues, religious beliefs and other ground realities prevailing in developing countries. Therefore, these factors should be given due attention in developing a measurement tool to put the responsiveness concept into practice.

- The responsiveness concept as used by WHO did not take into account the preventive, promotive and rehabilitative aspects of the health system. Ways and means should be explored to capture these aspects in measuring responsiveness. It should also reflect responsiveness of health providers to the needs of the programme. A shorter version of the questionnaire, which captures all eight domains of responsiveness, should be developed, using existing knowledge and experience of conducting surveys in a few countries.

- Weaknesses of the responsiveness survey both in terms of technical and logistic aspects could be improved through sharing of country experiences.

- The responsiveness survey frame should capture different groups of the population to include the users of both private and public hospitals and health institutions.

- In order to sustain this effort on measuring responsiveness, WHO should provide support for capacity strengthening activities (capability to compute, analyse and interpret) at the national and subnational levels.

■ The domains of responsiveness should be carefully reviewed to effectively cover various perspectives of responsiveness, taking into consideration different epidemiological and cultural scenarios of the individual countries, and especially covering various population groups.

■ As far as "respect for autonomy" is concerned, attention must be given to obtaining the right response on making decisions on one's own health and treatment. The individual's right to make decisions in health care including refusal of treatment and receiving informed consent are very important in the context of safeguarding human rights in the health care context. This also applies to the choice of health care institutions.

Dr Ravi P. Rannan-Eliya (Sri Lanka) provided a brief analysis of WHO's fairness in financing methodology and outlined in detail the following issues: the adequacy of concepts; the methods and data used in *The World Health Report 2000*; the methodology in country estimations; policy relevance and other alternatives.

Regarding the adequacy of concepts, the possible points to be considered relating to fairness in health are: fairness as implicitly or explicitly captured in the WHO's concept of fairness in financial contribution (FFC), i.e. fairness as horizontal equity, fairness as protection from catastrophic expenditures and fairness as progressivity in payments; notions of fairness rejected implicitly or explicitly by WHO in its concept of fairness in financing; fairness as progressivity in payment; fairness as equality of access or in utilization of services; and fairness as income redistribution or poverty alleviation.

In the context of Sri Lanka's perspective, he described fairness as horizontal equity, as protection from catastrophic expenditure, and as progressivity in payment, each having been an important national policy goal over a period of seventy years. Given Sri Lanka's good performance in health terms, other countries in the Region might take greater note of this. The WHO concept of fairness is of equal shares of ability to pay, not increasing shares, and it does not include the key goals that have played a part in Sri Lanka's long-term health success. Therefore, WHO's failure to accept the desirability of progressive payment is unfair and not consistent with Sri Lanka's own historical goals. The WHO thesis as to implicit goals was based on empirical evidence collected from a web survey of WHO staff, the questionable empirical reliability of which was evident.

Fairness is treated by many as involving equity in access and in utilization of services. WHO rejected this approach as being purely instrumental, although it is a fundamental concern of mainstream equity in health services research. It contradicts Sri Lankan social policy, which accepts equity in access as a basic social right of citizenship irrespective of health outcomes. Dr Rannan-Eliya illustrated this by referring to the continued provision of medical services by the Sri Lankan Ministry of Health to the members of the LTTE, the insurgent rebel group, even though it could be plausibly argued that overall social welfare was not served by this. The LTTE's right to Sri Lankan government health services was a basic right of citizenship and thus of fairness, and not merely a means to improving health status or social welfare. The WHO approach contradicts the fundamental linkage of access to social rights at the international level (such as in the 20/20 Declaration on Basic Social Rights) and also ignores the widely accepted arguments in philosophy and welfare economics for equity in access as an end in itself irrespective of equality in outcomes. Fairness in income redistribution or poverty alleviation is an important goal for many countries, but WHO, in its background paper misreads or misrepresents the rationale for this notion of equity in health finance literature by ascribing this goal as being derived purely from the tax literature.

Dr Rannan-Eliya then described the implications of the Sri Lankan perspective that the normative judgements in FFC are inconsistent with the health system goals of the Sri Lankan electorate/policy over 70 years. FFC does not measure important policy goals, such as equity of access and utilization of services, desirability of progressivity in payment system and impact on income redistribution.

He commented that there were problems with data and methods in *The World Health Report 2000*, and that it failed to adhere to the basic standards of integrity in the scientific process since it lacked full disclosure, which is the basis for scientific peer review. It also made inappropriate use of imputation and statistically unreliable methods. As a person asked to provide a commentary on the methods, the difficulty he faced was that the background papers had not been published and were not available for review. In fact, he had been informed by WHO/HQ just before the meeting that the relevant background papers had in fact not been completed. He expressed concern about this because it was acceptable for a private researcher to use such an approach, but WHO was different. It was not a private research agency, but was accountable to the Member Countries. He emphasized that WHO had to properly exercise its stewardship function.

The World Health Report 2000 study used actual country data to estimate fairness in financing in only 21 countries. It then used these data to estimate for the 170 other countries. He explained that the WHO defence of its imputation methods was that at least it was being transparent by publishing the confidence intervals in its estimates. However, if the WHO-published confidence intervals for the scores were derived from its prediction model, then these were almost certainly invalid, since the presumed prediction model showed evidence of poor fit. WHO has not published its prediction model, but a very similar model was presented by Paul Shaw at the PAHO consultation and WHO did not dispute it. He demonstrated this model on a slide and noted that the adjusted R-squared was only 0.07, and the regression diagnostics indicated poor model fit.

Moreover, knowing that the imputations are poor does not make their use any better when it is rankings that matter to countries. Most delegates and most SEAR countries were not bothered about the actual scores, but by their relative rankings. From this perspective, it was more important to know the confidence intervals for the rankings of countries. Since WHO had not published these, Dr Rannan-Eliya's office calculated the 80% confidence intervals using the data published in *The World Health Report 2000*. This was done using a Monte Carlo simulator in 30 000 trials. He then showed the estimated confidence intervals for the rankings of countries in fairness in financing and queried whether given the very large intervals obtained, the scores would be meaningful to policy-makers. In Sri Lanka's case, where the confidence interval for its ranking ranged from 49th position to 127th position, he argued that the estimated ranking published in the report would have no policy significance to policy-makers.

Dr Rannan-Eliya described the following problems that countries would face in implementing the WHO methodology for country studies: difficulties in estimating most taxes, e.g. capital taxes that are most progressive; reliance on surveys, which record only on a one month basis instead of a one year reference period in definition; lack of comparability between different datasets, and unavailability of reliable NHA estimates of out-of-pocket expenses in 75% of countries. These would create additional problems in interpreting the rankings of countries, even when data were not imputed.

He recommended that the conceptual basis of FFC be reviewed in addition to methods. WHO's data collection should more closely integrate with capacity building and improvement in permanent national data systems and incorporating existing equity initiatives. Rankings should not be published based on questionable imputations. WHO should establish standards of scientific disclosure to permit meaningful peer review.

After the above two presentations, the participants provided the following observations and comments:

- The most important issue in computing fairness in financial contribution across countries is the reliability and validity of data and also the data sources apart from methodological issues. In this context, all Member Countries should promote activities conducive to obtaining complete data/information including regular updating of the National Health Accounts. WHO should emphasize national and regional capacity building.

- The WHO Regional Office should collaborate with relevant WHO centres in promoting proper health financing policies and health sector reform activities, as they are inherently linked to fairness in financial contribution. Necessary evidence must be obtained by reviewing the results of studies carried out in the Region in the context of the developing countries' scenario.

Dr Anil Gumber (India) discussed the health equity scenario in India. He described the data required for computing fairness in financial contribution from household income and expenditure surveys, National Health Accounts and issues related to acquisition of data. He also pointed out measurement issues, such as how to arrive at effective income after adjusting for subsistence level (when the majority of the population barely meets the subsistence needs), when the share of direct taxes (usually progressive in nature) is small, difficulties in obtaining details of taxes paid by the households and their usage by the government, what constitutes the out-of-pocket payments for health care (direct medical, other direct expenditure, wage/income loss, borrowings, etc.) and household vs. individual concepts.

He emphasized that while considering fairness in financial contribution in India, the following issues are of importance: the private sector handling the major load of curative care (heterogeneous, large and widely dispersed, no regulatory mechanism, huge price and quality differences); accessibility problems in hilly, tribal and remote areas; a significant proportion of people not seeking care (mainly financial reasons); the reliance on the government sector is declining; government subsidies are not well-directed; health care prices are rising faster than general inflation; and rising income inequalities during 1990s.

As a response to the presentation, the participants expressed the general opinion that in considering equity issues and fairness in financial contribution, the role played by private sectors should be thoroughly analysed, and it should be decided how these could be incorporated into the computation of indices for fairness in financial contribution. Also, the issues raised by the presenter were endorsed, especially the rising of income inequalities versus health inequity.

EXPLAINING PERFORMANCE ASSESSMENT

Dr Than Sein (EIP-WHO/SEARO) outlined the major reform trends in the health sector, especially in relation to health care financing, provision of care, human resources and stewardship in health. He described in detail the reforms in collection and pooling of health care funds and in purchasing for health care. He stated that funds are raised from people according to their ability to pay and not according to needs and are spent according to needs and not ability to pay. He emphasized the necessity for expansion of coverage of the existing health insurance schemes (voluntary and mandatory) and promotion of various schemes for risk pooling, including community financing schemes and trust funds. Dr Than Sein pointed out that there is no single prescription for health care financing and that countries may build on their own experiences related to historical, political, socioeconomic, epidemiological and environmental situations.

Ms Kei Kawabata (WHO/HQ) made a presentation on health systems performance functions, especially in the area of developments in the context of macro-architecture of health systems, health financing, components of stewardship, health systems and provider performance. She defined the main goal of health systems performance as strengthening the health systems capacities to produce maximum possible health gain for the poor and vulnerable populations from investment of scarce resources in critical interventions, and ensuring fair distribution of benefits from such investments. She also mentioned that the challenges lying ahead in the area of stewardship are: to develop and execute a programme of work to strengthen national skills in policy analysis and strategic planning; assist ministries in designing enforceable legislation in criti-

cal areas, e. g. private delivery of services; support monitoring and evaluating performance, monitoring expenditure and health systems profiles.

Ms Kawabata discussed "effective coverage," which was defined as the proportion of the population who received effective health services out of the target population who needs those services. She then outlined the major tasks ahead, such as identification of critical health interventions that would produce a significant overall health gain in the population, particularly among the poor, and development of a planning and management tool using GIS that will help health system managers to incorporate data on effective coverage into the planning and management of health service delivery infrastructure. Ms Kawabata emphasized that in all these areas, WHO is trying to work in consultation with the Member Countries, the regional and country offices, and other relevant technical programmes whether they be international organizations, academics or research institutions.

Dr Christopher J.L. Murray (EXD-EIP, WHO/HQ) described the application of the HSPA framework at the subnational level. He explained in detail that the objectives of the subnational health systems performance assessment are: to monitor and evaluate the attainment of critical outcomes and the efficiency of components of the health system in a way that allows comparison over time and across components; to build a national evidence-base on the relationship between the design of the health system and performance; and to empower the public with relevant information.

Regarding stewardship, Dr Murray mentioned that subnational HSPA is a fundamental tool for effective stewardship. In a setting of decentralization, performance assessment may be one of the most effective tools for the central ministries of health. Subnational HSPA creates options for the government to use pluralistic provision.

Dr Murray identified types of subnational HSPA as geographic or administrative units (states, provinces or districts) and components of systems (public hospitals, private hospitals, public clinics, non-personal health services, etc.). In doing HSPA for subnational geographic and administrative units, the same concepts can be applied as for country health systems performance assessment. For small-area analysis, the course of acquiring information and the statistical stability of the measurements become important. It is crucial to develop affordable and robust measurement strategies for small-area analysis. Dr Murray stated that, regarding non-fatal health outcomes, population representative surveys with reduced sample size methods using new Bayesian tools, can be applied. He stressed that for ministries of health where subnational HSPA is to be a major tool for effective stewardship, country health information systems need to be redesigned to support this analysis on a routine basis. With reference to fairness in financial contribution, and subnational health accounts, central expenditures need to be attributed to geographic/administrative units for international compatibility. In doing geographic/administrative HSPA, existing registration systems such as vital registration, information from responsiveness exit surveys and population representative surveys are required. Conceptually, it is feasible to measure levels of health, responsiveness and catastrophic spending at the individual or household levels. However, inequalities in health and responsiveness cannot be measured at this level. Dr Murray re-emphasized that for the Ministry of Health, where subnational HSPA is to be a major tool for effective stewardship, health information systems need to be re-designed to support this analysis on a routine basis.

The participants debated on Dr Murray's presentation and provided the following comments and observations:

- Countries should consider carrying out HSPA at the subnational level, subject to resource availability. This would yield important information for evidence-based decision-making at the subnational level.

- It is important to study the relationship between different designs of health care systems and health systems performance.

- WHO should promote capacity building in HSPA, especially on small-area analysis, which could be useful for many purposes.

BUILDING BETTER EVIDENCE: ACTIVITIES IN THE SEAR

Dr Ravi P. Rannan-Eliya presented an overview of the current status of updating National Health Accounts (NHA) in the countries of Asia and the Pacific, including those of the South-East Asia Region. He recounted in detail the history and development of NHA from 1963 to the present. He mentioned the basic characteristics of the Asia-Pacific NHA: a largely local initiative (not driven by external donors); relatively good institutionalization (local ownership and integrated with national authorities); little reliance on external technical assistance; and low cost in running the systems (rely primarily on routine data systems and not on special surveys).

On the current status of NHA, he said that some developed or middle-income countries in the Asia-Pacific Region (OECD: Japan, Korea, Australia, SEAR: Sri Lanka, Thailand, WPR: China, Philippines) have permanent NHA systems with routine updating, while some countries (SEAR: Bangladesh, WPR: Hong Kong in China, Taiwan) were intending to update in the future. Some countries (SEAR: Indonesia, WPR: PNG, Samoa, Viet Nam, Malaysia, Mongolia) were constructing their NHA systems and most of the developing countries (SEAR: Bhutan, DPR Korea, India, Maldives, Myanmar, Nepal, WPR: Cambodia, Laos, Fiji, Vanuatu, Micronesia) had no official commitment to NHA.

Dr Rannan-Eliya also discussed issues relating to comparability, rapid adoption of OECD standards, methods for establishing NHA, lack of regional reporting systems, challenges in establishing permanent NHA systems, sharing of technical expertise, and concerns of policy makers regarding distribution of spending by source, socioeconomic groups and provinces.

The following generic issues were highlighted on updating and maintaining NHA:

- Comparability is difficult because of diverse national standards. In addition, there are differing concepts on boundaries, dimensions and classification systems.

- There are major problems in estimating private spending. Moreover, the quality and reliability of estimates are doubtful: there is a lack of standardized regional reporting systems; technical expertise to give guidance is not readily available; and it is very difficult to achieve a consensus of policymakers regarding the framework and contents of NHA.

Dr Ravi outlined the current activities of APNHAN (Asia-Pacific NHA Network), as well as the activities initiated under the Rockfeller Grant for the network to collaborate on regional standards. He also added a few activities on the EQUITAP initiative to develop protocols to extend OECD SHA to equity and mentioned the WHO NHA Producers' Guide together with the need of NHA for the WHO health systems performance assessment initiative.

Dr Ravi recommended that: coordination between WHO, APNHAN, countries and other development partners should be established; the WHO regional offices should take the lead in connecting countries and network; collaboration on joint funding proposals, such as potential availability of AIDS funding, is necessary; development of better methods to estimate private spending has to take place; sharing of expertise in implementing OECD SHA and of experience in institutionalization are crucial.

Following the presentation, the participants discussed and stated that:

- Development of better methods to estimate private spending on health will reinforce the health systems performance assessment methodology.

- WHO should promote standardized regional reporting systems on NHA. This could facilitate the computation of indices in health systems performance assessment.

Dr Somnath Chatterji (WHO/HQ) presented an overview of the WHO Multi-country Survey Study on Health and Responsiveness. He emphasized the importance of the need for cross-culturally comparable data, cross-population comparability, reliability and stability of applications, and novel techniques for cross-cultural comparability, such as vignettes and performance tests. He stressed on the need for a common survey instrument that has cross-cultural applicability, reliability, validity, easy response calibration and cross-population comparability. In addition to the classical psychometric criteria to make meaningful international and cross-population comparisons, the instrument should have: comparable response scales, or a common meter in different populations, i.e. the same response level corresponds to the same level of health in that domain; and evidence of equivalent metric properties should be shown by external calibration tests and other possible mechanisms. Dr Chatterji underlined the need to implement "cross-population comparability" criteria in the WHO Multi-country Survey Study, as well as uses of a comparable questionnaire in household surveys, telephone surveys, postal, e-mail or internet surveys.

After the presentation, the participants were of the general opinion that the development of a common survey instrument that will allow cross-population comparability is the priority activity. Emphasis should be given also to cross-cultural applicability.

Dr Myint Htwe (GPE, WHO/SEARO) summarized the specific activities of health information systems (HIS) in support of health systems performance assessment. He pointed out some practical aspects in reforming the national health information systems to support the health systems performance assessment

activities. The following issues required urgent attention: systematic review of the performance of existing HIS and phase-wise strengthening; strengthening the linkage between HIS and its subsystems; development of an information culture for health professionals; promotion of utilization of data for information for evidence-based decision-making; and development of a doable framework for WHO and country HIS focal points and institutions to work together for HSPA, i.e., promoting the activities of Enhancing the Health Systems Performance Initiative (EHSPI).

He outlined future directions of national HIS in support of HSPA, such as: a systematic review of the existing HIS and phase-wise strengthening; making the subsystems of the HIS complementary; making the HIS dynamic, user-friendly and responsive to needs; inculcating information culture; promoting utilization of data and information for evidence-based decision-making; conducting technical training workshops on HSPA methods; promoting subnational assessment of health systems performance; and developing doable framework for WHO and the country HIS focal points and institutions to work together for HSPA.

Dr Christopher J.L. Murray provided an outline on the activities of the WHO global Enhancing Health Systems Performance Initiative (EHSPI). He pointed out that a number of countries have indicated an interest to collaborate with WHO, to review their own health systems, to develop policies and strategies to improve performance, and to use the health systems performance assessment framework as a tool for analysing their health systems. He described in detail the national and global objectives of EHSPI.

National objectives are to have a better understanding of a system's overall performance, linking evidence to functions and actions to improve performance and a greater national capacity to monitor and improve performance. Global objectives are the refinement of the conceptual framework, methods, indicators, data and better international evidence-base for policy advice. Dr Murray also mentioned the current activities of EHSPI, which involve measurement of goals by nationals, technical support by WHO on data collection and analysis, as well as descriptions and functions of the organization, conduct of seminars to discuss preliminary findings, tentative identification of areas for future interaction and support by WHO.

The next steps in EHSPI are to give more emphasis on explaining performance functions, developing subnational applications, utilizing the findings and appropriate health system development, and establishing regional and interregional resource networks.

EHSPI activities are to be implemented collaboratively, among national policy-makers and researchers, staff of the WHO country offices, regional offices, HQ/EIP and other agencies and resource institutions.

EHSPI activities were fully endorsed by the participants. It was underlined that capacity building should go hand in hand when implementing the activities. There must be a balance between the actual application and practical thinking against the theoretical consideration.

GROUP WORK: FUTURE DIRECTIONS

The participants were divided into four groups for group work. Groups one and two were assigned to work on recommendations on the framework, design, data sources and data quality for health systems performance assessment. Group three was assigned to work on recommendations on the follow-up of EHSPI, including capacity building for health systems performance assessment. Group four was assigned to work on recommendations for strengthening the national health information systems to provide input for health systems performance assessment activities. The major recommendations and general opinion that came out from each group were as follows:

Group 1: Recommendations and General Opinion on the Framework, Design, Data Sources and Data Quality for Health Systems Performance Assessment

1. Framework
   a) Generally agreed with the concept of the framework.
   b) Disagreed with the aggregation and reporting of countries by ranking, using an overall index.
   c) Normative judgments are involved, but no global solution seems possible to sort this out.
   d) There is a notion against using high-level indicators or a composite, single summary measure. It could be reported using component indices separately.
   e) Mixed feelings for reporting of HSPA results every two years.

2. Health Status: DALE/HALE
   a) Agreed with the concept of inclusion of disability and morbidity in measuring health status as ideal goals.
   b) Problems with data sources were noted:
      ■ There may be resource constraints to collect morbidity data on a routine basis.
      ■ Alternatives for using existing data sources must be investigated.
      ■ Alternatives in using household surveys must be explored.
      ■ In collaboration with the Member Countries, WHO should develop a better instrument as an urgent priority.
      ■ Life expectancy at birth should continue to be used as a tool to compare countries and to recognize the desirability of proceeding at gradual and differing paces in different countries.
      ■ Countries should be supported towards an intensive routine data collection as a priority activity.

3. Distribution of Health Status
   a) Agreed with the concept.
   b) No disagreement on using child mortality as proxy for overall mortality, given that demographic and health surveys findings are available.
   c) Current measure of determining the distribution of health status is inadequate. It must include measurement of inequalities by population subgroup, such as socioeconomic situation and education.

4. Responsiveness
   a) Disagreed with the notion of universally legitimate expectations because it is paternalistic and the universal weighting of domains may not be feasible. Therefore, differential weightings by countries, based on survey responses, must be used.
   b) Some omissions in the survey were noted, e.g. measurement of the performance of non-medical services, such as public health programmes. It has to be made explicit that countries can incorporate additional questions to the responsiveness survey. Finally, utilization of services should be added.
   c) A practical problem regarding instrument feasibility in the field was that WHO needs to be more culturally sensitive.

5. Fairness in Financing
   a) The fairness definition should recognize equity in utilization and equity in respect of spending, and it should be measured as a separate intrinsic goal.

b) Progressiveness as increasing shares should be incorporated into the definition of the fairness in financing concept, not only in formula.

c) A single fairness in financing index should be replaced with multiple indices and statistics for different components of fairness.

6. Process Issues
   a) Failure to disseminate the results of work done under the health and responsiveness survey.
   b) WHO should focus on capacity-building as part of data collection, including involvement of nationals on training in data analysis. Efforts should not be simply to collect data for HQ.
   c) Better coordination with countries, national authorities and agencies is required.

Group 2: Recommendations and General Opinion on the Framework, Design, Data Sources and Data Quality for Health Systems Performance Assessment

1. Framework
   a) The composite index is acceptable subject to the following caveats: review the weighting of each component; define minimum requirement of data validity; compute the composite index and ranking only if data input for all components from a country satisfy the minimum validity criteria; for those countries that do not satisfy the minimum data validity criteria, work on a special programme to improve their data quality.
   b) WHO may clarify its position on health-for-all and health system performance indicators.
   c) WHO should provide five separate indices for policy actions at country level.
   d) Regarding the frequency of HSPA, some components, such as health could be assessed maybe every three to five years, as there would not be any significant and rapid changes in health outcome (unless epidemic or pandemic occurred). In addition, frequent assessment is required for responsiveness and fairness in financial contribution indicators.

2. Utilization of HSPA
   a) In the process of the HSPA exercises, it should be ensured that policy-makers participate in such a way that assessment outcome is brought into the policy agenda followed by subsequent actions.

3. National HSPA
   The components of health systems goals are acceptable:

a) Health: level and distribution.

b) Responsiveness: level and distribution (responsiveness domains should be reviewed to incorporate the full range of health systems activities, including community participation).

c) Fairness in financial contribution.

4. Small-Area HSPA
   a) At localized area level: where accurate estimates of health outcomes are inadequate (healthy life expectancy and distributions), only indicators on responsiveness and fairness in financial contribution are recommended. No composite indices would be feasible. Due to migration and rapid population mobility, subnational HSPA should be carefully planned.
   b) When conducting subnational HSPA, it is essential to focus on some key programmes as reflected by the disease burden or high degree of resource consumption, for example hospital sector and public health programmes.

5. Level of Health Indicators
   a) Where final health outcome indicators, such as healthy life expectancy, are inadequate, intermediate health indicators as proxies should be used, e.g. effective coverage. Efforts should be made to develop health outcome indicators.

6. Data Requirements
   Data sources
   a) A population-based survey may be required as the national health information systems have limited utility.
   b) National capacity building is needed to generate population-based descriptive epidemiological data.
   c) Health state valuation survey.
   d) Conduct a cross-sectional survey on disability at the same interval as global HSPA.

Group 3: Recommendations and General Opinion on Follow-up of EHSPI, Including Capacity Building for Health Systems Performance Assessment

1. Networking is essential for EHSPI: countries that are ready to participate in EHSPI should collaborate and the sharing of countries' experiences should be promoted.

2. Advocacy/collaboration: intersectoral collaboration with other sectors and local donors agencies.

3. Identifying focal points: appropriate institutions or persons should be identified in the countries and plans of action should be developed.

4. The private sector should be involved as well and an assessment should be made.

5. Technical support from other international agencies should be explored.

Group 4: Recommendations and General Opinion on Improvement of HIS in Countries to Provide Input for the Health Systems Performance Exercise

The following indicators may be considered for inclusion in the HSPA, and the national HIS should provide data to the extent possible.

1. Level of health
   a) Mortality rates: age- and disease-specific
   b) Morbidity: age- and disease-specific
   c) Maternal mortality ratio
   d) Infant mortality rate and neonatal mortality rate
   e) DALE/DALY/HALE
   f) Life expectancy
   g) Disease and disability prevalence

2. Distribution of health
   a) Immunization coverage
   b) Antenatal care
   c) Natal care, e.g. percentage of deliveries attended by trained personnel
   d) Growth monitoring
   e) Contraceptive prevalence rate
   f) Emergence of communicable diseases

3. Responsiveness
   a) Client satisfaction
   b) Use of facilities
   c) Availability of facilities
   d) Human resources for health
   e) Quality of care

4. Fairness in financial contribution
   a) Government health budget
   b) Contribution of NGOs/donors on health services
   c) Contribution from insurance
   d) Individual out-of-pocket expenditure

5. Measurement of health system efficiency
   a) Per capita expenditure
   b) Education/average years of schooling

Recommendations

■ Systematic review on performance of existing HIS should be made.

■ Data and information gaps should be identified and corrective measures taken.

■ The linkage between HIS and its subsystems should be strengthened.

■ HIS should be made dynamic, user-friendly and responsive to the needs of the country.

■ Evidence-based decision-making and management culture should be developed.

■ HIS should be strengthened to obtain data and information from the private sector, non-governmental organizations, and universities, including information on indigenous medicine, which is required for HSPA.

■ Information networks should be developed for sharing information with other agencies.

■ The system of obtaining National Health Accounts should be institutionalized.

■ Regular patient/client exit interviews should be carried out.

■ Periodic special surveys should be carried out.

■ The vital registration system should be strengthened.

Technical Workshop

Goodness and Fairness of Health Status

Dr Prasanta Mahapatra (India) presented datasets required for the computation of DALE and its proxy measure of equity using child mortality.

Dr Emmanuela Gakidou (WHO/HQ) made a presentation on conceptual issues relating to health inequalities. She described in detail health-related inequalities, such as group inequality (social classes, education groups, income groups, geographical areas) and individual inequality (individuals in a population). She stated that even if group inequality is zero, individual inequality could be large, but if individual inequality is zero, group inequality must be zero. She also spoke about measuring inequalities in health across individuals in a population, as health is a critical component of well-being. Determination of equality in health is therefore desirable, as it complements the social inequalities approach. In measuring equality, one should include information on fatal and non-fatal health outcomes and risks, as well as capture the entire experience of an individual from birth to death. The important fact is that it should be applicable to all countries and comparable across countries.

The two potential measures of equality are: healthy life span (duration of life for an individual adjusted for time spent in health states worse than full health) and healthy life expectancy (equivalent number of years in full health an individual born today can expect to live). Dr Gakidou pointed out that preference should be given to healthy life expectancy because the equality of healthy life span cannot be achieved. She briefly discussed the normative choices in selecting a measure of inequality. In this context, the following issues are to be sorted out by consensus: whether one should take relative or absolute inequality; the distribution of weight assigned to various points in the spectrum of inequality; and whether to compare people to the mean or to all other individuals in the population.

Discussions followed Dr Gakidou's presentation. Comments were made by the participants with regard to: consideration of utilization and effective coverage in measuring inequality; possibility of variation with respect to the choice of alpha and beta values; choice of family of measures between countries in calculating inequality index; and exercising caution in using mathematical figures because they may not be oriented towards practical actions.

The data sources that are required to measure child survival inequality are: demographic and health surveys, containing complete birth histories for nationally represented samples of women of reproductive age and variables such as mothers' education, assets, residence, and age. The different models used to estimate the distribution of risk of death, such as the extended beta–binomial model and random effects logit model were also explained. Dr Gakidou then focused on the covariates required to determine child survival mortality at the individual- and country-levels. She finally discussed the measurement of inequality in DALE, in which the need for individual records from census health surveys linked to death registries is emphasized. The survival analysis model and proportional hazards model can be used to determine inequality in DALE.

RESPONSIVENESS SURVEY

Dr Amala de Silva (Sri Lanka) made a presentation on vignettes used in responsiveness surveys. She described in detail the problems with self-reporting, e.g. that responses may be influenced by an individual's expectations, which are related to the individual's experiences. Responses are also sometimes affected by the wording of questions which are generally culture-sensitive. Gender, age and occupation may influence the response pattern heavily. Country-specific rating norms may depend on historical, political and cultural experience. Dr de Silva declared that vignettes were used to capture these national differences in attitude and rating patterns.

She defined responsiveness vignettes as hypothetical descriptions of individuals experiencing different states of responsiveness, which the respondents are asked to characterize on an ordinal scale. She gave several examples of vignettes and informed that cut-off points used in the vignettes could be determined by HOPIT i.e. hierarchical ordered probit model. HOPIT measures cut-off points for individuals or groups as well and adjusts for difference in these points.

Dr de Silva stressed that reliable and valid measurement is essential in applying vignettes in responsiveness surveys. It must be comparable and relevant across countries, within countries and stable over time. She concluded that the measurement technique used must be cost-effective and also able to monitor responsiveness of health systems. It is important to understand the determinants of responsiveness.

Ms Lipika Nanda (India) and Dr Agus Suwandono (Indonesia) shared their experiences in conducting responsiveness surveys in their respective countries. Ms Lipika Nanda spoke briefly on the experience of the health and responsiveness survey in Andhra Pradesh (AP), one of the states in India. She described in detail the stages of implementation of the survey, including the importance of meticulous planning before conducting the survey (translation of instrument, recruitment of surveyors, training of surveyors, team formation, use of feedback on results of pilot testing, retraining and some refinement before the main survey, imparting camping skills, groundwork before survey and printing the questionnaire). She mentioned that the most difficult part of the survey is data cleaning and issuing of missing information and unplausible data. Therefore, proper training and thorough review of the whole process are essential. Afterwards, Ms Nanda presented datasets obtained from the AP health system responsiveness survey.

Dr Agus Suwandono explained in detail the various practical steps of the survey carried out in Indonesia. He exposed many logistical and technical problems encountered in different phases of the study and the ways in which they were overcome. The experience he shared was very useful to his colleagues in the Member Countries before undertaking responsiveness surveys in their respective states. Dr Suwandono was of the opinion that conducting the survey for health systems performance assessment had resulted in improving the knowledge on new methods and techniques related to health surveys. It was therefore a good activity to strengthen the technical capability of health professionals. It stimulated more collaboration between the health staff and professionals from universities and the bureau of statistics.

The participants later commented on considering the possibility of using low-cost exit interview surveys and also using a "panel household" approach for routine monitoring of the distribution of health, responsiveness and fairness in financial contribution.

HEALTH CARE FINANCING—NATIONAL HEALTH ACCOUNTS

Dr Ravi P. Rannan-Eliya briefly commented on the methodological issues relating to updating and maintaining National Health Accounts (NHA). He described the framework by outlining the basis for structuring and conceptualizing NHA, boundaries, dimensions, classification, specifying minimal elements in NHA and reporting of results. He mentioned various choices of frameworks, estimation methods (household spending), institutional approaches, use of NHA in HSPA and policy, and the steps in health care financing studies with regard to the choice of framework. He enumerated the following current frameworks: US NCFA (1970s), SNA 1993 Satellite Accounts, Harvard approach (1993.1997.2000), OECD system of Health Accounts 2000 and NHA Producer's Guide (forthcoming).

He further clarified the criteria for selecting a framework, such as international comparability (requires common reporting framework, links to international standards), national relevance (relevant to local needs, consistent with the national health system and policy needs), and feasibility (obtaining data, institutional and financial resources required, sustainability and availability on an annual basis).

Regarding household expenditure, Dr Ravi P. Rannan-Eliya explained that it was often large and was dependent on survey data and therefore required exercise of judgement. He described sources of data for estimating household spending, e.g. household surveys, provider/industry data and national income accounts. He further elaborated on some basic principles of estimation and described reasons, methods

and caution for conducting household surveys, such as what to look for (reason for the survey, regularity, method, detail and specificity of questions, sampling versus non-sampling errors, potential to cross-check estimates), problems with household surveys and sampling and non-sampling errors in them.

The speaker then described the US survey experience and strategy for dealing with survey bias. He informed when new surveys have to be done and added that surveys should be regularly repeated. Routine surveys are preferred as data sources because they provide consistent time trends on spending and thus the non-sampling bias will remain fixed. Therefore, there will be more opportunities to estimate bias accurately. He emphasized that special surveys are more costly and are useful primarily for more detailed disaggregation of spending where the total spending level is already known, and are sometimes useful in estimating non-sampling bias in routine surveys.

Dr Rannan-Eliya pointed out that National Health Accounts are useful for WHO health systems performance assessment and for policy-makers. He recommended: promoting regional collaboration and coordination among the WHO regions and a network of institutions (SEARO/WPRO/EURO/ APNHAN/WHOCC for health economics); coordinated programmes to develop and share better methods; collaboration on the development of a regional health systems database containing lower-level systems indicators as in OECD; and establishing the WHO National Health Accounts database through initiatives of the regional offices of WHO.

Dr Viroj Tangcharoensathien made a presentation on *Universal Coverage: Experience from Thailand* and showed some datasets on health financing in Thailand. He discussed the objectives of universal coverage (UC): why it matters; the contextual environment of reform; alternative approaches for achieving UC; main features of UC; its financial feasibility; potential impact on demand and supply side; and potential risks.

Dr Tangcharoensathien pointed out that thirty per cent of the Thai population is uninsured and financial catastrophes due to illnesses are real issues. The sources of health financing are usually household cash and savings, borrowing from family networks and private sources. Therefore, families can easily fall into debt traps due to high medical bills. The speaker then focused on the detailed profile of the insured population in the context of low-income schemes for poor households. However, this scheme's coverage to the poor is inadequate and ineffective. He described the following three alternative approaches for achieving

UC. The conservative approach is a gradual expansion of each scheme where legislation will not be required, therefore the chance of reaching UC is remote. In the progressive approach, there will be a functional integration of different schemes and it requires legislation; the chance of reaching UC is high. In the "big bang" approach, a single fund will be created from different schemes that requires legislation, and the chance of achieving universal coverage is fast. Dr Tangcharoensathien then presented the pros and cons of the three approaches taking into consideration variables such as efficiency, equity, quality of care, choices and competition and cost containment. He commented on the political acceptability, and the managerial and technical feasibilities of these approaches in the context of the Thai situation. He described in detail the main features of universal coverage, which include co-packages, registration procedures, source of financing, system configuration, role of the private sector, purchaser role and payment methods.

BENCH-MARK OF FAIRNESS FOR HEALTH SYSTEMS REFORM

Dr Supasit Pannarunothai (Thailand) made a presentation titled *Benchmarks of Fairness for Health Systems Reform: a Tool for National and Provincial Health Development in Thailand*. He described in detail the development of benchmarks in Thailand (tools developed in the USA and tested in some developing countries in 1999). He also enumerated the elements of fairness (equity in health outcomes, access to all forms of health care, equity in health financing, efficiency in management and allocation, accountability and patient and provider autonomy).

The speaker listed the following bench-marks of fairness: intersectoral public health; financial barriers to equitable access; non-financial barriers to access; comprehensiveness of benefits and tiering; equitable financing; efficacy, efficiency and quality of health care; administrative efficiency; democratic accountability and empowerment; and patient and provider autonomy. He pointed out that in the Thailand case-study, there was wide agreement on the ethical framework of fairness despite large historical, political and cultural differences. Therefore, bench-marks are good policy tools at the national and local levels. According to Dr Pannarunothai, decentralization is happening and evaluation at the subnational level is important to mobilize the community to evaluate the health system of their province using bench-marks and to summarize the methodologies

in assessing health systems at the provincial level. Ten provinces have been selected for the bench-mark framework and there is a plan to expand this to 76 provinces in order to build up evidence-based information to facilitate discussion.

In conclusion, the speaker underlined that there was unequal access to health care, inefficient resource uses in the wealthiest health coverage scheme and unmet health needs because of financial barriers, payment schemes, different quality of service-providers and high cross-boundaries. He then mentioned that fine tuning of the co-package was required and that research was to be done as an integral part of UC development. The public and the media had to be well-informed and one had to achieve a balance of information from evidence versus vested interest groups. It was also noted that qualitative data were as important as quantitative data, and that judgement based on evidence was to be promoted. The results from phase two would suggest expansion to the whole country and apply to more countries, e.g. Viet Nam.

CONCLUSIONS AND RECOMMENDATIONS

- While an agreement was achieved on the overall concept of the framework for measuring health systems performance assessment developed by WHO, it was recommended that the Organization should further fine-tune the above-mentioned concept and method taking into consideration the sociocultural diversities of the countries and the broad definition of health.

- In order to generate reliable and valid information for measuring health systems performance, WHO should strengthen the capacity of the Member Countries, especially in data generation, compilation and analysis, devising policy instruments and analysis, and regular updating and maintaining of databases.

- WHO should organize a series of technical seminars, workshops and training programmes in order to familiarize the concept and methodologies of measuring health systems performance and the framework's strengths and limitations. It is crucial to be cautious about generalizations and making comparative analyses between countries that are different in various aspects.

- There should be continuous two-way dialogues among the countries, the regional offices and WHO headquarters for verification of relevant information required for assessment of health systems performance. The services of WHO collaborating centres and the network of national institutions should be utilized.

CLOSING SESSION

In his concluding remarks, on behalf of the participants, Dr Viroj stated that it is a big challenge in the Region to perform capacity building on different aspects of activities related to health systems performance assessment. The diagnostic part of the EHSPI requires full commitment from WHO and from the Member Countries. In this context, some institutional umbrellas (like health systems research institutes, or autonomous public health institutes, legally supported and funded by the government) are essential to help facilitate the initiation and implementation of the EHSPI activities.

Ms Kei Kawabata from WHO/HQ expressed the opinion that the exchange of the rich and concrete experiences of the Member Countries made the workshop very successful. She said that WHO headquarters would be fully involved in all activities related to health systems performance assessment, together with the WHO regional and country offices.

Dr Uton Muchtar Rafei, Regional Director, thanked the participants for their time and contributions to the success of the meeting. He declared that the observations, comments and recommendations made at this consultation were very important in determining the future directions of health systems performance assessment. He also noted that improving the performance of health systems would lead to improving the health status of the Region's people. The importance of the Enhancing Health Systems Performance Initiative was emphasized. In the speaker's view, the latter could not be carried out unless the ministries of health, the allied ministries and other relevant agencies, together with WHO, work in a very closely coordinated way. Dr Uton Muchtar Rafei assured the SEARO's fullest commitment in this endeavour. He further expressed his appreciation for the constructiveness and usefulness of the presentations, discussion points and technical issues deliberated during the last few days. He hoped that WHO headquarters would collate and crystallize all facts and issues discussed in the meeting before putting them forward to the peer review group, established by the Director-General, and that the global peer review group would take them seriously.

The progress of the work on health systems performance assessment carried out in the Region was pointed out and the speaker assured the participants that he would apprise the health ministers of their accomplishments. Dr Uton Muchtar Rafei mentioned that the health systems performance assessment was an ongoing process, continuous and dynamic. It had to adjust to the needs and requirements of the country situations. He urged the participants to communicate to SEARO or to WHO headquarters any new ideas, initiatives and suggestions that may come up after this meeting. In his words, innovative ideas and thoughts were always welcome and would be taken into consideration very seriously. The health information system is the backbone of generating the data and information required by the country for evidence-based decision-making. Dr Rafei urged the participants to review the status of the performance of the health information system *vis-à-vis* resource availability and requirement of the country for improving the overall health information system. SEARO would collaborate actively in this endeavour.

The speaker reiterated that WHO was trying its best to improve the performance of health systems through the scientific process. However, one caveat, which should always be kept in mind, is the balance between the actual application or practical thinking against the theoretical consideration. This is extremely important from the perspective of decision-making by high-level policy-makers.

NOTES

1 New Delhi, India, 18–21 June 2001

ANNEX 6.1
AGENDA

I. INAUGURAL SESSION

1. RD's Inaugural Address
2. Introduction of Participants
3. Nomination of Office Bearers

II. BUSINESS SESSION (FOR REGIONAL CONSULTATION: 18–19 JUNE 2001)

1. Background and Purpose of the Consultation:
   a) Overview of the developments since *The World Health Report 2000* and main elements of the framework, concepts and policy uses.

2. Measuring Performance: Comments on the Concept, Methods, Data Requirements and Uses of:
   a) Healthy Life Expectancy
   b) Health Inequalities
   c) Responsiveness
   d) Fairness in Financial Contribution

3. Explaining Performance: Linking Goals to Functions and Monitoring Reforms:
   a) Major reforms trend in the SEAR
   b) Current thinking on assessing functions
   c) Application of the framework at subnational level in order to monitor performance

4. Building Better Evidence: Activities in the SEAR:
   a) National Health Accounts
   b) WHO Survey Programme
   c) Health information systems in support of health systems performance assessment
   d) Enhancing Health Systems Performance Initiative (EHSPI)

5. Future directions (Group Work)

Closing of the First Part of the Consultation

III. BUSINESS SESSION (FOR TECHNICAL WORKSHOP: 20–21 JUNE 2001)

1. Goodness and Fairness of Health Status (DALE and its Proxy Measure of Equity Using Child Mortality). Datasets Required for Computation.

2. Responsiveness Survey: Concepts, Survey Instruments, Country Experiences.

3. Health Care Financing—National Health Accounts: Methodology/Updates.

4. Bench-mark of Fairness for Health System Reform (Thailand Case-Study).

IV. CLOSING SESSION

PROGRAMME OF WORK

08:45–09:15	I. Inaugural Session 1. RD's Inaugural Address 2. Introduction of Participants 3. Nomination of Office Bearers
09:30–11:00	II. Business Session 1. Background and Purpose of the Consultation a) Overview of the Developments Since *The World Health Report 2000* and Main Elements of the Framework, Concepts and Policy Uses [Dr Christopher J.L. Murray, Dr David Evans]

11:00–12:30	2. Measuring Performance: Comments on Concept, Methods, Data Requirement and Uses of:

11:00–12:30   2. Measuring Performance: Comments on Concept, Methods, Data Requirement
and Uses of:
a) Healthy Life Expectancy [Dr Prasanta Mahapatra and Dr Soewarta Kosen]
b) Health Inequalities [Dr Viroj Tangcharoensathien and Dr Than Tun Sein]

14:00–15:30   ...Continued
c) Responsiveness [Dr Agus Suwandono and Dr Amala de Silva]
d) Fairness in Financial Contribution [Dr Ravi P. Rannan-Eliya and
Dr Anil Gumber]

16:00–17:00   Recapitulation of the Main Agreed upon Points for the Day

19 JUNE 2001

09:00–10:30   3. Explaining Performance: Linking Goals to Functions and Monitoring Reforms
a) Major Reforms Trend in SEAR]Dr Than Sein and Dr Kumara Rai]
b) Current Thinking on Assessing Function [Dr Kei Kawabata]
c) Application of the Framework at Subnational Level in Order to Monitor Performance
[Dr Christopher J.L. Murray]

11:00–12:30   4. Building Better Evidence: Activities in SEAR
a) National Health Accounts [Dr Ravi P. Rannan-Eliya]
b) WHO Survey Programme [Dr Somnath Chatterji]
c) Health Information Systems in Support of Health Systems Performance Assessment
[Dr Myint Htwe]
d) Enhancing Health Systems Performance Initiative [WHO/HQ Staff]

14:00–15:30   5. Future Directions (Group Work)
Briefing for Group Work
Group 1–2: Recommendations on the Framework, Design, Data Sources and Data
Quality for Health Systems Performance Assessment
Group 3: Recommendations on Follow-Up of EHSPI Including Capacity Building for
Health Systems Performance Assessment
Group 4: Recommendations on Strengthening of National Health Information Sys-
tems to Provide Input for Health Systems Performance Assessment Activities

16:00–17:00   Presentation of the Group Work

Closing of the First Part of the Consultation

TECHNICAL WORKSHOP

20 JUNE 2001

09:00–10:30   III. Business Session
1. Goodness and Fairness of Health Status (DALE and its Proxy Measure of Equity
Using Child Mortality)—Datasets Required for Computation [Dr Prasanta
Mahapatra and Dr Chalapati Rao]

11:00–12:30   ...Continued

14:00–15:30   2. Responsiveness Survey: Concepts, Survey Instruments, Country Experiences [Dr Agus
Suwandono, Dr Amala de Silva, Ms Lipika Nanda]

15:30–16:30   ...Continued

21 JUNE 2001

09:00–10:30	3. Health Care Financing—National Health Accounts Methodology/Updates [Dr Ravi P. Rannan-Eliya and Dr Viroj]
11:00–12:30	4. Bench-mark of Fairness for Health System Reform Thailand Case-Study [Dr Supasit Pannarunothai]
14:00–15:00	IV. Closing Session

LIST OF PARTICIPANTS

Mr S.M. Shahjahan
Joint Secretary
Ministry of Health and Family
  Welfare
Dhaka
Bangladesh

Dr Enamul Karim
Consultant
Management Change Unit (MCU)
Dhaka
Bangladesh

Dr Syed Azizur Rahman
Assistant Chief (PRU)
Health Economics Unit
Ministry of Health and Family
  Welfare
Dhaka
Bangladesh

Dr Shahid Md Asib Nasim
Deputy Team Leader
Programme Coordinator Cell
  (PCC), HPSP
  Dhaka
Bangladesh

Mr Thinlay Dorji
Planning Officer, PPD
Thimphu
Bhutan

Mr Ugyen Wangdi
Information Officer
Ministry of Health
Thimphu
Bhutan

Dr Pak Jong Min
Director
Department of External Affairs
Ministry of Public Health
Pyongyang
Democratic People's Republic of
  Korea

Mr Jon Sang Chol
Interpreter
Ministry of Public Health
Pyongyang
Democratic People's Republic of
  Korea

Dr Prema Ramachandran*
Adviser (Health)
Planning Commission
New Delhi
India

Mr G.R. Patwardhan
Additional Secretary (Health)
Ministry of Health and Family
  Welfare
New Delhi
India

Dr S.P. Agarwal
Director-General of Health
  Services
Ministry of Health and Family
  Welfare
New Delhi
India

Dr P.K. Baliyar Singh
Officiating Director
Central Bureau of Health
  Intelligence
Ministry of Health and Family
  Welfare
New Delhi
India

Dr Jotna Sokhey
Additional Project Director
NACO
New Delhi
India

Mrs Urvashi Sadhwani
Additional Economic Adviser
Directorate-General of Health
  Services
Ministry of Health and Family
  Welfare
New Delhi
India

Dr L.S. Chauhan
ADG(IH)
Directorate-General of Health
  Services
Ministry of Health and Family
  Welfare
New Delhi
India

Dr Anil Gumber
Economist
National Council of Applied
  Economic
Research
New Delhi
India

Ms Lipika Nanda
Institute of Health Systems
Hyderabad
India

Dr A. Indrayan
Professor and Head
Department of Biostatistics
University College of Medical
    Sciences
New Delhi
India

Mr Sunil Nandraj
Senior Research Officer
CEHAT
Mumbai
India

Prof. Dr Azrul Azwar*
Director-General of Community
    Health
Ministry of Health and Social
    Welfare
Jakarta
Indonesia

Dr Sri Astuti Soeparmanto
Head/Director-General
NIHRD
Ministry of Health and Social
    Welfare
Jakarta
Indonesia

Dr Setiawan Soeparan
Chief
Bureau of Planning
Ministry of Health and Social
    Welfare
Jakarta
Indonesia

Ms Nasirah Bahaudin
Chief
Division of International
    Cooperation
Bureau of Planning
Ministry of Health and Social
    Welfare
Jakarta
Indonesia

Dr Hendrianto
Coordinator—Health and Health
    Responsiveness Survey
NIHRD
Ministry of Health and Social
    Welfare
Jakarta
Indonesia

Mr Arizal Ahnaf
National Bureau of Statistics
Jakarta
Indonesia

Dr Soewarta Kosen
Coordinator—Postal/Mail Survey
NIHRD
Ministry of Health and Social
    Welfare
Jakarta
Indonesia

Mr Bambang Hartono
Chief, Centre for Health Data
    and Information
Ministry of Health and Social
    Welfare
Jakarta
Indonesia

Dr Sarimawar Djaja
Researcher, Health Ecology
NIHRD
Ministry of Health and Social
    Welfare
Jakarta
Indonesia

Dr Sukanto Sumodinoto
Researcher, Health Service and
    Technology
NIHRD
Ministry of Health and Social
    Welfare
Jakarta
Indonesia

Dr Choliq Amin
Chief
Bureau of Finance
Ministry of Health and Social
    Welfare
Jakarta
Indonesia

Dr Budihardja
Provincial Health Office
Central Java
Semarang
Indonesia

Dr Sheena Moosa
Head of the Planning Section
Ministry of Health
Male
Maldives

Ms Shehenaz Fahmy
Assistant Director
Ministry of Health
Male
Maldives

Ms Fathimath Nasheeda
    Mohamed
Planning Officer
Ministry of Health
Male
Maldives

Dr Than Tun Sein
Director
Department of Medical Research
Ministry of Health
Yangon
Myanmar

Dr Phone Myint
Deputy Director
Department of Health Planning
Ministry of Health
Yangon
Myanmar

U Htay Win
Deputy Director
Department of Health Planning
Ministry of Health
Yangon
Myanmar

Dr B.D. Chataut*
Director General of Health
  Services
Ministry of Health
Kathmandu
Nepal

Dr Nilambar Jha
Associate Professor, Department
  of Community Medicine
B.P. Koirala Institute of Health
  Sciences
Dharan
Nepal

Dr K. C. S. Dalpatadu
Deputy Director-General of
  Health
Services (Planning)
Department of Health Services
Ministry of Health
Colombo
Sri Lanka

Dr Sunil Senanayake
Director (Health Information)
Ministry of Health
Colombo
Sri Lanka

Dr S.D. de Silva
Director
National Institute of Health
  Sciences
Kalutara
Sri Lanka

Dr Wiput Phoolcharoen
Director
Health Systems Research Institute
Ministry of Public Health
Nonthaburi
Thailand

Dr Niwat Lawpakdeekun
Dentist
Phrasamuthjaedee Community
  Hospital
Ministry of Public Health
Nonthaburi
Thailand

Dr Kanitta Bundhamcharoen
Bureau of Health Policy and
  Planning
Ministry of Public Health
Nonthaburi
Thailand

Dr Jadej Thammatuch-aree
Bangkruay Hospital
Ministry of Public Health
Nonthaburi
Thailand

Dr Prae Chittinanda
Bangyai Hospital
Ministry of Public Health
Nonthaburi
Thailand

Ms Sripen Tantivess
Division of Drug Control
Office of Food and Drug
  Administration
Ministry of Public Health
Nonthaburi
Thailand

Prof. Siripen Supakankunti
Director, Centre of Health
  Economics
Faculty of Economics,
  Chulalongkorn University
Bangkok
Thailand

Resource Group

Dr Prasanta Mahapatra
Director
Institute of Health Systems
Hyderabad
India

Dr Chalapati Rao
Faculty
Institute of Health Systems
Hyderabad
India

Dr Agus Suwandono
Secretary
National Institute of Health
  Research and Development
Ministry of Health
Jakarta
Indonesia

Dr Ravi P. Rannan-Eliya
Health Policy Programme
Institute of Policy Studies
Colombo
Sri Lanka

Dr Amala de Silva
University of Colombo
Colombo
Sri Lanka

Dr Supasit Pannarunothai
Head
Centre for Health Equity
Monitoring
Faculty of Medicine
Naresuan University
Phitanulok
Thailand

Dr Viroj Tangcharoensathien
Senior Policy Analyst
Health Systems Research Institute
Ministry of Public Health
Nonthaburi
Thailand

Country Offices

Dr George J. Komba-Kono
WHO Medical Officer (PHC)
Bangladesh

Dr T.S. Walia
Ag. WHO Representative
India

Mr Peter Pachner,
Technical Officer, WHO Country
  Office
Indonesia

Dr Stephanus Indradjaya
National Professional Officer
WHO Country Office
Indonesia

Prof. A.M. Das
WHO Technical Officer
(Health Planner)
Ministry of Health
Nepal

Dr Paramita Sudharto
WHO Public Health
Administrator (HSD)
Ministry of Health
Nepal

Dr A.S. Abdullah
Medical Officer
WHO Country Office
Sri Lanka

Dr Lokky Wai
WHO Management Officer
Ministry of Health
Sri Lanka

Dr Somchai Peeraprakorn
National Professional Officer
WHO Country Office
Thailand

WHO Secretariat

Dr Christopher J.L. Murray
Executive Director
Evidence and Information for
    Policy

Dr David B. Evans
Evidence and Information for
    Policy

Ms Kei Kawabata
Evidence and Information for
    Policy

Dr Phyllida Travis
Evidence and Information for
    Policy

Dr Emmanuela Gakidou
Evidence and Information for
    Policy

Dr Somnath Chatterji
Evidence and Information for
    Policy

Dr Ajay Tandon
Evidence and Information for
    Policy

Dr Piya Hanvoravongchai
Evidence and Information for
    Policy

WHO/SEARO

Ms Poonam Khetrapal Singh
Deputy Regional Director/
Director, Programme
    Management

Dr Than Sein
Director, Department of Evidence
    and Information for Policy

Dr N. Kumara Rai
Acting Director, Department of
    Health Systems and Community
    Health

Dr Myint Htwe
Regional Adviser
Evidence for Health Policy

Dr J. Leowski
Regional Adviser
Noncommunicable Diseases
    Surveillance

Dr Harry Caussy
Regional Epidemiologist

Dr S.P. Jost
Technical Officer
Health Systems Research

Dr Nihal Singh
Special Assistant
Evidence for Health Policy

Mr M. R. Kanagarajan
Administrative Assistant,
    Department of Evidence and
    Information for Policy

Ms Benita Dsouza
Secretary
Evidence for Health Policy

Mr R.K. Arora
Clerical Assistant
Evidence for Health Policy

* could not attend

Chapter 7

WESTERN PACIFIC REGIONAL CONSULTATION ON HEALTH SYSTEMS PERFORMANCE ASSESSMENT[1]

WHO REGIONAL OFFICE FOR THE WESTERN PACIFIC

SUMMARY

Representatives from ten countries and twelve technical experts convened to discuss the conceptual and methodological issues related to health systems performance assessment (HSPA); to describe various experiences regarding health systems performance; to identify other critical issues in its application, and to assess the linkage between health systems performance and the policy and managerial decision-making processes.

It was generally agreed at the regional consultation that HSPA provides an opportunity to review a country's health system and its improvement over time. How a country's health system compares with others requires an understanding of the historical, past development efforts and of the current conditions of health systems across countries. Some countries in the Region possess unique features, such as size, isolation, levels of economic and political development, diversity of health systems and human resources capacities, which may affect the results of assessment of their performance and yield meaningless inter-country comparisons and ranking. It was suggested that no ranking of countries be made in the subsequent *World Health Report*.

It was decided that the current HSPA methodology is complicated. The development of HSPA tools and methods will be more useful to the Member States if the objective of the assessment is for in-country use and if it is closely linked to health systems functions and managerial processes. The concept of responsiveness and its domains are culture-bound and vary with different socio-cultural settings. The fairness in financial contribution (FCC) index was less understood, especially in terms of what it ultimately measures. Suggestions were made to develop a few indicators, particularly at subpopulation levels, to illustrate various equity measures within the FFC index. The participants also cited the need to relate the summary indices with the provision and coverage of health services to capture various health care settings in countries, including traditional health systems.

The data requirements of HSPA pose problems for data collection. The information needs are not likely to be met by countries on a regular basis, as they involve huge resource trade-offs and capacity overload. There is clearly a need for simpler data sets and streamlined information requests from international partners. Simplification of tools and capacity-building support are needed.

According to the participants, the HSPA development processes have to be transparent. Second level HSPA work should not only take account of methodological issues, but also build on the Member States' health priorities and utilize the existing work on indicators going on in countries. For the latter to make an investment in HSPA, there has to be a buy-in process to foster ownership. The latter requires an understanding and agreement to the framework and methodologies. The research development process should include open peer review processes, easy and early availability of write-ups, with clear explanations on assumptions made and data limitation acknowledgements.

The Member States expressed the need to see greater collaboration among the development partners, especially with regards to information requests and the overall direction of health systems development. It was proposed that WHO in its stewardship role should initiate and facilitate this process. The Member States also want better coordination within WHO, especially in the areas of programme proposals, development of indicators, tools, methods, guidelines, consultations and communications on these new developments.

Background

Following the memorandum dated 13 March 2001 from the Director-General to "hear and reflect on the widest possible range of views and ideas on health systems performance assessment," the WHO Regional Office for the Western Pacific organized the Regional Consultation on Health System Performance Assessment (HSPA) in Manila from 3 to 5 July 2001. Representatives from ten countries and twelve technical experts gathered at the meeting with the following objectives:

- To discuss different conceptual and methodological approaches to assessing the performance of health systems.

- To take stock of different country and regional experiences in the Western Pacific on issues related to health systems performance assessment.

- To identify critical issues for furthering the conceptual and methodological development of a framework for measuring the performance of health systems that countries could apply on a regular basis and on which they could inform WHO periodically.

To discuss the linkage between health systems performance assessment practices and health systems policy and managerial decision-making processes.

Following the opening remarks by Dr Shigeru Omi, Regional Director, Mr John Goss, country participant from Australia served as Chairman, with Dr Nguyen Dang Vung, country participant from Viet Nam as Vice-Chair, and Dr Rozita Hussein, technical adviser from Malaysia as Rapporteur.

The participants were given the WHO background paper for the regional consultation on health systems performance assessment as reference material. The agenda of the regional consultation was designed to discuss the HSPA framework and methodology issues on the first day after the background presentation by Dr Christopher J.L. Murray, Executive Director, Evidence and Information for Policy. The next day saw country representatives and technical experts presenting their views on HSPA, especially in terms of its applicability to their respective country settings. Open plenary sessions followed to discuss the use of composite and multiple indicators in HSPA, as well as future

research and collaborative issues. On the third day, there was a presentation from Mr Orvill B. Adams, Director, Organization of Health Services Delivery, Evidence and Information for Policy, on the linkage of HSPA to policy and managerial decision-making processes in health systems. Discussions among the participants were followed by the summary presentation of the regional consultation. The regional consultation was undertaken as an open and frank dialogue.

This report provides a summary of the questions raised during the regional consultation. The report is divided as follows: the first part covers general observations on HSPA; the second discusses methodological issues related to WHO health systems performance assessment; the third examines the implications for future work on health systems performance assessment.

General Observations Regarding Performance Assessment

There has been a strategic shift and commitment from WHO to support the Member States in health systems performance assessment of their respective health care systems. This initiative was welcomed and supported by the Member States in the Western Pacific Region.

It was agreed that the assessment of health system performance and the way it improves over time is important for reviewing a country's health system. This evaluation has the potential to provide health policy and decision-makers with an impetus to consider and institute changes to improve the performance of their health care systems. Health systems performance assessments are a useful and necessary part of unravelling and measuring the "black box"—what happens between the inputs to health systems and the final outcomes achieved by countries. The tools developed within HSPA in general may therefore be useful for evidence-based decision-making, provided there is a consensus on the development and use of these tools across countries.

However, it must be noted that the comparison between the health systems of different countries requires an understanding of the historical, cultural, economic and social contexts, past development efforts, and current conditions of health systems across countries. Some of the countries in the Region are in the midst of reform initiatives and decentralization activities. Others are contemplating such reforms. The countries in the Western Pacific Region also possess unique features that may affect the results of assessments on their performance, such as size, distance and relative isolation, levels of economic and political development, diversity of health systems and human resource capacities. The various issues raised during the meeting were reflections of relevant health systems performance assessment issues in the context of the current health sector reform directions among the Member States.

METHODOLOGICAL ISSUES RELATED TO WHO HSPA

WHO HSPA FRAMEWORK AND METHODOLOGY

General

- There has not been a general consensus on the objective of HSPA as assumed by WHO in its publication, *The World Health Report 2000*. Although there was no dispute on the importance of health systems performance assessment for the Member States, it was believed that the main goal of the HSPA undertaken by WHO with its publication of *The World Health Report 2000* seemed to be inter-country comparison. The participants considered that the HSPA methods and tools would be more useful to the Member States if the assessment were extended to in-country use.

- It was generally agreed that the current WHO HSPA methodology was complicated and difficult to understand by policy-makers and researchers alike. There were strong requests for simpler methods and measures, which would illustrate the performance of health systems in a user-friendly fashion.

- The current methodology involves measuring attainment indicators for five goals and combining these into a composite index of health system performance. In this process, there has been an unfortunate mixing of new and recent conceptual and empirical developments in areas such as responsiveness with more advanced empirical research work on burden of disease and summary indices of population health. The resulting composite index of the WHO HSPA reveals the characteristics of research efforts in evolution, with all the problems that may be expected with a newly developing methodology. There were suggestions to concentrate only on the level and distribution of population health status measurement across countries within the WHO HSPA framework, while conceptual and method-ological development on the responsiveness and fairness of financial contribution elements progressed.

Responsiveness

- There are serious problems with regard to understanding the concepts of responsiveness and its domains, particularly given the very different socio-cultural settings of the various countries. It was decided that the domains measured for responsiveness were more reflective of the areas of concern for the developed countries and less so for the developing ones.

  Similarly, the weighting given to the distinct domains in developing the index for responsiveness would be different for different countries, particularly if the index reflected the health system policy priorities of the countries. The instruments developed for measuring these domains, as well as the health state preferences, suffer the same lack of understanding, agreement and acceptance by researchers from various countries.

  The development work undertaken by WHO may well solve some of these problems. However, since the instruments are still in the developmental phase and the third version is due to come out soon, there were suggestions that WHO should focus on cross-cultural development, acceptance and agreement of these instruments before trying to make comparisons across countries.

  Public health interventions and spending by governments did not seem to be reflected in the instruments and methodology developed to measure responsiveness. Although the contribution of public health activities would eventually be reflected in the level of health status and distribution, it was mentioned that having a fairly distributed and responsive public health system would go a long way towards improving the well-being of the population. As such, this needs to be measured under responsiveness.

Fairness in Financing

- Participants voiced a concern about the complexity of the fairness in financial contribution (FFC) index. They maintained that it was unclear what changes in the index might mean. The index at present includes measures of both horizontal and vertical equity, which make interpretation more difficult. Countries' low scores mainly result from extreme horizontal equity problems (catastrophic expenditures on health).

It was also discussed that the current FFC index relies on household survey data on income and expenditures. Data on government and employer sources of health care financing are implicitly included, but government subsidies, which are substitutes for income support, are not included so as to avoid possible double counting. The need to include non-monetary social support by households was noted.

It was necessary to go beyond the FFC index measuring the distribution of health financing contributions, to measuring the distribution of provision and coverage of health services. If there is an inequitable distribution of the provision of health services, this will show in the measurement of the equity of health outcomes, but equity of provision is such an important process indicator that it should be measured in its own right.

■ The need to measure the performance of the private, traditional and informal health care sectors was also raised during the discussion. Measurement should be made of resources in cash or in kind, spent on private providers, and also of services provided by traditional carers, such as birth attendants, healers and informal carers. This provision has an effect on the public provision of health services.

Data Issues

■ The data requirements of the current WHO health systems performance assessment pose problems for data collection. Problems with surveys related to the measurement of responsiveness and health state preferences were discussed. The understanding of various concepts measured in the questionnaires by respondents from different cultural backgrounds was one of the major issues raised by the participants. Issues regarding the reliability of responses, response rates to surveys and gaming were also discussed. The resource requirements of these surveys are extensive. The length of the questionnaires and the use of culture-bound vignettes were cited as causes for concern as well. Some of the participants declared that the introduction of vignettes had not improved the tool. In their opinion, the vignettes may in fact lead to more confusion in understanding the concept, resulting in responses that do not reflect a real comprehension. WHO is still assessing the validity of this methodology, including the use of vignettes.

The choice of data-collection methods will have a strong influence on the timing, frequency, and feasibility of the HSPA analysis and reporting. Household surveys are costly and in many instances can be organized only once every five or ten years. Postal surveys in developing Member States have a limited utility. The validity of the key informant survey instrument and method has yet to be established. The burden on countries in collecting data and developing significant analytical capacity in exchange for measuring marginal improvements in health system performance was at the centre of the discussion.

The suggestion that annual reporting is required to assist policy and decision-makers is dependent on the HSPA methodology being demonstrated as useful for strategic and operational policy and decision-making at the marginal level. There was a suggestion that the feasibility and appropriateness of biennial reporting should be investigated. Composite measures, without disaggregation to lower levels, will have less applicability and relevance to the successful management of factors directly within the bounds of control of a Minister/Ministry of Health.

■ The quality of data used for *The World Health Report 2000* was discussed. It was suggested that data quality issues be treated in a very transparent manner in future WHO HSPA undertakings. Information should be provided on the quality of data used for such calculations in a tabular format. This should indicate for each country the type and sources of data used, as well as give a score on the degrees of data quality, including whether the data are actual or an estimate.

Ranking Issues

■ In view of the various methodological problems cited, the ranking of countries based on the HSPA indices was discussed extensively. There was a general consensus (without dissent) that future reporting should not include rankings for the Member States. Opinions were expressed that countries should be grouped according to various criteria, such as development status, and that analysis should be provided without ranking. Although it was recognized that the information in any public WHO report of this nature would be used by others to rank countries, some participants stated that there was a difference between WHO ranking countries and others using it for that purpose.

■ Another major discussion revolved around translating the global strategy of HSPA into national and local action. If the WHO HSPA framework and methodology cannot be applied to subnational and subsystem settings of the Member States, it will be difficult for policy and decision-makers to use the current WHO methodology for health sector development within the countries.

COUNTRY VIEWS AND EXPERIENCES

■ A number of participants observed that the country ranks and scores attracted a lot of attention when *The World Health Report 2000* was released. This changed the focus from the main issues discussed in the report on improving the performance of health care systems. According to some participants, the lack of linkage between health systems performance and outcomes was one of the major limitations of use of the report's current HSPA framework. This hampered the seeking of guidance on how to improve health systems performance, as well as managerial policy and decision-making.

The World Health Report 2000 ranking of the countries' health systems performance without taking into account the very different resource bases, health conditions, historical influences and current developments in the systems, has been noted to be a major concern. At best, the WHO HSPA rankings elicited further queries on how to improve performance. At worst, some countries reported that the WHO HSPA rankings caused resentment because of the perceived negative and unjustified impressions of some countries' health system performance in the report.

■ Differences in the culture of policy and decision-making in various countries affect the use and applicability of a concept such as HSPA. In cases, in which politicians appear to be interested merely in the flow of resources to their constituencies, the applicability of the WHO HSPA methodology for intracountry comparison clearly becomes more important to them than the comparison itself. It was noted that judgements on health systems performance should be linked to the health system priorities of each country.

■ True ownership by countries of the HSPA process would be enhanced through clear understanding of and agreement with the framework, methodology and processes. The participants were concerned about the lack of a consultation prior to the official release of *The World Health Report 2000*. They suggested that the Member States should be consulted in the future development of the WHO HSPA and its related works. The future consultation process needs to be transparent.

■ Countries have expressed the need to place the WHO HSPA within the context of various health system reform efforts in health financing and decentralization. Delegation of health authority to lower administrative levels, such as states, provinces, or districts requires adapting the HSPA methodology to these levels in order to ensure that the assessment is meaningful within the context of health sector development in the Member States.

■ The current HSPA framework and methodology appear not to have taken into account previous and ongoing work and efforts within the countries on assessing the performance of their own health systems, and the development of health information and surveillance systems. Several countries had developed frameworks to monitor and evaluate health system performance using multiple indicators. A movement towards a multiple indicator-based HSPA system within the composite outcomes framework would be more in keeping with the countries' concerns for monitoring health system performance.

■ The information requirements of the WHO HSPA have been burdensome to the Member States. The information needs of the WHO HSPA are likely to involve resource trade-offs if they are to be met by the countries on a regular basis. Resources put into efforts on surveys should be balanced by investment needs in improving vital registration systems and reorienting routine health information systems. The resource constraints are not purely monetary or infrastructure related. In many developing countries in the Region, there are very limited numbers of trained staff and technical personnel to conduct such assessments. There is a significant problem of overloading the limited human resource capacity.

■ There is clearly a need for simpler data sets and streamlined information requests, especially from international partners, in addition to requests from the WHO regional offices and headquarters. Coordination of information requirements of donors and development partners in the Member States would reduce workloads.

■ Country-level capacities for HSPA are not sufficient. Some countries noted the lack of survey skills and a very limited capacity to carry out in-depth analysis and performance monitoring. Simplification of tools and capacity-building support are needed. The participants highlighted the Pacific island countries' requirements in these areas.

LINKS WITH POLICY AND MANAGEMENT PROCESSES

■ The participants in this Consultation strongly voiced the need for the HSPA framework to have direct relevance to policy and management decision-making. While research and development of the next level of indicators were recognized as potentially useful, the consultative process to develop them needs to be put in place. Future developments on the indicators of functions and intermediate goals were encouraged, provided that these indicators were relevant as inputs into intracountry assessments and management processes.

■ It was requested that WHO should review the existing in-country indicators in the Member States during the development and drawing-up of the next level of assessment tools. Some countries in the Region have institutionalized frameworks for these issues within their health information systems.

■ The use of a parsimonious set of indicators requires a prior agreement from the countries that these indicators indeed fit into their health system priorities and current direction. The development of standardized evaluation protocols for critical interventions should look into the current indicators used by the countries. Deliberate efforts should also be made to link the routine data collected by the Ministries of Health with these protocols.

■ Current work on the cost-effectiveness of critical interventions spans different types of interventions, from preventive to curative, and from public health to personal care services, e.g. from distribution of bednets, to seatbelt legislation, to insulin treatment. It is important to identify what can be considered sets of relevant critical interventions from the perspective of differences in health care systems. These sets of critical interventions must be agreed upon by the Member States and must be flexible to accommodate the priorities and needs of the countries with differing health needs and resources.

■ Given the current and future directions in health sector reform, the events in the private sector have to be examined. The countries in this Region are pluralistic. Focusing only on the public sector as the source of information or as the centre of the assessment will not capture a large and important part of the health system. In this connection, defining stewardship and the development of indicators for stewardship functions is important. The same applies to health care systems with strong and formally recognized traditional health sectors. Linking these providers' behaviour to responsiveness and quality of care was identified as potentially useful. WHO's technical expertise in developing mechanisms for governments to interact meaningfully with the private sector and traditional health practitioners, and also to gather reliable information from them, was discussed.

■ Policy work in the health sector can be informed by specific measures of affordability and access to health care services. The participants suggested that issues of cost containment and comparative pricing of health care services and commodities globally would provide practical information to policymakers.

■ The second-level WHO HSPA work processes and results must be communicated to the regions and the countries. The country experts should have the opportunity to review the data used and to carry out their own analysis in advance of the publication and dissemination of the findings. WHO has begun to send out preliminary data to the countries to enable such review. It was also suggested that research using methodologies not yet subjected to peer review should first be published as research reports, rather than in *The World Health Report 2000*. Only after the acceptance of the methodologies, should the findings be regularly featured in this report.

IMPLICATIONS FOR FUTURE WORK ON WHO HSPA AND RELATED AREAS

■ It is considered that health systems performance assessment is a valuable tool for health ministries in their efforts to improve the health of their population. The composite measures developed and the analyses conducted in the first phase of the WHO HSPA should be brought down to the subnational and (where appropriate) subpopulation group levels. In this context, the intracountry application of particular areas of the WHO HSPA methodology for Japan, as was demonstrated during the consultation, can serve as an example of the feasibility of such analysis, where reliable data are available. The presentation from Japan also demonstrated the value of time-series analysis. The meeting encouraged the future work on the WHO HSPA to make better use of the insights and tools from the management and policy sciences. At the same time, it clearly highlighted the need for good, disaggregated data beyond national totals and time-series data. Such data are not currently available for many countries in the Region. Neither are the skills needed to carry out such analyses. Extensive and intensive training in health economics is required.

■ Large investments in effort, time and resources are needed to undertake the WHO HSPA. For countries to make that level of investment, there has to be a buy-in process to ensure ownership. The latter requires understanding and agreement of the framework and methodologies. Hence, the future research development process of the WHO HSPA must be transparent. It should include open peer-review processes with both technical experts and country representatives, as well as easy and early availability of write-ups, with clear explanations on assumptions made and data limitations. The development of instruments and tools should progress gradually from pilot and small-scale studies in different settings to finalizing and stabilizing the instruments before applying them to more widespread and large-scale studies. An independent evaluation of the WHO HSPA initiative and programme would be helpful.

■ There should be a greater collaboration among the development partners, especially with regard to information requests and the overall direction for health systems development. It is proposed that WHO, in its stewardship role as the main global authoritative body on health issues, should initiate and facilitate this process. At the same time, WHO must have the commitment and capacity to perform the stewardship role of providing technical support to the countries that require and request it in improving their health systems.

■ The Member States want a better co-ordination within WHO, between different clusters and programmes at headquarters and between headquarters and the regional and country offices. Co-ordination is required in the areas of programme proposals, data requests, development of indicators, tools, methods and guidelines, consultations and communications of new developments. The Member States would like to see support for regional and subregional initiatives in capacity building, not just of personnel from the Member States, but also of WHO staff, in order to foster a close and continuous transfer of technology and skills building.

CONCLUSION

The Member States in the Western Pacific Region fully support the initiative to measure health system performance. This is reflected in the keenness of the countries to participate in and learn from the WHO health systems performance assessment initiative. Simultaneously, there is a recognition that the framework is only newly developed and still pushing forward the frontiers in some areas of research. While it is still in its evolutionary stage, the Member States want their concerns and constraints to be considered. To this end, the consultative process with the countries and the technical experts that has now been started is supported. It is the expectation of the Member States that such a process will continue throughout the development and finalization of the WHO HSPA framework, both in the initial phase and for the subsequent phases.

Through such consultations, it is expected that a manageable and relevant set of indicators and measurement tools will be developed that will not only take into account methodological issues, but will also incorporate the countries' priorities and inter and intracountry differences. It is hoped that these tools will be of use at the country-level with regard to management and policy.

The Member States look forward to the greater stewardship role of WHO in the coordination initiatives related to health and health care, at both inter and intra-agency levels. The Member States also look forward to a clear and committed role by WHO in helping the countries fulfil their potential to develop high-performing health care systems, as envisaged by the WHO HSPA initiative.

NOTES

1 Manila, Philippines, 3–5 July 2001

ANNEX 7.1

AGENDA

DAY 1

9:00–9:15	Opening Ceremony [Dr S. Omi, Regional Director, WHO/WPRO]
9:15–9:30	Introduction of the Regional Consultation on Health Systems Performance Assessment [Dr A. Ron, Director of Health Sector Development, WHO/WPRO]
9:30–10:15	Background Paper on Health Systems Performance Assessment Concept, Framework, Methods and Future Development [Presentation by Dr Christopher J.L. Murray, Executive Director, Evidence and Information for Policy Cluster, WHO/HQ]
10:15–10:30	Coffee Break
10:30–12:15	Plenary Discussion
12:15–13:45	Lunch Break
13:45–14:45	Health System Goals and Indicators
	Healthy Life Expectancy, Level and Distribution [Presentation by Dr M. Booth, New Zealand]
	Plenary Discussion
14:45–15:45	Responsiveness, Level and Distribution [Presentation by Dr K. Maskom, Malaysia and Dr G. Hiawalyer, PNG]
	Plenary Discussion
15:45–16:15	Coffee Break
16:15–17:15	Fairness in Financial Contribution [Presentation by Mr D. Bayarsaikhan, HCF/WPRO and Mr J. Goss, Australia]
	Plenary Discussion

DAY 2

9:00–9:10	Summary: Key Points Raised in Day 1
9:10–10:30	Views and Issues of WHO Health System Performance Assessment in Pacific Island Countries (Concept, Methods and Country Experiences)
	Panel of Presenters: Prof. Stowers, Samoa Dr G. Hiawalyer, Papua New Guinea Mr K. Mulo, Fiji Dr M. Dugue, Asian Development Bank
	Plenary Discussion
10:30–10:45	Coffee Break
10:45–12:15	Views and Issues of WHO Health System Performance Assessment in Asian Countries (Concept, Methods and Country Experiences)
	Panel of Presenters: Mr Jun Gao, China Dr Jae-Goog Jo, Republic of Korea Dr Nguyen Dang Vung, Viet Nam Dr M. Dayrit, Philippines Dr Masami Sakoi, Japan
	Plenary Discussion
12:15–13:45	Lunch Break
13:45–15:15	Composite Indices Versus Multiple Indicators on Health Systems Performance Assessment
	Open Forum:
	1. Potential Use and Impact of Composite Measurement Indicators on Health Sector Development Policy and Practice
	2. Use of Multiple Indicators in Health Systems Performance Assessment

15:15–15:30	Coffee Break	9:10–10:30	Linking Health Systems Performance Assessment and Health Systems Policy and Managerial Decision-Making Processes [Presentation by Mr Orville B. Adams, Evidence and Information for Policy Cluster, WHO/HQ]

15:30–17:15   Future Research and Development on Health Systems Performance Assessment (Research Issues and Collaborative Process Issues)

Panel of Presenters:
Dr T. Hasegawa, Japan (Research Issues)
Dr R. Hussein, Malaysia (Research Issues)
Dr D. Shuey, PMO/WPRO (Collaborative Process Issues)
Dr M. O'Leary, MO/WPRO (Pacific Perspective)

Plenary Discussion

Open Forum:
Country Reflections on HSPA as a Support for Health Systems Policy and Managerial Decision-Making Processes

10:30-11:00   Coffee Break

11:30–12:00   Summary of the Regional Consultation [Rapporteur and Dr Soe Nyunt-U, SAP/WPRO]

Day 3

9:00–9:10   Summary: Key Points Raised in Day 2

12:00–12:15   Closing Ceremony [Dr S. Omi, Regional Director]

List of Participants

Mr John Goss
Principal Economist
Australian Institute of Health and Welfare
GPO Box 570
Canberra City ACT 2601
Australia

Mr Jun Gao
Deputy Director
Center for Health Statistics Information
Ministry of Health
#1, Nanlu, Xizhimenwai
Xicheng District
Beijing 100044
China

Dr Pui-Yin Chiu
Principal Medical and Health Officer
Department of Health
21st Floor, Wu Chung House
213 Queen's Road East, Wan Chai
Hong Kong

Dr Masami Sakoi
Deputy Director
International Affairs Division
Minister's Secretariat
Ministry of Health, Labour and Welfare
1-2-2 Kasumigaseki, Chiyoda-ku
Tokyo 100-8916
Japan

Dr Kalsom Maskom
Principal Assistant Director
Planning and Development Division
Ministry of Health
14th Floor, Perkim Building
Ipoh Road
51200 Kuala Lumpur
Malaysia

Dr Mark Booth
Senior Analyst
Sector Policy Directorate
Ministry of Health
Level 1, Old Bank Chambers
Customhouse Quay
P.O. Box 5013
Wellington
New Zealand

Dr Gilbert Hiawalyer
Director
Monitoring & Research Division
Department of Health
P.O. Box 807
Waigani NCD
Papua New Guinea

Mario Villaverde
Director IV
Department of Health
San Lazaro Compound
Rizal Avenue, Sta Cruz
Manila
Philippines

Jae-Goog Jo
Director
Department of Health Research
Korea Institute of Health and
    Social Affairs
San 42-14, Bulgwang-dong
Eunpyung-gu
Seoul 122-705
Republic of Korea

Ms Pelenatete Stowers
Director of Nursing
Department of Health
Private Bag
Apia
Samoa

Dr Nguyen Dang Vung
Senior Officer
Health Policy Unit
Secretary of the High Level
    Committee on Health Policy
    and Strategy
Ministry of Health
138A Giang Vo St
Hanoi
Viet Nam

Dr Manuel Dayrit
Secretary of Health
Department of Health
San Lazaro Compound
Rizal Avenue, Sta Cruz
Manila
Philippines

Barry Borman
Manager, Analysis
Public Health Operating Group
Ministry of Health
P.O. Box 5013
Wellington
New Zealand

Dr Maryse Dugue
Health Specialist
Office of Pacific Operations
Asian Development Bank
P.O. Box 789-0980-Manila
6 ADB Avenue
1550 Mandaluyong City
Metro Manila
Philippines

Dr Toshihiko Hasegawa
Director
Department of Health Care Policy
National Institute of Health
    Services Management
1-23-1, Toyama, Shinjuku-ku
Tokyo 162-0052
Japan

Rozita Halina bte. Tun Hussein
Medical Officer in Research
Health Systems Research Division
Institute of Public Health
Ministry of Health
19 Changkat Tunku
50480 Kuala Lumpur
Malaysia

Dr Meng-Kin Lim
Associate Professor
Department of Community,
    Occupational and Family
    Medicine
Faculty of Medicine
National University of Singapore
MD3, 16 Medical Drive
Singapore 117597

Mr Kitione Mulo
Acting Director
Health Planning and Information
Ministry of Health
Box 2223
Government Building
Suva
Fiji

Ms Dontor Orkhon
Head
Division for Economics and
    Technology
Ministry of Health and Social
    Welfare
Ulaanbaatar
Mongolia

Kai-Hong Phua
Associate Professor and Head
Health Services Research
Department of Community,
    Occupational and Family
    Medicine
National University of Singapore
Faculty of Medicine
MD 3, 16 Medical Drive
Singapore 117597

Consultant

Dr Maria Cristina Bautista
Associate Professor
Ateneo de Manila University
Loyola Heights
Quezon City
Metro Manila
Philippines

Observers

Mr Tony Kingdon
Assistant Secretary
Policy and International Branch
Department of Health and
    Aged Care
Canberra, A.C.T. 2601
Australia

Mr Il Hoon Park
Administrative Officer
International Cooperation
    Division
Ministry of Health and Welfare
1, Joongang-Dong
Kwacheon City
Republic of Korea

WHO Secretariat

Dr Christopher J.L. Murray
Executive Director
Evidence and Information for
    Policy

Mr Orvill B. Adams
Evidence and Information for
    Policy

Dr Jie Chen
Special Representative of the
    Director-General

Dr Tessa Tan-Torres Edejer
Evidence and Information for
    Policy

Dr Ke Xu
Evidence and Information
    for Policy

Dr Alan D. Lopez
Evidence and Information for
    Policy

WHO/WPRO

Dr Aviva Ron
Director
Division of Health Sector
    Development

Dr Soe Nyunt-U
Scientist
Situation Analysis for Policy
Division of Health Sector
    Development

Yok-Ching Chong
Regional Adviser in Health
    Information
Division Health Sector
    Development

Dr Graham Harrison
Regional Adviser in Health
    Services
Division of Health Sector
    Development

ANNEX 7.2
REGIONAL DIRECTOR'S OPENING REMARKS AT THE REGIONAL CONSULTATION ON HEALTH SYSTEMS PERFORMANCE ASSESSMENT

Ladies and Gentlemen: a very good morning to you all, welcome to Manila and the Western Pacific Regional Office.

The World Health Report 2000 has brought health systems performance assessment to the forefront of the international health agenda. It has elicited great interest and debate among various stakeholders, within countries and among international organizations and institutions. The resolution taken during the 107th Session of the Executive Board of the World Health Organization called for this regional consultation to be held to enable WHO to assist countries in conducting health systems performance assessment on a regular basis within the spirit of understanding the goals and functions of health systems and the need for assessment of their performance.

The discussions in the next three days will be very critical in furthering the processes and tools for health sector performance assessment. Through various discussion sessions in this consultation, we will have the opportunity to voice our concerns about methodologies on one hand and linkages between assessment and policy on the other. This will provide the Member States with the best opportunity to influence the future framework and methodology of subsequent WHO work in this area.

You are probably all confronted by the complexity of the policy issues in the health sector in your day-to-day work in ministries of health or in other health sector endeavours. We all know that global solutions and prescriptions are likely to be altered when confronted by the realities and constraints of our different country settings. Living with these constraints is one thing, overcoming them and moving on to a better health system and better health status is another matter. To enable WHO to assist countries in the Region in making better policies that meet their health system goals, we invite you to participate fully in the discussions. The collective wisdom and experience in this room represents a good cross-section of the health system performance spectrum. I very much hope that you will provide comments from the perspective of your governments, and in addition, give us your comments as individuals with experience in health systems.

In the next two days and a half, we look forward to more intercountry sharing of experiences in health sector review and assessment, and to openness and reasoned debate on the matter. We will particularly appreciate your views on how the assessment can best serve you in policy development, implementation and monitoring to bring about the improvements you seek. With this encouragement to all our participants, I would like to declare this regional consultation meeting in session. I wish you all productive and frank discussions on the relevant aspects of the very important task of health systems performance assessment. I look forward to hearing your conclusions on Thursday. I also look forward to achieving a report of this regional consultation, which will provide very important input to the process of consultation outlined in the Executive Board Resolution.

Part III

EXPERT CONSULTATION REPORTS

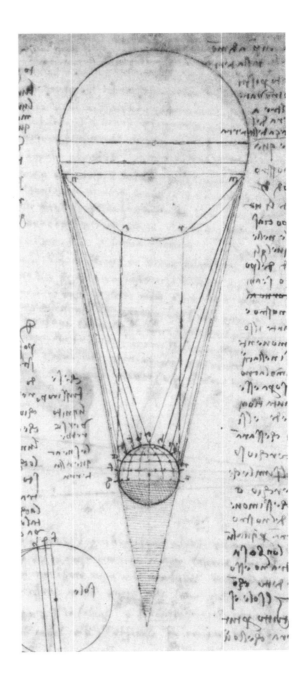

Chapter 8

Technical Consultation on Measurement of the Efficiency of Health Systems[1]

Introduction

This report is a summary of the major conclusions and recommendations of a meeting of experts on efficiency measurement organized by WHO and held in New Orleans, USA, on Monday, 8 January 2001. To maximize the potential participation of internationally renowned experts, the meeting was added at the end of the annual meetings of the American Economic Association. In addition to the three WHO staff members, the participants included major world experts on the measurement of economic efficiency. None had been involved in the preparation of *The World Health Report 2000* and the associated performance (efficiency) rankings. A list of participants and their affiliations, as well as the details of the agenda, can be found in Annex 8.1. The Rapporteur was Dr K. Kalirajan from the Australian National University who has published and consulted widely in this area.

Objectives and Agenda

There were two objectives of the meeting. The first was to collect the opinions of a group of recognized international experts on the approach taken by WHO to measure the efficiency of health systems. The second was to obtain their advice and suggestions on ways this work could develop in the future.

The meeting began with an outline by Dr Kalirajan of the recent developments in the estimation of economic efficiency, particularly those using frontier production technology. It was followed by a presentation of the work WHO has undertaken to measure and explain the performance of health systems, both for *The World Health Report 2000* and subsequently. Afterwards, three of the world's top experts (Profes-

sors William Greene, Subal Kumbhakar and C. A. Knox Lovell) responded formally to WHO's work taking into account the recent developments discussed earlier. Marijn Verhoeven presented an outline of the IMF's work in this area and its current plans. The rest of the agenda involved an open discussion by all participants of the WHO approach and the ways in which it could be developed in the future.

Main Conclusions and Recommendations

This section summarizes the conclusions for which there was general agreement.

On Frontier Production Functions

Appropriateness

There was general agreement that the frontier approach was an appropriate technique for measuring the efficiency of health systems. It has not been used widely in the health sector, apart from assessing the efficiency of hospitals, because economists have been uncertain about how to measure the outputs of the health sector and what the appropriate inputs to the production process are. Not only was it decided to be technically appropriate, but the participants were enthusiastic about the potential of the technique to address important practical policy questions, which would make a difference in the lives of many people.

Stochastic versus Deterministic Frontiers

There was a general consensus that given the nature of the data, stochastic frontier methods like those used by WHO were preferable to deterministic frontier methods for assessing health systems efficiency. The reason for this is that deterministic frontiers attribute all of the deviation from the frontier to inefficiency, whereas stochastic frontiers allow for the possibility that deviations from the frontier may also be due to random unobserved factors and measurement problems.

Estimating Efficiency for All Countries Together or for Subgroups of Countries

WHO had estimated efficiency for all countries together. The assumption was that the technologies available to all countries to improve health were the same and that the main limiting factor to their use was the availability of resources. Moreover, the appropriateness of the technologies does not differ by setting, i.e. the technology which provides the greatest possible benefit at the individual level in the treatment of cancer would be considered the best in all settings. If these arguments are accepted, the efficiency scores for all countries could be estimated together and there is no need to estimate them for subgroups of countries separately. This question was discussed extensively. Similar assumptions are unusual in the wider economic literature where the appropriateness of technologies differs across settings. It was agreed that the biological similarities between people mean that the assumption is appropriate to health and that resource availability is the major inhibitor of use. However, it was also suggested that there was value in estimating frontiers separately for selected subgroups of countries to check if the rankings of countries within the subgroups were consistent with the full ranking from the combined analysis.

Fixed-Effects Model

WHO estimated efficiency using a fixed-effects model based on panel data from 1993–1997. This was based on the strong recommendation of some of the published literature for estimation of frontiers using panel data. Take the function,

$$Y_{it} = \alpha + X'_{it}\beta + v_{it} - u_i \ ,$$

where X_{it} is a vector of inputs and v_{it} is the error term with mean zero. The term $u_i \geq 0$ is a random variable representing country-specific technical inefficiency. For the fixed effects model, this can be rewritten as:

$$Y_{it} = \alpha_i + X'_{it}\beta + v_{it} \ ,$$

where the new intercept $\alpha_i = (\alpha - u_i)$ is country-specific. The frontier intercept is represented by α and the u_i's are the country-specific inefficiencies. In order to ensure that all the estimated ui's are positive, the country with the maximum α_i is assumed to be the reference and is deemed fully efficient. Mathematically:

$$\hat{\alpha} = \max(\alpha_i)$$

and

$$\hat{u}_i = \alpha - \alpha_i \ .$$

This normalization ensures non-negative u_i's. Technical efficiency is defined as:

$$TE_i = \frac{E(Y_{it} \mid u_i, X_{it})}{E(Y_{it} \mid u_i = 0, X_{it})} \ .$$

In order to allow for the fact that health outcomes would not be zero in the absence of any factor of production, unlike in other sectors, WHO modified this equation by subtracting out the predicted minimum level of Y_{it} (denoted by M_{it}) from the numerator and denominator. Overall efficiency or E_i, is now:

$$E_i = \frac{E(Y_{it} \mid u_i, X_{it}) - M_{it}}{E(Y_{it} \mid u_i = 0, X_{it}) - M_{it}} \ .$$

This formulation is easy to estimate using standard statistical packages.

The experts pointed out that one possible problem with the fixed-effects approach is that the country-specific fixed effect might also include the influence of unmeasured determinants and not just efficiency. If there were missing explanatory variables, the form could overestimate the inefficiencies. On the other hand, if explanatory variables were included that were highly correlated with those already in the equation, the approach might well underestimate inefficiencies. (The question of which explanatory variables to include is discussed below.)

The meeting also suggested that a number of recent variations could be explored in the future. Professor Greene described how variable coefficient models have been developed that would allow greater flexibility in specifying the efficiency in a production function approach. One application would permit the error component associated with efficiency to be estimated as a random variable. An alternative form of the general approach described by Professor Green is the random coefficients model of the frontier itself, which has been developed by Dr Kalirajan.

Functional Form

It was suggested that there should be a formal test of whether regularity conditions for the translog form used by WHO are satisfied. Also, a test of the functional form across subsamples would be useful. This would entail a test to see if the estimated parameters of the translog function were the same for different subsamples of countries. Another possibility was to use "grade of membership" type models to subdivide the sample into subgroups for this testing. These models allow for endogenous determination of sample subgroups.

THE CHOICE OF INPUTS

Factors of Production

The choice of what variables should be included as inputs to the production process was discussed. WHO made a distinction based on the literature, between variables that were truly factors of production and those that might explain observed efficiencies. It used health expenditure per capita as the summary indicator of health system inputs and the average years of schooling of the adult population as the indicator of non-health system inputs to the production of health system outcomes. The group agreed that this distinction was appropriate. Only variables that are direct factors of production (such as labour and capital inputs in traditional economics) should theoretically go into the estimation of efficiency of the production process. Variables that might explain observed differences in efficiency should not be used as factors of production, but efficiency itself should be modelled as a function of those variables and kept separate from the factors of production. How this should be done is described later.

Given the availability of data across a large number of countries, the experts were of the opinion that health expenditure per capita was an appropriate way to summarize health sector inputs, while average years of schooling was also appropriate for non-health system inputs. Education could be considered a direct factor of production in the sense of available knowledge, or a proxy for other inputs, such as housing and nutrition, where data are not yet available for all countries and which would be highly correlated with it. Certainly, it would be preferable to measure

these other determinants directly, but it is not clear if they could be included if they are already very highly correlated with the existing factors of production. As mentioned earlier, this would lead to econometric problems with estimation.

Income per Capita

WHO explained that there is an extensive literature suggesting that major health improvements this century were highly correlated with improvements in the income per capita. This had led some experts to the conclusion that increases in income per capita should be included as a factor of production. An extreme form of this argument is that income per capita is the only determinant of health levels and that the health system has no impact on health. This can be shown to be incorrect in many ways, including the fact that the Preston curves, which plot income per capita against health outcomes in a given year, have moved up over the century, implying that there must be other factors influencing the health improvements.

These questions were discussed in relation to the need to keep the factors of production separate from possible correlates with efficiency. It was agreed that money by itself did not produce health. It is what the income purchases, for example food and housing, that produces health. Therefore, it is not theoretically correct to include income as a factor of production. If data were available, perhaps food (or nutritional intake) and housing could be used as factors of production. However, such data are not available for most countries. The group decided that the appropriate way to introduce income and a number of other variables such as geography, political institutions and so on, was as explanators of efficiency and not as factors of production.

Incorporating Factors Correlated with Efficiency

There are two ways to do this. WHO used a two-stage process described in the literature, in which efficiency scores were estimated from the production functions first. Subsequently, the estimated efficiencies were regressed on possible determinants. The participants recommended that the explanation of efficiency could be improved using the same maximum likelihood estimation process as used for the production function. In it, the component of the error term considered to be inefficiency is made a function of the possible correlates. This would be better econometrically than the method used by WHO and in this way income per capita could possibly be introduced. The new variable coefficients technology could also be used at this stage. None of the experts was certain about whether this would make a difference to the results obtained by WHO.

UNCERTAINTY ANALYSIS

The approach to uncertainty analysis used in the WHO report was considered novel and did not have theoretical problems. However, it was noted that information on the higher moments of the estimated outcome data (e.g. not just the mean and standard errors) had not been used and could probably be incorporated into the analysis. It was not possible to say at the meeting how this could be achieved as considerable work would be required to sort out the technical details of the process.

SMALL-AREA ANALYSIS

The experts were asked if they saw any theoretical problems of including subnational units in the estimation of the frontier. The rationale stated by WHO was that national efficiency is probably an average of different levels of efficiency achieved by subnational units, such as states or provinces. If data were available at this level, it would allow a better estimation of the "true" frontier. The experts did not see econometric or theoretical problems with this, but observed that the data quality at the subnational level was often lower than at the national level, and sometimes definitions used for variables differed across these units.

OTHER DISCUSSIONS

This section summarizes the discussions for which there was no general agreement or conclusion.

MIMIC MODELS

There was some discussion about whether the estimated efficiency scores could be incorporated into multiple-indicator-multiple-causes (MIMIC) type models, along with other possible factors believed to be indicators of efficiency, such as vaccine coverage rates, access, etc. A MIMIC type model would treat efficiency like an unobserved latent variable. One formulation of such a framework would model this latent efficiency variable as a function of observable exogenous determinants, as well as model the efficiency as a determinant of several observable effects (or indicators) of efficiency. There was no general agreement.

However, it was agreed that it would be useful to test if some of these other variables were correlated with the WHO efficiency scores.

PREFERENCE WEIGHTS

To construct the overall attainment index, WHO used fixed weights for all countries for the five indicators of system attainment. These weights were estimated from the responses given by a sample of people from many different countries and they represent the weights that people felt should be guiding policy. There was some discussion about whether these weights would vary across settings and cultures. It was agreed that this was an empirical question. WHO's best evidence at the moment was that they did not, but the large sample surveys now underway would provide updated information.

The experts pointed out that it was also possible to determine the weights, which were apparently used to guide policy in each country using data envelopment analysis (DEA) on the composite index. It is not clear if policy-makers really had those weights or if they had other preferences but were unable to achieve them. In any case, it would be possible to see if these implicit weights differed from the ones used by WHO. If so, the weights implied for each country could be used to recalculate attainment and the efficiency scores. These could be called "benefit of the doubt" efficiency scores: that is, the efficiency given the weights that appeared to be driving the country's policy rather than the weights that people think should be guiding policy.

As a technical nicety, constrained DEA would be preferable to unconstrained DEA, partly because it would be much easier for the programs to solve the algorithm. The other reason is that there is prior knowledge at least of the range into which the weights must fall. For example, it is not possible that the weight for health level is zero. In fact, it is unlikely that the weight for any specific component is zero. A way of setting the constraints would be to use surveys for eliciting preferences (as done by WHO), but to constrain the weights in the revealed preference analysis to be plus or minus x standard deviations from the mean of the surveys.

If the two sets of efficiency scores differ, it is not clear which one is more appropriate. This decision depends on the judgement about whether the people's or the policy-makers' expressed preferences should guide policy. It would be technically possible for WHO to provide the two types of efficiency estimates.

Minimum Frontier

The experts were not enthusiastic about the current method for estimating the minimum, but could not suggest an alternative given the data available. It was disputed whether the minimum really added anything to the analysis and it was suggested that the minimum adjustment could be made to the dependent and independent variables before doing the efficiency estimation rather than after, as in the WHO approach.

Notes

1 New Orleans, USA, 8 January 2001

ANNEX 8.1
AGENDA

9:00–9:30	Overview of Recent Developments for Measuring Efficiency [K. Kalirajan (Rapporteur), Australian National University]	
9:30–10:30	WHO's Measurement of Efficiency of Health Systems [C.J.L. Murray, D.B. Evans, A. Tandon, World Health Organization]	
10:30–11:00	Coffee Break	
11:00–11:45	Measuring Health System Efficiency Lead Discussants: S. Kumbhaker, University of Texas W. Greene, New York University	C.A. Knox Lovell, University of Georgia
11:45–12:30	General Discussion and Reactions	
12:30–2:00	Lunch Break	
2:00–2:45	Other Applications of Frontier Production Functions to Health [M. Verhoeven, International Monetary Fund]	
2:45–3:30	General Discussion	
3:30–4:00	Coffee Break	
4:00–5:00	Future Work on Efficiency of Health Systems	

LIST OF PARTICIPANTS

Prof. William Greene
Department of Economics
Stern School of Business
New York University
New York, NY 10012
USA

Prof. Subal Kumbhakar
Department of Economics
University of Texas
Austin, TX 78712
USA

Prof. C.A. Knox Lovell
Department of Economics
University of Georgia
Athens, GA 30602
USA

Prof. Kaliappa Kalirajan
Division of Economics
Research School of Pacific and
 Asian Studies
Australian National University
Canberra, ACT 0200
Australia

Marijn Verhoeven
International Monetary Fund
Washington, DC 20431
USA

Prof. Paul Wilson
Department of Economics
University of Texas
Austin, TX 78712
USA

Prof. Christopher Tong
Department of Economics
Hong Kong Baptist University
Hong Kong, SAR
China

Prof. Philip Grossman
Department of Economics
St Cloud State University
St Cloud, MN 56301
USA

* Accepted the invitation, but could
not attend at the last minute.

Prof. Jaume Puig-Junoy*
Research Centre for Health and
 Economics
Pompeu Fabra University
Barcelona
Spain

Dr Christopher J.L. Murray
Executive Director
Evidence and Information
 for Policy
World Health Organization
Geneva
Switzerland

Dr David B. Evans
Evidence and Information for
 Policy
World Health Organization
Geneva
Switzerland

Dr Ajay Tandon
Evidence and Information for
 Policy
World Health Organization
Geneva
Switzerland

Chapter 9

TECHNICAL CONSULTATION ON CONCEPTS AND METHODS FOR MEASURING THE RESPONSIVENESS OF HEALTH SYSTEMS[1]

INTRODUCTION

This report is a summary of the major comments and findings of a meeting of experts on responsiveness and related subjects held at WHO in Geneva, 13–14 September 2001. Careful planning preceded the consultation. In May 2001, WHO held a planning meeting to identify the criteria for the selection of respondents and to outline the consultation goals. The list of the technical consultation participants and the agenda are shown in Annex 9.1.

OBJECTIVES AND AGENDA

The main objective of the meeting was to canvass the experts' opinions on the concepts and measurement strategy proposed by WHO. These were described in the background reading materials sent to the participants before the consultation. The principal elements discussed in the above-mentioned materials were revisited in presentations prior to the discussions. This report is structured around the key topic areas and does not follow the chronological order of the agenda. The six major topic groupings are: conceptual issues, surveys, questionnaire, vignettes, other issues and future research.

MAIN CONCLUSIONS AND RECOMMENDATIONS

This section summarizes the key issues raised at the technical consultation. A detailed report of the technical consultation was sent to the participants immediately afterwards for comments and this document represents a summary of the main conclusions and recommendations, taking into account all comments received.

CONCEPTUAL ISSUES

Terminology and Definitions

As this is a new area, the domains and their definitions are still evolving. Several suggestions were made. It is clear that if terminology, such as that of the ethics or human rights literature, already exists, it should be applied wherever feasible. Otherwise, each concept should be formally defined and used consistently. This would be separate from the description of their characteristics for purposes of operationalization. Particularly relevant would be the terminology already existing in the human rights convention, which the majority of the Member States have ratified, such as rights to privacy, information, participation and non-discrimination.

Operationalizing Domains

It was suggested that a matrix be developed to organize the thinking around the items in a domain. It could be possible to identify operationable items at macro, meso and micro levels. For example, in the context of autonomy one can identify the involvement in decision-making regarding what health services are offered or how they are run as an item in this domain. This would be a "macro-level" item, whereas making a decision about the type of treatment would be a more micro-level type of involvement. For policy relevance, it was considered necessary that larger policy decisions in health systems, which may affect responsiveness, be looked into using this approach.

Elements within Specific Domains

Autonomy. The scope of this domain was much debated. One suggestion was to include the concept of "enablement" (empowerment) and self–care in autonomy. A second issue was whether the involvement of the community in resource decision-making should somehow be captured in this or another domain. Other issues were to include reference to information provided, as well as permission sought, under the notion of "informed consent" in autonomy. Parts of the discussion focused on individual autonomy versus the public good. Here the principles of limiting versus violating rights as applied in the field of human rights were discussed.

Communication. It was agreed to include "information on a healthy life style" as part of autonomy.

Social Support Networks. It was agreed that the present definition of social support networks needed to be expanded to include support for those under home care, community support and support to the family of the patients. This expanded definition would need a new title to include the notion of "family/community involvement" to avoid the sensitivity of using the term "support" in some cultures with the possible implication of interfering with social security activities.

Confidentiality. The right to privacy is an important human right. Unnoticed breaches of confidentiality need to be considered. These include access to one's own records under confidentiality. However, confidentiality is not a total control over one's personal information (for example, cases of child molesters where different social institutions are alerted of past offenders).

Prompt Attention. It was agreed that the definition of prompt attention should be expanded to include questions on how quickly people received routine care. Currently there is no distinction between the different types of care for which one could wait. Perhaps a distinction between emergency and non-emergency care could be introduced.

Dignity. It was agreed that the term "respect," which is currently used in some questions on dignity in the survey instrument should be applied to all questions in the English version. It is a clearer term for people to understand. For translation into different languages the most appropriate term would have to be found.

Non-discrimination was seen as an integral part of being treated with dignity.

Choice. It was agreed that the concept of choice requires further exploration. A lot of the participants shared the view that constraints arising from geographic access should be explored alongside the financial access ones.

Quality of Basic Amenities. There was a debate about whether this should be a domain because it might not be a priority of some governments given other more pressing concerns, such as staff availability. It was agreed that the quality of basic amenities is always a component of responsiveness, regardless of the circumstances, although its weight might differ according to the setting. After measuring this domain, governments can decide what policy actions to take depending on their priorities.

Distribution of Responsiveness

It was clear in the discussions that this was the most undeveloped area in the responsiveness work. In its measurement, WHO is trying to capture the degree of inequality existing in each country and in each domain based on the calibrated responses. Suggestions were received about ways to test whether discrimination is the cause of the observed inequalities in responsiveness by using population subgroups identified in the human rights literature, including age and sex groups.

Universally Legitimate Expectations

A concern was expressed that legitimate standards had to be agreed upon. It was explained that WHO's approach to establishing the norm is to let the overall preference of the respondents settle the range of processes or behaviours expected from the health system.

Responsiveness vs. Satisfaction

It was clarified that although the responsiveness work stems from the patient satisfaction literature, there is a clear distinction. Responsiveness measures what actually happens to people when they come in contact with the system rather than how satisfied they are or their opinions about their experiences. In some circumstances, it is conceivable that system responsiveness may actually lead to individual dissatisfaction.

MEASURING RESPONSIVENESS: THE SURVEY PROCESS

Sampling

All participants agreed on the importance of ensuring representative sampling when measuring responsiveness. A range of suggestions was made regarding the selection of respondents.

Capturing the Experiences of Children. The use of age 18 as the cut-off point was viewed as a problem. It was pointed out that the Convention on the Rights of the Child mandates the state parties to endorse children who are capable of having opinions of their own to be allowed to speak for themselves. This suggests a cut-off age of 12 or 14.

Including an Assessment of the Experiences of Non-Users of Personal Health Services. The inclusion of the non-users of personal health care services in the survey was considered important. In fact, 50% of the respondents from the first round of surveys in the WHO Multicountry Survey Study were non-users. Suggestions on ways to do this included interviewing them on possible reasons for non-use, which are related to responsiveness, and also on the non-personal health interventions, which benefit them. A last resort would be a more open opinion survey of non-users, but given that many reasons for non-use are unrelated to responsiveness, this would not be a particularly good way to analyse health system responsiveness.

Implementation Issues: Survey Modes

Exit Surveys. The advantage of exit surveys is that they are cheaper than household surveys, relative to the amount of data collected. However, the reporting of experience may be biased because the respondents are sensitive to the fact that they are still on the premises and they target only users of the service. Exit surveys may be particularly useful for special marginalized groups that are under-represented in a household survey, such as people who are HIV positive, those with tuberculosis, migrant workers and hill tribes.

Key Informant Surveys and Household Surveys. Responses from these different survey modes need to be compared. This process has already begun. Key informants may be able to provide information on some parts of health system responsiveness for which households are poorer informants, e.g. the confidentiality of medical records.

Subnational Survey Tools and Ensuring Policy Relevance. The need to develop practical subnational level survey tools that are relevant to both subnational and national policy-making was underlined.

Questionnaire: Content

Prevention, Promotion and "Response to Emergency" Care. It was agreed that prevention and health promotion aspects need to be included in as many of the domains as feasible. It was pointed out that while some aspects of prevention are not directly experienced by the individual and are difficult to capture in questionnaires, others, such as communication of health promotion messages could be included. Questions could be asked on the kind of advice given on smoking or HIV, for example, "Did you get information?", "Was it relevant?" and "Was it useful?"

The Inpatient-Outpatient Distinction. The discussion on whether this distinction was necessary revealed a range of opinions. The debate centred on the objectives of such disaggregation: for bench-marking or for policy formulation? It was suggested that for bench-marking it would be sufficient to consider hospital care in general, doing further disaggregation only if the findings were used for policy analysis. However, analyses of the first round of surveys suggest that there are significant differences between in and outpatient experiences. At the other end of the spectrum, there were suggestions about adding more inpatient questions connected to the different domains and formulating questions to relate to the various stages of hospitalization. Because only around 10% of the people surveyed in the Multicountry Survey Study population samples have had an inpatient experience in the past year, the number of observations of inpatient care was small. For this reason, a recall period of 2–5 years was considered more appropriate for inpatient care than 1 year. It would increase the number of observations and people are likely to remember inpatient experiences for much longer than outpatient contacts.

Questions to Increase the Analytic Scope or Precision. The range of suggestions included requesting information on: whether the institution named the "usual place of care" is public or private; the main reason for the visit (including whether it is a visit related to pregnancy or a need for contraception); introducing a wider range of examples of barriers to seeking care in addition to the financial barrier.

Questionnaire: Format and Wording

The Length and Complexity of Questions and Their Wording. Several approaches were suggested to address this issue. The simplest was to have the questionnaire edited by a non-health specialist, ensuring that standard dictionary definitions are used and that words open to various interpretations (such as "frequent" or "rare") are defined. Another suggestion was to use software that predicts the reading age of the respondents. Work to further clarify concepts and greater precision in domain titles will also help.

Translation. Attention was drawn to the need to use locally appropriate words, even where the basic language is the same.

Making the Questionnaire Easier to Follow. One suggestion was to include "don't know" and "no response" categories to avoid confusion. A second was to formulate questions in all domains using the continuum "never-to-always."

Questionnaire Length. It was observed that long questionnaires could have difficulty in obtaining ethical clearance and that the questionnaire would need to be shortened. WHO reported that one of the research strategy aims was to develop a short instrument, which could be incorporated easily as a module in other surveys run by countries.

Response Scales. Some of the survey specialists indicated that it would be useful to review how the use of scale has affected responses.

Questionnaire: Interpretation and Analysis

Specific comments were made on the uses of quantitative and cognitive testing to ascertain whether the wording problems were affecting the scores; how separate different domains are; how well respondents understand the complexly worded questions. Second, it was suggested that an analysis be developed on how the level of health system resources affects responsiveness. A question was raised about whether individual responses of experience could be aggregated to gain a health system rating.

VIGNETTES

A wide number of useful suggestions were received about ways to improve the responsiveness vignettes.

Vignette Formulation

The survey instrument asked the respondents to rate their last contact with the health system on the different domains of responsiveness. They were offered five possible response categories: very good, good, moderate, bad and very bad. For any given level in a domain, e.g. for autonomy, people categorize their experiences in different ways, with consistent variation observed by age, sex and country of residence, for example. This implies that their cut-points between the possible categorical responses differ. To establish how individuals use the categorical responses of "very good" to "very bad," a series of vignettes were devised for each domain covering the entire range of the latent or unobserved variable. For each vignette, respondents were asked to rate the experience described into the different categories of response. The responses on the set of vignettes for each domain could then be analysed to identify how cut-points on the latent scale systematically vary across individuals and communities. This information allows a more meaningful interpretation of each individual's responses for his or her own encounter with the health system.

In addition to the general recommendations about simplicity, brevity and care with translation of words in the vignettes, there was much discussion about how to adapt them to local situations and cultures, and how to make them less system-specific. The use of pictures and cartoons as a source of vignettes was suggested, as was having culturally equivalent substitutable phrases in some of them. It was pointed out that although local adaptation may affect cross-country comparability, it becomes necessary for even apparently simple phrases, such as "across the road" to suggest distance because roads differ in width between villages and towns. Where possible, generic terms, such as "greeted with affection," "spoken to with respect" should be used rather than describing specific gestures that are culturally sensitive, such as "shaking hands." With regard to wording, using a term like "your friend" is likely to be better than a hypothetical name or referring to a relative: the former distances the issue, while the latter may be culturally sensitive.

Content

As with the main questionnaire, several comments on missing elements and potentially misleading wording were made. For example, dignity vignettes mainly cover the issue of politeness and they all refer to actions of nurses alone. The disease mentioned in the vignette may influence the rating given and respondents may be more sympathetic to certain types of diseases. It may therefore be important to keep the "illness" constant. Some vignettes mix domains and this should be avoided. Problems like alcoholism and homelessness should not appear within the vignette, as these problems have stigma attached to them.

Other Steps to Improve Vignettes

Suggestions included: providing an explanation of their purpose at the beginning of the section; reducing the number of vignettes per domain if possible; using an educational expert to improve the presentation of the vignettes; switching the score order to have very good as five with very bad as one; having a visual scale shown to the respondent.

Different views on how to address cultural sensitivity were shared. One was to create a database of key words/key phrases to capture this (i.e. shake hands/kiss the cheek/hug) and system characteristics (hospital/health unit/clinic). Another was to avoid culturally specific references altogether.

Testing of Vignettes

Discussions about how to validate the relationship between self-report and vignettes resulted in a number of proposals:

- Structure the questionnaire so that self-reports are followed by vignettes, then followed again by self-reports to see if the self-report scores vary. This would suggest that the vignettes are making the individual take a wider or different perspective of the domains. Another suggestion was to ask individuals to paraphrase vignettes.

- Split vignette results by age to see if the difference that generally exists between young and old on self-reports is replicated.

- Examine whether high experience scores relate in any way to vignette scores.

- See whether there is a pattern in rating vignettes, i.e. if there are consistently harsh and mild raters.

- Observe whether any respondents in a country or population answer using the categories of "very good" or "very bad," as both extremes may be culturally unacceptable.

- Conduct standard psychometric tests on the vignettes, e.g. aiming for Kappa above 0.6.

- Use factor analysis to see if vignettes are loading appropriately.

- Perform more cognitive testing of vignettes (on a larger scale than previously).

- Decide on whether a rating of 1 to 5 is more desirable than the categorical variables ranging from "very good" to "very bad."

SUMMARY OF RECOMMENDATIONS ON FUTURE RESEARCH AND OTHER ACTIVITIES

CONCEPTUAL AND ANALYTIC WORK

- Improving the formal and operational definitions of domains is necessary. Further conceptualization of domains involving more in-depth analysis of the different domains to capture issues, such as cultural sensitivity, is necessary. Also, more work on responsiveness distribution focusing on defining different disadvantaged groups is needed.

- Analyses of responsiveness in the context of self-care and home care would be useful.

- Patient narratives, which provide insight into personal experiences, would be helpful in the further study of domains.

- Documenting the benefits to the country from the measurement of responsiveness would be useful.

- Involving the media and accreditation institutions for improving the awareness of responsiveness would be helpful.

SURVEY WORK

- In terms of instrument development, the following were recommended: thorough comparisons of the different modes of household surveys (face/postal, short/long versions) and between household and key informant surveys; development of methods for harmonizing the results gained through different modes, different sampling methods, and different sampling levels (national, state, provincial); developing in the future a survey instrument for institutional dwellers; analyses of non-users to gain an understanding of their characteristics.

- Additional sorts of surveys were suggested for particular purposes: running parallel surveys for youth and children; testing and developing the facility survey; using key informant surveys (perhaps using a pre-selected panel of key informants) to gain views on the aspects of public health that households may not experience, such as whether their patient records are made available to researchers. For example, conducting panel surveys, coverage of services could be usefully addressed in a module on service provision.

- The need to develop the survey module in such a way that it can be annexed to existing surveys was emphasized.

- It was recommended that a comprehensive data collection strategy be considered, involving providers and consumers through household, exit and facility surveys.

- An instruction pack for countries, explaining how to carry out surveys and training, as well as how to analyse results, is needed.

LINKING TO POLICY

There was an agreement on the need to share with the Member States the new data analysis methods developed for ensuring cross-population comparability of results. Issues and suggestions about ways to increase the government's role in measuring and improving responsiveness, and ways to communicate the findings to policy-makers, providers and consumers included:

- The value of involving providers in the entire discussion of responsiveness, not only the measurement step through surveys. This will raise awareness of and commitment to the new concepts and practices.

- Developing appropriate "reporting systems" to share findings with facilities and consumers.

- Undertaking analytical work on the sorts of incentives that lead to improved responsiveness. This would include looking at regulatory frameworks to investigate whether the existence of patients' rights and charters improves responsiveness, as well as studying the effect of legislation related to responsiveness issues.

NOTES

1 Geneva, Switzerland, 13–14 September 2001

ANNEX 9.1

AGENDA

13 SEPTEMBER 2001

Theme A: Responsiveness Concepts

8:30–8:40	Welcome [Christopher J.L. Murray]
8:40–8:55	Objectives of the Meeting [Kei Kawabata]
8:55–9:55	Responsiveness Concepts and Discussion [Amala de Silva]
	Discussion: What Is Our Understanding of Responsiveness
	Concepts, Problems with Them, Overlaps and Missing Dimensions
	Chair: Pedro Ferreira
9:55–10:20	Responsiveness Roots in Ethics [Reidar Lie]
10:20–10:30	Responsiveness Roots in Human Rights [Helena Nygren-Krug]
10:30–10:40	Summary of the Main Conceptual Issues
10:40–11:00	Tea Break

Theme B: Operationalizing Responsiveness

11:00–12:30	Results of WHO Responsiveness Surveys [Nicole B. Valentine]
	Discussion: What Are the Main Implications of the Results and the Remaining Challenges for Improving the Methods
	Chair: Leo Morales
12:30–13:45	Lunch Break
13:45–14:15	Responsiveness Items [Charles Darby]
14:15–15:30	Group Work A: What Items Best Exemplify the Responsiveness Domains and Are Most Cross-Culturally Applicable? What New Items Should Be Added? (Four Groups to Appoint Rapporteur to Report Back in Plenary)

15:30–16:00	Tea Break
16:00–17:00	Discussion and Summary of Findings in Plenary
	Chair: Sammy Gadalla
18:00–19:00	Reception in Cafeteria

14 SEPTEMBER 2001

Theme C: Use of Vignettes

8:45–9:15	Vignettes, Their Effectiveness and Proposed Strategies for Improvement [Nicole B. Valentine]
9:15–10:30	Group Work B: Go Through Sample of Vignettes and Self-Report Questions. What Works, Why and What Does Not and Why?
	(Four Groups to Appoint Rapporteur to Report Back in Plenary)
10:30–10:50	Tea Break
10:50–11:15	Discussion and Summary of Findings in Plenary
	Chair: Luis Justo

Theme D: Framing and Sampling

11:15–11:45	Introductory Questions: Different Options and Challenges [Angela Coulter]
11:45–13:00	Group Work C: What Is the Best Way to Introduce the Questionnaire to the Respondent in a Household Survey and What Sampling Biases Do We Need to be Aware of in Different Settings (e.g. Minorities, Institutionalized, Non-Users)
13:00–14:00	Lunch Break
14:00–14:45	Presentation and Discussion of Findings in Plenary
	Chair: T. Bedirhan Üstün

Theme E: Use of Data and Further Research

14:45–15:30	Discussion of Ways of Making Responsiveness Information Useful in Countries [Viroj Tangcharoensathien]

15:30–16:00	Tea Break
16:00–16:45	Discussion of Future Research Agenda Priorities:
	Chair: Abdelhay Mechbal
16:45–17:00	Summary and Closure of Meeting [Christopher J.L. Murray]

GROUP FACILITATORS AND NOTE-TAKERS

Group 1: Amala de Silva and Helena Nygren-Krug

Group 2: Charles Darby and Hedwig Goede

Group 3: Angela Coulter and Kei Kawabata

Group 4: Sammy Gadalla, Juan Pablo Ortiz and Jane Cottingham

Overall Conference Note-Taker: Amala de Silva

MATERIALS FOR THE PARTICIPANTS

Note on Description of Main Issues and Challenges with Annex Listing Revised Definitions

de Silva A, Murray CJL. *A framework for measuring responsiveness*. EIP Discussion Paper No. 32. Geneva, World Health Organization, 2000. (Original Conceptual Paper) URL:http://www3.who.int/ whosis/discussion_papers/discussion_papers.cfm#

Darby C et al. *World Health Organization (WHO): strategy on measuring responsiveness*. EIP Discussion Paper No. 23. Geneva, World Health Organization, 2000. URL: http://www3.who.int/ whosis/discussion_papers/discussion_papers.cfm#

LIST OF PARTICIPANTS

Dr John Campbell
GKT (Guy's King's and Thomas's) School of Medicine
Department of General Practice
5 Lambeth Walk
SE11 6 SP London
United Kingdom

Dr Angela Coulter
Picker Institute Europe
Oxpens Road
Oxford
OX1 1RX
United Kingdom

Charles Darby
Agency for Healthcare Research and Quality
6011 Executive Boulevard
Suite 200
Rockville, Maryland 20852
USA

Pedro Lopes Ferreira
Centro de Estudos e Investigação em Saúde
Faculdade de Economia
Universidade de Coimbra
Ave. Dias da Silva 165
3004-512 Coimbra
Portugal

Dr Samy Gadalla
Health Care International
35 Hadayek El Obour Bldgs.
Salah Salem Road
Cairo
Egypt

Dr Oyewusi Gureje
University of Ibadan
University College Hospital
PB 5116 Ibadan
Nigeria

Dr Maimunah A. Hamid
Health Systems Research Division
Ministry of Health
Malaysia
Jalan Bangsar
50590 Kuala Lumpur
Malaysia

Dr George van der Heide
Department of Health and Aged Care
Consumer Strategies Section
MDP 46
Canberra ACT 2601
Australia

Dr Luis F. Justo
Universidad Nacional del Comahue
Catamarca 140
(8324) Cipolletti
Rio Negro
Argentina

Prof. Reidar K. Lie
University of Bergen
N-5007 Bergen
Norway

Leo Morales
RAND/UCLA School of Medicine
10833 Le Conte Avenue
Room B-252 Factor Building
Box 951736
Los Angeles, CA 90095-1736
USA

Dr Fernando Muñoz
Centro Lationamericano de
   Investigación de Sistemas de
   Salud (CLAISS)
José Miguel de la Barra 412, Piso 3
Santiago
Chile

Dr Jamal Eddine Naji
57 Dufferin
H3X 2X8, Hampstead
Quebec
Canada

Dr Amala de Silva
Department of Economics
University of Colombo
Colombo
Sri Lanka

Dr Sukanto Sumodinoto
Health Technology and
   Information

Dr Agus Suwandono
Health Services Research and
   Development Center
JL. Percetakan Negara 23 A
10560 Jakarta
Indonesia

Dr Viroj Tangcharoensathien
Health Systems Research Institute
Ministry of Public Health
Nonthaburi 11000
Thailand

Dr David Whittaker
Health Services of Cape Town
5 Vale Road
7700 Rondebosch
South Africa

WHO Secretariat

Dr Christopher J.L. Murray
Executive Director
Evidence and Information
   for Policy

Dr Abdelhay Mechbal
Evidence and Information
   for Policy

Dr T. Bedirhan Üstün
Evidence and Information
   for Policy

Kei Kawabata
Evidence and Information
   for Policy

Nicole B. Valentine
Evidence and Information
   for Policy

Dr Hedwig Goede
Evidence and Information
   for Policy

Jane Cottingham
Technical Officer for Gender Issues

Helena Nygren-Krug
WHO Human Rights Research
   and Policy

Juan Pablo Ortiz
Evidence and Information
   for Policy

Richard Poe
Evidence and Information
   for Policy

Chapter 10

TECHNICAL CONSULTATION ON EFFECTIVE COVERAGE IN HEALTH SYSTEMS[1]

INTRODUCTION

A technical consultation on effective coverage in health systems was held in Rio de Janeiro, Brazil, from 27 to 29 August 2001. It was organized by the Cluster of Evidence and Information for Policy (EIP), WHO, in collaboration with the WHO Regional Office for the Americas and the Oswaldo Cruz Foundation, Brazil.

Thirty-five participants attended the meeting from the WHO regional offices, WHO headquarters, WHO Member States, various technical organizations and donor agencies. The participants were selected according to their practical experience in the field of health programme evaluation and monitoring, assessment of health service provision, health information systems, data collection and survey design.

The discussions focused on the following main themes:

■ Rationale for WHO's work on effective coverage.

■ Conceptual framework of measuring effective coverage.

■ Incorporation of equity dimension into the measurement of coverage.

■ Identification of interventions and indicators for the measurement of effective coverage.

■ Capacities of countries to carry out the measurement of effective coverage within the scope of their health information systems.

■ Approaches to improve data collection from private health care providers.

■ Future steps in the measurement of effective coverage.

RATIONALE FOR WHO'S WORK ON COVERAGE

At the regional consultations held since the 107th session of the Executive Board, it has been suggested that the assessment of effective coverage of a selected group of interventions be incorporated into the health systems performance assessment. Effective coverage does not measure the impact of a health intervention, which is often difficult to do, but does represent an intermediate step in achieving a health impact. Its usefulness as an intermediate goal lies in its direct link to the health system and in the fact that its measurement can reveal the impact of managerial practices and decision-making processes on the health service provision function at the local, regional and national levels.

WHO's work on effective coverage emphasizes scaling up international and country level responses to critical conditions that undermine people's well-being, with greater attention being given to the benefits of the investments made and to the distribution of those benefits among different socioeconomic groups. The work on effective coverage also supports WHO's current agenda for improving health systems performance:

■ Developing tools for evaluating health systems functions.

■ Focusing on the attainment of intermediate goals.

■ Making health systems performance measurement a tool for health planners and managers at the national and subnational levels.

■ Assisting countries in understanding the impact of their interventions on the population in most need.

■ Assisting countries in analysing and monitoring the performance of health care providers.

The participants stressed that WHO's work on the measurement of coverage must be consistent with the current assessment of health systems performance and complement and improve the information already collected by countries. Countries are finding the measurement of coverage useful and WHO needs to respond quickly to their interest.

Conceptual Framework for Measuring Effective Coverage

The principle background paper defined effective coverage as the proportion of the population in need of an intervention who have received an effective intervention. As a specific example, those considered to be effectively covered with a third dose of DTP (DTP-3) would have received three safe and correctly administered injections of a potent vaccine at the appropriate ages. The denominator of the percent effectively covered would be all children in the appropriate age group. It was stressed that the numerator of the coverage ratio should indicate the number of population units (individuals, houses, villages) receiving effective interventions, and the denominator should refer to the population that would need the type of services indicated in the numerator.

The background paper identified three main conceptual elements of effective coverage: access, utilization and effectiveness. Access was defined in terms of availability, accessibility, affordability and acceptability. Utilization was the combination of access and personal health behaviour. Effectiveness was considered a function of several variables, including efficacy, inputs (amount and quality of resources), quality assurance mechanisms (process of service delivery, provider performance), patient compliance and health behaviour, and external factors (environmental, biological, social, etc.).

The background paper distinguished effective coverage from the effectiveness of the intervention itself. For example, the effectiveness of DTP properly administered, is known to be high. However, unless the quality of the vaccine and the administration can be ensured, effective coverage with DTP even among those receiving the vaccine, might be low.

The participants suggested that the term *coverage with effective interventions* be used instead of *effective coverage*. They were of the opinion that *effective coverage* would best refer to the proportion of people for whom the health intervention had actually produced a desirable health outcome.

The background paper described five different aspects of coverage, which could be analysed in trying to determine where problems lay in achieving effective coverage. These are: availability coverage, accessibility coverage, acceptability coverage, contact coverage, and effective coverage.

Availability Coverage

- The proportion of people for whom sufficient resources and technologies have been made available.

- The ratio of resources to the total population in need.

- The proportion of facilities, which offer specific resources, drugs, technologies, etc.

Accessibility Coverage

- The proportion of people for whom health services are accessible in terms of their distance or travel time.

Acceptability Coverage

- The proportion of people for whom interventions are acceptable (cultural acceptability, beliefs, religion, gender, etc.).

- The proportion of people for whom health services are affordable.

Contact Coverage

- The proportion of the population that has contacted a health service provider.

Effective Coverage

- The proportion of the people who have received effective interventions.

The participants were in general agreement with this breakdown, but suggested that affordability be included as a separate domain, rather than as a dimension of acceptability coverage. It was also recommended that the role of the structural elements of health systems and their impact on coverage should be emphasized more. The importance of focusing on the health needs of the population and identifying them accurately was stressed as well, in order to select interventions appropriately and to avoid an excessively supply-oriented perspective of coverage.

While acknowledging the significance of measuring coverage with effective interventions as an intermediate goal of health systems, the participants also underlined the necessity of measuring the impact of those interventions.

INCORPORATION OF EQUITY DIMENSION INTO THE MEASUREMENT OF COVERAGE

The incorporation of an equity dimension into the measurement of coverage with effective interventions is necessary. It was suggested that the relationship between the asset and income distribution and the distribution of health services be further explored. The presentation of the World Bank (IBRD) demonstrated the relationship between the immunization coverage and the asset index in Tanzania and Malawi.

The IBRD's asset index approach to the study of equity in the distribution of health services employs the smallest feasible number of asset questions, which can be added to a household survey questionnaire. The index is applied to denominator data collected through a survey, and is used to divide a population into groups of equal size (for instance, quintiles) on the basis of wealth. The cut-off points for each group are established for each survey.

Some participants suggested that asset questions or some other variables associated with an individual's socioeconomic status be added to the clinical forms used for patients receiving certain interventions in facilities. Doing this for all patients could allow for constructing their socioeconomic profiles.

The participants discussed the issue of correlation between the asset index and income per capita. A concern was expressed that the asset index may not capture the socioeconomic differences in rich and middle-income countries, thereby limiting its applicability in the WHO methodology. In household surveys, the value given to certain assets by respondents of different social and cultural background would be different, therefore requiring calibration and adjustment of responses for better comparability. It was also mentioned that the use of quintiles for assessing economic status whether through income or asset index could be quite sensitive to the income distribution in the society, thus making discrete comparisons difficult. It was agreed that the issue of measuring the socioeconomic inequalities requires further methodological discussions in order to develop the best measurable descriptor of an individual's socioeconomic status.

IDENTIFICATION OF INTERVENTIONS FOR THE MEASUREMENT OF EFFECTIVE COVERAGE

The issue of selecting interventions and indicators for the measurement of coverage was intensely discussed. The measurement of coverage should be sensitive to the characteristics of different countries and locales, and the selection of interventions should reflect both country-specific and global perspectives. An objective assessment of the needs, for which effective interventions exist, should be the initial step in the process of identification of interventions.

The following criteria were proposed for the selection of interventions:

- Ability to produce a significant health gain in a relatively short time.

- The size of a health problem at the global and country levels.

- Evidence on the effectiveness of an intervention and its inherent credibility.

- Correspondence to the national health policies, priorities and objective needs.

- Balance between the different modalities of health care, from preventive to curative, and between the various types of illnesses: communicable, noncommunicable, life cycle related health conditions, etc.

- Cost-benefit ratio of obtaining information at the country level.

- Ability to link the global processes with the country priorities for the benefit of the latter.

The selection of indicators for the interventions would be guided by the following principles: internal and external validity of the indicator; feasibility of obtaining valid, reliable and comparable data for the numerator and the denominator; a parsimonious set of indicators.

Indicators should be chosen in such a way that would avoid the so-called "indicator creep": exclusive attention of policy-makers to the selected coverage indicators at the expense of other indicators and interventions not included in the indicator list. A good balance between the different health domains (preventive, curative) and illnesses could avert this problem.

It was further suggested that besides the measurement of coverage with effective interventions, the measurement of harmful practices (unsafe injections, over-use of antibiotics, sale of counterfeit drugs, etc.) would be useful, as well as in the assessment of the health service provision function.

In order to link the global and country-specific contexts, it was recommended that a core set of coverage indicators be selected for the global measurement, to which each country could add additional interventions according to its priorities. A selected group of interventions was chosen for detailed discussions, to get a cross-section of the critical data, the definitional and measurement issues that would be pursued in trying to estimate the coverage of effective health interventions.

COMMUNICABLE DISEASES

HIV/AIDS merits attention on several grounds: enormous health burden; possibility of producing significant health gain through effective preventive interventions; political commitment and increased international attention; significance of HIV/AIDS as an obstacle for socioeconomic development and the reduction of poverty.

Condom use was identified as the most sensible indicator of coverage with effective interventions against HIV/AIDS, given its preventive nature, effectiveness and wider availability. Despite the fact that condom use only indirectly captures HIV/AIDS programme activity, it was still considered to be the most concrete and feasible measure of HIV prevention at the population level.

There are other potential candidates (voluntary counselling and testing, management of opportunistic infections, mother to child transmission, anti-retroviral treatment), which represent different modalities of care. One of the major difficulties in measuring coverage with curative interventions in an HIV/AIDS programme is to ask individuals the question about their HIV positive status and to obtain an accurate response. It was suggested that the discussion with experts be continued in order to explore the potential of the interventions other than condom use, to contribute to the measurement of coverage.

Significant challenges were identified in the measurement of coverage in TB programmes. The evaluation of the TB programme relies on the service data for its indicators. An effective intervention against TB is the completion of a full course of treatment with sputum conversion. The cured status can be certified only by a doctor through sputum examination. This information is usually available only at health facilities, not in households, and the private sector is largely underrepresented in the service data. Furthermore, the TB treatment is long. If a survey captures a patient in the process of treatment, it cannot be assumed that effective intervention has taken place.

Besides the problem of the numerator, the measurement of coverage in TB programmes poses the denominator problem: in order to identify a true denominator a sputum examination has to be performed, which cannot be done in a survey. The only choice left is to ask an individual if he or she has ever been diagnosed with TB during the last 12 months and combine it with external data on TB incidence. The participants were of the opinion that in some cases, such as TB, the use of external data on incidence or prevalence of the health problem might be the only choice for a denominator figure.

NONCOMMUNICABLE DISEASES

Several possible candidates have been proposed for the measurement of coverage in noncommunicable diseases, such as diabetes mellitus, depression, angina pectoris, hypertension, cervical cancer, etc.

Most of the noncommunicable diseases share one characteristic: in order to ascertain the prevalence of needs in the population and validate the results of screening questionnaires, it is desirable to use reference tests. The reference test could be either a detailed diagnostic interview by a doctor or a lab test. However, it was decided that such tests are not always acceptable and affordable for the population. Moreover, they can be administered only to small samples and thus methods have to be streamlined, which would allow the generalization of a small sample observation to the entire population.

For the measurement of coverage with effective interventions in noncommunicable diseases, it is very important to focus on compliance to treatment regimen. Many noncommunicable illnesses are chronic conditions and require either long-term or lifetime treatment. In this situation, the only definition of effective intervention would be the compliance to treatment.

For certain noncommunicable diseases, the most effective intervention is prevention or early diagnostic screening, for instance for cervical cancer. However, it was noted that data on these types of preventive interventions are very poor.

LIFE CYCLE RELATED INTERVENTIONS

The specific nature of this group of interventions and their integrated character makes the selection of an appropriate indicator difficult. Two main challenges were identified: to capture as many dimensions of integrated programmes as possible and to be parsimonious in selecting interventions.

One of the advantages of life cycle interventions was a "normative denominator": all people in a specific age and physiological cycle of their life. However, for specific interventions, a selection of specific subgroups might be required, for instance pregnant women at risk of perinatal complications.

The participants also acknowledged the difficulty in obtaining valid information from the respondents when the questions relate to certain lifestyle practices, such as sexual practices, contraceptive use, etc.

IMMUNIZATION

The participants recognized the importance of childhood immunization as an effective intervention that should be measured in the context of health service coverage. However, the immunization coverage figures do not tell the full story. There is a need for additional information about the quality of the intervention. A parallel surveillance system might be useful to monitor the quality of services through looking at the morbidity and mortality from infectious diseases. For example, measles mortality can reveal the quality of the immunization programme.

Although DTP coverage is not the best tracer of health system performance, its use as a proxy still can be justified on the grounds that DTP3 requires three visits to a health care facility and by one survey it is possible to obtain enough information to judge the difference between contact and effective coverage.

There are many biases and pitfalls in service data and mass immunization campaigns are not usually captured by service statistics, which raises the need for validating the data from time to time with representative surveys.

The participants discussed a case study on the estimation of valid immunization coverage in Bangladesh based on the 1997 Demographic and Health Survey (DHS). A statistical method of estimation of valid immunization from crude immunization figures was presented. The method was based on predictive probability assessment of valid immunization among the children whose immunization status has been confirmed by history. It was agreed that the methodology should be further tested and tried on different samples.

CAPACITIES OF COUNTRIES TO CARRY OUT THE MEASUREMENT OF EFFECTIVE COVERAGE WITHIN THE SCOPE OF THEIR HEALTH INFORMATION SYSTEMS

Capacities for measuring effective coverage should be decentralized to the national and subnational levels. The measurement of coverage should first serve the purpose of improving management and enhancing performance and then be used for global comparisons.

The measurement of coverage at the country level should offer capacity building opportunities for improving the performance of the health information system locally. Capacity building efforts should focus on methodological issues, as well as on the use of coverage information for decision-making and management. A thorough inventory of the existing data and data collection instruments in countries should be made in order to avoid duplication of efforts in the measurement of coverage.

The participants raised the issue of the scarcity of financial resources required for building strong health information systems, which would incorporate both service-generated data and surveys (whenever necessary) in routine reporting.

APPROACHES TO IMPROVE DATA COLLECTION FROM PRIVATE HEALTH CARE PROVIDERS

Another topic of discussion was improving data collection from private providers. Although there were no definite strategies, some interesting suggestions were made:

- Refine the definition of private health care providers.

- Develop an inventory of all private providers by categories and location at subnational levels.

- Map the population coverage of each private entity.

- Identify incentive mechanisms and make them work for improving reporting from private providers.

- Develop regulatory procedures, which through contractual agreements or licensing rules will define data reporting requirements for private providers.

The key for improving reporting from private providers is to design incentives that outweigh the burden of reporting.

Future Steps in the Measurement of Effective Coverage

The participants discussed the future steps that WHO should take in order to operationalize the measurement of coverage with effective interventions.

The development of a survey module was suggested as the first step in transforming the concept of effective coverage into an assessment and monitoring tool. WHO's survey on health and health system responsiveness was considered a potential instrument that could accommodate a coverage module.

The latter should focus on core health care interventions, selected according to the criteria proposed by the meeting. It should be tested in several countries before being applied on a global scale. The module should be flexible in order to be adapted to the various priorities in different countries.

The participants touched upon the issue of using small samples for estimating the event in the population. This was considered particularly important at the subnational level. It was agreed that statistical techniques and methodology be further streamlined and tested, which would allow the use of small samples for obtaining valid, reliable and comparable estimates.

Key Messages

- The measurement of coverage with effective interventions is a valuable complement to WHO's work on enhanced health systems performance.

- Measurements of coverage should optimally include a measurement of the distribution of coverage by various socioeconomic groups, recognizing that coverage of many health interventions tends to be systematically lower in those with lower socioeconomic status. An appropriate asset index should be developed for assessing the population's true economic status via household surveys. The results of

such assessment could be used as dummy variables for describing the distribution of health services in the population.

- The measurement of coverage should focus on a selected set of interventions to be chosen according the following criteria:
  a) Ability to produce a significant health gain in a relatively short time.
  b) The size of a health problem at the global and country levels.
  c) Evidence on effectiveness of an intervention and its inherent credibility.
  d) Correspondence to the national health policies, priorities and objective needs.
  e) Balance between the different modalities of health care, preventive to curative, and between the various types of illnesses: communicable, noncommunicable, life cycle related health conditions, etc.
  f) Cost-benefit ratio of obtaining information at the country level.
  g) Ability to link the global processes with the country priorities for the benefit of the latter.

- The measurement of coverage should accommodate both the country-specific and the global perspectives by accommodating a core module of interventions. Each country should be able to select interventions and indicators according to its needs and add them to the core module.

- Besides measuring coverage at the national level through large samples, it is necessary to design appropriate techniques for using small samples for measuring coverage at the subnational level.

- The measurement of coverage should avoid concentration on vertical programmes. It should keep the health system (at the subnational or national level) as a unit of assessment and use the interventions as tracers of the performance of health service provision.

- The measurement of coverage should become a management tool and aid strategic planning and the decision-making process at the subnational and national levels.

- The measurement of coverage should enhance the capacity of the national health information systems and improve the validity, reliability and comparability of the routinely reported data.

- In the process of the measurement of coverage, WHO should offer countries opportunities for capacity building.

- Improving data collection from the private sector should be an important task for WHO and countries in strengthening the health information systems.

- WHO's work on coverage should be carried out in close cooperation with WHO regions and Member States.

NOTES

1 Rio de Janeiro, Brazil, 27–29 August 2001

Annex 10.1
List of Participants

Ms Jenny Amery
Senior Adviser for Latin America
and the Caribbean
Department for International
Development (DFID)
94 Victoria Street
London, SW1E 5JL
United Kingdom

Dr George Bicego
Research Coordinator
Demographic and Health
Research Division (MEASURE
DHS +)
ORC Macro International, Inc.
11785 Beltsville Drive
Calverton, MD 20705-3119
USA

Dr Trena M. Ezzati-Rice
Chief, Survey Design Staff
National Center for Health
Statistics, CDC
6525 Belcrest Road, Rm 915
Hyattsville, MD 20782
USA

Dr Davidson Gwatkin
Principal Health and Poverty
Specialist
Room G3-036
The World Bank
1818 H Street, N.W.
Washington, D.C., 20433
USA

Dr Ralph Henderson
Special Facilitator
1098 MConnell Drive
Decatur, GA 30033-3402
USA

Dr Lalit Kant
Senior Deputy Director General
Indian Council of Medical
Research
Ansari Nagar, Post Box 4911f
New Delhi 110029
India

Dr Ilmo Keskimäki
Research Fellow, Academy
of Finland
National Research and
Development
Centre for Welfare and Health
(STAKES)
P.O. Box 220
00531 Helsinki
Finland

Dr Carlos Montoya-Aguilar
Professor of Public Health
Alberto Henkel 2337
(Providencia)
Santiago
Chile

Participants from Brazil

Dr Célia M. Almeida
DAPS/ENSP/FIOCRUZ

Dr Jarbas Barbosa da Silva
CENEPI/FUNASA/MS

Dr Rita Barradas Barata
FM Sta Casa

Dr José Carvalho de Noronha
Presidente ABRASCO

Dr Leticia Krauss
DAPS/ENSP/FIOCRUZ

Dr Célia Landmann Szwarcwald
DIS/CICT/FIOCRUZ

Dr Silvia Porto
DAPS/ENSP/FIOCRUZ

Dr Elba Cristina Rego Lima
GM/MS

Dr Cláudio Salm
Assessor do MS

Dr Paulo Santa Rosa
Sec. Exec. /MS

Dr Cláudia Travassos
DIS/CICT/FIOCRUZ

Dr Joaquim Valente
DEMQS/ENSP/FIOCRUZ

Dr Francisco Viacava
DIS/CICT/FIOCRUZ

Dr Alícia Ugá
DAPS/ENSP/FIOCRUZ

Dr João Yunes
FSP/SP e MS

WHO Country Office

Dr Jacobo Finkelman
Señor Representante da
OPAS/OMS
Caixa Postal 08 729
CEP: 70912-970
Brasília, DF
Brazil

Ms Makhamokha Mohale
Support to Health Systems
  and Services Development
  (HSD/HSR)
AFRO
Parirenyatwa Hospital
P.O. Box BE 773
Harare
Zimbabwe

Dr Prosper Tumusiime
Support to Health Systems
  and Services Development
  (HSD/HSR)
AFRO
Parirenyatwa Hospital
P.O. Box BE 773
Harare
Zimbabwe

Dr Daniel Lopez-Acuña
Director
Division of Health Systems and
  Services Development (HSP)
AMRO/PAHO
525 23rd Street, N.W.
Washington, DC
USA

Dr Cesar Gattini
Regional Adviser on Health
  Services
Division of Health Systems and
  Services Development (HSP)
AMRO/PAHO
525 23rd Street, N.W.
Washington, DC
USA

Dr Hernán Montenegro
Regional Advisor on Hospitals
  and Health Management
Division of Health Systems and
  Services Development (HSP)
AMRO/PAHO
525 23rd Street, N.W.
Washington, DC
USA

Dr Belgacem Sabri
Director
Health Systems and Community
  Development (DHS)
EMRO
WHO Post Office
Abdul Razzak Al Sanhouri Street
Naser City
Cairo 11371
Egypt

Ms Ainna Fawcett-Henesy
Regional Adviser
Health Systems Management
  (HSP/HSM)
EURO
8, Scherfigsvej
DK-2100 Copenhagen Ø
Denmark

Dr U Myint Htwe
Regional Adviser
Evidence for Health Policy (EIP)
SEARO
World Health House
Indraprastha Estate
Mahatma Gandhi Road
New Delhi 110002
India

WHO Secretariat

Mr Orvill B. Adams
Evidence and Information for
  Policy

Dr Patrick Berckmans
Evidence and Information for
  Policy

Dr Cynthia Boschi-Pinto
Department of Child and
  Adolescent Health and
  Development (CAH)

Dr Mario Dal Poz
Evidence and Information for
  Policy

Dr Hilary King
Department of Management of
  Noncommunicable Diseases
  (MNC)

Dr Fabio Luelmo
Stop TB Initiative (STB)

Dr Christopher J.L. Murray
Executive Director
Evidence and Information for
  Policy

Dr Bakhuti Shengelia
Evidence and Information for
  Policy

Dr Michel Thieren
Evidence and Information for
  Policy

Dr T. Bedirhan Üstün
Evidence and Information for
  Policy

Ms Lara Vaz
HIV/AIDS

Chapter 11

TECHNICAL CONSULTATION ON STEWARDSHIP[1]

INTRODUCTION

This report is a summary of the major conclusions and recommendations of a meeting of experts on the stewardship function of health systems. *The World Health Report 2000* proposes a comprehensive framework for health systems performance assessment, which identifies the goals of health systems and the four main functions that contribute to their attainment. These four main functions are provision, resource generation, health financing and stewardship. The Director-General's introduction to the report defines stewardship as "the careful and responsible management of the well-being of the population" and calls it "the very essence of good government." The report also claims that stewardship is "arguably the most important" of the four health systems functions and that "it ranks above and differs from the others" (p. 119). Nevertheless, it has been difficult to arrive at a detailed, operational definition of stewardship, which can be used in identifying how countries might strengthen stewardship and improve their health systems performance. The report identified three principal components of stewardship: formulating health policy, exerting influence, collecting and using intelligence (p. 122).

The Technical Consultation on Stewardship in Health Systems was organized by WHO and held in Geneva, Switzerland on 10–11 September 2001. A list of the participants and their affiliations, as well as details of the agenda, can be found in Annex 11.1.

OBJECTIVES AND AGENDA

The consultation was part of a broader programme of similar meetings, which followed the publication of *The World Health Report 2000*. There were two objectives of the meeting. The first was to obtain the opinions of a group of renowned international experts on refining the *The World Health Report 2000's* definition of stewardship and decomposing stewardship to more tangible elements for its better assessment in a particular country. The second was to receive the experts' advice and suggestions for the WHO work program in this area in order for the Organization to better support countries.

The meeting began with an update on WHO work on stewardship. Several experts presented a variety of perspectives on this function, including views from business management, studies of social capital, control of corruption and health system design. The rest of the agenda involved specific working groups, as well as open discussions on how WHO can move ahead with a relevant program of work on the stewardship of health systems.

MAIN CONCLUSIONS AND RECOMMENDATIONS

This section summarizes the conclusions and the key discussions surrounding the issues raised at the technical consultation.

REFINING THE DEFINITION OF STEWARDSHIP

The efforts to come to a consensus on the definition of stewardship focused on its relationship with "governance" and its normative content. There was a general agreement that stewardship incorporates much of what is described as (public) governance. The participants shared the view that stewardship differed from governance more in its style or approach to particular tasks than in its scope. More specifically, stewardship was described as "good," "ethical," "inclusive" or "proactive" governance (recognizing the fact that such terms might have culturally-specific interpretations). In describing stewardship, the participants referred to it metaphorically as a combination of three elements: glue that holds the elements of the health system together, oil that keeps it running smoothly, and energy that gives it (ethical) direction and momentum. In addition to its ethical content and relationship to governance, stewardship was also seen as the function that "embeds" the health system in the society. Therefore, the stewardship function needs to internalize and reflect the cultural and political context, the broader societal norms, and to reach out to address the interactions between the health system and other aspects of society. The scope of effective stewardship needs to extend beyond the conventionally defined boundaries of the health sector.

Despite the key role of stewardship at the heart of effective health systems, it was noted that stewardship does not equate to centralized control. A key element of this function is fostering a culture of self-determination and self-direction among individuals and organizations in the system within an overall framework of agreed on norms and values.

Several participants commented that the term stewardship does not translate well into languages other than English and that previous translations by WHO have not accurately reflected the concept. It was suggested that another, more universally recognizable title for the function be identified.

Decomposing the Elements of Stewardship

The participants agreed that some form of descriptive characterization (or classification) of approaches to stewardship would be useful. Initially, this might be based on a fairly simple listing of specific stewardship tasks. By identifying which tasks are carried out in individual countries (and possibly how and by whom they are carried out), it should be possible to describe different countries' approaches to the stewardship function. It may then also be feasible to distinguish "clusters" of stewardship tasks, which broadly define "styles" of stewardship.

In small group discussions, the participants produced a list of possible stewardship tasks, most of which fit into the three-part classification noted earlier (see Table 11.1).

This provisional list needs to be revised in light of the further research and empirical investigations at the country level to develop a list that is both comprehensive and appropriate in multiple cultural settings. Furthermore, the appropriate boundaries between stewardship and other functions have to be clarified (for example: Does "health education" belong to stewardship or is it more appropriately seen as part of the service provision function? Should "management and

Table 11.1   Tasks of the stewardship function

Formulating health policy	*Exerting influence*	*Collecting and using intelligence*
■ Policy analysis.	■ Consensus building inside and outside the health sector.	■ Intelligence gathering.
■ Policy formulation with involvement from stakeholders and civil society groups.	■ Synchronization of health players.	■ Monitoring and evaluation of public health.
■ Development of an overarching national health plan.	■ Strategic institution building.	■ Encouraging the dialogue between communities and the health system.
■ Defining a vision for health.	■ Regulation and enforcement.	■ Communication.
■ High-level investment and resource allocation decisions.	■ Promulgation of an overarching national health plan.	
■ Establishing shared values and the ethical base for a health action.	■ Promoting a vision for health.	
■ Policy evaluation and correction.	■ Promoting and strengthening shared values and the ethical base for a health action.	
	■ Creating incentives.	
	■ Consumer education.	
	■ Establishing and institutionalizing transparency in management.	
	■ Advocating for healthy public policies in other sectors.	

development of human resources" be considered an element of the resource generation function?).

Other ways to classify the stewardship tasks were discussed. One proposal focused on domains, such as: stewardship of health system functions, strategic management of the health system and stewardship of factors in the broader social, political, and economic environment within which the health system operates.

ASSESSING THE EFFECTIVENESS OF STEWARDSHIP AT THE COUNTRY LEVEL

The participants agreed that effective stewardship should have a broad focus and a long-term view; it should be ethically driven and diverse. Stewardship needs a broad focus because it is not simply about managing a central ministry of health. Nor is its scope limited to those services that are directly funded, managed or delivered by the state. Effective stewardship involves influencing other players, in the private sector and in fields other than health, to bring about positive change. Stewardship needs a long-term view because it is not limited to addressing the challenges of today. It seeks to develop lasting solutions, to build the capacity to solve the problems of the future, to foster continuous improvement. Stewardship needs to be ethically driven because it requires that the interests of citizens be placed above those of the people or organizations in positions of power. A good steward behaves as a servant, not a master, of the citizenry. Finally, stewardship is diverse since it can involve a wide range of different interventions and actions. In some cases, it might include direct delivery of services to the end-users (i.e. citizens or health service consumers). In other cases, it can involve indirect forms of action, such as advocacy, regulation setting or communication.

The participants were asked to propose indicators and measures of good stewardship. Proposals were largely qualitative in nature (e.g. "transparency and effective communication," "free of corruption" or "even-handedness and respect for democratic and legal processes"), although some were more immediately measurable (such as "stability of institutions, personnel and policy settings," as proposed by Veenstra and Lomas).

The need to consider the broader societal context in any assessment of stewardship effectiveness was also raised. Is it possible to have effective steward-ship in an environment of poor public governance at the national level?

POSSIBLE APPROACHES TO FUTURE WORK

The overall objective of the future work in this area is to help countries improve the performance of their health systems by means of more effective stewardship. In order for this to be achieved, it will first be necessary to develop a clearer understanding of the relationships between the different approaches to stewardship, the resultant effectiveness of the stewardship function and the performance of health systems.

The meeting emphasized the need for empirical research into stewardship and governance in health, including in particular descriptive studies of the stewardship tasks, approaches and styles. There was disagreement over the degree to which such research could be comparative given the large differences in the country-specific contexts. However, the value of comparative research was acknowledged, as long as it is carried out in a participatory manner and in a way that encourages the sharing of experience among countries. Involvement of both academics and health officials from the countries concerned has proven effective in similar exercises and could be valuable in this context.

Any approach to assessing stewardship and stewardship effectiveness should be both practical and multiculturally acceptable. In order not to overburden governments, it should be as simple as possible and aim for direct relevance to decision-making at the country level.

Concerns were expressed at the prospect of WHO seeking simply to "measure" stewardship or stewardship effectiveness in countries. Relevance at the country level was seen as a prerequisite for success. In order to achieve relevance, however, it may be necessary to adopt different approaches, fine-tuned to the needs and situations of individual countries. There are also opportunities to learn from work that has already been carried out by WHO and other international organizations in the fields of stewardship and/or good governance, as well as from experience in other sectors.

NOTES

1   Geneva, Switzerland, 10–11 September 2001

ANNEX 11.1

AGENDA

10 SEPTEMBER 2001

09:30–11:00	Welcome [Dr C.J.L. Murray, Executive Director, EIP/WHO]
	Introductions
	Overview of Stewardship [P. Davies, WHO]
11:00–11:30	Coffee Break
11:30–13:00	Views on Stewardship: Plenary Discussion
	Observations on the Stewardship Function [R. Saltman]
13:00–13:45	Lunch Break
13:45–15:00	Scope of Stewardship: Plenary Discussion
15:00–15:30	Coffee Break
15:30–17:00	Stewardship Tasks: Group Work

11 SEPTEMBER 2001

08:30–09:00	Review of Day 1
09:00–10:30	Governance and Social Capital [G. Veenstra]
	Recognizing Good and Bad Stewardship: Plenary Discussion
10:30–11:00	Coffee Break
11:00–12:30	Stewardship Theory [L. Donaldson]
	Pre-conditions for Effective Stewardship: Group Work
12:30–13:30	Lunch Break
13:30–15:00	Corruption in Health: a Failure of Stewardship? [A. Martiny]
	Bench-Marks for Good and Bad Stewardship: Plenary Discussion
15:00–15:30	Coffee Break
15:30–16:45	Personal Reflections on Issues Discussed at the Meeting [S. Nitayarumphong, F. Aboulhassani]
	Next Steps: Suggestions for a Programme of Work: Group Discussion
16:45–17:00	Closing Session

LIST OF PARTICIPANTS

Dr Farid Aboulhassani
Ministry of Health and Medical
   Education,
Tehran
Iran

Dr Luis Bohigas
Ministerio de Sanidad y Consumo
Madrid
Spain

Prof. Lex Donaldson
Australian Graduate School of
   Management
Universities of New South Wales
   and Sydney
Australia

Dr Gillian Durham
Ministry of Health
Wellington
New Zealand

Prof. Lucy Gilson
University of the Witwatersrand
Johannesburg
South Africa
London School of Hygiene and
   Tropical Medicine
United Kingdom

Prof. Yoshinori Hiroi
Chiba University
Japan

Dr Kimmo Leppo
Ministry of Social Affairs
   and Health
Helsinki
Finland

Dr Anke Martiny
Transparency International
   (Deutschland)
Munich
Germany

Dr Fernando Munoz
Latin American Centre for Health
   Systems Research
Santiago
Chile

Dr Sanguan Nitayarumphong
Ministry of Public Health
Nonthaburi
Thailand

Dr Claes Örtendahl
Senior Health Systems Analyst
Karolinska Institute
Sweden

Prof. Richard B. Saltman
Emory University
Atlanta, GA
USA

Dr Rubèn Torres
Fundacion Isalud
Buenos Aires
Argentina

Prof. Gerry Veenstra
The University of British
   Columbia
Vancouver, BC
Canada

WHO Regional Office

Dr Miguel Kiasekoka
WHO—DSD, AFRO

Dr Daniel Lopez Acuña
WHO—AMRO/PAHO

Dr Myint Htwe
WHO—SEARO

Mr Graham Harrison
WHO—WPRO

WHO Secretariat

Dr Christopher J.L. Murray
Executive Director
Evidence and Information for
   Policy

Dr Abdelhay Mechbal
Evidence and Information for
   Policy

Ms Kei Kawabata
Evidence and Information for
   Policy

Dr Dominique Egger
Evidence and Information for
   Policy

Dr William D. Savedoff
Evidence and Information for
   Policy

Ms Geneviève Pinet
Evidence and Information for
   Policy

Ms Anneli Milen
Evidence and Information for
   Policy

Dr Philip Davies
Evidence and Information for
   Policy

Ms Liz Ollier
Facilitator

Chapter 12

Technical Consultation on Statistical Strategies for Cross-Population Comparability[1]

Introduction

This report is a summary of the major conclusions and recommendations of a meeting of experts on statistical methods for enhancing the cross-population comparability of survey data. The consultation was organized by WHO and held in Cambridge, Massachusetts, USA, on 1–2 October 2001. In addition to the four WHO representatives, the participants included psychometricians, statisticians and social scientists who had substantial experience with survey data analysis. A list of the participants and their affiliations, as well as details of the agenda, can be found in Annex 12.1.

Background

The WHO Multi-country Survey Study uses self-report data for assessing non-fatal health in populations, as well as the responsiveness of health systems. These self-report data take the form of ordered categorical (ordinal) responses. One key analytical issue is that these self-report ordinal responses are not comparable across populations primarily because of response category cut-point shifts. Conceptualizing the observed responses as resulting from a mapping between an underlying unobserved latent variable (for example, ability on the underlying domain of mobility) and a set of categorical responses, cut-points are threshold levels on the latent variable, which characterize the transition from one observed categorical response to the next. If cut-points differ systematically across populations or even across socio-demographic groups within a population, then the observed ordinal responses are not cross-population comparable since they will not imply the same level on the underlying latent variable that we are trying to measure (Figure 12.1).

Another way of characterizing this problem is that for the same level of the latent variable on any given domain, the probability of an individual responding in any given response category is different across populations. The issue of cross-population comparability is not limited to health surveys. It is of equal relevance to self-report surveys on responsiveness of health systems, as well as to numerous other questions that rely on ordinal responses. In psychometric parlance, this is known as differential item functioning (DIF).

One example of self-report health data from the WHO Multi-country Survey Study on Health and Responsiveness 2000–2001 on the domain of mobility is: "Overall in the past 30 days, how much difficulty did you have with moving around?" Respondents are asked to classify themselves using one of five response categories: "1 = Extreme/Cannot do; 2 = Severe

Figure 12.1 Mapping from unobserved latent variable to observed categorical response categories

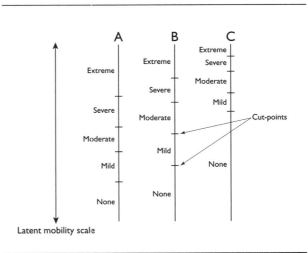

difficulty; 3 = Moderate difficulty; 4 = Mild difficulty; 5 = No difficulty."

OBJECTIVES AND AGENDA

There were two objectives for the meeting. The first was to obtain the opinions of a group of experts on the approach taken by WHO in enhancing the cross-population comparability of survey results. The second was to obtain advice and suggestions on the future directions for this work.

The meeting began with an outline of standard statistical models used in the analysis of ordinal variables. The focus was on the ordered probit model (widely used by economists, political scientists and other social scientists) and the partial credit model (widely used by psychometricians). A simulated data set was used where the observed response categories were generated from two hypothetical countries having different mean values of the latent variable as well as differences in the response category cut-points. The country with the higher level of the latent variable was also assumed to have higher expectations for its population's health, such that in the end, the distributions of the observed categorical responses across three self-report questions did not look very different for the two countries. It was demonstrated that the use of standard techniques, such as the ordered probit and the partial credit model, which do not allow for response category cut-point differences in estimation, could lead to misleading inferences regarding the underlying latent variable when such differences were present in the data generating mechanism.

This was followed by a presentation of the work WHO has undertaken in terms of introducing methodological innovations to address the issue of cross-population comparability. The work revolves around the use of vignettes to assess cut-point differences across socio-demographic groups. A vignette is a description of a concrete level of ability on a given domain, which respondents are asked to evaluate in addressing the main overall question for that domain and using the same categorical response scale. Vignettes are used to fix the level of ability, such that any variations in responses are attributed to variations in response category cut-points.

More specifically, modifications to the ordered probit model and the partial credit model were introduced. These modifications utilize information from responses to vignettes to calibrate self-report responses to both the main and auxiliary questions (if any), so as

to make the estimates of the underlying latent variable cross-population comparable. These models, namely the hierarchical ordered probit (HOPIT) model and the hierarchical partial credit model (HPCM), modify the basic structure of the ordered probit model and the partial credit model in order to allow for cut-point shifts and "difficulty" parameter shifts, respectively, based on the individual responses to vignettes.

A presentation by Dr Jakob Bjorner from the National Institute of Occupational Health in Denmark followed. Dr Bjorner elaborated on the models psychometricians use for analysing ordinal data and their application to health surveys. He also talked about DIF and methods used to test for it in psychometric analysis. The speaker highlighted the different sources of DIF, especially in the context of cross-language research. These included: differences in the translation/interpretation of response choices; differences in the translation/interpretation of items; the fact that the relation between the items and the underlying construct may vary across populations, and that the meaning of the underlying construct may vary. Dr Bjorner elaborated on the basic structure of several models, including the basic Rasch model, the logistic item response theory model, the normal-ogive item response theory model, etc. He discussed the estimation of these models and presented a test of DIF using the conditional Rasch model. The basic idea behind the test of DIF is that if the Rasch model were to be re-estimated in each subgroup, the estimates should be the same as in the total population. A test can be constructed using the combined likelihood over subgroups with the likelihood for the total population model.

Issues relating to unidimensionality, as well as goodness-of-fit were also considered. The results from using alternative calibration methods, such as the use of measured tests, were presented. There was a detailed discussion of the conditional estimation procedure implemented in the dichotomous Rasch model and the polytomous partial credit model. The meeting ended with a presentation of the results obtained from applying these methods to health and responsiveness data from the recent WHO Multicountry Survey Study.

MAIN CONCLUSIONS AND RECOMMENDATIONS

This section summarizes the discussions and conclusions, for which there was a general agreement.

ON THE NEED FOR CROSS-POPULATION COMPARABILITY

There appeared to be a general agreement on the need to correct survey results in order to make them cross-population comparable. The problem is especially pertinent since WHO Member States span a wide spectrum of levels in health status and socioeconomic development.

ON EXISTING METHODS FOR CROSS-POPULATION COMPARABILITY

The problem is well-known and has been addressed before, but there is no satisfactory solution to it. For example, psychometric analysis is typically based on large "item" (i.e. question) banks and one way to deal with DIF is to eliminate questions that exhibit DIF. It was acknowledged that this would not be applicable in the context of the WHO Survey Study given the small number of questions related to each of the domains in health and in responsiveness (typically ranging from one to five questions in each domain).

ON THE USE OF VIGNETTES

There was a consensus that the methods proposed by WHO based on the use of vignettes were novel and interesting. Using the simulated data, these methods are demonstrably superior to standard statistical methods, such as the ordered probit and the partial credit models, in terms of recovering estimates of the underlying latent variable.

ON GOODNESS-OF-FIT

The problem of assessing the goodness-of-fit for categorical response models was discussed. The methods used by WHO based on receiver operating characteristic (ROC) curves were presented. The ROC analysis was undertaken for all ordinal responses in one step. It was agreed that a better method would be to perform the ROC analysis using success in predicting one categorical response at a time. It was also suggested that a detailed examination of the existing methods for assessing goodness-of-fit was merited.

ON THE USE OF RESPONSE CATEGORIES

One of the problems highlighted was the "stacking" of response categories, in that most respondents in most WHO survey countries were answering "no difficulties" to the self-report questions, especially in the health domains. There was a general agreement that the wording of the questions should be re-examined and adjusted, with the goal of making better assessments of less-than-perfect states of health.

OTHER DISCUSSIONS

This section summarizes the suggestions made for developing the methods and analysis further.

ON VIGNETTES

Suggestions were made on testing the assumption of fixed abilities for vignettes across countries. Both the HOPIT and the HPCM are premised on the assumption that vignettes are fixing ability on a given domain across countries, and that any differences are attributed to response category cut-point shifts. One way to test this assumption is to allow each vignette to vary in turn by country to assess the validity of the assumption using cross-country data. Another suggestion was to ask survey respondents to indicate which vignette they most resemble on a particular domain.

ON LATENT VARIABLE DIFFERENCES

The methods presented by WHO assume that both the vignettes and the self-report questions are based on the same underlying latent variable. It was suggested that this assumption could be relaxed by allowing a multidimensional latent variable formulation of the model that allowed for different latent variables for vignettes and for self-reports, but at the same time permitted some degree of correlation between the two measures.

NOTES

1 Cambridge, MA, USA, 1–2 October 2001

Annex 12.1
Agenda

9:00–10:30   Introduction. Problem of Cross-Population Comparability and Differential Item Functioning (DIF), and WHO's Strategies for Dealing with the Problem: Vignettes, HOPIT/CHOPIT, Measured Tests [Christopher J.L. Murray, Ajay Tandon, Joshua A. Salomon, T. Bedirhan Üstün]
World Health Organization

10:30–11:00   Coffee Break

11:00–12:00   Applications, "*in-silica*" Experiment, Examples on Domains of Health from WHO Survey Programme [Christopher J.L. Murray, Ajay Tandon, Joshua A. Salomon, T. Bedirhan Üstün, World Health Organization]

12:00–12:30   General Discussion and Reactions

12:30–2:00   Lunch Break

2:00–3:30   IRT and DIF Presentation. Discussion [Jakob Bjorner, National Institute of Occupational Health, Denmark]

3:30–4:00   Coffee Break

4:00–5:00   General Discussion and Reactions

2 October 2001

9:00–10:30   Other Topics
Unidimensionality of Domains, Model fit, Applications to Responsiveness

10:30–11:00   Coffee Break

11:00–12:30   Closing Remarks and Discussion

List of Participants

Dr Betty Bergstrom
Vice President
Program Management and
  Psychometric Services
Computer Adaptive Technologies,
  Inc.
1007 Church Street
Evanston, IL 60201
USA

Dr Juergen Rehm
Professor, Addiction Research
  Institute
University of Zurich
Konradstr. 32
CH 8031 Zurich
Switzerland

Dr Eugene Laska
Nathan S. Kline Institute for
  Psychiatric Research
Statistical Sciences and
  Epidemiological Division
140 Old Orangeburg Road
Orangeburg, NY
USA

Dr Cees A. W. Glas
Faculty of Educational Science
  and Technology
Department of Educational
  Measurement and Data
  Analysis
University of Twente
Enschede
Netherlands

Dr Gary King
Professor, Department of
  Government
Harvard University
34 Kirkland Street
Cambridge
USA

Dr Jakob Bjorner
Senior Researcher
National Institute of
  Occupational Health
Lersoe Park Allé 105, DK-2100
  Copenhagen
Denmark

Dr Rafael Di Tella
Harvard Business School
Soldier Field
Boston MA 02163
USA

Dr Larry Ludlow
Educational Research, Measure-
    ment, and Evaluation, Chair
Boston College
Lynch School of Education
140 Commonwealth Avenue
Chestnut Hill, MA 02467-3813
USA

Dr Paul Gertler
Haas School of Business
University of California
Berkeley, CA 94720
USA

Dr Jin Pihuan
Department of Health Statistics
Shangai Medical University
138 Yi Xue Yuan Road
Shangai 200032
China

Dr Leo S. Morales
UCLA Assitant Professor
Division of General Internal
    Medicine and Health Services
    Research
School of Medicine
911 Broxton Plaza, Room 103
Los Angeles, CA 90024
USA

WHO Secretariat

Dr Christopher J.L. Murray
Executive Director
Evidence and Information for
    Policy

Dr T. Bedirhan Üstün
Evidence and Information for
    Policy

Dr Joshua A. Salomon
Evidence and Information for
    Policy

Dr Ajay Tandon
Evidence and Information for
    Policy

Chapter 13

TECHNICAL CONSULTATION ON FAIRNESS IN FINANCIAL CONTRIBUTION[1]

BACKGROUND

This report is a summary of the major conclusions and recommendations of the Technical Consultation on Fairness in Financial Contribution organized by WHO and held in Geneva, Switzerland on 4-5 October 2001. In addition to the WHO headquarters and regional staff, the participants included international experts on the measurement of inequality and health financing from each of the WHO regions. None had been involved in the preparation of *The World Health Report 2000*. A list of the participants and their affiliations, as well as details of the agenda, can be found in Annex 13.1. The meeting covered nine sessions over two days and ranged from broad conceptual issues to specific technical problems of measurement. Different participants were invited to chair each session.

OBJECTIVES AND AGENDA

The meeting had two objectives: to exchange views on the different conceptual approaches to measuring the fairness in financial contribution and to obtain the participants' advice and suggestions on the ways, in which WHO work in this area could be developed in the future.

INTRODUCTION

The consultation started with an overview by Dr Christopher J.L. Murray of the recent developments in the WHO concept and measurement of fairness in financial contribution. The focus was on the rationale for the construction of the conceptual framework and the improvement of the methodology. The presentation followed the topics outlined in the background paper, which was delivered to the participants in advance.

THE FFC CONCEPT

WHO's concept of fairness in financial contribution is based on the principle of equal burden. Given a society that raises x% of GDP for its health system, the burden of each household should be equal. The burden is measured as the ratio of the household's total payments to the health system to its capacity to pay. This constitutes the household's financial contribution (HFC). The distribution of household financial contributions across households is summarized in the index of fairness in financial contribution (FFC).

DEVELOPMENT OF THE FFC CONCEPT AND DATA COLLECTION SINCE *THE WORLD HEALTH REPORT 2000*

After the publication of *The World Health Report 2000*, it was argued that the actual food expenditure might not capture the subsistence income of a household, as certain non-subsistence food items are inevitably included in food expenditure. To respond to the argument, the international absolute poverty line (food poverty line) was adopted as a proxy of subsistence expenditure. This change improved the international comparability of the results.

To assess the consistency of the distributional rankings, alternative summary measures of the HFC distribution were explored. These included the Theil's index, the Atkinson's index, the mean logarithmic deviation and different variants of the FFC index. There seemed to be a high rank order correlation between these summary measures.

A decomposing analysis of the FFC index was undertaken. Three components were distinguished:

catastrophic expenditure (extreme horizontal inequality), moderate horizontal inequality and vertical inequality. Empirical results where the vertical effect was separated from the FFC index indicated that this component seemed to have a rather small impact on overall inequality. Separating the effect of extreme horizontal inequality showed that catastrophic health care payments (over 40% of capacity to pay) explained the main part of the variations in FFC indices in the lower FFC countries and moderate horizontal inequality was the main reason for the unfairness in the higher FFC countries.

Surveys are currently available for 74 countries. In addition, for some countries time series data are available, providing a total of 98 data points. The database will be expanded as relevant microdata from countries that undertaking periodic household income and expenditure surveys becomes available.

Main Issues Highlighted at the Meeting

Defining Household Financial Contribution (HFC)

Issues concerning the household financial contribution were discussed separately for the numerator and the denominator.

The Numerator

The Definition of Health Expenditure. The general concern that health expenditure should be made as comparable as possible across countries was raised by several participants. Certain items, such as cosmetic products and plastic surgery, should not be included in health expenditure, whereas expenditure for medical treatment in long-term care facilities should be taken into account.

Conclusions and Recommendations. No consensus was reached on this issue. On one hand, it was discussed that only the part of health care expenditure that goes to finance basic services should be taken into account in the comparisons. On the other hand, no uniform definition of basic services exists and information on expenditure for the institutionalized population is rarely available. The information contents of the datasets have to be analysed case by case in order to arrive at as uniform definitions as possible. The WHO National Health Accounts classifications have been used for this purpose.

Government Non-Tax Revenue. Questions were raised by some Member States about how to assign government non-tax revenue, such as oil revenue, diamond revenue or donations to households. Three approaches were proposed in the meeting. The first one was to assign the same absolute amount of money to each household. This approach raised the issue of the varying impact on rich versus poor households of the same absolute amount of money. The second proposal was to assign the same proportion of each household's capacity to pay and to add it in both the numerator and the denominator. The third alternative would be to assign the same proportion of capacity to pay to each household, but only add this proportion in the numerator.

Conclusions and Recommendations. There was some preference for the second of the above approaches. The arguments against the third approach were that adding non-tax revenue only to the numerator would increase the proportion of health spending to capacity to pay. This would increase the number of households facing catastrophic payments, although the FFC score will remain the same. It was agreed that analyses using different approaches would be performed to see the distributional effects of each incidence assumption.

The Medical Saving Account. The participants also discussed how to treat medical saving accounts in the calculation of HFC. There was a suggestion that these could be treated like social security contributions. However, it was noted that whereas social security contributions are normally fully spent in the current year, only a small portion of the medical saving account is used for the same amount of time.

Conclusions and Recommendations. It was decided that without knowing the details of the specific financing system, it was difficult to provide advice and recommendations.

The Denominator

Discussions on the denominator focused on three main issues: the choice of using income or expenditure to measure the capacity to pay, the definition of subsistence expenditure and the application of the international poverty line.

Income vs. Expenditure. The argument for using income instead of expenditure to proxy effective income came from the OECD countries where the household income data were obtained from a registration system, which was more reliable than the survey expenditure data. It was observed that the purchase of certain consumer durables could generate large variations in expenditure. The same argument applied to discussions on the treatment of household savings and borrowing.

Conclusions and Recommendations. It was concluded that there is a trade-off between using income or expenditure in the denominator. It is a matter of choosing between two approaches and each has its pros and cons. The pros are that expenditures are generally considered to be less prone to short-term variation than transitory income and more reflective of longer-term economic status. Another advantage is that collecting these data is more straightforward and reliable, particularly in developing countries. The cons are as stated above. As data have to be collected from both developed and developing countries on a comparable basis, WHO prefers to continue using expenditure data for all countries. Nevertheless, various alternatives will be explored as possible proxies when data are of poor quality or not available.

The Definition of Subsistence Income and the Poverty Line. In his presentation, Dr van Doorslaer demonstrated formally the distributional impact of deductions from capacity to pay. Along the lines proposed by the WHO, deducting subsistence expenditure from the total household expenditure will have a progressive impact if the deduction is income inelastic. In this sense, the distribution of capacity to pay will comprise an element of progressivity and the hypothetical distribution of equal HFCs would be progressive with respect to the pre-payment income/expenditure distribution. This formulation helps to discern that when the food poverty line is used instead of actual food expenditure, more progressivity will be introduced into the measure. However, the speaker expressed his concern about the ability of the summary FFC measure to distinguish between these two progressivity components. As these effects are combined into one composite measure, one cannot say whether the vertical effect comes from the health payment or from the subsistence deduction.

At a more specific level, different views were expressed as to what should be included in household subsistence expenditure. Some participants argued that the poverty line should include basic spending on medical service, while others suggested it should only include basic food if it is adjusted using food purchasing power parities. In addition to the discussions on

the definition of subsistence expenditure, operational issues on applying the food poverty line in HFC calculation were raised. The first question was how to measure the household capacity to pay if the actual food expenditure or total expenditure is under the poverty line. The participants agreed that part of the reason for this problem might come from data error. Households may have under-reported their actual food expenditure for various reasons. However, apart from the data error, 1.3 billion people in the world are still living under the absolute international poverty line. This means that some households under the poverty line actually have these low expenditures.

Conclusions and Recommendations. There was an agreement that in general the switch from using actual food expenditure to the poverty line was well justified. However, this will increase the number of observations with negative non-subsistence expenditure. The present approach to deal with these cases is to substitute household capacity to pay by actual household non-food expenditure.

SUMMARIZING THE HFC DISTRIBUTION

Distributional Characteristics of the FFC Index

A concern about the ability of the FFC index to address vertical equity and progressivity was raised during the meeting. In this context, it was suggested that the measure could gain from an explicit demonstration of who is affected by the deviations from the norm. This would involve the inclusion of a socioeconomic dimension to the notion of fairness in the burden of payments. It was also pointed out that because of its sensitivity to the right hand tail of the distribution, the current FFC measure combines both the distributional dimension and the threshold dimension of inequality into one composite index. It was suggested that these two components could be analysed separately: one analysis addressing the number of households facing catastrophic payments and the other measuring the deviations of the HFCs from the norm of proportionality. However, it was argued that the summary measure should capture the tail in the distribution if catastrophic expenditure is a concern.

Dr Murray proposed that the concept of the distribution of health system contributions could roughly be divided into two approaches: one examining the effect of health system payments on the distribution of income and levels of poverty, and one examining health system payments in terms of the burden on households and catastrophic payments (Table 13.1).

The income space approach focuses on the income distribution changes and examines how many households are pushed under the poverty line because of health payment. The burden space approach is to discover the distribution of health payment burden across the population and to examine the extent of households facing catastrophic health spending. Both approaches begin by examining the distribution of the direct and indirect contributions to the health system in isolation of the distribution of its benefits. The various views that were expressed in this section will be described in more detail below, where the discussions and conclusions associated with each topic will be presented separately.

Decomposing the FFC Index

The decomposition analysis demonstrated that the FFC index is rather sensitive to horizontal inequalities and it captures the impact of extreme (catastrophic) health spending. While it was argued that particularly in the OECD countries, vertical inequities are perhaps a more pressing policy concern than catastrophic payments, it was acknowledged that in all countries the economic consequences of extreme health care payments are of primary concern.

No consensus was reached over what represents the best available approach to measure the distribution of health payments in a health financing system. However, there was an agreement that each approach emphasizes different important aspects of the distribution of the financial burden to households and each should be considered. The discussions were helpful in offering a better understanding of the differences and similarities of the various approaches, which have been recently used to measure the distribution of payments in health financing systems.

Understanding the Macro Determinants of FFC

In order to better understand the macro determinants of FFC and to link the analysis to policy-making, the determinants of the variation in FFC scores across

countries were explored. These included governmental size, the Gini coefficient, out-of-pocket payment, the share of total health expenditure and the risk sharing properties of the financing system. The participants argued that risk sharing has already been built into FFC and should not be included in the regressions. It was suggested that other factors, such as epidemiological transition, poverty incidence, system reform, historical variables and supply side variables might be worth exploring. Several useful suggestions on how to further improve the analysis were presented. These concerned both model design and estimation techniques.

OTHER ISSUES DISCUSSED

Country Case Analyses

Three participants were invited to make presentations on the results based on their own data analysis. They came from Mexico, South Korea and Australia. First, Dr Knaul made a presentation on a policy application of the FFC measure in Mexico. The FFC and catastrophic payments have been used in the context of the Seguro Popular Project to assess the potential benefits of extending the coverage of universal health insurance in the population. The analysis showed that the greatest benefits could be achieved by insuring the poorest households, small cities, rural areas, as well as nominally small expenditures, such as medications and ambulatory care (doctor visits). Next, Dr Yang presented the FFC results for South Korea in the period 1996–2000. There seemed to be an improvement in the FFC scores after 1998, despite the worsened economic situation. This could at least partly be explained by the government's efforts to decrease the share of private financing in the overall health financing. Finally, Dr Goss from Australia demonstrated several ways in which the health financing burden and the FFC index could be partitioned into components showing the effects of different services and the contribution to the FFC index at various income levels.

The country exercises were rather illustrative and the participants expressed further constructive opinions on how to make the whole analysis more useful for policy-makers.

Time Frame of the Survey

The recall period of the surveys was of concern to the participants. They discussed the advantages and disadvantages of long versus short recall period concerning the measurement of catastrophic expenditure.

Table 13.1   The dimensions of health system contributions

Space	Distribution	Threshold
Income	Change of income distribution	Poverty impact: the difference in the headcount before and after the health payment
Burden	Distribution of the financing burden	Percentage of households facing catastrophic spending

To better link to the policy process in the developing countries, a short recall period might be better than a long one. However, in the developed countries, a long recall period may capture catastrophic spending better. Apart from this, a short recall period will have a smaller memory bias than a long one, while a long one may capture impoverishment better. Questions on the comparison of different recall period data were also raised, but no clear suggestions were made on this issue. Dr Knaul kindly agreed to explore various empirical strategies to observe the sensitivity of the different recall periods.

Time Lag Problems

Negative out-of-pocket payments could occur in some households because of the time lag of the insurance reimbursements. For the same reason, negative direct tax might be expected from income registration data. However, with register data there is usually sufficient time between the execution of the survey and its release to bring the registers up to date. The participants suggested two solutions: to delete the observations with negative values or to set the negative value at zero. There was no discernible preference for either option.

Notes

1   Geneva, Switzerland, 4–5 October 2000

ANNEX 13.1
AGENDA

4 OCTOBER 2001

09:30–10:00	Introductions and General Information about the Meeting [K. Kawabata, Coordinator, EIP/WHO]
10:00–11:00	Overview of FFC Measurement [Dr C.J.L. Murray, Executive Director, EIP/WHO; Dr K. Xu, EIP/WHO]
11:00–11:30	Coffee/Tea Break
11:30–12:45	Alternative Rationales for the Construction and Definition of FFC
	Chair: Dr Andrew Jones
12:45–14:00	Lunch Break
14:00–15:30	Policy Oriented In-Depth Analysis and Capacity Building for the Member States

1. In-Depth Analysis on Catastrophic Expenditure (Example, Lebanon)
2. The Subnational Analysis
3. The Time Series Analysis
4. Local Capacity Building

Case Studies: Mexico (Felicia Knaul), South Korea (Bong-Min Yang), Australia (John Goss)

Chair: Dr Rozita Halina Tun Hussein

15:30–15:45	Coffee/Tea Break
15:45–17:00	Defining Household Financial Contribution (HFC)

1 The Numerator of HFC
2. The Denominator of HFC
3. The Estimation of Food Purchasing Parities (Food PPP) for All Member States

Chair: Mr John Goss

17:00–18:00	Summarizing the HFC Distribution

1. Distribution of HFC
2. Alternative Summary Measures

Chair: Dr Supasit Pannarunothai

5 OCTOBER 2001

8:30–10:00	Decomposition of the FFC Index: Vertical Equity and Horizontal Inequality

1. Impact of Health System Contribution on Income Redistribution
2. Separation of Vertical Effect from the FFC Index
3. Separation of Extreme Horizontal Effect from the FFC Index

Chair: Dr Eddy van Doorslaer

10:00–10:15	Coffee/Tea Break
10:15–11:30	Further Steps and Challenges in Refining the Methodology

1. Distribution of Government Non-Tax Revenue, Oil, etc.
2. Distribution of Employers' Contribution to Private Health Insurance
3. Medical Saving Account

Chair: Dr Zilvinas Padaiga

11:30–12:45	Data Issues

1. Low-cost Survey Data
2. Techniques of FFC Estimation from Incomplete Data Sets
3. Understanding the Macro Determinants of FFC

Chair: Dr Jürgen John

12:45–14:00	Lunch Break
14:00–15:00	Closing Session

List of Participants

Mr Zainal Andidine Massonde
Ministry of Planning, Moroni
Comores

Dr Kadama
World Bank Health Project
Ministry of Health, Entebbe
Uganda

Dr Derek J. Hudson
Phaleng Consultancies (Pty) Ltd.
Botswana

Dr Felicia Knaul
FUNSALUD, Fundacion Mexicana
   para la Salud
Mexico

Mr Zine Eddine El Idrissi Moula
Royaume du Maroc, Ministere
   de la Sante
Morocco

Dr Hossein Salehi
c/0 WHO Tehran
Iran

Dr John Jurgen Heimo
Institute of Health Economics
   and Health Care
Germany

Prof. Zilvinas Padaiga
Kaunas University of Medicine
Lithuania

Dr Eddy van Doorslaer
University of ERASMUS,
   Rotterdam
Netherlands

Prof. Andrew Jones
University of York
United Kingdom

Prof. Sudhir Anand
St Catherine's College, Oxford
United Kingdom

Dr Supasit Pannarunothai
Asociated Institute: Centre for
   Health
University of Naresuam
Thailand

Dr Htwe Myint
India

Mr Sunil Nandraj
India

Mr John Goss
Australian Institute of Health
   and Welfare
Australia

Prof. Bong-Min Yang
Seoul National University
Republic of Korea

Dr Rozita Halina Tun Hussein
Institute of Public Health, MOH
Malaysia

WHO Secretariat

Dr Christopher J.L. Murray
Executive Director
Evidence and Information for
   Policy

Dr Ke Xu
Evidence and Information for
   Policy

Ms Kei Kawabata
Evidence and Information for
   Policy

Chapter 14

Technical Consultation on the Measurement of Health Inequalities[1]

Introduction

This report is a summary of the major conclusions and recommendations of a meeting of experts on the measurement of health inequalities organized by WHO and held in Geneva, Switzerland, on 7–8 November 2001. In addition to the WHO headquarters representatives, the participants included economists, statisticians, public health professionals and other social scientists who had substantial experience in measuring health inequalities. Details of the agenda, a list of the participants and their affiliations, as well as a list of the invited participants who could not attend, can be found in Annex 14.1.

Background

The World Health Organization framework for the assessment of health systems performance identified three intrinsic social goals to which health systems contribute: population health, responsiveness of the health system and fairness in the financial contributions of households to the health system. The goal of population health is defined as improving the average level of health and the distribution of health across individuals, i.e. reducing inequalities in health.

Levels of health were assessed using disability adjusted life expectancy, now renamed healthy life expectancy (HALE). WHO argued that logically, health inequalities should be measured as the distribution of healthy life expectancy across individuals. Because of the limitations of data and methods, for *The World Health Report 2000* health inequality was assessed by measuring the distribution of the probability of survival across children.

A parametric model was used to estimate the distribution of the probability of surviving to age two. This distribution was then summarized with the following measure of inequality:

$$II[3,.5] = \frac{\sum_{i=1}^{n}\sum_{j=1}^{n}\left|s_i - s_j\right|^3}{2n^2 \bar{s}^{0.5}}$$

where s_i is the expected survival time of a child i from birth to age 2, and $\bar{s}$ is the average survival time in the population. The measure is based on comparing each child to every other child in the population. It gives a large weight to the tails of the distribution as all differences are raised to the power of 3 in the numerator and is a relative measure as the mean is included in the denominator. This measure was selected based on the responses to an internet survey, which included questions on the normative choices involved in the selection of an inequality measure. In *The World Health Report 2000* estimates of equality in child survival were reported to preserve the consistency with the reporting on the other four goals of health system, which were all on a positive scale (i.e. a higher number is better). Equality in child survival was simply estimated as one minus the inequality index (II) presented above.

Data on child survival came from complete birth histories available through the Demographic and Health Surveys (DHS) programme. For the developed countries child survival data from small geographical areas, such as counties or municipalities, were used. Since the publication of *The World Health Report 2000*, new methods have been developed for the measurement of child survival inequality and the study of its determinants, as well as for the measurement of inequality in healthy life expectancy.

Objectives and Agenda

There were two objectives of the meeting: to obtain the opinions of a group of experts on the approach taken by WHO in measuring health inequalities and to receive their advice and suggestions on ways this work could develop in the future.

The meeting began with an overview of the conceptual framework used by WHO in the measurement of health inequalities, including a discussion of different measures of inequality borrowing on the literature from other fields. A presentation on the methods used to measure child survival inequality in *The World Health Report 2000* and the subsequent analysis of the decomposition of this measure into its potential determinants followed. Afterwards, the potential methods that could be used to extend the measurement to adult survival were discussed, including models for aggregated data that could serve in the formulation of reasonable approximations, where individual-level data are not available. Subsequently, Dr Hasegawa from Japan and Dr Varavikova from the Russian Federation presented their work on using small-area data to look at trends in mortality and health status in their countries. There was a presentation of WHO's work on estimating health states across the Member States in a comparable way and on the ways in which inequality in health states could be measured. The rest of the agenda involved an open discussion, inspired by a presentation by Dr Wolfson, on ways in which age-sex specific information on the distribution of health states and risks of death could be combined in the estimation of the distribution of healthy life expectancy. The final session specifically addressed how to best summarize the bivariate distribution of health and income, and how WHO could best quantify the health of the poor, particularly in low- and middle-income countries.

Main Conclusions and Recommendations

This section summarizes the conclusions, for which there was general agreement.

Quantity of Interest: Inequality in HALE

There was a general consensus that since WHO is reporting the average levels of health in terms of healthy life expectancy, its measure of inequality in health should also reflect variation in HALE. The measure of inequality should be constructed in such a way that contributions of socioeconomic factors, as well as specific diseases, such as HIV/AIDS and tuberculosis, can be calculated. Decomposability of the inequality measure into contributions from various components was an attribute that was deemed essential by all participants. (Due to the nature of most inequality measures, additive decomposability is usually not feasible.) An agreement was reached on the need for a measure that can be presented to policy-makers in a simple way. Inequalities in health between males and females were also discussed. It was generally agreed that a special focus should be given to the differences between the two sexes and particular attention should be paid to cases where biological causes could not explain the differences observed.

Inequalities across Individuals versus Social Groups

It was generally agreed that the two approaches to the measurement of health inequalities answer fundamentally different questions and are complementary, rather than conflicting. There was a consensus on the premise that differences in health across individuals are interesting in their own right and that differences across social groups are also interesting and worth measuring. The WHO measure of inequality should be a complement, not a replacement, for existing measures. WHO has been reporting routinely on the average levels of health for countries. Reporting on inequalities in health within countries should be routine as well.

Voluntary and Genetic Risks

The feasibility of excluding voluntary and/or genetic risks from the calculation of inequalities in healthy life expectancy was considered. The group agreed that given the questionable boundaries which qualify a risk as voluntary or purely genetic, these should not be excluded from the estimation.

Measure of Inequality

The discussion around the measure that should be used to summarize the distribution of the quantity of interest was not conclusive. However, there was general agreement on the fact that no single measure of inequality would reflect all the important attributes of the distribution of health and that a combination of measures may need to be calculated to encompass the concerns about inequality. It was decided that WHO needed to use a single measure in its final estimation of health system attainment and that such a measure did not need to reflect the average level of health, as the latter is reported separately by WHO. The participants suggested the consideration of simpler measures, such as the interquartile range (e.g. for expected life lengths from a period survival curve), if after further study it was shown to reflect the right dimensions of variability in health.

Measurement of Child Survival Inequality

The methods used in *The World Health Report 2000* and the new models developed since its publication were discussed. The individual-level random effects logit model was preferred to the extended beta-binomial because it can be used to study the effect of individual-level covariates. Some participants suggested that other specifications of the distribution of the random effect should be explored.

Decomposition of the Inequality Index

The currently used methods for allocating the index of inequality into the effects of potential determinants were discussed. The present method for assets and education involved removing the effect of variation in assets and variation in education and recalculating the index. For the variable that is the health system proxy, the results presented were the effect of an increase in access to 100% (thus increasing the average level and removing the effect of variation in access). It was proposed that the decomposition analysis also be performed by increasing the level of education by 1 year for every mother and removing the effect of variation in access to health services without affecting the average level. There was further discussion on what the variable labelled "access to health services" meant. It was agreed to capture different things in different countries: from the pure effect of immunization on child health in some settings to access to health services in other settings, as well as other possible factors not specifically related to the health system. It was suggested that additional variables, which might capture the access to health services available (such as antenatal care and type of birth attendant for women of reproductive age), be considered in the analysis as well.

Models for Adult Inequality

The methods currently used to estimate the distribution of mortality risk in older age groups involve survival analysis models correcting for additional variation not captured by the available covariates. The discussion focused on a few models and it was suggested that in addition to controlling for community-level effects with the extra term in the model, it would be interesting to add some of the community-level variables in the model, where they are available. In the setting of the USA, where the current data are available but the geocodes are randomized, the potential to add community-level variables in the model is limited. However, in the future analysis of data without this limitation, community-level variables, such as income inequality, availability of health services or health expenditure, will be added to the model. The main drawback of the proposed methods was data availability.

Small-Area Data

Data from small geographical areas was proposed as one of the potential ways to estimate the distribution of risk of mortality in adult age groups. These data-sets are more readily available for a large number of countries and can be more easily collected for the developing countries than individual-level data. The relationship between small-area data and individual-level data for the US was presented. This relationship needs to be researched in more detail. If it is found that there is a systematic relationship between individual-level data and small-area data for several countries, then small areas could be used in the approximation of the distribution of mortality risks for countries where individual-level data are not available. The presentations from the Russian Federation and Japan supported the hypothesis that looking at variations across administrative areas reveals variations that could be useful in policy formulations. The group discussed the fact that data from different countries would be at different levels of aggregation (or administrative districts) and there might be problems with the comparability of results across countries. The best strategy seemed to be to collect data at the smallest level of aggregation possible for each country. It is important to test this strategy by using data from multiple levels of geographic aggregation within one (or more) countries and compare them to estimates from individual-level data.

INEQUALITY IN HEALTH STATES

Preliminary results on the distribution of health states by age and sex from the analysis of the WHO Multi-country Survey Study on Health and Responsiveness 2000–2001 were presented. The value of looking at variations in health states was viewed separately from looking at inequality in healthy life expectancy. It was noted that the use of the term "inequality" in this context might not be adding any analytical value. The trends depicted in health states are often not consistent with those seen in risk of death. Therefore, it was considered useful to look at each independently, prior to combining them into a single metric of inequality in healthy life expectancy. It was observed that while for mortality the quantity of interest is risk of death, for health states the quantity examined is the outcome, which is the current health state.

CORRELATING RISKS OF ILL-HEALTH ACROSS AGES

The discussion on how to combine all the pieces of information that feed into inequality in healthy life expectancy was led by Dr Wolfson who proposed a variant of a micro-simulation model. This would estimate HALE for a hypothetical population, for example of 1 million individuals. In this model, individuals would be exposed to a set of mortality and ill-health risks throughout their lifetime. By setting the correlation of their health risks across ages at one, the upper bound of inequality could be estimated. As the correlation of health risks across ages is unlikely to be 1, one way to estimate the true value is to use the correlation of mortality rates across ages in small areas to approximate it. Before it is used, this approach should be applied to real data from a country with both small-area data and longitudinal mortality follow-up data (such as the UK) to confirm its validity.

HEALTH OF THE POOR

The new approach of WHO to measure permanent income in the World Health Survey was discussed at length. It was agreed that it would be very useful to have cross-comparable measures of health and of permanent income in the same instrument, as that would allow for a much improved measurement of health of the poor. Current approaches to measuring health of the poor are not necessarily comparable across countries and are limited to those countries with good data on income. The World Health Survey would lead to much better information on poverty and permanent income in the developing countries and in cross-population comparable estimates of health of the poor. This approach was deemed as very important for WHO to pursue in its next round of measurement. It was emphasized that the method should first be clarified by distinguishing which of the three quite different applications are intended: a measure of poverty, a means of ranking individuals by socioeconomic status within countries, or a measure most likely to have causal significance. These three objectives will not necessarily lead to the same choice of measure.

OTHER DISCUSSIONS

This section summarizes the discussions for which there was no general agreement or conclusion.

USE OF TERM "INEQUALITY"

There was a long discussion on the use of the term "inequality" in the field of public health. The dispute was about whether the term "health inequalities" should be reserved to mean "inequalities in health across groups defined by social, demographic or geographical characteristics," as it has been used for some time by several researchers in the field, or whether it should be used in the same way as in other fields of social and physical science, which would imply that "inequalities in health" means differences in health across individuals. Examples of other fields mentioned included economics, political science, education and biology. It was agreed that the name would need to be specified, so that it is clear to all readers what it is measuring. The attendees shared the view that the name chosen by WHO must be clarified sufficiently in order for the goals of all researchers to be accomplished.

MEASURE OF INEQUALITY

The discussion on which summary measure of a distribution to use as the measure of inequality did not arrive at a concrete conclusion. The merits of different measures were considered and measures such as the interquartile range of a distribution were proposed. One proposal was that WHO should calculate and report both relative and absolute indices of health inequality. It was agreed that in the context of health system performance assessment, one measure of inequality had to be selected for the calculation of the index of attainment. Any single measure should be accompanied by complementary measures (for example, indices of both absolute and relative inequalities). Some participants suggested that in the short run, WHO should report inequality in health using simple indicators, such as the interquartile range and differences by socioeconomic status. Simultaneously, the Organization has to develop data and methods for more complex indicators that would, for example, consider partial orderings of distributions according to the Lorenz criterion. It was also suggested that WHO should make available both the summary indicator ultimately chosen, as well as other indicators and the underlying distribution to interested researchers.

Finally, some participants proposed that different indicators of health inequality might be more relevant for some countries than others. For example, for high-income countries it might be more useful to compare them on a measure that might not be applicable or of interest to low-income countries.

Notes

1 Geneva, Switzerland, 7–8 November 2001

ANNEX 14.1
AGENDA

7 NOVEMBER 2001

9:00–10:30	Conceptual Framework for the Measurement of Health Inequality
	Chair: Anton Kunst
	Presenter: Christopher J.L. Murray
10:30–11:00	Coffee Break
11:00–12:30	Measures of Health Inequality
	Chair: Anton Kunst
	Presenter: Emmanuela Gakidou
12:30–2:00	Lunch Break
2:00–3:30	Inequality in Child Survival: Measurement and Determinants
	Chair: El Fatih El Samani
	Presenter: Gary King
3:30–4:00	Coffee Break
4:00–5:30	Inequality in Adult Survival: Models for Individual-Level Data
	Chair: El Fatih El Samani
	Presenter: Emmanuela Gakidou

8 NOVEMBER 2001

9:00–10:30	Inequality in Adult Survival: Models for Small-Area Data
	Chair: Than Tun Sein
	Presenters: Alan Lopez, Elena Varavikova, Toshihiko Hasegawa
10:30–11:00	Coffee Break
11:00–12:30	Inequality in Health States
	Chair: Than Tun Sein
	Presenter: Ajay Tandon
12:30–2:00	Lunch
2:00–3:30	Inequality in Healthy Life Expectancy: Combining Health States with Risks of Death, and Risks of Ill-Health across Ages
	Chair: Michael Marmot
3:30–4:00	Coffee Break
4:00–5:30	Health of the Poor: How to Best Summarize the Bivariate Distribution of Health and Income
	Chair: Michael Marmot
	Presenter: Michael Wolfson

LIST OF PARTICIPANTS

Prof. Sudhir Anand
St. Catherine's College
Oxford University
OX1 3U3
United Kingdom

Dr Toshihiko Hasegawa
Director, Department of Health Care Policy
National Institute of Health Services Management
1-23-1, Toyama
Shinjuku-ku, Tokyo 162-0052
Japan

Tanja A.J. Houweling, MA
Department of Public Health
Faculty of Medicine and Health Sciences
Dr. Molewater Plein 50
P.O. Box 1738
3000 DR Rotterdam
Netherlands

Dr Gary King
Centre for Basic Research in the Social Sciences
Harvard University
34 Kirkland Street, RM.2
Cambridge, MA 02138
USA

Dr Anton Kunst
Department of Public Health
Faculty of Medicine and Health Sciences
Erasmus University
PO Box 1738
3000 DR Rotterdam
Netherlands

Prof. Sir Michael Marmot
Head of Department
Department of Epidemiology and
    Public Health
University College London
1-19 Torrington Place
London WC1E 6BT
United Kingdom

Dr El Fatih Zeinelabdin El
    Samani
The WHO Representative
P.O. Box 11365-3597
Tehran
Iran

Dr Than Tun Sein
Director
Department of Medical Research
Yangon, Myanmar
c/o WHO Representative,
    Myanmar

Dr Elena Varavikova
Monitoring of Health Losses Unit
Room 323
Central Research Institute of
    Information and Organization
    of Public Health
Dobrolubova 11
127254 Moscow
Russian Federation

Dr Michael Wolfson
Assistant Chief Statistician,
Analysis and Development
    Branch, Statistics Canada
24th Floor, R.H. Coats Building
Ottawa, Ontario
Canada K1A 0T6

WHO Secretariat

Dr Christopher J.L. Murray
Executive Director
Evidence and Information
    for Policy

Dr David B. Evans
Evidence and Information
    for Policy

Mr Brodie D. Ferguson
Evidence and Information
    for Policy

Dr Emmanuela Gakidou
Evidence and Information
    for Policy

Ms Margaret Hogan
Evidence and Information
    for Policy

Dr Alan D. Lopez
Evidence and Information
    for Policy

Dr Abdelhay Mechbal
Evidence and Information
    for Policy

Dr Ajay Tandon
Evidence and Information
    for Policy

List of Invited Participants
Who Could Not Attend

Dr Mustapha Azelmat, Ministry
    of Health, Morocco
Dr Norberto Dachs, WHO-AMRO
Dr Eddy van Doorslaer, Erasmus
    University
Dr Timothy Evans, Rockefeller
    Foundation
Dr Davidson Gwatkin,
    World Bank
Dr Andrew Jones, York University,
    United Kingdom
Dr Rene Loewenson, EQUINET
Dr Johan Mackenbach, Erasmus
    University
Dr Geoff Rowe, Statistics Canada
Dr Than Sein, WHO-SEARO
Dr Viroj Tangcharoensathien,
    International Health Policy
    Program, Thailand
Dr Martin Tobias, Ministry of
    Health, New Zealand

Chapter 15

WHO MEETINGS OF EXPERTS ON MEASURING AND SUMMARIZING HEALTH[1]

INTRODUCTION

This report is a summary of the major conclusions and recommendations of the following meetings of experts on measurement of health and summary measures of population health organized by WHO and held over the last two years to support the development of summary measures or reporting on average levels of population health for the WHO Member States:

- Conference on Summary Measures of Population Health, Marrakech, Morocco, 6–9 December 1999

- 1st Preparatory Working Group Meeting on Measuring Health Status, Geneva, Switzerland, 2–3 August 2000

- 2nd Preparatory Working Group Meeting on Measuring Health Status, Geneva, Switzerland, 4–5 September 2000

- Meeting of Committee of Experts on Measurement and Classification for Health, Geneva, Switzerland, 11–12 September 2000

- Joint ECE/WHO Expert Meeting on Measuring Health Status, Ottawa, Canada, 23–25 October 2000

In addition to the WHO staff members, the participants at these meetings included experts on the measurement of population health from all WHO regions and senior representatives of national and international health statistical agencies. A full list of the participants and their affiliations, as well as details of the agendas for the meetings, can be found in the Annexes.

SUMMARY MEASURES OF POPULATION HEALTH

Summary measures of population health (SMPH) are measures that combine information on mortality and non-fatal health outcomes. The interest in these measures has been rising in recent years and the calculation and reporting of various measures have become routine in a number of settings. With the proliferation of work on summary measures, there has been an increasing debate about their application in public health, ranging from the ethical implications of the social values incorporated in these measures, through technical and methodological issues regarding the formulation of different measures, to concerns about distributive justice and the use of summary measures in resource allocation. Given these developments and the diverse opinions about the construction and use of summary measures, the World Health Organization's Global Programme on Evidence for Health Policy convened a conference in Marrakech, Morocco, on 6–9 December 1999, to provide a forum for discussion and debate over the scientific, ethical and policy issues around SMPH.

The Conference brought together over 50 internationally recognized experts from a range of disciplines, including population health analysts, statisticians, epidemiologists, health economists, health policy-makers, philosophers and ethicists.

USES OF SUMMARY MEASURES OF POPULATION HEALTH

There are a variety of uses of SMPH. These range from comparisons of the health of populations or of the same population over time, quantifying health inequalities, incorporating the effects of non-fatal outcomes in measuring overall population health, setting priorities for health services delivery and planning, to guiding research and development in the health sector, improving professional training, and analysing the benefits of health interventions for use in cost-effectiveness studies.

BASIC CONCEPTS

Given this array of potential uses of summary measures, the conference considered some of the basic concepts underlying their definition and construction. How broadly, for example, should the concept of "health" be defined? Should SMPH try to measure well-being as distinct from, and in addition to, health, and if not, are these two concepts really separable? Quite apart from such philosophical considerations, how should well-being be measured and what are the critical concerns, such as additivity, in measures of well-being? An important issue raised was the need for summary measures to reflect both distributional and overall level concerns. There was a general consensus that summary measures should not try to simultaneously assess both the level of health and the inequalities in it. Separate measures are preferable.

HEALTH EXPECTANCIES, HEALTH GAPS AND CAUSAL ATTRIBUTION

Summary measures of population health fall into two broad categories: health expectancies and health gaps. A wide range of health expectancies have been proposed since the original notion was developed. The conference reviewed the basic characteristics of health expectancy measures, including the implications of the methods used to calculate life expectancy (period or cohort) and the methods used to estimate health expectancies (prevalence-rate life tables, multistate life tables). Of key concern were the consequences of using different definitions and measurements of health status in the calculation of health expectancies, and perhaps most importantly, the implications of basing health expectancy measures on dichotomous versus multistate valuations of health states.

Of the different summary measures that have been widely used, none includes information on both incidence and prevalence. There are longstanding arguments in health statistics about the relative merits of incidence-based and prevalence-based measures, but simple evaluative criteria suggest that summary measures should include information on both for the purpose of comparing the health of different populations. The conference debated the necessity for inclusion of both types of information and the implications for the construction and measurement of SMPH.

While less easily interpreted, health gap measures are critical to understanding the comparative importance of disease, injuries and risk factors for population health levels. Over the past 50 years, a variety of health gap measures have been proposed and calculated. Health gaps extend the notion of mortality gaps to include time lived in health states worse than ideal health. Several aspects of health gap measures were discussed, such as the choice of implicit or explicit population targets and the goals for health gaps. Normative choices for health gap measures were provided. The implications of the age-dependent characteristic of gap measures, which is not an issue for health expectancies, were also discussed, and criteria were advanced and debated for desirable properties of health gap measures.

Given the fact that one of the fundamental goals in constructing summary measures is to identify the relative magnitude of different health problems, including diseases, injuries and risk factors, an appropriate framework is required that would be both coherent and readily interpretable. There are two dominant traditions in the widespread use of causal attribution: categorical attribution and counterfactual analysis. In categorical attribution, an event like a death is attributed to a single cause according to a defined set of rules (in this case the International Classification of Diseases). In counterfactual analysis, the contribution of a disease, injury or risk factor to the overall disease burden is estimated by comparing the current levels of a summary measure with the levels that would be expected under some alternative hypothetical exposure scenario. Discussion focused around the relative advantages and disadvantages of these two approaches and the implications for comparability of using the two approaches in the same analysis.

HEALTH STATUS DESCRIPTION AND CLASSIFICATION

Standardized, multidimensional assessments of health states are increasingly being used to describe a population's health status, quite apart from the need for such data in summary measures. Well known examples include the SF-36, Nottingham Health Profile, Quality of Wellbeing Scale and WHO-DAS II, but there are many others. Yet all efforts at measuring health state valuations and the subsequent calculation of severity weights incorporated within a summary measure of population health depend on using meaningful, complete and comprehensible health state descriptions. Two key issues in describing health states were discussed: what constitutes a complete description of a health state and how to convey this information effectively to an individual undertaking the valuations? WHO's work on a comprehensive classification scheme, the ICF (or ICIDH-2) was discussed as well. The presentations and discussion identified the need for a stronger theoretical and methodological basis to: explain and potentially adjust for gaps between self-reported health and observed health status measures or medical diagnosis; explain and potentially adjust for systematic patterns of deviations between self-reported health status and selected socioeconomic and cultural factors; and enhance the cross-population comparability of measures of health status from surveys using standardized calibration techniques.

HEALTH STATE VALUATION

Any summary measure of population health requires, by definition, the quantification or explicit valuation of states of health worse than perfect health. There has been extensive debate in the health economics literature on a number of fundamental issues relating to health state valuation, including: whose values should be used, e.g. individuals in health states, the general public, healthcare providers or household members carrying for individuals in health states; what type of valuation approaches should be used, such as the standard gamble, time trade-off, person trade-off or visual analogue; how should health states be presented for the elicitation of valuations, that is, with what type of description and what level of detail, including some selection of domains; what range of health states from mild to severe are to be valued at the same time; and what combination of valuation questions and type of deliberative process should be used. While there were conflicting views on some of these issues, many of the participants agreed that the empirical basis for the calculation of summary measures would be improved considerably through the collection of population-based data on individual valuations of a wide range of health states.

Regardless of the resources available, it is clearly not feasible to measure health state valuations in a population for every possible health state. For the calculation of summary measures of population health, a predictive model, which allows one to impute health state valuations from information on health status associated with a particular state, would be clearly desirable. To date, there have been at least four published

attempts to develop systems that can be used to map from levels on a set of domains of health status to valuations of health states described along these domains: the Quality of Well-Being (QWB) scale, the Disability and Distress Scale, EuroQol and the Health Utilities Index (HUI). The characteristics of such approaches, as well as a broader research agenda for developing new methods, were debated at the conference.

One of the major substantive issues relating to health state valuation is the question of variation in values within and across populations. There are a number of compelling reasons why health state valuations might be expected to vary between populations that have different cultural beliefs on disease causation, individual responsibility, fatalism, social roles and functioning or expectations for well-being, etc. Further, individual variation in valuations according to age, sex, education, income and other sociodemographic variables might be expected. To date, however, there is little empirical evidence that health state values vary markedly within and across populations. This may simply be a function of insufficient power to detect these differences or of the paucity of comparable data on health state valuations. On the other hand, it is possible that the contributions of the different domains of health to the overall valuation of a health state are similarly viewed across populations, but what differs between populations are the health status characteristics associated with a given disease state. Concepts and methods for modelling the determinants of variation in health state valuations within and between populations were presented and discussed.

GOODNESS, FAIRNESS AND SOCIAL VALUE CHOICES

A key concern in the use of summary measures for resource allocation is that policies and programmes are chosen based on several considerations, not only on the concern to maximize health outcomes. Optimizing the health of populations is but one option and others may be, and generally are, better supported by moral arguments. Should we give moral priority to the worst-off? Or should we attach greater significance to large benefits than to the sum of many small gains, with life-saving interventions counting most of all? Or might we give less importance to life extension past a normal life span, thus attaching greater moral weight to achieving what has been described as "fair innings." Two methodological issues that have broad implications for measurement are cutting across these moral choices. One issue is whether our judgments on these moral trade-offs should be explicitly incorporated into the summary measures themselves, via weighting, or whether they should be regarded as an altogether separate set of considerations in the allocation debate. Another issue is whether these issues of resource allocation should ideally be settled by processes of democratic deliberation and the elicitation of the public's values, or by the best of moral argumentation and theory. Several presentations were made to guide and encourage the debate around this moral arithmetic.

The calculation and specification of summary measures of population health also involves a number of explicit social value choices. One key issue is whether or not to differentially weight healthy years of life lost at different ages and if so, on what basis. Even if most people consider the period of young adulthood (for example, the early childbearing years) as more valuable than years lived at the beginning or end of life, this view may be objectionable if the basis is the societal value of young adults compared to other people. Secondly, the choice of a discount rate for health benefits, even if technically desirable, may entail morally unacceptable allocations between generations. Are there other widely held values and on what basis should we decide to incorporate social values into the summary measure? Or should we keep them distinct? If they are to be incorporated, should these values be determined at local/national level for country analyses and/or at the international level for cross-national comparisons? There was an extensive debate on similar social value choices, as well as on their application in summary measures.

OUTCOMES OF THE CONFERENCE

One key objective of WHO, in addition to advancing the technical work on summary measures, has been to promote greater transparency and understanding of the inputs to calculate these measures and their appropriate application. The Marrakech conference provided a unique opportunity to challenge existing notions and to advance the conceptual and methodological research agenda concerning SMPH and their use. Leading experts from a range of disciplines addressed the current state of the work, beyond basic concepts and uses, covering the conceptual frameworks for measurement of population health, the description and valuation of health states, as well as social values and ethical considerations. Given the expected heterogeneity as far as the latter are concerned, the meeting fostered a debate about conceptual, technical and practical concerns, and addressed a number of implications for the use of summary measures.

The various papers presented at the Marrakech meeting, supplemented by additional chapters that arose from the discussion or were commissioned to fill important gaps in the debate, have been published in an edited, peer-reviewed volume by WHO in 2002.[2] This book represents a milestone in the evolution of health metrics and contributes substantially to the ongoing development and use of SMPH. A draft version was provided as a background document to support the discussion of SMPH and the development of appropriate recommendations by the WHO Committee of Experts on Measurement and Classification for Health (See Section 4).

MEASURING HEALTH STATUS

Following the Marrakech conference on SMPH, WHO undertook expert consultations on the measurement of health status during 2000, leading to a Meeting on Measuring Health Status held in Ottawa on 23–25 October 2000. This meeting was jointly sponsored by WHO Headquarters and the United Nations Statistical Commission and Economic Commission for Europe (UN/ECE), and hosted by Statistics Canada.

Two preparatory working group meetings of experts on measuring health status were held in Geneva during August and September 2000 to prepare for the Ottawa meeting.

The main objectives of the Ottawa meeting were:

- To review briefly the major health policy and related considerations driving the need for internationally comparable population health status information.

- To share information on and review the status and direction of a number of key initiatives currently underway, regarding the development of health status measures, particularly in relation to international comparability.

- To discuss new approaches for the collection and analysis of such data.

- To present a proposal from WHO for a generic framework for internationally comparable health status measurement based on the ICF (ICIDH-2).

- To develop specific approaches and actions leading to a broadened consensus on a framework, as well as concrete actions for its adoption and implementation.

Background

For several years, the Conference of European Statisticians (CES) has had as its objective in the area of health statistics "To develop a comprehensive and coherent system of health statistics capable of supporting policy analysis and decision-making in the field of health, particularly monitoring the inputs, outputs and outcomes of the health care system in both monetary and non-monetary terms." In pursuit of this objective, a Joint UN/ECE-WHO Meeting on Health Statistics (CES/AC.38/1998/3) was held on 14–16 October 1998 in Rome. This meeting strongly recommended that the Conference encourage international organizations involved in health statistics to increase their cooperation and coordination in those areas of health data collections and research not yet adequately coordinated. The meeting further suggested that the Conference give a higher priority to the area of health statistics and that its work programme focus more on the conceptual issues of measurement, classifications, standardization and harmonization of data.

As a result, the agenda of the Conference of European Statisticians (CES) meeting on 14–16 June 1999 in Neuchatel devoted an hour to discussing issues in health statistics. This meeting concluded that the area of health should be a priority area and that coordination should be further encouraged in international health work and data collection. Furthermore, intellectual leadership should be promoted to advance conceptual issues of measurements and classifications. Finally, a health monitoring system capable of supporting policy analysis and decision-making in the field of health should be the long-term goal of the Conference's work. The meeting also endorsed an international experts conference in Ottawa in 2000 to follow up the October 1998 Joint UN/ECE-WHO Rome meeting.

In December 1999, the OECD, with the sponsorship of the US Department of Health and Human Services, organized a meeting on the implications of disability for ageing populations. Among the conclusions of this meeting were that policy-oriented discussions were seriously hampered by the lack of internationally comparable data and that development of valid and comparable statistical measures (based on a coherent and agreed upon conceptual framework), as well as further analysis of the primary topic of the meeting, should be top priorities of the OECD.

Objectives of the Ottawa Meeting

In early 2000, it was decided to enhance the scope of the Ottawa Meeting to move beyond review and discussion of the existing initiatives in order to capitalize on the efforts underway at WHO Headquarters to develop a generic framework for health status assessment with a particular focus on cross-population comparability. Measures of health that are valid and comparable cross-nationally necessitate not only a common conceptual approach, but also common operational methods. In practice, this translates to a common process for data collection, analysis and reporting of core measures of health, whether at the global, regional or national level. Reviews of the existing methods by several organizations and groups, such as the OECD, REVES, WHO/HQ, WHO/EURO and EC, had revealed an array of data collection approaches and instruments, different methods to analyse and report multidimensional profiles or indicators of health status, and a lack of interpretation guidelines for the obtained estimates. These issues seriously hamper the comparison of the collected data and substantially limit the utility of these data for health policy. With regard to the increasing priority of assessing trends in health status and linking them as outcomes of health policy, it was decided that the Ottawa meeting should address this fundamental objective.

Preparatory Working Group Meetings

Two preparatory Working Group Meetings were held in Geneva on 2–3 August and 4–5 September 2000, to consider these issues and to advise on the preparation of the agenda and agenda papers for the Ottawa Meeting. The agendas for these preparatory meetings and the participants in them are listed in Annex 15.2.

Joint UN/ECE and WHO Meeting on Measuring Health Status, Ottawa, 23–25 October 2000

The meeting was attended by 41 experts from the following countries: Australia, Canada, Denmark, France, Italy, Netherlands, France, New Zealand, Spain, United Kingdom and United States. Eurostat, OECD, World Bank, Inter American Development Bank, WHO/EURO, WHO/PAHO and the United Nations Statistical Division were represented as well. The agenda of the meeting and the participants in it are listed in Annex 15.3.

The meeting concluded that enhancing cross-population comparability of health status is important and that it raises significant issues for the use of health status data within countries, especially those with ethnically or culturally diverse populations. The meeting considered the WHO framework a major step towards the meaningful connection of health status assessment to health policy, and recommended development of operational standards and transparent methods of analysis.

The candidate domains for inclusion in the standardized health state measurement instrument were discussed in detail and six of the 21 domains were singled out to form a shorter profile as the basis of SMPHs: mobility, self-care, social functioning, pain, affect, and cognition.

The meeting examined the utility of various methods for assessing cross-population comparability of survey item responses. The strong assumptions necessary to use methods such as Rasch analysis and Differential Item Functioning were highlighted in the discussion, leading to the recognition of the inability to assess cross-population comparability without external criteria. WHO speakers presented new methodological work in this area using measured tests and vignettes to provide external calibration of self-response items.

The meeting ended with a discussion of the need for methodological advances and systematic collection of evidence on how to test and adjust for cross-population comparability.

MEASUREMENT AND CLASSIFICATION FOR HEALTH

In order to prepare a draft of recommendations on the measurement and classification of health status for the consideration of the WHO Executive Board and the 2001 World Health Assembly, WHO convened a Committee of Experts on Measurement and Classification for Health, which met in Geneva on 11–12 September 2000. The agenda and the members of the Committee of Experts are shown in Annex 15.4.

The Committee of Experts considered the following three components of a common health-reporting framework:

■ WHO Family of International Classifications on Health.

■ Operational Systems of Data Collection on Health States of Populations.

■ Summary Measures of Population Health.

The Committee of Experts made a series of recommendations on the development of these components of a common framework for reporting on population health status.

WHO FAMILY OF INTERNATIONAL CLASSIFICATIONS ON HEALTH

The International Classification of Impairments, Disabilities and Handicaps (ICIDH) was created in 1975 (WHA Resolution 43.24) to report the consequences of diseases and the needs of individuals. ICIDH was used in several countries for field trial purposes and a revision process was commenced in 1995 to address various issues, including the need to use ICIDH as a framework for the reporting of the health status of populations. Over the five years between 1995 and 2000, several collaborating centres, governmental and non-governmental organizations have taken part in the revision and field-testing of three successive versions of the classification. Following an extensive consultation process during this five year period (not documented here), the Pre-final Version of the ICIDH Revision 2 was examined by the Committee of Experts, who recommended its endorsement by the WHO Executive Board and the World Health Assembly.

Renamed the International Classification of Functioning, Disability and Health (ICF), this classification was endorsed by the World Health Assembly in May 2001 as a member of the WHO family of international classifications on health[3].

OPERATIONAL SYSTEMS FOR DATA COLLECTION ON HEALTH STATES OF POPULATIONS

Building on the work of the Ottawa meeting and on the results of pilot applications of a standardized health status survey module in the general population of several Member States, the Committee of Experts concluded that cross-population comparability is an essential requirement for reporting on health for the WHO Member States, in addition to cross-cultural applicability, reliability and validity. It recommended that the Member States use an explicit strategy to establish cross-population comparability, which be incorporated into the common instrument design for each health domain. Finally, it recommended that a subset of core health domains selected from ICF form the basis of the development of this common survey instrument for measuring health states in general populations (see Appendix 9 of ICF).

Summary Measures of Population Health

The Committee of Experts deliberated on the need for standardized summary measures of population health that are sensitive to both mortality and non-fatal health outcomes to report on the average level of population health for the WHO Member States. The experts concluded that the comparison of levels and distribution of population health for the Member States requires a positive summary measure of population health, healthy life expectancy, whereas reporting on the causes of loss of population health to inform policy formation and evaluation requires health gaps measures. The Committee also recommended that:

- Since both the distribution of health within populations and the level of health are important, separate summary measures should be used to report on the two.

- Since health state valuations are a critical input to the reporting of both health expectancies and health gaps, health state valuations should be measured in population-representative samples in each Member State.

- WHO, in consultation with the Member States and the appropriate expert networks, should develop guidelines and standards for the calculation and reporting of summary measures of population health for purposes of international comparison.

Notes

1 Conference on Summary Measures of Population Health, Marrakech, Morocco, 6–9 December 1999; 1st Preparatory Working Group Meeting on Measuring Health Status, Geneva, Switzerland, 2–3 August 2000; 2nd Preparatory Working Group Meeting on Measuring Health Status, Geneva, Switzerland, 4–5 September 2000; Meeting of Committee of Experts on Measurement and Classification for Health, Geneva, Switzerland, 11–12 September 2000; Joint ECE/WHO Expert Meeting on Measuring Health Status, Ottawa, Canada, 23–25 October 2000.

2 Murray CJL et al., eds. *Summary measures of population health: concepts, ethics, measurement and applications.* Geneva, World Health Organization, 2002.

3 World Health Organization. *International Classification of Functioning, Disability and Health (ICF).* Geneva, World Health Organization, 2001.

Annex 15.1
Conference on Summary Measures of Population Health
Marrakech, Morocco, 6–9 December 1999

Agenda

6 December 1999

Opening Ceremony

Dr Abdelouahed El Fassi, Minister of Health, Morocco

Session I: Uses of Summary Measures of Population Health

Chair	Dr J. Marks, CDC, USA
Speaker	Dr P. van der Maas, Erasmus University Rotterdam, Netherlands
Discussants	Dr G. Mooney, University of Sydney, Australia
	Dr P. Mahapatra, HACA Bhavan, Hyderbad, India

Session II: Basic Concepts and Data Inputs for Summary Measures of Population Health

Chair	Dr J. Marks, CDC, USA
Speaker	GPE/WHO
Discussants	Dr D. Brock, Brown University, USA
	Dr J. Richardson, Australia

Session III: Health Expectancies

Chair	Dr E. Crimmins, University of Southern California, USA
Speaker	Dr C. Mathers, Australian Institute of Health and Welfare, Australia
Discussants	Dr J.M. Robine, INSERM, France
	Dr E. Sondik, NCHS, USA

Session IV: Health Gaps

Chair	Dr E. Crimmins, University of Southern California, USA
Speaker	GPE/WHO
Discussant	Dr A. Hyder, Johns Hopkins University, USA
	Dr J. Barendregt, Erasmus University Rotterdam, Netherlands

7 December 1999

Session V: Incidence and Prevalence Issues in Summary Measures of Population Health

Chair	Dr M. Wolfson, Statistics Canada
Speaker	Dr J. Barendregt, Erasmus University Rotterdam, Netherlands
Discussants	Dr J. Broome, University of St Andrew's, UK GPE/WHO

Session VI: Decomposition of Summary Measures of Population Health into Contributions of Different Diseases, Injuries and Risk Factors

Chair	Dr M. Wolfson, Statistics Canada, Canada
Speaker	Dr S. Greenland, University of California, USA
Discussants	Dr C. Mathers, Australian Institute of Health and Welfare, Australia GPE/WHO

Session VII: Health Status Descriptions and Classification Approaches

Chair	Dr A. Mechbal, WHO/EMRO
Speaker	Dr I. McDowell, University of Ottawa, Canada
Discussants	Dr D. Feeny, University of Alberta, Canada
	Dr M.L. Essink-Bot, Erasmus University Rotterdam, The Netherlands GPE/WHO

Session VIII: Self-Reported versus Observed Measures of Health

Chair	Dr A. Mechbal, WHO/EMRO
Speaker	Dr D. Thomas, RAND/UCLA, USA
Discussants	Dr A. Sebai, American University of Beirut, Lebanon GPE/WHO

8 DECEMBER 1999

Session IX: Overview of Methods and Valuation Instruments

Speaker	Dr M. L. Essink-Bot, Erasmus University Rotterdam, Netherlands
Discussants	Dr P. Mahapatra, HACA Bhavan, Hyderbad, India
	Dr J. Richardson, Centre for Health Program Evaluation, Australia GPE/WHO

Session X: Modelling the Relations between Health Status Domains and Health State Valuations

Chair	Dr P. van der Maas, Erasmus University Rotterdam, Netherlands
Speaker	Dr P. Dolan, University of Sheffield, UK
Discussants	Dr D. Feeny, University of Alberta, Canada
	Dr C. Mathers, Australian Institute of Health and Welfare, Australia

Session XI: Determinants of variance in health state valuations

Chair	Dr P. van der Maas, Erasmus University Rotterdam, Netherlands
Speaker	Dr J. Sommerfeld, University of Heidelberg, Germany
Discussants	Dr P. Dolan, University of Sheffield, UK GPE/WHO

Session XII: Goodness: Conceptual and Ethical Issues

Speaker	Dr J. Broome, The University of St Andrew's, UK
Discussants	Dr E. Nord, National Institute of Public Health, Norway
	Dr D. Hausman, University of Wisconsin, USA

9 DECEMBER 1999

Session XIII: Fairness and Equity

Chair	Dr D. Wikler, WHO
Speakers:	Dr F. Kamm, New York University, USA GPE/WHO
Discussants	Dr D Brock, Brown University, USA
	Dr F. Peter, Harvard Center for Population and Development Studies, USA

Session XIV: Social Value Choices in Summary Measures of Population Health

Chair	Dr D. Wikler, WHO
Speaker	Dr A. Tsuchiya, University of York, UK
Discussants	Dr J. Richardson, Centre for Health Program Evaluation, Australia
	Dr J. Barendregt, Erasmus University Rotterdam, The Netherlands
	Dr N. Dachs, Pan American Health Organization, USA

Review and Closing Session

	Dr J. Marks, CDC, USA
	Dr A. Mechbal, WHO/EMRO

LIST OF PARTICIPANTS

Dr Jan Barendregt
Department of Public Health
Faculty of Medicine
Erasmus University of Rotterdam
Netherlands

Dr Dan W. Brock
Professor of Philosophy and
  Biomedical Ethics
Director, Center for Biomedical
  Ethics
Dept. of Philosophy
Brown University
Providence
USA

Dr J. Broome
Department of Moral Philosophy
The University of St Andrews
Fife
United Kingdom

Dr Eileen M. Crimmins
Andrus Gerontology Center
University of Southern California
Los Angeles
USA

Dr MS. Concha
ACHS
Holanda 1555
Departamento 202
Providencia, Santiago
Chile

Dr P. Dolan
Reader in Health Economics
Sheffield Health Economics
    Group
Department of Economics
University of Sheffield
Sheffield
United Kingdom

Dr M. L. Essink-Bot
Department of Public Health
Erasmus University Rotterdam
Netherlands

Dr David Feeny
Merck Frosst Chair
Faculty of Pharmacy and
    Pharmaceutical Sciences
University of Alberta
Edmonton
Canada

Dr Dan Hausman
Chair
Department of Philosophy
University of Wisconsin
Madison, WI
USA

Dr Adnan A. Hyder
Research Associate
Department of International
    Health
School of Hygiene and Public
    Health
Johns Hopkins University
Baltimore
USA

Dr Erik Nord
National Institute of Public
    Health,
Oslo
Norway

Dr Frances M. Kamm
Department of Philosophy
New York University
USA

Dr Soewarta Kosen
National Institute of Health,
    Research and Development
Jakarta
Indonesia

Dr M. McKenna
National Center for Chronic
    Diseases, Prevention and
    Health, CDC
Atlanta
USA

Mr Gaetan Lafortune
Health Policy Unit
Organization for Economic Co-
    operation and Development
    (OECD)
Paris
France

Dr Jim Marks
National Center for Chronic
    Diseases, Prevention and
    Health, CDC
Atlanta
USA

Dr Colin D. Mathers
Principal Research Fellow
Australian Institute of Health and
    Welfare
Canberra
Australia

Dr Prasanta Mahapatra
Director
The Institute of Health Systems
Hyderabad
India

Dr Ian McDowell
University of Ottawa
Epidemiology and Community
    Medicine
Ontario
Canada

Dr Sander Greenland
Topanga, California
USA

Dr Catherine Michaud
Senior Research Associate
Burden of Disease Unit
Harvard Centre for Population
    and Development Studies
Cambridge, MA
USA

Dr Gavin Mooney
Director, Social and Public Health
    Economics Research Group
    (SPHERE)
Department of Public Health and
    Community Medicine
University of Sydney
Australia

Dr Jeff Richardson
Director, Health Economics Unit
Centre for Health Program
    Evaluation
West Heidelberg, Victoria
Australia

Dr J-M. Robine
INSERM Démographie et Santé
Montpellier
France

Dr Abla Mehio Siai
American University of Beirut
Faculty of Health Sciences
Department of Epidemiology and
    Biostatistics
Beirut
Lebanon

Dr Edward J. Sondik
Director
National Center Health Statistics
Hyattsville, Maryland
USA

Dr Johannes Sommerfeld
Department of Tropical Hygiene
    and Public Health
Ruprecht-Karls University of
    Heidelberg
Germany

Dr Duncan Thomas
RAND/UCLA
Santa Monica, California
USA

Dr Aki Tsuchiya
Centre for Health Economics
(RISS)
University of York
United Kingdom

Dr Paul Van Der Maas
Department of Public Health
Erasmus University Rotterdam
Rotterdam 3000 DR
Netherlands

Dr Theo Vos
Public Health and Development
Department of Human Services
Victorian Government
Melbourne
Australia

Dr Michael Wolfson
Director General
Analysis and Development
Statistics Canada
Ottawa, Ontario
Canada

WHO Secretariat

Dr Christopher J.L. Murray
Executive Director
Evidence and Information for
  Policy

Ms Gabriella M. Covino
Evidence and Information for
  Policy

Dr N. Dachs
Regional Office for the Americas/
  Pan American Sanitary Bureau

Dr David B. Evans
Evidence and Information for
  Policy

Mr Jeremy A. Lauer
Evidence and Information for
  Policy

Dr Alan D. Lopez
Evidence and Information for
  Policy

Dr Rafael Lozano
Evidence and Information for
  Policy

Mr Kim Moesgaard-Iburg
Evidence and Information for
  Policy

Dr Abdelhay Mechbal
Evidence and Information for
  Policy

Dr Ouakrim
Regional Advisor EIP
Eastern Mediterranean Regional
  Office

Dr B. Sabri
Regional Advisor
Eastern Mediterranean Regional
  Office

Dr Ritu Sadana
Evidence and Information for
  Policy

Mr Joshua A. Salomon
Evidence and Information for
  Policy

Dr Tessa Tan Torres Edejer
Evidence and Information for
  Policy

Dr T. Bedirhan Üstün
Evidence and Information for
  Policy

Dr Daniel Wikler
Evidence and Information for
  Policy

Annex 15.2
Preparatory Working Group Meetings on Measuring Health Status
Geneva, Switzerland, 2–3 August, 4–5 September 2000

Agenda

2–3 August 2000

I. Review and Discuss WHO Draft Framework on Health Status Assessment

II. Review of Strengths and Limitations of Item Response Theory

III. New Approaches to Improving Comparability of Health Status Data across Countries

IV. Design Issues for Proposed WHO Standardized Health Status Measurement Instrument

4–5 September 2000

I. Introduction and Update on Draft WHO Recommendations

II. Overview of First Working Group Meeting

III. Design of Standardized Health Status Module

Background and Criteria for Selection of Domains and Items

Background and Selection of Observed Calibration Tests: Physical Locomotion, Cognitive and Vision Tests

IV. Selection of Domains and Items

Domains, Items, ICIDH Classification and Relation to Existing Instruments

Domains for Health Status Assessment vs. Domains for Health State Valuations

V. Cross-Population Comparability

Current Status of New Statistical Methods (IRT with Exogenous Calibration)

Calibration Techniques: Vignettes and Reference Populations

Calibration Techniques: Observed Tests

VI. Preparation of Working Papers for Ottawa Meeting

List of Participants

Dr Jordi Alonso
Head, Health Services Research
  Unit
Institut Municipal d'Investigacio
  Medica (IMIM)
Barcelona
Spain

Dr Gouke Bonsel
Department of Social Medicine/
  Public Health
University of Amsterdam
Netherlands

Dr Jacques Bonte
EUROSTAT
Luxembourg

Dr Marijke W. de Kleijn de
  Vrankrijker
TNO
Leiden
Netherlands

Dr Jeff Koplan
Director
Centers for Disease Control and
  Prevention
Atlanta
USA

Dr Edward J. Sondik
Director
National Center Health Statistics
Hyattsville, Maryland
USA

Prof. Alan Tennant
Rheumatology and Rehabilitation
    Research Unit
University of Leeds
Leeds
United Kingdom

Dr Michael Wolfson
Director General
Analysis and Development
Statistics Canada
Ottawa, Ontario
Canada

WHO Secretariat

Dr Christopher J.L. Murray
Executive Director
Evidence and Information for
    Policy

Dr Somnath Chatterji
Evidence and Information for
    Policy

Dr Alan D. Lopez
Evidence and Information for
    Policy

Dr Colin D. Mathers
Evidence and Information for
    Policy

Dr Ritu Sadana
Evidence and Information for
    Policy

Dr T. Bedirhan Üstün
Evidence and Information for
    Policy

Annex 15.3
Joint UNECE/WHO Meeting on Measuring Health Status
Ottawa, Canada, 23–25 October 2000

Agenda

23 October 2000

Official Opening

Ivan Felligi, Chief Statistician, Statistics Canada

Session I: The Uses of and Needs for Population Health Status Measures

Chair	Michael Wolfson, Statistics Canada
Speakers	Ed Sondik, National Centre for Health Statistics, USA
	Michael Decter, Chairman of the Canadian Institute for Health Information
	John Fox, Chief Statistician, Department of Health, United Kingdom
	Marleen De Smedt, Eurostat

Session II: Roundtable on National Initiatives

Chair	Alan D. Lopez, WHO
Speakers	Healthy People 2000 (retrospective) and 2010 (prospective): Jennifer Madans, NCHS, USA
	Institute of Medicine Work, and Other Initiatives: Marthe Gold, NYLI, USA
	Gary Catlin, Statistics Canada
	Richard Madden, Director, Australian Institute of Health and Welfare, Australia
	Vittoria Buratti, Italian National Statistical Institute (ISTAT)
	Niels K. Rasmussen, Danish Institute for Clinical Epidemiology (DICE)
	Siobhan Carey, Office of National Statistics UK (ONS)
	Martin Tobias, Ministry of Health of New Zealand

Jean-Louis Lanoe, Institut National de la Statistique et des Etudes Economiques (INSEE), France

Session III: International Agencies' Initiatives

Chair	Gary Catlin, Statistics Canada
Speakers	Marleen De Smedt, Eurostat
	Pieter Kramers, National Institute of Public Health and the Environment, Netherlands
	Anatoli Nossikov, WHO/EURO
	Norberto Dachs, WHO/PAHO
	Manfred Huber, OECD
	Margaret Mbogoni, UNSD
	Margaret Rothman, Johnson and Johnson

Session IV: Towards a Framework for Measuring Population Health Status

Chair	Ed Sondik, NCHS, USA
Speakers	Michael Wolfson, Statistics Canada
	Christopher J.L. Murray, WHO/GPE
	T. Bedirhan Üstün, WHO/GPE
	Alan D. Lopez, WHO/GPE

24 October 2000

Session V: Critical Review of the Comparability of Surveys and Data

Chair	Richard Madden, Australian Institute of Health and Welfare
Speakers	Marleen De Smedt, Eurostat— European Survey
	Gaetan Lafortune, OECD— OECD Survey
	Niels Rasmussen, EURO— REVES Experience
	Ritu Sadana, WHO/HQ— WHO Analysis

Session VI: Use of Existing Standardized Health Status Measures at the National Level

Chair   John Millar, CIHI, Canada

Speakers   Siobhan Carey, ONS, United Kingdom

               Jean-Marie Berthelot and Julie Bernier, Statistics Canada

Session VII: Comparability of Health Status Assessment Methods

Chair   Marijke de Kleijn-de-Vrankrijker, TNO Prevention and Health, Netherlands

Speakers   John Ware, Quality Metric, Inc, USA

               Alan Tenant, University of Leeds, United Kingdom

Gouke Bonsel, University of Amsterdam, Netherlands

Session VIII: New Methodological Approaches towards Cross-Population Comparability. External Calibration

Chair   Gouke Bonsel, University of Amsterdam, Netherlands

Speakers   Christopher J.L. Murray, WHO/GPE

25 OCTOBER 2000

Session IX: Perspectives on Health Status Assessment and the WHO Common Framework: Discussion

Chair   Michael Wolfson, Statistics Canada

Speakers   Ed Sondik, USA

               John Fox, United Kingdom

LIST OF PARTICIPANTS

Richard Madden
Director
Australian Institute of Health and Welfare
Canberra
Australia

Julie Bernier
Health Analysis Modelling Group
Social and Economics Studies Division
Statistics Canada
Ottawa
Canada

Jean-Marie Berthelot
Health Analysis Modelling Group
Social and Economics Studies Division
Statistics Canada
Ottawa
Canada

Gary Catlin
Health Statistics Division
Statistics Canada
Ottawa
Canada

Michael Decter
Canadian Institute for Health Information (CIIII)
Lawrence Decter Investment Counsel Inc.
Toronto
Canada

David Feeny
Faculty of Pharmacy and Pharmaceutical Sciences
University of Alberta
Edmonton, Alberta
Canada

Ivan Fellegi
Chief Statistician of Canada
Statistics Canada
Ottawa
Canada

Anil Gupta
Microsimulation Modelling and Data Analysis Division
Health Canada
Canada

Lan McDowell
Department of Epidemiology and Community Medicine
University of Ottawa
Ottawa
Canada

John Millar
Research and Population Health
Canadian Institute for Health Information (CIHI)
Ottawa
Canada

Janice Miller
Canadian Institute for Health Information (CIHI)
Ottawa
Canada

Louise Ogilvie
Canadian Institute for Health Information
Ottawa
Canada

Sylvain Paradis
Quantative Analysis and Research
   Section
Stragetic Policy Directorate
Health Canada
Ottawa
Canada

Daniel Tremblay
Santé Québec
Institut de la statistique
   du Québec
McGill College
Montreal, Québec
Canada

Michael Wofflon
Assistant Chief Statistician
Analysis and Development Field
Statistics Canada
Ottawa
Canada

Niels Rasmussen
National Institute of Public
   Health
Copenhagen
Denmark

Jean-Louis Lanoe
INSEE
18 Boulevard Adolphe Pinard
Paris
France

Vittoria Buratta
Department of Social Statistics
ISTAT (Italian National Statistical
   Institute)
Rome
Italy

Viviana Egidi
Director
Department of Social Statistics
ISTAT (Italian National Statistical
   Institute)
Rome
Italy

Gouke Bonsel
Department of Social Medicine
   and Public Health
University of Amsterdam
Amsterdam
Netherlands

Marijke de Kleijn-de-Vrankrijker
TNO Prevention and Health
Leiden
Netherlands

Pieter Kramers
Deputy Head, Department of
   Public Health Forecasting
National Institute of Public
   Health and the Environment
Bilthoven
Netherlands

Martin Tobias
Ministry of Health
Wellington
New Zealand

Jordi Alonso
Head, Health Services Research
   Unit
Insitut Municipal d'lnvestigacio
   Medica (IMIM)
Barcelona
Spain

Siobhan Carey
Office for National Statistics
London
United Kingdom

John Fox
Director of Statistics
Department of Health
London
United Kingdom

Paul Kind
Outcomes Research Group
Centre for Health Economics
University of York
York
United Kingdom

Alan Tennant
Rheumatology and Rehabilitation
   Research Unit
University of Leeds
Leeds
United Kingdom

Steven Cohen
Center For Cost and Financing
   Studies
Agency for Healthcare Research
   and Quality
Rockville, MD
USA

Dennis Fryback
Preventive Medicine
Program in Population Health
University of Wisconsin-Madison
Madison, Wisconsin
USA

Marthe R. Gold
Department of Community
   Health and Social Medicine
City University of New York
   Medical School
New York, NY
USA

Michael Wolfson
Director General
Analysis and Development
Statistics Canada
Ottawa, Ontario
Canada

Marjorle S. Greenberg
Data Policy and Standards
National Center for Health
   Statistics
Hyattsville, Maryland
USA

Jennifer H. Madans
National Center for Health
   Statistics
Hyattsville, Maryland
USA

William Marton
Office of the Assistant Secretary
  for Planning and Evaluation
U.S. Department of Health and
  Human Services
Washington, DC
USA

David McQueen
National Center for Chronic
  Disease Prevention and Health
  Promotion
Centers for Disease Control and
  Prevention
Atlanta, Georgia
USA

Gregory Pappas
Deputy Director
Macro International
Calverton, MD
USA

Margaret Rothman
Health Economics
Johnson and Johnson
Titusville, NJ
USA

Joint UNECE/WHO Secretariat

Lene Mikkelsen
ECE Statistical Division
United Nations, Geneva

Dr Alan D. Lopez
Evidence and Information for
  Policy

Dr Christopher J.L. Murray
Executive Director
Evidence and Information for
  Policy

James Schuttinga
National Institutes of Health
Office of Science Policy
Bethesda, MD
USA

Edward Sondik
National Center for Health
  Statistics (NCHS)
Hyattsville, Maryland
USA

Lois M. Verbrugge
Institute of Gerontology
University of Michigan
Ann Arbor, Michigan
USA

John Ware
QUALITYMETRIC, Inc.
Lincoln, RI
USA

International Organizations

Margaret Mbogoni
United Nations Statistics Division
New York, NY
USA

Marleen De Smedt
Statistics on Health and Safety
Statistical Office of the European
  Communities
European Commission—Eurostat
Luxembourg

Manfred Huber
OECD Health Policy Unit
Directorate for Education,
  Employment, Labour and
  Social Affairs
Paris
France

Gaetan Lafortune
OECD Health Policy Unit
Directorate for Education,
  Employment, Labour and
  Social Affairs
OECD
Paris
France

Deon Filmer
The World Bank
Washington, DC
USA

Anatoly Nossikov, M.D.
Health Information Unit
World Health Organization
Regional Office for Europe
Copenhagen
Denmark

Norberto Dachs
Public Policy in Health Program
Pan-American Health
  Organization
Washington, DC
USA

Jose Antonio Mejia-Guerra
MECOVI-lDB
Inter American Development Bank
Washington, DC
USA

Dr Ritu Sadana
Evidence and Information for
  Policy

Dr T. Bedirhan Üstün
Evidence and Information for
  Policy

Annex 15.4
Meeting of Committee of Experts on Measurement and Classification for Health
Geneva, Switzerland, 11–12 September 2000

Agenda

I. Provisional Agenda

II. Introduction of Participants

III. Election of Chairperson, Vice-Chairperson, Rapporteur

IV. WHO Family of International Classifications for Health: ICIDH Beta-2 Draft

V. Concepts and Operational Methods for Health Status Measurement

VI. Principles and Indicators for Summarizing Population Health

VII. Recommendations and Next Steps

VIII. Closure of Meeting

Associated Documents

Document 1. *Measuring and Reporting on the Health of Populations*

Document 2: *WHO Family of International Classifications on Health*

Document 3: *Survey Measurement of Health Status of Populations*

Document 4: *Summary Measures of Population Health—Requirements and Standards*

Background Annex: *ICIDH-2 Pre-final Draft Short Version*

List of Participants

Dr Farid Abolhassani
Director General
Ministry of Health and Medical
  Education
Primary Health Care Department
Teheran
Iran

Dr Jacob Adetunji
Sociology Department
Bowling Green State University
Bowling Green
USA

Dr Debbie Bradshaw
Burden of Disease Unit
Medical Research Council
Tygerberg
South Africa

Dr Marisol Concha-Barrientos
Project Director, ACHS
Professor Universidad de Chile
Adviser, Ministry of Health
Santiago
Chile

Dr Peter M. Kilima
Regional Representative
International Trachoma Initiative
Dar es Salaam
Tanzania

Dr Katarzyna Kissimova-Skarbek
Head of the Department of
  Health Economics, Finance and
  Accounting
School of Public Health
Krakow
Poland

Dr Jeff Koplan
Director
Centers for Disease Control and
  Prevention
Atlanta
USA

Dr Soewarta Kosen
National Institute of Health
  Research and Development
Jakarta
Indonesia

Dr M. Laaziri
Directeur de la Planification et
  des Ressources Financières
Ministère de la Santé
Rabat
Morocco

Prof. Ruy Laurenti
Head, WHO Collaborating
  Centre for Classification of
  Diseases in Portuguese
School of Public Health
University of Sao Paulo
Sao Paulo
Brazil

Dr Prasanta Mahapatra
Director
Institute of Health Systems
Hyderabad
India

Dr Paul Van Der Maas
Department of Public Health
Erasmus University Rotterdam
Rotterdam
Netherlands

Dr Kenji Shibuya
Department of Hygiene and
  Public Health
Teikyo School of Medicine
Tokyo
Japan

Dr Martin Tobias
Ministry of Health
Wellington
New Zealand

WHO Secretariat

Dr Christopher J.L. Murray
Evidence and Information for
  Policy

Dr Somnath Chatterji
Evidence and Information for
  Policy

Dr Alan D. Lopez
Evidence and Information for
  Policy

Dr Colin D. Mathers
Evidence and Information for
  Policy

Dr Ritu Sadana
Evidence and Information for
  Policy

Dr T. Bedirhan Üstün
Evidence and Information for
  Policy

Part IV

METHODS
AND
EMPIRICISM

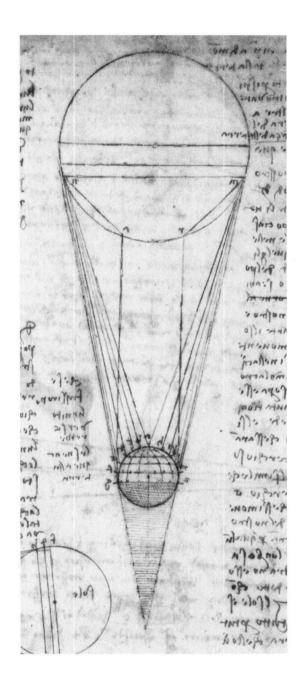

Chapter 16

NATIONAL HEALTH ACCOUNTS: CONCEPTS, DATA SOURCES, AND METHODOLOGY

JEAN-PIERRE POULLIER, PATRICIA HERNANDEZ, KEI KAWABATA

INTRODUCTION

Major technological advances, demographic transition, changing patterns in burden of disease, and rising incomes have increased the need and demand for health services around the world. By 2000, almost a third (57 of 191) of the countries that were then members of WHO devoted more than 7% of their entire GDP to health. This includes low-income as well as middle and high-income countries.

In many OECD countries the most pressing issue in health financing is how to provide the current level of care efficiently. In many developing countries the issue is how to equitably and efficiently make available a minimum set of interventions that address the increased incidence and prevalence of communicable diseases such as HIV/AIDS, malaria, and tuberculosis, while at the same time face the challenges of the growth of non-communicable diseases associated with the demographic transition. In these countries, the demand for health services exceeds the capacity of the government to finance them despite the availability of external assistance, so a high proportion of total health expenditure is paid out-of-pocket by households. This puts households at risk of catastrophic spending and possible impoverishment (1).

As early as the 1960s, WHO responded to a growing desire by health ministries to better understand patterns of health spending in their countries and to learn from the experiences of other countries. It undertook a six-country comparative study of health expenditures and, in 1963, used the findings to publicize the importance of regular, standardized health expenditure reviews (2). A further study of 14 developing countries was completed and published in 1967 (3). During the same period, the US government was preparing to enact legislation providing publicly funded health insurance for the elderly and the poor.[1] Anticipating the need for a tool that allowed comparison of the financial performance of those programmes with the predominant private-sector insurance programmes, policy analysts revived the health accounts framework first developed in the 1930s (4) and began producing annual estimates of "national health expenditures," starting in 1966.

Today, only the member states of the Organisation for Economic Co-operation and Development (OECD)[2] report health expenditures in a standardized manner on an annual basis. Globally, more than 60 countries have undertaken one or more exercises in health accounting, although they are not all available internationally. A limited amount of information for a limited set of countries is reported annually in the World Development Indicators of the World Bank. Since 2000, WHO has been reporting more detailed information on its Member States each year in its *World Health Report*.

In 2000, the OECD published its manual *A system of health accounts* (5). It provided a framework for National Health Accounts (NHA) producers who wished to use the OECD standardized approach developed over 15 years. This manual represents a milestone in the establishment of an international standard for NHA, but its primary audience is that of high-income countries, excluding some considerations specific to developing countries. One example is the role of external resources such as donor funds in financing care. In an effort to encourage other countries to produce NHA, the United States Agency for International Development (USAID), the World Bank (WB), and the World Health Organization (WHO) jointly sponsored the development of a complementary manual, *A guide to producing National Health Accounts: with special applications for low and middle income countries* (6). It is denoted by the term PG (producer's guide) in the subsequent text. The remainder of this chapter highlights key concepts from the PG that guide the development of estimates of health expenditure reported by WHO.

Concepts

Purpose

National Health Accounts (NHA) systematically trace all the resources that flow through the health system in a country in a given year. They are presented as a set of tables or matrices which identify who pays for health, how much is paid, through what intermediary, what the payment is spent on, and who benefits. As NHA are designed to be comprehensive, consistent, standardized, and recurrent, they are valuable tools for monitoring a country's health resource flows over time.

The primary purpose is to provide a useful policy tool for policy-makers, which shows the complex interactions that occur from the moment funds are allocated to the health system, to the moment they reach a beneficiary. NHA transcribe them into a traceable flow. This enables governments to monitor the impact of their policies, to assess the effect of health system reforms, and generally to play their stewardship role. It encourages transparency and accountability.

There are other uses of NHA. For example, international comparisons of the level and structure of health expenditure can be used to assess questions of health systems performance. In addition, external funding agencies that provide resources in the form of grants (e.g. donor agencies) or loans (e.g. international financial institutions) require more accountability from intermediary financing agents and executing institutions. The need to be able to document resource flows is ever more important in developing countries. NHA tables can demonstrate whether donor funds resulted in a net increase in overall health expenditures, and if this increase reached the targeted population such as the poor. Since the proliferation of donor-specified projects has sometimes exacerbated health system inefficiencies, donor coordinated support through Sector-wide approach (SWAPs), Poverty Reduction Strategy Papers (PRSPs), and other broad budget support programmes have been encouraged. However, before such programmes could be implemented, clear mechanisms for accountability were essential. NHA have played a key role in enabling the monitoring and evaluation of this accountability.

Although NHA are essential for evidence-based policy-making, they are not sufficient. NHA remain a measurement tool, and do not replace the need for other types of information and discretionary decisions by policy-makers.

Basic Principles of NHA

NHA are constructed to disaggregate complex interactions into a sequence of discrete tables, in which all agents and transactions of the health care system are uniquely classified. When properly constructed, the accounts fit into the larger system of social economic accounts.

Both the OECD manual and the USAID/WB/WHO PG embody most of the principles of the System of National Accounts 1993 of the United Nations (SNA93) (7). National Health Accounts follow the accounting principals of national accounting. By and large, NHA should be comparable with the equivalent information in SNA93. There are, however, some important differences. On the one hand, National Health Accounts tend to focus on the production and consumption of goods and services in the economy as a whole, and are useful to policy-makers interested in tracing the factors of production, regardless of whether they are consumed locally or exported. On the other hand, National Health Accounts are more concerned with consumption of, and financing or payment for, health goods and services in the economy, and are useful to policy-makers interested in tracing the financial value of the resources used to pay for health care for the population.

Adapting from the PG (6), NHA are:

- *comprehensive*, covering the whole health system and all entities which act in or benefit from this system;

- *consistent*, using the same definitions, concepts, and principles for each entity and each transaction measured;

- *comparable across time and space*, allowing evaluation of changes in health expenditure over the years and of differences in experience among various geopolitical entities;

- *compatible with other aggregate economic measurement systems*, so that health expenditure can be examined in an overall economic context;

- *timely*, providing accurate and useful information when policy-makers need it;

- *accurate*, so that policy-makers can safely use the resulting information to make sound decisions;

- *sensitive to policy concerns*, giving information with the level of detail needed for good macroeconomic planning;

- *replicable*, ensuring the openness necessary for users to assess the validity of the figures they contain and for analysts to update and extend them.

NHA reflect a sequence of identities:

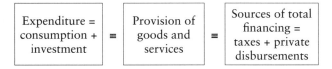

The nominal value (or, in its absence, the imputed value) of the total resources spent in a health system equals the sum of the value of all goods and services produced, which in turn equals the sum total of the resources provided to the health system.

DEFINITIONS AND CATEGORIZATIONS WITHIN NHA

Boundaries of a Health System

The PG defines the boundaries for the measurement of expenditures to be included in National Health Accounts to encompass all expenditures for activities whose primary purpose is to improve health during a defined period of time, regardless of the type of the institution/entity providing or paying for the health activity. This is consistent with the definition of the health system used by WHO (8). The OECD SHA manual restricts the definition to activities based on medical technology. The broader definition of the PG permits the inclusion of services by traditional healers as well as intersectoral activities whose primary intent is to improve health, for example, the enactment of seat belt legislation.

TIME-FRAME

NHA capture expenditure over a twelve-month period, based on a calendar year, unless otherwise stated. Expenditure is recorded based on national currency, current prices, and on an accrual basis, i.e. when resources are consumed and not when actual payments are made. For a situation analysis, an NHA-type exercise that covers only one year produces valuable finan-

cial information. For policy planning, monitoring, and evaluation, time series information is critical. Health accounting must become routine before it can be used regularly with confidence for policy-making.

Categorizing Health Expenditures

A full set of health accounts can be presented in a myriad of ways depending on what information is being sought by the policy-maker. Building on the OECD manual and the priorities defined in many NHA studies undertaken globally, the PG presents the six most common dimensions that policy-makers desire from health expenditure data. They are:

- Financing sources—institutions or entities that provide the funds used in the system by financing agents. The purpose is to distinguish between public funds, private funds, and funds provided by sources external to a country such as a donor. Public funds include those raised by all levels of government through taxes. Private sources include employer and household funds and those provided by nonprofit institutions serving individuals;

- Financing agents—institutions or entities that channel funds provided by financing sources and use these funds to pay for, or purchase, the activities inside the health accounts boundary. Based on the OECD International Classification for Health Accounts classification for financing agents (ICHA-HF), the latter are categorized into public and non-public sector institutions. The former includes all levels of government, social security funds, and parastatal organizations, for example. The latter comprises private health insurance, nongovernmental organizations, firms, and households through their out-of-pocket payments. There is usually a difference between the funds provided by entities which appear in the financing source matrix, e.g. households, and those channelled through the same entities that act as financing agents;

- Providers—entities that produce the activities included in the health accounts boundary. The classification proposed in the PG is based on the OECD International Classification for Health Accounts classification scheme for providers (ICHA-HP) and includes public and private hospitals, clinics, nursing homes, community health centres, independent physicians, etc., as well as the provision and administration of public health programmes;

- Functions—the types of goods and services provided and activities performed within the health accounts boundary, including inpatient services, ambulatory services, public health interventions, etc. Health related functions such as training of health personnel and health research are included here;

- Resources—often referred to as "line items," these are the factors or inputs used by providers or financing agents to produce goods and services consumed, or the activities conducted in the system. Resources include labour, pharmaceuticals, medical equipment, etc.; and

- Beneficiaries—the people who receive the goods and services or benefit from the activities of the health system. They can be categorized in a number of different ways, including by age and sex, socioeconomic status, health status, and location (6).

Some additional characteristics of NHA are important to note. First, the NHA matrices link the flow of funds between two dimensions for a given year. In many cases, a single type of expenditure can be associated with a number of categories simultaneously. Households, for instance, are the source of funds for three categories of financing agents—social medical insurance, private medical insurance, and out-of-pocket payments. Second, the dimensions to be analysed depend on predefined national priorities. It is not necessary to include all possible matrices in a particular NHA exercise; the extent of comprehensiveness depends entirely on the policy-maker's needs and availability of resources. If only aggregate level information is required, it would be an inefficient use of scarce resources to undertake surveys to identify expenditures by beneficiary groups.

Even a minimal set of aggregate level information can be very informative for local decision-making or cross-country comparisons. Since 2000, WHO has presented annually basic information about health expenditures in all its Member States in its *World Health Report*. It shows total and per capita health expenditures in the US and in international dollars, as well as expenditure as a proportion of GDP. It also presents indicators on financing agents with selected information on financing sources (9). As more information becomes available, additional matrices will be provided.

Data Sources

Before a team embarks on building National Health Accounts, it must have a good sketch of the country's health system and the actors within it. A data plan can then be established in relation to the scope of the study. A lot of the data are often found "off the shelf." However, only a small portion will be located at the Ministry of Health. Steering committees involving the multiple actors in the health system and sensitization campaigns are useful means to identify data from a wider range of sources.

Selected International Sources

- United Nations Population Division. *World population prospects: the 2002 revision population database* (10)

- International Monetary Fund. *International financial statistics* (11)

- International Monetary Fund. *Government financial statistics yearbook* (12)

- United Nations. *National accounts statistics: main aggregates and detailed tables* (13)

- Annex 5, *The World Health Report* provides aggregate data for all Member States of WHO, by financing source—external, public, private (14)

- Organisation for Economic Co-operation and Development *OECD Health Data 2002* (15)

- Household survey reports including those compiled by the International Labour Organization (ILO) (16)

- The Living Standard Measurement Survey and Poverty Survey reports of the World Bank (WB) (17)

- International Monetary Fund, World Bank, and other regional bank country and sector reports (sometimes with limited circulation)

- Economic Commission for Latin America and the Caribbean (ECLAC) (18)

Selected National Sources

- National Health Accounts reports where they exist. In many cases these provide detailed information for an earlier year as a base from which to extrapolate. More than 30 non-OECD countries have produced such reports at least once.

■ Other important national sources include statistical yearbooks; expenditure reports of the Ministry of Finance, Ministry of Health, social security institutions, and international funding agencies; existing NHA exercises; national reports of selected industries such as private medical insurance and the pharmaceutical sector; NGO reports; academic studies; household expenditure surveys; censuses; and administrative records. Information contained in the Ministry of Health will need to be supplemented by the activities of other government departments related to the health sector in order to obtain a complete picture of total government expenditure. This would include, for example, expenditure in social security agencies.

These disparate sources of national and international data are not always consistent and must be reconciled to produce valid and reliable information about a country's health expenditure. This step is facilitated by establishing a network of experts who can help to validate and combine different, sometimes conflicting, sources of information.

An additional problem is that sometimes the only data available for specific categories are either incomplete or outdated, and standard projection accounting techniques using extrapolation will be required. WHO is developing a library of estimates using these techniques, and countries that have not developed their own NHA can utilize this library as they begin their work. In the future, uncertainty intervals around the figures reported by WHO will be gradually introduced to clearly indicate the variation in the reliability of the data.

Selected Uses

The World Health Report 2000 identified stewardship as a key function in generating good health systems performance. Stewardship requires both intelligence and vision. Detailed information on health financing enables policy-makers to organize a strategic vision around information on the levels of resources available and their utilization. It helps them to better monitor the implementation of interventions and to evaluate the outcome of the policies adopted. The flow-of-funds information contained in NHA permits policy-makers to identify whether financing is in line with policy priorities, and to determine where effective levers for policy change lie. This might be at the national or subnational level. Selected examples are provided in this section.

Under the Guatemalan Peace Agreements negotiated in the mid-1990s, an explicit target was to increase public spending from 0.87% of GDP in 1995 to 1.31% by the year 2000. NHA information was necessary to set the targets and to monitor compliance. The changes for the 1996–2000 plan included the channelling of two-thirds of public resources to preventive care and enabled the monitoring of targeted health improvements in targeted population groups (*19*).

The NHA studies for Egypt and Morocco revealed the heavy reliance on household out-of-pocket expenses in financing the health system. In Morocco this stimulated a national policy debate on health insurance reform (*20*). Lebanon's NHA study showed a relatively high level of health expenditure as a percentage of GDP, but a relatively low level of health measured in terms of healthy life expectancy[3] in comparison to its neighbouring countries. This led to a concerted government action designed to improve the efficiency with which health expenditures were used to improve health (*21*).

The Sri Lanka National Health Accounts study showed the importance of having good evidence on private versus public sector activities in both financing and provision. Figure 16.1 shows that most government expenditure goes to fund inpatient care and very little to fund outpatient care, while non-governmental expenditure is concentrated on outpatient curative care and on pharmaceuticals (*22*). Government subsidy of inpatient care, which is of relatively high cost, might explain why a relatively low proportion of households in Sri Lanka face financial catastrophe because of health expenditures and the healthy life expectancy of the population is one of the highest in South-East Asia, at the age of 61 (*23*).

Spending trends by function and by health condition are particularly relevant for many OECD countries where cost containment has become a national priority. A study in the Netherlands identified expenditure by functions (hospital inpatient care, nursing home inpatient care, inpatient psychiatric care, and other services for mentally disabled people) and by demographic and health characteristics (by age and sex, and by 34 diagnostic groups). As in many other OECD countries, health costs in the Netherlands rise exponentially after the age of 50. Furthermore, all mental disorders together accounted for 28.4% of the total health expenditures. Based on this evidence, any policies to restrain expenditure would have to take into account the increasing longevity of the population and the risks of disability particularly associated with

Figure 16.1 Private and public health expenditures by function, Sri Lanka

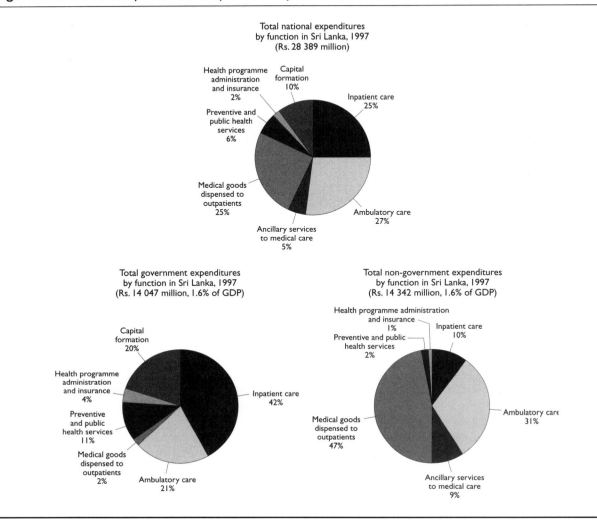

mental conditions (*24*). As many developing countries also enter into a stage of demographic transition, distributional analysis could simulate the impact of such changes on the health financing system in the forthcoming years.

NHA tables showing the beneficiaries of health expenditure are valuable for addressing questions of equity and effectiveness. Beneficiary groups can be disaggregated by disease category or by interventions received. As major epidemics burden the capacity of a large number of poor countries to finance their health systems, external providers of funds are looking at efficient ways to channel funds to address specific diseases. A NHA study on Rwanda in 1998 showed that while 10% of all health expenditures were spent on prevention and treatment of HIV/AIDS, more than 90% of these came from out-of-pocket payments by

seropositive patients and their families (*25*). Although bilateral and international agencies financed half of all health expenditure, only 6% was targeted specifically at HIV services and activities, despite the over 11% of the population expected to be seropositive. Most of these funds were channelled to prevention.

The Rwandan review concluded that, while national funding should continue to emphasize support for prevention, there was an urgent need to address the high burden of out-of-pocket costs of the seropositive individuals. In addition, the low utilization rate by the poor because of their inability to pay for care had to be corrected. USAID/PHR/WHO responded by evaluating prepayment schemes in a pilot region to determine if they could alleviate the burden that financing care placed on the poor and the sick. This highly subsided pilot programme helped to increase the utilization rate fivefold (26). A number of financing studies on HIV/AIDS in Latin America (ONUSIDA/SIDALAC)[4] have similarly demonstrated the usefulness of National Health Accounts in monitoring the effectiveness of interventions targeted to address the HIV epidemic.

Beneficiary analysis can also identify geographical inequality by demonstrating that some regions are disproportionately penalized over others in the allocation of public funds. Mexico's political strategy, like in many countries where universal coverage has not been achieved, was to ensure that limited public resources benefit the poor. A careful review using NHA data revealed that contrary to the policy intention, public resources designed to provide services for the uninsured population disfavoured the states with greater epidemiological challenges. Figure 16.2 shows clearly the inequality in the distribution of per capita expenditure on health. Health spending in the northern states is almost nine times higher than in the southern states. Within the states, urban areas are favoured over rural areas (27).

There has been a growing international concern about the effectiveness of international aid, particularly as debt servicing has resulted in net outflows, rather than net inflows of resources, in a number of countries. NHA data can be used to monitor compliance with the Poverty Reduction Strategies (PRSP) developed under the Heavily Indebted Poor Countries initiative (HIPC).[5] In fact, debt relief negotiations were facilitated in five countries under the HIPC initiative because they had undertaken NHA studies. This was considered proof of these countries' capacity to contin-

uously monitor the impact of their poverty reduction programmes funded under the debt relief agreement. NHA can also be used to monitor the impact and sustainability of programmes such as those funded by the Global Alliance for Vaccines Initiative (GAVI) and the newly created Global Fund for AIDS, Tuberculosis and Malaria (GFATM).

Finally, NHA can provide useful comparative information across countries. For example, a study comparing Denmark, France, Germany, Sweden, the United Kingdom, and the USA found wide variation in expenditures between categories of resources such as physicians, nurses, drugs, and equipment. It provided valuable insights into how countries that rely less on advanced equipment and drugs and more on personnel can still achieve high levels of health (28).

Conclusion

As the evidence grows on the importance of health for individual and societal well-being, as well as for economic development, national authorities and the global community are injecting new resources for health. In some cases, the additional resources, although welcome, pose immense strains on the capacity of the health system to provide services efficiently. Governments and their international partners are looking at ways to better ensure that scarce resources are spent efficiently and reach the intended beneficiaries. It is an opportune time for those countries that have not yet done so to embark on National Health Accounts. Expenditure flows need to be transparent from their

Figure 16.2 Per capita expenditure on health by region in Mexico, 1995

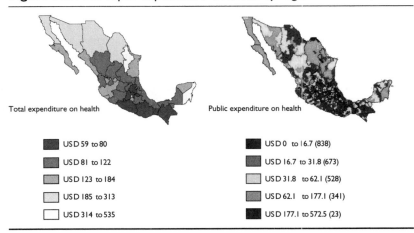

Total expenditure on health

- USD 59 to 80
- USD 81 to 122
- USD 123 to 184
- USD 185 to 313
- USD 314 to 535

Public expenditure on health

- USD 0 to 16.7 (838)
- USD 16.7 to 31.8 (673)
- USD 31.8 to 62.1 (528)
- USD 62.1 to 177.1 (341)
- USD 177.1 to 572.5 (23)

Source: Frenk, Julio and Gonzalez, E. Strategic Use of National Health Accounts in Mexico. Keynote Speech at NHA Symposium at IHEA Conference, York, July 2001. URL: http://www.phrproject.com

source through the production chain to the beneficiaries. Close monitoring of these flows at all stages can help to inform policy-makers on a timely basis. To monitor flows, however, NHA should be institutionalized and repeated regularly, preferably on an annual basis, although one-time efforts also demonstrate the usefulness of NHA as a policy tool.

NHA information can provide evidence and justification to argue for more external funding for health and health system actors. For example, the Ministry of Health can make a case for more resources from the central authorities. The evidence can permit timely adjustments in the allocation of funds related to health policy reforms to enhance the efficiency or equity in the use of resources. Finally, a transparent system for monitoring the flow of funds can make the providers and consumers of funds more accountable.

A final word of caution, however, is that NHA is only a tool, albeit an important one, for policy-makers. The resulting information must be combined with evidence on how the resources are translated into the key outcomes that people value, and how the different functions of the health system are being performed, for the development of policy. However, without the evidence provided by NHA, it is difficult even to begin the debate about the efficiency and equity of the health system.

NOTES

1 These programmes are known as Medicare, a federal insurance programme for people over the age of 65 years, people permanently unable to work because of disability, and people with end-stage renal disease; and Medicaid, which is jointly administered by the federal government and each of the State governments and insures against health care costs principally of low-income people.

2 OECD members include most of the high-income countries in Europe, Australia, Canada, Japan, Korea, Mexico, New Zealand, and the United States of America. URL: http://www.oecd.org.

3 HALE—healthy life expectancy reported by WHO for all its Member States, is the length of time a newborn child can expect to live in equivalent good health.

4 ONUSIDA/SIDALAC is a UNAIDS/AIDS programme for Latin America.

5 HIPC—Heavily Indebted Poor Countries: a term used by the International Monetary Fund and the World Bank coordinated initiative which identified a number of HIPC countries with good governance to be considered for debt relief.

REFERENCES

(1) Xu K et al. Understanding household catastrophic health expenditures: a multi-country analysis. In: Murray CJL, Evans DB, eds. *Health systems performance assessment: debates, methods and empiricism.* Geneva, World Health Organization, 2003.

(2) Abel-Smith B. *Paying for health services: a study of the costs and sources of finance in six countries.* Public Health Papers No. 17. Geneva, World Health Organization, 1963.

(3) Abel-Smith B. *An international study of health expenditure and its relevance for health.* Public Health Papers No. 32. Geneva, World Health Organization, 1967.

(4) The Committee on the Costs of Medical Care. *Medical care for the American people*, Table 5. Chicago, The University of Chicago Press, 1932. URL: http://www.ssa.gov/history/RICE.html

(5) Organisation for Economic Co-operation and Development. *A system of health accounts.* Paris, Organisation for Economic Co-operation and Development, 2000.

(6) United States Agency for International Development, World Bank, World Health Organization. *A guide to producing National Health Accounts: with special applications for low and middle income countries.* Geneva, World Health Organization, 2003.

(7) Organisation for Economic Co-operation and Development, International Monetary Fund, World Bank. *System of national accounts 1993.* Brussels, Luxembourg, New York, Paris, Washington, DC, CEC, IMF, OECD, UN, WB, 1994.

(8) Murray CJL, Frenk J. A framework for assessing the performance of health systems. *Bulletin of the World Health Organization*, 2000, 78(6):717–731.

(9) Poullier JP et al. Patterns of global health expenditures: results for 191 countries. In: Murray CJL, Evans DB, eds. *Health systems performance assessment: debates, methods and empiricism.* Geneva, World Health Organization, 2003.

(10) United Nations Population Division. *World population prospects: the 2002 revision population database.* 2003. URL: http://esa.un.org/unpp/

(11) International Monetary Fund. *International financial statistics yearbook.* Washington, DC, International Monetary Fund, 2002.

(12) International Monetary Fund. *Government financial statistics yearbook.* Washington, DC, International Monetary Fund, 2002.

(13) United Nations. *National accounts statistics: main aggregates and detailed tables, 2000.* New York, United Nations, 2002.

(14) World Health Organization. Statistical Annex Table 5: Selected National Health Accounts Indicators for all Member States, Estimates for 1995 to 2000. *The World Health Report 2002. Reducing Risks, Promoting Healthy Life*. Geneva, World Health Organization, 2002:202–217.

(15) Organisation for Economic Co-operation and Development. *OECD health data 2001: a comparative analysis of 30 countries*. Paris, Organisation for Economic Co-operation and Development, 2002.

(16) International Labour Office. *Household income and expenditure statistics No. 4*. Geneva, International Labour Office, 1995.

(17) World Bank. *Living Standards and Measurement Study (LSMS)*. URL http://www.worldbank.org/html/prdph/lsms/index.htm

(18) Economic Commission for Latin America and the Caribbean (ECLAC). *Statistical yearbook for Latin America and the Caribbean 2002*. Santiago, United Nations, 2003.

(19) Finkelman J, Rivera T, Victoria D. *El proceso de transformación de la salud en Guatemala*. Guatemala, World Health Organization, Regional Office for the Americas/Pan American Health Organization, 1996.

(20) Ministère de la Santé, Royaume du Maroc. *Comptes nationaux de la santé 1997/98*. Rabat, Ministère de la Santé, Royaume du Maroc, 2001.

(21) Ministry of Health Lebanon. *Lebanon National Health Accounts: Executive Summary* (Working Draft). Ministry of Health, Lebanon, 2000.

(22) Ministry of Health, Institute of Policy Studies. *Sri Lanka National Health Accounts: Sri Lanka national health expenditures 1990–99*. Colombo, Institute of Policy Studies, 2001.

(23) Dorabawila T et al. *WHO fairness in financing study: estimates for Sri Lanka 1995/96 using WHO methodology*. Colombo, Institute of Policy Studies of Sri Lanka, 2001.

(24) Meerding WJ et al. Demographic and epidemiological determinants of healthcare costs in Netherlands: cost of illness study. *British Medical Journal*, 1998, 317: 111–115.

(25) Schneider P et al. *Rwanda National Health Accounts 1998*. Bethesda, Abt Associates. Partnerships for Health Reform Project, 2000.

(26) Schneider P et al. *Paying for HIV/AIDS services*. UNAIDS Best Practice Collection. Geneva, UNAIDS, UNICEF, UNDP, UNFPA, UNDCP, ILO, UNESCO, WHO, World Bank, 2001.

(27) Fundación Mexicana para la Salud. *National Health Accounts: inequidad en México, 1990–1996*. Mexico D.F., Fundación Mexicana para la Salud, 1998.

(28) Anell A, Willis M. International comparison of health care systems using resource profiles. *Bulletin of the World Health Organization*, 2000, 78:770–778.

Chapter 17

Patterns of Global Health Expenditures: Results for 191 Countries

Jean-Pierre Poullier, Patricia Hernandez, Kei Kawabata, William D. Savedoff

Introduction

Inadequate funding for health services is often cited as a major constraint for governments to be good stewards of their countries' health systems. Yet in most cases, the data to support such claims are lacking. Making progress on a variety of health policy questions requires good national data on the sources and uses of funds in the health system, preferably comparable across countries. With such data, it is possible to begin answering questions related to the best ways to allocate limited resources towards improving health, or what level of funding is needed in particular epidemiological and demographic contexts.

The World Health Report 2000 contained National Health Accounts (NHA) information for the 191 Member States of the World Health Organization (WHO); this information has been updated and expanded in the subsequent *World Health Reports*. The methods and concepts underlying these data are described elsewhere (1). This chapter reviews the latest available data to show the general patterns of health spending in the world. It begins with the very high levels of world spending on health that are, however, very unequally distributed. It then considers the patterns of health status relative to health expenditures, along with the magnitude of private health spending. It concludes with a discussion of external resources, the magnitude of those resources, and the countries to which they are primarily directed.

A World of Difference

Health Spending is High and Unequal

The figures on world health spending in 2000 show that expenditures were very high, higher than in previous estimates (2). In 2000, the world spent an estimated I$3.6 trillion on health goods and services out of an estimated total world income of I$43.8 trillion.[1] Thus, health spending represented some 8.1% of global GDP, which comes to an average expenditure per person of I$588 on health services. But this average varied significantly across countries and across regions,[2] ranging from only I$88 per person in Africa to I$2 347 in the OECD countries.

Per capita income approximates the amount of resources available for consumption of different goods and services, and health spending is one important use of these resources. Although health spending does not necessarily have to rise with income (countries have plenty of other things to spend on), it turns out that it is highly correlated with per capita national income. In 2000, the correlation of income and health spending was 0.96 (significant at the 0.01% level), and a simple regression in logs of expenditure on income yields an elasticity of 1.2. In other words, a 1% difference between countries in income is associated with a 1.2% difference in health spending.

Comparisons across countries have limitations in predicting how much more any particular country will spend on health as its income rises. In other studies that use panel data, the elasticity of health spending to income is shown to be close to 1 (3). These studies rely exclusively on data from OECD countries that have among the highest incomes in the world, so the income elasticity of health spending may or may not be greater for countries with lower income levels.

The share of national income that countries spend on health is greater for higher income countries (Table 17.1 and Figure 17.1). Health spending as a share of GDP ranges from about 1% to 13%. The higher shares are found in Europe, the Americas, and in some oil producing countries. The lowest shares are found in

Table 17.1   Health spending by income groups and regions

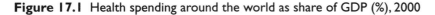

Group or region	Total health expenditure (millions)		Per capita health expenditure		Share of GDP (%)
	FX rates	I$	FX rates	I$	
GDP p.c.					
< 1 000	3 350	9 385	8	24	3.4
1 000–2 200	40 893	108 744	24	65	4.5
2 200–7 000	143 510	482 515	60	203	5.0
> 7 000	2 693 591	2 953 025	1 686	1 849	9.4
Region					
Africa	20 434	55 968	32	88	5.5
Americas	104 073	221 613	251	535	7.8
Middle East	55 765	96 525	116	200	4.6
E. Europe and C. Asia	37 495	115 687	106	327	5.4
OECD	2 552 728	2 650 294	2 261	2 347	9.9
S. Asia	42 727	116 879	28	76	4.0
Asia & Pac.	68 056	296 629	46	200	5.1
Total	2 881 279	3 553 594	477	589	8.1

Note: The columns headed "FX rates" present figures that are converted from local currency into United States dollars at official exchange rates. The columns headed "I$" present figures converted from local currency at purchasing power parity rates.

Figure 17.1   Health spending around the world as share of GDP (%), 2000

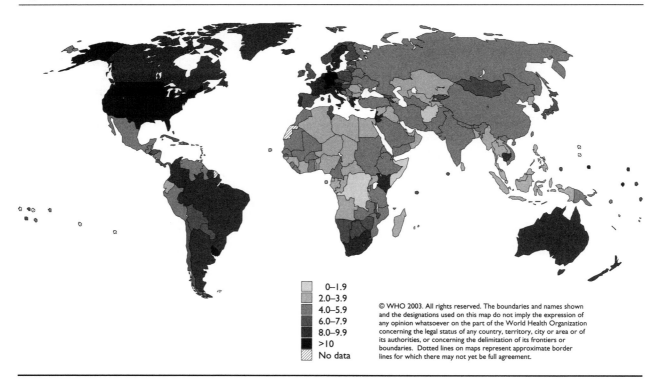

0–1.9
2.0–3.9
4.0–5.9
6.0–7.9
8.0–9.9
>10
No data

Africa and in some Asian countries. Measured health spending as a share of GDP in OECD countries ranged from near 7% in the United Kingdom and Ireland, to 13% in the United States. On the other hand, one-fourth of the countries in the world, most of which are poor, spend less than 4% of GDP on health. Only a few middle-income countries can be found in this latter category, such as Oman and Singapore. The relationship between the share of GDP spent on health and income is not as strong as the relationship between spending and income, but it is still significant and positive, with a simple correlation coefficient of 0.47.

NHA estimates for 2000 show that health spending is highly unequal. The OECD countries spend the most on health per person. These countries contain 19% of the world's population, but account for over 89% of world spending on health. By contrast, the poorest 80% of the world's population accounted for only 11% of the world health expenditures.

Looking across regions, the disparities are apparent (Figure 17.2). At the one extreme, Africa contains 11% of the world's population, yet accounts for only 1% of the world's health spending. In Asia and the Pacific (the region including China), 25% of the world's population accounts for only 2% of world health spending.

Health spending across countries is more unequally distributed than income. This contrasts with the distribution of health spending across households within countries which, although unequal, is often more equitably distributed than household income.[3] While the interquartile distribution across countries for income is estimated to be 7.4, the interquartile distribution for health spending is 9.5.

HEALTH SPENDING AND HEALTH OUTCOMES

Countries that spend little on health also have poorer health conditions. The median healthy life expectancy (HALE) in the 91 countries that spend less than I$200 per capita on health was only 47 years in 2000 (4). However, the range is also very wide. The lowest quartile of countries in terms of healthy

life expectancy, have HALEs below 39 years, while the top quartile have HALEs over 56 years. Above the I$200 per capita spending level, there is much greater convergence. Among the 63 countries spending between I$200 and I$850 per person on health, three-quarters have healthy life expectancies above 57 years. Among the 37 countries spending over I$850, the range is even smaller, with three quarters of them enjoying HALEs of over 67 years, with a maximum of 74 years in Japan.

Although health spending can affect health conditions, it is important to note that the efficiency with which countries are able to transform their spending into better health outcomes varies significantly. While a more complete model of health determinants would be necessary to properly make such comparisons, it is still instructive to look at the rough differences in health between countries with similar levels of health spending (Figure 17.3). In fact, many countries fall drastically below the levels of health attained by their peers.

Four distinct patterns emerge from the data when looking at health and health spending. The first group of countries, in the lower left corner, contains those that spend less than I$60 per capita on health. The great majority of these countries fall below the mean regression line, and of those below the line, more than two-thirds are from Africa. The countries in the middle range of spending, by far the largest group, are densely scattered around the mean, and there is no clear pattern. Here, there may be lessons as to why countries with similar spending levels and disease bur-

Figure 17.2 Inequality in health spending and income by region, 2000

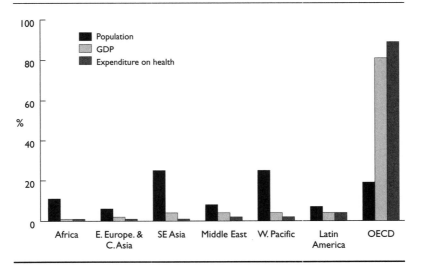

Figure 17.3 Healthy life expectancy and health spending, 2000

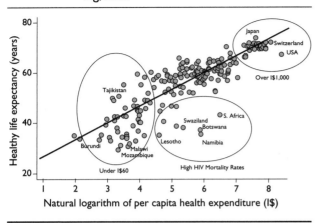

dens have such different health outcomes. The third group spends at levels comparable to others in this middle range, but stands out for being substantially below the mean regression line in terms of health outcomes. Understandably, these countries include those facing the highest mortality from HIV/AIDS. Finally, at the upper end are countries with health expenditures over I$1 000 per capita that generally cluster close to the mean. They include all the high-income OECD and Eastern European countries. The figure suggests that, among high spending countries, those that spend more do not gain much more health when measured by healthy life expectancy. The USA, and, to some degree, Switzerland, are countries with high spending levels and estimated HALE below the mean regression line.

When looking at the relationship between spending and health status, then, three broad patterns emerge. First, among the lowest spending countries, higher spending appears to be associated with signifi-

cant improvements in health status. Second, even at very low levels of per capita spending, some countries achieve better health than others, suggesting that there may be an opportunity for public policy to make a difference. Third, among high spending countries, additional spending bears little relationship to improvements in healthy life expectancy. This may be part of the reason behind the concern in wealthier countries for cost containment.

THE COMPOSITION AND STRUCTURE OF HEALTH SPENDING

In order to understand why some countries achieve better health conditions with otherwise similar levels of per capita spending, it is necessary to analyse how those funds are mobilized, pooled, allocated, and applied. In their current state, the NHA data produced by WHO are most useful for analysing how funds are mobilized and pooled. However, as the data collection process improves in scope and precision, it will be possible to go into more depth on all aspects of health financing.

In global terms, public spending on health exceeds private spending. Together, tax-based and social security-based funding represent about I$1.7 trillion, compared to about I$1.4 trillion of private spending. Out-of-pocket spending alone accounts for some I$742 million—almost as much as is spent through social insurance—while external funding is negligible (Table 17.2 and Figure 17.4).

The estimates of public expenditure on health range from as low as 11% to almost 100% of all health spending. The wealthier and healthier countries tend to rely more heavily on public sources of funds as a share of total spending. However, countries and

Table 17.2 Share of total spending on health by type and region, 2000 (%)

	Social security	Tax	External resource	Private insurance	Out-of-pocket	Others	Total
Africa	5.1	38.0	4.2	24.8	24.1	3.8	100
Americas	14.7	33.2	0.7	15.3	35.6	0.5	100
Middle East	9.0	45.9	0.5	1.8	38.8	4.0	100
E. Europe & C. Asia	23.1	48.6	1.8	0.9	24.5	1.1	100
OECD	29.7	29.2	0.0	19.7	16.6	4.7	100
S. Asia	1.8	19.8	2.7	1.0	74.1	0.5	100
Asia & Pacific	16.3	20.8	0.6	0.3	59.3	2.8	100
World	27.8	29.7	0.2	18.3	19.7	4.4	100

Note: The relatively high private insurance shares are influenced by a few countries with large health expenditures — South Africa in Africa and the USA in OECD and world figures.

Figure 17.4 Composition of world spending on health, 2000

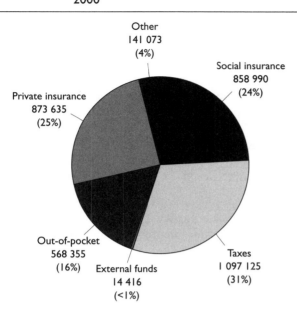

Figure 17.5 Public share of health spending by income group

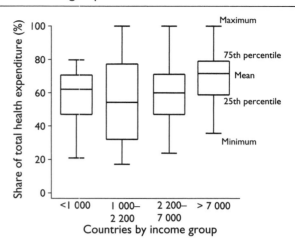

regions vary significantly along this dimension, and not only as a consequence of differences in income.

One way of looking at this wide range of public commitment to health expenditure is to compare countries in groups with similar per capita income levels. All income categories have shares of public expenditure on health that range from less than 20% to over 80%, with the exception of the highest spenders who range from a low near 40% to many countries reaching close to 100%. The interquartile range is virtually the same for the first and third categories (less than I\$1 000 per capita and between I\$2 200 and I\$7 000 per capita), while it is the largest for countries that have per capita incomes between I\$1 000 and I\$2 200 (Figure 17.5). In fact, public expenditure on health as a share of total health spending is poorly correlated with per capita GDP, showing a relatively low correlation coefficient of 0.33, even if it is statistically different from zero.

This pattern is consistent with the notion that public spending dominates in the lowest income countries by default—people have so little income that there is little effective demand to support an active private sector—or because of a significant amount of external resources. By contrast, among countries that spend somewhat more, a lower share of public spending can indicate an active private sector or a policy of limited public involvement. In the highest spending brackets, the public share of expenditure on health converges

at a relatively high level. Except for a few cases (e.g. the United States and Switzerland), public spending essentially replaces private spending.

Focusing on the three major sources of health spending, tax-financed spending, social security spending, and private spending, shows clear differences in the structure of health systems (Table 17.2). South Asia is the region with the largest private sector share and virtually no reliance on social security systems. Africa and the Middle East also rely heavily on private financing, but appear to have larger public tax-based (or externally supported) sources. In Asia and the Pacific region, private spending is also high, but the public share has a significant portion in social security (driven almost exclusively by China). The Americas rely heavily on private financing as well, though somewhat less than other developing regions. Much of the difference is accounted for by a significant reliance on social insurance systems. It is only in Europe and the OECD that health systems depend very little on private financing, and rely instead on significant shares of both social security and tax-based funding.

Among countries with large public shares of health spending, there are few differences in terms of health outcomes whether the public funds derive from taxes or social security contributions. In this regard, it appears impossible to infer that one type of public financing system is better than the other. It is also clear from the data that most countries in Europe have a mix of all three kinds of financing. Hence, policy debates that assume a country's health system exclusively follows a tax-based or social security based model are oversimplified.

The commitment of the public sector to health financing can also be inferred from the share of total government spending dedicated to health. Public spending on health as a share of total government spending ranges from as low as 2% to as high as 32%. No OECD country has a share that is less than 9%, with Greece and Turkey having the lowest ratios. Even among countries that spend very little on health, about one-third spend more than 10% of the governmental budget on it.

PRIVATE SPENDING

Private health spending is overwhelmingly paid out-of-pocket. In fact, in most countries, the share of private health insurance in total health expenditure is insignificant. Prepaid private insurance accounts for more than 5% of private health expenditure in only about one-fourth of the world's countries. In those countries where prepaid private insurance has some significance,[4] the prepaid share of this private spending averages only 24%, while private spending as a whole accounts for an average 10% of all health spending. These countries are quite varied and include 5 African countries, 16 Latin American countries, 5 Eastern Mediterranean countries, and 16 European countries, in addition to Thailand, Canada, the United States, Australia, New Zealand, and South Korea.

Private insurance tends to be a luxury of either high-income countries or high-income households within low-income countries. The importance of private insurance in total health spending depends significantly on the health system's structure. In some countries private insurance is considered an integral part of the health system, subject to regulation. In others, it is viewed as a luxury good and either tolerated or encouraged. However, in most countries, private insurance is simply one more segment of a fragmented health system. The importance of private insurance, then, depends on the domestic level and distribution of income, as well as on public policy.

The bulk of private spending is paid out-of-pocket at the time of service. The most problematic aspect of high shares of health financed through out-of-pocket spending is that the burden falls on a small portion of households in any given year, and, relative to income, the burden is much heavier for the poor than for the rich. Out-of-pocket spending accounts for a much greater share of health expenditures in poor countries than in rich ones (Figure 17.6). This is dramatic in the case of regions with very high private shares of spending, e.g. South Asia. However, it is also large in all middle- and low-income countries.

More than any other fact, the high level of out-of-pocket spending in low- and middle-income countries stands out as one of the most troubling issues for public policy. Finding ways to reduce citizens' exposure to large and uncertain health costs is increasingly a major facet of public debates, forced to center stage by NHAs that show how out-of-pocket spending often dwarfs, or at least matches, health spending in the public sector.

EXTERNAL RESOURCES

Given the poor health conditions in the world's poorest countries, it is particularly relevant to understand how much external funding is being supplied, how it is being allocated, and whether it is effective. Beginning such analyses is now possible because *The World Health Report 2001* (4) introduced estimates of external resources on health as a percentage of expenditure on health, a practice continued in *The World Health Report 2002* (5).

There is a growing need for bilateral and multilateral agencies to increase their financial support to the health systems in low-income and high disease burden countries (6). Additionally, there is a growing concern among countries that provide grants and loans that their funds be targeted to the most needy populations and be applied effectively. Aggregate NHA data cannot answer all of these questions. Nevertheless, by reporting this information, a few general patterns can be discerned.

The information on external funding was largely obtained from the OECD Development Assistance

Figure 17.6 Out-of-pocket share of health spending by income

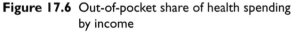
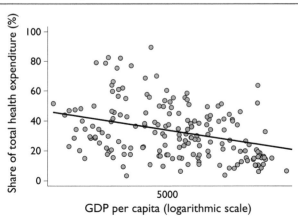

Committee (7) and supplemented by recipient country data. Although these figures remain tentative, the available information would indicate that externally funded assistance accounts for about I$14.4 billion compared to the I$2.7 trillion spent by OECD countries in 2000. This represents only a tiny fraction of health spending by high-income countries, a mere 0.5%. Such a limited amount of transfers makes virtually no dent in the large world inequalities in health spending discussed earlier.

Most external funding goes to countries with large populations. For example, the top three recipients of external funds for health are India (I$1 585 million), the Russian Federation (I$1 883 million), and Indonesia (I$1 205 million), accounting for almost one-quarter of all foreign resources. In other cases, countries seem to have been picked out for special assistance because they are recovering from war (e.g. Bosnia and Herzegovina) or fighting with very severe disease

burdens (e.g. Uganda). Political attachments between particular countries probably also play a role.

In per capita terms, external assistance is largest in smaller countries, ranging from a few pennies per person in many countries to over I$25 per capita in Barbados and Suriname (Table 17.3). By region, the highest level of external funding on a per capita basis goes to Eastern Europe and Central Asia. In general, external funds are only a few dollars per person and are a fraction of the resources mobilized by local governments and paid out-of-pocket by the population. Among the poorest countries, such as Tanzania, Zimbabwe, and Bolivia, out-of-pocket spending is twice the level of per capita external funding. In countries such as Cambodia and Sri Lanka, this reaches extremes, with out-of-pocket spending being respectively 6.5 and 20 times larger than external funding.

If Europe, the USA, and Canada transferred only 0.5% of their health spending (less than 0.1% of GDP)

Table 17.3 External resources, consumption, and health spending, selected countries, 2000 (I$ per capita)

Country	GDP	Out-of-pocket spending on health	External financing for health	Public expenditure on health
Bhutan	1 549	6	27	58
Bolivia	2 368	36	15	114
Cambodia	1 363	84	13	27
China	3 852	124	0	75
El Salvador	4 427	215	9	167
Estonia	9 123	110	2	427
Fiji	4 911	67	24	126
Guatemala	4 075	86	9	92
Haiti	1 094	12	18	27
India	1 461	58	2	13
Indonesia	3 121	59	6	20
Kyrgyzstan	2 426	56	18	90
Lesotho	1 580	18	6	82
Malawi	500	9	16	18
Mauritius	9 591	144	5	186
Mozambique	697	5	13	19
Nepal	1 224	42	5	19
Papua New Guinea	3 567	14	32	130
Russian Federation	7 621	95	13	293
Rwanda	774	12	10	20
Sri Lanka	3 303	60	3	59
Suriname	4 347	63	60	238
Uganda	932	13	13	14
United Republic of Tanzania	457	12	5	13
Zambia	866	14	7	30
Zimbabwe	2 331	38	13	73

to Africa, it would represent an additional I$25 per capita, 5 times larger than the current amount of external aid. To achieve the same increase, Africans would have to transfer an additional 1.5% of GDP or increase public spending on health by more than 60%.

National income is so low in many recipient countries that, even when external funding is small, it may represent a significant share of total health expenditure. For example, in 66 countries, external assistance represents over 10% of estimated total health expenditures. In the 20 countries that are most dependent on external funding, these foreign sources represent between one-third and three-quarters of all public spending on health, demonstrating the importance and responsibility of external agencies and governments in public health policy decisions.

The pattern of external financing does not necessarily reflect greatest need. While the twenty countries with the highest HIV mortality rate are all from the African continent, only six of these are among the top 20 recipients of external funding. The Global Fund established under the auspices of the United Nations to combat AIDS, Malaria, and TB may begin to rectify this imbalance.

Conclusions

National Health Accounts data are beginning to make it possible to provide evidence in an internationally comparable framework that is relevant to decision-making and to the monitoring of health systems performance. The data for 1998 confirm that health spending in the world is quite high and very unequally spread, with substantial concentration of health spending in the richest countries, both in absolute and per capita terms.

While higher health spending is associated with better health, this relationship presents an enormous variation. Thus, public policy may be able to play a role in improving the effectiveness with which resources are transformed into better health, even in countries that spend relatively little in this area.

The structure of health systems, as shown by the main health financing agents, varies widely across regions, with higher income countries generally displaying higher shares of public spending. Conversely, the share of health spending that is paid out-of-pocket is inversely related to income, a situation that exacerbates the unequal burden of health spending across households within countries. The NHA data also show that external resources represent a tiny fraction

of total health spending. Even so, the ability to raise funds is so low in many countries that these foreign inflows may represent enormous shares of public or total expenditure on health.

This brief overview of patterns found in National Health Accounts data demonstrate that it is possible to gain important insights into the way health systems operate, the priorities established by national policies, and the effectiveness of public policy through cross-country and cross-regional comparisons. WHO and its Member States need to continue to improve and institutionalize the process of NHA generation in order to develop a broader and more robust evidence base for guiding policy decisions and health system monitoring in the future.

Acknowledgements

The authors are indebted to Christopher J.L. Murray for the impetus and many insights in this chapter. They would also like to give special thanks to Chandika Indikadahena, Takondwe Mwase, Piya Hanvoravongchai, and Riadh Zeramdini for their technical assistance and inputs.

Notes

1 The "international dollar" (I$) is used to represent a currency unit which is meant to have the same purchasing power in a given economy that a US$1 will have in the US. Using official exchange rates, the figures would be US$2.9 trillion, US$31.6 trillion, and 9.1%, respectively.

2 The regions used in this chapter seek to group relatively similar countries in broad income and/or geographic categories. The OECD countries are grouped together as one region. Africa refers mainly to sub-Saharan countries. The Middle East category includes Northern African countries through to Pakistan and Afghanistan in the east. Europe and Central Asia includes the non-OECD European countries and the former Soviet Republics of Central Asia. South Asia comprises 10 countries, including India and Indonesia, while Asia and Pacific encompasses China, the Philippines, and the Pacific Island countries.

3 Within countries, health spending is generally more equitably distributed across households than is income, in contrast to the variation across countries reported in the text. For example, in Brazil, where the ratio of average health expenditure in 1997 was 6 to 1 across income quintiles, it was over 20 to 1 for average income. In Ecuador, the range of health spending between the top and bottom deciles is no more than 4 to 1, while for income the range is more than 40 to 1 (8).

4   For the purposes of this chapter, "significant prepaid private insurance" is taken to include countries in which private insurance accounts for more than 5% of total private spending.

REFERENCES

(1)   Poullier JP, Hernandez P, Kawabata K. National Health Accounts: concepts, data sources, and methodology. In: Murray CJL, Evans DB, eds. *Health systems performance assessment: debates, methods and empiricism*. Geneva, World Health Organization, 2003.

(2)   World Bank. *World development report. Investing in health*. New York, Oxford University Press, 1993.

(3)   Gerdtham U-G, Jönsson B. International comparisons of health expenditure. In: Culyer AJ, Newhouse JP, eds. *Handbook of health economics*. Amsterdam, New York, Elsevier, 2000.

(4)   World Health Organization. *The World Health Report 2001. Mental Health: New Understanding, New Hope*. Geneva, World Health Organization, 2001.

(5)   World Health Organization. *The World Health Report 2002. Reducing Risks, Promoting Healthy Life*. Geneva, World Health Organization, 2002.

(6)   Commission on Macroeconomics and Health. *Macroeconomics and health: investing in health for economic development*. Geneva, World Health Organization, 2001.

(7)   OECD Development Assistance Committee. *International development statistics. AID at a glance for recipient countries and territories*. Paris, Organization for Economic Co-operation and Development, 2001.

(8)   Pan American Health Organization. *Investment in health: social and economic returns to health*. Washington, DC, Pan American Health Organization, 2001.

Chapter 18

MONITORING THE HEALTH FINANCING FUNCTION

WILLIAM D. SAVEDOFF, GUY CARRIN, KEI KAWABATA, ABDELHAY MECHBAL

APPROACH

Every health system collects, manages, and spends funds. In order to contribute to good health, the financial part of health services presumably needs to generate sufficient funds, effectively pool risk, and be allocated to services in ways that are consistent with encouraging good performance.

To monitor the financing function, it is necessary to measure the function's performance along all these dimensions. Drawing on "Who pays for Health Systems?," Chapter 5 of *The World Health Report 2000,* this chapter proposes a limited set of indicators that are key to understanding the financing function. Many of the indicators are reported by international organizations (e.g. tax effectiveness), can be calculated from existing surveys (e.g. out-of-pocket spending share from expenditure surveys), or require additional questions on existing surveys. On the other hand, there are numerous indicators that will only be available if new surveys are undertaken. In some areas, methodological work will be necessary to arrive at definitions before indicators can even be identified and selected—notably for those dimensions related to intermediate institutions.

Choosing indicators of financing function performance is particularly difficult because the relevant data differ in relation to the structure of the financing system itself. Financing systems that rely on general revenues channelled into public provision require collecting data on the efficiency of public administration; while systems relying on separate insurance pools might need data on the competitiveness of the market. If the systems divided easily into a small number of categories, the data collection effort could be distinct for each category. However, few systems cleanly fit into distinct categories. Almost all involve some combination of collection, pooling, and purchasing mechanisms. The fact that these multiple combinations interact and mutually influence each other introduces additional complexity that requires specific kinds of information.

In this early stage of defining indicators, WHO is considering a variety of alternatives and paying attention to existing efforts to collect data on health financing functions. Such alternatives include work at PAHO/AMRO and the European Observatory on country profiles, and current studies in EMRO that aim to summarize a subset of intraregionally comparable indicators upon its completion. Country-specific studies that are collecting data on the financing function will also be taken into account.

INDICATORS

The proposed indicators tell us broadly about external conditions that affect the financing system (e.g. national income), as well as the financing function's structure (e.g. number of pools) and its behaviour (e.g. share of public spending allocated to health). Many of these indicators do not have a clear ordering of what is "good" or "bad." Therefore, it would additionally be useful to have a few summary indicators that provide cardinal measures of how well the financing function is being performed. Three such summary or "target" indicators will be identified below—one each for assessing collection, pooling, and purchasing.

Following *The World Health Report 2000,* the proposed indicators will be divided among those related to collection, pooling, and purchasing. This can be expanded in stages, as demonstrated in Figure 18.1. A summary of the indicators discussed here can be found in Table 18.1.

Figure 18.1 The process of developing indicators for the financing function

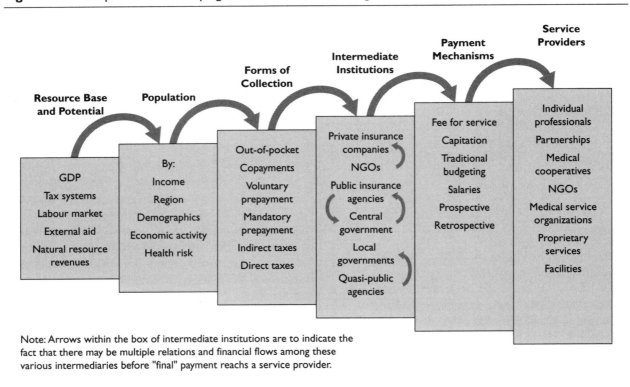

Note: Arrows within the box of intermediate institutions are to indicate the fact that there may be multiple relations and financial flows among these various intermediaries before "final" payment reaches a service provider.

COLLECTION

To evaluate the effectiveness of the financing function in collecting resources, performance has to be measured relative to the potential for raising funds. Thus, the first set of indicators is aimed at measuring the resources potentially available to the system, the conditions that influence how difficult it might be to mobilize these resources, and the broader budget constraint faced by policy-makers in the public sector. In addition to more general macroeconomic data (e.g. GDP per capita) which are readily available, specific indicators of interest would include:

■ The formal sector share of GDP.

■ Natural resource revenues as a share of total public sector income.

The size of the formal sector is a rough indicator of the ease with which governments can tax or enforce mandatory contributions, since the formal sector economy is legally registered and visible to government agencies in ways that the informal economy is not. This does not mean that resources cannot be mobilized from the informal sector, nor does it mean that tax compliance in the formal sector is universal. Rather,

it is meant to provide an indicator that reflects international differences in the constraints facing governments in raising revenues. Natural resource revenues also represent a relatively easy source of public sector income that distinguishes the politics of health sector spending in certain countries from others. These indicators would need to be created through judicious use of data from the IMF and the ILO, and cross-checked with other country-specific studies.

■ Public sector expenditures as a share of GDP.

■ External health sector aid as a share of total GDP.

The first of these indicators measures the share of national income effectively captured and utilized by the public sector. In a sense, this represents the public sector's budget constraint when allocating resources between different public demands. Countries with large external aid have additional public resources to work with, but they may be subject to conditions set by donors or multilateral lenders.

■ The share of public health expenditures in total public expenditure.

■ Total health expenditure (per capita level and share of GDP).

Table 18.1 Indicators for the financing function

Indicators	Purpose
Revenue collection	
■ The formal sector share of GDP	Potential resources available to finance public health spending
■ Natural resource revenues as a share of total public sector income	
■ Public sector spending (% of GDP)	To measure resources specifically available to the public sector
■ External health sector aid (% of GDP)	
■ The share of public health expenditures in total public expenditure	To measure public sector allocation decisions, additional resources, and potential constraints
■ Per capita health expenditure and share of GDP	
■ The share of total health expenditures that are prepaid	A broad measure of financial protection against out-of-pocket expenses
Pooling	
Means and distributional measure of:	Measures of the scale, depth of financial coverage, and existence of compensatory mechanisms across pools
■ Share of copayments to total health expenditure in each pool	
■ Membership in each pool, and	
■ Per capita spending in each pool	
■ Share of administrative expenses out of total spending	These two indicators require more work. The first aims to measure the efficiency of pool management. The second aims to measure the effectiveness of compensatory mechanisms.
■ Average ratio of transfers to estimated shortfall (or surplus) of need (conditional on health risk of affiliated population	
Purchasing	
■ Share of pool expenditures accounted for by "active purchasing"	This and other indicators require more work, aimed at characterizing the pool–purchaser relationship
■ Number of purchasers	To characterize the structure of interactions between purchasers and providers
■ Mean and distribution of total expenditure across purchasers	
■ Mean and distribution of the number of providers who are contracted or hired by each purchaser	
■ Share of total funds spent with different payment mechanisms (e.g. salaries, fee-for-service, capitation)	To measure the financial incentives embedded in payments to providers

The first represents the amount of public resources that, within the overall public budget, are allocated to health. The measure needs to comprise all levels of government and all public institutions, including national and subnational expenditures, as well as public agencies (such as social security institutions). The second measure incorporates all other sources of health spending, whether private or external. This information should be available through National Health Accounts.

In addition, it is necessary to have information about the distribution of payments into the health system across individuals and households. At the household level, this information is already being calculated by WHO in the form of the fairness in financial contribution index. Beyond that key outcome indicator, it is important to have information on the forms

of such payments and special sources of funding. The proposed indicator is:

■ The share of total health expenditures that are prepaid (as against those which are paid out-of-pocket at the time of service).

This indicator provides a first approximation of the degree to which the population is insured against major health costs. When a large share of health spending is prepaid, it is less likely to find individuals paying large amounts out-of-pocket at the time of service.

Two of these measures, per capita health spending and the share of prepayment, would make good target indicators of this subfunction's performance. Per capita spending tells us whether the collection system is generating a great deal or very few resources; while the share of prepayment provides information about the degree to which the population is insured against catastrophic spending in the aggregate.

POOLING

There are various institutional arrangements at the level of pooling and managing funds that affect the performance of the health financing system. At one extreme, there are systems which effectively function as one large pool that insures almost all citizens for necessary services. At the other extreme, there are countries with many different pools, sometimes overlapping, along with a large share of the population with no explicit attachment to any particular insurance mechanism. For this intermediate level, it is extremely difficult to identify indicators that would be both relevant and comparable across many countries.

Progress in this area will have to begin by generating a more precise definition of pools. One problem in identifying the number, size, and types of pools is that there is frequently a wide gap between what insurance institutions report and the coverage they effectively provide. WHO is considering an approach to defining pools on the basis of estimating the probability that a given individual's health service needs will be insured by a given pool. Out of this distribution of probabilities, nominal boundaries can be drawn between pools in terms of 1) number of individuals "covered," 2) the depth of coverage (i.e. what share of the health costs are reimbursed or paid for by the pool), and 3) by interventions (i.e. some pools may cover only rare high cost interventions, while others are comprehensive).

After a workable definition of pools is agreed upon, it will be important to measure several characteristics that affect the pools' abilities to manage risks, share risks across pools, and insure individuals. Therefore, some relevant indicators will include the mean and a distributional measure of the following three indicators:

- Share of copayments to total health expenditure in each pool.

- Membership in each pool.

- Per capita spending in each pool.

The means of these three indicators provide proxies of the depth of insurance coverage, the average scale for managing risk, and the average resources applied to health services. The distributional measures provide information regarding the distribution of insurance depth, size, and spending between the different institutions. The distributional measures are valuable for evaluating the efficiency of the system in relation to such features as the efficient scale for managing risks, or, where pools compete with one another, the competitiveness of the market. But the distributional information is also important for evaluating the effect of the financing mechanism on equity.

In particular, the distribution of per capita spending may give some indication of the degree to which compensatory mechanisms smooth out spending over different populations. However, the interpretation of the indicator is only straightforward in cases where populations and their associated health risks are relatively homogeneous across the various pools. This is rarely the case. Therefore, further work will be necessary to improve this indicator by generating information of spending relative to "need," i.e. relative to the actual health risks associated with the pool's affiliated population.

It is also desirable to have a more direct measure of the existence of compensating mechanisms and their effectiveness in redressing imbalances across pools. In this regard, it may be necessary to develop a measure of the net financial transfers to (or from) a pool relative to an estimate of the expected financial shortfall (or surplus) conditional on the composition of its population. The average of this ratio across pools would indicate the degree to which the compensatory mechanism implicitly or explicitly transfers funds into and out of pools in proportion to their needs.

Beyond these measures, it is important to have some indication of the effectiveness of accountability mechanisms. In systems with competition among pools, some measure of "market" competitiveness will be required (e.g. barriers to entry); whereas in systems with single or a limited number of non-competing pools, indicators will have to focus on measures related to governance or effective public administration. The share of funds spent on administration instead of direct service provision is potentially useful in this regard. However, it will require significant efforts to develop standard definitions of what constitutes "administrative" costs in ways that will provide relevant comparisons across countries with very different structures and accounting systems. With a more precise definition of pools, some new proposals may emerge. It is likely that these indicators will have to be composite indices relating to a variety of institutional characteristics.

It would be helpful to have two summary measures of pooling. One related to efficiency, such as the amount of resources applied directly to services; and one related to financial protection and equity, such as the average ratio of transfers to the financial shortfalls (or surpluses), the denominator being estimated in relation to the health risks of the associated population.

PURCHASING

When we reach the level of purchasing, the picture clears up somewhat because it is easier to identify "purchasers" than it is to identify pools. "Purchasers" are public and private agencies that spend money to provide services directly or to purchase services for their beneficiaries. Respondents in household or provider surveys are more likely to be able to give a clear answer to the question of who provided a service and who paid for it, than they are to the question of who they are insured by or to which pooling institutions they are affiliated.

However, the first step of relating pools to purchasers is not simple. In some cases, pools and purchasers are one and the same. At one extreme, individuals who pay directly for services or medications out-of-pocket are not pooled at all and are themselves the purchasers. At the other extreme, are pools that directly provide health services to their affiliated population or purchase services for it. In between, there are mixed arrangements. Some of the mixed arrangements are institutional—as when a pool contracts with an insurance agency or specialized purchasing agency to contract services. Other mixed arrangements occur when the purchasing decision itself is broken up into different pieces—as when a pool negotiates or sets fees for different services, but leaves the choice of provider to the insured individual. More work is required to identify appropriate indicators of the relationship between pools and purchasers.

Once the purchasers are identified, the selection of indicators is considerably easier. Some basic structural indicators should include:

- Number of purchasers.

- Mean and distribution of total expenditure across purchasers.

- Mean and distribution of the number of providers who are contracted or hired by each purchaser.

These indicators provide information about the number and distribution of key actors involved in the purchasing phase of financing. Systems in which there are few purchasers and many providers are likely to have more monopsonistic features, while those with many purchasers and few providers are likely to exhibit other kinds of dynamics. In systems with very few purchasers and a few major providing institutions, the dynamics are likely to be ruled by patterns of "gaming," bargaining, negotiation, or bilateral monopoly. Any one of these patterns will have different implications for the system's distribution of benefits and efficiency.

- Share of total funds allocated by inputs (e.g. salaries and traditional budgets), by outputs (e.g. fee for service) or by covered individuals (e.g. capitation).

It is well known that different forms of payment generate different financial incentives for payers and providers. These incentives are embedded within other forms of regulation or professional norms that may alter or offset their impact. However, they still exert a pronounced pressure on decision-making in the health system.

Further work will be necessary to derive standard definitions for conceptually distinct forms of payment, and to address the fact that most health systems rely on a complex mix of these payment mechanisms. For example, in a single social insurance plan, a district might receive a capitated payment that it then pays in salaries to personnel in primary care facilities, but pays specialists with prenegotiated fees per service. Or personnel might be paid in salaries and service-related bonuses.

At this point, the indicators of the financing function begin to overlap with the indicators related to provision. Coordination is envisioned in the collection of indicators for all four functions. However, the close interaction between financing and provision will require special attention to developing common data collection instruments, definitions, and sources.

NEXT STEPS

The proposed set of indicators is a starting point for discussion of the best way to measure the financing function. Some of the unresolved issues that will have to be addressed in this process include:

- How best to define a "pool" and who is a "member" of a pool?

- How to address the scope of services that are covered by the pool?

- How to incorporate institutional factors, such as restrictions that keep purchasers from selecting an exclusive list of providers or constrain risk selection?

- How best to address people who are not "covered" for financial reasons: define membership as share of total population (and uncovered is residual); include an additional indicator; rely on the coverage indicator being prepared separately? The difficulty here is to measure the impact of the system on people who do not spend on health services due to poverty and are either not in a pool or are in a pool that does not pay for services they need.

- Should the progressivity/regressivity of resource generation in the public sector be measured independently of the financial burden distribution?

- How to address the separation and overlap of decisions, such as when individuals choose providers and insurance companies pay?

The next steps in this process are to submit a proposed matrix of indicators for discussion among experts and policy-makers, to begin collecting and organizing available data in a usable format, and to identify potential sources and procedures for collecting new financing system data.

Chapter 19

Developing Health Financing Policies[1]

William D. Savedoff, Guy Carrin

Introduction

The objective of this chapter is to suggest elements of what could eventually be incorporated into policy on health financing. It is written so as to build on the framework and analysis of *The World Health Report 2000* in two important ways. First, it takes as given that the overarching goals of the health system—and in this particular case, health financing—are to contribute to better health, responsiveness, and fairness in financing. Second, it adopts the conceptual model of health financing that traces the flow of funds from collection, through pooling and purchasing.

From these starting points, the chapter takes as a basic premise that policy options with regard to health financing should be evaluated in terms of how effective they are at attaining the overarching goals. It seeks to be pragmatic by showing how different policies may or may not be the most effective way to reach those goals in various contexts, and by explicitly recognizing that difficult trade-offs will arise. Thus, the chapter presumes that by understanding the varied effects of policies in different contexts and upon different goals, it will be possible to provide better guidance to WHO Members. Through such understanding, policy advice can be better adapted to the particular nature of a country's health system, which is conditioned, in turn, by its history, social institutions, governance, political processes, wealth, and culture.

Concepts, Principles and Evidence

A good health financing system contributes to improved health conditions by generating enough resources to adequately finance the health system. It also affects health conditions by modifying the incentives faced by those who pay and those who receive funds with respect to the provision and utilization of health services. But financing systems also affect a variety of social goals other than improving health conditions, namely: solidarity (fairness in paying for the health services relative to income), financial protection (giving individuals claims on the health system that protect them from catastrophic health expenditures in case of illness), and accountability (responsible use of funds).

This chapter presents the concepts comprising the health financing function, along with guiding principles and evidence from existing studies. It aims to illustrate both the advantages and disadvantages of different institutional arrangements used by countries to finance their health systems. Which particular arrangements will be best suited to a particular country or context cannot be determined *a priori* on the basis of theoretical reasoning. Moreover, the current state of evidence is generally too limited to control for the full complexity of health financing systems, the range of institutional arrangements, their interactions among themselves and with the national context. Therefore, the following discussion should be seen primarily as an effort to organize the varying mechanisms and possible relationships, leading towards a proposal for collecting the kinds of evidence that will allow more rigorous testing of some of the emerging hypotheses.

For the purpose of understanding how health financing works, it is useful to conceptually separate the financing function into three parts: collection, pooling, and purchasing[2] (1).

COLLECTION

The effectiveness and impact of different ways of mobilizing funds to support the health system are generally analysed from one of two perspectives: public finance and political economy. From the public finance perspective, the best practices in collecting tax revenues or mandatory insurance premiums for health are very similar to those for collecting obligatory payments for other uses. The form of collecting revenues is thought to be separable from the decision-making over allocation, and therefore there would be no definitive reason that health should be treated differently from other important social services such as education. The same characteristics and benefits of a sound tax system in general will also apply to any tax specifically oriented for the health sector (2).

Arguments in favour of distinguishing health service financing from other forms of taxation or collection rely primarily on arguments of a political or social nature. For example, countries may find it easier to increase revenue collection if citizens are told that payments will be exclusively reserved to fund health services. Also, many countries have pre-existing institutions, such as workers' health insurance funds, that already distinguish health service payments from other contributions. In such cases, countries may find it less costly and/or politically easier to adapt or expand the existing mechanisms for raising revenues. General principles of effective revenue collection from both these perspectives can be applied to a variety of questions that emerge when analysing or changing health system financing.

Earmarked taxes and mandatory contributions dedicated to health insurance can sometimes assure a regular source of additional revenue for a particular function, but they can also reduce flexibility over time in allocating public funds to the best possible use. Earmarked taxes sometimes reduce the accountability of agencies to whom the funds are allocated when those revenues are determined by factors independent of the number or quality of services provided (e.g. share of total payroll) (3;4).

"Sin taxes" are sometimes earmarked for specific health promotion efforts. They deserve special mention because they have two additional characteristics that other earmarked sources may lack. On the one hand, studies have shown that "sin" taxes are effective in reducing the demand for harmful substances, such as tobacco and alcohol, by raising the price closer to its true social cost and increasing the price faced by consumers. On the other hand, if these taxes become

an important source of revenues, they can generate a conflict of interests for public officials. For example, in the United States, after the nationally negotiated "tobacco settlement," it has been argued that many states are less interested in reducing smoking because they now have a strong financial interest in preserving the industry which provides them with large revenues (5;6).

Payroll taxes, along with many other forms of mandatory contribution, can be an effective way to generate resources for the health sector for several reasons: they can be inexpensive to administer and they can be utilized to pursue redistributive aims. Redistribution tends to be limited, however, since contributions are levied against labour income and normally do not touch returns to capital. Redistribution is also limited to a relatively privileged part of the work-force in many developing countries because the formal sector on which such mandates are placed, is often relatively small. In addition, such contributions are easier to evade than indirect taxes in countries with a large informal sector. Unless explicit policies are implemented to achieve universal coverage, such revenue systems may create an exclusive link between claims to health services and employment in ways that pit haves against have-nots.

For many of the reasons mentioned above, general taxes may be preferable as sources of revenue since they are collected from a broader tax base, may be more difficult to evade, and can encompass the full population in pursuing redistributive aims. Nevertheless, general taxes can be at odds with redistributive aims, as in those cases where consumption taxes are not designed well and fall more heavily on lower income groups, and may generate diffuse accountability since the funds pass through broader national allocation systems.

Since the health sector may utilize a significant amount of domestic resources, it is important to be aware that revenue collection for health services may create problems for other parts of public policy. For example, in small open economies where growth of labour productivity is modest, taxing labour may reduce employment or lead to greater informalization of the economy.

Therefore, collection policies that rely on taxes or mandatory contributions need to address issues common to all fiscal revenue mechanisms, such as: the most effective marginal tax and contribution rates; ease of evasion; positive and negative incentives to enhance compliance; discrimination in collection; relative importance of taxes or contributions based on labour, land, capital, or trade; and disincentive effects of user fees or co-payments. Collecting can also be a costly process and should be as efficient as possible. This means that the administrative costs of collecting taxes, contributions, premiums, user fees or co-payments are another element in making decisions.[3]

Collection mechanisms can be, but do not necessarily have to be, directly connected to the goals of solidarity and financial protection. If they are not connected, then the collection function can focus on mobilizing resources in the most efficient manner. Other policies can be developed independently to redistribute income and insure against catastrophic expenses. However, most countries do choose to link collection with solidarity and financial protection, and therefore, aim to collect from contributors in proportion to their capacity to pay. To the extent that a country chooses to link these goals, the literature supports three general policy recommendations.

First, countries should try to minimize large out-of-pocket payments (including both co-payments and deductibles), either by minimizing out-of-pocket finance generally, or by using prepayment to cover large expenses so that out-of-pocket spending is not catastrophic. The world's wealthier countries, particularly European countries and Japan, have already largely achieved these aims. For example, out-of-pocket spending represents less than 20% of total health expenditure in Canada, Germany, Denmark, and the UK. Concomitantly, in these same countries, less than 0.5% of households in a survey reported medical expenses that took more than 40% of their non-subsistence income. At every level of national income, countries vary considerably regarding the share of out-of-pocket spending in total health expenditures and the share of population exposed to very high medical expenses. Among lower middle-income countries, one survey estimates that 27% of spending is being paid out-of-pocket and 5% of households are paying catastrophic medical expenses in Azerbaijan. In Indonesia, a survey has shown the corresponding figures to be 72% and 7.7%. Among the OECD countries, both Portugal and Greece have substantial shares of out-of-pocket spending (23% and 38%, respectively) and households facing catastrophic expenditures (4.8% and 2.4% of households, respectively).

The second strategy for countries that choose to link collection with solidarity and financial protection is that funds should be collected through progressive means—unless those instruments affect the capacity to generate and apply funds. Where this is achieved, it is often accomplished by financing health through progressive general taxation. Even in systems that rely heavily on proportional payroll taxes, progressivity is often introduced through transfers into the health system from more progressive general taxes. In Europe, progressive rate structures are the dominant source of progressivity of gross and net tax liabilities in health systems that rely on general taxes, such as Australia, Italy, and Spain, as well as systems that rely on social insurance, such as France and the Netherlands (7).

But even if progressivity is desirable, it has to be evaluated relative to any negative impact it may have on the main objective of collection, which is raising funds. There are cases such as Guatemala, in which the income tax is highly progressive, but it generates so little income (due to evasion) that there is little to spend on public health services. By contrast, Chile's overall tax burden is less progressive, but a larger share of national income is available for public expenditures that have generated more equitable health outcomes. This highlights the potential trade-off between progressivity and effectiveness of collection[4] (8).

The third implication of trying to link collection with the goals of solidarity and financial protection is that policies should attempt to reduce links between contributions and the ability to access and utilize health services (paying attention again to the impact on generating funds). At one extreme, out-of-pocket payments at the time of service necessarily link the payment with the individual receiving a health service. In this kind of payment, the direct link to receiving a benefit is what makes individuals willing to part with their money. With prepaid plans, whether private or public, the benefit that people receive is less circumscribed and less certain. Prepayment gives the individual access to some unidentified service at some time in the future if needed. Depending on the kind of institution, the prepayment may be required for access to particular services. This is commonly the case for social security institutions. In other cases, prepayment is necessary for being indemnified, as in many private health plans. But in other cases, prepayment may not explicitly confer benefits that differ from those who do not pay. This is generally the case for systems relying on general taxes or social security systems when they must serve unaffiliated individuals. It is in these latter systems where the solidaristic ideal of each person receiving benefits based on need and paying based on income is most likely to be achieved. However, as the link between payment and access to benefit weakens, the ability to mobilize funds and enforce accountability is diminished.

Other issues arise where prepayments are voluntary. This occurs less in wealthy countries where voluntary prepayment is generally restricted to small and complementary shares of total health spending. It is much more common in middle-income countries that have developed insurance markets, such as Brazil, or that have promoted explicit programmes, such as the voluntary health card that Thailand had introduced in the 1980s. And it is also increasingly common in low-income countries like the D.R.Congo's Bwamanda Health Insurance scheme (9).

Voluntary prepayment, whether for insurance or direct access to a health service provider network, eliminates the concerns with evasion that plague mandatory systems. The more successful schemes also benefit from mutual trust that has been built up between managers and members. Accountability is further enforced through the individuals' ability to withdraw if they are dissatisfied. They can also be scaled to capacity to pay since wealthier people are generally willing to spend a higher share of their income on health insurance than lower income groups. However, they generate a variety of problems unless strong regulatory mechanisms are put in place. Some of these problems include differential access to health services and in the case of insurance schemes, adverse selection and risk selection. The Chilean health reform in the 1980s allowed individuals to "opt out" of the social security fund and purchase private insurance. This has been accompanied by significant improvements in health services, but also by an excessive profusion of unstandardized and incomplete insurance contracts (10).

It is critical to recognize that in choosing how to finance the health system, no country starts from a blank slate. Existing systems of taxation, social security institutions, fee structures, and the organization of medical service providers and insurers have all developed out of a historical process conditioned by experiences of colonialism, nation building, labour movements, wars, and technological change. Out of this, citizens already have developed beliefs and expectations regarding the proper ways to pay for health care, and countries have established administrative mechanisms for revenue collection or user fees. The costs and difficulties of altering social institutions and of creating new ones must be an integral part of any discussion about health financing policy.

Therefore, a first step in any policy discussion requires collecting, disaggregating and analysing the sources of health sector spending so as to understand who pays and under what conditions (e.g. mandatory or voluntary), and not just how much is paid. In many cases, this requires information about the general tax and mandatory contribution systems, even if the health system has little influence over them. There is also a need for more and better information about out-of-pocket spending, its distribution across the population and over time, what it is spent on, who is paid, and why people rely on this method of obtaining services. From this basis, it is possible to develop policies that mobilize sufficient resources, reduce the incidence of catastrophic spending, and improve the incentives faced by payers and payees alike.

FUND POOLING

Good pooling contributes to improving health conditions by sharing resources effectively between individuals, so that people can get access to services when needed. Pooling of funds means that financial resources in the pool are no longer tied to a particular contributor. Healthy people will necessarily pay in more to the pool than they receive in terms of health services, while the unhealthy will receive more.

Financing systems that do not include some kind of pooling force individuals who face large medical expenses to effectively "self-insure," using up their own resources (e.g. savings, assets, medical savings accounts), borrowing, or drawing upon household and extended familial networks. There are several reasons that public policy may be justified in trying to replace this kind of "self-insurance" with effective pooling mechanisms. First, individuals may be willing to pay a small fee if it will reduce the likelihood of having to pay large sums of money in the event of an accident or major ailment (when the mechanism is credible). If there is such a demand but effective insurance markets are lacking, then some collective approaches (whether public or private) to insurance can improve social and economic welfare. Second, in most countries, it is considered unfair for individuals to suffer catastrophic financial losses for adverse health problems. Pooling makes it possible to reduce the incidence of such catastrophic events. Finally, when individuals need to rely on their own resources, it affects health status in several ways: individuals may not seek medical care that would improve their own health; if infectious, such untreated illnesses could harm those around them; and unprotected losses of labour income can affect the health of other family members.

Decisions about the "right" kind of pooling are extremely difficult because they touch on fundamental ethical questions that have no simple answers. For example, should pooling health system funds (which transfer resources from the healthy to the sick) also be used to redistribute income from the richer to the poorer? Income redistribution can be achieved at the revenue collection stage (as discussed above), but only if the claims to services are also structured in particular ways—either by pooling the rich and poor together for purchase of similar services or by separating rich and poor with explicit subsidies from the "richer" pool to the "poorer" one.

Another issue arises regarding whether there should be separate fund pools for personal and non-personal health services. If separate, how will each of them be governed, and if combined, how can an appropriate allocation to each category be assured. This is a critical issue, but one about which very little has been written, and which requires significantly more research.

A fundamental question for public policy towards pooling is whether there should be one national pool or many separate ones. A single national pool has the advantage of size, a single administrative system, virtually no adverse selection, and the potential to provide highly equitable access to services and promote efficient allocation of resources. But single national pools may also have disadvantages including diseconomies of scale, weak incentives for controlling costs, and potentially diverting resources or services based on inappropriate criteria or political pressures. Most examples of single pools in the world are either small countries, like Costa Rica, or are financed through general taxes, such as Norway or Oman.

Having a number of separate pools is by no means a panacea, but it can present some advantages. Having separately managed pools introduces the possibility of new tools for accountability, such as bench-marking among purely public agencies or through competition among public, private or mixed entities. If they have the appropriate scale, they might be less costly to administer and be more effective at adjusting to the heterogeneous needs of their populations.

However, separately managed pools present a number of additional questions and problems. First, is whether individuals choose among pools or are assigned by some criteria (e.g. place of residence, type of employment, risk category). When individuals can choose among pools, problems of moral hazard and adverse selection by clients and risk selection by the insurers can emerge, although these problems are attenuated when membership in some pool is mandatory. Good systems of risk-equalization can also significantly address these problems. Administrative

costs may also increase due to spending on advertising or multiple registration systems (11).

In countries such as Argentina and Thailand, individuals are assigned into pools which have no explicit mechanism to cross-subsidize or compensate funds that enrol riskier or lower income individuals (although recent reforms are changing this). In other countries, such as the Netherlands, Germany, and Colombia, individuals may be assigned to specific pools or choose them, but in all events, there is an explicit mechanism to integrate the pools into a larger scheme providing some degree of broader risk-sharing and/or income redistribution. In Japan too, an explicit mechanism assures that pools with poorer members, and even those with higher than average expenditures, are compensated (12). Another example is the Belgian social health insurance system, in which the population can choose to insure with one of the six mutual health funds (and one auxiliary public fund). A national health insurance oversight agency applies risk equalization, thereby keeping certain mutual health funds from running deficits while others run surpluses (13). Canada is a good example of a country with multiple pools (defined by Province) that function within a larger national funding scheme (14).

An important example of voluntary multiple pools has emerged in recent years in many developing countries, variously labelled "community insurance" or "micro-insurance"(15). These are generally voluntary schemes, organized at the village, community, municipal, or district level that allow individuals to pay in small premiums in return for coverage of unexpected health expenditures.

These small pooling arrangements are attractive in mobilizing revenues that might not otherwise be forthcoming for national plans lacking credibility or towards which communities do not feel solidarity. They can also be attractive for public policy in terms of improved governance, particularly in decentralized systems, because local participants are usually involved in overseeing, directing and shaping the character of the health plan and use of funds. Finally, this approach has been proposed as a transitional instrument, building experience with insurance mechanisms so that in future years larger scale and more efficient systems can be put in place. Many health systems currently providing universal coverage started out with small disparate pools that provided only partial coverage, including countries as different as Germany and Uruguay.

Even the strongest proponents recognize the limitations of community and micro-insurance. For example, in poor communities it may simply be impossible to raise sufficient funds to afford any reasonable kind of health service coverage. Furthermore, local governance can be effective, but it can also be corrupt or subject to manipulation by local elites. Finally, the pools may simply be too small to assume substantial risk. Each of these drawbacks can be compensated by national policy—whether providing subsidies, regulating and monitoring administration, or providing public or private reinsurance—as has been analysed and proposed for voluntary schemes in Africa and Asia (*16*). Nevertheless, in cases where these national compensatory policies can be effectively implemented, it is worth questioning why a proper insurance scheme with broader coverage cannot be enacted.

Any mandatory criteria for pooling individuals will have implications for the epidemiological profile of members, the risks faced by the pool, and consequently its average costs. This in turn will affect individuals' satisfaction with the pool. For example, healthy people who have ended up in a relatively high-risk and high-cost pool may feel they are unfairly burdened.

In any case, the existence of multiple pools requires a proactive role by the government in setting rules for membership criteria, whether pools can reject members, valid criteria for setting premiums, any mechanisms for reinsurance or transfers between pools, and the degree to which pools can differ in contribution requirements or services provided. These rules cannot be set independently of one another, but have to be coherent with the ways providers, individuals, and pool managers will respond and behave (*17;18*).

Regardless of whether there is one pool or many, the financial solvency of the pool needs to be assured. This requires some governance or oversight mechanism to monitor the financial risks of the funds that are managed, the liquidity of the pool relative to potential demands for funds, and in the case of multiple pools, rules for bankruptcy and insolvency. Often, a good communication strategy is important to assure that beneficiaries' expectations do not exceed the institution's financial capacity to respond. Due to the largely public nature of most health system financing, political processes are a factor in assuring financial solvency. This needs to be considered whether allocating funds to complement shortfalls in social insurance contributions, to cover the expenses of a general tax-funded health system, or to adequately subsidize subpopulations who are excluded on the basis of income or location.

As in the case of collection, most countries already have a variety of mechanisms for pooling funds inside or outside the health sector. In some countries, notions of insurance are widespread and the idea of creating health funds is quite acceptable. In other countries, the concept of sharing risk outside of the family or village may not be well established or the level of trust in those managing the funds may be very low. Many cultural, political and social factors affect the acceptability and credibility of a pooling system, and need to be taken into consideration when making policies in this area.

Therefore, decisions about the best way to pool funds must begin with an analysis of any existing system with regard to who (if anyone) is pooled and how many, along with the criteria for membership, capacity to manage risk, and mechanisms for establishing contributions and access. Analysis can determine how risk is actually spread between groups, and whether the pools are large enough to manage risk or whether they need access to reinsurance. The mechanisms by which fund managers are held accountable must be examined through the composition and selection of a board of directors and their interests, or through analysing market structure and competitivity. The relative power of pooling agencies in relation to service providers must also be considered.

Any proposals for change need to address the ways in which pool membership affects access to services, whether pools are culturally and politically accepted and supported, whether they are financially sustainable, and whether pool managers have the necessary information systems, training, and tools to manage the collection and use of funds.

PURCHASING[5]

Good purchasing contributes to health sector policy goals by assuring that funds are allocated and used effectively. "Purchasing" is the process through which revenues that have been pooled are allocated to providers, public or private, to deliver a set of interventions to particular groups of individuals. Therefore, the term purchasing as used here, refers to a wide spectrum of spending decisions, ranging from budgeting in hierarchical bureaucracies to contracts between purchasers and independent providers, and even encompassing individual transactions between clients and providers. By looking at all these financial allocation relationships together, it is possible to learn about better ways of making the process more effective in producing good health outcomes.

Purchasing is an extremely important interface between financing of the health system and provision. It is where evidence on the costs and effects of interventions can have an influence. It is also a key element among the many factors that condition the behaviour and choices of health service providers. For example, in the literature analysing the determinants of health spending, the only institutional factors that have been regularly and demonstrably influential are those affecting the payment of health service providers. Other institutional factors, such as the public share of spending or the presence of a social insurance system, have not demonstrated a robust relationship with health spending or outcomes (19;20).

A great deal has been learned about the process of purchasing health services. Much of the literature analyses the impact of asymmetric information and uncertainty on the methods of buying health services. Such methods range from fee-for-service to fixed salaries, and capitation[6] (18;21;22). In a seminal article, Kenneth Arrow (1963) argued that due to the particularities of health services, societies have necessarily evolved a variety of non-market methods to compensate for market failures—including professional ethics and basic trust between patient and physician. These non-market aspects of decision-making by health service providers must be incorporated in any analysis of the impact of allocating financial resources, through whatever mechanisms, to health providers.

A large literature has also developed specifically around the question of financial allocation within the public sector. This ranges from modernizing public administration to so-called internal markets and performance contracts. Jérôme-Forget et al. provide an overview of internal market mechanisms in Canada, the United States, Sweden, the Netherlands, and Britain (23). Since the early 1990s, health policy discussions in developing countries have often revolved around determining a "basic package" of health services using cost-effectiveness and burden of disease information to develop a strategy regarding which interventions the public sector should prioritize (24).

The structure of collection and pooling has an impact on the choice of who purchases. Most directly, in the case of out-of-pocket payments, it is the individual who purchases services. When governments finance health services out of general tax revenues, they may contract providers directly under a Ministry of Health or transfer those funds to private or public agencies under certain terms, in which case those agencies will do the purchasing. In social security systems with mandatory payroll or income contributions, the choice between direct hiring and contracting out must be made.

One of the most common ways to purchase health services is through purchasing inputs. Traditional budgeting is a widespread example of this: the government or insurer contracts a certain number of doctors, nurses, and administrators on salary, and builds and equips facilities. This is administratively simple, but requires effective public administration to assure that funds are used wisely and produce the kinds of health services needed.

Another way of purchasing is service based. This has the advantage of only paying for services or goods that were actually provided, but it also encourages overprovision. In a context of limited access and low productivity, such a payment mechanism may be quite beneficial. In other contexts, however, it can contribute to a rapid escalation of costs. It can be administratively simple or costly depending on the amount of controls that are necessary to assure that only appropriate services are provided and reimbursed. However, it does have an interesting advantage for managing the health system in that it can generate extensive information on patterns of utilization, service provision, and epidemiology.

Finally, purchasers can try to buy health outcomes directly. This is difficult because the determinants of health conditions are multiple and uncertain. Furthermore, health outcomes are difficult to measure despite current advances (i.e. health states, DALY reductions, etc.). Nevertheless, there have been efforts to focus on outcomes by using capitation schemes in which the purchaser contracts with medical service providers for maintaining the health of each affiliated person in return for a per person payment. The United States has a range of organizations that contract all or some portion of insurance coverage under capitation schemes, but low-income countries have also experimented with such arrangements. For example, in the mid-1990s, Guatemala began to purchase basic health services from NGOs on a capitated basis. This was credited with extending very basic health services over a four-year period to an additional three million Guatemalans who had never before had access to such services at all (25). Capitation payment for hospital based outpatient and inpatient services was also used in the ORT health plus project, a community-based health insurance scheme in the Philippines (26).

In all cases, "prices" of some kind, whether for inputs, outputs or outcomes, need to be negotiated or set. The price setting process can have significant effects on service provision and cost. For example, when providers set prices and submit bills to a third party insurer, there are few incentives to use inputs efficiently. In other cases, services are priced *ex ante*, generally through negotiation between payers and providers. In this case, the efficiency incentives are greater, but so are incentives to avoid treating patients who are more costly to serve than the prenegotiated fee.

Price setting through any kind of negotiated process is difficult because the purchaser may have little information about the cost of providing health services, particularly in comparison with the providers. Furthermore, even if the costs of providing particular services were known, the actual determinants of health beyond the specific services provided are uncertain and difficult to attribute to specific interventions. There are many experiences of price setting systems throughout the world, and a constantly evolving set of alternative formulas. For example, Canada has a long experience in setting budgets (for hospitals) and fees (for physicians) with the goal of providing care and containing costs. To this effect, most of the provinces have worked with hard budgets, and in the past, overruns were even compensated via claw-backs (27).

Ethical issues arise when attempting to calculate health costs—whether or not different groups should be averaged together or costed separately. Protocols and guidelines are often developed as approximations to identifying the kinds and quality of services that ought to be provided in different circumstances. These protocols or guidelines can then be used by the purchaser to assess whether providers fulfilled their obligations, regardless of the payment system involved.

Every country has a variety of experiences with different service purchasing schemes. Out-of-pocket fee-for-service spending is often the most widespread. However, most countries also have some doctors who are paid on salary, and increasingly, countries are turning to bonuses or performance contracts with providers or provider organizations. Policies in this area need to balance the risks of overprovision and underprovision (risks associated with fee-for-service and capitation, respectively). They need to consider the impact of payment mechanisms on the mix of services provided[7] (28–32). And they need to design changes in collaboration with other mechanisms for assuring quality, such as the development of protocols, medical training reforms, and peer review.

Medical professionals and their various associations play a unique role both in how the health system performs and in the debates over health system policy. They can collaborate in defining protocols and peer review, organizing service provision and identifying service categories, as well as pricing inputs and linking them to services. But they also play political roles and promote their interests, just as other interested social actors, such as politicians, consumer groups, and businesses (33). For this reason, there is growing interest in understanding how these various groups interact in recent processes of health system reform. Efforts have been made to determine the best ways to incorporate these different social actors so as to select the best policies. The fact that health sector financing involves money makes it a central focus of many of these discussions.

Conclusion

It is apparent that financing, through the collection, pooling, and purchasing subfunctions, is bound to have a strong impact on the fairness in financial contribution to the system and some effect on a country's health outcomes and responsiveness. Changes to the financing system must take into account the existing financing mechanisms and social institutions that have developed historically, along with people's beliefs and expectations about paying for health services. The incentives generated by financial flows at every level of the system need to be recognized and, where possible, modified to improve the responsiveness and effectiveness of service provision.

Abstracting from specific circumstances, systems that rely on general taxes and offer universal access appear to have many advantages for achieving goals of mobilizing resources, while offering the potential for solidarity and financial protection, because they can minimize out-of-pocket spending, reduce the incidence of catastrophic spending, separate the link between contribution and utilization, and minimize distortions in the economy. However, these systems are not without their problems: quality and access concerns in wealthy countries or limited coverage and inefficiency in poorer ones. That is why many countries choose to develop and rely on financing systems based on social insurance or mandatory private insurance, and many of these have demonstrated that they can also be successful. The lack of strong evidence to associate any specific financing system with clear improvements in health outcomes and financial equity assures us that there are better and worse ways to make any particular financing system perform. Utilizing principles such as those summarized here and those found in the wider literature, is the best way currently available for countries to guide their systems towards a better performance. Through collecting more and better data, future research may be able to provide more definitive guidance.

REFERENCES

(1) World Health Organization. *The World Health Report 2000. Health Systems: Improving Performance.* Geneva, World Health Organization, 2000.

(2) Musgrave RA, Musgrave PB. *Public finance in theory and practice.* London and New York, McGraw Hill, 1989.

(3) Brett C, Keen M. Political uncertainty and the earmarking of environmental taxes. *Journal of Public Economics*, 2000, 75(3).

(4) Buchanan J. The economics of earmarked taxes. *Journal of Political Economy*, 1963, 71:457–469.

(5) Chaloupka FJ, Warner KE. *The economics of smoking.* NBER Working Paper No. W7047. Cambridge, MA, NBER, 1999.

(6) Bulow J, Klemperer P, Centre for Economic Policy Research. *The tobacco deal.* London, Centre for Economic Policy Research, 1999.

(7) Wagstaff A, van Doorslaer E. What makes the personal income tax progressive? A comparative analysis for fifteen OECD countries. *International Tax and Public Finance*, 2001, 8(3):299–316.

(8) Inter-American Development Bank. *Facing up to inequality in Latin America: economic and social progress in Latin America: 1998–1999 report.* Washington, DC, distributed by the J. Hopkins University Press for the Inter-American Development Bank, 1998.

(9) Criel B. District-based health insurance in sub-Saharan Africa. *Studies in Health Services Organisation and Policy*, vol. 10. Antwerp, Belgium, Institute of Tropical Medicine, 1998.

(10) Sánchez H, Zuleta G, eds. *La hora de los usuarios.* Washington, DC, Inter-American Development Bank, 2000.

(11) Fielding J, Thomas R. Can managed competition solve problems of market failure? *Health Affairs*, 1993, 12.

(12) Ministry of Health and Welfare. *Outline of social insurance in Japan.* Tokyo, Ministry of Health and Welfare, 1999.

(13) European Observatory on Health Care Systems. *Health care systems in transition.* Belgium, 2000. URL: http://www.observatory.dk

(14) Blomqvist AG. *Limits to care: reforming Canada's health system in an age of restraint.* Toronto, C.D. Howe Institute, 1994.

(15) Dror DM, Jacquier C. Micro-insurance: extending health insurance to the excluded. *International Social Security Review*, 1999, 52:71–97.

(16) Carrin G, Desmet M, Basaza R. Social health insurance development in low-income developing countries: new roles for Government and Nonprofit Health Insurance Organizations in Africa and Asia. In: Scheil-Adlung X, ed. *Building social security: the challenge of privatisation.* London, Transaction Publishers, 2001.

(17) Enthoven A. *Theory and practice of managed competition in health care finance.* North Holland, 1988.

(18) Robinson JC. Theory and practice in the design of physician payment incentives. *The Milbank Quarterly*, 2001, 79.

(19) Gerdtham U-G, Jönsson B. International comparisons of health expenditure. In: Culyer AJ, Newhouse JP, eds. *Handbook of health economics.* Amsterdam, Elsevier, 2000.

(20) Culyer AJ, Newhouse JP. *Handbook of health economics*, 1st ed. Amsterdam, Elsevier, 2000.

(21) Barnum H, Kutzin J, Saxenian H. Incentives and provider payment methods. *International Journal of Health Planning and Management*, 1995, 10:23–45.

(22) Feldstein MS. *Economic analysis for health service efficiency. Econometric studies of the British National Health Service.* Amsterdam, North-Holland Pub. Co., 1967.

(23) Jérôme-Forget M, White J, Wiener JM, eds. *Health care reform through internal markets.* Montreal, Quebec and Washington, DC, Institute for Research on Public Policy and The Brookings Institution, 1995.

(24) World Bank. *Investing in health.* Washington, DC, World Bank, 1993.

(25) Nieves I, La Forgia GM, Ribera J. Large-scale government contracting of NGOs to extend basic health services to poor populations in Guatemala. In: Rösenmoller M, ed. *Challenges for health reform: reaching the poor.* Barcelona, Estudios y Ediciones, S.A., 2000: 117–131.

(26) Ron A. NGOs in community health insurance schemes: examples from Guatemala and the Philippines. *Social Science & Medicine*, 1999, 48(7):939–959.

(27) Barer ML, Lomas J, Sanmartin C. Reminding our Ps and Qs: medical cost controls in Canada. *Health Affairs*, 1996, 15(2):216–234.

(28) Newhouse JP. An iconoclastic view of health cost containment. *Health Affairs*, 1993, 12(1):152–171.

(29) Gruber J, Wise D. *An international perspective on policies for an aging society.* NBER Working Paper No. W8103. January, 2001. URL: http://papers.nber.org/papers/W8103

(30) Andrade R, Alcázar L. Induced demand and absenteeism in Peruvian hospitals. In: Di Tella R, Savedoff WD, eds. *Diagnosis corruption: public hospitals in Latin America.* Washington, DC, Inter-American Development Bank, 2001.

(31) Tussing AD, Wojtowycz MA. The Cesarean decision in New York State, 1986. Economic and noneconomic aspects. *Medical Care*, 1992, 30:529–540.

(32) Tussing AD, Wojtowycz MA. The effect of physician characteristics on clinical behavior: Cesarean section in New York State. *Social Science & Medicine*, 1993, 37:1251–1260.

(33) Murrillo MV, Maceira D. *Social sector reform in Latin America and the role of Unions.* Research Department Working Paper Series, WP-456. Washington, DC, Inter-American Development Bank, 2001.

NOTES

1 This chapter is virtually identical to inputs provided for the Scientific Peer Review Group on Health Systems Performance Assessment Meetings of December 2001. It draws on earlier drafts by Philip Musgrove and has benefited from comments by Christopher J.L. Murray, Kei Kawabata, and Abdelhay Mechbal.

2 See *The World Health Report 2000* for a fuller characterization of health system functions.

3 For more information about theory and evidence on public financing, see Musgrave and Musgrave, 1989.

4 For a more detailed discussion, see Chapter 8 in Inter-American Development Bank, 1999.

5 "Purchasing" as used here, refers not only to explicit purchases from private entities, but also to management processes that allocate funds to providers within public agencies.

6 For recent discussions of payment mechanisms, see Barnum et al., 1995 and Robinson, 2001. For an earlier and more schematic treatment, see Feldstein, 1967.

7 The system of indemnity insurance in the US during the 1960–1980 period created incentives for a rapid development of advanced, and often costly, technology. See Newhouse J. *Health Affairs*, 1993, 12(1):152–171 for an iconoclastic view of health cost containment, which has recently received some support in Gruber J, Wise D. *An international perspective on policies for an aging society*. NBER Working Paper No. W8103. January, 2001. The evidence of excessive service provision under fee-for-search is quite apparent and shocking in the case of Cesarean deliveries (*30–32*).

Chapter 20

Beyond Access and Utilization: Defining and Measuring Health System Coverage

Bakhuti Shengelia, Christopher J.L. Murray, Orvill B. Adams

Introduction

Much has been published on the assessment of health systems, particularly on the provision of health services (*1–9*). Delivery of health interventions to individuals in need is a critical pathway through which health service provision can contribute to social objectives, such as improving population health and reducing health inequalities. This natural focus on the delivery of interventions has earned the measures of utilization and access a prominent role in the health policy literature (*10–15*). Provision of health services can be evaluated more comprehensively through the measure of coverage. It provides a stronger basis for identifying the contribution of health services to major health system goals, such as population health. The time lag between health system actions and coverage as their intermediate outcome is shorter than that between health system actions and their final outcomes. A long time lag in the latter case makes it difficult to attribute outcomes to actions (*16;17*). Using coverage as a metric of health service provision may help to overcome this challenge.

In this chapter, we begin with the common-sense notion that health systems should deliver as much health gain to the population as achievable with the existing resources and knowledge. We build the conceptual and analytical framework for defining and measuring health system coverage on the rich and extensive literature on utilization and access (*14;18–20*). Our framework aims at understanding and measuring the contribution of factors such as geographic access, resource availability, cultural acceptability, financial affordability, and quality of care to health system coverage.

This chapter is organized into five sections. In sec-

tion two, we briefly discuss some important issues raised in the literature on utilization, access, and intervention-specific coverage. In the third section, the key concepts of coverage, health gain, efficacy, effectiveness, and effective coverage are introduced and formally defined for a single intervention. In section four, coverage of a single intervention is expanded to health system coverage. Operationalization of these concepts and the associated measurement strategies are presented next. The final section presents a discussion of some implications and directions for further work.

Background

The extensive existing literature reflects the importance of utilization and access as metrics of health service provision (*3;8;15;21–32*). In this chapter we focus attention on four topics: concepts of utilization and access, intervention versus health system coverage, individual versus population coverage, and *ex post* and *ex ante* perspectives of coverage.

Concepts of Utilization and Access

Concepts of utilization were the dominant approach in the 1960s and 1970s. Utilization is often defined as the quantity of health care services and procedures used (*19*). Studies on health service utilization frequently extend beyond measuring the quantity of health services used, and focus on the determinants of utilization. Several conceptual frameworks of the determinants of utilization have been proposed (*3;15;21;24;32;33*). These frameworks identify with important variations individual, community, and health system factors. Economic studies by Gerlter, van der Gaag and others (*11;34–45*) have further advanced the measurement of health care utilization. They provide examples of modelling demand functions for health care using variables such as price of care, travel time and the opportunity costs linked to it, patient's income, perceived quality of care, provider behaviour, etc. *(11;31;46-61)*. Such models give useful information about the elasticity of demand for different types of health services. They help predict the response of consumer health-seeking behaviour to changes in key demand factors that result from various policy actions.

Studies on access compared with those on utilization focus more on health system characteristics (supply factors) rather than a patient's health-seeking behaviour (demand factors). Several theoretical models exist for describing access *(8;62-67)*. Some of these models view access as a fit between predisposing factors on one side, and enabling and health system factors, on the other *(8;19)*. Predisposing factors include an individual's perception of an illness, as well as population-specific cultural, social, and epidemiological factors. Enabling factors include the means available to individuals for using health services. Health system factors comprise resources, structures, institutions, procedures, and regulations through which health services are delivered.

Despite numerous studies measuring access, utilization, and demand for health services, the literature is rather scarce about the models for quantifying the contribution of various health system factors, including access factors, to population health, one of the final goals of health systems. Such models could prove extremely useful in identifying specific constraints in health service delivery and could be strong policy tools for effective stewardship.

INTERVENTION VERSUS HEALTH SYSTEM COVERAGE

Programme managers focused on the delivery of interventions such as childhood immunization, DOTS for tuberculosis, antenatal care, and cervical cancer screening, have extensively analysed and reported on their coverage *(27;56;68-73)*. In this literature, coverage is defined simply as the proportion of the population in need of an intervention that actually received the intervention *(13;32;74-78)*. Formally:

$$C_j = \frac{N_j}{M_j} \qquad [1]$$

where N_j is the number of people who received intervention j, and M_j is the total population who needed the intervention.

There is a significant body of literature attempting to examine determinants of coverage for different single interventions *(27;56;68-71;77;79-82)*. A key challenge remains: can the intervention-specific concept of coverage be linked to a health system perspective on access and utilization without losing details of the information about the intervention? Clearly, the content and effectiveness of interventions that health systems deliver under different types of services matter, and not just the total volume of services. Because the health system characteristics are important determinants of service delivery, we believe that health system coverage in its entirety offers much more information for the assessment of health systems performance than the coverage of specific interventions.

INDIVIDUALS VERSUS POPULATION

Utilization, often measured as a continuous variable, has been reported and analysed *(3;9;21;23;24;26;30; 49;52;65;83-85)* at both the individual and the population levels. Intervention-specific coverage is usually reported at the population level as a dichotomous variable. Analyses of the determinants of access have mostly been undertaken at the aggregate level. We believe it is useful to define concepts and measures of coverage that are meaningful for individuals as well as for populations. Conceptual consistency between these two levels will allow for decomposition of coverage by intervention or population groups, allowing for a comprehensive assessment of inequalities in coverage *(69;81;86-92)*.

Ex Post and *Ex Ante* Perspectives

Data on coverage of specific interventions, utilization of health services, or access are naturally reported *ex post* (after the fact). The common-sense notion of coverage, however, is of an anticipatory or *ex ante* (before the fact) character. Individuals believe that they are covered by the health system if they will receive the appropriate interventions when they need them in the future. The mismatch between this common-sense notion of individual coverage and the convenience of measuring it *ex post* can be fixed by thinking of coverage in probabilistic terms (probability of receiving an intervention when needed).

COVERAGE FOR A SINGLE INTERVENTION

In this section, we formalize definitions for the following: coverage for an intervention at the individual level, health gain, efficacy, effectiveness, quality, and effective coverage.

COVERAGE

Based on the discussion in the previous section, we propose a formal definition of coverage. At the individual level, coverage can be defined as the probability of receiving a necessary health intervention, conditional on a health care need. As this quantity is defined at the individual level as a probability, it should be confined to a discrete time interval, such as one year. We present the advantages of defining coverage in this way later in the paper.

We can aggregate coverage across a group of individuals by taking into account the probability of each individual requiring the intervention. In notation:

$$C_j = \frac{\sum_i C_{ij} d_{ij}}{\sum_i d_{ij}} \qquad [2]$$

where C_{ij} is the probability of individual i receiving intervention j conditional on having a health condition that would benefit from intervention j, and d_{ij} is the probability of the health condition requiring intervention j for individual i. Summing across individuals and taking into account the probability of different individuals requiring an intervention means that at the population level, C_j will equal the traditional measure of population coverage defined above (Equation [1]).

FROM COVERAGE TO EFFECTIVE COVERAGE

The link between the coverage of key interventions and the level of population health is mediated by the extent to which interventions deliver the potential health gain possible with the available technology. In order to identify the extent to which health systems are delivering at their potential, the definition of coverage must encompass not only simply delivering an intervention, but also delivering the potential health gain achievable through the intervention. To expand the definition of coverage, we must first formalize the concepts of health gain, efficacy, effectiveness, and quality.

Health Gain

Usually health gain is defined on the basis of the counterfactual (assumed scenario) of receiving an intervention. Therefore, it is difficult, if not impossible, to directly observe it at the individual level. Nevertheless, the concept and notation will be helpful in the development of these ideas. Expected health gain from intervention j for individual i can be defined as the difference between the healthy life expectancy of individual i receiving needed intervention j and the counterfactual healthy life expectancy of the same individual without receiving intervention j.

$$HG_{ij} = HALE_{ij} - HALE_i \qquad [3]$$

where $HALE_{ij}$ is the healthy life expectancy for individual i with intervention j, and $HALE_i$ is the healthy life expectancy for individual i without intervention j.

In cases where there is an externality associated with delivering an intervention to individual i, this definition is not sufficient. For example, treatment of an individual with smear-positive pulmonary tuberculosis will decrease the risks of transmission of tuberculosis to the rest of the population. Likewise, in cases of herd immunity, high levels of immunization coverage may decrease the risk of disease for the rest of the population. Health gain from delivering intervention j to individual i, should be generalized to include all changes in healthy life expectancy for all individuals in the population. Fortunately, this distinction is quantitatively important for a very limited number of interventions. For the sake of simplicity, in the rest of the chapter, we will assume that there are no such externalities. This assumption does not alter any of the arguments and concepts presented below.

Efficacy

In clinical trials on efficacy individuals who have co-morbidities or belong to certain age groups are often excluded. Further provider performance is carefully monitored and maintained at its best. One way of representing the notion of efficacy is to relate it to health gain where providers are behaving optimally, they have all technologies available, and patients adhere to the treatment regimen. This is shown in the following notation:

$$Efc_j = \frac{\sum_{i=1}^{l} HG_{ij} | X_i \neq excl.criteria, P_{jk} = P_{opt}, Y_{ij} = 1, R_{jk} = 1, \forall k = 1, \dots k}{l} \qquad [4]$$

where HG_{ij} is the health gain for individual i from intervention j; P_{jk} is the performance of a provider, in terms of technical quality of the intervention, and taking into account available resources; P_{opt} is the optimum performance of the provider; Y_{ij} and R_{jk} are indices of adherence and resource availability which are equal to 1 when ideal; X_i is the set of individual characteristics; and l is the number of individuals without the excluding criteria (comorbidities, certain age groups, exposure to risk factors, etc.).

It should be noted that health gain is not a standard unit of efficacy. Traditionally efficacy is expressed in terms of reduction in mortality and morbidity (case fatality rate, mortality rate, incidence rate, etc.), survival within a specific time interval, reduction of intensity and frequency of clinical symptoms, etc. It is difficult to compare the efficacy of different types of interventions if they are expressed in different units. This problem can be overcome by using health gain as a unit of efficacy. This also is more practical because in the end, all other traditional units imply the improvement of healthy life expectancy, which captures both fatal and non-fatal health outcomes.

Effectiveness

In reality, due to the individual comorbidities, individual behaviour, and provider performance, the potential health gain represented by efficacy is often not achieved. In the cost-effectiveness and quality of care literature, the actual health gain which is a fraction of efficacy, is referred to as effectiveness (93;94). Formally, the effectiveness of intervention j at the individual level can be defined as an average individual health gain from the intervention. Formally it can be represented by the following notation:

$$Eft_j = \frac{\sum_{i=1}^{N} HG_{ij}}{N}, \qquad [5]$$

where HG_{ij} the health gain for individual i *with intervention j*, and N is the population size.

Effective Coverage

When the average individual in a population says that he/she is covered by the health system for treatment of depression, he/she most likely means that if he/she gets clinical depression he/she will receive appropriate treatment. This common-sense notation is a reflection of many factors including the quality of care and financial, physical, and cultural access to providers.

Effective coverage measures the expected health gain from intervention j relative to the potential health

gain possible with the optimal performance of providers in a given health system. Effective coverage of an individual with intervention j can be represented by the following notation:

$$EC_{ij} = \frac{HG_{ij}C_{ij}}{(HG_{ij}|P_k = P_{opt}, Y_{ij} = 1, R_{jk} = 1, \forall k = 1, \ldots)} \qquad [6]$$

where HG_{ij} is the expected health gain from intervention j for individual i; C_{ij} is the probability of receiving effective intervention j for individual i conditional on the presence of a health problem; P_k is the provider performance; and P_{opt} is the optimal provider performance possible with available resources; Y_{ij} and R_{jk} are indices of compliance and resource availability, respectively, which are set to 1 when ideal.

As with coverage, effective coverage can be simply aggregated across individuals by taking into account the probability that they will need an intervention:

$$EC_j = \frac{\sum_{i=1}^{n} HG_{ij}C_{ij}d_{ij}}{\sum_{i=1}^{n}(HG_{ij}|P_k = P_{opt}, Y_{ij} = 1, R_{jk} = 1, \forall k = 1, \ldots)d_{ij}} \qquad [7]$$

Examination of the equation for coverage with an intervention j [2] and the equation for effective coverage [7] reveals that effective coverage is simply coverage multiplied by the fraction of potential health gain that has been achieved with the intervention. This brings the notion of coverage closer to the health impact of service provision.

MULTIPLE DETERMINANTS OF EFFECTIVE COVERAGE

It would be useful to develop a measure of effective coverage that captures multiple factors related to health systems or individuals (16;17). An individual's coverage can be affected by several factors, such as the cost of seeking care, physical proximity to the provider, availability of medical technology and human resources, and sociodemographic characteristics. In a given health system, it is likely that individuals with similar characteristics encounter similar experiences in seeking care for the same health problem. Therefore, by looking at the *ex post* coverage of a group of individuals with shared characteristics, we may be able to predict the coverage of similar individuals who do not have the health problem currently, but may require a health intervention in the future.

The multicausal nature of effective coverage for individual i with intervention j can be represented in the following function:

$$EC_{ijk} = f(B_{jk}, I_i, Y_{ij}, Q_{ijk}, Z_{jik}, R_{jk}, HG_{ij}, P_{ijk}) \quad [8]$$

where EC_{ijk} is effective coverage; B_{jk} is the price of the intervention j offered by provider k to the individual i; I_i is an individual's disposable income; Y_{ij} is adherence to a recommended treatment regimen, Q_{ijk} is the physical access (expressed in units of travel time) of individual i to provider k delivering intervention j; Z_{jik} is cultural acceptability of intervention j offered by provider k to individual i; R_{jk} is the available technology needed to deliver intervention j by provider k; HG_{ij} is health gain; and P_{ijk} is provider performance as defined previously. We use this formulation to introduce some important counterfactual constructs, but it is not an exhaustive catalogue of the determinants that can influence effective coverage.

In the previous section we discussed the conceptual framework of effective coverage as an intermediate goal of health system performance, and a measure of the health service provision function. In order to make the measurement of effective coverage more operational, we propose a framework in which the gap between actual and maximum effective coverage is decomposed into seven components (78):

- Resource availability gap

- Physical accessibility gap

- Affordability gap

- Cultural acceptability gap

- Provider-related quality gap

- Adherence gap

- Strategic choice gap

Each of these concepts is a function of individual and health system factors.

Resource Availability Gap

The resource availability gap demonstrates if sufficient amounts of resources and technologies are available to deliver an intervention. This might include the number of health facilities, the number of personnel, and the availability of technology (drugs, equipment, etc.) (74;77;78). For an individual i, availability gap with intervention j can be defined as the probability of not receiving the intervention if the only limiting factor were the availability of the technology to providers

for delivering the intervention, i.e. the counterfactual situation.

This can be represented as:

$$Av_{ij} = 1 - EC_{ijk}|(B_{jk} = 0, Z_{jik} = \theta, Q_{ijk} = 0, P_{ijk} = P_{opt}, \\ Y_{ij} = 1) \forall k, k = 1, \dots, n \quad [9]$$

This conditional expression says that resource availability coverage is the difference between ideal effective coverage, which would equal 1, and effective coverage of individual i with intervention j if all providers were offering the intervention free of charge ($B_{jk} = 0$), all providers were located in the immediate proximity to the individual thereby requiring zero travel time ($Q_{ijk} = 0$), the cultural acceptability of the intervention offered by all providers were equal to a certain acceptable value θ of the latent variable of "cultural acceptability," providers were delivering the intervention optimally, individuals were fully adhering to treatment, and the most effective intervention were selected among possible choices for the given health condition. The only constraint would be the availability of the intervention. Measurement of the resource availability gap would require estimation of the relationship between effective coverage and the variables in equations [8]–[9]. The practical implications for data collection and estimation are discussed below.

Physical Accessibility Gap

The physical accessibility gap measures the extent to which an intervention is physically accessible to the population. For example, it is well known that the utilization of health care facilities declines as the distance to the provider increases (30;95). Time is another factor of accessibility related to distance and transportation facilities. In fact, travel time to a health facility and the waiting time to see a health professional seem to be more associated with the consumers' perception of accessibility of services than with distance (58).

The accessibility gap for individual i for intervention j can be defined in a way similar to the resource availability gap: it is the difference between ideal effective coverage and effective coverage of individual i with intervention j, given that there are no constraints in terms of affordability, cultural acceptability, resource availability, provider quality, adherence, and the choice of the right intervention. The only constraint is physical access. The formal notation of physical accessibility gap can be constructed as that of the resource availability gap.

Affordability Gap

Affordability depends on the amount of an individual's disposable income for health, and also on the way health care finance is organized within a country. For simplicity, we will consider the price of an intervention at the point of use as the only constraint for effective coverage. Thus, the affordability gap is the gap between ideal effective coverage and effective coverage of individual i with intervention j, given that there are no constraints in terms of cultural acceptability, physical access, availability of resources, provider performance, adherence, and the choice of the most effective intervention. The formal notation of affordability gap can be constructed as that of the technology availability gap.

Cultural Acceptability Gap

The cultural acceptability gap measures the extent to which services are culturally acceptable to the population. Even if resources are available and accessible, they may not be used if they are not acceptable to the population.

Cultural acceptability includes non-monetary factors such as beliefs, religion, gender, type of facility and responsiveness of health services (64). Information about the cultural acceptability gap is essential in enabling policy-makers to better understand the use of services.

The acceptability gap for individual i can be defined as the difference between ideal effective coverage and effective coverage with intervention j given there are no constraints other than cultural acceptability. The formal notation of acceptability gap can be constructed as that of the resource availability gap.

Provider-related Quality Gap

Given available resources, we can examine the limitations on coverage due to sub-optimal performance of providers. It is important to note that on an absolute scale, technical quality will be a function of provider behaviour and available resources. Limitations of resources are captured in availability coverage, but the decrement in coverage due to provider performance is not reflected in any of the previous counterfactual measures. We label this concept as provider-related quality gap. Formally, provider-related quality gap can be defined as the differences between ideal effective coverage and effective coverage of individual i with intervention j, given the providers have all necessary resources and technologies to deliver the intervention, and there are no constraints in terms of physical access, cultural acceptability, affordability, adherence, and the right choice of an intervention. The only constraint is the ability of providers to use the available technologies and resources for producing health gain in an individual. The notation of provider-related quality gap can be constructed as that of resource availability gap.

Adherence Gap

Adherence to the treatment regimen for chronic diseases is an important condition for the realization of the potential health gain from an intervention. The difference between the full potential effective coverage and the effective coverage when the only constraint is adherence to the treatment regimen can be defined as the adherence gap. Formally it can be represented by a notation similar to that of the resource availability gap.

Strategic Choice Gap

Usually there are various strategies that one can choose from to address a certain health condition. The effectiveness of those strategies might differ and so can the health gain realized through their implementation. The strategic choice gap can be defined as the difference between the maximum effective coverage of interventions, the best feasible strategy for a given health condition, and the maximum effective coverage with intervention j, the intervention actually selected.

DECOMPOSING GAPS IN EFFECTIVE COVERAGE

The counterfactual concepts of availability, accessibility, affordability, acceptability, adherence, and provider-related quality can be used to decompose the gaps in effective coverage into their components. Identification of the main factors contributing to limitations in effective coverage would be extremely useful for policy analysis. If the relationship between the variables such as price, distance, etc. in equation [9] is linear, the decomposition of the gaps in coverage is additive. It is likely, however, that in reality multiple factors interact with each other, and thus the relationship between effective coverage and each of the variables in equation [9] is not linear. For policy discourse, however, it is often difficult for health policy stakeholders and the media to accept that causes are not additive. In these cases, as in the analysis of risk factor data, it may be useful to use Shapley values or similar approaches to show non-additive causes (96;97).

HEALTH SYSTEM COVERAGE

So far we have formalized the concept of effective coverage for an individual or groups of individuals for a specific intervention. The contribution of different factors such as accessibility or acceptability can be precisely defined and analysed. If we believe that there are systemic factors that underlie coverage of different interventions, such as how financing is structured or how health system providers are paid, it is important to link effective coverage with a specific intervention to more general coverage of the health system.

The statement "I am covered by the health system" can be taken to mean that if "I get sick the health system will take care of me and provide appropriate interventions." In the context of effective coverage, this notion can be captured as expected health gain from all needed interventions divided by potential health gain from those interventions, where the potential health gain is based on a system that is accessible, affordable, acceptable, available, and of high quality. The formalization of effective coverage of a health system, henceforth referred to as health system coverage, for multiple interventions would be:

$$EC = \frac{\sum_{j=1}^{n} HG_j EC_j d_j}{\sum_{j=1}^{n} (HG_j | P_k = P_{opt}, R_{jk} = 1, \forall k = 1, ...) d_j} \quad [10]$$

where HG_j is the total health gain from intervention j for the entire population. The numerator of this ratio is the expected total health gain from all interventions delivered by the system. The denominator is the total potential health gain if the system has resources, and provider performance, acceptability, affordability, and accessibility are equal to their maxima. The latter three are implicitly captured because the denominator assumes that coverage with each intervention is 100%, a condition that can only take place if each of these constraints is lifted.

The same logic that applies to a single intervention can be applied to the overall health system—what percentage of potential health gain is the system delivering? Having calculated health system coverage, we can define availability, accessibility, affordability, acceptability, and provider-related quality coverage at the health system level. The formalization of these counterfactuals follows the same format as for a single intervention.

We have defined health system coverage in terms of multiple interventions that can contribute to potential health gain for the population. While this is appropriate at a conceptual level, an important task at the stage of measurement and implementation will be to define health system coverage in terms of a specific set of interventions. Effective coverage with such a set of interventions can be thought of as a proxy for the effective coverage of the overall health system. A set of interventions used in any practical implementation of this concept is likely to differ across populations because of epidemiological, demographic, and health system variations.

Effective coverage for a set of interventions can also be defined at the level of an individual. We first aggregated coverage across individuals for a specific intervention and then across interventions. We can also aggregate across interventions for individuals so that overall inequalities in health system coverage can be studied and the contribution of different social, economic and cultural factors to these inequalities can be measured and defined.

MEASUREMENT STRATEGIES

In this section we discuss some practical aspects of measuring health system coverage. First we focus on data requirements for estimating health system coverage and its counterfactual components. We then elaborate on the selection of interventions to include in measuring coverage.

DATA REQUIREMENTS FOR ESTIMATING EFFECTIVE COVERAGE

In order to estimate the effective coverage of an intervention, and consequently health system coverage, the following data are required: 1) coverage of individuals with the intervention, which is defined above as the probability of receiving a necessary health intervention conditional on the need for that intervention; 2) efficacy and effectiveness of the intervention expressed in health gain; and 3) individual risk of developing a health condition requiring the intervention.

Individual Coverage

Individual coverage which is defined in probabilistic terms in our framework cannot be directly observed. Two main measurement challenges need to be addressed: how to estimate coverage when the need for a health intervention is of a probabilistic nature, and how to estimate the probability of receiving an intervention from *ex post* information which is directly observable.

For certain health interventions the need is defined based on directly observable objective characteristics such as age, sex, and exposure to certain risk factors. Examples of this include all pregnant women needing antenatal care during their pregnancy, or all children needing complete vaccinations before their first birthday. However, for many other interventions the need is based on the presence of an adverse health condition, which can be identified with certainty only through clinical diagnostic procedures. However, this is not feasible for measurement at the population level. For this purpose it is more appropriate to use results of symptomatic screening, which determines the presence of a health care need with only a certain level of probability. The probability of having a set of symptoms, given the presence of an adverse health condition, can be combined with prior knowledge of the prevalence of the disease in the population in order to estimate the distribution of the posterior probability of an adverse health condition. This can be accomplished through Bayesian analysis which allows us to define need for a health intervention as a probability rather than as a dichotomous variable (*98*).

The probability of receiving an intervention given the presence of a need for it, C_{ij}, can be predicted by using a multivariate logistic regression model. The model will relate the *ex post* information, which is the occurrence of an intervention (a dichotomous event) among individuals with a health care need, to a set of explanatory variables that characterize the individuals, households, and communities. All variables that are thought to have an effect on the probability of receiving the intervention will be included in the model. The parameter estimates of each variable will then be used to predict the probability of receiving the intervention (C_{ij}) for each individual. The accuracy of the model will depend on the quality of the covariate data.

Three possible data sources exist to estimate individual coverage, service delivery registries, population surveys, and epidemiological estimates of disease prevalence. Each source has its advantages and disadvantages. Service data usually are inexpensive and can provide a wide range of information that is difficult to obtain from surveys. However, service data may have disadvantages as well, such as under-representation of the private sector, incentive-driven reporting (leading either to over-reporting or under-reporting), and sometimes cross-country incomparability due to

different medical practices and reporting procedures (*99*).

The major advantage of population-based surveys is their ability to capture events which occur beyond the public sector, that are not always available through service data. This is especially true for developing countries. Population surveys enable the use of short symptomatic screening tools needed to identify individuals with health conditions. Also, surveys can generate a more comprehensive set of explanatory variables that can better predict the probability of receiving an intervention.

Epidemiological estimates of disease prevalences are readily available. These data are useful as informative priors for determining the probability of health conditions in individuals based on symptomatic screening.

Health Gain

Estimates of the effectiveness of different interventions can be obtained from cost-effectiveness studies. These studies use different units of effectiveness (per cent decrease in occurrence of symptoms, per cent reduction of case fatality rate, disability-adjusted life years or life years gained, etc.). For comparability across different interventions it is necessary to transform these units into healthy life expectancy (HALE) (*17;18*). Counterfactual analysis can allow projections of potential health gain from interventions for an individual or a population group (*100–107*). Expected health gain can be estimated from the potential health gain by adjusting it for individual level parameters such as age, sex, and adherence to treatment, as well as system level parameters such as quality of care and provider performance.

Health Risk

The individual probability of developing a certain health condition d_{ij}, health risk, can be obtained through modelling based on sex and age-specific prevalence/incidence estimates, and individual level variables collected in population surveys. We propose using a Bayesian approach to the estimation of the individual health risk (*98*). Age and sex-specific prevalence of a health condition can provide an initial idea about its distribution in the population—this is a prior distribution referred to simply as a "prior." The information obtained from a survey on the distribution of the condition among individuals, linked with the information such as their age, sex, employment status, income, education, and exposure to risk factors, can be used to model a more accurate distribution of the condition in the population—this is referred to as a likelihood estimation. Using Bayes theorem, a posterior distribution of the individual health risk, d_{ij}, can be determined from the combinatory estimate of the prior and likelihood distributions.

Data for the Counterfactuals of Effective Coverage

In order to decompose effective coverage into the five determinants discussed above (section Coverage for a Singe Intervention) through counterfactual analysis, the following data are required: time necessary to reach a health care provider delivering the intervention (including waiting time), availability of resources by the health care provider, the price of the intervention at the point of delivery, the cultural acceptability of the intervention and the provider behaviour, and the technical quality of services.

These data can be obtained from household surveys. Provider surveys can give additional information, particularly in relation to the quality of services and availability of resources.

Information about travel time, prices, availability of resources and cultural acceptability of interventions should be obtained from both individuals who have received the intervention and if possible, those who have not. The latter may provide useful insights about the extent to which these factors have prevented them from receiving the intervention.

Provider surveys can serve to supplement household surveys by providing data on the availability of resources and on the quality of services.

SELECTION OF INTERVENTIONS

Selection of interventions is a critical step in the measurement of health system coverage. As discussed in section IV, Health System Coverage, the set of interventions which will serve as a proxy for the entire health service delivery, can be designed so that it reflects region-specific population characteristics and health system priorities. We propose the following criteria for selection of interventions:

- Evidence of effectiveness of an intervention and ability to produce a significant health gain.

- Disease and economic burden from a health condition that can benefit from the intervention.

- Correspondence and consistency to national health priorities.

- Balance between preventive and curative care and between communicable, non-communicable and life cycle related health conditions.

- Low cost of obtaining information at the regional level.

DISCUSSION

The conceptual framework proposed in this paper for measuring health system coverage has significant policy implications.

Health system coverage measures outcomes occurring within a short time after actions taken in health service provision. This will prevent judgement about the performance of health systems by the results of policies implemented in the relatively distant past, which can reduce the political sensitivity of health systems performance assessment (16;17).

Health system provision frameworks for measuring access and utilization have focused mostly on the types of services (primary care services, hospital admissions, outpatient visits, maternal health services, etc.) rather than on specific interventions. These frameworks have been concerned mainly with the total volume of services delivered to individuals, sometimes disaggregated by age, sex, and socioeconomic groups. The contribution of access factors, such as distance to providers and cost of seeking care, to health system goals has been studied usually in a qualitative context and rarely quantified. In contrast, the framework of effective coverage described here is concerned with specific interventions and their contribution to achieving health gain. It combines the health intervention perspective with the health system perspective, and provides for a quantification of the impact that various individual and system components have on health system goals. The framework is novel in that it allows for decomposition of the gap between the maximum potential and expected health gains into its causes for the purposes of policy analysis.

The effective coverage framework is a useful management tool because it expands the assessment of health service provision beyond the measurement of access and utilization, and offers a more comprehensive way to trace the degree to which health systems implement activities and the level of impact these have on population health. The framework can help health system managers to identify bottlenecks in health service provision and design appropriate strategies.

Health system coverage as conceptualized in this chapter, is an outcome variable that assesses the effi-

230

Health Systems Performance Assessment

ciency of utilization of various input categories of health services provision. Efficiency can be measured by the amount of effective coverage achieved with different input units. We also recommend to include health system coverage in the frontier production function implemented by WHO for measuring health system efficiency (108). Efficiency in this context would measure how well a health system is performing in terms of achieving its goals, including coverage, compared to the maximum it could achieve with the available inputs.

The framework for measuring health system coverage is applicable at both the national and subnational levels. It can be adapted to the interests of subnational policy-makers and managers by selecting the interventions that reflect local priorities. National estimates of health system coverage can be used for estimating subnational level coverage if they are supplemented with a small set of subnationally representative data.

The World Health Report 2000 of the World Health Organization (WHO) (21) argues that the equality of the distribution of health system achievements, referred to as health system goals, is as important as the average level of those achievements. The inequality of health service provision has been less frequently studied than the inequality of health outcomes. Our concept of effective coverage facilitates the study of inequality at the individual level because it looks at the probability of being covered by the health system. This is advantageous to more traditional methods of measuring coverage at the aggregate level, where inequalities studies are limited to comparisons of large subgroups.

One of the important steps in the assessment of health system coverage is the selection of interventions. Ideally all possible interventions would be included in the assessment, but this is neither practical nor necessary. However, in selecting interventions it is crucial that they actually produce significant health gain and are high contributors to the burden of disease.

Currently there is much focus on scaling up global efforts against the diseases of indigent populations. Substantial financial resources are being mobilized for investing in health systems to fight HIV/AIDS, tuberculosis and malaria. With such investments, monitoring the health systems performance in delivering effective interventions against these diseases will become an imperative. Effective coverage seems a promising indicator for such monitoring.

Availability of valid, reliable, and comparable data is critical for the assessment of health system coverage. These data are often not available in many country health information systems, or are often of substandard quality (99). Health service statistics rarely contain detailed information about the sociodemographic characteristics and economic status of users. We believe that nationally representative population surveys, if developed via rigorous scientific methodology, can provide quality data to supplement the statistics generated by the health service delivery system. The discussion about the burden that information gathering and analysis imposes on countries is frequent in public health debates (16;17;99). Combined collection of different types of data through multimodular instruments may actually reduce this burden, improve the quality of data, and allow for a more comprehensive analysis of health service provision.

The concepts and the framework for measuring coverage proposed in this paper require empirical testing. We understand that some of the approaches suggested here can be further developed and refined based on empirical applications. Limitations in data availability currently may render some of the estimation infeasible. The next immediate steps will include gathering strong empirical evidence to test the framework with feedback from the public health community.

REFERENCES

(1) Andersen R, Fleming GV, Aday LA et al. Evaluating the Municipal Health Services Program. *Annals of the New York Academy of Sciences*, 1982, 387:91–110.

(2) World Health Organization. *National assessments of health care coverage and of its effectiveness and efficiency*. Document SHS/83.7. Geneva, World Health Organization, 1983.

(3) Andersen R et al. Health status and medical care utilization. *Health Affairs*, 1987, 6:136–156.

(4) Dabis F et al. Monitoring selective components of primary health care methodology and community assessment of vaccination, diarrhœa, and malaria practices in Conakry, Guinea. *Bulletin of the World Health Organization*, 1989, 67:675–684.

(5) World Health Organization. *Tools and methods for health system assessment: inventory and review*. Document WHO/ARA/98.4. Geneva, World Health Organization, 1998. URL: http://whqlibdoc.who.int/hq/1998/WHO_ARA_98.4.pdf

(6) McColl A et al. Performance indicators for primary care groups: an evidence based approach. *British Medical Journal*, 1998, 317:1354–1360.

(7) Gomez-Dantes O et al. Assessment of a health program

for the non-insured population. *Revista de Saude Publica,* 1999, 33:401–412.

(8) Aday LA, Andersen R. A framework for the study of access to medical care. *Health Services Research,* 1974, 9: 208–220.

(9) Begley CE, Aday LA, McCandless R. Evaluation of a primary health care program for the poor. *Journal of Community Health,* 1989, 14:107–120.

(10) Hurst J, Jee-Hughes M. *Performance measurement and performance management in OECD health systems.* Labour market and social policy—occasional papers No 47. 2001. URL: http://www.olis.oecd.org/OLIS

(11) Sawano K. Access to hospital and the demand for ambulatory care services in Japan. (In Japanese. With English summary.) *Osaka Economic Papers,* 2001, 50: 26–40.

(12) Fox PD. Access to medical care for the poor. *Medical Care,* 1972, 10.

(13) Taylor GD, Aday LA, Andersen R. A social indicator of access to medical care. *Journal of Health & Social Behavior,* 1975, 16:39–49.

(14) Andersen R, Aday LA. Access to medical care in the U.S.: realized and potential. *Medical Care,* 1978, 16: 533–546.

(15) Patton MQ. *Utilization focused evaluation.* Beverly Hills, Sage Publications, 1978.

(16) World Health Organization/AFRO. *Background Document of Regional Consultation on Health Systems Performance Assessment.* Harare, World Health Organization/AFRO, 2001. URL: http://www.who.int/health-systems-performance/regional_consultations/afro_backgroundfr.pdf

(17) World Health Organization/AMRO. *Background Document of Regional Consultation on Health Systems Performance Assessment.* Washington, DC, World Health Organization/AMRO, 2001. URL: http://www.who.int/health-systems-performance/regional_consultations/amro_background.pdf

(18) Aday LA. The impact of health policy on access to medical care. *Milbank Memorial Fund Quarterly—Health & Society,* 1976, 54:215–233.

(19) World Health Organization. *Health care—an international study report of the World Health Organization. International Collaborative Study of Medical Care Utilization.* London, Oxford University Press, 1976.

(20) World Health Organization. *The World Health Report 2000. Health Systems: Improving Performance.* Geneva, World Health Organization, 2000.

(21) Abbs AA, Walker GJ. Determinants of the utilization of maternal and child health services in Jordan. *International Journal of Epidemiology,* 1986, 15:404–407.

(22) Gumber A, Berman P. *Measurement and pattern of morbidity and utilization of health services: a review of recent health interview survey in India.* Ahmedabad, Ahmedabad Gujarat Institute of Development Research, 1995.

(23) Habib OS, Vaughan JP. Determinants of health services utilization in southern Iraq: a household interview survey. *International Journal of Epidemiology,* 1986, 15: 395-403.

(24) Haddad S, Fournier P. Quality, cost and utilization of health services in developing countries. A longitudinal study in Zaire. *Social Science & Medicine,* 1995, 40: 743–753.

(25) Hall J. *Measuring outcomes of health services.* Westmead Centre, Westmead, Australia Dept. of Community Medicine, 1984.

(26) Leslie J, Gupta GR. *Utilization of formal services for maternal nutrition and health care.* Washington, DC, International Center for Research on Women, 1989.

(27) Malison MD. Estimating health service utlization, immunization coverage, and childhood mortality a new approach in Uganda. *Bulletin of the World Health Organization,* 1987, 65:325–330.

(28) Morton AM, Loos C. Does universal health care coverage mean universal accessibility? Examining the Canadian experience of poor, prenatal women. *Women's Health Issues,* 1995, 5:139–142.

(29) Regidor E et al. Socioeconomic differences in the use and accessibility of health care services in Spain. *Medicina Clinica,* 1996, 107:285–288.

(30) Stock R. Distance and the utilization of health facilities in rural Nigeria. *Social Science & Medicine,* 1983, 17: 563–570.

(31) Thomas JW, Penchansky R. Relating satisfaction with access to utilization of services. *Medical Care,* 1984, 22:553–568.

(32) World Health Organization. *Health services concepts and information for national planning and management experiences based on the WHO/International Collaborative Study of Medical Care Utilization.* Geneva, World Health Organization, 1977.

(33) Rosenstock IM. Why people use health services. In: White KL et al., eds. *Health services research: an anthology.* Washington, DC, Pan American Health Organization, 1992:366–382.

(34) Gertler P, van der Gaag J. *The willingness to pay for medical care: evidence from two developing countries.* Baltimore and London, Johns Hopkins University Press for the World Bank, 1990.

(35) Richardson J. Supply and demand for medical care: or,

is the health care market perverse? *Australian Economic Review*, 2001, 34:336–352.

(36) Deb P. A discrete random effects probit model with application to the demand for preventive care. *Health Economics*, 2001, 10:371–383.

(37) Bockstael NE. The use of random utility in modelling rural health care demand: discussion. *American Journal of Agricultural Economics*, 1999, 81:692–695.

(38) Grytten J, Carlsen F, Skau I. The income effect and supplier induced demand: evidence from primary physician services in Norway. *Applied Economics*, 2001, 33: 1455–1467.

(39) Gertler P. Insuring consumption against illness. *American Economic Review*, 2002, 92:51–76.

(40) Gertler P, Locay L, Sanderson WC. Are user fees regressive? The welfare implications of health care financing proposals in Peru. *Journal of Econometrics, Special Issue on Topics in Development Economics*, 1987, 36:67–88.

(41) Hakkinen U. The production of health and the demand for health care in Finland. *Social Science & Medicine*, 1991, 33:225–237.

(42) Benzeval M, Judge K. The determinants of hospital utilisation: implications for resource allocation in England. *Health Economics*, 1994, 3:105–116.

(43) Gertler PJ. Strategies for pricing publicly provided health services. In: Schieber GJ, ed. *Innovations in health care financing: proceedings of a World Bank conference, March 10–11, 1997*. Discussion Paper No. 365. Washington, DC, World Bank, 1997.

(44) Nocera S. The demand for health: an empirical test of the Grossman Model using panel data. In: Zweifel P, ed. *Health, the medical profession, and regulation. Developments in health economics and public policy*, vol. 6. Boston, Kluwer Academic Publishers, 1998.

(45) Blundell R, Windmeijer F. Identifying demand for health resources using waiting times information. *Health Economics*, 2000, 9:465–474.

(46) Wennberg JE, Barnes WA, Zubkoff M. Professional uncertainty and the problem of supplier induced demand. *Social Science & Medicine*, 1992, 16:811–824.

(47) Gertler PJ. A latent variable model of quality determination. *Journal of Business & Economic Statistics*, 1988, 6:97–104.

(48) Gertler PJ. *A decomposition of the elasticity of Medicaid nursing home expenditures into price, quality, and quantity effects*. National Bureau of Economic Research Working Paper No. w1751. Cambridge, MA, National Bureau of Economic Research, 1985. URL: http://www.nber.org/.

(49) Stoller EP. Patterns of physician utilization by the elderly: a multivariate analysis. *Medical Care*, 1982, 20: 1080–1089.

(50) Gertler PJ. A latent-variable model of quality determination. *Journal of Business & Economic Statistics*, 1988, 6:97–104.

(51) Deolalikar AB. The demand for health services in a developing country: the role of prices, service quality, and reporting of illnesses. In: Ullah AG, Giles DEA, eds. *Handbook of applied economic statistics. Statistics textbooks and monographs*, vol. 155. New York, Base, Hong Kong, Dekker, 1998:93–117.

(52) Vernon AA et al. Changes in use of health services in a rural health zones in Zaire. *International Journal of Epidemiology*, 1993, 22:S20–31.

(53) Bevan G. Ways of seeing: explaining variations in use of acute hospital services. *International Journal of Epidemiology*, 1995, 24:103–108.

(54) Gulliford MC et al. Social environment, morbidity and use of health care among people with diabetes mellitus in Trinidad. *International Journal of Epidemiology*, 1997, 26:620–627.

(55) Lwanga SK, Abiprojo N. Immunization coverage surveys—methodological studies in Indonesia. *Bulletin of the World Health Organization*, 1987, 65(6): 847–853.

(56) Monteith RS et al. Use of maternal and child health services and immunization coverage in Panama and Guatemala. *Bulletin of Pan American Health Organization*, 1987, 21:1–15.

(57) Chapman RD, Gous AG. Determining aspects of primary health care coverage in urban and rural areas of the Orange Free State. *South African Medical Journal*, 1991, 80:501–504.

(58) Melnyk KA. Barriers to care: operationalizing the variable. *Nursing Research*, 1990, 39:108–112.

(59) Wiener JM, Engel J. *Improving access to health services for children and pregnant women*. Washington, DC, Brookings Institution, 1991.

(60) Thaddeus S, Maine D. Too far to walk: maternal mortality in context. *Social Science & Medicine*, 1994, 38: 1091–1110.

(61) Stuart H. Access to physician treatment for a mental disorder: a regional analysis. *Social Psychiatry & Psychiatric Epidemiology*, 2000, 35:61–70.

(62) Andersen RM et al. Exploring dimensions of access to medical care. *Health Services Research*, 1983, 18: 49–74.

(63) Beck RG. Economic class and access to physician services under public medical care insurance. *International Journal of Health Services*, 1973, 3.

(64) Penchansky R, Thomas JW. The concept of access: definition and relationship to consumer satisfaction. *Medical Care*, 1981, 19:127–140.

(65) Phillips KA et al. Understanding the context of healthcare utilization: assessing environmental and provider-related variables in the behavioral model of utilization . *Health Services Research*, 1998, 33:571–596.

(66) Phillips RLJ. Using geographic information systems to understand health care access. *Archives of Family Medicine*, 2000, 9:971–978.

(67) Donabedian A. *Aspects of medical care administration.* Cambridge, Harvard University Press, 1973.

(68) Mobarak AB. *Study on coverage, effectiveness and efficiency of rural health delivery service in Egypt.* Cairo, Ministry of Health of Egypt, 1980.

(69) Ries P. Health care coverage by sociodemographic and health characteristics. *Vital & Health Statistics—Series 10: Data from the National Health Survey,* 1987:1–69.

(70) World Health Organization. *Coverage of maternity care: a listing of available information,* 4th. Document WHO/RHT/MSM/96.28. Geneva, World Health Organization, 1997.

(71) Bos E, Batson A. *Using immunization coverage rates for monitoring health sector performance: measurement and interpretation issues.* Health, Nutrition & Population, Washington, DC, World Bank, 2000. URL: http://www1.worldbank.org/hnp/

(72) World Health Organization. *Global Tuberculosis Control.* Geneva, World Health Organization, 2001. URL: http://www.who.int/gtb/publications/globrep00/index.html

(73) Tonglet R et al. Evaluation of immunization coverage at local level. *World Health Forum*, 1993, 14:275–281.

(74) Tanahashi T. Health services coverage and its evaluation. *Bulletin of the World Health Organization*, 1978, 56:295–303.

(75) Hogarth J. *Glossary of health care terminology.* Copenhagen, World Health Organization/EURO, 1975.

(76) Knippenberg R. The Bamako Initiative: experiences in primary health care from Benin and Guinea. *Children in Tropics*, 1990, 184/185.

(77) World Bank. *Better health in Africa.* Washington, DC, World Bank, 1994.

(78) World Bank. Technical Note No. 5: *Assessing health sector performance.* Washington, DC, World Bank, 2001. URL: http://www.healthsystemsrc.org/Pdfs/HNP_tecnnote5a.pdf

(79) World Health Organization. *Measurement of coverage, effectiveness and efficiency of different patterns of health care.* Document SHS/78/1. Geneva, World Health Organization, 1978.

(80) World Health Organization. *Background paper on the measurement of coverage, effectiveness and efficiency of different patterns of health care.* Document SHS/79.4. Geneva, World Health Organization, 1979.

(81) Montoya-Aguilar C, Marin-Lira MA. International equity in coverage of primary health care examples from developing countries. *World Health Statistics Quarterly*, 1986, 39:336–344.

(82) Lever P. Management by targets: is coverage an adequate measure for health care? *Health Policy*, 1994, 14:356–359.

(83) Berk ML, Bernstein AB, Taylor AK. The use and availability of medical care in health manpower shortage areas. *Inquiry*, 1983, 20:369–380.

(84) Howard KI et al. Patterns of mental health service utilization. *Archives of General Psychiatry*, 1996, 53:696–703.

(85) Lagoe RJ, Arnold KA, Littau SA. Analyzing hospital admission rates at the community level. *Journal of Nursing Care Quality*, 1999, Spec. No:25–39.

(86) Aday LA, Andersen RM. Equity of access to medical care: a conceptual and empirical overview. *Medical Care*, 1981, 19:4–27.

(87) Bin Juni MH. Public health care provisions: access and equity. *Social Science & Medicine*, 1996, 43:759–768.

(88) Goddard M, Smith P. *Equity of access to health care.* York, University of York, Center for Health Economics, 1998.

(89) Carr D et al. *Guide to country-level information about equity, poverty, and health available from multi-country research programs.* Health, Nutrition and Population Division, Washington DC, World Bank, 1999.

(90) Kinman EL. Evaluating health service equity at a primary care clinic in Chilimarca, Bolivia. *Social Science & Medicine*, 1999, 49:663–678.

(91) Waters HR. Measuring equity in access to health care. *Social Science & Medicine*, 2000, 51:599–612.

(92) Gwatkin D et al. *Socio-economic differences in health, nutrition and population.* Washington DC, Health, Nutrition and Population Division, World Bank, 2000.

(93) Maxwell RJ. Dimensions of quality revisited: from thought to action. *Quality of Health Care*, 1992, 1:171–177.

(94) Brook RH, Lohr KN. Efficacy, effectiveness, variations, and quality. Boundary-crossing research. *Medical Care*, 1985, 23:710–722.

(95) Haynes R et al. Effects of distances to hospital and GP surgery on hospital inpatient episodes, controlling for needs and provision. *Social Science & Medicine*, 1999, 49:425–433.

(96) Bilbao JM. The Shapley value for games on matroids: the static model. *Mathematical Methods of Operations Research*, 2001, 53:333–348.

(97) Moulin H. *Cooperative microeconomics: a game-theoretic introduction*. Princeton, Princeton University Press, 1995.

(98) Gurrin LC, Kurinczuk JJ, Burton PR. Bayesian statistics in medical research: an intuitive alternative to conventional data analysis. *Journal of Evaluation in Clinical Practice*, 2000, 6:193–204.

(99) Lippeveld T, Sauerborn R, Bodart C, eds. *Design and implementation of health information systems*. Geneva, World Health Organization, 2000.

(100) Hutubessy RCW et al. Stochastic league tables: communicating cost-effectiveness results to decision-makers. *Health Economics*, 2001, 10:473–477.

(101) Flay BR. Efficacy and effectiveness trials (and other phases of research) in the development of health promotion programs. *Preventive Medicine*, 1986, 15: 451–474.

(102) Field PA. Effectiveness and efficacy of antenatal care. *Midwifery*, 1990, 6:215–223.

(103) Franklin C. Effectiveness and efficacy—which is which? *Critical Care Medicine*, 1994, 22:1335–1336.

(104) Clarke GN. Improving the transition from basic efficacy research to effectiveness studies: methodological issues and procedures. *Journal of Consulting and Clinical Psychology*, 1995, 63:718-725.

(105) Evans TG, Murray CJ. A critical re-examination of the economics of blindness prevention under the Onchocerciasis Control Programme. *Social Science & Medicine*, 1987, 25:241–249.

(106) Mathers CD et al. *Estimates of DALE for 191 countries: methods and results*. EIP Discussion Paper No. 16. Geneva, World Health Organization, 2000. URL: http://www3.who.int/whosis/discussion_papers/discussion_papers.cfm#

(107) Murray CJL et al. Development of WHO guidelines on generalized cost-effectiveness analysis. *Health Economics*, 2000, 9:235–251.

(108) Evans DB et al. *The comparative efficiency of national health systems in producing health: an analysis of 191 countries*. EIP Discussion Paper No. 29. Geneva, World Health Organization, 2000. URL: http://www3.who.int/whosis/discussion_papers/discussion_papers.cfm#

Chapter 21

PROVISION OF PERSONAL AND NON-PERSONAL HEALTH SERVICES: PROPOSAL FOR MONITORING

ORVILL B. ADAMS, BAKHUTI SHENGELIA, BARBARA STILWELL,
ITZIAR LARIZGOITIA, ANDREI ISSAKOV, SYLVESTER Y. KWANKAM,
FERDINAND SIEM TJAM

INTRODUCTION

The provision function refers to the combination of inputs into a production process that takes place in a particular organizational or home setting, and that leads to the delivery of a series of interventions.

The inputs for health service provision are human resources, physical capital, and consumables. The outputs are personal and non-personal health services (Figure 21.1). Personal health services are delivered individually. They can be of therapeutic, rehabilitative or preventive nature, and may generate positive externalities. Non-personal health services are actions applied either to collectives (e.g. mass health education) or to the non-human components of the environment (e.g. basic sanitation) and usually produce significant positive externalities or reduce possible negative externalities from individual or collective actions (1).

The goal of health service provision is to improve health outcomes in the population and to respond to people's expectations, while reducing inequalities in both health and responsiveness. The health care needs of the population should be met with the best possible quantity[1] and quality of services produced at minimum costs.

Types of inputs in health service provision largely determine production costs. The organizational structure and processes determine quantity and quality of outputs for a given quantity of inputs. The quantity and quality of services and their distribution, together with other health system and non-health system factors, determine how much health gain can be achieved in the society.

In order to assess health service provision, we can focus on three areas: a) health system inputs, b) organizational structure and processes, and c) the quantity and quality of personal and non-personal health services in relation to the health care needs of the population. The outcomes of the health service delivery process will be captured by the measurement of the overall level and the distribution of health.

Inputs have direct implications for the cost of production. Some inputs are easily varied, such as drugs, other medical supplies, and health care personnel[2], while other types of inputs, such as structures and expensive equipment, are fixed in the short run and cannot be varied. In the long run all inputs become variable inputs (2–4).

The production of the resources that will be used later as inputs in the service delivery process can be considered as a domain of the resource generation function. The management of inputs and their deployment in the production process can be considered a domain of the service provision function. The management and deployment of inputs could be assessed and monitored through: a) the recurrent costs of service provision, b) the physical availability of inputs, c) the skill-mix of health care personnel, and d) utilization of medical equipment and structures.

Figure 21.1 Health service provider

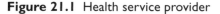

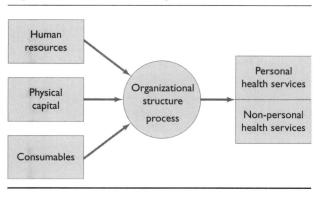

Given the scarcity of resources, it is vital to use the available inputs in such a way that could maximize the quantity and quality of outputs. This largely depends on the way the health service delivery systems are structured and organized, and the way processes are carried out. The organizational structure of the system and the process of health service delivery could be assessed through: a) the level and type of autonomy and integration, and b) incentive structures.

Knowing the degree and locus of autonomy and the extent of integration in the health service delivery system will help in understanding how decisions are made about the deployment of different mix of inputs; how providers respond to market signals, public regulations, or expectations of consumers and the society; and how efficient the links between the different levels and domains of health service delivery are.

Incentive structures have an impact on the way health care providers behave or can be expected to behave in different settings.

The outputs of the health service provision process can be monitored by the degree to which systems achieve effective coverage of the population with critical health interventions. Effective coverage of a health system can be defined as the ratio of the realized health gain from a set of interventions (weighed by the health risk) over the total potential health gain possible if providers performed at their optimal level for a given health system. This applies to both personal and non-personal health interventions. The outcomes of the service provision function will be reflected on the overall level and distribution of the health of the population.

Provider performance measures the contribution of the professional actions of providers to the outputs and outcomes of service provision. In a sense, provider performance measures the direct consequences of providers' professional actions for individual patients. The assessment of provider performance helps understand to what extent one can attribute the outputs and outcomes of health service provision to the professional actions of providers. For instance, effective coverage of a population with health services is determined by factors such as accessibility, availability, affordability, and acceptability, all of which are influenced by elements of provider performance. The assessment of provider performance can inform policy decision with the evidence on the expected or the actual contribution of providers' professional actions into the attainment of the intermediate and final goals of health systems.

The framework for the assessment of the health service provision function is described graphically in Figure 21.2.

RECURRENT EXPENDITURES

Recurrent expenditures, as mentioned above, are most closely associated with variable inputs. The bulk of recurrent expenditures is composed of variable costs that are directly related to the scale of production and to how much output is produced (4;5). They include salaries and wages, drugs and other supplies, utilities,

Figure 21.2 Assessment of health service provision

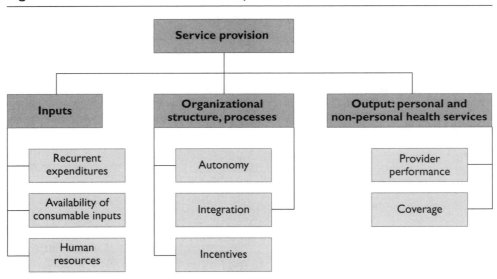

operating costs of structures and equipment, etc. Proportions of these different elements as part of total recurrent expenditures vary from country to country (3;4;6). Usually the wage bill and expenditures on pharmaceuticals and supplies constitute the bulk of recurrent expenditures (4;7;8). Table 21.1 shows the expenditure shares to salary and drugs and supplies in eight Latin American and Caribbean countries. In all except one country (Peru), the salary and drugs shares exceed all other shares. However, the costs of operation and maintenance of physical assets might also reach significant proportions depending on the magnitude of the stock of physical assets and maintenance practices (3–6).

Usually the maintenance of structures and equipment is considered a part of recurrent expenditures. In relation to human resources the equivalent of maintenance could be continuing education and training. However, since the purpose of maintenance is to sustain productivity and quality of assets regardless of the amount of their utilization, we suggest assessing the maintenance costs under the framework of resource generation. At the same time, another component of recurrent costs, operating costs, which are directly linked to the intensity of the utilization of assets, could be assessed under the framework of service provision. This division is suggested only for the purpose of conceptual classification of different measurements of health system functions, and does not necessarily represent established accounting norms and standards.

Measurement of different elements of recurrent costs could provide a reasonable estimation of the input mix used in the production of health services. The data on recurrent expenditures can be obtained from national health accounts. From a long list of potential indicators, the following key indicators could be suggested for indirect assessment of the use of inputs:

- The share of recurrent expenditures as a per cent of total health care spending.

- The share of the wage bill as a per cent of total recurrent expenditures.

- The share of expenditures on drugs and other medical supplies as a per cent of total recurrent expenditures.

- Operating costs of structures and equipment as a per cent of total recurrent expenditures.

In relation to the last indicator, it should be noted that the life cycle costs of physical capital are often neglected, and problems associated with this are not sufficiently perceived. Given the importance of medical technologies for the delivery of health services, life

Table 21.1   Expenditure shares to salary and drugs and supplies in eight LAC countries

| Country | Agency | Per cent of expenditure | | | |
		Salary	Drugs and supplies	All other	Total
Bolivia	Ministry of Health	58.3	8.8	32.9	100
	Social Insurance Organization	44.7	21.2	34.1	100
Dominican Republic	Ministry of Health	66.9	16.6	16.5	100
	Social Insurance Organization	71.3	16.5	12.2	100
Ecuador	Ministry of Health	72.2	4.7	23.1	100
	Social Insurance Organization	50.3	29.3	20.4	100
El Salvador	Ministry of Health	47.3	11.5	41.2	100
	Social Insurance Organization	51.3	20.6	28.1	100
Guatemala	Ministry of Health	52.0	21.1	26.9	100
	Social Insurance Organization	50.0	30.9	19.1	100
Mexico	Ministry of Health	47.9	12.3	39.8	100
	Social Insurance Organization	74.4	9.0	16.6	100
Nicaragua	Ministry of Health	37.7	23.5	38.8	100
	Social Insurance Organization	35.7	50.2	14.1	100
Peru	Ministry of Health	11.1	8.2	80.7	100
	Social Insurance Organization	28.0	9.4	62.6	100

Source: (7)

cycle cost analysis as part of investment decision-making process requires more attention.

AVAILABILITY AND UTILIZATION OF DRUGS AND OTHER MEDICAL SUPPLIES

With a set of essential drugs, vaccines, and other consumables (needles, bandages, etc.) the majority of communicable and non-communicable diseases can be successfully treated, prevented or controlled. The availability of quality consumables is therefore a crucial factor in health service provision and an important determinant of the effectiveness of the services provided. There is evidence that reform processes in the health sector and economic changes have profound effects on the access and use of drugs (9).

The following indicators can be proposed for measuring the availability of drugs in the health service provision system:

■ The proportion of health care facilities and central/regional stores or warehouses that have essential drugs in stock.

This indicator will measure the current availability of drugs to treat common health problems in health facilities and supply depots. A list of 10–15 key essential drugs or health items for common health problems is needed.

■ The average number of stock out days for 10–15 essential drugs during a certain period (number of days in a year or half year).

This indicator will measure the historical availability of drugs to treat common health problems.

The data for these two indicators can be obtained from facility surveys. The monitoring of these indicators has already been tested (10;11).

SKILL-MIX

Health care is labour intensive. The cost of labour accounts for a high proportion (sometimes reaching 70% or more) of total costs (7;12;13). The following graph (Figure 21.3) shows the variation in the numbers of different types of health professionals employed in OECD countries.

The wide variation is evident: what is not known is how this variation affects service provision and health outcomes. To confuse matters further, there is no consensus about what is meant by skill-mix or personnel mix. The term skill-mix can refer to the mix of posts in the establishment; the mix of employees in

Figure 21.3 Physicians, nurses, and dentists per 1 000 population, in selected OECD countries, 1998

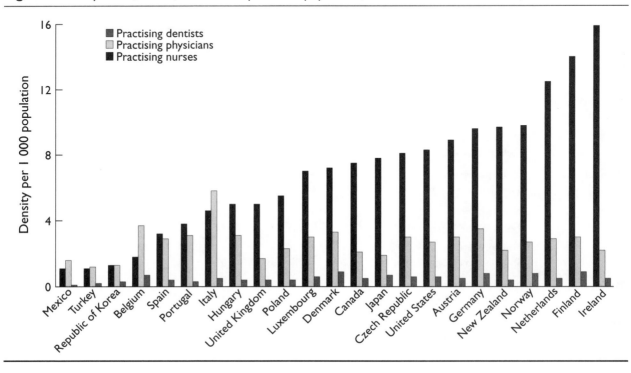

a post, or alternatively the combination of activities that comprise each role, rather than the combination of different professionals, as is shown in the table above (*12;13*).

The effectiveness of a particular skill-mix of health care personnel could be measured both by its costs and by the effect it has on patient outcomes. It is possible to evaluate skill-mix by directly linking skill-mix ratios, costs of inputs, and outcomes (*14*), though most existing studies are descriptive (*12*). In the comprehensive assessment of the health system functions and goal attainment, the measurement of direct or indirect determinants and results of skill-mix will be helpful in understanding the implications of different types of skill-mix for effective health service delivery.

For the assessment of skill-mix, the following indicators are proposed:

- The ratio of skilled to unskilled staff per unit of health gain.

- The ratio of nurses to doctors per unit of health gain.

UTILIZATION OF STRUCTURES, MEDICAL EQUIPMENT, AND INFORMATION TECHNOLOGIES

It is not only the physical availability of structures and technology which is important, but also the extent to which they are utilized. Empty hospital beds and idle technologies are a frequent picture in many places. While systematic evidence is lacking, two documented examples serve to illustrate the situation. In Georgia, a hospital survey showed that in 1996 the average bed occupancy was as low as 15%, and almost 30% of the X-ray imaging equipment had been idle for more than four months (*15*). In one Latin American country the stock of equipment was valued at around US$5 billion, 40 per cent of which (worth almost US$2 billion) was not functional (*16*).

The utilization of Information and Communication Technology (ICT), is playing an increasingly important role in health. Greater application of ICT has the potential for dramatic reduction in medical errors, more knowledgeable workers, greater worker retention, improved patient care at the point of care, improved health system management, and evidence-based care through best practices (*17*). The movement to wireless and mobile Internet applications will lead to migration from desktop platforms to wireless and mobile configurations, with a significant impact on future health care delivery systems (*18*).

The Agency for Healthcare Research and Quality (AHRQ) reviewed 455 studies relating to Telemedicine programmes, 362 of which were in the United States. Thirty medical specialists were represented (*19*). Their report shows that Telemedicine is a growth technology which can be used for clinical benefit.

Although more studies are needed, available evidence indicates that telemedicine can be beneficial. Simple call centres that provide health information and advice to callers demonstrate the demand for such services (*20*). Studies in a large urban home health agency in the United States show that telehomecare resulted in significant cost savings: an episode of care for diabetic patients cost $87 327 with telehomecare compared to $232 872 for hospitalized patients (*21*). One study shows that Dobutamine stress tele-echo-cardiography avoided unnecessary hospitalization of 72% of patients with suspect coronary health problems. In another study, 23% of unnecessary transfers of cardiac patients were avoided. And in a third study, telecardiology led to a 5.4-day reduction in the length of hospital stay in neonatal ICU patients (*22*).

The following indicators can be proposed for the assessment of the utilization of structures, equipment, and health technologies:

- Bed occupancy rate at first referral level, to include both public and private facilities.

Bed occupancy has been commonly used in health services assessment. The information can be obtained from provider surveys.

- The proportion of medical equipment underutilized.

We propose obtaining information from provider surveys about the proportion of medical equipment that has been idle in the past month. (Duration to be determined through key informant surveys.)

AUTONOMY

The literature on decentralization in health systems identifies a number of different constructs (*23*). The main stated objective of the different forms of decentralization resulting in different degrees of autonomy of decision-making is to place the locus of decision-making closer to the point where decision becomes operative (*24*). Decentralization in health systems can be viewed from both stewardship and service provision points of view. At the macro level, when decentralization entails deconcentration of power from central offices to peripheral offices of the same administrative structures (i.e. Ministry of Health), or devolution of responsibility and authority from central offices of the Ministry of Health to separate administrative structures, it seems more appropriate to view these processes from the lenses of the stewardship function. In these situations, the decentralization of power and decision-making affects the way health systems are steered as a whole.

At the micro level, decentralization may have more direct implications for the service provision function when decision-making is delegated to semiautonomous agencies (i.e. hospitals, provider networks, etc.) usually with boards of directors representing separate corporate interests, or when the shift of decision-making is combined with privatization, creating contractual relationships between public entities and private providers. Therefore, within the domain of the service provision function, we should focus on these types of decentralization and autonomy.

In reviewing five country case studies of hospital autonomy (Kenya, Zimbabwe, Ghana, India, and Indonesia), Govindaraj and Chawla (25) identified two major organizational models of provider autonomy: the corporate, individual facility model, found in four countries, and the parastatal, multi-facility model found only in India. Govindaraj and Chawla were impressed by the parastatal model, as it means that the government only has one organization to deal with, it is simpler to monitor and regulate one organization instead of many smaller units, and one organization requires only one good management team (25). The parastatal model they discuss has 162 hospitals and 9 646 beds.

However, Govindaraj and Chawla also point out that individual leadership may be the key to success of autonomy. They note that some managers were able to bring about significant improvements in their hospital sites, while others were not, despite similar positions of autonomy for the hospitals. They propose that improved management structures may be more important than autonomy.

It has been suggested that the autonomy of service providers may lead to technical and allocative efficiency for the following reasons: a) the incentive structures and other reforms that usually accompany autonomy; b) the assumption of greater responsibility by autonomous providers; and c) the greater freedom of autonomous providers to choose their optimal production function (25–27). However, when autonomy is not associated with incentive structures, or the incentives are inadequate, potential benefits of autonomy

may not be realized. Furthermore, autonomy may lead to a loss of benefits of economies of scale and scope (28).

Autonomy is expected to increase accountability because when vested with greater authority, providers may respond to local community needs better. This, in turn, is expected to increase public support and acceptance, as well as community participation in hospital decision-making. However, it is also quite possible that freedom from central control can allow hospitals to pursue their self-interest or the interests of local politicians (26–28).

Evidence on the benefits of autonomy is controversial (23;24;27;29). Often investment in autonomy in public sector hospitals has not yielded many of the hoped-for benefits in terms of efficiency, quality of care, and public accountability, with rare exceptions.

Autonomy can be assessed along two dimensions: the type of policy and management decisions relevant to operating hospitals, and the extent to which decisions are made at the central level (24;25;27). This is displayed in the matrix in Figure 21.4.

We propose the following measures to capture information on the degree of autonomy:

- The proportion of institutional providers who have full autonomy in human resource management and labour market issues.

The ability to hire and release health care workers is one of the most critical elements in the management of health services. The wage bill is often estimated to be between 50 and 70 per cent of the total health expenditures (13). In order to change the balance between different inputs, the manager at the institutional level must have this authority both legally and in practice. In countries where all government workers are part of the civil service and are bound by rules of a Civil Service Commission, the decentalization of human resource management to the individual institutional level has proven to be difficult. Ghana is an example of a country in the process of separating the link between health service workers and the civil service. This measure can be captured by provider surveys and validated through random national policy analysis. Autonomy will be assessed by the review of the national legal frameworks and management and labour market procedures actually carried out at the provider level.

- The proportion of institutional providers with an autonomous budgeting process.

The ability to develop budgets autonomously is important as it allows institutional health care pro-

Figure 21.4 Matrix of decision autonomy

Nature of autonomy—policy and management functions	Extent of autonomy				
	Fully centralized	Some autonomy			Fully decentralized
Identification of organizational goals					
Strategic management & administration					
Procurement					
Staffing decisions and human resource management					
Investment decisions					
Financial management					
Revenue generation					

Adapted from (25)

viders to better reflect the current and required capacities in their budgets, in addition to the needs of the population to whom they provide services. As with the previous indicator, a comparative analysis will be carried out between the legal position and what is done in practice.

■ The proportion of institutional providers with the authority to independently contract external services.

Sometimes it is much more efficient for institutional providers to contract certain services out, such as laundry, provision of food, some diagnostic procedures, rather than perform those functions themselves. The ability to find the best contractor and contract those services out could enable institutional providers to better respond to market forces, and reduce production costs.

■ The proportion of institutional providers who can autonomously decide on the type and volume of services to provide.

The ability to choose the volume and type of services enables health care providers to better respond to market signals and the needs of the populations whom they serve. It will also help them to better align their activities with their capacities.

These indicators can be obtained from provider surveys.

INTEGRATION

Integration has been defined in a variety of different ways (30–32). The following working definition can be used: Integration is a variety of managerial or operational changes to health systems to bring together inputs, organization, management, and delivery of particular service functions. Integration aims to improve the efficiency and quality of service provision. Integration is a way to provide an optimum level of care. The integration of health services is the process of bringing together common functions within and between organizations to solve common problems, by developing a commitment to a shared vision and goals, and by using common technologies and resources to achieve these goals (33).

Various examples of integration include a) the integration of service tasks within a given setting (multi-purpose clinics providing primary health care together with antenatal and infant care; pharmaceutical stores used for other purposes, i.e. condoms; etc.); b) the integration of management and support functions (i.e. comprehensive planning for family health, rather than separate planning for single-purpose programmes; in-service staff training designed to upgrade staff skills in several areas of a service responsibility in a single course rather than many short, specialized courses; collecting and sharing health information, etc.); c) the integration of organizational components (integration of the efforts of different resource providers operating at various administrative levels through coordinating mechanisms such as health committees or councils; making district hospitals an integral part of the district health service instead of discrete institutions, so that district hospitals serve not only as referral centres, but also as resources for support services, etc.).

Integrated health care is believed to have the following advantages (*31;32*):

■ Allows the delivery of a range of services selected to suit national health policies and local needs.

■ Incorporates inputs from different components of the health system.

■ Allows multipurpose use of resources.

■ Makes it easier to respond to user needs.

■ Allows a more holistic approach to health.

For example, in Zambia, local hospitals have taken the initiative to improve the vertical and horizontal integration of health services. The hospital partners included all health centres and charity institutions in the district, and all "vertical" programmes were under the jurisdiction of the district medical officer. The strategy was based on joint planning, problem solving, and decision-making. This initiative led to: better community support for action decided by the "health development group" and spearheaded by the local hospital; better visibility of the district at the level of regional and central government and donors; and a better bargaining position on the part of the regional health authorities for necessary funds and supplies (*31;32*).

The World Health Report 2000 distinguishes between three types of integration: vertical, horizontal, and virtual (*30*).

Vertical integration usually denotes a hierarchical structure in which one level of care provision takes directions from a higher level. The norms that must be followed may lead to lack of ability of a facility at a lower level of the hierarchy to respond to local conditions.

Horizontal integration occurs when different organizational structures with no hierarchical relationships are involved in the delivery of care to the same individual or population. They may be integrated through the use of common managerial structures.

Virtual integration uses communication technology and other systems to share information between providers quickly, and without cumbersome controls. *The World Health Report 2000* argues that this is particularly valuable for referrals and can help to include

nongovernmental providers who have proved hard to integrate under other organizational approaches.

Integration in health service delivery can be assessed by examining a) planning and budgeting processes; b) internal organization; c) staff roles and responsibilities; d) training; e) supervision; f) logistics and vehicles; g) management information systems and monitoring; h) and client services (*31*).

For the assessment of integration in health service delivery the following indicator is proposed:

■ The proportion of local health care facilities in which management and delivery of a selected set of essential services are fully integrated.

This indicator will provide information about the provision of an integrated primary health care package of services versus an approach of service provision through vertical programmes.

It will be necessary to develop criteria for selecting services which will serve as tracers of the assessment of integration. The degree of full integration can be assessed along the eight elements of integration discussed above (*31*). The data for this indicator can be obtained from provider surveys. The potential of population surveys to supplement the information from provider surveys should also be explored.

PROVIDER INCENTIVES

Incentives can be characterized as all the rewards and deterrents that providers face within the organizations in which they work, within the institutions under which they operate, within the existing systems of provider payment, and in relation to the specific interventions they provide (*30*). Literature on incentives is primarily focused on the impact of specific incentives on individual provider behaviour, especially that of physicians. There is a noticeable preoccupation among researchers with financial incentives. There is a need for more evidence of how a range of non-financial incentives affect motivation, including factors such as loyalty to an employer, perceptions of control or empowerment in the job environment, and professional satisfaction from the job.

From the point of view of an individual provider, incentives can be classified as financial (pay, pensions, different allowances, subsidies, etc.) and non-financial (flexible working hours, holidays, educational opportunities, career perspective, etc.). From the point of view of the organizational behaviour (institutional providers), *The World Health Report 2000* distinguishes between internal and external incentives. Internal incentives include: rights to make autonomous decisions, accountability, financial responsibility for losses and right to profit, unfunded mandates. External incentives refer to methods used by the health system as a whole to control the activities of health care organizations (institutional providers). Regulation is used, for example, to place limits on the right to make autonomous decisions so that the public interest is not jeopardized (30).

In the analysis of institutional provider behaviour in relation to economic incentives, it is very important to look at the specific methods of provider payment and options providers have to deal with financial risk associated with providing care, and the health risk of the population whom they serve. Providers have different options to reduce or control their financial risk: a) to select low health risk populations (if the institutional provider and the payer/insurer are the same entity), which is called cream skimming; b) to shift the financial risk associated with the provision of services to other providers (increased referrals between providers), and c) to reduce production costs by skimping on the services provided or deploying a cheaper combination of inputs without reducing the intensity and quantity of services. The ability and propensity of providers to choose any of these strategies depends on the integration of different functions (purchasing, insuring, service provision) and different types of services (preventive, curative, primary, secondary, tertiary).

The economic approach to incentives for purchasing health services was discussed in *The World Health Report 1999* and *The World Health Report 2000* under the heading of "strategic purchasing." The focus there was on purchaser-provider relationships, and the objective was to develop relationships in which appropriate packages of health care services could be purchased. In these relationships capitation or fundholding and contracting involve risk sharing in the sense that the provider agrees to accept responsibility for providing a negotiated bundle of services according to agreed standards of care at a fixed rate; the purchaser undertakes to finance care for insured populations and to be accountable to the public (or clients if the purchaser is a social security plan or private insurer).

The motivation of individual health care providers is a strong factor determining their behaviour. Motivation is directly linked to financial and non-financial incentives. Bennet and Franko (34) propose a conceptual framework for analysing individual provider motivation.

■ Individual level determinants: individual needs, expectations of outcomes or consequences of work activities.

■ Organizational context: salary, benefits, human resource management systems, feedback about performance, and organizational culture.

■ Social and cultural context: community expectations and feedback.

The following measures are proposed to provide policy-makers with insights into the type and nature of both the individual and institutional provider incentives in order to assess their impact on the health service provision function.

■ The proportion of health care providers by different mode of payment, salary, capitation, fee-for-service, or blended payments.

This measure will provide information to test the behaviour of providers in relation to outcome measures such as coverage and responsiveness. Barnum et al. (35) provide the following description of advantages and disadvantages of different payment methods (Table 21.2).

■ The proportion of individual providers who hold both public and private sector jobs.

In countries where individual providers have the opportunity to work in both the public and private sector, there is a conflict between their public sector obligations and their private sector activity. In Egypt, most physicians work multiple jobs and earn their income from different sources (36). As surveyed in the national provider survey, only 11% of Egyptian physicians in private practice reported having only one job. Of the 89% holding more than one job, about 60% reported having a government or a public sector position in addition to their individual private practice. This example suggests that motivation and incentives assessment is needed in order to account for the multiple objectives of individual providers.

■ Motivation of health care providers.

This measure would be similar in its nature to the measure of the responsiveness of the health system to patients' legitimate expectations. While motivation is not easy to measure, several domains of individual provider motivation can be developed based on the typology of incentives. Each domain would

Table 21.2   Incentives

Payment method	Main advantages	Main disadvantages
Budget	Allows strong central control Predictable expenses	No direct financial incentive for efficiency Provider may under-provide services
Capitation	Predictable expenses Provider has incentives to operate efficiently Eliminates supplier-induced demand Low administrative costs	Financial risk may "bankrupt" provider
Fee-for-service	Increase health system productivity	Cost-escalating: strong incentives for supplier-induced demand Higher administrative costs
Case-based	Strong incentive to operate efficiently	Provider has incentives to select low-risks within case categories Case-based payment less suitable for outpatient care

carry different weight, which can be determined by provider surveys. It would be possible to develop a composite measure of individual provider motivation and its distribution among public and private sectors, inpatient and outpatient facilities, rural versus urban settings (5).

The data for the above proposed indicators of incentives can be obtained from health care provider surveys.

PROVIDER PERFORMANCE

The provision of health services is the combination of inputs in a production process that takes place in a particular organizational setting and that leads to the delivery of a series of interventions (1). In order to assess the impact of provider performance on the provision of health services and on the performance of health systems, a number of key determinants of the quality of performance within the health system will have to be addressed. They will include: knowledge and skills of health care providers, satisfaction with care received; effectiveness of process, degree of public participation; quality of educational institutions; quality of medical education, methods of improving quality - development of accreditation processes.

Provider Performance Assessment was initially developed for acute hospitals in several developed countries, such as the United States, Canada, the United Kingdom and Australia (37;38). In recent years, however, it has been expanded to encompass other types of care, such as various forms of long-term care and primary care. The development of specific instruments has, for the most part, followed in-country extensive and complex consultation processes, including academic and scientific research. This process takes

into consideration a series of issues such as the relevance of the measure combined with specific objectives of the provider unit, the technical characteristics of the measure or its scientific soundness (supported on clinical evidence, reproducible, valid, accurate), and its feasibility (at a reasonable cost, allowing for confidentiality, logistically feasible, precisely specified, and measurable).

A great deal of work remains to be done before we are in a position to propose measures that will be comparable across countries and give policy-makers the information they need to assess the performance of providers. This is a critical area of work and is being pursued actively.

COVERAGE

The degree to which the health system carries out critical activities that have an impact on people's health can be examined through determining how effectively populations are covered by health interventions (39;40).

Effective coverage of a health system can be defined as the expected health gain from intervention *j* relative to the potential health gain possible with the optimal performance of providers in a given health system. Effective coverage of an individual with intervention *j* can be represented by the following notation:

$$EC_j = \frac{\sum_{i=1}^{n} HG_{ij} C_{ij} d_{ij}}{\sum_{i=1}^{n} (HG_{ij} | P_k = P_{opt}, Y_{ij} = 1, R_{jk} = 1, \forall k = 1, \ldots) d_{ij}}$$

where HG_{ij} is the expected health gain from intervention j for individual i; C_{ij} is the probability of receiving effective intervention j for individual i conditional on the presence of a health problem; d_{ij} is individual health risk (probability of developing a health condition requiring intervention j); P_k is the provider performance; P_{opt} is the optimal provider performance possible with available resource; Y_{ij} and R_{jk} are indices of compliance and resource availability respectively which are set to 1 when ideal.

At the health system level effective coverage would be an aggregation of intervention-specific effective coverage:

$$EC = \frac{\sum_{j=1}^{n} HG_j EC_j d_j}{\sum_{j=1}^{n} (HG_j | P_k = P_{opt}, R_{jk} = 1, \forall k = 1,\ldots) d_j}$$

The gap between the maximum and actual effective coverage can be described in terms of seven possible causes: resource availability gap, physical accessibility gap, affordability gap, cultural acceptability gap, provider-related quality gap, adherence gap, and strategic choice gap.

RESOURCE AVAILABILITY GAP

Resource availability gap can be represented by the following notation:

$$Av_{ij} = 1 - EC_{ijk} | (B_{jk} = 0, Z_{jik} = \theta, Q_{ijk} = 0, P_{ijk} = P_{opt},$$
$$Y_{ij} = 1) \forall k, k = 1, \ldots, n$$

This conditional expression says that resource availability coverage is the difference between the ideal effective coverage, which would equal 1, and the effective coverage of individual i with intervention j if all providers were offering the intervention free of charge ($B_{jk}=0$), all providers were located in the immediate proximity to the individual thereby requiring zero travel time ($Q_{ijk}=0$), the cultural acceptability of the intervention offered by all providers were equal to a certain acceptable value θ of the latent variable of "cultural acceptability," providers were delivering the intervention optimally, individuals were fully adhering to treatment, and the most effective intervention were selected among possible choices for the given health condition. The only constraint would be the availability of the intervention.

PHYSICAL ACCESSIBILITY GAP

Accessibility gap for individual i for intervention j can be defined in a way similar to the resource availability gap. It is the difference between the ideal effective coverage and the effective coverage of individual i with intervention j given that there are no constraints in terms of affordability, cultural acceptability, resource availability, provider quality, adherence, and the choice of the right intervention. The only constraint is physical access. The formal notation of physical accessibility gap can be constructed as that of resource availability gap.

AFFORDABILITY GAP

Affordability gap is the gap between the ideal effective coverage and effective coverage of individual i with intervention j, given that there are no constraints in terms of cultural acceptability, physical access, availability of resources, provider performance, adherence, and the choice of the most effective intervention. The formal notation of affordability gap can be constructed as that of technology availability gap.

ACCEPTABILITY GAP

Acceptability gap for individual i can be defined as the difference between the ideal effective coverage and the effective coverage with intervention j given there are no constraints other than cultural acceptability. The formal notation of acceptability gap can be constructed as that of resource availability gap.

PROVIDER-RELATED QUALITY GAP

Formally, provider-related quality gap can be defined as the difference between the ideal effective coverage and the effective coverage of individual i with intervention j, given the providers have all necessary resources and technologies to deliver the intervention, and there are no constraints in terms of physical access, cultural acceptability, affordability, adherence, and the right choice of an intervention. The only constraint is the ability of providers to use the available technologies and resources for producing health gain in an individual. The notation of provider-related quality gap can be constructed as that of availability gap.

ADHERENCE GAP

Adherence to the treatment regimen for chronic diseases is an important condition for the realization of

Table 21.3 Matrix for the assessment and monitoring of health service provision function

Concept	Question	Indicator	Potential source(s)
Recurrent expenditures	How efficiently are the inputs used in the production function, estimated through the magnitude and composition of recurrent expenditures?	The share of recurrent expenditures as a % of total health care spending	Facility surveys National Health Accounts
		The share of the wage bill as a % of total recurrent expenditures	Facility surveys National Health Accounts
		The share of expenditures on drugs and other medical supplies as a % of total recurrent expenditures	Facility surveys National Health Accounts
		Operating costs of structures and equipment as a % of total recurrent expenditures	Facility surveys, National Health Accounts
Availability and utilization of drugs and other medical supplies	Are the necessary supplies available to deliver services and sustain the patient flow?	The proportion of health care facilities and central/regional stores or warehouses that have essential drugs in stock	Facility surveys
		The proportion of expired essential drugs in facilities, warehouses and private retail outlets	Facility surveys
		The proportion of generic drugs in the essential drug stock of facilities	Facility surveys
		The expenditure on drugs and other medical supplies as a % of total health expenditure	National Health Accounts
Skill-mix	How efficiently different types of health care personnel are used?	The ratio of different categories of health care personnel per 100 hospital beds	Provider surveys Labour force surveys The Ministry of Health The Ministry of Labour Professional registries
		The proportion of health care personnel costs in the total cost of one inpatient day	Facility surveys
Utilization of structures, medical equipment, and information technologies	How different physical resources are utilized?	Bed occupancy rate	Facility surveys
		The proportion of medical equipment underutilized	Facility surveys
		The proportion of health care providers who keep conputerized patient records	Provider surveys Facility surveys
Autonomy	Where the locus of decision-making power lies and how it affects different management functions?	The proportion of institutional providers who have full autonomy in human resource management and labour market issues	Provider surveys Facility surveys
		The proportion of institutional providers with an autonomous budgeting process	Provider surveys Facility surveys
		The proportion of institutional providers with the authority to independently contract out services	Provider surveys Facility surveys
		The proportion of institutional providers who can autonomously decide on the type and volume of services to provide	Provider surveys Facility surveys
Integration	How well those tasks and functions are brought together that require the similar capacities, address the similar issue, and can benefit from economies of scale and scope	The proportion of primary care facilities in which health services are fully integrated	Facility surveys

continued

the potential health gain from the intervention. The difference between the full potential effective coverage and the effective coverage when the only constraint is the adherence to the treatment regimen can be defined as the adherence gap. Formally it can be represented by a notation similar to that of resource availability gap.

STRATEGIC CHOICE GAP

Usually there are various strategies one can choose from to address a certain health condition. The effectiveness of those strategies might differ and so can the health gain realized through their implementation. The strategic choice gap can be defined as the difference between the maximum effective coverage of intervention s, the best feasible strategy for a given health condition, and maximum effective coverage with intervention j, the intervention actually selected. The maximum effective coverage for both interventions can be defined as counterfactual constructs. Formally strategic choice gap can be represented by the following notation:

$$SG = (EC_{isk} - EC_{ijk}) | (B_{s,jk} = 0, Z_{s,jik} = \theta, Q_{s,jik} = 0,$$
$$P_{s,jik} = P_{opt}, Y_{s,ji} = 1, R_{s,jk} = 1) \forall k, k = 1, \dots, n)$$

We propose to measure effective coverage through household surveys. For this purpose a coverage module is being designed, which will be added to WHO's World Health Survey, and will be piloted in several countries before rolling it out on a global scale. More detailed description of the coverage measure and its conceptual framework is provided in Chapter 20 of this book.

NOTES

1 Appropriate quantity should be determined by the needs of population.

2 Health care personnel is less variable than drugs and consumables. However, at the institutional provider level, skill-mix can be varied. The extent to which this is possible is determined by the degree of autonomy of health care provider institutions.

Table 21.3   Matrix for the assessment and monitoring of health service provision function *(continued)*

Provider incentives	How incentives facing health care providers determine their motivation?	The proportion of health care providers by different modes of payment	Providers surveys
		The proportion of individual providers who hold both public and private sector jobs	Provider surveys
		The proportion of professional income monthly derived from private sources for the individual providers engaged in public sector	Provider surveys
		Motivation of health care providers	Provider surveys
Provider performance	How can providers' professional actions explain the outputs and outcomes of service delivery?	Patient satisfaction	Population surveys Exit surveys
		Medical mistakes	Provider surveys Population surveys
		Hospital readmission	Facility surveys Population surveys
		Return to operating theatre	Facility surveys Population surveys
		Prescription patterns	Providers surveys Population surveys
Effective coverage	How well health systems meet health care needs of the population?	The proportion of the population in need of interventions, who receive effective interventions	Population surveys (WHO's World Health Survey)

REFERENCES

(1) Murray CJL, Frenk J. A famework for assessing the performance of health systems. *Bulletin of the World Health Organization*, 2000, 78(6):717-732.

(2) Folland S, Goodman AC, Stano M. *The economics of health and health care,* 2nd ed. Upper Saddle River, Prentice Hall, 1997.

(3) UNICEF. Problems and priorities regarding recurrent costs. *Policy Review*, 1988.

(4) World Health Organization. *Recurrent costs in the health sector.* Document WHO/SHS/NHP/89.9. Geneva, World Health Organization, 1989.

(5) Club du Sahel. *Recurrent costs in the Sahel to take off.* Paris, Club du Sahel-OECD, 1981.

(6) Working Group on Recurrent Costs. *Recurrent costs of development programs in the countries of the Sahel: analysis and recommendations.* Ouagadougou, Haute-Volta, CILSS, Paris, Club du Sahel-OECD, 1980.

(7) Berman P et al. *Health care financing in eight Latin American and Caribbean nations: the First Regional National Health Accounts Network.* Washington, DC, Partnerships for Health Reform Project, 1999. URL: http://www.lachealthaccounts.org/files/480_16hsrpres8studies.pdf

(8) World Bank. *Health expenditures, services and outcomes in Africa, basic data and cross-national comparisons, 1990-96.* Human Development Network, Washington, DC, World Bank, 1999.

(9) Cederlof C, Quick JD. *Impact of economic factors on use of medicines: concepts and evidence on selected issues.* Presented at the International Conference on Improving the Use of Medicines, Chian Mai, Thailand, 1997.

(10) Rational Pharmaceutical Project. Management Sciences for Health. *Rapid pharmaceutical management assessment: an indicator-based approach.* Washington, DC, Management Sciences for Health, 1995.

(11) Brudon-Jakobowicz P, Rainhorn JD, Reich MR. *Indicators for monitoring national drug policies: a practical manual.* Geneva, World Health Organization, 1994.

(12) Buchan J. Determining skill mix. *Human Resources for Health Development Journal*, 1999, 3(2).

(13) Buchan J, Ball J, O'May F. *Determining skill mix in the health workforce: guidelines for managers and health professionals.* Document WHO/EIP/OSD/00.11. Geneva, World Health Organization, 2000.

(14) Needleman J et al. *Nurse staffing and patient outcomes in hospitals: final report US Department of Health and Human Services.* Washington, DC, US Department of Health and Human Services, 2001.

(15) Abt Associates. *Hospital financing study for Georgia.* Bethesda, Abt Associates, Partnerships for Health Reform Project, 1999.

(16) World Health Organization. *Interregional meeting on the maintenance and repair of health care equipment.* Document WHO/SHS/NHP/87.5. Geneva, World Health Organization, 1987.

(17) US President's Information Technology Advisory Commission. *US President's Information Technology Advisory Commission 2001 Report: Transforming Health Care through Information Technology.* Washington, DC, 2001.

(18) Laxminarayan S, Istepanian RS. UNWIRED E-MED: the next generation of wireless and internet telemedicine systems. *IEEE Transactions on Information Technology in Biomedicine*, 2000, 4(3):189-193.

(19) Agency for Healthcare Research and Quality (AHRQ). *Telemedicine for the Medicare population.* Evidence Report/Technology Assessment No. 24. Washington, DC, Agency for Healthcare Research and Quality, 2001.

(20) Wootton R. Recent advances in telemedicine. *British Medical Journal*, 2001, 323(8):557-560.

(21) Dansky KH et al. Cost analysis of telehomecare. *Telemedicine Journal and E-Health*, 2001, 7(3):225-232.

(22) Roine R, Ohinmaa A, Hailey D. Assessing telemedicine: a systematic review of the literature. *Canadian Medical Association Journal*, 2001, 165(6):765-771.

(23) Janovsky K, Travis P. *Decentralization and health systems change: a framework for analysis.* Document WHO/SHS/NHP/95.2. Geneva, World Health Organization, 1998. URL: http://whqlibdoc.who.int/hq/1995/WHO_SHS_NHP_95.2.pdf

(24) Bossert T. Decentralization. In: Janovsky K, ed. *Health policy and systems development: an agenda for research.* WHO/SHS/NHP/96.1. Geneva, World Health Organization, 1996.

(25) Govindaraj R, Chawla M. *Recent experiences with hospital autonomy in developing countries - what can we learn?* International Health Systems Group Working Paper. Boston, Harvard School of Public Health, 1996.

(26) Austin JE. Autonomy revisited. *Public Enterprise*, 1984, 5(3):247-253.

(27) Data for Decision Making Project, Harvard University. *Improving hospital performance through policies to increase hospital autonomy.* Boston, Harvard University, 1995.

(28) World Bank. *Public hospitals in developing countries: resource use, cost, and financing.* Population and

Human Resources Division, Washington, DC, World Bank, 1992.

(29) Collins C. Decentralisation. In: Janovsky K, ed. *Health policy and systems development: an agenda for research*. WHO/SHS/NHP/96.1. Geneva, World Health Organization, 1996.

(30) World Health Organization. *The World Health Report 2000. Health Systems: Improving Performance*. Geneva, World Health Organization, 2000.

(31) Management Sciences for Health (MSH). *Managing integrated services*. The Manager's Electronic Resource Center, Management Sciences for Health, 1998.

(32) Schierhout G, Fonn S. *The integration of primary health care services: a systematic literature review*. Durban, Health Systems Trust, 1999.

(33) World Health Organization. *Health systems development and integrated health care*. Geneva, World Health Organization, 1999.

(34) Bennet S, Franko LM. *Public sector health worker motivation and health sector reform: a conceptual framework*. Technical Paper 1. Bethesda, Abt Associates, Partnerships for Health Reform Project, 1999.

(35) Barnum H, Kutzin J, Saxenian H. Incentives and provider payment methods. *International Journal of Health Planning and Management*, 1995, 10:23-45.

(36) Berman P. *Understanding supply side: a conceptual framework for describing and analyzing the provision of health care services with an application to Egypt*. Boston, Harvard School of Public Health, 1999.

(37) Commonwealth Department of Health and Family Services. *National leadership through performance assessment*. Occasional Papers Series No. 1. Canberra, Commonwealth Department of Health and Family Services, 1997.

(38) NHS Executive. *The NHS performance assessment framework*. NHS Executive, 1999. URL: http://www.doh.gov.uk/nhsexec/nhspaf.htm

(39) World Health Organization/AFRO. *Background Document of Regional Consultation on Health Systems Performance Assessment*. Harare, World Health Organization/AFRO, 2001. URL: http://www.who.int/health-systems-performance/regional_consultations/afro_backgroundfr.pdf

(40) World Health Organization/AMRO. *Background Document of Regional Consultation on Health Systems Performance Assessment*. Washington, DC, World Health Organization/AMRO, 2001. URL: http://www.who.int/health-systems-performance/regional_consultations/amro_background.pdf

Chapter 22

Inequalities in Coverage: Valid DTP3 and Measles Vaccination in 40 Countries

Saba Moussavi, Bakhuti Shengelia, Ajay Tandon, Neeru Gupta, Christopher J.L. Murray

Introduction

Global interest in inequalities in health and its determinants has increased in recent years (*1–9*). This interest reflects both the persistence of inequalities between social groups in mature welfare states (*10*) and the growing concern with inequalities in developing countries (*11*). The usual focus of work on inequalities is on outcomes, in this case, health. However the important role of health interventions in improving health makes inequalities in service provision also a subject of considerable interest. Social group differences in the coverage of certain interventions have been reported for a number of countries (*3;4;12–23*). Given that effective coverage is a further refinement of measuring health service provision, it is a natural extension to explore inequalities in effective coverage.

Following Gakidou et al. (*24;25*), we focus on the total inequality in effective coverage of an intervention. Total inequality is a function of between-group inequality and within-group inequality. By assessing the total inequality of effective coverage, we are able to make meaningful comparisons across populations even when the social, economic or ethnic groupings that reveal the greatest difference may vary across countries. For example, in one country inequalities in the coverage of childhood immunization may be largely a function of income, whereas in another country they may be due to race or ethnicity. Total inequality measures facilitate easy decomposition of the results into between-group and within-group measures, allowing exploration of the contribution of a range of factors to inequality.

Shengelia et al. (*26*) present the definition of coverage as the probability of an individual receiving an intervention. Coverage so defined is an *ex ante* probability rather than an *ex post* realization. From an *ex post* perspective, individuals who need an intervention have either received it or not. One cannot measure total inequality *ex post*, whereas it is possible to study between-group differences if sample size permits. However, given that the coverage construct is *ex ante*, total inequality in the probability of immunization can be assessed and ultimately decomposed into between-group and within-group inequality. Effective coverage extends the construct one step further to take into account the fraction of potential health gain possible through an intervention that is actually provided.

In this chapter, we examine inequalities in the coverage of valid measles vaccinations and three doses of diptheria-tetanus-pertussis vaccine (DTP3) as measures of effective coverage. These interventions warrant attention in there own right, as they are important components of global efforts to immunize children. Measles immunization saves a considerable number of lives per year (*27;28*) and could save many more if coverage were improved. Measles immunization is also one of the 48 indicators of the Millennium Development Goals. Further, through the efforts of the Global Alliance for Vaccines and Immunizations, these interventions have received renewed policy attention in recent years. Because DTP3 and measles coverage information has been collected systematically over many years through household surveys such as the Demographic and Health Surveys (DHS), it is feasible to explore total inequality across a range of countries and over time.

Data and Methods

Data Sources

Empirical data were obtained from fifty-one DHS conducted over the period of 1990–2000 in various developing and transitional countries (with some countries having two surveys, but conducted in different years). Tables 22.1 and 22.3 contain the full list of these surveys, the year and the countries where the surveys were implemented.

DHS is one of the largest programmes collecting quantitative data on population, health and nutrition in the developing world. The DHS uses a two-stage sampling scheme, with selection at the first stage of primary sampling units or clusters followed by random selection of households within each cluster (29). All mothers of reproductive age from the selected households are asked to show the interviewer the health cards of children born in the five years (or sometimes three years) prior to the survey. The date of each vaccine is documented for all eligible children (under five years of age) (30). If no card is presented, the interviewer asks the mother to recall all vaccinations without specifying dates.

Statistical Methods

The degree of inequality in vaccination coverage was based on the extent of within-country variation in the estimated probability of receiving a valid DTP3 or measles vaccination. The extent of variation in estimated probabilities for a given country was summarized using several inequality indices (detailed later). Country rankings of inequality using each of these indices were compared for consistency.

The validity of DTP3 and measles vaccination coverage was assessed based on whether or not the vaccinations adhered to WHO's recommended schedule (27). However, given that the WHO schedule is not universally followed, a more flexible timetable was allowed for maximizing cross-population comparability. For DTP3, validity was determined if three doses of the vaccine were completed by 12 months of age, the first having been administered not earlier than six weeks of age and the two subsequent doses at a minimum of four weeks apart. For measles, validity was determined if one dose of the vaccine was delivered no earlier than nine months of age but by 15 months of age. Only children surviving up to 12 months of age are considered in the analysis to avoid the issue of censored observations.

Validity of vaccinations based on the above-mentioned schedule was assessed from the dates reported on health cards for those survey respondents who had this information. However, for some in the survey who had vaccinations as per mother's recall, this documented information to assess validity was not available. Possible reasons include situations where: a) the health card was lost, misplaced, or stored in a health facility rather than in the household, b) the health card was issued, but the date not recorded or improperly recorded, and c) the health card was never issued, even though the children were vaccinated. For this group of respondents, the probability of having a valid vaccination was predicted from estimates based on those who did have documented information. This out-of-sample prediction may be biased if the group that had documented information is markedly different from the group that did not (i.e. the two samples differ in a systematic way). However, previous analyses of these data have suggested that this problem of sample selection is not a major concern (31).

The probability of having a valid vaccination was estimated for those who had documented information using a random-effects probit model. The probit model assumes that there is an unobserved latent index measuring the household's proclivity for having a valid vaccination, y^*, which is a function of several measured covariates ($X\beta$) at the individual level, such as mother's age and education, children's birth order and sex, as well as household socio-demographic characteristics such as rural-urban residence:

$$y^* = X\beta + u + \varepsilon,$$

where $u \sim N(0, \sigma_u^2)$ denotes the household-level random effect capturing systematic unobserved variation due to factors affecting the likelihood of having a valid vaccination, and $\varepsilon \sim N(0,1)$ is the standard statistical error term. For each child i in the household, vaccination validity ($y_i = 1$ valid, and $y_i = 0$ not valid) is observed from documented information such that:

$$y_i = 1 \quad \text{if } y^* \geq 0$$
$$y_i = 0 \quad \text{if } y^* < 0.$$

Hence,

$$\Pr(y_i = 1) = \Pr(y^* \geq 0) = \Pr(X\beta + u + \varepsilon \geq 0)$$
$$\Pr(y_i = 0) = \Pr(y^* < 0) = \Pr(X\beta + u + \varepsilon < 0)$$

Given the assumption of normality for the random effect and for the error term, these probabilities are easily derived. Parameters of the probit model were estimated using maximum likelihood methods. These estimated parameters were then used to predict the probability of having valid vaccination for those without documented information.

The covariates used in the model to estimate the probability of vaccination were chosen partly because their measurement and definition were fairly consistent across countries, thus facilitating cross-national comparisons. While mother's education and place of residence refer to characteristics reported at the time of the survey, given the relatively short interval between interview and outcome of interest (vaccination status among children born in the last three or five years), these variables can generally be considered to appropriately reflect the characteristics at the time of service utilization. It should be noted that in Kazakhstan and Uzbekistan, almost all mothers (99%) had at least some secondary education, hence, secondary and above secondary education were the categories used in the estimation model. Beyond these parameters, household-level and community-level factors can contribute to a child's probability of being vaccinated. The underlying concept is that individuals are not passive acceptors of health interventions; rather their surrounding environment contributes to their attitudes and behaviours.

Summary Measures of the Distribution

The distribution of the probability of valid DTP3 or measles vaccination is highly informative. It can be cumbersome, however, to compare the inequality of a range of distributions by simple visual inspection. In many fields, the standard approach to this problem is to summarize each distribution using some type of inequality index (24;25;32–37). The choice of an inequality index is a normative choice and not a statistical one.

Elsewhere in this volume, Gakidou et al. provide a simplified framework for understanding the value choices embedded in some of the more commonly used inequality indices (24;25). For this chapter, we use four different measures that belong to the two families described in Gakidou et al. We present four measures of inequality. From the family of interindividual measures, we use the Gini coefficient which is a scalar independent measure of inequality. In other words, if every person's value is multiplied by a scalar, the Gini coefficient is unaffected. From the family of individual-mean differences, we present three different indices, two of which are the variance and the coefficient of variation that is simply the square root of the variance divided by the mean. The fourth measure places greater emphasis on the tails of the distribution by cubing the absolute differences between each individual and the mean. The summation of the cubed differences is divided by the mean value, which for convenience we label the IMD3. The cube root of this

quantity is then taken to return the index to natural units. This is demonstrated in the following formula:

$$IMD(\alpha, \beta) = \frac{\sum_{i=1}^{n} |y_i - \bar{y}|^3}{n\bar{y}^{-1}}$$

Results

Tables 22.3A and 22.3B provide for every survey included in the analysis the coefficients and 95% confidence intervals for each of the covariates and the random effect, as well as the per cent of households reporting vaccination for more than one child. The significance of covariates differ depending on the survey (results not shown). In general, the direction of the coefficients for both valid DTP3 and measles coverage is as expected, with mother's education and urban residence positively associated with valid vaccination coverage. Higher birth order and maternal age less than 20 and greater than 35 years are overall negatively associated with valid vaccination coverage. Gender was significant in only seven countries, with a positive association between being male and probability of vaccination coverage.

The most important source of variation in the estimated probabilities, however, stems from the random effect, the systematic variation in the probability of valid DTP3 and measles vaccination across households that is not related to the covariates in the model. Information content to estimate the magnitude of the random effect comes only from households that report on the vaccination status of more than one child. In the random effect probit model, the latent variable ranges from negative to positive infinity. Tables 22.3A and 22.3B indicate that there is a considerable range and uncertainty in the magnitude of the random effect. Where the uncertainty is large, this may be due to the relatively small number of households in the survey reporting vaccinations for more than one child. To illustrate, in the Bangladesh 1993/1994 survey, the random effect is quite large for both DTP3 (2.5) and measles (2.1). However, the 95% confidence interval range is also quite large, in fact the largest of all surveys, indicating a high level of uncertainty in estimation. As expected, only 11% of households report vaccination status for more than one child in the Bangladesh 1993/1994 survey. This indicates that there are not enough households with multiple children in the sample to provide a precise estimation of the systematic differences among households. Alternatively, a similarly large random effect is found in the Indonesia 1994 survey for both DTP3 and measles, however, with a much tighter confidence interval range. The per cent of households reporting vaccinations for more than one child in this survey, 43%, is considerably higher than in Bangladesh, thus allowing for a more stable estimate of the higher level contributions to the probability of effective coverage.

Figure 22.1 illustrates four cases of the distributions of valid DTP3 generated by the model. For the Rwanda 1992 survey (Figure 22.1A), the distribution of the probability of coverage is nearly normal with a mean of 0.63 and a small standard deviation 0.06. In contrast, Kazakhstan 1999 (Figure 22.1B) also has a fairly normal distribution, but with a higher mean of 0.71 and a larger standard deviation of 0.1, which is reflected in the spread of probabilities. A completely different distribution spread is seen in Zambia 1992 (Figure 22.1C), with a mean of 0.56, but with children distributed proportionately across the spectrum from almost zero to 100% probability of valid vaccination. Indonesia 1997 (Figure 22.1D) demonstrates a case of extreme inequality, exhibiting a bimodal distribution with a large group of children with almost no probability of valid DTP3 vaccination and another large group with almost 100% probability.

Table 22.1 provides for each survey the summaries of the distribution of the probability of vaccination, using the four inequality indices for both DTP3 and measles. The variance can range from a minimum of zero to a maximum of 0.25. The average variance across countries is 0.09 for both measles and DTP3. Within the estimated distributions of the variance of DTP3, a tremendous range of inequality exists, from very low levels around 0.01 in Kenya 1998/99, Tanzania 1996, Nicaragua 1997, and Kazakhstan 1999, to values of 0.19 in Bangladesh 1993/94 and Indonesia 1994, or only slightly lower, 0.18, in Indonesia 1997 and Philippines 1993. The range of variances is slightly

Figure 22.1   Distribution of the probability of valid DTP3

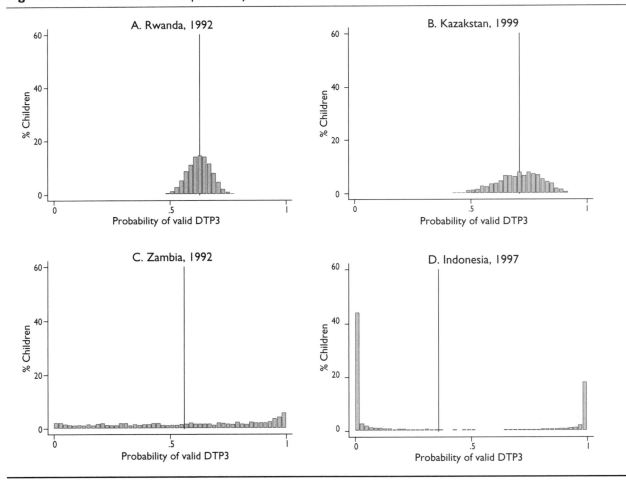

Table 22.1 Summary table of the four inequality indices for DTP3 and measles

Country	Survey year	Variance index DTP3	Variance index Measles	Individual mean cubed DTP3	Individual mean cubed Measles	Coefficient of variation DTP3	Coefficient of variation Measles	Gini coefficient DTP3	Gini coefficient Measles
Bangladesh	1993/1994	0.19	0.14	0.60	0.52	1.10	0.72	0.54	0.49
Bangladesh	1996/1997	0.14	0.13	0.53	0.49	1.68	1.01	0.50	0.44
Benin	1996	0.09	0.12	0.45	0.45	1.58	0.74	0.43	0.38
Bolivia	1998	0.13	0.07	0.59	0.44	1.44	0.73	0.63	0.48
Brazil	1996	0.10	0.03	0.41	0.24	0.71	0.38	0.29	0.13
Burkina Faso	1993/1994	0.07	0.12	0.54	0.47	0.93	0.87	0.62	0.42
Burkina Faso	1998	0.06	0.11	0.55	0.51	0.57	0.67	0.66	0.50
Central African Republic	1994/1995	0.04	0.07	0.40	0.41	0.47	0.47	0.45	0.42
Colombia	1995	0.14	0.09	0.48	0.38	1.85	1.12	0.39	0.25
Comoros	1996	0.13	0.08	0.50	0.40	0.69	0.48	0.47	0.39
Cote d'Ivoire	1994	0.06	0.07	0.42	0.39	0.57	0.39	0.46	0.37
Dominican Republic	1996	0.14	0.06	0.59	0.35	1.15	0.79	0.60	0.30
Egypt	1995/1996	0.14	0.12	0.48	0.43	0.66	0.49	0.34	0.29
Ghana	1993/1994	0.16	0.15	0.56	0.50	2.50	1.27	0.74	0.44
Ghana	1998/1999	0.10	0.08	0.46	0.38	0.68	0.56	0.41	0.30
Guatemala	1995	0.10	0.07	0.51	0.39	1.03	0.64	0.54	0.34
Guatemala	1998/1999	0.09	0.08	0.46	0.38	1.88	1.21	0.45	0.32
Guinea	1999	0.07	0.08	0.57	0.52	1.93	1.45	0.69	0.57
India	1992/1993	0.12	0.10	0.61	0.62	0.54	0.38	0.67	0.71
Indonesia	1994	0.19	0.18	0.64	0.62	1.00	0.61	0.60	0.60
Indonesia	1997	0.18	0.19	0.63	0.62	0.93	0.67	0.63	0.56
Kazakhstan	1999	0.01	0.05	0.13	0.29	0.32	0.70	0.07	0.17
Kenya	1993	0.04	0.06	0.26	0.32	0.50	0.65	0.21	0.21
Kenya	1998/1999	0.01	0.17	0.17	0.51	0.19	0.76	0.14	0.37
Madagascar	1992	0.10	0.08	0.51	0.43	0.50	0.42	0.54	0.44
Malawi	1992	0.04	0.02	0.28	0.20	0.31	0.23	0.20	0.12
Mali	1995/1996	0.03	0.07	0.42	0.44	0.29	0.37	0.56	0.47
Morocco	1992	0.08	0.13	0.38	0.44	0.93	1.18	0.31	0.31
Mozambique	1997	0.16	0.13	0.53	0.48	0.65	0.47	0.48	0.41
Namibia	1992	0.03	0.03	0.18	0.26	0.30	0.28	0.30	0.25
Nicaragua	1997/1998	0.01	0.04	0.53	0.60	0.32	0.41	0.16	0.15
Niger	1998	0.05	0.10	0.53	0.60	0.58	0.62	0.66	0.68
Nigeria	1990	0.06	0.08	0.63	0.60	0.78	0.62	0.77	0.70
Pakistan	1990/1991	0.07	0.06	0.59	0.53	0.65	0.34	0.72	0.65
Paraguay	1990	0.08	0.06	0.53	0.42	1.12	0.84	0.60	0.47
Peru	1991/1992	0.14	0.06	0.52	0.34	0.86	0.38	0.48	0.27
Peru	1996	0.11	0.08	0.46	0.37	0.69	0.55	0.40	0.25
Philippines	1993	0.18	0.18	0.57	0.55	0.69	0.64	0.52	0.46
Philippines	1998	0.14	0.21	0.49	0.58	0.71	0.73	0.43	0.48
Rwanda	1992	0.00	0.03	0.07	0.23	0.29	0.93	0.05	0.11
United Republic of Tanzania	1996	0.01	0.06	0.15	0.32	0.77	1.36	0.13	0.20
United Republic of Tanzania	1999	0.05	0.11	0.32	0.42	0.31	0.44	0.28	0.28
Togo	1998	0.08	0.10	0.46	0.52	0.88	0.66	0.49	0.55
Turkey	1998	0.12	0.09	0.56	0.42	0.57	0.39	0.59	0.36
Uganda	1995	0.14	0.11	0.56	0.49	0.86	0.78	0.55	0.48
Uzbekistan	1996	0.01	0.01	0.17	0.14	0.29	0.23	0.12	0.08
Yemen	1991/1992	0.03	0.08	0.44	0.62	0.65	1.33	0.62	0.73
Zambia	1992	0.10	0.01	0.40	0.16	0.89	0.30	0.31	0.12
Zambia	1996/1997	0.05	0.02	0.30	0.18	0.61	0.32	0.21	0.11
Zimbabwe	1994	0.10	0.17	0.41	0.51	0.65	0.80	0.26	0.34
Zimbabwe	1999	0.08	0.09	0.37	0.39	0.64	0.61	0.25	0.24

wider for measles from 0.01 in Zambia 1992 and Uzbekistan 1996, to 0.21 in the Philippines 1998.

As expected, the variance values correlate well with the graphical representations of the distributions, with the lowest variance values for DTP3 inequalities seen in the countries with normal distributions, Rwanda (<0.01) and Kazakhstan (0.01), and the higher variance values seen in countries with bimodal or almost uniform distributions, Zambia 1992 (0.1) and Indonesia 1997 (0.18).

Inequality, as assessed by the variance, demonstrates considerable temporal stability in countries with pairs of surveys. For the 10 countries with two surveys included in this analysis, the correlation coefficient of the variances for DTP3 in the first survey compared to the second survey, is 0.81. The consistency of results between two different datasets for the same country corroborates that the model is detecting a real phenomenon captured through the selected covariates and the household-level random effect. The correlation for the variance of measles over time is much lower, 0.57; however, there is one notable outlier for measles. In Kenya 1993, the variance for measles is estimated to be 0.06 and for Kenya 1998/1999, the variance is 0.17, a marked increase in inequality. Excluding Kenya, the correlation coefficient of the variances for measles coverage between the first and second surveys increases to 0.71. With the exception of Kenya, the temporal stability in these inequality measurements suggests that inequalities in coverage may be slow to change. It will be of interest to investigate further what factors contribute to the huge increase in inequality in valid measles coverage during the five years in Kenya.

Figure 22.2 shows a comparison of the estimated variance for valid DTP3 and measles. Inequality for the two vaccinations has a correlation coefficient of 0.57. In the relationship shown, again there is one notable outlier, Kenya 1998/99, where variance for DTP3 is very low, 0.01, and variance for measles is high, 0.17. Excluding this outlier, the correlation for the other countries is 0.66. The relatively high correlation suggests that a similar set of individual, household, socioeconomic, and health system factors has a strong influence on inequality in DTP3 and measles coverage. Using the variance as a metric of inequality, there appears to be no significant difference in the extent of inequality seen for DTP3 in comparison with measles. This similarity is surprising, given that in some countries a campaign strategy is used for measles, and the health system infrastructure required

to support three valid doses of DTP3 may be more extensive than for a single dose of measles.

Four countries consistently have the highest levels of inequality both for measles and valid DTP3: Ghana, Indonesia, Philippines, and Bangladesh. The latter three also exhibit this pattern over time. A second tier of countries with high levels of inequality in valid vaccination coverage span three regions and include Mozambique, Egypt, Uganda, Colombia, and India. At the other end of the spectrum, the countries that appear to have the lowest levels of inequality include Zambia, Tanzania, Kazakhstan, Namibia, Malawi, Nicaragua, and Rwanda. This consistency, seen in the higher and lower levels of inequality between valid DTP3 and measles coverage, suggests that similar exogenous factors influence extreme levels of inequality in both vaccinations. We also looked at the relationship between the Gini coefficient for income and the Gini coefficient for vaccination coverage for the surveys with both data available (results not shown). One would expect that inequalities in valid vaccination coverage are due to the system level factors which are contributing to the inequalities in income, and these two types of inequalities are related. Poor people may have less probability of receiving effective intervention, and thus high inequalities in income would correlate with high inequalities in effective coverage. However, our initial comparison showed no apparent systematic relationship. This observed phenomenon might be due to the nature of the immunization programmes. They are often campaign driven. This could mask the

Figure 22.2 Comparison of DTP3 and measles inequality variance index

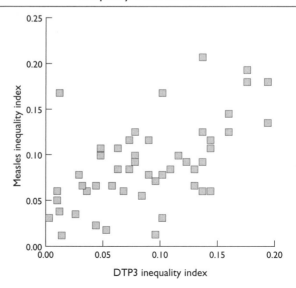

relationship between the income inequality and the inequality in health system access, when the latter is measured only through vaccination coverage.

As a measure of inequality, the variance exhibits translation independence, which means that adding a constant to every child's probability of vaccination will not change the variance. It is a measure of absolute as opposed to relative inequality. Table 22.1 also presents three other measures of inequality: the coefficient of variation, the IMD3, and the Gini coefficient. All three of these include the mean level of vaccination coverage in the denominator so that raising every child's probability of vaccination by the same amount will reduce these relative measures, thus giving the appearance of less inequality. Table 22.2 provides the Spearman's rank order correlation coefficients matrix comparing all four measures for both valid DTP3 and measles. Not surprisingly, the three relative measures of inequality (Gini coefficient, IMD3, and the coefficient of variation) are all highly correlated for both valid DTP3 and measles. The correlation of the variance with these three is lower as it is an absolute measure, dropping to 0.37 for DTP3 when compared to the coefficient of variation.

DISCUSSION

In this first exploration of the inequality in vaccination coverage, we have demonstrated that it is possible to capture systematic variation in the probability of vaccination for children as a function of a limited set of covariates, as well as systematic variation across households due to a range of unmeasured covariates. There are several potential areas of concern in the application of the model that require further investigation: the choice of covariates, selection bias, and community-level effects.

As undertaken in the analysis of the inequality of child mortality in this volume, a measure of household permanent income in the analysis can provide much insight. As discussed in Ferguson et al. (38), questions incorporated in most DHS on the ownership of assets and household services such as electricity, can be used to estimate household permanent income. While including permanent income in future work can provide a more comprehensive understanding of inequalities in valid vaccination coverage, the work on child mortality inequalities (39;40) suggests that inclusion or exclusion of the permanent income variable does not bias the estimate of inequality. This is because the household-level random effect expands to capture the effect of permanent income, if it is not included in the model.

For both DTP3 and measles, where information on the schedule of vaccinations used to assess validity is available for only a subset of respondents with a card, selection bias could have an effect on the estimates of inequality. Murray et al. (31) have explicitly

Table 22.2   Correlation of inequalities indices for probability of being covered for DTP3 and measles (Spearman's rho)

	DTP3 (Spearman's rho)			
	Individual mean cubed	Variance index	Coefficient of variation	Gini coefficient
Individual mean cubed	—	—	—	—
Variance index	0.68**	—	—	—
Coefficient of variation	0.80**	0.37**	—	—
Gini coefficient	0.82**	0.45**	0.96**	—
	Measles (Spearman's rho)			
	Individual mean cubed	Variance index	Coefficient of variation	Gini coefficient
Individual mean cubed	—	—	—	—
Variance index	0.58**	—	—	—
Coefficient of variation	0.85**	0.71**	—	—
Gini coefficient	0.98**	0.56**	0.85**	—

** with significance level of $p < .05$

Table 22.3A Measles: estimated covariates and random effect from probit model

		Child's gender			Residence			Mother's education Primary			Secondary +		
Country and survey year		β	95% CI		β	95% CI		β	95% CI		β	95% CI	
Bangladesh	1993/1994	0.34	−0.19	0.87	0.02	−0.60	0.65	1.20	−0.37	2.70	2.30	−0.34	4.90
Bangladesh	1996/1997	0.47	0.22	0.72	0.28	−0.12	0.69	1.10	0.72	1.40	1.80	1.20	2.30
Benin	1996	−0.03	−0.20	0.13	−0.05	−0.25	0.15	0.58	0.33	0.84	1.30	0.73	1.80
Bolivia	1998	−0.01	−0.14	0.13	0.07	−0.10	0.23	0.55	0.30	0.81	0.83	0.54	1.10
Brazil	1996	−0.04	−0.16	0.08	0.26	0.11	0.42	0.35	0.12	0.59	0.56	0.30	0.82
Burkina Faso	1993/1994	−0.09	−0.19	0.02	0.47	0.33	0.61	0.17	−0.01	0.36	0.84	0.53	1.10
Burkina Faso	1998	0.02	−0.11	0.15	1.20	0.95	1.40	0.59	0.33	0.85	0.72	0.31	1.10
Central African Republic	1994/1995	−0.09	−0.28	0.10	0.61	0.36	0.86	0.25	0.04	0.47	0.74	0.40	1.10
Colombia	1995	0.06	−0.11	0.23	0.12	−0.09	0.33	0.92	0.49	1.40	1.30	0.81	1.80
Comoros	1996	0.25	−0.06	0.56	−0.07	−0.43	0.29	0.19	−0.20	0.57	0.82	0.24	1.40
Cote d'Ivoire	1994	0.05	−0.09	0.13	0.63	0.46	0.80	0.56	0.38	0.75	1.00	0.75	1.30
Dominican Republic	1996	0.03	−0.13	0.18	0.20	0.02	0.37	0.40	0.13	0.66	0.80	0.49	1.10
Egypt	1995/1996	0.05	−0.07	0.17	0.43	0.27	0.60	0.48	0.31	0.66	0.92	0.73	1.10
Ghana	1993/1994	−0.28	−0.57	0.01	0.71	0.29	1.10	0.59	0.22	0.96	1.40	0.53	2.30
Ghana	1998/1999	0.01	−0.15	0.17	0.38	0.17	0.60	0.37	0.13	0.60	0.79	0.57	1.00
Guatemala	1995	0.01	−0.11	0.12	−0.06	−0.22	0.11	0.44	0.30	0.59	0.64	0.35	0.92
Guatemala	1998/1999	−0.04	−0.18	0.10	0.12	−0.08	0.31	0.38	0.21	0.55	0.86	0.54	1.20
Guinea	1999	−0.07	−0.17	0.04	0.05	−0.10	0.20	0.43	0.31	0.56	0.55	0.28	0.82
India	1992/1993	0.21	0.14	0.28	0.41	0.32	0.50	1.00	0.89	1.10	1.60	1.50	1.80
Indonesia	1994	−0.06	−0.20	0.08	0.62	0.42	0.83	0.99	0.70	1.30	2.10	1.60	2.50
Indonesia	1997	−0.10	−0.29	0.09	0.57	0.29	0.85	1.20	0.69	1.70	2.50	1.80	3.30
Kazakhstan	1999	−0.10	−0.32	0.13	−0.20	−0.44	0.04				0.06	−0.25	0.37
Kenya	1993	−0.12	−0.25	0.00	−0.05	−0.29	0.19	0.37	0.20	0.55	0.76	0.52	1.00
Kenya	1998/1999	0.05	−0.22	0.33	0.60	0.01	1.20	0.23	−0.24	0.70	0.85	0.16	1.50
Madagascar	1992	−0.02	−0.16	0.11	0.25	0.06	0.43	0.38	0.18	0.58	0.91	0.65	1.20
Malawi	1992	0.09	−0.05	0.23	0.35	0.16	0.55	0.37	0.21	0.52	0.88	0.46	1.30
Mali	1995/1996	0.08	−0.06	0.22	0.60	0.41	0.78	0.32	0.10	0.55	1.00	0.65	1.40
Morocco	1992	−0.03	−0.14	0.19	1.40	1.20	1.70	0.51	0.18	0.85	0.40	−0.02	0.83
Mozambique	1997	−0.09	−0.27	0.10	1.60	1.00	2.10	0.60	0.33	0.86	0.81	0.19	1.40
Namibia	1992	−0.02	−0.17	0.12	0.23	0.05	0.41	0.26	0.05	0.47	0.47	0.22	0.72
Nicaragua	1997/1998	−0.06	−0.16	0.03	0.03	−0.08	0.14	0.42	0.30	0.55	0.59	0.42	0.75
Niger	1998	−0.06	−0.25	0.14	1.50	1.00	1.90	0.55	0.21	0.89	0.35	−0.12	0.81
Nigeria	1990	−0.05	−0.21	0.11	0.85	0.62	1.10	1.00	0.80	1.30	1.60	1.20	1.90
Pakistan	1990/1991	0.24	0.07	0.42	0.29	0.09	0.48	0.51	0.21	0.82	1.40	1.10	1.80
Paraguay	1990	−0.12	−0.28	0.04	0.32	0.13	0.52	0.72	0.22	1.20	1.10	0.58	1.70
Peru	1991/1992	0.03	−0.07	0.14	0.57	0.44	0.70	0.13	−0.06	0.31	0.35	0.14	0.56
Peru	1996	−0.06	−0.15	0.03	0.39	0.28	0.51	0.40	0.24	0.57	0.86	0.66	1.10
Philippines	1993	−0.19	−0.37	−0.02	0.05	−0.16	0.26	1.90	1.30	2.60	2.45	1.80	3.10
Philippines	1998	0.03	−0.18	0.24	−0.18	−0.45	0.09	3.00	2.10	3.90	3.80	2.80	4.80
Rwanda	1992	0.10	−0.04	0.23	0.08	−0.15	0.32	0.21	0.06	0.36	0.50	0.15	0.85
United Republic of Tanzania	1996	−0.08	−0.20	0.04	0.42	0.24	0.60	0.61	0.46	0.76	0.88	0.52	1.20
United Republic of Tanzania	1999	0.07	−0.13	0.27	0.48	0.18	0.77	0.51	0.26	0.77	1.10	0.58	1.60
Togo	1998	−0.05	−0.22	0.13	0.65	0.39	0.91	0.49	0.27	0.71	1.10	0.72	1.50
Turkey	1998	0.10	−0.13	0.34	0.59	0.27	0.92	1.40	0.88	1.90	1.80	1.20	2.40
Uganda	1995	0.04	−0.10	0.19	0.26	0.06	0.45	0.43	0.24	0.62	1.20	0.87	1.50
Uzbekistan	1996	0.03	−0.20	0.25	−0.10	−0.33	0.14				−0.01	−0.37	0.35
Yemen	1991/1992	0.06	−0.12	0.23	1.50	1.10	1.80	0.64	0.33	0.96	1.10	0.55	1.60
Zambia	1992	−0.04	−0.14	0.06	0.12	0.00	0.23	0.38	0.24	0.52	0.65	0.46	0.85
Zambia	1996/1997	−0.04	−0.14	0.06	0.12	−0.00	0.24	0.17	0.03	0.32	0.46	0.27	0.65
Zimbabwe	1994	0.03	−0.31	0.37	0.16	−0.30	0.62	0.13	−0.40	0.67	0.88	−0.09	1.90
Zimbabwe	1999	−0.07	−0.25	0.10	0.42	0.16	0.69	0.10	−0.24	0.44	0.27	−0.11	0.66

	Maternal age					Birth order						Random effect			% Households with > 1 eligible child
	20–34			35+			2nd–3rd			4th+						
β	95% CI		β	95% CI		β	95% CI		β	95% CI		σ	95% CI			
42	−0.26	1.10	0.73	−0.34	1.80	−0.32	−0.96	0.32	−0.89	−1.90	0.07	2.50	0.66	9.50	11%
42	0.09	0.75	−0.01	−0.66	0.65	−0.24	−0.56	0.07	−0.66	−1.10	−0.23	1.90	1.40	2.50	45%
04	−0.25	0.34	−0.13	−0.51	0.25	0.07	−0.21	0.34	0.15	−0.14	0.44	0.78	0.50	1.20	17%
24	0.01	0.47	0.36	0.05	0.67	−0.19	−0.38	0.01	−0.49	−0.72	−0.26	0.98	0.78	1.20	62%
35	0.17	0.53	0.45	0.18	0.73	−0.24	−0.40	−0.10	0.59	−0.80	−0.38	0.73	0.54	0.97	46%
49	0.29	0.70	0.70	0.45	0.98	−0.45	−0.65	−0.25	−0.56	−0.76	−0.35	0.77	0.64	0.92	60%
29	0.05	0.53	0.39	0.08	0.70	−0.06	−0.29	0.16	−0.22	−0.47	0.03	0.88	0.70	1.10	60%
14	−0.15	0.43	0.13	−0.31	0.56	−0.35	−0.60	−0.06	−0.31	−0.63	0.01	0.87	0.55	1.40	23%
41	0.15	0.66	0.27	−0.12	0.67	−0.30	−0.51	−0.10	−0.35	−0.64	−0.05	1.10	0.82	1.50	46%
01	−0.50	0.49	−0.11	−0.75	0.52	−0.43	−0.89	0.02	−0.52	−1.00	−0.01	0.97	0.41	2.30	32%
22	−0.02	0.45	0.15	−0.17	0.48	−0.27	−0.52	−0.03	−0.33	−0.59	−0.06	0.80	0.58	1.10	16%
34	0.11	0.56	−0.02	−0.43	0.39	−0.35	−0.54	−0.16	−0.66	−0.93	−0.40	0.80	0.59	1.10	58%
31	0.10	0.52	0.32	0.02	0.61	−0.18	−0.36	−0.01	−0.49	−0.70	−0.29	1.20	1.10	1.40	60%
28	−0.18	0.74	0.26	−0.35	0.86	−0.29	−0.69	0.12	−0.49	−0.95	−0.02	1.30	0.68	2.60	16%
33	0.04	0.62	0.32	−0.06	0.69	−0.37	−0.61	−0.13	−0.44	−0.7	−0.17	0.89	0.65	1.20	49%
23	0.04	0.42	0.15	−0.11	0.42	−0.21	−0.39	−0.03	−0.20	−0.40	0.00	0.94	0.79	1.10	70%
22	−0.01	0.44	0.26	−0.06	0.57	−0.20	−0.41	0.01	−0.44	−0.68	−0.19	0.93	0.76	1.10	69%
32	0.15	0.50	0.30	0.06	0.54	−0.10	−0.26	0.06	−0.19	−0.37	−0.00	1.10	0.85	1.40	54%
48	0.38	0.59	0.49	0.29	0.69	−0.34	−0.43	0.26	−0.80	−0.91	−0.68	1.40	1.20	1.50	42%
78	0.51	1.10	0.93	0.55	1.30	−0.42	−0.61	−0.23	−1.20	−1.40	−0.89	1.90	1.60	2.40	43%
60	0.26	0.95	1.20	0.69	1.80	−0.42	−0.66	−0.18	−1.50	−1.90	−1.10	2.30	1.80	3.00	38%
34	−0.04	0.72	0.19	−0.36	0.73	0.05	−0.20	0.29	0.25	−0.15	0.64	0.95	0.59	1.50	36%
27	0.04	0.49	0.08	−0.20	0.38	−0.47	−0.68	−0.26	−0.76	−0.99	−0.52	0.85	0.68	1.10	66%
57	0.03	1.10	0.27	−0.41	0.94	−0.59	−1.10	−0.08	−1.30	2.20	−0.51	1.70	0.81	3.40	23%
39	0.16	0.62	0.48	0.17	0.79	−0.29	−0.50	−0.08	−0.29	−0.52	−0.05	0.96	0.78	1.20	69%
07	−0.32	0.18	−0.10	−0.42	0.22	0.02	−0.23	0.27	−0.23	−0.50	0.04	0.60	0.37	0.96	24%
12	−0.13	0.36	0.23	−0.10	0.55	−0.08	−0.32	0.17	−0.30	−0.58	−0.03	0.95	0.68	1.30	22%
12	−0.22	0.46	−0.01	−0.42	0.40	0.11	−0.14	0.35	−0.10	−0.37	0.16	1.20	0.96	1.50	62%
24	−0.06	0.55	0.38	−0.04	0.80	−0.28	−0.58	0.03	−0.53	−0.89	−0.17	1.20	0.72	2.00	15%
22	−0.03	0.47	0.22	−0.10	0.55	−0.13	−0.35	0.08	−0.21	−0.45	0.03	0.68	0.50	0.92	56%
27	0.13	0.42	0.37	0.16	0.59	−0.13	−0.27	0.01	−0.29	−0.46	−0.13	0.79	0.66	0.94	56%
47	0.12	0.82	0.80	0.32	1.30	−0.19	−0.52	0.15	−0.44	−0.82	−0.06	1.30	0.90	1.90	23%
07	−0.19	0.34	0.46	0.09	0.83	−0.04	−0.29	0.20	0.07	−0.20	0.34	1.30	1.00	1.60	69%
31	0.02	0.61	0.13	−0.28	0.54	−0.31	−0.56	−0.06	−0.42	−0.69	−0.15	1.10	0.81	1.40	67%
45	0.16	0.73	0.61	0.24	0.98	−0.23	−0.45	−0.00	−0.60	−0.86	−0.34	0.88	0.67	1.20	65%
40	0.23	0.58	0.41	0.17	0.65	−0.24	−0.38	−0.09	−0.48	−0.65	−0.03	0.79	0.63	0.98	58%
46	0.31	0.61	0.48	0.28	0.69	−0.28	−0.41	−0.15	−0.44	−0.60	−0.29	1.00	0.85	1.20	53%
35	−0.11	0.70	0.35	−0.09	0.80	−0.36	−0.61	−0.11	−0.92	−1.20	−0.61	1.70	1.40	2.00	66%
59	0.15	1.00	0.69	0.13	1.20	−0.23	−0.50	0.05	−0.78	−1.10	−0.43	2.20	1.80	2.60	63%
17	−0.15	0.49	0.23	−0.14	0.60	−0.01	−0.24	0.22	−0.28	−0.51	−0.05	0.87	0.66	1.10	64%
08	−0.30	0.13	0.02	−0.27	0.31	−0.06	−0.26	0.15	−0.19	−0.41	0.03	0.91	0.74	1.10	60%
58	0.20	0.95	0.38	−0.11	0.87	−0.56	−0.92	−0.20	−0.62	−1.00	−0.22	1.20	0.93	1.60	62%
32	−0.03	0.66	0.34	−0.10	0.77	−0.15	−0.44	0.15	−0.30	−0.61	0.01	1.10	0.82	1.60	15%
04	−0.33	0.42	0.92	0.24	1.60	−0.17	−0.44	0.10	−0.83	−1.30	−0.38	0.80	0.39	1.60	46%
34	0.11	0.57	0.41	0.07	0.76	−0.28	−0.51	−0.06	−0.49	−0.76	−0.23	1.10	0.89	1.40	55%
00	−0.39	0.39	0.08	−0.59	0.76	0.13	−0.16	0.42	0.18	−0.18	0.55	0.57	0.20	1.60	22%
01	−0.33	0.35	−0.03	−0.45	0.40	−0.39	−0.68	−0.11	−0.39	−0.70	−0.09	1.30	1.10	1.60	76%
01	−0.16	0.18	−0.05	−0.29	0.18	−0.09	−0.26	0.07	−0.10	−0.29	0.08	0.41	0.26	0.66	67%
25	0.08	0.42	−0.00	−0.24	0.23	−0.26	−0.43	−0.10	−0.39	−0.58	−0.20	0.55	0.40	0.76	66%
24	−0.41	0.90	0.35	−0.53	1.20	−0.20	−0.77	0.37	−0.33	−1.04	0.39	2.00	0.74	5.20	15%
58	0.29	0.88	0.67	0.24	1.10	−0.20	−0.47	0.07	0.49	−0.49	−0.82	1.20	0.86	1.50	40%

Table 22.3B DTP3: estimated covariates and random effect from probit model

Country and survey year		Child's gender			Residence			Mother's education					
								Primary			Secondary +		
		β	95% CI		β	95% CI		β	95% CI		β	95% CI	
Bangladesh	1993/1994	0.15	−0.17	0.47	−0.12	−0.59	0.35	1.20	0.32	2.05	1.60	0.37	2.84
Bangladesh	1996/1997	0.26	0.08	0.45	−0.10	0.39	0.19	0.70	0.45	0.94	1.14	0.79	1.49
Benin	1996	0.08	−0.10	0.27	−0.01	−0.24	0.22	0.23	−0.04	0.50	0.67	−0.18	1.20
Bolivia	1998	−0.08	−0.24	0.08	0.33	0.12	0.54	0.58	0.26	0.90	1.20	0.80	1.55
Brazil	1996	−0.19	−0.15	0.12	0.35	−0.17	0.54	0.43	0.15	0.72	0.70	0.40	1.01
Burkina Faso	1993/1994	0.02	−0.12	0.15	1.32	1.10	1.50	0.41	0.19	0.62	0.80	0.47	1.10
Burkina Faso	1998	−0.03	−0.18	0.12	1.50	1.20	1.80	0.75	0.46	1.00	0.65	0.26	1.00
Central African Republic	1994/1995	0.03	−0.15	0.21	0.69	0.44	0.93	0.39	0.18	0.61	0.81	0.49	1.12
Colombia	1995	0.03	−0.13	0.20	0.12	−0.09	0.33	0.74	0.30	1.20	1.33	0.84	1.80
Comoros	1996	−0.19	−0.54	0.17	−0.29	−0.74	0.16	0.62	−0.80	1.20	0.65	0.03	1.30
Cote d'Ivoire	1994	0.11	−0.04	0.25	0.64	0.46	0.82	0.39	0.21	0.56	0.62	0.36	0.88
Dominican Republic	1996	−0.11	−0.30	0.08	0.20	0.03	0.43	0.65	0.26	1.04	1.40	0.92	1.90
Egypt	1995/1996	0.15	0.03	0.28	0.63	0.45	0.81	0.54	0.36	0.73	0.90	0.69	1.10
Ghana	1993/1994	0.07	−0.21	0.34	0.93	0.40	1.50	0.61	0.21	1.00	1.20	0.31	2.01
Ghana	1998/1999	0.12	−0.04	0.28	0.31	0.09	0.53	0.30	0.06	0.55	0.50	0.29	0.71
Guatemala	1995	0.01	−0.11	0.12	−0.06	−0.22	0.11	0.44	0.30	0.59	0.64	0.35	0.92
Guatemala	1998/1999	−0.04	−0.18	0.10	0.12	−0.08	0.31	0.38	0.21	0.55	0.86	0.54	1.20
Guinea	1999	0.05	−0.11	0.21	0.86	0.62	1.10	0.24	−0.07	0.56	0.59	0.23	0.95
India	1992/1993	0.25	0.18	0.32	0.45	0.37	0.54	1.10	0.98	1.20	1.80	1.60	1.90
Indonesia	1994	0.01	−0.15	0.16	0.90	0.66	1.10	1.10	0.75	1.40	2.10	1.70	2.50
Indonesia	1997	−0.04	−0.19	0.12	0.64	0.41	0.86	0.78	0.44	1.10	1.70	1.30	2.20
Kazakhstan	1999	−0.05	−0.23	0.13	−0.16	−0.35	0.03				−0.07	−0.31	−0.18
Kenya	1993	0.00	−0.11	0.11	−0.13	−0.33	0.07	0.28	0.12	0.44	0.51	0.31	0.72
Kenya	1998/1999	0.07	−0.08	0.21	−0.32	−0.55	−0.09	0.11	−0.14	0.36	0.16	−0.12	0.45
Madagascar	1992	0.03	−0.11	0.17	0.48	0.28	0.68	0.61	0.37	0.85	1.30	1.00	1.60
Malawi	1992	−0.03	−0.17	0.11	0.10	−0.08	0.28	0.42	0.26	0.58	0.19	−0.16	0.54
Mali	1995/1996	−0.04	−0.17	0.10	1.10	0.82	1.30	0.30	0.09	0.51	0.99	0.65	1.30
Morocco	1992	0.06	−0.08	0.20	0.87	0.68	1.10	0.41	0.15	0.67	0.21	−0.09	0.52
Mozambique	1997	−0.03	−0.23	0.16	1.60	1.10	2.10	0.65	0.36	0.93	0.75	0.13	1.40
Namibia	1992	−0.01	−0.14	0.13	0.00	−0.16	0.17	0.41	0.20	0.61	0.55	0.31	0.78
Nicaragua	1997/1998	−0.01	−0.09	0.07	0.04	−0.05	0.13	0.29	0.18	0.39	0.36	0.23	0.50
Niger	1998	0.11	−0.06	0.27	1.70	1.30	2.10	0.30	0.05	0.56	0.46	0.08	0.84
Nigeria	1990	−0.05	−0.22	0.12	0.98	0.74	1.20	1.10	0.86	1.40	1.50	1.20	1.80
Pakistan	1990/1991	0.17	−0.01	0.34	0.19	−0.02	0.40	0.85	0.52	1.20	1.10	0.75	1.40
Paraguay	1990	0.01	−0.31	0.06	0.56	0.32	0.81	0.81	0.20	1.40	1.40	0.76	2.10
Peru	1991/1992	0.05	−0.07	0.17	0.89	0.71	1.10	0.32	0.08	0.56	0.68	0.41	0.95
Peru	1996	−0.02	−0.11	0.06	0.53	0.42	0.65	0.36	0.20	0.52	0.80	0.61	0.99
Philippines	1993	−0.12	−0.29	0.05	−0.02	−0.23	0.18	1.50	0.90	2.10	2.00	1.40	2.60
Philippines	1998	−0.07	−0.22	0.07	0.15	−0.02	0.33	1.90	1.40	2.50	2.50	1.90	3.10
Rwanda	1992	0.09	−.004	0.18	0.04	−0.11	0.19	−0.00	−0.11	0.10	−0.05	−0.26	0.16
United Republic of Tanzania	1996	0.01	−0.09	0.10	0.18	0.05	0.31	0.04	−0.08	0.15	0.26	0.02	0.50
United Republic of Tanzania	1999	−0.08	−0.23	0.08	0.01	−019	0.21	0.15	−0.04	0.35	0.40	0.08	0.73
Togo	1998	0.18	0.02	0.34	0.46	0.24	0.67	0.18	−0.01	0.37	0.72	0.38	1.10
Turkey	1998	0.01	−0.22	0.25	0.68	0.34	1.00	1.10	0.61	1.50	1.30	0.74	1.80
Uganda	1995	−0.04	−0.21	0.13	0.20	−0.02	0.43	0.50	0.26	0.73	1.30	0.88	1.60
Uzbekistan	1996	−0.02	−0.22	0.18	0.00	−0.21	0.22				−0.25	−0.58	0.08
Yemen	1991/1992	0.01	−0.04	0.24	0.90	0.69	1.10	0.43	0.17	0.68	1.10	0.63	1.50
Zambia	1992	−0.01	−0.13	0.12	0.47	0.31	0.62	0.55	0.36	0.73	1.10	0.79	1.30
Zambia	1996/1997	−0.00	−0.11	0.11	0.43	0.29	0.57	0.29	0.13	0.45	0.76	0.54	0.98
Zimbabwe	1994	−0.03	−0.26	0.19	0.09	−0.21	0.39	0.40	0.03	0.77	0.94	0.40	1.50
Zimbabwe	1999	0.04	−0.12	0.19	0.27	0.05	0.49	0.13	−0.18	0.43	0.19	−0.15	0.53

	Maternal age				Birth order				Random effect		% Households with > 1 eligible child
	20–34		35+		2nd–3rd		4th+				
β	95% CI	β	95% CI	β	95% CI	β	95% CI	σ	95% CI	
26	−0.22 0.75	0.16	−0.66 0.99	−0.14	−0.60 0.33	−0.16	−0.71 0.40	2.10	0.87 4.90	11%
20	−0.04 0.44	−0.09	−0.58 0.41	−0.12	−0.35 0.12	−0.38	−0.69 −0.07	1.30	0.99 1.80	45%
01	−0.34 0.32	−0.25	−0.69 0.19	−0.19	−0.50 0.11	0.04	−0.29 0.36	1.10	0.74 1.50	17%
27	0.01 0.54	0.53	0.16 0.90	−0.22	−0.44 0.01	−0.64	−0.92 −0.37	1.40	1.20 1.80	62%
45	0.25 0.66	0.58	0.26 0.90	−0.27	−0.44 −0.11	−0.86	−1.10 −0.63	1.10	0.93 1.40	46%
42	0.17 0.67	0.55	0.22 0.87	−0.34	−0.57 −0.11	0.42	−0.83	1.10	0.92 1.30	60%
36	0.08 0.63	0.54	0.19 0.89	−0.16	−0.41 0.09	−0.38	−0.65 −0.11	1.10	0.86 1.40	60%
22	−0.07 0.51	0.34	0.09 0.76	−0.16	−0.45 0.12	−0.13	−0.44 0.18	0.73	0.41 1.30	23%
56	0.31 0.82	0.46	0.07 0.85	−0.37	−0.57 −0.17	−0.68	−0.97 −0.39	1.30	1.00 1.70	46%
11	−0.47 0.68	0.54	−0.24 1.30	−0.42	−0.92 0.07	−0.39	−0.93 0.15	1.30	0.60 2.80	32%
32	0.08 0.56	0.28	−0.06 0.61	−0.09	−0.33 1.50	−0.11	−0.36 0.15	0.90	0.67 1.20	16%
44	0.16 0.72	0.71	0.17 1.20	−0.27	−0.50 −0.04	−0.71	−1.00 −0.38	1.50	1.20 1.90	58%
29	0.07 0.51	0.42	0.11 0.73	−0.13	−0.30 0.05	−0.56	−0.77 −0.34	1.40	1.30 1.70	60%
12	−0.49 0.49	−0.17	−0.82 0.48	−0.01	−0.52 0.32	−0.02	−0.49 0.45	1.50	0.81 2.90	16%
30	−0.00 0.60	0.33	−0.06 0.72	−0.23	−0.47 0.01	−0.42	−0.70 −0.14	1.10	0.83 1.40	49%
23	0.04 0.42	0.15	−0.11 0.42	−0.21	−0.39 −0.03	−0.20	−0.40 0.00	1.20	1.00 1.40	70%
22	−0.01 0.44	0.26	−0.06 0.57	−0.20	−0.41 0.01	−0.44	−0.69 −0.19	1.10	0.88 1.30	69%
07	−0.34 0.21	−0.09	−0.47 0.29	−0.02	−0.29 0.25	−0.09	−0.39 0.21	0.39	−0.07 0.85	54%
49	0.39 0.59	0.45	0.26 0.64	−0.24	−0.33 −0.16	−0.71	−0.83 −0.60	1.40	1.20 1.50	42%
85	0.57 1.10	0.99	0.59 1.40	−0.33	−0.53 −0.14	−1.30	−1.60 −1.00	2.30	1.90 2.70	43%
63	0.35 0.91	1.10	0.65 1.50	−0.42	−0.62 −0.22	−1.30	−1.60 −0.96	1.90	1.60 2.40	38%
07	−0.38 0.24	−0.04	−0.49 0.41	0.13	−0.07 0.33	0.35	0.02 0.67	0.51	0.24 1.10	36%
07	−0.12 0.25	−0.19	−0.45 0.08	0.07	−0.11 0.24	0.07	−0.13 0.26	0.70	0.55 0.89	66%
16	−0.08 0.40	0.06	−0.30 0.41	−0.22	−0.44 −0.01	−0.29	−0.53 −0.04	0.48	0.15 1.50	23%
44	0.19 0.69	0.70	0.35 1.00	−0.17	−0.40 0.05	−0.27	−0.52 −0.02	1.20	0.95 1.40	69%
06	0.19 0.30	0.09	−0.22 0.41	−0.08	−0.32 0.16	−0.18	−0.44 0.08	0.75	0.54 1.00	24%
09	−0.16 0.33	0.16	0.17 0.48	−0.09	−0.33 0.16	−0.03	−0.30 0.23	0.70	0.42 1.20	22%
08	−0.20 0.37	−0.04	−0.39 0.31	−0.01	−0.22 0.20	−0.10	−0.32 0.12	0.91	0.72 1.20	62%
13	−0.20 0.45	0.32	−0.13 0.77	0.03	−0.28 0.34	−0.20	−0.55 0.15	1.50	0.96 2.20	15%
45	0.22 0.68	0.56	0.25 0.86	−0.28	−0.47 −0.08	−0.20	−0.42 0.03	0.67	0.50 0.89	56%
25	0.13 0.36	0.36	0.18 0.54	−0.14	−0.25 −0.02	−0.20	−0.33 −0.07	0.50	0.39 0.65	56%
39	0.10 0.68	0.45	0.07 0.84	−0.35	−0.64 −0.05	−0.32	−0.63 −0.01	0.89	0.57 1.40	23%
18	−0.10 0.46	0.34	−0.05 0.73	0.09	−0.16 0.34	0.08	−0.20 0.36	1.30	1.00 1.60	69%
48	0.16 0.80	0.48	0.04 0.91	−0.21	−0.46 0.05	−0.53	−0.81 −0.25	1.30	0.99 1.60	67%
79	0.43 1.20	1.10	0.65 1.60	−0.36	−0.62 −0.11	−0.82	−1.10 −0.51	1.10	0.83 1.50	65%
44	0.23 0.65	0.53	0.24 0.81	−0.30	−0.47 −0.13	−0.65	−0.85 −0.44	1.30	1.10 1.50	58%
28	0.14 0.42	0.37	0.18 0.56	−0.21	−0.32 −0.09	−0.36	−0.50 −0.22	1.10	0.98 1.30	53%
47	0.12 0.82	0.45	0.01 0.89	−0.16	−0.40 0.07	−0.80	−1.10 0.51	1.80	1.50 2.10	66%
81	0.51 1.10	0.84	0.46 1.20	−0.35	−0.55 −0.15	−0.71	−0.94 −0.47	1.30	1.10 1.60	63%
08	−0.14 0.29	0.06	−0.20 0.31	−0.09	−0.24 0.06	−0.15	−0.31 0.00	0.35	0.19 0.65	64%
10	−0.06 0.26	0.08	−0.14 0.30	0.01	−0.14 0.17	0.03	−0.14 0.20	0.49	0.35 0.68	60%
13	−0.15 0.40	0.09	−0.28 0.47	−00.09	−0.34 0.16	−0.11	−0.38 0.16	0.81	0.61 1.10	62%
28	0.03 0.60	0.12	−0.27 0.51	−0.25	−0.52 0.03	−0.15	−0.43 0.13	1.00	0.74 1.40	15%
46	0.08 0.85	1.00	0.31 1.70	−0.37	−0.60 −0.01	−1.20	−1.60 −0.66	1.30	0.91 2.00	46%
26	−0.01 0.53	0.46	0.05 0.87	−0.22	−0.48 0.03	−0.37	−0.67 −0.07	1.50	1.10 1.80	55%
05	−0.30 0.41	0.51	−0.13 1.10	0.33	0.06 0.61	0.09	−0.24 0.41	0.51	0.17 1.60	22%
02	−0.29 0.26	−0.18	−0.51 0.16	−0.23	−0.47 0.01	−0.19	−0.44 0.06	0.86	0.67 1.10	76%
24	0.02 0.45	0.02	−0.28 0.31	−0.05	−0.26 0.15	−0.03	−0.26 0.20	1.00	0.83 1.20	67%
08	−0.10 0.26	−0.19	−0.44 0.06	0.03	−0.21 0.14	−0.10	−0.30 0.09	0.81	0.66 1.00	66%
41	0.01 0.81	0.22	−0.30 0.73	−0.07	−0.42 0.27	0.15	−0.25 0.55	1.20	0.64 2.30	15%
53	0.27 0.79	0.67	0.29 1.00	−0.11	−0.34 0.12	−0.28	−0.57 0.00	1.00	0.75 1.30	40%

modelled selection bias, using the Heckman probit model for valid DTP3 in assessing overall average levels of valid DTP3 vaccination. Correction of any potential selection bias did not substantively change the results. We suspect, therefore, that the results presented here would not be altered greatly by using a selection model.

In the model estimation, the household-level random effect is capturing systematic variation in the probability of childhood vaccination across households. This will logically include variation due to unmeasured household covariates and community-level effects that influence households within each community. Given the nature of vaccination programmes, households in communities with no physical access to the health system, including vaccination programmes, will have a zero or near-zero probability of vaccination. Likewise, in some communities, all children will be fully vaccinated. On the latent variable used in the probit model, the random effect is normally distributed with mean zero and the variance estimated by the model. If there are substantial numbers of households with a zero or 100% probability of vaccination, the variance of the random effect will be very large to accommodate this pattern. An alternative specification of the model would be to include fixed effects by community. However, this cannot be estimated in the setting of zero or 100% coverage. Ideally, exogenous information on the geographical coverage of vaccination programmes could be used to create a community-level variable capturing the presence of the programmes. Further work on this is necessary to best formulate how to capture this community-level effect.

Table 22.3 clearly illustrates that in populations where there are few children per household due to lower fertility rates and thus few households with vaccination information on more than one child, the uncertainty in the household-level random effect can become very large. Alternative measurement strategies may be required to estimate inequality in vaccination coverage in low fertility populations.

In this chapter, we have used four different indices to summarize distributions of inequality of vaccination coverage. We have focused on the variance in much of the presentation of the results. While there is a strong relationship between the various measures of inequality, one important issue is the choice between a measure of absolute inequality in the probability of vaccination such as the variance and a relative measure such as the coefficient of variation. This choice is normative and should be based on a broad discussion of how communities and decision-makers view the implied value judgements. For vaccinations, however, inequality of coverage that is distributed from 10% to 30% with a mean of 20%, does not seem to be four times more unequal than a distribution from 70% to 90% with a mean of 80%. In the absence of a more systematic investigation of population views on this question, we have focused on the variance as it is an absolute measure of inequality.

This analysis clearly demonstrates that considerable variation exists in inequality in valid vaccination coverage across countries. The temporal stability of the estimates of inequality using this approach strengthens the validity of the model results. Nearly constant levels of inequality over periods of three to five years, are a clear reminder that the combination of socioeconomic and health system factors which explain coverage inequalities, is slow to change. It will be important in future work to explore more formally the contribution of different factors, including physical access, to coverage inequalities. Using cases where the DHS has been undertaken two or three times, we may be able to explore the impact of country policies on reducing inequalities in effective coverage.

References

(1) Acheson D. Inequalities in health. Report on inequalities in health did give priority for steps to be tackled. *British Medical Journal*, 1998, 317(7173):1659.

(2) Barker J. Inequalities—whose health for all? *Health Visit*, 1990, 63(7):232–233.

(3) Gwatkin DR et al. *Socio-economic differences in health, nutrition, and population in the Central African Republic*. HNP/Poverty Thematic Group of the World Bank, Washington, DC, World Bank, 2000. URL: http://www.worldbank.org/poverty/health/data/car/car.pdf

(4) Gwatkin DR et al. *Socio-economic differences in health, nutrition, and population in Benin*. HNP/Poverty Thematic Group of the World Bank, Washington, DC, World Bank, 2000. URL: http://www.worldbank.org/poverty/health/data/benin/benin.pdf

(5) Reading R et al. Do interventions that improve immunisation uptake also reduce social inequalities in uptake? *British Medical Journal*, 1994, 308:1142–1144.

(6) Gakidou E, King G. Measuring total health inequality: adding individual variation to group-level differences. *International Journal of Equity in Health*, 2002, 1(3).

(7) Mackenbach JP. Socioeconomic inequalities in health in The Netherlands: impact of a five year research pro-

gramme. *British Medical Journal*, 1994, 309(6967): 1487–1491.

(8) Mackenbach JP, Gunning-Schepers LJ. How should interventions to reduce inequalities in health be evaluated? *Journal of Epidemiology and Community Health*, 1997, 51(4):359–364.

(9) Marmot M et al. Social inequalities in health: next questions and converging evidence. *Social Science & Medicine*, 1997, 44(6):901–910.

(10) Acheson, D. *Independent inquiry into inequalities in health*. London, The Stationery Office, 1998.

(11) Anand S et al. Measuring disparities in health: methods and indicators. In: Evans T et al., eds. *Challenging inequities in health: from ethics to action*. New York, Oxford University Press for the Rockefeller Foundation, 2001:49–67.

(12) Reading RF, Openshaw S, Jarvis SN. Measuring child health inequalities using aggregations of Enumeration Districts. *Journal of Public Health Medicine*, 1990,12(3/4):160–167.

(13) Krieger N. Inequality, diversity, and health: thoughts on "race/ethnicity" and "gender". *Journal of the American Medical Women's Association*, 1996, 51(4):133–136.

(14) Krieger N, Fee E. Measuring social inequalities in health in the United States: a historical review, 1900–1950. *International Journal of Health Services*,1996, 26(3): 391–418.

(15) Krieger N, Chen JT, Selby JV. Comparing individual-based and household-based measures of social class to assess class inequalities in women's health: a methodological study of 684 US women. *Journal of Epidemiology and Community Health*, 1999, 53(10):612–623.

(16) Lee PR, Moss N, Krieger N. Measuring social inequalities in health. Report on the Conference of the National Institutes of Health. *Public Health Reports*, 1995,110(3): 302–305.

(17) Bicego G, Ahmad O. *Infant and child mortality*. Demographic and Health Surveys Comparative Studies No. 20. Calverton, Macro International Inc., 1996. URL: http://www.measuredhs.com/pubs/

(18) Boerma JT, Sommerfelt AE. Demographic and Health Surveys (DHS): contributions and limitations. *World Health Statistics Quarterly*, 1993, 46(4):222–226.

(19) Curtis SL. *Assessment of the quality of data used for direct estimation of infant and child mortality in DHS-II surveys*. Calverton, Macro International Inc., 1995.

(20) Gotpagar KB. Differentials in the maternal age at first and last births in DHS data. In: Srinivasan K, Mukerji S, eds. *Dynamics of population and family welfare*. Bombay, Himalaya Publishing House, 1993:41–56.

(21) Macro International Inc. *An assessment of the qual-*

ity of health data in DHS surveys. Calverton, Macro International Inc., 1993.

(22) Stanton C, Abderrahim N, Hill K. An assessment of DHS maternal mortality indicators. *Studies in Family Planning*, 2000, 31(2):111–123.

(23) Sullivan J, Rutstein S, Bicego G. *Infant and child mortality*. Demographic and Health Surveys Comparative Studies No. 15. Calverton, Macro International Inc., 1994. URL: http://www.measuredhs.com/pubs/

(24) Gakidou E, King G. Measuring total health inequality: adding individual variation to group-level differences. In: Murray CJL, Evans DB, eds. *Health systems performance assessment: debates, methods and empiricism*. Geneva, World Health Organization, 2003.

(25) Gakidou E, Murray CJL, Frenk J. A framework for measuring health inequality. In: Murray CJL, Evans DB, eds. *Health systems performance assessment: debates, methods and empiricism*. Geneva, World Health Organization, 2003.

(26) Shengelia B, Murray CJL, Adams OB. Beyond access and utilization: defining and measuring health system coverage. In: Murray CJL, Evans DB, eds. *Health systems performance assessment: debates, methods and empiricism*. Geneva, World Health Organization, 2003.

(27) World Health Organization. *Immunization policy*. WHOGPV/GEN/95.03 REV. 1. Global Programme for Vaccines and Immunizations, Geneva, World Health Organization, 1996.

(28) Guerin N. Assessing immunization coverage: how and why? *Vaccine*, 1998, Suppl. 16:S81–S83.

(29) Boerma JT, Bicego GT. The quality of data on child immunisation in DHS-I surveys. In: DHS Methodological Reports. *An assessment of the quality of health data in DHS-I surveys*. Calverton, Macro International Inc., 1994.

(30) ORC Macro. *Model "A" questionnaire*. MEASURE DHS+ Basic Documentation. Calverton, ORC Macro, 2001.

(31) Murray CJL et al. Validity of reported vaccination coverage in 45 countries. In: Murray CJL, Evans DB, eds. *Health systems performance assessment: debates, methods and empiricism*. Geneva, World Health Organization, 2003.

(32) Xu K et al. Summary measures of the distribution of household financial contributions to health. In: Murray CJL, Evans DB, eds. *Health systems performance assessment: debates, methods and empiricism*. Geneva, World Health Organization, 2003.

(33) Murray CJL et al. Assessing the distribution of household financial contributions to the health system: concepts and empirical application. In: Murray CJL, Evans DB, eds. *Health systems performance assessment: debates,*

methods and empiricism. Geneva, World Health Organization, 2003.

(34) Sen A. *Inequality reexamined*. Cambridge, Harvard University Press, 1992.

(35) Kakwani N. On the estimation of income inequality measures from grouped observations. *The Review of Economic Studies*, 1976, 43(3):483–492.

(36) Kakwani N, Wagstaff A, van Doorslaer E. Socioeconomic inequalities in health: measurement, computation, and statistical inference. *Journal of Econometrics*, 1997, 77(1):87–103.

(37) Nygard F, Sandstrom A. Income inequality measures based on sample surveys. *Journal of Econometrics*, 1989, 42(1):81–95.

(38) Ferguson BD et al. Estimating permanent income using indicator variables. In: Murray CJL, Evans DB, eds. *Health systems performance assessment: debates, methods and empiricism*. Geneva, World Health Organization, 2003.

(39) Gakidou E, King G. *An individual-level approach to health inequality: child survival in 50 countries*. EIP Discussion Paper No. 18. Geneva, World Health Organization, 2001. URL: http://www3.who.int/whosis/discussion_papers/discussion_papers.cfm#

(40) Gakidou E, King G. Determinants of inequality in child survival: results from 39 countries. In: Murray CJL, Evans DB, eds. *Health systems performance assessment: debates, methods and empiricism*. Geneva, World Health Organization, 2003.

Chapter 23

Validity of Reported Vaccination Coverage in 45 Countries

Christopher J.L. Murray, Bakhuti Shengelia, Neeru Gupta, Saba Moussavi, Ajay Tandon, Michel Thieren

Introduction

There is a rising interest globally in outcomes assessment of health programmes. Donor-supported initiatives like the Global Alliance for Vaccines and Immunizations (GAVI), which provides aid to countries for strengthening their immunization programmes, and the Global Fund to Fight AIDS, Tuberculosis and Malaria, have an imperative to monitor results. GAVI rewards countries monetarily according to the increases in the absolute number of children vaccinated and is testing methodological approaches to achieve this (1–3). With this increasing focus on outcomes monitoring and its important policy and operational implications, it is necessary to verify the quality of the estimates used to evaluate the performance of health programmes (4). In this chapter we address the quality of data currently used to monitor outcomes of immunization programmes.

Two main sources exist for assessing the coverage of immunization programmes worldwide: health service delivery records and household-based surveys (5;6) Countries are requested to report their vaccination coverage estimates annually to the World Health Organization (WHO) and to the United Nations Children's Fund (UNICEF) using the WHO/UNICEF Joint Reporting Form on Vaccine Preventable Diseases. For convenience in this chapter, we refer to these as "officially reported data" (7;8). The methods and strategies for collecting and reporting these data are specific to each country. The source of data for official reports can include service registries, surveys, or a combination of both. The target population for assessing vaccination coverage can also vary, considering either annual number of births, infants surviving to their first year of life, or children of a given age range. Further, a country may change its methodology for obtaining estimates from year to year (3;9). The lack of standardization in data sources and methods of collection decreases the comparability of officially reported data across countries and over time. Officially reported data tend to be the primary source of information for assessing vaccination coverage (3;8), and thus it is essential to analyse their validity.

Immunization is also an important model for many other health programmes. There has been a long investment in developing information systems in many countries to support programme implementation, monitoring, and evaluation. A careful assessment of the validity of coverage estimates collected from service providers will have important implications for improving the accuracy of health information systems.

The main objective of our analysis is to assess the validity of officially reported vaccination coverage data by comparing them to the best available "gold standard." Nationally representative household-based surveys such as the Demographic and Health Surveys (DHS), one of the largest programmes collecting quantitative data on population, health, and nutrition in the developing world, can serve as a potential gold standard. Using DHS has advantages for conducting comparative analysis since the surveys use standardized instruments, training, data collection, and data processing (10). Studies which have extensively validated the DHS methodology and examined the quality of DHS vaccination data, have found little evidence of systematic bias (11;12). Further, as data compiled through the DHS are generally nationally representative, they capture vaccinations delivered by both the private and public sectors, whereas officially reported data are often reflective of only the latter (3).

DTP3 and measles vaccinations are most often used globally to monitor childhood vaccination coverage levels and trends (3;5). In this chapter, we focus on

DTP3 and compare the officially reported DTP3 coverage with that from the DHS.

METHODS

We used vaccination data from 67 DHS collected in forty-five countries during the period 1990–2000. Surveys were excluded if the data were not nationally representative, if officially reported data were not available for the corresponding years, or if the surveys followed a local calendar system for date-related information.

The DHS used a two-stage sampling scheme, with selection at the first stage of primary sampling units or clusters followed by random selection of households within each cluster (*13*). From the selected households that participated, all mothers aged 15–49 years were asked to show the interviewer the health cards of children born in the five years (or sometimes three years) prior to the survey (*10*). The interviewer documented the date each vaccine was received. If no card was presented, the interviewer asked the mother to recall all vaccinations, and, when appropriate, the number of doses received, without asking for dates.

For this analysis, we selected the proportion of children receiving DTP3 vaccination as an indicator of vaccination coverage. The numerator was the number of children who received three doses of DTP, according to a modified schedule recommended by WHO (*7*). Since WHO's schedule is not universally followed, we allowed for a more flexible timetable to maximize cross-national comparability: three doses of DTP vaccine to be completed by 12 months of age, with the first dose administered not earlier than one month of age and the two subsequent doses at a minimum of four weeks apart. Vaccinations administered according to this schedule are here referred to as valid vaccinations.

The denominator of our indicator was the population of children surviving until 12 months of age for each birth cohort in the five (or sometimes three) years prior to the survey. Since children under 12 months of age may not have completed all vaccinations, they were excluded to avoid problems of censored observations. We estimated vaccination rates for each cohort representing a full calendar year prior to the survey's administration.

Different approaches exist for interpreting DTP3 coverage rates from survey data. One approach considers only valid vaccinations that are documented with a health card (herein after referred to as *documented*

valid vaccination). This can result in underestimation of total valid vaccinations because undocumented valid vaccinations cannot be captured. Cards are not always presented at the time of interview because of loss, misplacement, storage at health facilities or elsewhere, or other survey-related procedures (*11*). Another approach considers all vaccinations regardless of the schedule of administration and the presence of documentation (herein after referred to as *crude* vaccination). Such interpretation, while more inclusive than the former, also does not reflect total valid coverage because it does not differentiate between valid and invalid vaccinations.

In response to the limitations of the two aforementioned interpretations, we developed a method for estimating total valid vaccinations from the survey data. A probit model with sample selection (also known as the Heckman probit model in the literature) was used to model the probability of a DTP3 vaccination being valid. The model accounts for the differential likelihood of having documented vaccination information among respondents (*14;15*); that is, it accounts for the fact that respondents who have documented information may be a non-random subsample of all respondents. The model checks for the correlation between the error terms of the equations (not shown here) which are used for predicting the two probabilities, i.e. the probability of having valid immunization and the probability of having documented vaccination information. The presence of a correlation means that the possession of a documented history of vaccination affects the prediction of the validity of vaccination. In such case, the model corrects for systematic differences between the two groups of respondents so that predicted probabilities for respondents do not have a selection bias (*16*).

In the four surveys where sample selection was found not to bias the probability of valid vaccination, a probit model without sample selection was used to model the probability of a DTP3 vaccination being valid among children with documented information on vaccination.

Several studies have examined socio-demographic influences on vaccination status (*17–21*). Drawing on this literature, a number of mother-, child-, and household-related variables were tested for an association with having documented information on vaccination and with the validity of vaccination. The variables that showed statistically significant associations were used to model the probability of having a documented vaccination (the probability of inclusion in the sample from which the probabilities of valid vaccinations were estimated), and the probability of valid vaccinations among those with documented vaccinations. The predicted probability of valid vaccination with adjustment for sample selection was then applied to children with undocumented vaccination status. Total valid DTP3 vaccination coverage rates were constructed from the sum of the predicted and documented valid vaccinations. All rates were weighted at the cluster level to reflect the DHS sampling design.

Survey data are not impervious to systematic errors. The above-described method does not account for potential recall bias due to memory lapses or event omission. Current evidence on the quality of data from maternal recall is not straightforward. Some studies suggest low accuracy of mothers' recall of vaccinations (22–24). Other studies indicate high levels of accuracy, with between 83% and 98% of vaccinations recalled correctly by mothers (25–27).

In order to check for any potentially significant bias, we compared DTP3 vaccination rates for countries that had data available from two consecutive surveys conducted three years apart. This allowed comparing confidence intervals for the coverage rate for the same birth cohort from two sources different essentially in terms of the period of mothers' recall. Such surveys with overlapping cohort data were available for Bangladesh, Indonesia, and the United Republic of Tanzania. We also compared the differences between the officially reported and the total valid immunization rates from DHS among cohorts in order to see if recall bias was introducing a cohort effect.

Countries generally reported vaccination rates based on the calendar year (28), whereas we estimated total valid rates from the DHS by birth cohort. In order to compare the two rates, the officially reported rates were adjusted to simulate a cohort-based schedule, assuming uniform distribution of births and DTP3 vaccinations across the calendar year. Based on DTP3 vaccination schedule it was assumed that children under the age of three months normatively would not be able to complete their vaccinations. Therefore, in any given calendar year the birth cohort from the previous year would receive 3/12 more DTP3 vaccinations than the birth cohort of the same calendar year. This implied attributing, to a given birth cohort, 4.5/12 (37.5%) of DTP3 vaccinations from the same calendar year and 7.5/12 (62.5%) of vaccinations from the following calendar year.

Comparisons were made of cohort-specific rates between the two sources using ordinary least squares regression. We also performed time-trend analysis for officially reported and DHS coverage data for those countries that had two surveys conducted at least three years apart. All statistical procedures were conducted using the Stata software package (29).

RESULTS

ESTIMATES OF DTP3 COVERAGE FROM DEMOGRAPHIC AND HEALTH SURVEYS

The total valid DTP3 rates range from 11% to 77% across countries (Figure 23.1). As expected, the total valid vaccination rates by birth cohort fell between the crude rates, which ranged from 17% to 92%, and the documented valid rates, which ranged from 2% to 74%. The large cross-national diversity in vaccination coverage was not surprising, given the wide differentials in socio-demographic characteristics and degrees of health system development. For example, levels of education ranged from 3% of mothers having attained some secondary schooling in some countries, to over 99% in others.

Figure 23.1 indicates that large differences existed between the estimates of crude and documented valid vaccination coverage, in some countries as high as 65 percentage points. Much of the disparity between these two rates was due to whether the verification of DTP3 vaccination was based on predominantly mothers' recall or health cards. There did not appear to be a universal pattern in terms of the magnitude of the difference between the total valid and crude or between total valid and documented valid estimates.

Figure 23.1 DTP3 immunization coverage rates by birth cohort (1985–1998) from the DHS, 45 countries (sorted by increasing total valid immunization rates)

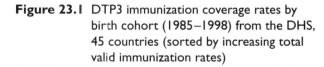
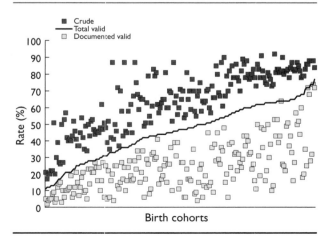

Comparisons of Officially Reported and DHS Coverage Estimates

Our analysis pointed to systematically high officially reported DTP3 coverage rates, as compared to total valid estimates from the DHS. As Figure 23.2 indicates, 90.7% of the DTP3 rates by birth cohort from officially reported data lay above the equivalence line; 55.4% of these data points were at least 20 percentage points higher (with 75.5% at least 10 percentage points higher). According to the observed trend, 20.9% officially reported coverage would be expected at 0% total valid coverage from DHS (95% CI: 14.4%, 27.4%; $R^2 = 0.531$). A few exceptions were found (7% of cohorts) when officially reported estimates were some 1-16% lower than DHS estimates.

Officially reported DTP3 rates were compared with crude rates from the DHS. Although the difference was smaller than that between officially reported and total valid DTP3 rates, the results (not shown) suggested that 16.3% officially reported coverage could be expected at 0% crude coverage rate according to DHS (95%CI 7.5%, 25.3%; $R^2 = 0.408$). Part of this difference in the pattern of over-reporting may be attributable to the fact that crude vaccination rates, like officially reported rates, may not take into consideration adherence to the recommended schedule for administration.

We examined the relationship of officially reported estimates with the difference between these and total valid vaccination estimates from the DHS. Figure 23.3 shows that with each percentage point increase in officially reported DTP3 rates, the degree of their over-reporting increased on average by 48% (95% CI 41.1%, 54.7%; $R^2 = 0.49$). In other words, high values of officially reported DTP3 rates had a greater likelihood of corresponding to lower DHS estimates.

Checking for Recall Bias

The officially reported rates were compared to total valid vaccination rates from DHS separately for each cohort. If differences between the officially reported rates and the DHS estimates increased from the youngest to the oldest cohort, this would suggest a systematic internal bias in the DHS. However, our results did not show any statistically significant difference among cohorts (results not shown).

The comparison of coverage rates for the same cohort with overlapping data from two consecutive surveys did not indicate a recall bias in any of the three countries. Significant differences in the coverage figures reported for the same cohort would suggest bias; Figure 23.4 shows that the rates from the two sources consistently fell within the 95% confidence interval. Thus, any potential differences in rates due to recall were within the surveys' sampling error range, which corroborates with the findings of other studies (*12*). However, availability of more surveys with overlapping cohort-based data might have allowed for greater robustness of this analysis.

Figure 23.2 DTP3 vaccination rates by birth cohort (1985–1998), according to source of data, 41 countries

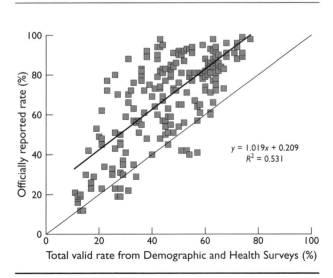

Figure 23.3 Differences in DTP3 vaccination rates by birth cohort (1985–1998), according to source of data, 45 countries

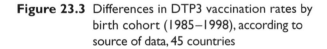
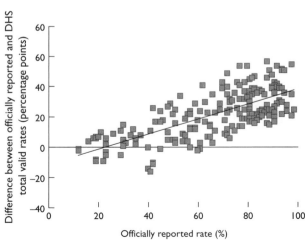

CHANGES OVER TIME IN ESTIMATES FROM DHS VERSUS ROUTINE SOURCES

The comparison of changes over five-year periods between officially reported DTP3 coverage rates and the DHS rates did not present a strong pattern (Figure 23.5). We would expect that if officially reported data are reflective of those from the "gold standard" DHS, then changes over time would be similar for both. The analysis showed a weak relationship between the changes seen in the officially reported rates and the corresponding DHS estimates (coefficient 0.21, $R^2 = 0.02$). These results infer that using officially reported data could be misleading for assessing changes in vaccinations over time.

DISCUSSION

Officially reported levels of vaccination coverage are highly informative if they are low. However, if reported coverage is high, total valid coverage in the population may in fact be rather low. More disturbingly, changes in official coverage are not at all correlated with changes in the total valid level of coverage in the population. What can explain these huge differences?

Four main factors probably account for most of them. First, information collected through service providers often records all vaccinations, not just those that have been delivered according to the recommended schedule. In other words, they tend to report on crude coverage rather than on total valid coverage,

even though the latter is the relevant policy variable. As illustrated above, however, there is a substantial difference even between crude coverage and officially reported data. Second, officially reported vaccination coverage data in most countries only record vaccinations delivered in public sector providers. Those delivered by non-governmental organizations or other private providers are not included. This should in principle bias official reports down, not up. Third, weak information systems can lead to the transmission of inaccurate information from the periphery to the centre in many health systems. Fourth, where vaccination coverage is related to financial or non-monetary incentives for health workers or supervisors, figures may in some cases be intentionally inflated.

Further analysis is needed to understand the relative importance of these four factors to the difference between officially reported and gold standard assessments of vaccination coverage. One significant initiative sponsored by GAVI and WHO is a series of Data Quality Audits (DQA). DQA verify the number of reported vaccinations per country. A verification factor is calculated based upon the proportion of reported DTP3 vaccinations during the previous year that could be verified. The verification factor in eight countries, where the first series of DQAs has been conducted, ranged from 40% to 87% (with ±30% confidence interval). DQAs pointed to several weaknesses in information systems, including low timeliness and completeness of reporting, inconsistent computer filing procedures, dual reporting systems, lack of writ-

Figure 23.4 Comparison of total valid DTP3 vaccination rates for overlapping birth cohorts across two successive DHS surveys in three countries

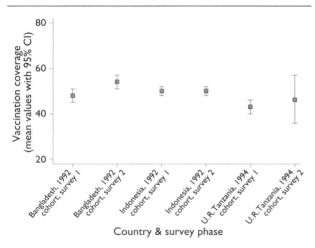

Figure 23.5 Quinquennial change in coverage rates for DTP3 by birth cohort (1986–1998), according to source of data, 16 countries

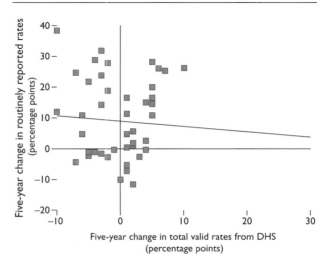

ten policies, poor data storage, insufficient analysis and feedback, and confusion in denominator use (3). Due to the limited number of DQAs conducted to date (eight countries in 2000 and 12 in 2001), unavailability of the official reports from the last series of DQAs, and no time overlap between DQAs and the data analysed in our study, we could not validate our findings with the findings of the DQAs.

It would have been interesting to explore the extent to which the variation in the methods for compiling the officially reported coverage rates can explain the differences between the latter and the DHS estimates. However such analysis was not possible because the WHO/UNICEF Joint Reporting Forms for Vaccine Preventable Diseases available to us did not specify the source of officially reported coverage rates.

A promising avenue for further analysis is to try and identify the factors that predict or explain the difference between coverage as assessed by service delivery registries and household surveys. Factors such as the presence and magnitude of incentive payments or the extent of vertical or horizontal management of immunization programmes would be potential ones to be included in a multivariate analysis. These studies may provide clues as to how information collected from service providers can be used as an input to valid and reliable assessments of vaccination coverage.

These findings support the WHO recommendation that all national programmes monitor coverage of vaccination periodically through household surveys (30). Experience has shown that household surveys have the advantage of capturing the activities of all actors in the health system, both in the public and the private sector. Our analysis of the quality of vaccination data obtained in the DHS, as many other studies examining the extent of maternal recall bias, suggested high reliability of survey findings (22–27), corroborating their potential role as a validating tool for routine data. Surveys that collect comprehensive information about coverage with critical health interventions and other important aspects of health systems performance, i.e. WHO's World Health Surveys, can produce significant economies of scale and lower marginal costs of data collection. It will be to the detriment of health programme monitoring and health systems performance assessment, if in the efforts to strengthen national health information systems such surveys are not considered an essential source of routinely collected information together with the service delivery records.

We believe that these findings have implications for efforts to collect information on the coverage of other health interventions. Globally, the efforts to gather valid and reliable information on vaccination coverage to support programme implementation and monitoring of progress have been among the most extensive in public health. Despite this impressive investment, changes in coverage based largely on data collected from public sector service providers are uncorrelated with changes in coverage as detected in household surveys. This complete lack of information content in reported changes means that efforts to expand the scope of information on the coverage of health interventions must be based on careful validation studies. The coverage of health interventions is essential information for decision-makers; tools developed to monitor coverage for other interventions must be based on strategies that are likely to be valid.

Acknowledgements

The authors wish to thank their colleagues from the WHO Department of Vaccines and Biologicals, in particular the Vaccine Assessment and Monitoring team, for kind collaboration in providing routine vaccination coverage figures used in the present analysis, as well as other information in improving our understanding of the childhood immunization programme. We also thank Macro International for providing permission to use the Demographic and Health Surveys for this research. We wish to acknowledge the contributions of Jason Trickovic for research assistance, and Elena Varavikova for useful comments.

References

(1) Wittet S. Introducing GAVI and the Global Fund for Children's Vaccines. *Vaccine*, 2000, 91(4–5):385–386.

(2) Brugha R, Starling M, Walt G. GAVI, the first steps: lessons for the Global Fund. *The Lancet*, 2002, 359: 435–438.

(3) The LATH Consortium. *Immunization data quality audit evaluation report. Final report.* Deloitte Touche Tohmatsu Emerging Markets, Euro Health Group, Liverpool Associates in Tropical Health, 2001.

(4) Guerin N. Assessing immunization coverage: how and why? *Vaccine*, 1998, 16 (Suppl):S81–S83.

(5) UNICEF. *Routine immunization: estimates on immunization coverage 1980–1999.* UNICEF Statistics 2001. URL: http://www.childinfo.org/eddb/immuni/database.htm.

(6) Cutts FT, Waldman RJ, Zoffman HMD. Surveillance for the Expanded Programme on Immunization. *Bul-*

letin of the World Health Organization, 1993, 71(5): 633–639.

(7) World Health Organization. Immunization policy. Publication No. WHOGPV/GEN/95.03 REV 1. Global Programme for Vaccines and Immunizations, Geneva, World Health Organization, 1996.

(8) World Health Organization. Informal meeting on issues of immunization data and monitoring/management of adverse events. Publication No. WHO/V&B/99.06. Department of Vaccines and Biologicals, Geneva, World Health Organization, 1999.

(9) Borgdoff MW, Walker GJA. Estimating vaccination coverage: routine information or sample survey? Journal of Tropical Medicine and Hygiene, 1988, 91:35–42.

(10) ORC Macro. Model "A" questionnaire. MEASURE DHS+ Basic Documentation series. Calverton, MD, ORC Macro, 2001.

(11) Boerma JT, Bicego GT. The quality of data on child immunisation in DHS-I surveys. An assessment of the quality of health data in DHS-I surveys. DHS Methodological Reports. Calverton, MD, Macro International Inc., 1994.

(12) Brown J et al. Assessment of the quality of estimates of child immunization coverage from population-based surveys. MEASURE Evaluation Working Paper series. Chapel Hill, NC, University of North Carolina at Chapel Hill, 2002.

(13) Macro International Inc. Sampling manual. DHS-III Basic Documentation series. Calverton, MD, Macro International Inc., 1996.

(14) Heckman JJ. Sample selection bias as a specification error. Econometrica, 1979, 47:153–162.

(15) Van de Ven WPMM, Van Praag BMS. The demand for deductibles in private health insurance: a probit model with sample selection. Journal of Econometrics, 1981, 17:229–252.

(16) Berk RA. An introduction to sample selection bias in sociological data. American Sociological Review, 1983, 48:386–398.

(17) Singh R et al. Immunisation status of children of parents belonging to various educational groups. Indian Journal of Pediatrics, 1976, 43(340):118–124.

(18) Angelillo IF et al. Mothers and vaccination: knowledge,

attitudes, and behavior in Italy. Bulletin of the World Health Organization, 1999, 77(3):224–229.

(19) Lewis T et al. Influence of parental knowledge and opinions on 12-month diptheria, tetanus, and pertussis vaccination rates. American Journal of Diseases of Children, 2002, 142(3): 283–286.

(20) Bennet P, Smith C. Parents attitudinal and social influences on childhood vaccination. Health Education Research, 1992, 7(3):341–348.

(21) Bhattacharya N. Immunization: parental knowledge and attitude in relation to low income and literacy. Indian Journal of Public Health, 1990, 34(4):220.

(22) Suarez L, Simpson DM, Smith DR. Errors and correlates in parental recall of child immunizations: effects on vaccination coverage estimates. Pediatrics, 1997, 99(5): 1–5.

(23) Ramakrishnan R et al. Magnitude of recall bias in the estimation of immunization coverage and its determinants. Indian Pediatrics, 1999, 36:881–885.

(24) Valadez JJ, Weld LH. Maternal recall error of child vaccination status in a developing nation. American Journal of Public Health, 1992, 82(120):120–122.

(25) George K, Victor S, Abel R. Reliability of mother as an informant with regard to immunisation. Indian Journal of Pediatrics, 1990, 57(4):588–590.

(26) Gareaballah ET, Loevinsohn BP. The accuracy of mother's reports about their children's vaccination status. Bulletin of the World Health Organization, 1989, 67(6): 669–674.

(27) Langsten R, Hill K. The accuracy of mother's reports of child vaccination: evidence from rural Egypt. Social Science & Medicine, 1998, 46(9):1205–1212.

(28) World Health Organization. WHO vaccine preventable diseases monitoring system: 2000 global summary. Publication No. WHO/V&B/00.32. Department of Vaccines and Biologicals, Geneva, World Health Organization, 2000.

(29) StataCorp. Stata statistical software release 7.0: user's guide. College Station, TX, Stata Corporation, 2001.

(30) World Health Organization. The EPI coverage survey. Training for mid level managers. Publication No. WHO/ EPI/MLM/91.10. Expanded Programme on Immunization, Geneva, World Health Organization, 1991.

Chapter 24

Human, Physical, and Intellectual Resource Generation: Proposals for Monitoring

Orvill B. Adams, Mario R. Dal Poz, Bakhuti Shengelia,
Sylvester Y. Kwankam, Andrei Issakov, Barbara Stilwell,
Pascal Zurn, Alexandre Goubarev

Introduction

To perform efficiently, health systems require the combination of a large number of properly balanced physical and technical resource inputs. Policy-makers must address a number of questions, which include:

- What is the most cost-effective balance between different types of productive resources[1] and how to reach this balance?

- What investment strategy to use (i.e. to train new nurses or to recruit from outside of the country; to build a new hospital or to provide incentives for the private sector to invest in hospitals; etc.).

The main points that need to be emphasized in the discussion on the resource generation function are the following:

- The link between health care resources and population health is not well understood.

- Investment decisions have long-term implications for health systems.

- Investment decisions in health systems are subject to the political influence of different stakeholders.

- There is significant variation among countries in terms of their investment patterns and resource profiles.

- Investment decisions affect the geographic distribution of health care resources and services.

- Investment decisions in health systems affect other systems as well.

Economists distinguish between capital, investments, and depreciation. Capital refers to the existing stock of productive assets (human resources, physical capital, and knowledge). Investment is a flow and refers to additions to capital. Depreciation is also a flow and refers to subtractions from capital as the value of productive resources decreases over time. The adjustment of capital stock usually occurs slowly over time (*1*).

The resources are produced by a diverse group of organizations: universities and other educational institutions, research centres, and companies producing specific technologies such as pharmaceutical products, devices, and equipment. Investment decisions are often made outside those organizations (especially if the organizations are public) and involve a variety of stakeholders for whom investment decisions may entail changes in the distribution of financial, technical, and political power (*2;3*).

The link between health care resources and population health is not well understood. However, it is needless to argue that the stock of assets and their composition, as inputs to the production of health, are important elements in the performance of health systems. In the short run, capital stock is sunk costs (fixed inputs) and there is little one can do about it. In the short run, a deficit in stock can be a real constraint to the delivery of services, while on the other hand, excess capacities, requiring regular maintenance, can drain financial resource from health systems. In the long run, capital stock becomes variable inputs, therefore allowing amelioration of current problems in the future through effective investment planning.

Investments in human and physical capital are usually of a long-term nature. The analysis of the census and Labour Force Survey (1991) in the UK estimated expected working lives of between 19 and 22 years for nurses and 26 and 29 years for doctors[2] (*4*). Unfortunately, the data on expected working lives (worklife tables) of health care personnel for most countries are not available, which precludes the comprehensive analysis of expected lifetime costs associated with human resources and comparison of such costs across countries. Worklife tables would also be quite useful in the planning of human resource generation and in the comparative cross-country analysis of recurrent lifetime costs of health care personnel. The lifetime of productive assets is an important concept as it has implications for maintenance and operating costs of the assets.

The current efficiency of health systems is often a result of past investment decisions. In Georgia, between 1990 to 1999 public health expenditure as a per cent of GDP fell from 3% to 0.5%, an almost sixfold decrease, while the number of physicians per 10 000 population remained almost unchanged at 49, and hospital beds per 10 000 population declined from 9.7 to 4.8, a twofold reduction. Past investment decisions responsible for current excess capacities make it difficult for Georgia to maintain its health system in the condition of dramatically declining financial resources (5).

Investment decisions have an impact on the type of services provided, the geographic distribution of services, and the political power of the providers—the power and influence of the health care providers who are the direct beneficiaries of investments will increase with investments. On the other hand, the investment decisions themselves are often influenced by local politics and driven by strong groups of stakeholders.

Investments in capital such as a new hospital could have a significant impact on the economy in the area where the hospital is to be located. Local politicians, professional groups, and unions all have their own interests in such decisions. Once built, hospitals are difficult to close. The public often associates with institutions in its area and views the potential loss of these institutions as the loss of a personal and community good.

Countries differ significantly in terms of the availability of different resources, which reflects their investment patterns. For example, in 1991 Denmark had 2.5 MRI units per million population, the UK had 1.1, and the USA had 10.1. In the same year, the USA had almost five times as many CT scanners per 1 million population as Denmark. Figure 24.1 demonstrates the differences in resource profiles of various OECD countries based on hospital beds per 1 000 population, MRI units, and CT scanners per 1 million population according to the data from 1997 (6).

Figure 24.2 shows the variation of the total health employment per 1 000 population in different OECD countries (6).

Countries show significant variations also in terms of the amount of investments they make in their health systems. Figures 24.3 and 24.4 represent the comparison of different OECD countries in terms of total health expenditure (THE) as a per cent of GDP and the total investment in medical facilities as a per cent of THE (6).

Figure 24.1 Availability of health technology, 1997

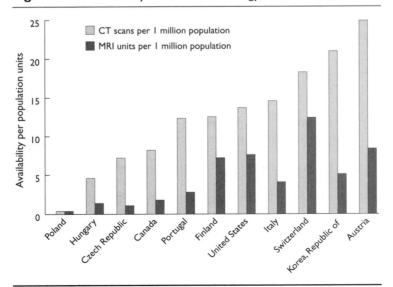

Source: *OECD Health Data (6)*

As can be seen on these graphs, OECD countries with lower total health expenditure as a per cent of their GDP invest more in medical facilities as a per cent of their total health expenditure.

Unfortunately the data on resource profiles and investments in health systems are hardly available from developing countries, despite the importance of such data for policy decisions.

Strong public stewardship is necessary to guide investment in health systems. Policy-makers and managers require tools to assist them in monitoring the impact of investment decisions on the delivery of health services and the performance of the health system.

The resource generation function is closely linked with the service provision one. The boundaries between these two functions might not always be clear. Figure 24.5 schematically represents the relationship between the resource generation and service provision functions.

Figure 24.2 Total health employment per 1 000 population, 1997

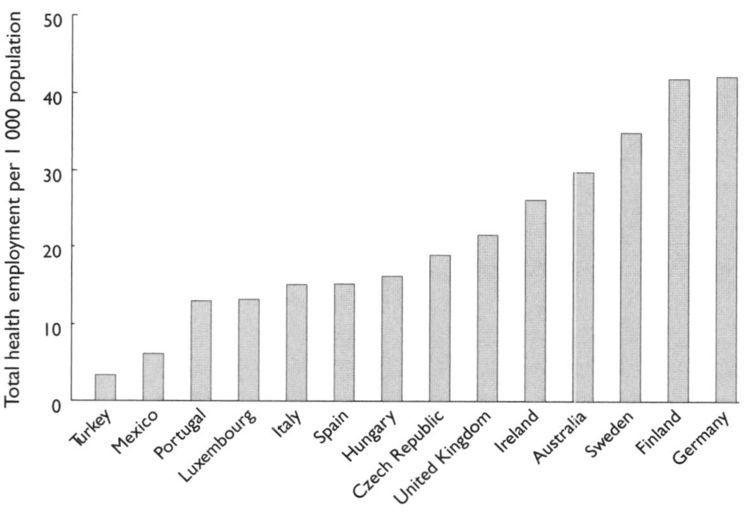

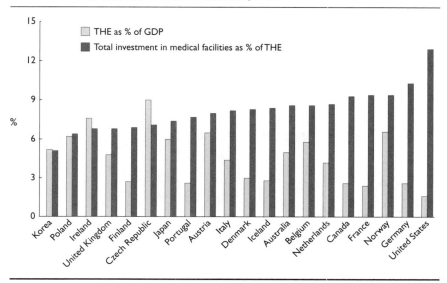

Source: *OECD Health Data (6)*

Figure 24.3 Comparison of the total health expenditure (THE) and total investment in medical facilities, 1998

Source: *OECD Health Data (6)*

The products of the resource generation function become inputs in the process of service provision.

HUMAN RESOURCES FOR HEALTH

As stated in *The World Health Report 2000*, human resources are the "most important of the health system's inputs" (7). Drawing from the wider definition of health systems from *The World Health Report 2000*, human resources can be defined as the stock of all individuals engaged in the promotion, protection, or improvement of the health of the population. This would include both private and public sectors, and different domains of health systems such as personal curative and preventive care, non-personal public health interventions, health promotion, and disease prevention.

This broad definition of human resources is supported and accepted both in management science and practice, and in the literature relating to health systems assessment (8;9). However, considering different elements of planning, production, retention, and recruitment of health personnel for the health systems workforce, a more sophisticated typology of human resources is desirable. Table 24.1 sets out two types of human resources, their description, and the current challenges which Member States face in human resource generation and provision.

Figure 24.4 Comparison of total health expenditure (THE) and total investment in medical facilities, 1998

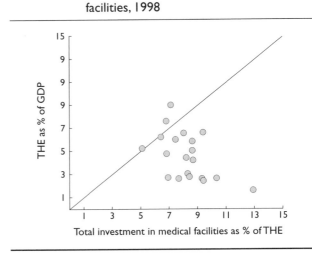

Source: *OECD Health Data* (6)

The classification of human resources is based on the primary intent of their professional education and training. Those human resources actually engaged in the health system can be referred to as health system work-force or health work-force, including both health professionals and non-health professionals.

The issue of human resources concerns both the resource generation and service provision functions. The production of human resources (education), main-

Figure 24.5 The link between resource generation and service provision functions

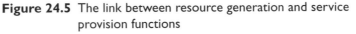
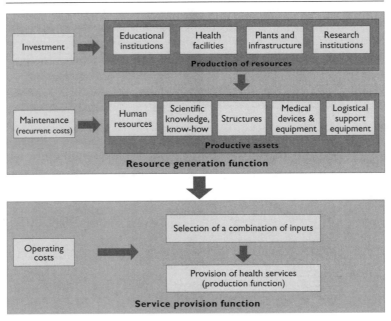

Table 24.1　Classification of human resources for health systems

Type	Description	Challenges
Health professionals	Health professionals generated by the health care system either in full or in part. Includes doctors, nurses, midwives, psychologists, pharmacists, dentists, and others.	The health system expects to employ 90% of the health care providers which it generates. If this expectation is not met, shortages will follow. Competition for health care providers may be external – migration from developing to developed countries for example, or internal – from the public to the private sector.
Non-health professionals	Those workers of the health care system who are not health professionals.	The health system must compete in the wider labour market to employ non-health professionals. In the UK, for example, managers were recruited to health services from industry, but to do so a substantial raise in the salary levels of managers (in order to compete with salaries in other sectors) is required.

tenance of their quality and productivity through continuous education and training, determination of the size and composition of the workforce at the macro level, regulation of the education of health care providers and of professional practices (licensing, accreditation, etc.), can be considered elements of the resource generation function.

Deployment of human resources, selection of an appropriate skill-mix for the production of health services, distribution of the work-force between different levels of the health service provision system, setting up incentives structures for health personnel, and human resources management can be considered elements of the service provision function. In this case, human resources could be regarded as inputs into the health production function.

Three types of costs are associated with human resources for health systems: a) investment costs spent on their production (capital expenditures on educational facilities, expenditures on training and education), b) maintenance costs (continuing education), and c) salaries and other benefits paid or offered to human resources. According to accounting norms, maintenance costs of all types of productive assets, together with operating costs (salaries and other benefits in the case of human resources), constitute the recurrent costs. The division between continuing education (above referred to as maintenance) and salaries is proposed only for delineating the resource generation and service provision functions for assessment and monitoring purposes, and therefore such a division is artificial. We suggest including continuing education (maintenance of human resources) in the assessment and monitoring of the resource generation function on the premise that continuing education is a means of maintaining productivity and quality of human resources. Salaries are the cost of the utilization of human resources as inputs in the service provision process. Therefore, we suggest looking at salaries and

other incentives for human resources within the scope of the services provision function.

There are a variety of levels and points at which the costs of human resources can be measured. In order to annuitize the costs of education and training for health care personnel, Netten and Knight (1999) suggest measuring the costs of the initial investment in training and then estimating the return on investment over time using the number of full-time equivalent years that a health professional produces over the course of his or her employment, but also taking into account the costs of career breaks and early retirement (4). According to the estimation of Netten et al. Equivalent Annual Costs (investment cost) of full-time equivalent nurse and doctor in the UK are £4 735 and £21 215 respectively.

Dahlen and Bolmsjo (1996) include a variety of additional costs that need to be factored into the total cost of employment. Among those are the cost of recruiting the employee, the costs associated with the initial training period for any employee to learn the system in which he or she works, and the cost of health benefits and any other payments that may be mandated on the part of the employer (10). Absenteeism, illness, and rehabilitation are additional costs of employment that Dahlen and Bolmsjo suggest need to be taken into consideration.

The total stock and composition of human resources reflect the trends in the development of health systems. In the 1950s and early 1960s, the main human resource concern in sub-Saharan Africa was to train a cadre of senior professionals to staff the new "centres of excellence." Auxiliary health workers were neglected. By the late 1960s and early 1970s, concern shifted to preventive health care and access to rural health services. This created a need for more nurses and auxiliary health workers. However, despite the shift of emphasis from hospitals to health centres, hospitals and physicians retained their central and dominant roles and even expanded their share of national health budgets (*11*).

Comparison of different regions and countries shows striking differences in the stock and the composition of human resources. For instance, in 1995 in sub-Saharan Africa the average number of physicians per 1 000 population was 0.3, while in the OECD Member European countries it was 2.9 (*6;12*). Figures 24.6A and 24.6B show the sharp regional disparities in terms of the distribution of health professionals. The

distribution of physicians is unequal across regions and populations. In the African Region, the overall density is the lowest with a few exceptions such as Algeria, Mauritius, Seychelles, and South Africa. The European Region has the highest density overall with three exceptions: Albania, Bosnia, and Turkey. In the Americas, countries with the highest density are Cuba, Uruguay, and St. Lucia, followed by Canada and the United States with the second highest category (150–299 per 100 000 inhabitants). Similar trends can

Figure 24.6A Distribution of countries by physicians per 100 000 inhabitants

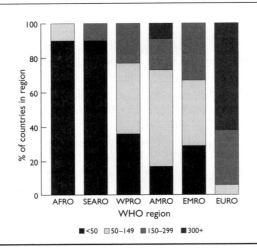

Source: WHO, *HFA Database*

Figure 24.6B Distribution of countries by nurses per 100 000 inhabitants

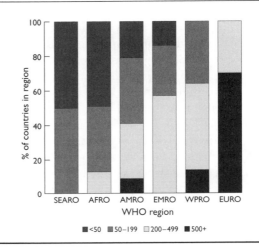

Source: WHO, *HFA Database*

Figure 24.7 Comparison of the number of health care personnel in selected African countries, 1996

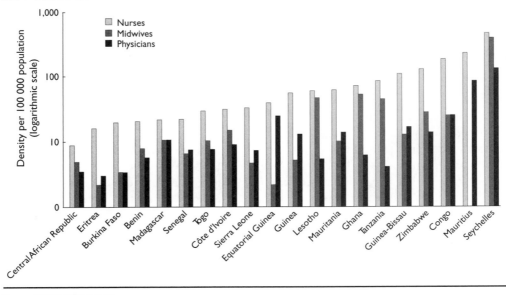

Source: WHO, *HFA Database*

be found in the distribution of nurses, but the differentials in density across countries and regions are less sharp.

The data on the profile of the stock of human resources in developing countries are hardly available, calling for intensive work to generate such data. It is expected that there is a huge variation in the availability of different types of human resources. However, the evidence on the effect of different compositions of human resources on health systems performance is not yet available. Figure 24.7 shows the availability of different types of health care personnel per 100 000 population in some African countries for which the data were available in the WHO, HFA database.

As we can see, the availability of doctors and midwifes in these African countries varies significantly. While generally more nurses are available than doctors, the variation in the availability of nurses is higher (standard deviation values for nurses, doctors, and midwives are 100.9, 79.18, and 86.25 respectively).

Similar data for some European countries are displayed in Figure 24.8.

The graph reveals the greatest variation in the nurse population ratio (standard deviation values for nurses, doctors, and midwives are 474.38, 106.09, and 68.91 respectively). The difference in the availability of doctors and nurses is better represented in Figure 24.9.

Migration of human resources is becoming an issue of increasing importance for many countries. Migration refers to the flow of health workers from one work location to another, though it does not necessarily imply from one country to another. Migration of health staff from rural to urban areas, for example, is an issue of concern in many developing countries (*13*). There are mixed views on the effects of migration on countries depending on whose perspectives are studied—that of the donor country, the recipient country or the migrating individual. It is impossible to assess the impact of migration objectively without clear evidence, of which there is little currently available. The effect which migration has on a country is related to

Figure 24.9 Comparison of the number of nurses to the number of doctors in Europe, 1998

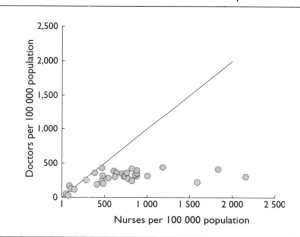

Source: WHO, *HFA Database*

Figure 24.8 Comparison of the number of health care personnel in selected European countries, 1998

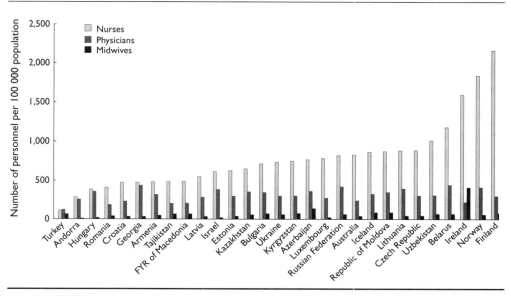

Source: WHO, *HFA Database*

the relative needs and loss of health personnel in that country, the impact being greatest where needs and loss are both high. For example, in Zimbabwe, there are high vacancy rates in nursing positions, while nurses from Zimbabwe are being actively recruited to the UK, USA, Canada, and New Zealand (*14*) .

Migration of health work-force from developing countries to developed ones can be viewed as a growing problem, exacerbating shortages and producing a disproportionately adverse impact on developing countries with relatively poor health status and few economic resources (*15*). Ojo (1990) explored the detrimental effects of migration of health personnel from sub-Saharan Africa (*13*). He calculated the cost of emigration of physicians from Nigeria by estimating the resources invested to produce a medical university graduate. He included in the costs: 1) living cost 2) educational fees, regardless of who paid them, and 3) earnings foregone while in school. He calculated that the cost of producing a medical graduate in 1988 in Nigeria was $30 000, and that the cost of losing 400 graduates a year was therefore $12 000 000. Ojo does not calculate remittances returning to the country, and does not explain how he arrives at his figures. Clearly, this example shows that there is a cost to migration for exporting countries, which can be detrimental both economically and in terms of the capacity of that country's health system to function.

Remittances, the portion of international migrant workers' earnings sent back from the country of employment to the country of origin, play a central role in the economies of many labour-sending countries, and have become a focal point in the ongoing debate concerning the costs and benefits of international migration for employment.

The main sources of official data on migrants' remittances are the annual balance of payments records of countries, which are compiled in the *Balance of Payments Yearbook* published by the International Monetary Fund (IMF). Global estimates of official remittance flows based on these balance of payments statistics suggest that remittances increased from $43.3 billion in 1980 to $70 billion in 1995 (*16*). Although the data based on migrants' remittances have several deficiencies (for a review see (*17–19*)), they suggest that for a number of countries the level of remittances is very significant in proportion to the country's merchandise exports. As Table 24.2 shows, in Bangladesh, remittances were equivalent to about 44% of total merchandise exports in 1993; in India, about 13% in 1990; in the Philippines, about 22% in 1993; and in Pakistan, about 24% in 1993.

Despite the fact that emigration of health care personnel is quite high from certain countries, there are hardly any data available on the contribution of immigrant health workers in the flow of remittance into the exporting countries.

Without more accurate information about the costs and benefits of migration, its full impact remains unclear.

Evidence from the UK suggests that the number of nurses entering the country and being registered for work is increasing. Table 24.3 shows admissions of

Table 24.3   Admissions of non-UK qualified nurses to the nursing register, 1990–1998

Method of admission	1990/91	1993/94	1997/98
EEC arrangements	813 (24.4%)	456 (20.2%)	1 439 (33.2%)
Other	2 518 (75.6%)	1 802 (79.8%)	2 894 (66.8%)

Table 24.2   Flow of workers' remittances and its share in imports and exports of goods in selected labour exporting countries

	1980			1985			1990			1993		
	Remit-	As a % of		Remit-	As a % of		Remit-	As a % of		Remit-	As a % of	
Countries	tances	Exports	Imports	tances	Exports	Imports	tances	Exports	Imports	tances	Exports	Imports
Bangladesh	286	36.1	12.2	502	50.2	22.0	779	46.6	23.9	1 004	44.1	28.2
India	2 715	32.7	19.5	2 427	25.6	16.1	2 263	12.4	9.7	—	—	—
Indonesia	—	—	—	61	0.3	0.5	166	0.6	1.2	346	0.9	1.2
Korea, Rep. of	100	0.6	0.5	265	1.0	1.0	597	0.9	0.9	605	0.7	0.8
Pakistan	2 108	82.1	38.7	2 573	97.2	43.8	2 175	40.4	26.9	1 602	23.7	17.2
Philippines	613	10.6	7.9	805	17.4	15.8	1 460	17.8	12.0	2 542	22.3	14.4
Sri Lanka	139	13.1	7.5	233	17.7	12.7	369	19.9	15.9	551	19.8	15.6
Thailand	348	5.4	4.2	809	11.5	9.6	774	3.4	2.6	—	—	—

Source (*20*)

non-UK qualified nurses to the nursing register from 1990–1998 (21).

For the planning and management of human resources, policy-makers need to have answers to at least the following questions: what is the stock of current human resources, what is the total cost of annual investments, and what is the ratio of productive resources over the total stock of human resources.

The following indicators can be proposed for the assessment and monitoring of the production of human resources.

■ Total annual investments in human resources as a per cent of total health expenditure.

The total annual investment ideally should include not only the expenditures on health education, but also the costs of continuing education and other forms of professional training, which can be considered as maintenance of the quality and productivity of human resources. It should cover both public and private sectors. The feasibility of obtaining such detailed expenditure categories from the National Health Accounts should be explored.

■ The ratio of the number of new graduates from the health educational institutions over the total stock of health care personnel by different professions.

This indicator will measure the replacement rate of human resources, and can help in the projection analysis. The data can be obtained from academic institutions and Ministries of Health and Education.

■ The total stock, composition, and distribution of human resources.

The measurement of the total stock of human resources should focus on the total number and the number of different categories of health care personnel per population units. Information should also be collected on the geographic distribution of human resources (inequality of human resource distribution) within the country, gender and age balance in the health work-force, distribution of human resources between the public and private sectors, level and type of education, and degree of engagement in the health labour force (full and half-time equivalent).

Geographic distribution of human resources has many implications in terms of access to health care. Many countries experience shortage of health care personnel in rural and remote areas.

One of the key determinants of labour market behaviour is age. In the US and the UK, for example, the nursing and midwifery work-forces experience noticeable "ageing."

In the US, the average age of registered nurses increased by more than four years between 1983 and 1998 (22;23). An "ageing" work-force has a number of significant employment policy implications, chief of which is deciding how to replace the loss in labour force as many nurses will retire around the same time. Buerhaus et al (2000) predict that in the United Sates the RN workforce will be 20% below projected requirements by 2020 (22).

Assessing gender balance in the health work-force is also interesting, as it may reveal the extent to which women and men have equal opportunities in education and career choice. However, in health care, gender can be important for other reasons too. For example, communication patterns between physicians and patients during the medical visit reveal behavioural gender differences and varying satisfaction levels depending on the physician's gender. The communication style of female physicians often includes slightly more focus on the patient's emotional and psychosocial concerns, more positively toned communications, and a more egalitarian style reflected in increased levels of patient participation (24;25). Nurses have often attributed their poor pay and conditions to the fact that nursing is a female-dominated profession, in which the work nurses do is seen simply as women's work, and not given a high market value (26).

The distribution of providers between the public and private sectors is important for estimating the relative size of each sector. Also, it might be a useful variable for explaining some of the outcomes of the health service provision function, such as coverage, provider performance, etc. In some countries, the estimation of the size of the private provider sector by the amount of private expenditure on health might lead to overestimation, because a large proportion of health care personnel employed in the public sector see patients on the terms of private practice, and therefore a significant share of private payments goes to public providers. For this reason, the direct measurement of the size of the private/public provider sectors might be more useful than its estimation by the amount of private spending.

The data on the total stock, composition, and distribution of human resources can be obtained from labour force surveys, censuses, provider surveys, national Ministries of Health or Labour, professional associations, etc. There are several examples of relevant provider surveys, such as the National Sample Survey of Registered Nurses in the USA. The history of labour force surveys starts in 1940 in the USA. In Europe, the first labour force survey was conducted in France in 1950.

The census is currently widely used by many countries and international agencies (UN, ILO, OECD, European Union and others). Besides the characteristics of households, families, and so on, the census presents some variables concerning work-force analysis, such as workforce characteristics like employment, hours of work, remuneration, social security, etc.

Some of the examples of the usage of the census data include the following:

In 1997, US Bureau of the Census provided detailed data on employment in health care and social assistance settings at the state and sub-state levels (27). In 1998, US Bureau of the Census, which covers a nationally representative sample of more than 100 000 individuals, collected data on employment of registered nurses (28). The European Community Household Panel study (ECHP) profiles labour market experiences in the European Union (29).

Even among countries that have a very good and long tradition of gathering census data, there is a large disparity in the way occupation data classification is coded. Only a few countries are employing detailed occupational descriptions with three or four digits, as defined by the International Standard Classification of Occupations (ISCO-88) (30).

Clearly, more development is needed on the use of labour force and provider surveys as methods for assessing and monitoring human resource generation in health systems.

■ Migration of human resources.

Indicators to capture migratory flows could include numbers of foreign health workers entering a country or seeking admission to a professional register and numbers of health workers leaving a country or migrating from rural to urban areas.

The data on migration of health work-forces could be obtained from professional registries, labour force surveys, providers surveys, and special bodies of government dealing with immigration issues.

PHYSICAL CAPITAL

Physical resources together with human resources are an important part of health systems capital, which has been defined in *The World Health Report 2000* as existing stock of productive assets. In the literature, physical resources normally encompass three broad categories: buildings/structures with auxiliary facilities (power generators, water pumps, etc., depending on local conditions); medical equipment; and logistics including supply systems, transport, warehouses, and logistic facilities. Physical resources are often referred to as health system infrastructure and technology or equipment. Physical resources provide the material platform on which the delivery of care rests. Quality and numbers of staff, as well as availability of drugs and consumables, are of little value without adequately built and equipped facilities, just as the latter by themselves are of little utility without the former.

Physical resources represent a significant investment for the health sector. This investment is constantly increasing, reflecting technological progress. The graph below (Figure 24.10) represents the trend in total per capita investment in medical facilities (in PPP terms) in OECD countries from 1980 to 1999.

This graph demonstrates a considerable variation between different OECD countries in terms of per capita total investments in medical facilities. As the investment increases over time, the variation between the countries also increases. The country that has experienced the highest increase in per capita investment is Norway. As we have demonstrated in the introductory section, the OECD countries with lower total health expenditure as a per cent of GDP tend to invest more in medical facilities as a per cent of total health expenditure.

Health authorities are confronted with a bewildering array of choices when making difficult decisions on investment in medical equipment. The number of different types, brands, and models of medical devices offered on the world market in 1994 was estimated at 750 000, produced by some 10 000 manufacturers (31). The same source estimates that the number of makes and models had almost doubled by the year 2000. This unprecedented pace of technology development and transfer has, in many instances, far exceeded the capacity of health systems to track the innovations and to put in place adequate support systems for use of new technology. Monitoring innovations is important as technological progress strongly influences the economic and clinical lifetime of physical capital: old

Figure 24.10 Trends in total per capita investments in medical facilities in PPP terms

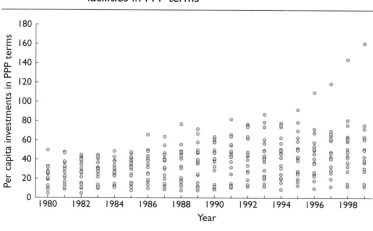

Source: *OECD Health Data, 2001 (6)*

investments quickly become outdated as new and improved technologies emerge.

New investment is a critical activity for adjusting capital stock and creating new productive assets. Information on such investment is essential for policy-makers as they make decisions about the allocation of resources now, as opposed to investments that will support the provision of health services in the future. Past sustained investment has resulted in adequate stock in most industrialized nations permitting in some cases lower capital investment now than about 15 or 20 years ago (7).

Acquiring physical resources is only one step of the many that make up the capital assets management function, and requires that attention be given to the overall technology life cycle. The expenditure plan should therefore be based on life cycle costing, which takes into account factors such as maintenance, repair, operation, and depreciation. Experts suggest, based on service records at facility level, that the annual allocation for maintenance in relation to replacement cost should be about 5–15% for medical equipment, 2–3% for buildings and plants, and 5% for vehicles (32;33). Most medical equipment needs to be replaced within five to 20 years depending on the type and the way it is handled. Reasonable estimates of the combined annual costs for equipment maintenance and replacement, based on documented experience from development agencies, are 20–25% of the current purchase (34). As an illustration, the replacement value of medical equipment in the NHS acute trusts in England is around £3 billion, with some £220 million spent annually on

acquiring new equipment and replacing old, and a further £120 million spent on maintenance (35).

The situation in developing countries where information systems are weak and data not readily available merits special attention. These countries account for only an estimated 10% of the world medical equipment market (36). But the small share of expenditure on infrastructure and equipment is estimated, from formal and informal reports, to be as high as 40 to 50% of the total public health budget in some developing countries.[3] Equivalent figures are typically not more than 5% among OECD countries (7).

The acquisition of physical resources should be driven by health/clinical necessity. To maximize the utility of these resources, countries need to monitor factors which influence their use within the context of their specific delivery systems or services. While it may be interesting to have a large number of indicators, given the complex issues involved in planning and managing physical resources, a parsimonious set that provides insights into the operation of the health system may be more feasible for health systems performance. The following measures are proposed:

■ Annual new investment in health facilities as a per cent of the total health expenditure.

This measure would be designed to capture the decisions that are made each year to invest in new capital. These decisions are not made in isolation from other investments (expenditures) in the same year. The ratio of annual investments in health facilities as a proportion of total health expenditures will provide the policy-maker with information on the allocation of resources.

■ The annual expenditure on maintenance as a percentage of annual investment in health facilities.

This measure will provide information on the state of productivity of the asset. The ratio of annual investment in maintenance as a proportion of total investment in health facilities will give information on the balance between investment and maintenance. Annual investment in maintenance can also be expressed as a proportion of total stock of equipment and physical plants (replacement costs) in the system. This will provide information that can be used in estimating the productive life of the capital stock. The hypothesis is that a country with a lower ratio of investment in maintenance to capital stock will have a higher degree of inefficient use of the capital stock.

■ Total stock of health facilities (current value) in the system as a proportion of GDP.

This measure aims at collecting information on the value of existing facilities in the system, and can be used as a proxy for the total investment the country has made. Over time, it can show the changing worth of physical investments in the country.

KNOWLEDGE

Growth in the available knowledge or advances in technology, such as new drugs, can substantially increase the capacity of human resources to solve health problems, and thereby improve the performance of health systems (7).

New knowledge is created from investments in research and development. There is a need to build alliances between researchers, decision-makers, users, and fund providers in the identification and formulation of problems for research, believing that early collaboration will result in a better utilization of the results. Recent studies which have focused on the use of new knowledge in clinical practice have also concluded that perceived relevance of the knowledge to the user is vital in changing behaviour (37). Involving stakeholders in the process of production of knowledge appears to be a method of improving its application and, ultimately, the quality of health care (38). Investing in the generation of knowledge has, therefore, two major components: investment in

research and development, and investment in use of the findings (39).

Health research takes place in a number of settings: universities, hospitals, research institutes and centres, industrial laboratories, and government facilities. Funding for research can come from the private sector, from the public sector or through joint ventures. In developing countries, funding for research may also come from donor countries.

Concern over the level, balance, and return on research investment has become high on the policy agenda of many countries. Buxton et al. (40), in discussing research in the United Kingdom, suggest that the direct opportunity cost of substantial investment of NHS funding is spending on patient care. NHS research is expected to generate returns through improvements in health and welfare, and thus there is pressure to justify the total allocation of resources to research, as opposed to health services.

Without investments in knowledge, health systems will lag behind in the application of new and appropriate technology in the provision of health services. *The World Health Report 2000* argues that new knowledge has contributed to shifting the boundaries between hospitals, primary health care, and community care. Further vaccines have altered the strategy and costs of tackling epidemic diseases such as measles and poliomyelitis, and new vaccines will continue to necessitate rethinking to ensure an efficient mix of inputs in national health strategy.

For the assessment and monitoring of the generation of knowledge, the following measures can be proposed:

■ The total annual investment in research and development.

Linking annual investment to total health expenditures will give an indication of the allocation decisions being made by countries. Given the nature of investments in research and development, it will be important to separate out investments by the public sector and the private sector. In the future, it will also be useful for policy-makers to have comparable information on the distribution of investments in knowledge.

A number of countries and research consortia (e.g. Global Forum on Health Research) are currently engaged in trying to define good measures of health research. The data on investments in research and development could be obtained from National Health Accounts, various government sources, and donor agencies.

There is a growing body of evidence that certain mechanisms are more likely than others to bring about individual and organizational change in the way that new knowledge is used in policy development and in practice (37;41). Investment in knowledge generation must be accompanied by changing methods of knowledge dissemination, application, and use, so that assessing the investment in knowledge must also include an assessment of what measures are taken to ensure knowledge is relevant. The two suggested here are a review of professional development and continuing education methods, and the process of involving stakeholders in the generation of the research agenda.

Conclusions

In this chapter we argued that resources are crucial components of the health system. However, there is little systematic evidence on the impact of investment decisions on the performance of health systems. The data for many countries on various aspects of the resource generation function are scarce, making it difficult to perform cross-country comparisons. The link between health care resources and population health is not well understood. This chapter suggests that: 1) investment decisions have long-term implications for health systems; 2) investment decisions in health systems are subject to the political influence of different stakeholders; 3) there is significant variation among countries in terms of their investment patterns and resource profiles; 4) investment decisions affect the geographic distribution of health care resources and services; and 5) investment decisions in health systems affect other systems as well.

We discussed two categories of resources for health systems: human resources and physical capital.

We defined human resources as the stock of all individuals engaged in the promotion, protection, or improvement of the health of the population. For the assessment and monitoring of human resource generation we proposed the following measures:

- Total annual investments in human resources as a per cent of the total health expenditure.

- The ratio of the number of new graduates from health educational institutions over the total stock of health care personnel by different professions.

- The total stock, composition, and distribution of human resources.

We defined physical capital as a combination of three broad categories: buildings/structures with auxiliary facilities (power generators, water pumps, etc., depending on local conditions); medical equipment; and logistics including supply systems, transport, warehouses, and their logistic facilities.

For the assessment and monitoring of the generation of physical capital we proposed the following measures:

- Annual new investment in health facilities as a per cent of total health expenditure.

- The annual expenditure on maintenance as a percentage of annual investment in health facilities.

- Total stock of health facilities (current value) in the system as a proportion of GDP.

For the assessment and monitoring of the investments in knowledge generation, we propose to measure total annual investment in research and development.

Notes

1 For the purposes of this chapter the term "resources" is used synonymously to "productive assets," and it does not include financial resources.

2 The approach for estimating expected working life is similar to worklife tables produced to predict labour force participation and lost earnings capacity. The expected working life is the sum of the full- and part-time years over the entire working life adjusted for mortality, emigration, and proportion of people qualified at different ages. The following formula is used for the estimation of working life:

$$E = \sum q_i[(p_{fti}Y_{fti} + p_{pti}Y_{pti})(1 - m_i)],$$

where q_i is the proportion of professionals qualified by age i, p_{fti} is the proportion of professionals in full-time work at age i, p_{pti} is the proportion of professionals in part-time work at age i, Y_{pti} is the expected part-time working year at age i, Y_{fti} is the number of full-time working years in age group i, and m_i is the probability of dying between the age of qualification and age i.

3 The anecdotal nature of some of the references in this section stems from the dearth of statistics regarding expenditure on, and quality and state of, physical resources in developing countries. We are left with formal and informal reports as the primary source of data, in trying to draw attention to the problems of physical resources in these countries.

REFERENCES

(1) Anell A, Barnum H. The allocation of capital and health sector reform. In: Saltman R, ed. *Critical challenges for health care reform in Europe.* Copenhagen, WHO/ EURO, 1996.

(2) Mills A. Health care reforms in developing countries. *Informing and Reforming,* 1998, 5:2–5.

(3) Reich M. The politics of health sector reform in developing countries: three cases of pharmaceutical policy. In: Berman P, ed. *Health sector reform in developing countries: making health development sustainable.* Boston, Data for Decision Making (DDM), Harvard University, 1995.

(4) Netten A, Knight J. Annuitizing the human capital investment costs of health service professionals. *Health Economics,* 1999, 8:245–255.

(5) Abt Associates. *Hospital financing study for Georgia.* Bethesda, Abt Associates, Partnerships for Health Reform Project, 1999.

(6) Organisation for Economic Co-operation and Development. *OECD Health Data,* 2001. Paris, Organisation for Economic Co-operation and Development, 2001.

(7) World Health Organization. *The World Health Report 2000. Health Systems: Improving Performance.* Geneva, World Health Organization, 2000.

(8) Cassels A, Janovsky K. Management development for primary health care: a framework for analysis. *International Journal of Health Planning and Management,* 1991, 6:109–124.

(9) World Health Organization. Achieving the right balance: the role of policy making processes in managing human resources for health problems. In serial: *Issues in Health Services Delivery.* Document: WHO/EIP/OSD/00.2. Geneva, World Health Organization, 2000. URL: http:// whqlibdoc.who.int/hq/2000/WHO_EIP_OSD_00.2.pdf

(10) Dahlen P, Balmsjo GS. Life-cycle cost analysis of the labor factor. *International Journal of Production Economics,* 1996, 46:459–467.

(11) Vaughan JP. *Health personnel development in Sub-Saharan Africa.* Population and Human Resources Department, Washington, DC, World Bank, 1992.

(12) Peters D et al. *Health expenditures, services and outcomes in Africa, basic data and cross-national comparisons, 1990–96.* Human Development Network, Washington, DC, World Bank, 1999.

(13) Ojo KO. International migration of health manpower in Sub-Saharan Africa. *Social Science & Medicine,* 1990, 31:631–937.

(14) Mutizwa-Magiza D. *The impact of health sector reform on public sector health worker motivation in Zimbabwe.*

Major Applied Research 5, Working Paper 4 . Bethesda, Abt Associates, Partnerships for Health Reform Project, 1998.

(15) Global Advisory Group on Nursing and Midwifery. *Report of the Sixth Meeting Geneva, 19–22 November 2000. Executive Summary.* Geneva, World Health Organization, 2001.

(16) Russell S. Migrant remittances and development. *International Migration: Quarterly Review,* 1992, 30:267–287.

(17) Athukorala P. The use of migrant remittances in development: lessons from the Asian experience. *Journal of International Development,* 1992, 4:511–529.

(18) Brown PC. *Consumption and investments from migrants' remittances in the South Pacific. Report to the International Labour Office.* Geneva, International Labour Office, 1995.

(19) Swami G. *International migrant workers' remittances: issues and prospects.* World Bank Staff Working Paper 481. Washington, DC, World Bank, 1981.

(20) International Labour Organization. *Migrant worker remittances, micro-finance and the informal economy: prospects and issues.* Working Paper No. 21. Geneva, International Labour Organization, 1999. URL: http:// www.ilo.org/public/english/employment/finance/papers/ wpap21.htm

(21) Hardill I, MacDonald S. Skilled international migration: the experience of nurses in the UK. *The Journal of the Regional Studies Association,* 2000, 34(7). URL: http:// www.regional-studies-assoc.ac.uk

(22) Buerhaus PI, Staiger DO, Auerbach DI. Implications of an ageing registered nurse workforce. *Journal of the American Medical Association,* 2000, 283:2948–2954.

(23) Buchan J. The greying of the UK nursing workforce: implications for employment policy and practice. *Journal of Advanced Nursing,* 1999, 33:818–826.

(24) Roter DL, Hall JA. How physician gender shapes the communication and evaluation of medical care. *Mayo Clinic Proceedings,* 2001, 76:673–676.

(25) Hall JA, Roter DL. Medical communication and gender: a summary of research. *Journal of Gender-Specific Medicine,* 1998, 1:39–42.

(26) Salvage J, Heijnen S. *Nursing in Europe: a resource for better health.* WHO Regional Publications, European Series No. 74. Copenhagen, WHO/EURO, 1997.

(27) U.S. Census Bureau. 2001. URL: http://www.census.gov

(28) Buerhaus PI, Staiger DO, Auerbach DI. Implications of an ageing registered nurse workforce. *Journal of the American Medical Association,* 2000, 283:2948–2954.

(29) Fisher K et al. *Examining flexible labour in Europe: the first three waves of the ECHP.* ISER Working Paper

2000-29. Institute for Social & Economic Research, University of Essex, 2000.

(30) Hoffmann E. *International statistical comparisons of occupational and social structures: problems, possibilities and the roles of ISCO-88*. Geneva, International Labour Organization, 1999. URL: http://www.ilo.org/public/english/bureau/stat/download/iscopres.pdf

(31) Nobel JJ. The universe of medical devices. In: Van Gruting CWD, ed. *Medical devices: international perspectives on health and safety*. Elsevier Science, 1994.

(32) World Health Organization. *Maintenance and repair of laboratory, diagnostic imaging, and hospital equipment*. Geneva, World Health Organization, 1994.

(33) World Health Organization, Medical Research Council of South Africa. *Report of the workshop on health care technology in sub-Saharan Africa: challenges and collaboration possibilities*. Cape Town, Medical Research Council of South Africa, 1994.

(34) Bloom G, Temple-Bird C. Medical equipment management. In: Lankinen KS et al., eds. *Health and disease in developing countries*. London, Macmillan, 1994.

(35) National Audit Office. *The management of medical equipment in NHS acute trusts in England*. National Audit Office Press Notice, 1999.

(36) Issakov A. Health care equipment: a WHO perspective. In: Van Gruting CWD, ed. *Medical devices: international perspectives on health and safety*. Elsevier Science, 1994.

(37) National Health Service. National Health Service Centre for Reviews and Dissemination. *Effective Health Care Bulletin*, 1999, 5.

(38) Pan American Health Organization. *Strategies for utilization of scientific information in decision-making for health equity*. Washington, DC, Pan American Health Organization, 2001. URL: http://www.paho.org/English/HDP/hdr/MEX-final.pdf

(39) Leininger CJ, Seaman LH. Selecting clinical quality improvement projects: getting a bigger return for your investment. *Top Health Information Management*, 2000, 20:27–34.

(40) Buxton M, Croxson B, Hanney S. *Assessing the payback for health R&D: from ad hoc studies to regular monitoring*. HERG Research Report No. 27. Health Economics Research Group (HERG), Brunel University, 1999.

(41) Muir Gray JA. *Evidence-based health care*. Edinburgh, Churchill Livingstone, 1997.

Chapter 25

Towards Better Stewardship: Concepts and Critical Issues

Phyllida Travis, Dominique Egger, Philip Davies, Abdelhay Mechbal

Introduction

The World Health Report 2000 (*1*) identified four core functions that all health systems carry out in some way, regardless of how they are organized or where they are. They were financing, resource generation, service delivery, and stewardship. In order to explain attainment of health system outcomes and efficiency, greater understanding of these four health system functions is required. This chapter focuses on the function of stewardship.

The report broadly defined stewardship as "the careful and responsible management of the well-being of the population," and in the most general terms as "the very essence of good government." Stewardship is the responsibility of the government, usually through the Ministry of Health. This does not mean that the government needs to fund and provide all interventions. Certain stewardship tasks may themselves be delegated to other actors. Who the latter are depends on how the health system is organized.

Responsibilities for different aspects of stewardship may be divided (intentionally or otherwise) between central and subnational health authorities, local government, other ministries such as finance, planning, civil service commissions, audit commissions, parliamentarians, professional associations, ombudsmen, inspectorates, insurance funds, other purchasing agents (sometimes including donors), and even some providers. However, a country's government, through its health ministry, remains the "steward of stewards" for the health system, with a responsibility to ensure that they collectively provide effective stewardship.

Stewardship has similarities to the notion of public governance, but as envisaged by WHO is more specifically focused on the state's role in taking responsibility for the health and well-being of the population, and guiding the health system as a whole. It influences the ways other health system functions are undertaken. In addition, it "embeds the health system in wider society" (*2*). In characterizing stewardship, the report identified three broad "tasks" of health system stewardship: providing vision and direction for the health system, collecting and using intelligence, and exerting influence through regulation and other means. It asserted that how well or poorly a government executes its stewardship role can influence all health system outcomes.

Many countries are searching for ways to understand and improve different aspects of health system stewardship. Building on previous work with related concepts, work is now under way to develop practical ways to assess stewardship, by analysing different approaches and then exploring the relationships with attainment in the various health system goals. Efforts will be made to develop approaches that allow comparisons between health systems so that relevant lessons can be shared.

This chapter reports current WHO work on stewardship. Section two reviews related work in health and other sectors. Section three presents WHO's current thinking on "domain/sub-functions" of stewardship. The final section discusses WHO's ideas on how to assess stewardship and outlines future work.

Characterizing Stewardship: Related Work in Health and Other Sectors

What are the essential things stewards should be doing in order to influence the behaviour of health system actors? Although the word itself has not previously been much used in relation to health systems, the importance of many of the activities thought to contribute to effective stewardship has long been written about (*3–5*). As a first step in the current programme of work, related concepts from health and other sectors are being reviewed in detail. Solid evidence is relatively scarce, but there is quite a lot of convergence in prevailing notions of what constitutes "good" stewardship, especially from the fields of public health and work on more general governance. Other recent input into WHO's work on stewardship comes from the Policy-Makers Forum and the WHO Meeting of Experts on the Stewardship Function in Health Systems held in September 2001 (*2*).

CONCEPTUAL ISSUES

The ways that stewardship or its related concepts are characterized can be divided broadly into two groups (*6–13*). There are those that characterize *what should be done*, and those concerned with *how things should be done*. In general, the public health literature pays more attention to identifying a wide range of concrete *desirable activities* of ministries of health in "guiding" the system (grouped into broad categories such as policy and planning, regulation, monitoring, and evaluation). It also often refers to how things should be done: many analysts suggest that, for example, participatory and transparent processes or, put another way, many of the current notions of "good governance," are desirable achievements in themselves.

In WHO's current efforts to develop a coherent framework to assess all four functions, a rigorous attempt is being made to avoid conceptual overlap between functions. For this reason, there are some similarities and distinctions worth making between stewardship as conceptualized in the WHO health systems performance assessment framework, the related concept of the steering role of ministries of health, and "core" or "essential" public health functions (EPHF) (*14;15*). The only real difference between the literature on the steering role and stewardship is that the steering role documents are specifically devoted to the roles of health ministries in different processes of health sector reform, whereas stewardship is a function of the whole health system, and its assessment involves considering more than the ministries of health. With regard to the essential public health functions, many of them do contain key elements of stewardship. However, the scope of stewardship is broader. It includes ensuring oversight, regulation, and accountability of all actors involved in any of the four health system func-

tions—including financing and all aspects of resource generation. Stewardship also excludes those aspects of essential public health functions which more appropriately come under provision or resource generation—for example, human resource development and training in public health.

The governance literature contains a range of definitions of governance. A number are based on what Armstrong (*16*) refers to as "high order tasks," some of which are similar to the stewardship tasks defined in *The World Health Report 2000*, such as the capacity to formulate and implement sound policies. But much of the literature puts greater emphasis on more abstract core characteristics of good governance which it is desirable to achieve. For example, the Commonwealth's paper on governance (*10*) identifies transparency, accountability, and participation as key elements of good governance. Kaufmann et al. (*13*) identify six aspects of governance (voice and accountability, political instability and violence, government effectiveness, regulatory burden, rule of law, and graft) which reflect different aspects of the process of government selection, the capacity of the state to implement sound policies, and the respect—of the citizens and the state—for the rules which govern their interactions.

Some people view governance as almost synonymous with the function of stewardship. In part, this depends on which definition of governance is used. We suggest that there are important distinctions regardless of the definition used. Both stewardship and governance are in part about the way things are done: the principles of governance permeate all social systems including health. The quality of governance affects the environment within which health systems operate, and the stewards of the health system have a responsibility to ensure the health system operates according to governance principles. But both stewardship and governance are also associated with sets of actions. There are many actions carried out in the name of governance whose primary intent is not to improve health, for example the process by which governments are replaced. By contrast, we argue that the actions of stewardship are all about improving health. It is true that in the course of their work, stewards of the health system may wish to influence aspects of governance that affect the population's health and well-being, much like they might wish to influence education or environmental issues. But stewardship, as one of the core functions of the health system, is a distinct entity.

Approaches to the Assessment of the Stewardship Function

There are also different views on how to articulate the stewardship function for assessment purposes. One is to start by simply describing what is being done in the name of stewardship, and only determine what might be considered "good" by analysing their association with differences in the performance of intermediate goals or outcomes. Those that favour this view do so on the grounds that they believe it is not currently possible to make any reasonable judgement about the content or quality of stewardship activities because inadequate evidence exists.

Another approach is to start by characterizing some core components of stewardship based on current views, propose some notions of "good" performance in these areas, and then investigate whether these are justified, again by examining their association with intermediate goals and outcomes. Those that favour this view do so on the grounds that there is sufficient experience to justify suggesting which are the key responsibilities and what constitutes good performance in each. The concern about whether these are the core components of stewardship that matter, and whether stewardship itself matters, can, and will still be, put to the test. This approach does not presuppose that certain instruments are used, simply that certain responsibilities are carried out effectively. There are many, sometimes conflicting and often unproven, views about effective instruments, strategies, and mechanisms.

With this second approach, how much certainty can there be that one has the core components of stewardship roughly right to start with? What evidence exists that the components of stewardship being proposed, largely based on prevailing wisdom, make any difference to outcomes? A more extensive literature review, especially of the political science literature, needs to be carried out, but as a start the work of Dollar and Pritchett (17) is informative, because it showed that "good policies" and "good institutions" are important determinants of aid effectiveness. Dollar and Pritchett used various markers of success, for example, GDP per capita growth. They found that in countries with sound policies and institutions, external aid was more effective. How did they decide how to judge what were "good" policies and "good" institutions? Good institutions were judged by governance measures: strength of rule of law, quality of public bureaucracy, and pervasiveness of corruption. Good policies were assessed by examining what were considered to be desirable results: low inflation, small fiscal imbalances, and open trade regimes.

The Domains/Sub-functions of Stewardship

Based on the above review, WHO is attempting to identify a small number of core domains/sub-functions that collectively are thought to constitute effective health system stewardship that leads to better outcomes. It builds on the definition of stewardship presented in *The World Health Report 2000*, and the work of Moran (8), who identified three core elements of a concept he calls "governing in health": making authoritative decisions, creating the means to put those into effect, and creating support for them.

Ideally the sub-functions should be defined in a way that avoids any conceptual overlap between them, and that between them cover all aspects of stewardship.

Who are stewards trying to influence, and how? They are aiming at influencing the behaviour of a wide range of players: those involved in provision, financing or generation of other resources; the behaviour of the stewards themselves; users or consumers; and non-health system actors whose actions affect health. Multiple policy levers and instruments are therefore used in the execution of stewardship.

Six domains/sub-functions of stewardship are presented here for discussion. They are constructed from prevailing notions of what constitutes the function of stewardship. Some are primarily concerned with market failures common to health systems, and others are more concerned with addressing potential public sector failure. There may be questions about both the categories and their content, and these domains/sub-functions are expected to further evolve after a wide debate. Their definition, their contribution to effective stewardship, the effectiveness of different instruments and approaches within these domains/sub-functions, and the links to intermediate goals and outcomes can all be investigated.

- Generation of intelligence

- Formulating strategic policy framework

- Ensuring tools for implementation: powers, incentives, and sanctions

- Building coalitions/building partnerships

- Ensuring a fit between policy objectives and organizational structure and culture

■ Ensuring accountability

What follows is an attempt to describe the core attributes of each domain/sub-function more concretely.

GENERATION OF INTELLIGENCE

This domain/sub-function is justified on the assumption that intelligence contributes to more informed decisions and thus to better health system outcomes.

Which actors require intelligence for effective stewardship? Those with stewardship responsibilities at all levels of the health system.

One could also argue that part of this sub-function of stewardship is to ensure that all health system actors—not just stewards—have access to the information they need to make their contribution to health system outcomes, i.e. including information for consumers/users of the system, ensuring providers get the information on new products they need, etc. The production of this information would be part of resource generation.

What sort of intelligence is required? Intelligence is broader than information. It implies identifying and interpreting essential knowledge for making decisions from a range of formal and informal sources—routine information, research, the media, opinion polls, pressure groups, etc. Although there is no universal agreement on what is essential, the areas listed below are commonly cited. Differences remain in the level of detail considered desirable.

What scope of intelligence is required? Three broad categories are suggested below.

We propose that stewards should have access to reliable, up-to-date information on:

■ *Current and future trends in health and health systems performance.* For example, on levels, trends, and inequalities in key areas such as national health expenditures, human resources, health system outcomes, health risk factors, vulnerable groups, coverage, provider performance, and organizational or institutional challenges in provision, financing, resource generation, and stewardship.

■ *Important contextual factors and actors.* The political, economic, and institutional context; the roles and motivation of different actors; user and consumer preferences; opportunities and constraints for change; and events and reforms in other sectors with implications for the health sector.

■ *Possible policy options, based on national and international evidence and experience.* For example, intelligence on different policy tools and instruments for similar problems, on their effects in different settings, and on managing change. It includes information on relatively specific matters such as cost-effective interventions, and on possible institutional arrangements for different functions.

Part of the investigation of the relationship between better intelligence and better overall stewardship, and between that and better outcomes, may involve trying to more systematically explore which sorts of intelligence really seem to influence and help decision-makers and improve decisions.

FORMULATION OF A STRATEGIC POLICY FRAMEWORK

This second sub-function is included on the grounds that the provision of a clear sense of vision and strategic direction for the health system contributes to better stewardship and thus better health system outcomes.

Here, the analysis is not of the technical content of particular policies, which will clearly vary between countries. It is more concerned with ascertaining whether government takes a broad, inclusive view of its responsibilities; the extent to which it is really addressing the health system's major policy issues; whether it has developed a vision of how the system should develop; and if it is monitoring progress, and is able to adjust its policies and strategies to new developments (*18*).

The key components to consider in monitoring this domain/sub-function are whether there is:

■ *Articulation of health system goals and objectives* (medium- and longer-term), based on reliable intelligence, and governing values, ethics, principles, etc.

■ *Clear definition of roles* of public, private, and voluntary sector actors in financing, provision, resource generation, and stewardship functions.

■ *Identification of policy instruments and institutional arrangements* required to achieve improvements in financing, provision, resource generation, stewardship, and thus health system goals.

■ *Outline of feasible strategies* for making required changes.

■ *Guidance for prioritizing health expenditures,* based on realistic resource and needs assessment. It would include decisions or priorities for major capital investments and investments in human resource development.

- *Outline of arrangements to monitor performance* and effects of change.

One thing to consider further is whether one should look for explicit evidence of certain features which, though implicit in the WHO goals, may deserve special emphasis: attention to addressing inequalities as well as levels of health and responsiveness, and protection of consumers, vulnerable groups, and the poor.

When thinking about how to arrive at answers to these questions, it is not sufficient to look merely for the existence of policy documents or plans, as these do not always address major policy issues. The assessment of the policy agenda and direction also comes from assessing statements and debates in parliament, the media, etc.; from asking a range of key players for their understanding of current goals and directions; and from observing how these concerns and intentions are being linked to action—for example, through budget allocations or changes in regulation. This has implications for the design of an assessment instrument and the ways people are selected to be part of that assessment.

Effective policy formulation includes assessment of the feasibility of change, which links back to the sort of intelligence that needs to be generated and making use of it.

Ensuring (Formal) Tools for Implementation: Powers, Incentives, and Sanctions

This third sub-function is justified on the grounds that a key element of stewardship is ensuring the implementation of policies designed to achieve health system goals. One part of that capacity to implement policy has to do with the stewards having and exercising the powers to guide the behaviour of different actors. Two other aspects of capacity to implement are addressed in the domains/sub-functions of "coalition building"; and "ensuring a fit between policy and organizational structure and culture."

We present here the argument that good stewardship involves ensuring that stewards have the powers to do their jobs, and also to ensure that others do theirs. More elegantly:

- Stewards have powers commensurate with their own responsibilities, and these powers are used properly.

- Stewards set and ensure enforcement of fair rules, incentives, and sanctions that are in line with the health system goals, for actors involved in provision, financing, and resource generation.

- Stewards ensure that the rights and responsibilities of users/consumers are defined and that mechanisms to protect consumers are exercised fairly.

By regulatory framework, we refer to a spectrum of rules, procedures, laws, decrees, codes of conduct, standards, etc., that exist to guide a health system.

Ensuring Stewards' Powers Are Commensurate with Responsibilities

In any state, even federal ones, the national government remains the "steward of stewards." However, the division of stewardship responsibilities is dispersed, in different ways, across all states. Local actors generally acquire more stewardship responsibilities with the various forms of decentralization that can occur. Examples of mismatches between responsibilities held and the powers provided to meet them are not uncommon at any level of the system.

- A central ministry of health may be expected to ensure implementation of the national health policy, but have few powers to do so in a situation where health funds go directly from treasury to the local authorities, and another agency hires and fires health staff.

- A law may be passed giving district councils formal responsibility for all local health services, but not giving them any control over either money or staff.

- It may be stated policy to decrease inequalities in health funding between regions, but the existing rules for determining resource allocation give little margin for change.

Questions will need to help identify where there are serious mismatches.

Stewards Set and Enforce Rules, Incentives, and Sanctions for Other Actors

This involves examining whether appropriate tools and rules to influence the behaviour of other actors actually exist, are used, and are contributing towards achieving the health system goals.

The question of whether the mix of rules, incentives, and sanctions that exist together constitute an effective regulatory framework can be approached in a number of ways.

One is to consider the common forms of market failure to which health systems are prone and whether there are effective safeguards in place against them. For example, what are the mechanisms in place to ensure the provision of pure public goods, or to compensate for the common problem of asymmetric information between patient and provider or provider and payer.

Another is to consider the different health system goals, examine the available evidence on the biggest perceived problems in terms of aligning the behaviour of actors towards those goals, and look for the regulations and incentives that current evidence suggests are effective in addressing them. For example, considering health inequalities, responsiveness or fairness in financial contribution.

Assessing effective regulation faces a number of challenges. There can be both too much and too little regulation. The same instruments can have different effects in different settings. There can also be conflicts and contradictions between sanctions or incentives, and between these and the health system goals they are supposed to support. A key element of any assessment, for which it will be hard to devise measures, is to assess the coherence of effects of the different regulatory instruments.

Matters to assess include:

■ *The scope of the existing regulatory framework.* In some countries, there are key aspects of the health system that seem to be largely outside the boundaries of current regulation (*19*). For example, are major policy areas such as private providers, drug manufacturers, consumer protection, road safety, and tobacco addressed?

■ *Enforcement and effects of sanctions and incentives.* A critical issue to assess when trying to explain the operation of this domain/sub-function would be the capacity that exists to actually enforce incentives and sanctions. There are many examples where existing laws and regulations are ignored because there are no mechanisms for detection or effective sanctions against evaders. For example, in a supposedly free at the point of care system, informal payments may be widespread. Drug quality control rules may exist, but no capacity exists to detect whether these are observed by manufacturers.

Much more work is required to develop appropriate questions, but they might address issues such as whether quality standards for health facilities, individual providers or manufacturers (accreditation, licensing) are enforced; whether codes of conduct for health workers exist and are enforced; and whether rules about out-of-pocket payments exist and are observed.

As mentioned earlier, a key element is to assess the coherence of effects of different regulatory instruments. Are these best judged through assessment of other functions or outcomes?

BUILDING AND SUSTAINING PARTNERSHIPS

This domain/sub-function is justified on the assumption that there are many factors that impact on health either directly or indirectly, and over which stewards have little or no formal authority. The steward cannot influence such factors by acting alone, and must involve other actors if positive change is to occur (*20–22*). To be fully effective therefore, stewards need to build and maintain a wide variety of relationships. This sub-function is thus an important complement to other, more formal, ways of exerting influence through regulation, legislation, and similar means as discussed above.

Relationships can be characterized by their type, the parties they involve, and the purposes they serve:

■ *Types of partnerships* vary along a spectrum of formality from loose affiliations at one extreme to legally binding partnerships at the other. They may also be bilateral or multilateral. Stewards need to be able to form relationships of many different types. In some cases, a relationship may involve little more than communication of key messages or networking among individuals. In others, the steward may need to establish coalitions or alliances with other players within or outside the health sector to achieve the desired goals (*23;24*). The amount of time and resources required to establish and maintain relationships will also vary significantly depending on their nature.

■ *The parties involved in partnerships* will be determined by the purpose of the relationship. They might include professional associations, patient or consumer groups, other ministries (especially ministries of finance and the civil service), private enterprises involved in service delivery, organizations such as medical schools and the pharmaceutical industry that play a role in resource generation, research foundations, politicians in national and local government, insurance funds, NGOs, regulatory bodies, donors, and many others. In order to decide who to involve in relationships, the steward should have a good understanding of the main influences on health and the positions, connections, and motivations of the different stakeholders who have (formal or informal) ability to influence them (25–27). An effective steward will be versatile and pragmatic in establishing and maintaining relationships, recognizing that many important determinants of health lie outside the health system itself, and that action on a broad front is often needed to achieve sustainable health gains.

■ *The purposes for which partnerships need to be established* include specific one-off events or issues, regular and repeated tasks, and ongoing activities. Examples of one-off tasks might include development of new policy and legislation, a media campaign or a large-scale reform initiative. Regular and repeated tasks could encompass planning or budget setting, while possible examples of ongoing activities are routine monitoring of service quality and consumer satisfaction. In all of these areas, relationships might need to be established to ensure success.

In assessing how this sub-function is carried out, it will be important to consider whether the steward has the right relationships with the right players both within and outside the sector. If senior health officials are isolated from, or not respected by, their peers in other ministries, in the wider sector, in key professional bodies, private enterprises, etc., then their ability to exercise effective stewardship may well be compromised.

An essential requirement for building and maintaining relationships is effective communication. Effective communication with the general public and with health sector organizations is a critical part of developing, and developing support for, both popular and unpopular policies and strategies. It can be done in various ways—directly through media campaigns, or more indirectly through representative groups and opinion leaders.

Communication is also fundamental to health promotion activities. Within the WHO framework, however, health promotion is more properly regarded as a form of service provision. Approaches to, and effectiveness of, that particular form of communication should thus be considered alongside other aspects of service delivery.

CREATING A FIT BETWEEN POLICY OBJECTIVES AND ORGANIZATIONAL STRUCTURE AND CULTURE

This is the third of the stewardship domains/sub-functions related to implementation capacity. It is included on the grounds that part of effective stewardship is to ensure that the overall architecture of the health system fits with policy objectives, and that there are clear linkages and lines of communication. It involves being able to remove essentially structural constraints to equitable and efficient resource use, and to assure a supportive management culture.

Lack of organizational congruence may arise for many reasons. For example, it may arise because there has been no recognition of the need to complement separation of functions with organizational change. It may arise from the failure to establish structures that have been approved by law, i.e. health boards have been approved in law but not created in practice. It may arise from the creeping duplication that may occur when a new structure is established and an existing one with similar responsibilities is not removed or retooled. It may arise when districts are expected to deliver care in an integrated way, while vertical programmes continue to employ staff and obtain earmarked funds. It may arise when reporting channels between organizations are not altered to fit new lines of authority and accountability.

Assuming that actors have clearly defined functions and responsibilities (this comes under the policy formulation domain/sub-function) and the means to carry them out, one would be interested in the following:

■ The extent to which organizational arrangements minimize overlap, undesirable duplication, or fragmentation.

■ Whether any intended separation or integration of functions and responsibilities is reflected in organizational arrangements.

■ Whether clear and operational lines of communication and reporting exist. For example, do organizational linkages facilitate exchange of information and communication, e.g. between people responsible for capital and recurrent budgeting; between people identifying health needs and those planning resources; between people financing and providing services; and between programmes?

Part of the effectiveness of stewards will be determined by the management culture within the system and the government's credibility in the eyes of other health actors (28). The following are suggested as important contributing factors:

- Policy stability and institutional memory, for example, through staff continuity and records.

- A supportive management culture: fostering and communicating successful innovation and experiment, reducing patronage, and rewarding good performance.

- The quality of bureaucracy—judged by the amount of unnecessary "red tape," institutional rigidity, irregular payment, and the competence of civil servants.

- Resources are available to identify and build stewardship skills and management capacities to carry out responsibilities.

Ensuring Accountability and Answerability to the Population

Accountability is considered a sub-function here on the grounds that it is a stewardship responsibility to ensure that all health system actors (public and private, providers, payers, producers of other resources, stewards) are held accountable for their actions. Accountability to the population is also a means of influence for the population, since it creates a way of balancing the powers accorded directly or indirectly by them to other health system actors.

Accountability helps detect and therefore reduce waste or other misuse of resources, malpractice, or negligence. In addition, good stewardship involves ensuring that mechanisms for accountability are fair and do not exclude particular groups.

One could examine the extent to which

- other health system actors are held accountable to stewards as proxies or representatives of the population (or are accountable directly to the public);

- stewards are themselves held accountable to the population for which they are responsible.

Ensuring Accountability: the Instruments

A wide variety of potential instruments, channels, and mechanisms exists—political, bureaucratic, technical, financial, the media. The government as a whole is the ultimate steward, and much health system accountability will be dependent on the general government mechanisms that exist: for reducing corruption, for ensuring transparency in the execution of different social system functions, and for allowing public scru-

tiny of governmental actions. However, it is possible to envisage differences in the extent to which different ministries facilitate or enforce these general principles of good governance in their own sector.

There are also health system specific procedures and mechanisms for accountability, which may be able to operate even in an unfavourable wider climate—for example, disciplinary procedures for doctors.

What Are the Commonly Cited Markers of Strong/Weak Accountability?

- Existence of rules about publishing plans, reports, codes of conduct, financial accounts, fee schedules, etc.

- Their actual publication, availability, and wide dissemination in a comprehensible form.

- Existence of independent watch-dog committees—political or administrative—with oversight powers: facility boards, health authority committees, e.g. ombudsman, audit commissions, parliamentary committees.

- Access to political representatives.

- Operation of self-audit, e.g. through professional bodies.

- Operation of other sorts of NGOs, representing different interest groups (both users and producers or providers).

- Through the existence of a free popular and scientific press.

Given the multitude of instruments, all of which may vary in effectiveness, questions will need to be devised which capture the desirable attributes and execution of the "sub-function" independently of the organization(s) involved.

Proposed Strategy for Monitoring Stewardship

Methodological Options and Challenges

Analyses of health policies and systems are done using many different methodological approaches. They cover a spectrum from descriptive case-studies to measurement. All have value and limitations. The case-study approach uses largely qualitative information and aims at comparison by using a common framework for analysis (28–30). Comparative case-studies can be valuable in investigating what exists, and also how and why, which helps when considering the relevance of findings to other settings. However, the number of case-studies conducted is usually small, and this limits investigations of causality. The lack of rigorously standardized approaches and measurement also limits the comparability of results.

There is an increasing body of work to measure governance, in which quantitative data on different attributes of policies, systems, and institutions have been gathered, usually through surveys. Subject to the usual limitations of survey techniques in different national and cultural settings, such approaches can potentially offer more comparable data. Information from other sources is likely to be needed to interpret findings.

Existing Tools

Because it is a new construct, there are no tools for looking at all aspects of stewardship. Attempts to assess the components of stewardship have been made from several disciplinary perspectives. An extensive review of literature is under way.

Within the health field, the most recent and comprehensive is the "Essential Public Health Functions" (EPHF) instrument (14). This was developed as part of a wider programme of work examining the steering role of health ministries, and presents a comprehensive list of questions and indicators for eleven essential public health functions carried out by the National Health Authority, some of which are aspects of stewardship. There are 48 indicators, plus around 120 measures leading to almost 700 specific questions. Most questions are answered on a simple yes/no basis to indicate the presence or absence of a particular feature (resource, practice, organizational entity, etc.) in the country concerned. Such answers are then scored 1 or 0 respectively. For each of the 11 EPHFs a composite measure is obtained by adding the scores for all relevant questions (all are weighted equally). Function-specific scores are expressed as percentages of the maximum possible. The resulting set of 11 percentages (one for each EPHF) is then displayed graphically to provide a profile of perceived strengths and weaknesses in the country's performance of the EPHFs. So far this instrument has been applied in 20 countries. The respondents are groups of key actors from the whole public health spectrum, who meet for a three-day workshop. Feedback on the instrument has been widely solicited from public health specialists and other users, but psychometric testing to establish the validity and reliability of the instrument has not yet been conducted. It was not designed for cross-population comparability. To the extent that there is an overlap between the EPHFs and the elements of stewardship identified in this paper, this approach can be seen to represent one way of assessing health system stewardship.

Outside the health sector, the World Bank's recent work analysing governance in different countries (13) is informative. Kaufmann et al. analysed more than 300 governance indicators compiled from a variety of sources (polls of experts and surveys) for over 150 countries. These were used to examine three elements of governance: the process of government selection, the ability to formulate and implement sound policies, and the respect of citizens and the state for institutions which govern interactions. Six aggregate measures of governance were constructed. The relationships of each of these aggregate indicators to three development outcomes (per capita income, infant mortality, and adult literacy) were then tested statistically.

Over the last year, WHO has itself been exploring which aspects of governance appear to be associated with WHO's two measures of health system efficiency (31). Two of the six indices of governance published by Kaufmann et al. were considered in detail. The analysis showed that both the health and overall efficiency measures are strongly positively correlated with the index of government effectiveness. There is also a positive but less strong correlation between a second index, the index of voice and accountability, and the two health system efficiency measures.

WHO's Recent Work on Health and Responsiveness

WHO's experience with the definition and measurement of health and responsiveness has stimulated debate about whether these approaches could also be adapted to the assessment of stewardship.

As part of the programme of work on stewardship, WHO proposes to develop a generic survey instrument that would include questions under each of the domains/sub-functions of stewardship. Such an instrument could be administered to selected key actors involved in different health system functions. There are also some aspects of stewardship where the perceptions of households would be important.

The intention is to phrase the questions in a way that they can be answered using ordered categorical response scales, for example, from "never" to "always" or "very strong" to "very weak," or using a continuous thermometer scale (*13*).

There is some relevant experience with surveys of governance. A preliminary overview of governance tools reviewed by the World Bank suggests ways of asking questions. For example, the quarterly country risk assessments produced by Standard and Poor's DRI/McGraw-Hill (*13*) ask respondents questions such as: "rate from 1 to 10 any changes in environmental regulations that reduce investment."

An instrument developed by the European Bank for Reconstruction and Development was used to survey local public officials, private firms, academics, lawyers, and other experts. Box 25.1 contains a sample question on effectiveness of regulation.

Any list of questions is likely to be long in the first instance. One important aspect of the development of any instrument will be to make it as short as possible by going through a process of systematic item reduction once it has been field tested. Further work to more thoroughly define domains/sub-functions is of course required in the first instance. There will also be a more extensive review of existing survey tools and experts collecting information on related concepts.

One of the key challenges in the analysis and interpretation of survey data across populations is the comparability of answers to questions that use ordered categorical response scales. This is because of differences in the ways individuals understand and use available responses for a given question. If one imagines a continuous scale of possible responses, different individuals will make the transition from one categorical response (for example from "never" to "rarely") at different "cut-points."

WHO has developed the concept of vignettes as a component of survey instruments for health and responsiveness, that allows adjustment for response category cut-point differences in ordinal self-reported data in order to improve the comparability of data (*32*). A vignette is a description or "story" of an experience that respondents are asked to evaluate using a categorical response scale (see Box 25.2). A vignette is always related to one of the main questions about personal experience (for example, state of health or experience with responsiveness) in a survey, which the respondent has also been asked to answer.

For each vignette, the respondent is asked the corresponding main question in the survey: in the above example this is "How much difficulty did Rob have moving around?" and the response categories are the same as those used for the self reports, from 1) extreme difficulty, 2) severe, 3) moderate, 4) mild, 5) no difficulty.

In summary, there is much work to be done in the area of stewardship. There is further conceptual work to more rigorously characterize stewardship, delineate its sub-functions, and develop tools and methods to assess it. There is analytic work required to explore the links between the organization and operation of the stewardship function and different health system outcomes in various settings. Finally, there is a need to identify effective ways to strengthen the stewardship function in different national health systems, and ways for WHO to contribute effectively to this process.

Box 25.1   The effectiveness of legal rules on banking

Score definition

1. Legal rules governing financial institutions and markets are usually very unclear and often contradictory. The regulatory support of the laws is rudimentary. Supervisory mechanisms are either non-existent or poor. There are no meaningful procedures in place to make financial laws and regulations fully operational.

2. Legal rules are somewhat unclear and contradictory. Supervision of banking activities exists on an ad hoc basis. But there are few if any meaningful procedures in place to enforce the law.

3. Although legal rules governing banking are reasonably clear, regulatory and supervisory support of the law may be inconsistent so as to create a degree of uncertainty. Although the regulator may have engaged in corrective actions against failing banks, enforcement problems still exist.

4. Legal rules governing banking activities are easily ascertainable. Banking laws are generally well-supported administratively and judicially, particularly regarding the efficient functioning of enforcement measures against failing institutions and illegal practices. For example, the regulator has taken corrective action against individuals, but could still benefit from more systematic and rigorous enforcement. Courts have the authority to review enforcement decisions.

5. Regulators possess comprehensive enforcement powers and exercise authority to take corrective action on a regular basis. Examination of securities intermediaries and licensing is frequent, as is the use of corrective action, such as prosecution for insider dealing, revocation of licenses, and liquidation of insolvent banks.

Box 25.2   Examples of vignettes

Vignette 1: [Rob] is able to walk distances of up to 200 metres without any problems but feels breathless after walking one kilometre or climbing more than one flight of stairs. He has no problems with day-to-day physical activities, such as carrying food from the market.

Vignette 4: [Margaret] feels chest pain and gets breathless after walking distances of up to 200 metres, but is able to do so without assistance. Bending and lifting objects such as groceries produces pain.

References

(1) World Health Organization. *The World Health Report 2000. Health Systems: Improving Performance.* Geneva, 2000.

(2) World Health Organization. *Report on WHO meeting of experts on the stewardship function in health systems.* Document HFS/FSR/STW/00.1. Geneva, 2002.

(3) World Health Organization. *Strengthening ministries of health for primary health care. Report of a WHO Expert Committee.* WHO Technical Report Series No. 766. Geneva, 1988.

(4) Londoño JL, Frenk J. Structured pluralism: towards an innovative model for health system reform in Latin America. *Health Policy and Planning,* 1997, 41:1–36.

(5) Pan American Health Organization. World Health Organization, *Steering role of the ministries of health in the processes of health sector reform.* Document CD40/13. Washington, DC, 1997.

(6) Murray CJL, Frenk J. A framework for assessing the performance of health systems. *Bulletin of the World Health Organization,* 2000, 78(6):717–731.

(7) Saltman RB, Ferroussier-Davis O. The concept of stewardship in health policy. *Bulletin of the World Health Organization,* 2000, 78(6):732–739.

(8) Moran M. *Governing the health care state; a comparative study of the United Kingdom, the United States and Germany.* Manchester, Manchester University Press, 1999.

(9) United Nations Development Programme. *Public sector management, governance, and sustainable human development.* Discussion Paper No. 1. New York, 1995.

(10) Commonwealth Secretariat. *Promoting good governance: principles, practices and perspectives.* London, 2000.

(11) Organisation for Economic Co-operation and Development. *Participatory development and good governance.* Co-operation Guidelines Series. Paris, 1995.

(12) Organisation for Economic Co-operation and Development. *Shaping the 21st century: the contribution of development co-operation.* Paris, 1996.

(13) Kaufmann D, Kraay A, Zoido-Lobatón P. *Governance matters.* Policy Research Working Paper No. 2196. Washington, DC, World Bank, 1999.

(14) *Public health in the Americas. Instrument for performance measurement of essential public health functions.* Washington, DC, Pan American Health Organization, World Health Organization, Centers for Disease Control and Prevention, Centro Latino Americano de Investigación en Sistemas de Salud, 2001.

(15) WHO Regional Office for the Western Pacific. *Project operating guideline: the structure and sustainable delivery of essential public health functions in the Western Pacific Region.* Manila, 2001.

(16) Armstrong J. *Stewardship and public service. A discussion paper prepared for the Public Service Commission of Canada.* Canada, Canadian Public Service Commission, 1997.

(17) World Bank. *Assessing aid: what works, what doesn't, and why.* New York, Oxford University Press, 1998.

(18) Cassels A. *A guide to sector-wide approaches for health development: concepts, issues and working arrangements.* Document WHO/ARA/97.12. Geneva, World Health Organization, 1997.

(19) Bennett S et al. Carrot and stick: state mechanisms to influence private provider behavior. *Health Policy and Planning,* 1994, 9(1):1–13.

(20) Walt G. *Health policy, an introduction to process and power.* Johannesburg, Witwaterstrand University Press, 1994.

(21) Robinson R, Le Grand J. *Evaluating the NHS reforms.* UK, King's Fund Institute, 1994.

(22) Quick JD, Musau SN. *Impact of cost sharing in Kenya: 1989–1993. Effects of the Ministry of Health Facility Improvement Fund on revenue generation, recurrent expenditures, quality of care, and utilization patterns.* Boston, Management Sciences for Health, 1994.

(23) Mizrahi T, Rosenthal BB. Complexities of coalition building: leaders' successes, strategies, struggles, and solutions. *Social Work,* 2001, 46:63–78.

(24) Sabatier PA. An advocacy coalition framework of policy change and the role of policy-oriented learning therein. *Policy Sciences,* 1988, 21:129-168.

(25) Brugha R, Varvasovsky Z. Stakeholder analysis: a review. *Health Policy and Planning,* 2000, 15(3):239–246.

(26) David J, Zakus L, Lysack CL. Revisiting community participation. *Health Policy and Planning,* 1998, 13(1): 1–12.

(27) Paalman M. How to do (or not to do)…media analysis for policy making. *Health Policy and Planning,* 1997, 12(1):86-91.

(28) Grindle MS, ed. *Getting good government: capacity building in the public sectors of developing countries.* Cambridge, Harvard University Press, 1997.

(29) European Observatory in Health Care Systems. *Health care systems in transition: production template and questionnaire.* Copenhagen, 2000.

(30) Organisation for Economic Co-operation and Development. *Improving the performance of health care systems: from measures to action (a review of experiences in*

four OECD countries). Document DEELSA/ELSA/WP1(2001)6. Paris, 2001.

(31) Evans DB et al. Determinants of health system performance: second-stage efficiency analysis. In: Murray CJL, Evans DB, eds. *Health systems performance assessment: debates, methods and empiricism.* Geneva, World Health Organization, 2003.

(32) Salomon JA, Tandon A, Murray CJL. *Using vignettes to improve cross-population comparability of health surveys: concepts, design, and evaluation techniques.* EIP Discussion Paper No. 41. Geneva, World Health Organization, 2001. URL: http://www3.who.int/whosis/discussion_papers/discussion_papers.cfm

Chapter 26

QUANTIFYING INDIVIDUAL LEVELS OF HEALTH: DEFINITIONS, CONCEPTS, AND MEASUREMENT ISSUES

JOSHUA A. SALOMON, COLIN D. MATHERS, SOMNATH CHATTERJI,
RITU SADANA, T. BEDIRHAN ÜSTÜN, CHRISTOPHER J.L. MURRAY

INTRODUCTION

The measurement of health, in a way that is comparable over time and across populations, is an essential requirement for the evaluation of health policies, assessment of intervention effectiveness, and measurement of the efficiency of health systems (1). Without meaningful measures of health, it would be impossible to appraise whether health systems are achieving their primary goals, namely improving population health levels and reducing health inequalities. The World Health Organization (WHO), through its commitment to annual reporting on average levels of population health for its 191 Member States (2;3), to routine assessment of the global burden of disease (4), and to regular evaluation of health systems performance (5), has recognized the fundamental need for cross-population comparable data on health and various other categories of evidence for health policy. Towards this end, WHO has developed new approaches to address the problem of interpersonal comparability of self-reported data on health status obtained from interviews or surveys, as well as new methods to describe, measure, and value health states. In 2000–2001, WHO undertook a Multi-country Survey Study involving 71 surveys in collaboration with 61 Member States using a standardized health survey instrument together with new statistical methods for enhancing the comparability of self-reported health measures (6;7). Results from this study provided strong evidence that the methods improve cross-population comparability and were used to guide the development of the World Health Survey, which commenced in 2002.

Based on extensive consultation and consensus building, one of the core functions of WHO is to standardize concepts and terminology relating to health.

One major shift in recent decades has been the realization that information on both mortality and health as a living state are required in order to describe health at the individual or population levels. Elsewhere, we have examined the conceptual, methodological, and empirical basis for summary measures of individual and population health, which explicitly combine information on mortality with information on the full spectrum of health experiences of individuals (8;9). The tradition of time-based summary health measures (such as healthy life expectancy (10) or Disability-Adjusted Life Years (11), among others) require aggregation, in some way, across different moments in an individual's life. Murray et al. (9) have proposed three distinct alternatives for the choice of time perspective used in these measures: a) an instantaneous, "snapshot" view of health; b) health over the entire life span; and c) current health and future prospects. Regardless of the time perspective that is chosen, or the numerous methodological considerations demanded by various different types of measures, an elemental requirement of any summary measure is the need to describe and quantify the health state level of an individual at a particular moment in time.

This paper outlines the foundations for the conceptualization, definition, description, and measurement of health that guides WHO's work in this area, which has resulted in widespread debate and consultation (5;12–14). Section 2 begins with an overview of issues and historical developments in the definition of health. Section 3 outlines a conceptual framework for quantifying levels of health for individuals and populations. In Section 4, a number of important measurement challenges are discussed, including the selection of key dimensions or domains of health to be measured, the problem of cross-population comparability, and methodological concerns regarding the derivation of summary indices of health state levels. Finally, we conclude with the elaboration of several consensus points, remaining challenges, and a brief discussion of the continuing research agenda.

Defining Health

Historical efforts to define health have typically been concerned with two major objectives: 1) articulating ideals of health that may serve as targets or goals to which individuals and societies may aspire; and 2) defining the scope and boundaries of health. The latter objective has resulted in considerable debate between proponents of relatively broad definitions of health encompassing wide-ranging aspects of human welfare, advocates for narrow definitions that emphasize a more biomedical view, and numerous more shaded views falling somewhere between these two extremes.

In 1941, Henry Sigerist, considering health in the context of human welfare, stated that "[a] healthy individual is a man who is well-balanced bodily and mentally, and well-adjusted to his physical and social environment. He is in full control of his physical and mental faculties, can adapt to environmental changes, so long as they do not exceed normal limits, and contributes to the welfare of society according to his ability. Health therefore is not simply the absence of disease; it is something positive, a joyful attitude towards life, and a cheerful acceptance of the responsibilities that life puts upon the individual" (*15*). This notion of health was endorsed by the President of the First World Health Assembly of WHO, Dr Andrija Stampar from the School of Public Health in Zagreb, who played a crucial role in drafting the definition of health in the preamble to the WHO Constitution. In this document, the founders of WHO famously defined health as "a state of complete physical, mental and social well-being and not merely the absence of disease or infirmity." This definition was preceded by a declaration that "...the following principles are basic to the happiness, harmonious relations and security of all peoples" and followed by the statement that the "health of all peoples is fundamental to the attainment of peace and security..." (*16*).

In the broadest terms, the 1947 definition set forth a lofty ideal for health as an integral component of well-being and, further, expressed the notion that good health is a necessary condition for attaining the high-

est possible levels on all other aspects of well-being. In defining health in terms of an ideal, the WHO Constitution provided a first building block for an operational definition of health. Over the half-century since the WHO definition was set forth, there have been continuing efforts to develop more precise conceptualizations of health that may be linked to operational measures (*17–20*). Often, however, operational approaches to measuring health, e.g. using standardized questionnaires or interviews, have not been based on an explicit and clear conceptualization of health. In a comprehensive review covering 30 years, Hansluwka (*21*) concluded that the challenge remained to develop appropriate measures that are comparable, yet reflect the multidimensional nature of health.

An important line of debate has revolved around the distinction between health and well-being. In the 1970s and 1980s, a number of critics argued that health is a component of well-being, not identical to it, and that the WHO definition medicalized non-health elements of everyday life (*22–26*). In attempts to define health more narrowly than well-being, two contrasting positions often have been adopted: the descriptivist and the normativist. The former argues that health and disease are concepts that can be specified in a value-neutral manner purely in terms of statistical deviation from typical levels of biological functioning (*27*), a position adopted by many bioethicists (*28;29*). The normativist position, as elaborated by Nordenfelt (*30*), relates health to an individual's ability to realize one's vital goals. It thus makes health an inherently evaluative notion since an individual must achieve health in order to achieve happiness or well-being. In this latter view, health is conceptualized in terms of integrated human functioning within a social context, and is culturally relative (*31–33*). Others argue that health has some intrinsic value and on pragmatic considerations may be focused on and differentiated from other aspects of well-being (*34*).

That some core notion of health exists across populations despite sociocultural variation on the determinants and experience of health, is consistent with current thinking on common values (*35;36*). This is more than a matter of face validity, which is certainly important. As the international technical agency in health, WHO has an implicit obligation to characterize health in a way that accords with the common understanding of health around the world. Even without embracing either the purely descriptivist or normativist positions, there seems to be a powerful intuitive notion that health is not identical to well-being.

Across all populations and cultures, some distinction is made between health and other aspects of well-being (37;38). In addition to health, education, economic security, environmental quality, and peace are usually considered as some of the important components of well-being (39).

We may also gain some understanding of intuitive notions about the scope of health by appealing to common views of what may be characterized as health interventions, and by examining the range of responsibilities of health ministries. *The World Health Report 2000* defined the health system to include all actors, institutions, and resources that undertake *health actions*, i.e. all actions whose *primary intent* is to improve health (2). This is a broader definition than the health actions typically under the direct control of a Ministry of Health, and encourages the stewards of the health system to focus on the delivery of key personal and non-personal health services, as well as to be effective advocates for intersectoral activity on a range of actions aimed specifically at improving health. If health were to be defined as broadly as well-being, this would imply that the health system includes all areas of human activity—such as education, industry, tourism, and agriculture, among others (5). Consequently, there would no longer be any operational distinction between the health system and any other system, and so ministers and ministries of health would need to be held accountable for all areas of human activity.

As ongoing debates about the scope of health proceed, we may identify several basic consensus points that have emerged:

- that health is a separate concept from well-being, and is of intrinsic value to human beings as well as being instrumental for other components of well-being;

- that health is comprised of states or conditions of functioning of the human body and mind, and therefore any attempts to measure health must include measures of body and mind function; and

- that health is an attribute of an individual person, although aggregate measures of health may be used to describe populations.

One of the most critical implications of this consensus view is that there is a clear distinction between health itself and its determinants and consequences. In the spirit of the definition set forth in the WHO Constitution, we do not equate health with diseases or diagnostic categories, but rather recognize a causal chain through which risk factors are determinants of diseases, and diseases in turn are determinants of health states. Factors, both physical and behavioural, that cause changes in health cannot themselves be construed as measures of health. For example, tobacco use may lead to respiratory problems. In such situations the risk factor of tobacco needs to be understood as distinct from the health outcomes to which it contributes. To understand how we may act to improve health, we must be able to separate the actual health states in which people live from the factors that influence these health states—only then can we examine the relationships between health and its determinants and intervene in this causal chain. This distinction is reflected in the evolution of the WHO family of classification systems, which includes the International Classification of Diseases and Related Health Problems (ICD) and the International Classification of Functioning, Disability and Health (ICF).

The ICD was originally developed to classify causes of mortality for common international use, but has since been extended to include diagnoses and causes of morbidity, as well as a wide variety of signs, symptoms, abnormal findings, complaints, and social circumstances that may be reasons for contact with a health service but do not qualify for a formal diagnosis (40). Over the last several decades, it has become clear that risk factors, diagnostic causes, and mortality events are inadequate indicators of the health impact of diseases, injuries and more distal determinants, the utilization of resources or the need for services. Thus, efforts to characterize more precisely the relevant attributes of a particular state of health have led to a gradual shift in focus away from diagnostic descriptions alone and towards an understanding of health in terms of functioning and disability expressed in different domains.

WHO, in recognition of this need, published the International Classification of Impairments, Disabilities and Handicaps (ICIDH) in 1980 to provide a framework for the study of disablement (41). Since its publication nearly two decades ago, the ICIDH has been used extensively across the world and translated into several languages internationally. The ICIDH was published as a prototype rather than a true classification system, and the conceptualization embodied in the ICIDH evolved dramatically through the development of its second incarnation, now called the International Classification of Functioning, Disability and Health, or ICF (42). The ICF provides a formal framework for cataloguing the multiple domains of health.

The Conceptual Basis for Quantifying Health

In this section, we consider the conceptual basis for the quantification of health levels. A common theme that has emerged from efforts to develop operational definitions of health is the view of health as an intrinsic, multidimensional attribute of individuals. This intuitive understanding of health crosses cultural boundaries, such that when we talk about a person's health, we are understood to be referring to his or her levels on the various components or domains of health. In other words, our conceptual framework focuses on the *health state* of an individual. A description of the health state of the individual thus consists of a series of values indicating levels on domains such as mobility, pain, hearing, and seeing.

The quantification of health levels requires cardinal measures of health that allow for meaningful interpersonal comparisons. The simplest comparisons are those in which only one domain is considered. On a single domain, ordinal comparisons are usually straightforward; for example, most people would agree that somebody with monocular blindness is healthier than a person with binocular blindness, *ceteris paribus*. The challenge of aggregating across different individuals requires that we go beyond the level of ordinal comparisons such that we can make meaningful comparisons of differences between two health levels. In other words, we require measures with interval-scale properties.

As a starting point, each domain must specify a sufficiently coherent construct to allow for quantification along a single scale. Such a scale may be observable or latent. If it is not possible to construct a single measurement scale for a domain, that is an indication that the domain includes more than one important health construct. For example, inclusion of colour blindness in the domain of vision will probably lead to measurement difficulties, since colour blindness cannot be measured or reported on the same scale as visual acuity. If colour blindness turned out to be an important aspect of health for description or measurement, then it would be necessary to include it in a health state description as a separate domain.

What Are We Measuring in Domains of Health?

The ICF replaced the concepts of *disability* and *handicap* in the ICIDH with the concepts of *capacity* and *performance*. *Capacity* refers to an individual's ability on a domain as it would be manifested in a uniform environment (or set of environments)—for example, the ability to walk 100 metres on a level, well-lit, non-slippery surface. *Performance* describes an individual's ability on a domain as it is manifested in his or her current environment. The gap between capacity and performance therefore reflects the impact of an individual's actual environment (and perhaps motivation) relative to the uniform environment. Both performance and capacity may be measured either with or without an individual's personal aids. Unlike performance, which is directly observable, measurement of capacity requires either changing the environment of the individual or carrying out a counterfactual analysis—asking what the individual's performance would be in an environment other than the actual one.

Given this distinction between capacity and performance, which construct do we aim to capture in conceptualizing levels of health for measurement? To the extent that performance reflects an individual's unique environmental setting, which may vary widely over time and as individual circumstances change, it is probably not congruent with most notions of health. If a person cannot climb stairs in her usual environment because the stairs are too steep, most people would not say that her health state had changed if the stairs were modified to be less steep. Likewise, we would not want to characterize the same cognitive impairment differently in two individuals simply because they have different vocations that call upon different types of cognitive tasks, and would not say that an individual with a hearing impairment is healthier simply because he avoids noisy gatherings. These examples point to a common-sense understanding of health that does not correspond to performance because it excludes the idiosyncrasies of an individual's environment. This is consistent with the notion of health as an attribute of individuals rather than environments (though environments may have causal influence on a person's health state). Note that here we clearly part company with those who would equate health with well-being or overall quality of life, since these latter constructs clearly do depend on local environmental barriers and facilitators.

The notion of capacity corresponds more closely to the common-sense interpretation of health by defining external environmental factors in a uniform way. More precisely, we believe that capacity *with* an individual's currently available treatment interventions (e.g. therapeutic drugs) and personal aids is the most appropriate construct. The latter requires clarification on two important issues: the boundary between personal aids and environmental factors, and the specification of the normative environment.

On the question of personal aids and treatments, there are certain factors outside the naked individual that many societies commonly understand to improve health states along relevant domains. These include specific classes of drugs that compensate for an individual's health problems, as well as personal aids such as pacemakers, glasses, and hearing aids. For example, an individual may have normal blood pressure if relevant drugs are available and consumed, but high blood pressure without these drugs. We believe that most people would consider the person's health to have changed through the use of the drugs. Some may argue that only those personal aids that directly change a person's physiology should be taken into account. This argument would imply, for instance, that a laser operation to modify the cornea of a vision-impaired individual would improve health, but that provision of contact lenses or glasses would not; similarly, a human hand transplant would improve health, but a bionic hand, no matter how sophisticated, would not. We believe that such distinctions are inappropriate. Drawing the boundary to include those interventions that change physiology and exclude those that substitute or compensate for physiological impairments would omit many health system interventions that are commonly perceived to improve health. Stated another way, defining health too narrowly will mean that many health system interventions such as pacemakers, certain dietary supplements and drugs, or contact lenses and glasses, will not result in health improvements, but only in well-being improvements.

This issue is closely related to the question of how health domains are defined. For example, if the function for the vision domain relates to "seeing," then it makes no sense to distinguish corneal modification from contact lenses in terms of their health impacts. On the other hand, if the function for the vision domain relates to the refractive properties of the eyeball only, then corneal modification improves health whereas contact lenses do not. We argue that the common-sense notions of health embodied in health system activities in most societies reflect broader domains of human functioning, such as seeing, hearing and mobility, rather than narrow domains of physiological function. Appealing to common-sense notions of health, a reasonable distinction may be made between interventions that are specific to a person, and those that stay with the environment. Defining the boundary between personal aids and environmental factors in this way—more broadly than by the physiological

criterion—an individual with near vision problems would be understood to gain in health through either a laser operation or the provision of contact lenses or glasses, but not through an increase in the font size of all print in the person's local environment.

The distinction we propose here leaves us with personal interventions (drugs, implanted devices, external devices and aids) that improve capacity in a health domain and are available to individuals in the wide range of environments that they are likely to encounter, i.e. interventions that are essentially within individual control rather than environmentally determined. The Global Burden of Disease Study (43) drew the line at simple aids that should in principle be available to all people (including simple crutches, non-powered wheelchairs, glasses, and standard hearing aids). This distinction relates also to the issue of the boundaries of good health that will be discussed in the following section. Improvements in domain capacity above a certain threshold are not seen as health improvements. Thus, for example, though a car improves mobility, it exceeds the mobility threshold above which improvements are no longer considered as health gains.

Having identified capacity with personal aids as the relevant construct, it is necessary to specify the normative external environment in which capacity is contextualized. Should the normative environment for assessment of capacity be a global standard, or should it vary across different regions or countries? For example, should the normative uniform environment for assessment of mobility include a global standard provision of ramps for wheelchairs, or should the standard for developed countries reflect the greater provision of ramps (so that the health improvement resulting from providing a wheelchair to a person with paraplegia would be greater in developed than in developing countries)? We would argue that a single global standard should be used for all health domains in the interests of comparability. Thus, in the vision domain, provision of an appropriate pair of glasses would result in the same health improvement in all settings, and would not depend on the average level of illumination at night in different countries.

THE BOUNDARIES OF GOOD HEALTH

Another issue that needs to be addressed in operationalizing a definition of health is whether all increments and decrements on a domain are understood as improvements and losses of health, respectively, or whether there is some threshold above which increments and decrements are not perceived as changes in a person's health state. For example, should one consider a person with an IQ of 180 as being healthier in the domain of intellectual functioning than another individual with an IQ of 150? Or should one say that the former is not necessarily healthier by virtue of a capacity that exceeds some norm for cognitive excellence? This is of relevance to the construction of measures of population health that are congruent with common notions of health and also common perceptions of the intrinsic value of health (for example, health may be perceived as a basic right or a human right, and societies as having some moral obligation to direct resources towards the improvement of health). We believe that the concept of a threshold for full health accords better with commonly held societal views of health than an allowance for unbounded improvements in domain capacities to be considered as improvements in health. The "supra-health" levels are perhaps better referred to as talent.

As used in the ICF, disability no longer refers to limitations of performance or capacity in a set of domains defined solely in terms of tasks or activities, but is an umbrella term also embracing impairments in domains of body functions and structures, and referring to decrements below some domain-specific norm. While we could specify separate cut-points on the domain scale for loss of health and for disability, there seems to be no compelling reason not to use the same cut-point and equate disability in a domain with less than full health in that domain (Figure 26.1). Because the ICF includes a larger set of health-related domains that go beyond direct domains of health, disability can refer to limitations of performance in either health domains or non-health domains in the ICF. Thus, a person could have disability (on non-health domains) but full health (by having no decrements on any health domain). The

converse, however, is not true: if a person has less than full health, then the person by definition also has disability.

Some have argued that the cut-point for full health can be identified purely in biological terms by examining the statistical distribution of functioning in the domain (*27*). Others have argued that the judgment of whether one individual is healthier than another can only be understood in terms of the ability to realize one's vital goals (*30*). It seems clear to us that the domain threshold for full health is a normative choice: there is no criterion that would allow us, *a priori*, to choose a particular point on the population distribution of domain capacity as representing the threshold for full health. Further, this normative choice should reflect common perceptions that health is both intrinsically valuable and instrumentally valuable to human beings. We therefore suggest that the identification of thresholds for domain capacity should be empirically-based and linked to health state valuations (see below). In intuitive terms, the threshold for a particular domain is the level of capacity below which people generally recognize decrements as departures from excellent health.

COMBINING DIMENSIONS IN HEALTH STATE VALUATIONS

We have thus far been discussing conceptualizations of levels within a single domain of health. More complicated conceptually is the problem of comparing overall health levels associated with multidimensional health states. If we imagine that an individual's health may be described in terms of a vector of levels on the numerous domains that constitute health, we refer to overall judgments about the health level associated with this health state as *health state valuations*. Health state valuations are measured on a cardinal scale that ranges from zero (for a state equivalent to death) to unity (for a state of ideal health). The mapping between multiple domains of health and health state valuations reflects the relative weights that individuals place on different domains of health, which may include complex interactions between levels on various domains.

By assigning a single number to an individual's health state in reference to ideal health, health state valuations allow aggregation of individual health levels over time and comparisons of health across individuals, and provide the critical link that allows the non-fatal health experience of individuals to be combined with information on mortality in summary measures of population health (*8*). These weights for-

Figure 26.1   Health and disability in a single health
                 domain

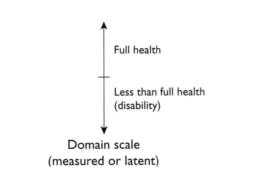

Full health

Less than full health
(disability)

Domain scale
(measured or latent)

malize the intuitive notions that health levels lie on a continuum and that we may characterize an individual as being more or less healthy than another at a particular moment in time. Health state valuations quantify departures from perfect health, i.e. the reductions in health associated with particular health states. It is important to emphasize that these weights *do not* measure the quality of life of people with disabilities and *do not* measure the value of persons to society.

In fact, there have been a variety of different conceptual interpretations of health state valuations for use in different applications, which has led to considerable confusion in defining the basis for measuring and understanding these valuations, and health itself. It is useful for us to contrast our conceptual definition of health state valuations with these other concepts.

Utility

Some health economists have explicitly defined health state valuations as measurements of the utility associated with health states (44;45). As Richardson (46) and others have noted, however, utility has been defined somewhat circularly as the quantity that is maximized when individuals make choices that obey the axioms of expected utility theory, which offer a set of principles relating to preferences under uncertainty. The use of the standard gamble technique for elicitation of valuations is linked to the axiomatic foundations of expected utility theory, but it is well appreciated that the standard gamble invokes both assessments of health levels associated with different states as well as attitudes towards risk and uncertainty (46;47). The notion of utility in the context of health state valuations, therefore, conflates our concept of health with the separate concept of risk aversion, which we do not believe is relevant for characterizations of health levels in measures of individual or population health (9). It is reasonable to assume that health state utility, as measured through the standard gamble, is related monotonically to the level of health (48), but responses to the standard gamble cannot be interpreted directly as quantifications of health levels.

Quality of Life, Well-being and Health-related Quality of Life

The term quality of life (QoL) has been used widely in various social science contexts to refer to the overall, subjective appraisals of happiness or satisfaction experienced by individuals (49). In this sense, it is a subjective notion, something "felt" or experienced, and should thus probably be distinguished from "goodness" or utility.

In health, the term QoL often has been used in a more particular way to refer to a multidimensional construct relating to symptoms, impairments, functional status, emotional states, and what we have labelled as health domains (50;51). This use of QoL is clearly inconsistent with the general use of the term, so health researchers have taken to referring to this construct as "health-related QoL" (HRQoL). To the extent that an individual's HRQoL is conceived of as a vector of levels on "health-related" dimensions of life, it is similar to our conceptual framework for measuring health, albeit with less precisely articulated boundaries. There is considerable confusion in the HRQoL literature, however, regarding the actual meaning of this construct. The most common understanding of HRQoL equates it to "subjective [health-related] well-being" in contrast to objective "health status" (52;53). The HRQoL literature abounds with statements that two people with the same "health status" may have quite different health-related quality of life.

Where HRQoL is viewed as a summary measure of the contribution of an individual's health to his or her overall well-being, rather than as a multidimensional descriptive measure, conceptual problems emerge from the fact that well-being is not clearly separable into independent health and non-health components, as Broome has convincingly argued (54). In other words, when we compare the well-being or "quality of life" of individuals with different health levels, these relative comparisons may change depending on their levels on non-health dimensions of well-being. Because well-being is not separable into a health and non-health component that are independent, a measurement strategy for HRQoL conceived in this way would require that all components of well-being be measured along with overall well-being (if that were possible) in order to determine empirically the causal relationships with levels on health domains given particular levels on non-health aspects of well-being.

Health Level

We avoid these difficulties if we consider a health state valuation to provide a scalar cardinal index of the overall level of health associated with a multidimensional health state, defined in terms of a set of numbers quantifying capacity on each domain scale (e.g. level of mobility, level of self-care, level of affect, level of pain, and level of cognition). In this conceptualization, health state valuations pertain strictly to the components of health, not to broader sets of components of well-being, or the contribution of health to well-being, or the felt sensation or satisfaction associated with a particular state of health.

Unlike the notion of utility, we do not believe that it is necessary to define this construct explicitly in terms of choices or preferences. Almost everybody can agree that a person with one amputated leg is healthier than a person with two amputated legs, all else being equal, without resorting at all to either the language of choice or to statements about the overall well-being of either person. While this is a simple case of a dominance ordering (because the difference is in the level of only one domain), the same intuitive notions apply to more complicated examples: if we say that somebody with a mild sore throat is, *ceteris paribus*, healthier than somebody with two broken arms, perhaps not everybody would agree, but most everybody can at least understand our statement through some common-sense notion of health. Indeed, this common-sense notion extends beyond ordinal comparisons, for example, allowing us to say that going from perfect vision to myopia is a smaller change in health than going from myopia to quadriplegia. In all of these cases, we submit that there is an intuitive understanding of the concept of *quantities of health* that is not based on the concept of choice.

It is important to distinguish between the tools that are used to elicit judgments about health levels and the conceptual definition of the construct itself. Although we will return to this question below in our discussion of measurement issues relating to the elicitation of health state valuations, we introduce an example of this distinction here. One of the common elicitation techniques used in survey research on health state valuations is the *time trade-off*, which asks individuals to choose between different hypothetical scenarios that involve choices between improved health levels and reduced longevity (55). On the face of it, this technique appears to parallel closely the notion of summary health measures that are based on equivalence between length of life and levels of health. The similarity of the framing, however, does not imply that an individual's *preferences* over different combinations of health levels and longevity are the actual phenomena of interest, which we can illustrate with an example. Imagine that we ask survey respondents whether they would be willing to give up any time at the end of their lives in order to avoid living with a mild hearing impairment. Some respondents may be unwilling to sacrifice any longevity to avoid this minor health problem, even though they acknowledge that the state of

having a mild hearing impairment represents a lower level of health than a state with no hearing impairment, all else being equal (indeed, empirical research confirms this finding; see, for example, Robinson et al. (56)). In this case, it is the judgment that the hearing impairment represents a decrement from perfect health that interests us, not the preferences that result from the combination of this judgment with numerous other considerations. In other words, the preferences that we may infer from techniques such as the time trade-off are likely to depend, at least in part, on assessments of health levels, but they may also reflect a range of other values and considerations that are distinct from the measurement of health levels.

MEASUREMENT ISSUES

Having defined a conceptual framework for quantifying the health of individuals or populations, it is necessary to develop a valid, reliable, and comparable way to operationalize the measurement of health. This requires the enumeration of a set of core domains that are necessary and sufficient to describe health states for measurement purposes; methods to measure levels of capacity on each of these domains; and methods for eliciting judgments about overall health levels associated with different multidimensional states, or aggregating across capacity levels on multiple domains.

WHICH DOMAINS TO MEASURE

During the last three decades, there has been general acceptance of an approach to describing health states of individuals in terms of multiple domains of health, and in developing self-report instruments that seek information on each of these domains. Existing health state measurement instruments have differed considerably in their content, however, in an attempt to arrive at a set of domains that covers the universe of health adequately. They have often combined domains of physiological function with other domains of well-being.

The first standardized health state measurement instruments generally focused on capturing the most severe states, particularly among older age groups and individuals living in long-term care institutions. Measures such as the Activities of Daily Living (ADLs) emphasized performance in different areas, for example eating; getting in and out of bed; getting around in the home; and dressing, bathing or using the toilet (57). The levels of performance in these areas were considered to be proximate descriptions of the severity of health states in terms of the level of assistance required by persons in these states.

These early instruments were enlarged to apply to a broader group of individuals and included questions covering Instrumental Activities of Daily Living (IADLs), such as heavy housework; light housework; laundry; shopping for groceries; getting around outside the home; travelling; managing money; taking medicine; and telephoning (58). Typically, ADL questions are relevant to the most severe health states because of their focus on basic physical and cognitive functions, while IADL questions provide more sensitive discrimination at less severe levels of health. However, as IADL questions are based on normative roles and activities, the responses are more prone to cultural and gender biases, both within and across populations. As a result, IADL questions may not all be applicable to everyone within populations. For example, in a survey of the elderly in four Western Pacific countries, the IADL question "can you prepare your own meals," was only asked to women (59).

The second wave of health state measurement instruments was developed with clinical and general populations in mind, and combined self-assessments on different dimensions of health and performance in different activities and roles (50;51;60;61). Standardized general health state profiles that have been used internationally by multiple research groups include the Quality of Well-Being Scale (62); the McMaster Health Index (63); the Sickness Impact Profile (64); the Nottingham Health Profile (65); the Health Utilities Index Mark 3 (66); EuroQol EQ-5D (67); Short-Form 36 Health Survey (68); the WHO Quality of Life (WHOQOL-BREF) Assessment Instrument (69); and the WHO Disability Assessment Schedule-II or WHODAS-II (70).

Additional health state descriptive instruments that have been used within primary health settings include the Quality of Life Index (71); the Functional Status Questionnaire (72); COOP Charts for Primary Care Practice (73); and the Duke Health Profile (74). Disease-specific measures are more often used in clinical trials or with individuals receiving specialized treatments.

The challenge for standardizing health state descriptions is to include all domains considered to be important in terms of societal health goals and in terms of health state valuations. The set of domains used for measurement must be as exhaustive as possible within the practical constraints of data collection mechanisms, as well as generally acceptable as capturing the content of the ordinary meaning of health. At the same time, to reduce respondent burden, we must identify a parsimonious set of domains of health that minimize overlap or redundancy, which occurs if the measured level on one domain can be largely explained by measurement of one or more other domains.

We may distinguish three categories of domains that can be considered in the design of a health state descriptive system (Figure 26.2):

■ core domains of health that almost all people agree upon as important to the direct measurement of health (common examples shown in bold),

■ domains of health that most people agree are direct measures of health, but that might not provide substantial information additional to the core domains, and

■ other domains that are not strictly components of health but serve as good proximate measures of the experience of health (labelled as indirect measures of health).

In outlining a conceptual definition of health, we emphasized the distinction between health and the consequences or impacts of a state of health on the well-being or other aspects of the life of an individual, especially if these are mediated through the physical or social environment. While this distinction is critical for conceptual clarity, we note that in some instances the best or only *measurable* phenomena pertaining to levels on some domains may in fact be consequences that are outside the realm of health, a consideration that needs to be kept in mind when operationalizing domains of health. Thus, amongst the domains listed in Figure 26.2, some of the domains labelled as indi-

Figure 26.2 Domains of health

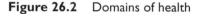

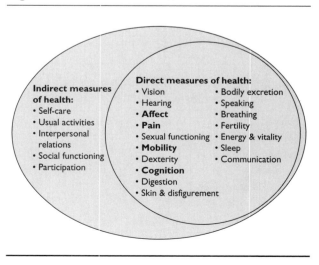

rect measures of health, while not strictly defined as its components, may serve as useful proxy indicators of health in a parsimonious measurement instrument.

Sadana (75) has reviewed the domains included in the commonly used standardized health status assessment instruments, and WHO has undertaken a survey development programme to establish a core set of generic domains to describe health states (6). Although most previous health measurement efforts have been led by researchers in North America and Europe, WHO has collaborated with groups throughout the world to develop a generic health measurement module with broad applicability. Selection of domains has been guided by the following key criteria:

■ valid in terms of intuitive, clinical, and epidemiological concepts of health,

■ linked to the conceptual framework of the ICF,

■ amenable to self report, observation, or direct measurement,

■ comprehensive enough to capture the most important aspects of health states that people value, and

■ cross-population comparable.

Although there may be a large level of agreement on many of the core health domains included in a measurement instrument, we acknowledge that any selected subset of domains will be contested by some. Affect, cognition, mobility, pain, and self-care have been included in almost all generic measures of health states. These domains served as the starting point for development of the health measurement module in the WHO Household Survey programme. The current health state descriptive module in the ongoing World Health Survey (Box 26.1) is the product of several iterations of instrument development based on empirical data collection and analysis, but we rec-

---

Box 26.1	Domains of health in the World Health Survey, 2002–2003

Mobility

Self-care

Pain and discomfort

Cognition

Interpersonal activities

Vision

Sleep and energy

Affect

---

ognize that the choice of domains and items used to measure capacity on these domains may continue to evolve over time.

Given the choice of a set of domains for measurement, simple summary graphs may be used to describe levels on these multiple dimensions in different populations. For example, Figure 26.3 presents findings from the first round of the WHO Household Survey programme for six health domains in selected countries and surveys (76).

MEASURING PERFORMANCE OR CAPACITY

Ideally, it would be made explicit in the measurement process whether the quantity of interest is capacity or performance. We have argued above that the relevant construct should be capacity with available personal aids. As an example of the operationalization of this construct, the World Health Survey health measurement module includes the following questions for the domain of vision:

Q2070. Do you wear glasses or contact lenses? (If respondent says YES to this question, preface the next two questions with "Please answer the following questions taking into account your glasses or contact lenses.")

Q2071. In the last 30 days, how much difficulty did you have in seeing and recognizing a person you know across the road (i.e. from a distance of about 20 meters)? (None/Mild/Moderate/Severe/Extreme or cannot do)

Q2072. In the last 30 days, how much difficulty did you have in seeing and recognizing an object at arm's length or in reading? (None/Mild/Moderate/Severe/Extreme or cannot do)

In practice, there may be a high degree of correlation between performance and capacity on some domains, and it may not always be necessary to make these subtle distinctions in self-report questions. For domains comprised of more complex tasks, such as usual activities and self care, it may be more practical to measure performance rather than capacity with or without usual aids.

TOWARDS CROSS-POPULATION COMPARABILITY

Because the most widely collected data relating to health domain levels are categorical self-reported data, the fundamental challenge of cross-population comparability emerges from differences in the way different individuals use categorical response scales. Efforts to

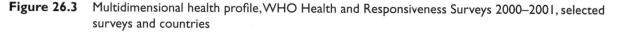

Figure 26.3   Multidimensional health profile, WHO Health and Responsiveness Surveys 2000–2001, selected surveys and countries

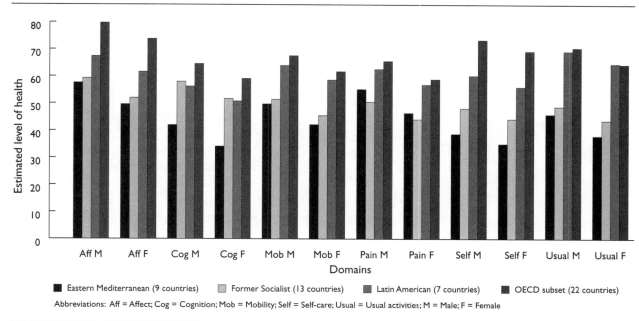

Abbreviations: Aff = Affect; Cog = Cognition; Mob = Mobility; Self = Self-care; Usual = Usual activities; M = Male; F = Female

ensure linguistic equivalence of questions across different settings may improve the psychometric properties of these questions in terms of traditional criteria such as reliability and within-population validity, but they will not resolve problems stemming from non-comparability in the interpretation and use of response categories. There has been great progress over the past three decades in developing health status measurement instruments that are reliable and demonstrate within-population validity (*63–68*). Even with these advances, however, results obtained using these instruments often are not comparable across populations (*77*), or across different socioeconomic subgroups within populations (*78*). Thus, cross-population comparability represents a more stringent criterion for evaluation of measurement instruments, beyond the traditional concepts of reliability and validity. The difference between comparability on the one hand and validity and reliability on the other can be illustrated with two thermometers, one of which is Celsius, the other Fahrenheit. Both thermometers give valid and reliable measurements of temperature. However, 26 degrees on one thermometer is not comparable to 26 degrees on the other. Comparability is fundamental to the use of survey results for development of evidence for health policy but has been under-emphasized in instrument development.

Empirical examples suggesting that self-reported categorical data on health lack cross-population comparability abound (*79*). A number of different studies have pointed to likely differences in the use of response categories on self-reported assessments of general health, morbidity, or levels on particular domains of health. For example, in Australian national health surveys comparing the self-reported health status of Aboriginals with that of the general population, only around 12% of the Aboriginal population characterized their own health status as fair or poor, while more than 20% of the general population rated their health in these low categories. By any other major indicator of mortality and morbidity, the Aboriginal population fares much worse than the general population, which suggests that there may be important differences in the interpretation of categorical responses in the different subpopulations due to shifts in response category cut-points (*80*). Similarly, residents of the state of Kerala in India—which has the lowest rates of infant and child mortality and the highest rates of literacy in India—consistently report the highest incidences of morbidity in the country (*81;82*).

The problem of comparability can be conceptualized in terms of response category cut-point shifts across populations, across subgroups within a population, or within the same population over time. Figure 26.4 illustrates the primary challenge of

Figure 26.4 Latent variable for a health domain: an illustration for mobility

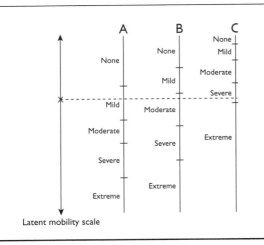

Latent mobility scale

using self-reported levels on a health status domain (even when reliability and within-population validity have been well established). For each domain, there is some true or latent scale for it that is, by definition, unobserved (column 1 in Figure 26.4). Imagining a self-reported survey question that asks respondents how much difficulty they have walking up stairs and offers five response categories ("no difficulty," "mild difficulty," "moderate difficulty," "severe difficulty," and "extreme/cannot do"), we can represent response patterns in different populations in terms of the location of response category cut-points, which are levels of mobility at which an individual will shift from one response category to another. The lowest cut-point in the figure shows the transition from answering "extreme/cannot do" to "severe difficulty." In population B, the response category cut-points are shifted relative to those in population A so that a higher level of mobility is associated with each of the response categories. Population C shows a third example with even further shift in the cut-points. The implication is dramatic. The same level on the latent mobility scale would be characterized as "mild difficulty" in population A, "moderate difficulty" in population B, and "severe difficulty" in population C. In this example, survey results may be reliable and valid within each population, but they cannot be compared across populations without adjustment.

We can hypothesize that cut-points may vary between populations because of different expectations for domains of health. They are likely to vary both within and between cultural groups. The cut-points for older individuals may shift as their expectations for a domain diminish with age. Men may be more likely to

deny declines in health so that their cut-points may be systematically shifted as compared to women. Contact with health services may influence expectations for a domain and thus shift cut-points (*81;83–86*). Response category cut-point shift can make crude comparisons of results across populations nearly meaningless, even when exactly the same questions are used, as illustrated by some of the examples already provided.

Strategies for enhancing the comparability of self-reported health measures demand the augmentation of both existing instruments for data collection and existing statistical models for data analysis (*79*). Standard statistical models for ordinal data, such as the ordered probit model, cannot allow for variation in response category cut-points. Adaptations of these standard models to incorporate systematic cut-point shifts in relation to some defined set of covariates, such as country, age, sex, and education, have been described elsewhere (*7;87*). Anchoring vignettes have been developed as a new component of survey instruments used in conjunction with the new statistical models to position self-reported responses on a common, interpersonally comparable scale (*88*). An anchoring vignette is a description of a concrete level on a given health domain that respondents are asked to evaluate with the same questions and response scales applied to self-assessments on that domain. Vignettes fix the level of ability on a domain so that variation in categorical responses is attributable to variation in response category cut-points. The key objective underlying the anchoring vignette strategy is to elicit responses from subjects for hypothetical levels on a given domain that reflect individual norms and expectations for health in approximately the same way that the self-ratings do for the subjects' own health levels.

The anchoring vignette approach to improving cross-population comparability of self-reported health survey data has been implemented in the WHO Multi-country Survey Study through 71 surveys in collaboration with 61 Member States (*6*). Findings from these surveys provide clear evidence that self-report health data are not comparable without adjusting for such biases (*76*). These new data, together with comprehensive analyses of epidemiological data for all regions of the world, and new life tables for all WHO Member States, have enabled us to calculate healthy life expectancy for 191 countries for the year 2000 in a way that is comparable across countries (*10*).

Measurement Issues Regarding Health State Valuations

The two primary measurement challenges relating to health state valuations concern 1) developing methods for eliciting numerical assessments of overall health levels associated with multidimensional states that have meaningful interval-scale properties; and 2) understanding valuation functions, which formalize the mapping between levels on multiple domains of health and overall health state valuations.

Above, we described a conceptual basis for health state valuations that is not framed in terms of choice or preferences. While not necessary for the conceptualization of health state valuations, preferences nevertheless often provide a convenient way to elicit information on these valuations. Choice-based elicitation techniques, such as the standard gamble and time trade-off methods, allow inference about levels of health by having respondents weigh changes in these levels against other quantities, e.g. mortality risks or length of life (47;55;89). There are two major drawbacks to the use of these methods, however. Firstly, these techniques have been designed to be implemented among highly educated respondents, as they rely on abstract and cognitively demanding thought experiments. A more feasible valuation tool for respondents across a wide range of levels of educational attainment is the simpler visual analogue scale (VAS), which has been implemented in diverse cultural settings, including India, Tanzania, Colombia, Cambodia, and the Philippines, and has been demonstrated to have higher reliability than other methods (90;91). Secondly, none of the elicitation methods offers a direct measure of the quantity of interest (overall health level), because responses on each method are also influenced by other considerations such as risk aversion (in the standard gamble), time preference and threshold effects (in the time trade-off), and distributional concerns (in the person trade-off) (48).

Based on these two sets of concerns, data collection on health state valuations in the WHO household survey programme has been based on a two-tiered strategy. Because the visual analogue scale appears to be most feasible for use in community-based surveys, the 10 large sample surveys that included a health state valuation module elicited valuations for a range of health states using this technique. Based on long-standing results from both psychophysics and psychometrics, however, it is necessary to rescale valuation results obtained through visual analogue scales in order to obtain interval-scaled valuations for construction of summary measures. This rescaling should be empirically-based and therefore requires a second avenue of data collection using deliberative protocols based on multiple states and multiple valuation methods. Using an analytical approach described elsewhere (48), responses from multiple elicitation methods may be used to model the way that underlying core values inform all of the different methods, by explicitly accounting for the other unrelated values (risk aversion, etc.) that inform method-specific responses. The relationship between visual analogue scale values and these estimated core values can then be used to adjust VAS responses for scale distortions. This approach has been implemented in the WHO survey programme in groups with higher levels of educational attainment.

The second major measurement challenge regarding health state valuations is the derivation of mapping functions that capture the relationship between a set of domain scores describing a particular health state and the overall valuation of that state. These *valuation functions* reflect the relative weights individuals place on different domains in arriving at summary judgments about the level of health associated with a multidimensional state. It is worth noting that the characterization of the valuation function as a weighting function does not limit consideration to strictly linear functions. In fact, the function may include a complex structure of interactions between different domains. Because there are no compelling normative arguments to guide us on the relative importance of various health domains to overall levels of health (is a certain level of pain more important than a certain level of mobility?), it is recommended that valuation functions be derived empirically.

Estimated valuation functions are useful in predicting health state valuations where only domain-specific scores are available and in ensuring comparability in the health state values assigned to different individuals who have identical levels on all domains. The latter objective is one argument for using a common global valuation function applied in every setting, although there is also interest in understanding the extent to which valuation functions vary across countries or subnational population groups. Despite assertion by some commentators that there is extreme heterogeneity of valuations for given health states, empirical evidence suggests otherwise. Valuation studies carried out with deliberative small groups from a wide range of different countries have found surprising consistency in valuations across cultures (92). More recently, valuation studies carried out as part of the WHO Multicountry Survey Study (6) also have found remarkable consistency in health state valuations. This result is not, perhaps, a major surprise, given the fundamental importance of the core health domains to all human beings, irrespective of their social or socioeconomic circumstances. It is possible that there may be more heterogeneity in values around well-being outcomes than health outcomes, although there is little empirical basis for this supposition. Given the fundamental importance of the core health domains for the achievement of the goals that people commonly value, we believe that valuation of health states for summary measures of population health is not only meaningful, but operationally achievable. WHO will continue to pursue an ambitious range of health state valuation studies in representative population samples in diverse settings, in order to examine variation in valuations across and within countries.

DISCUSSION AND CONCLUSIONS

The conceptual framework for health outlined here supports the consensus view that health is more than a matter of the absence of specific disease or injury. It is also the presence of certain threshold levels of ability to carry out physical and mental actions and tasks. In summary,

- *Health* is an attribute of individuals, which is best operationalized as a multidimensional set of domains.

- To obtain meaningful information on health and health interventions, the *boundaries and scope* of health must be defined by identifying a set of core domains of health.

- The *threshold* for loss of health in any given domain reflects societal norms or standards.

- Health state description and measurement must be distinguished from 1) subjective evaluations of health; 2) consequences of health states; and 3) environmental impacts on health and other proximate or distal determinants of health.

In keeping with the above conclusions, we propose that for measurement purposes, health be understood as a multidimensional phenomenon that can be sufficiently described by a core set of health domains, each characterized by a single cardinal scale of capacity (measured or latent, and including currently available personal aids). The overall level of health associated with the set of abilities (or capacities) on the core health domains may be characterized by a cardinal

scale of health state valuations. These valuations quantify level of health, not quality of life, well-being, or utility.

People with the same health, defined in this way, may experience considerable differences in total well-being primarily due to differences in other determinants of well-being (including social, economic, environmental and individual factors), as well as the interaction of their health with other individual or environmental determinants of well-being. We thus distinguish between health itself and the consequences or impacts of a state of health on the well-being or other aspects of the life of an individual, especially if these are mediated through the physical or social environment. For example, an individual, because of cognitive impairments, may be socially isolated, with few friends or other interpersonal relationships. Although the various mental functions required to acquire and maintain relationships are components of health, the lack of relationships is a well-being consequence of a health state, not a loss of health *per se*.

Some may argue that health should be understood solely in terms of a person's perception or reported experience. While some domains of health, such as pain, certainly require subjective assessment, this does not mean that response categories to self-report questions should be assumed to be comparable across population groups (so that self-reported "mild pain" is assumed to refer to the same health state in all population groups). The WHO Household Survey Study has provided clear evidence of cut-point shifts for such response categories across populations, even within countries at similar levels of development. The survey evidence shows that people in more developed countries tend to use more severe labels to describe the same level of capacity in a health domain (76). Similarly, comparisons of self-report data for domains amenable to observation or direct measurement have shown that perceptions may vary widely for a given health state (78). Thus, while we may depend on individuals to describe the experiences of a particular health state on certain key domains, the interest of comparability demands that raw self-reported health ratings be mapped onto a common scale, for example through the anchoring vignette approach we have described.

Reidpath et al. (93) have argued that health state valuations as used in the Global Burden of Disease Study do not appropriately take into account differences in well-being resulting from the social, economic, and environmental context. It should be clear from our discussion above that those contextual aspects which result in lower capacities in health domains (for example, if paraplegics in developing countries experience more pain due to inadequate pain control than those in developing countries) will be reflected in lower overall health state valuations. On the other hand, contextual factors which result solely in worse experience in non-health domains of well-being would not imply lower overall health state valuations, which we believe is appropriate.

Our focus on cardinal scales of capacity in each health domain may be misperceived as taking a "medical model" approach to the conceptualization of health by restricting attention to "loss of health" rather than positive aspects of health. In fact the cardinal scale for a health domain has no intrinsic directionality—higher values are associated with better health and lower values with lesser health, and these relationships are symmetric. The existence of a normative threshold above which all levels of domain capacity represent full health is an empirical question which we have argued may be addressed through health state valuation studies.

There may also be concern that the exclusion of health determinants from our conceptualization of health will direct people's attention to treatment interventions rather than primary prevention interventions, and to pathology rather than broader social and environmental determinants. Given that our definition of health focuses explicitly on the domains of health rather than its determinants, whether distal risk factors such as cholesterol and blood pressure or proximal determinants such as disease and injury, it does not privilege interventions that act at any particular level of the causal web. The relationship of both classes of determinants to health states is amenable to empirical study, as long as the measurement of the determinants is not incorporated into or confounded with the measurement of the health states.

With regard to measures of health on a set of multiple domains, besides the challenge of cross-population comparability, it is necessary to arrive at a parsimonious set that reflects the breadth of individual health. Initial results from WHO surveys suggest that besides the core domains of pain, affect, cognition, mobility, and self-care, additional domains such as vision, sleep and energy, and interpersonal activities may be sufficient to capture major variations in the health of individuals. Using these domains as the basis for descriptions of health states allows detailed data collection on key components of individual health and, in conjunction with empirical and analytical work on health state valuations, provides a basis for assigning numerical values to different health states. It is worth reiterating that this conceptualization of health is clearly narrower than the concept of well-being, but broader than a restrictive definition of health that concerns only the physiological and mental functioning of the naked individual.

With the WHO Household Survey Programme, WHO has measured health state valuations in a larger and more diverse group of people than in any previous study, and has assembled the largest available empirical evidence base on variations in health state valuations. This will enable a) quantification of the actual range of variation in health state valuations; and b) assessment of the impact of these variations on comparative judgements of levels of population health. Thus far, this work has indicated minimal cross-country differences, but we await further results from additional countries.

The development of multi-domain health state measurement instruments, together with statistical techniques to ensure the comparability of self-report data across populations, and the development of techniques to elicit health state valuations from the general population, will for the first time enable us to truly measure, and compare, the health of populations across the world. This is a key input to the public policy process as comparable measurement of population health levels creates possibilities of investigating broad determinants at national and cross-national level, and of assessing the achievements of health systems.

ACKNOWLEDGEMENTS

The authors gratefully acknowledge helpful discussions with Jerome Bickenbach, Dan Brock, John Broome, David B. Evans, Dan Hausman, Ajay Tandon and Dan Wikler, and support from the National Institute on Aging (P01-AG17625).

REFERENCES

(1) Murray CJL, Frenk J. A framework for assessing the performance of health systems. *Bulletin of the World Health Organization*, 2000, 78(6):717–731.

(2) World Health Organization. *The World Health Report 2000. Health Systems: Improving Performance.* Geneva, World Health Organization, 2000.

(3) World Health Organization. *The World Health Report 2001. Mental Health: New Understanding, New Hope.* Geneva, World Health Organization, 2001.

(4) Murray CJL et al. *The Global Burden of Disease 2000*

project: aims, methods and data sources. EIP Discussion Paper No. 36. Geneva, World Health Organization, 2001. URL: http://www3.who.int/whosis/discussion_papers/discussion_papers.cfm#

(5) World Health Organization. *Proposed strategies for health system performance assessment. Summary document.* Geneva, World Health Organization, 2002. URL: http://www.who.int/health-systems-performance/peer_review_docs/Final%20SPRG%205.pdf.

(6) Üstün TB et al. WHO Multi-country Survey Study on Health and Responsiveness 2000-2001. In: Murray CJL, Evans DB, eds. *Health systems performance assessment: debates, methods and empiricism.* Geneva, World Health Organization, 2003.

(7) Tandon A et al. Statistical models for enhancing cross-population comparability. In: Murray CJL, Evans DB, eds. *Health systems performance assessment: debates, methods and empiricism.* Geneva, World Health Organization, 2003.

(8) Murray CJL, Salomon JA, Mathers CD. A critical examination of summary measures of population health. *Bulletin of the World Health Organization,* 2000, 78(8): 981–994.

(9) Murray CJL, Salomon JA, Mathers CD. The individual basis for summary measures of population health. In: Murray CJL et al, eds. *Summary measures of population health: concepts, ethics, measurement and applications.* Geneva, World Health Organization, 2002:41–51.

(10) Mathers CD et al. Healthy life expectancy in 191 countries, 1999. *The Lancet,* 2001, 357(9269):1685–1691.

(11) Murray CJL, Acharya AK. Understanding DALYs (disability-adjusted life years). *Journal of Health Economics,* 1997, 16(6):703–730.

(12) Almeida C et al. Methodological concerns and recommendations on policy consequences of the World Health Report 2000. *The Lancet,* 2001, 357(9269): 1692–1697.

(13) Murray CJL, Frenk J. World Health Report 2000: a step towards evidence-based health policy. *The Lancet,* 2001, 357(9269):1698–1700.

(14) Navarro V. World Health Report 2000: responses to Murray and Frenk. *The Lancet,* 2001, 357(9269):1701–1702.

(15) Sigerist HE. *Medicine and human welfare.* New Haven, Yale University Press, 1941.

(16) World Health Organization. *Constitution.* Geneva, World Health Organization, 1948.

(17) World Health Organization. *Measurement of levels of health: report of a study group.* Technical report series No. 137. Geneva, World Health Organization, 1957.

(18) Breslow L. A quantitative approach to the World Health Organization definition of health: physical, mental and social well-being. *International Journal of Epidemiology,* 1972, 1(4):347–355.

(19) Chen MK, Bryant BE. The measurement of health—a critical and selective overview. *International Journal of Epidemiology,* 1975, 4(4):257–264.

(20) Moriyama IM. Problems in the measurement of health status. In: Sheldon EB, Moore WE, eds. *Indicators of social change: concepts and measurements.* New York, Russell Sage Foundation, 1968.

(21) Hansluwka HE. Measuring the health of populations: indicators and interpretations. *Social Science & Medicine,* 1985, 20(12):1207–1224.

(22) Mechanic D. Health and illness in technological societies. *Studies/Hastings Center,* 1973, 1(3):7–18.

(23) Zola IK. In the name of health and illness: on some socio-political consequences of medical influence. *Social Science & Medicine,* 1975, 9(2):83–87.

(24) Crawford R. Healthism and the medicalization of everyday life. *International Journal of Health Services,* 1980, 10(3):365–388.

(25) Mishler EG. Viewpoint: critical perspectives on the biomedical model. In: Mishler EG, ed. *Social contexts of health, illness, and patient care.* Cambridge, Cambridge University Press, 1981.

(26) Callahan D. The WHO definition of "health." In: Beauchamp TL, Walters L, eds. *Contemporary issues in bioethics,* 2nd ed. Belmont, Wadsworth, 1982.

(27) Boorse C. Health as a theoretical concept. *Philosophy of Science,* 1977, 44:542–573.

(28) Ladd J. The concepts of health and disease and their ethical implications. In: Gruzalski B, Nelson C, eds. *Value conflicts in health care delivery.* Cambridge, Ballinger Publishing, 1982.

(29) Wachbroit R. Health and disease, concepts of. *Encyclopedia of Applied Ethics,* 1998, 533–538.

(30) Nordenfelt L. *On the nature of health: an action-theoretic approach.* Dordrecht, Reidel, 1987.

(31) Guttmacher S. Whole in body, mind & spirit: holistic health and the limits of medicine. *Hastings Center Report,* 1979, 9(2):16–21.

(32) Jones K, Moon G. *Health, disease and society.* London, Routledge and Kegan Paul, 1987.

(33) Helman C. *Culture, health, and illness,* 2nd ed. London, Wright, 1990.

(34) Brock DW. The separability of health and well-being. In: Murray CJL et al., eds. *Summary measures of population health: concepts, ethics, measurement and applications.* Geneva, World Health Organization, 2002:115–120.

(35) Doyle L, Gough I. *A theory of human need.* London, Macmillan, 1991.

(36) Bok S. *Common values.* Columbia, University of Missouri Press, 1996.

(37) Deutsch E. *Introduction to world philosophies.* Upper Saddle River, Prentice-Hall, 1997.

(38) Scharfstein BA. *A comparative history of world philosophy from the Upanishads to Kant.* Albany, State University of New York Press, 1998.

(39) Dasgupta P. *An inquiry into well-being and destitution.* Oxford, Clarendon Press, 1993.

(40) World Health Organization. *International Classification of Diseases and Related Health Problems —Tenth Revision (ICD 10).* Geneva, World Health Organization, 1992.

(41) World Health Organization. *International Classification of Impairments, Disabilities, and Handicaps.* Reprint 1993. Geneva, World Health Organization, 1980.

(42) World Health Organization. *International Classification of Functioning, Disability and Health (ICF).* Geneva, World Health Organization, 2001.

(43) Murray CJL, Lopez AD, eds. *The global burden of disease: a comprehensive assessment of mortality and disability from diseases, injuries, and risk factors in 1990 and projected to 2020.* Cambridge, Harvard University Press, 1996.

(44) Torrance GW. Toward a utility theory foundation for health status index models. *Health Services Research,* 1976, 11(4):349–369.

(45) Torrance GW et al. Multiattribute utility function for a comprehensive health status classification system. Health Utilities Index Mark 2. *Medical Care,* 1996, 34(7):702–722.

(46) Richardson J. Cost utility analysis: what should be measured? *Social Science & Medicine,* 1994, 39(1):7–21.

(47) Froberg DG, Kane RL. Methodology for measuring health-state preferences—II: scaling methods. *Journal of Clinical Epidemiology,* 1989, 42(5):459–471.

(48) Salomon JA, Murray CJL. A multi-method approach to measuring health state valuations. *Health Economics,* 2003 (forthcoming).

(49) Gill TM, Feinstein AR. A critical appraisal of the quality of quality-of-life measurements. *The Journal of the American Medical Association,* 1994, 272(8): 619–626.

(50) Patrick DL, Erickson P. Concepts of health-related quality of life. In: Patrick DL, Erickson P, eds. *Health status and health policy quality of life in health care evaluation and resource allocation.* New York, Oxford University Press, 1993:76–112.

(51) McDowell I, Newell C. *Measuring health: a guide to rating scales and questionnaires,* 2nd ed. New York, Oxford University Press, 1996.

(52) Gold MR et al. *Cost-effectiveness in health and medicine.* New York, Oxford University Press, 1996.

(53) Testa MA, Simonson DC. Assessment of quality-of-life outcomes. *New England Journal of Medicine,* 1996, 334:835–840.

(54) Broome J. Measuring the burden of disease by aggregating well-being. In: Murray CJL et al., eds. *Summary measures of population health: concepts, ethics, measurement and applications.* Geneva, World Health Organization, 2002: 91–113.

(55) Torrance GW. Measurement of health state utilities for economic appraisal. *Journal of Health Economics,* 1986, 5(1):1–30.

(56) Robinson A, Dolan P, Williams A. Valuing health status using VAS and TTO: what lies behind the numbers? *Social Science & Medicine,* 1997, 45(8):1289–1297.

(57) Katz S et al. Studies of illness in the aged. The index of ADL: a standardized measure of biological and psychosocial function. *The Journal of the American Medical Association,* 1963, 185:914–919.

(58) Lawton MP, Brody EM. Assessment of older people: self-maintaining and instrumental activities of daily living. *Gerontologist,* 1969, 9(3):179–186.

(59) Andrews GR et al. *Aging in the Western Pacific.* Manila, Philippines, World Health Organization Regional Office for the Western Pacific, 1986.

(60) Bowling A. *Measuring health: a review of quality of life measurement scales.* Buckingham, Open University Press, 1991.

(61) Bowling A. *Measuring disease: a review of disease specific quality of life measurement scales.* Buckingham, Open University Press, 1995.

(62) Fanshel S, Bush JW. A health-status index and its application to health services outcomes. *Operations Research,* 1970, 18(6):1021–1065.

(63) Chambers LW et al. Development and application of an index of social function. *Health Services Research,* 1976, 11(4):430–441.

(64) Bergner M et al. The sickness impact profile: conceptual formulation and methodology for the development of a health status measure. *International Journal of Health Services,* 1976, 6(3):393–415.

(65) Hunt SM et al. The Nottingham Health Profile: subjective health status and medical consultations. *Social Science & Medicine,* 1981, 15:221–229.

(66) Feeny D et al. Multi-attribute health status classification systems: health utilities index. *PharmacoEconomics,* 1995, 7(6):490–502.

(67) Brooks R. EuroQol: the current state of play. *Health Policy*, 1996, 37(1):53–72.

(68) Ware JE et al. *SF-36 health survey manual and interpretation guide.* Boston, Nimrod Press, The Health Institute, New England Medical Center, 1993.

(69) WHOQOL Group. The World Health Organization quality of life assessment: development and general psychometric properties. *Social Science & Medicine*, 1998, 46(12):1569–1585.

(70) World Health Organization. *Disability assessment schedule, version 3.1a (WHODAS-II).* Geneva, World Health Organization, 1999.

(71) Spitzer WO et al. Measuring the quality of life of cancer patients: a concise QL-Index for use by physicians. *Journal of Chronic Diseases*, 1981, 34(12):585–597.

(72) Jette AM et al. The functional status questionnaire: reliability and validity when used in primary care. *Journal of General Internal Medicine*, 1986, 1(3):143–149.

(73) Nelson EC et al. Assessment of function in routine clinical practice: description of the COOP chart method and preliminary findings. *Journal of Chronic Diseases*, 1987, 40(Suppl. 1):S55–S63.

(74) Parkerson JGR, Broadhead WE, Tse CK. The Duke health profile: a 17 item measure of health and dysfunction. *Medical Care*, 1990, 28(11):1056–1072.

(75) Sadana R. Development of standardized health state descriptions. In: Murray CJL et al, eds. *Summary measures of population health: concepts, ethics, measurement and applications.* Geneva, World Health Organization, 2002:315–328.

(76) Sadana R et al. *Describing population health in six domains: comparable results from 66 household surveys.* EIP Discussion Paper No. 43. Geneva, World Health Organization, 2002. URL: http://www3.who.int/whosis/discussion_papers/discussion_papers.cfm#

(77) Sadana R et al. Comparative analyses of more than 50 household surveys on health status. In: Murray CJL et al, eds. *Summary measures of population health: concepts, ethics, measurement and applications.* Geneva, World Health Organization, 2002:369–386.

(78) Iburg KM et al. Cross-population comparability of physician-assessed and self-reported measures of health. In: Murray CJL et al, eds. *Summary measures of population health: concepts, ethics, measurement and applications.* Geneva, World Health Organization, 2002:433–448.

(79) Murray CJL et al. Cross-population comparability of evidence for health policy. In: Murray CJL, Evans DB, eds. *Health systems performance assessment: debates, methods and empiricism.* Geneva, World Health Organization, 2003.

(80) Mathers CD, Douglas RM. Measuring progress in population health and well-being. In: Eckersley R, ed. *Measuring progress: is life getting better.* Collingwood, Victoria, CSIRO Publishing, 1998:125–155.

(81) Murray CJL, Chen LC. Understanding morbidity change. *Population and Development Review*, 1992, 18(3):481–503.

(82) Sen A. Health: perception versus observation. *British Medical Journal*, 2002, 324(7342):860–861.

(83) Caldwell J, Caldwell P. What have we learnt about the cultural, social and behavioral determinants of health? From selected readings to the first health transition workshop. *Health Transition Review*, 1991, 1(1):3–20.

(84) Johansson SR. The health transition: the cultural inflation of morbidity during the decline of mortality. *Health Transition Review*, 1991, 1(1):39–68.

(85) Johansson SR. Measuring the cultural inflation of morbidity during the decline of mortality. *Health Transition Review*, 1992, 2(1):78–89.

(86) Riley JC. From a high mortality regime to a high morbidity regime: is culture everything in sickness? *Health Transition Review*, 1992, 2(1):71–78.

(87) King G et al. Enhancing the validity and cross-cultural comparability of measurement in survey research. *American Political Science Review*, 2003 (forthcoming).

(88) Salomon JA, Tandon A, Murray CJL. *Using vignettes to improve cross-population comparability of health surveys: concepts, design, and evaluation techniques.* EIP Discussion Paper No. 41. Geneva, World Health Organization, 2001. URL: http://www3.who.int/whosis/discussion_papers/discussion_papers.cfm#

(89) Krabbe PFM, Essink-Bot M, Bonsel GJ. The comparability and reliability of five health-state valuation methods. *Social Science & Medicine*, 1996, 45:1641–1652.

(90) Shibuya K. *Quantifying the economic impact and health consequences of disease: implications for the studies on smoking* [Doctoral Thesis]. Boston, Harvard School of Public Health, 1999.

(91) Sadana R. Measurement of variance in health state valuations in a Phnom Penh, Cambodia. In: Murray CJL et al. eds. *Summary measures of population health: concepts, ethics, measurement and applications.* Geneva, World Health Organization, 2002:593–618.

(92) Murray CJL, Lopez AD. Progress and directions in refining the global burden of disease approach: a response to Williams. *Health Economics*, 2000, 9(1):69–82.

(93) Reidpath DD et al. *Social, cultural and environmental contexts and the measurement of the burden of disease. An exploratory comparison in the developed and developing world.* Report to the Global Forum for Health Research. Melbourne, Key Centre for Women's Health in Society, 2001.

Chapter 27

Alternative Summary Measures of Average Population Health

Colin D. Mathers, Joshua A. Salomon, Christopher J.L. Murray,
Alan D. Lopez

Introduction

To measure the level of population health in the Performance Framework, we need to choose an appropriate summary measure of population health (SMPH). Improving population health, level and distribution, is the defining goal to which health systems contribute (1). Without being able to measure health, the most important outcome of the health system, it is impossible to know if health policies are working—if levels of health are improving and inequalities are being reduced. Health policy is not aimed only at reducing mortality. Substantial resources are devoted to reducing the incidence of conditions that cause ill health but not death, and to reducing their impact on people's lives. Therefore, it is important to capture both fatal and non-fatal health outcomes in any measure of population health.

The epidemiologic transition, characterized by a progressive rise in the average age of death in virtually all populations across the globe, has necessitated a serious reconsideration of how the health of populations is measured. Average life expectancy at birth is becoming increasingly uninformative in many populations where, because of the non-linear relationship between age-specific mortality and life expectancy at birth, significant declines in death rates at older ages have produced only relatively modest increases in life expectancy at birth. At the same time, there is considerable uncertainty in many populations as to whether—and to what extent—gains in life expectancy have been accompanied by improvements in health status (2–8). Such considerations are critical for the planning and provision of health and social services. Separate measures of survival and of health status among survivors, while useful inputs into the health

policy debate, need to be combined in some fashion if the goal is to provide a single, holistic measure of overall population health.

This chapter reviews summary measures of average population health (SMAPH), explains the reasons for choosing healthy life expectancy, and examines possible developments in SMAPH for future health system performance analyses and other applications.

Background

In the last two decades, considerable international effort has been put into the development of summary measures of population health that integrate information of mortality and non-fatal health outcomes, and international policy interest in such indicators is increasing (9–13). The concept of combining population health state prevalence data with mortality data in a life table to generate estimates of expected years of life in various health states (health expectancies) was first proposed in the 1960s (14;15). An informal international research network, the Network on Health Expectancy (Réseau Espérance de Vie en Santé or REVES) was established in 1989 with objectives including the harmonization of calculation methods and identification of the conditions necessary for comparison of health expectancy estimates, both across populations and over time (11;16–19).

During the 1990s, disability-free life expectancy (DFLE) and related measures were calculated for many countries (7;20–22). DFLE has been recommended as a summary measure of population health and reported for OECD countries since 1993 in its health database (8;23). Because DFLE incorporates a dichotomous weighting scheme for health states, the threshold definition of disability has a dramatic effect on the results (*24*). Wilkins and Adams (*25*) suggested a more sensitive weighting scheme based on the severity of functional limitations, leading to the health-adjusted life expectancy approach.

Murray and Lopez (*26*) published disability-adjusted life expectancy (DALE) estimates for the eight regions of the world based on the estimates of severity-weighted disability prevalence developed in the Global Burden of Disease Study (*27–31*). Health-adjusted life expectancy has also been calculated for Australia and Canada (*32–36*). The United States of America has adopted a public health policy goal to increase health-adjusted life expectancy (referred to as expected years of healthy life or YHL) and has used health-adjusted life expectancy to measure the progress towards this goal (*37–40*).

Another type of summary measure, Disability-Adjusted Life Years (DALYs) has been used in the Global Burden of Disease Study (*26–31;41*) and in a number of National Burden of Disease Studies (*32;42–50*). The DALY is the best known example of a "health gap" summary measure, which quantifies the gap between a population's actual health and a defined goal (*51*).

Reflecting the rising interest in summary measures of population health in the academic and policy communities, the United States' Institute of Medicine convened a panel on summary measures and published a report that included recommendations to enhance public discussion of the ethical assumptions and value judgements, establish standards, and invest in education and training to promote use of summary measures (*10*). More recently, WHO convened a conference of experts across a range of disciplines including descriptive epidemiology, public health, health economics, philosophy, and ethics to discuss issues around the conceptual, technical, and ethical basis for summary measures of population health. A book addressing these issues based in part on the papers presented at the WHO conference was published in 2002 (*13*).

Interest in summary measures relates to a range of potential uses. Murray, Salomon and Mathers (*12*) identified eight of these:

- Comparing the health of one population to the health of another population.

- Comparing the health of the same population at different points in time.

- Identifying and quantifying overall health inequalities within populations.

- Providing appropriate and balanced attention to the effects of non-fatal health outcomes on overall population health.

- Informing debates on priorities for service delivery and planning.

- Informing debates on priorities for research and development in the health sector.

- Improving professional training curricula in public health.

- Analysing the benefits of health interventions for use in cost-effectiveness analyses.

Broad interest and use of summary measures in the policy arena demonstrate the recognition of their value at the practical level for many of these purposes. *The World Health Report 2000* used healthy life expectancy as a summary measure of the level of population health in Member States in order to provide a comparative assessment of levels of health, and as a component of the composite health system goal performance measure (*1*). Over time, successive reporting on healthy life expectancy will provide evidence of progress towards achieving global goals for improving health.

A TYPOLOGY OF SMAPH

HEALTH EXPECTANCIES AND HEALTH GAPS

Summary measures of population health can be divided into two classes: *health expectancies* and *health gaps*.

These two classes of measures are in principle complementary (Figure 27.1). The bold curve in Figure 27.1 is an example of a survivorship curve $S(x)$ for a hypothetical population. The survivorship curve indicates, for each age along the horizontal axis, the proportion of an initial birth cohort that will remain alive at that age. The area under the survivorship function is divided into two components: A which is time lived in full health and B which is time lived at each age in a health state less than full health. The familiar measure of life expectancy at birth is simply equal to A + B (the total area under the survivorship curve).

A health expectancy is generally of the form:

$$\text{Health expectancy} = A + f(B) \qquad [1]$$

where $f(\cdot)$ is a function that weights time spent in B by the severity of the health states that B represents. When a set of health state valuations are used to weight time spent in health states worse than ideal health, the health expectancy is referred to as a health-adjusted or disability-adjusted life expectancy. Another type of health expectancy is exemplified by disability-free life expectancy in which time spent in any health state categorized as disabled is assigned arbitrarily a weight of zero, and time spent in any state categorized as not disabled is assigned a weight of one (i.e. equivalent to full health).

In contrast to health expectancies, health gaps quantify the *difference* between the actual health of a population and some stated norm or goal for population health. The health goal implied by Figure 27.1 is for everyone in the entire population to live in ideal health until the age indicated by the vertical line enclosing area C at the right.[1] In the specific example shown, the normative goal has been set as survival in full health until age 100. By selecting a normative goal for population health, the gap between this goal and current survival, area C, quantifies premature mortality. A health gap is generally of the form:

$$\text{Health gap} = C + g(B) \qquad [2]$$

where $g(\cdot)$ is a function that weights time spent in B by the severity of the health states that B represents. Note that because health gaps measure a negative entity, namely the gap between current conditions and some established norm for the population, the weighting of time spent in B is on a reversed scale as compared to the weighting of time spent in B for a health expectancy. More precisely, full health is 1 in a health expectancy, whereas death or a state equivalent to death is 1 in a health gap.

Years of life lost measures are all measures of a mortality gap, or the area between the survivorship function and a target survivorship function (area C in Figure 27.1). Mortality gap measures were first suggested in 1947 by Dempsey (52) and potential years of life lost has been used extensively as a population health indicator since its first calculation by Romeder and McWhinnie (53). These all measure the gap in years between age at death and some arbitrary standard (typically 65 or 75 years). Murray (51) and others (54;55) have since proposed and calculated a variety of health gaps.

Health gaps are very convenient for disaggregating population health into the contribution of different causes. Time-based health gap measures also offer the possibility of using a common metric for population health and for the outcomes of interest in randomized control trials, in cohort studies, and in some health services administrative datasets. A common metric is the key to linking economic evaluations of interventions, monitoring of health system outcomes, and the overall health burden attributable to diseases, injuries, and risk factors in the population (56).

HEALTH STATE EXPECTANCIES AND DISABILITY-ADJUSTED LIFE EXPECTANCIES

We can categorize health expectancies into two main classes: those that use dichotomous health state weights and those that use health state weights for a more disaggregated set of health states. Examples of the first class include:

- *Disability-free life expectancy.* This health expectancy gives a weight of 1 to states of health with no disability (above an explicit or implicit threshold) and a weight of 0 to states of health with any level of disability above the threshold. Other examples of this type of health expectancy include active life expectancy, independent life expectancy, and dementia-free life expectancy.

- *Life expectancy with disability.* This is an example of a health expectancy which gives 0 weight to all states of health apart from one specified state of less than full health (in this case, disability above a certain threshold of severity). If health state 3 in Figure 27.2 is "moderate disability," then the segment of the area under the survival curve corresponding to health state 3 represents life expectancy with moderate disability. Other examples of this type of health expectancy include handicap expectancy, severe handicap expectancy, and unhealthy life expectancy.

Figure 27.1 Survivorship function for a population

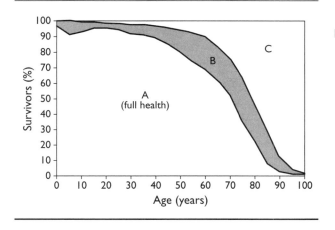

Examples of the second type of indicator include:

■ *Health-adjusted life expectancies.* These have been calculated for Canada and Australia using population survey data on the prevalence of disability at four levels of severity together with more or less arbitrary severity weights (*33–35*). Canada has also produced the first estimates of health-adjusted life expectancy based on population prevalence data for health states together with measured utility weights (*36*).

■ *Disability-adjusted life expectancy.* This was calculated for the Global Burden of Disease Study using disability weights reflecting social preferences for seven severity levels of disability (*27*). DALE has also been calculated for Australia using prevalence data from the Australian Burden of Disease Study (*32*) and preference weights derived from the Global Burden of Disease Study and a Dutch study using similar valuation methods (*57*).

■ *Healthy life expectancy.* This has been calculated by WHO for all 191 Member States for the years 1999 through 2001 using methods that combine information from nationally representative population surveys and from the Global Burden of Disease 2000 project, in order to maximize cross-population comparability (*58*).

TERMINOLOGY

In the mid-1990s, REVES developed a set of recommendations for terminology (*59*). With the development of health gap measures in the 1990s, there has been some shift in the use of these terms, and health expectancy is now used to denote the general class of summary measures that relate to the area under the survival curve. Also, following the feedback from Member States and to better reflect the inclusion of all states of health in the calculation of healthy life expectancy, the name of the indicator used by WHO to measure healthy life expectancy was changed from disability-adjusted life expectancy (DALE) to health-adjusted life expectancy (HALE) in *The World Health Report 2001*.

WHO has adopted the following terminology:

Health expectancy (HE): Generic term for summary measures of population health that estimate the expectation of years of life lived in various health states.

Health state expectancy: Generic term for health expectancies that measure the expectation of years lived in a single specified health state (e.g. disability-free).

Health-adjusted life expectancy (HALE): General term for health expectancies that estimate the expectation of equivalent years of good health based on an exhaustive set of health states and weights defined in terms of health state valuations.

Disability-adjusted life expectancy (DALE): Term used for HALE calculated based on DALY estimates from a burden of disease study.

Healthy life expectancy: WHO implementation of a cross-population comparable HALE, using population-based health state preferences.

CRITICAL APPRAISAL OF SMAPH

MINIMAL CRITERIA FOR SMAPH

Murray, Salomon and Mathers (*12*) proposed a set of desirable properties for evaluating summary measures of average population health (SMAPH) based on common-sense notions of population health of the following type:

> If two populations are identical in every way except that infant mortality is higher in one, then we expect that everybody would agree that the population with the lower infant mortality is healthier.

They suggested a minimal set of desirable properties for summary measures that will be used to compare the health of populations:

Figure 27.2 Survivorship function for four health states

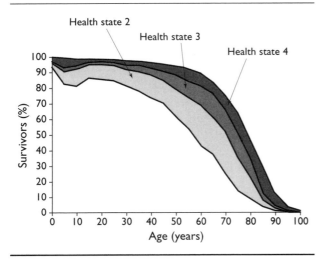

Criterion 1: If age-specific mortality is lower in any age group, *everything else being the same*, then a summary measure should be better (i.e. a health gap should be smaller and a health expectancy should be higher).[2]

Criterion 2: If the age-specific prevalence of some health state worse than ideal health is higher, *everything else being the same*, a summary measure should be worse.

Criterion 3: If the age-specific incidence of some health state worse than ideal health is higher, *everything else being the same*, a summary measure should be worse.

Criterion 4: If the age-specific remission for some health state worse than ideal health is higher, *everything else being the same*, a summary measure should be better.

Criterion 5: If the severity of a given health state is worse, *everything else being the same*, then a summary measure should be worse.

Mathers (*60*) has assessed health expectancies against these five criteria. All health expectancies meet criterion 1. Health expectancies based on prevalence data (for example, those calculated using Sullivan's method) meet criteria 1 and 2 but fail criteria 3 and 4 (until prevalence rates change to reflect the change in transition rates). Health expectancies based on transition rates (for example, those calculated using the multistate life table method) meet criteria 1, 3, and 4 but fail criterion 2. Health-adjusted life expectancies (HALEs) meet criterion 5, whereas health expectancies using dichotomous health state weights (e.g. disability-free life expectancy) do not. Table 27.1 summarizes these conclusions.

The dichotomous weighting scheme in health state expectancies such as DFLE means that the summary indicator is not sensitive to changes in the severity distribution of disability within a population (criterion 5). The overall DFLE value for a population is largely determined by the prevalence of the milder levels of disability, and comparability between populations or over time is highly sensitive to the performance of the disability instrument in classifying people around the threshold. For this reason, Murray, Salomon, and Mathers (*12*) concluded that health state expectancies are not appropriate for use as SMPH, and that HALE is the most appropriate form of health expectancy for use as a SMPH.

There has been considerable discussion among the experts consulted about whether it is possible or desirable to construct a health expectancy that simultaneously meets criteria 2 and 3, i.e. is sensitive to differences in both incidence and prevalence. Barendregt (*61*) and Mathers (*60*) both have proposed forms of population health expectancy which meet both criteria, but these are considerably more complex and less comprehensible than the usual period-based Sullivan health expectancies. We return to this issue in the sections on the "Individual Basis for SMAPH" and "Incidence-based Healthy Life Expectancy: a Proposal," below.

OTHER DESIRABLE PROPERTIES

Murray, Salomon and Mathers (*12*) proposed two other desirable attributes of summary measures that are to be used to inform policy discussions. These are not attributes based on arguments about whether a population is healthier than another, but rather on practical considerations:

- Summary measures should be comprehensible and feasible to calculate for many populations. Comprehensibility and complexity are different. Life expectancy at birth is a complex abstract measure but it is easy to understand. Health expectancies are popular because they are also easily understood.

- Summary measures should be linear aggregates of the summary measures calculated for any arbitrary partitioning of subgroups. Many decision-makers, and very often the public, desire information that is characterized by this type of additive decomposition. In other words, they would like to be able to answer what fraction of the summary measure is related to health events in the poor, in the uninsured, in the elderly, in children, and so on. Additive decomposition is also often appealing for cause attribution.

Most health expectancies satisfy the first attribute. However, they cannot be additively decomposed in

Table 27.1 SMPH criteria met by various forms of health expectancies

	Health state expectancies Dichotomous weights (e.g. DFLE)	Health-adjusted life expectancies Polytomous weights (e.g. HALE)
Prevalence-based measures	1, 2	1, 2, 5
Transition-rate based measures	1, 3, 4	1, 3, 4, 5

respect to causes or population subgroups. Health-adjusted life expectancies are additively decomposable into health expectancies for specified levels of disability severity (see above). This form of decomposition may be useful in understanding which levels of disability severity are contributing most to changes in population health. Health state expectancies should thus be understood as a decomposition of a HALE summary measure, rather than as SMPH in themselves. This interpretation is consistent with the usual ways in which families of health state expectancies are presented for a population (62;63).

In general, health gaps can be decomposed into the contribution of various causes in a more intuitive and easily communicated fashion than health expectancies. DALYs are additive across causes to give the total health gap for a population. A health expectancy such as HALE and a health gap such as the DALY thus fulfil different needs for SMPH to summarize and report on trends and achievements in population health across countries.

THE CALCULATION OF HEALTHY LIFE EXPECTANCIES

A key step in the construction of a health expectancy or a health gap is comparing time lived in a health state worse than full health with time lived in full health (in health expectancies), and with time lost due to premature mortality, compared to a normative goal (in a health gap). Two sets of issues are common to both health expectancies and health gaps: the conceptual framework and measurement strategy to describe health states and the conceptual framework and measurement strategy to value time spent in health states, as discussed elsewhere (64–66).

MEASUREMENT OF HEALTH STATES

DFLE estimates based on self-reported health status information are not comparable across countries due to differences in survey instruments and cultural differences in reporting of health (7;24;67). Analyses of over 50 national health surveys for the calculation of healthy life expectancy in *The World Health Report 2000* identified severe limitations in the comparability of self-report health status data from different populations, even when identical survey instruments and methods were used (68). We have demonstrated how these comparability problems relate not only to differences in survey design and methods, but also much more fundamentally to unmeasured differ-

ences in expectations and norms for health (67;69). For example, response categories for a given survey item on a domain such as mobility may have very different meanings across different cultures, across socioeconomic groups within a society, across age groups or between men and women. During the past five years, WHO has embarked on large-scale efforts to improve the methodological and empirical basis for the measurement of population health, and has initiated a data collection strategy consisting of household and/or postal or telephone surveys in representative samples of the general populations using a standardized instrument together with new statistical methods for correcting biases in self-reported health (70;71).

VALUING HEALTH STATES

In order to use time as a common currency for measuring the health impact of living years in various states and for life lost due to premature mortality, we must numerically value time lived in non-fatal health states. The health state valuations used in DALY and HALE calculations represent quantifications of the overall health levels associated with different states. They range from 0 representing a state of good or ideal health, to 1 representing states equivalent to being dead. These weights do not represent the lived experience of any disability or health state, or imply any societal value of the person in a disability or health state (64,66).

ENSURING COMPARABILITY ACROSS POPULATIONS

A fundamental requirement for SMAPH for reporting on levels of health for WHO Member States is cross-population comparability (67). In the broadest sense, comparability is required not only across countries, but also within countries and over time. In constructing estimates of healthy life expectancy for 191 countries for the year 2000 (71), we sought to address these methodological challenges regarding comparability of health status data across populations and cultures (58). Because comparable health status prevalence data are not yet available for all countries, a three-stage strategy was used to estimate severity-weighted health state prevalences for countries in a way that maximizes cross-country comparability:

■ Firstly, data from the Global Burden of Disease 2000 Study (72) were used to estimate severity-adjusted disability prevalences by age and sex for all 191 countries.

- Secondly, data on health state prevalences and health state valuations from the WHO Multi-country Survey Study on Health and Responsiveness 2000–2001 (70) were used to make independent estimates of severity-adjusted disability prevalences by age and sex for 55 countries.

- Finally, for the survey countries, "posterior" prevalences were calculated using Bayesian methods to combine the survey prevalences with the "prior" GBD 2000-based prevalences. The relationship between the GBD 2000-based prevalences and the survey prevalences among the survey countries was then used to adjust the GBD 2000-based prevalences for the non-survey countries.

THE INDIVIDUAL BASIS FOR SMAPH

Much of the literature on SMAPH has grown out of the demographic and epidemiologic traditions, which take a population perspective as their starting point. For some uses such as measuring inequalities in health across individuals or measuring the health of individuals in clinical settings or intervention trials, it is important to formulate SMAPH in terms of the health of a set of individuals. Many of the challenges in constructing a SMAPH are intimately related to the linkage between population and individual health measures. Distinctions between incidence and prevalence perspectives, or period and cohort perspectives, for example, can be recast in terms of different choices as to the set of individuals (real or hypothetical) whose health is aggregated into a population measure. Recent efforts have been made to develop formal expressions of population health as aggregations of individual health measures (74–77). Previously, we have attempted to set out a systematic framework for characterizing the individual basis for summary measures of population health (77). We summarize some of this framework here as a basis for the discussion in the section entitled: "Incidence-based Healthy Life Expectancy: a Proposal."

IS PERSON A HEALTHIER THAN PERSON B?

Imagine a casual conversation in which one participant says that John is healthier than Jack. What is the common-sense meaning of this statement? How does the use of the phrase "is healthier than" correspond to various measures of individual health? We believe that there are at least three more precise formulations of the question "Is person A healthier than person B?"

- Taking into account only *current* levels in various domains of health, is person A in a better state of health than person B?

- After both person A and person B have died, will person A have lived a healthier life overall than person B?

- For the remainder of their lives, will person A have a healthier life than person B?

We believe that the last question may be closest in meaning to the common usage of the phrase "is healthier than."

EX ANTE, EX INTERIM, AND EX POST PERSPECTIVES

It is easy to confound the three questions asked about person A and person B with the vantage point in time when the question is asked. In fact, however, the time perspective constitutes a separate dimension along which different characterizations of individual health may be distinguished.

Question 1 which asks about individual health states can only apply to a particular moment in time, since it refers only to the state of health of an individual at that moment in time.

Health over the entire life span (question 2) can be asked from three different vantage points in time:

- The *ex post* perspective reviews the life spans of person A and person B after they have both died.

- The *ex ante* perspective compares the expected life spans of person A and person B at birth, before any of the health events have been realized, based on a comparison of the risks of being in different health states (including death) at different ages for person A and person B. Such an *ex ante* view of health over the life span is used in the framework for measuring health inequality presented by Gakidou et al. (78)

- The *ex interim* perspective is located at an intermediate vantage point. Accounting for the actual health states lived in from birth until now and risks of being in different health states from now into the future. It is interesting to note that Williams (79) has proposed an *ex interim* view of life expectancy as the basis for assessing inequality.

Question 3, which asks whether person A or person B will have a healthier life from now forward, is by its formulation an exclusively *ex ante* view. For two individuals evaluated at the (same) moment of birth, question 3 is identical to the *ex ante* formulation of question 2. At all other ages, this question differs from question 2 by ignoring past differences in health and focusing only on the health of individuals from the present until death. This question is probably closest in spirit to the common usage of the phrase "is healthier than."

The three questions and the three time perspectives lead to five different variants of the simple question "Is person A healthier than person B?" (Table 27.2). Murray et al. (77) present formal specifications for each of these five variants and discuss the implications for SMAPH. Here we consider only the implications for average population health expectancies.

EX ANTE HEALTHY LIFE SPAN

We assume that the health state of an individual at a particular moment in time can be characterized completely in J domains (64). For each domain, we assume further that the level for an individual may be characterized on a cardinal scale. We postulate that there is some valuation function such that any combination of levels on the J domains can be translated to a single cardinal value on a scale anchored by 1 (complete health) and 0 (a state comparable to death) (66).

More formally, we represent the valuation of a health state as follows:

$$h_i(t) = f\big(y_{1i}(t), y_{2i}(t), \ldots, y_{Ji}(t)\big) \qquad [3]$$

where $h_i(t)$ is the valuation of an individual i's health state at time t and $y_{Ji}(t)$ is the level for individual i on domain j at time t. This formulation assumes for simplicity that the valuation function $f(\cdot)$ mapping between levels on the J domains is the same for all individuals.

Rather than asking "*Did* person A live a healthier life than person B?" we can ask the question from birth, "*Will* person A live a healthier life than person B?". The answer to this question, *ex ante*, is a probabilistic statement, as both persons face some uncertain distribution of different life span paths of health. To formalize the *ex ante* view, we need to capture the probability distribution of individuals being in differ-

ent health states at different ages. Because states of health at one age cannot be completely independent of states of health at other ages, we can formulate the *ex ante* view as a distribution of probabilities of different healthy life spans under different possible states of the world:

$$EAHL_i = \sum_{s \in \Omega} r(s) \int_0^\infty h_i(s, a)da \qquad [4]$$

where Ω is the universe of all possible states of the world and $r(s)$ is the probability of a particular state s. Gakidou et al. (78) have used this type of formulation as the conceptual basis for the measurement of population health inequality.

EX INTERIM AND FUTURE HEALTHY LIFE SPAN

There is another perspective: given the past experience of health from birth until the present for person A and person B, combined with their prospects for health in the future, which person will have the healthier life span overall. This *ex interim* perspective combines the realization of health risks from birth to the present with an *ex ante* view of health risks from now until death. The *ex interim* healthy life span for an individual at age x is:

$$EIHL_i(x) = \int_0^x h_i(a)da + \sum_{s \in \Omega} r(s) \int_x^\infty h_i(s, a)da \qquad [5]$$

The final option which asks whether person A or person B will live a healthier life from now forward, is the one that is perhaps closest to the common usage of the phrase "is healthier than." In fact, a number of web sites (for example, *LongToLive.com* or various "life expectancy calculators") will provide a computation of future health prospects based on a particular risk factor profile input by an individual. Parallels to the two families of SMPH can also be formulated to answer this question for a person. Health expectancy for an individual can be defined as:

$$HE_i(x) = \sum_{s \in \Omega} r(s) \int_x^\infty h_i(s, a)da \qquad [6]$$

Table 27.2 Different questions and time perspectives for describing individual health

	Ex post	Ex ante	Ex interim
Current health	(no time dimension)	(no time dimension)	(no time dimension)
Life span health	Ex post healthy life span and ex post health gap	Ex ante healthy life span and ex ante health gap	Ex interim healthy life span and ex interim health gap
Future health		Health expectancy and health gap	

This differs from the *ex interim* healthy life span because it ignores previous health experience from birth until the present.

The future health formulation of the question is probably closest to the vernacular notion of individual health, which may have important implications for aggregate-level comparisons, where we ask whether population A is healthier than population B. Although some currently used population health measures account for at least part of the future stream of health consequences, none of the available measures incorporates the health prospects formulation of individual measures in a comprehensive way. Depending on the intended application, new summary measures of population health may be required in order to capture the same aspects of individual health reflected in this view.

FROM INDIVIDUAL TO POPULATION LEVEL HEALTH EXPECTANCY

In the previous section, we outlined a formalization of individual health, which provides a basis for constructing aggregate health expectancies for populations. In principle, the population health expectancy defined as the average of all the *future* individual health expectancies for the people comprising the population at a given point of time satisfies all five criteria for SMAPH. This is because the future individual health expectancies are dependent not only on current and future transition rates (incidence), but also on the current health status (prevalence) of each individual. *Future* individual health expectancies require assumptions about future incidence, remission, and mortality rates that the individuals will face, whereas currently computed period health expectancies provide a measure based only on currently measurable aspects of health. For this reason, we may choose to define and estimate individual health expectancies by assuming that future incidence, remission, and mortality rates that the individuals will face reflect the current health conditions only. This would be an analogue of the well known period life expectancies and health expectancies. We can then calculate a population-based aggregate health expectancy which satisfies the five criteria.

Suppose that the current prevalence of each health state h in the population aged x is $prev_{hx}$. The period health-adjusted life expectancy $HALE_{hx}$ for an individual in health state h at age x can be calculated from the current transition rates observed in the population in the usual way (this assumes that the individual faces

the transition risks at each future age observed for that age group in the current population). $HALE_{hx}$ is a measure of the conditional expectation of equivalent years of good health for an individual specified to be in health state h at age x.

The average health-adjusted life expectancy at age x for the actual prevalence distribution of individuals in the population is thus:

$$HALE_x = \sum_h prev_{hx} * HALE_{hx} \qquad [7]$$

where the prevalences are defined so that at each age x,

$$\sum_h prev_{hx} = 1 \qquad [8]$$

A summary measure for the population could then be based on some aggregation of the individual *future* expectancies at each age, such as a simple average across all individuals in the population:

$$\overline{HALE} = \frac{\sum_x \left(n_x * \sum_h prev_{hx} * HALE_{hx} \right)}{\sum_x n_x} \qquad [9]$$

where n_x is the number of individuals aged x. This aggregate measure would reflect both incidence and prevalence and would be age-structure dependent. This summary measure would satisfy all five criteria and would also be easily interpretable as the average expected years of good health (averaged across all people in the actual population), assuming current transition rates remain unchanged.

A summary measure independent of age structure could also be constructed by age-standardizing the age-specific health expectancies. If p_x is the proportion of people aged x in the standard reference population, then the standardized summary measure is:

$$\overline{\overline{HALE}} = \sum_x \left(p_x * \sum_h prev_{hx} * HALE_{hx} \right) \qquad [10]$$

This measure reflects current prevalence rates in a population, as well as current incidence, remission, and mortality transmission rates. Its calculation would require substantially more information than is currently available for most populations. It does not, however, require substantially more information than is already required to calculate HALE using the multi-state life table method or microsimulation techniques.

INCIDENCE-BASED HEALTHY LIFE EXPECTANCY: A PROPOSAL

The prevalence-based healthy life expectancy that has been used by WHO to measure the level of attainment of health in *The World Health Report 2000* reflects to some extent the impact of past health system activity (and other health determinants), as well as the current health system activity. If efficiency is to be related to current health system resource usage for a given reference year, then estimating efficiency would require controlling for all possible non-health system determinants and the impact of health actions taken in the past. This approach would be very difficult to implement practically, as current health system actions are generally highly correlated with those in recent previous years (which would need to be controlled). This would also risk exclusion of the impact of broad long-term public health actions, where the impact of this year's effort is not easily separable from efforts in surrounding years.

Several of the regional consultations on the health systems performance assessment framework discussed this issue, and it seems clearly preferable to base the SMAPH for the level of health goal on current health conditions in the population, to the extent possible. The HALE in *The World Health Report 2000* analysis uses current prevalence estimates for countries. These reflect past exposures to risk factors as well as current exposures and risks. For some risk factors, such as smoking, current incidence of conditions like lung cancer and disabling COPD depends on exposures 20 to 30 years past.

Moving to a population-averaged future HALE as discussed in the previous section, would not solve this problem, since future HALE for people who were smokers 20 years ago will reflect that past exposure. In order to maximize the impact of current health activities, we propose that the concept of a period health expectancy be extended so that HALE is based on current incidence rates (where these reflect current risks) and current health risks rather than on current health state prevalences.

If sufficient data were available, the correct approach to implement this would be to use a multi-state life table based on the current observed period transition rates between all health states (and death). The period concept would need to be extended so that where current transition rates (such as lung cancer mortality) reflect past exposure to risks (tobacco smoking), they would be adjusted to reflect current exposures to risk (i.e. to assume that the current preva-

lence of smoking by age and sex had applied at all past times). Note that whereas a true period measure must be based on incidence rates (transition rates) for health states, it should reflect prevalence (rather than incidence) of relevant risk exposures, since it is the prevalence of exposure that determines risk of transition between health states.

Clearly, the data demands to implement the multi-state life table approach are not possible to fulfil at present. We propose a simplified approach, involving modifications that can be implemented to the current methodology for the calculation of healthy life expectancy. Five steps are proposed:

■ Inclusion in the GBD 2000 of prevalence estimates based on current transition rates (so-called "incidence-based" prevalences) as well as the observed prevalence rates. These two types of prevalence estimates would differ only for causes where there was evidence of a non-equilibrium state for the disease model, due to time trends in incidence, remission or case fatality, e.g. HIV/AIDS in many regions. GBD-based prior estimates would be calculated using prevalences derived from currently estimated incidence rates (rather than the currently observed prevalences). For many diseases, such as HIV/AIDS, use of current incidence rather than prevalence would ensure that current risk factor profiles were taken into account.

■ For selected risk factors where there are long lags to health outcomes, estimation of incidence and mortality for the population would be based on a counterfactual assumption that the population had been exposed to current levels of the risk factor for a long time in the past. The GBD 2000 comparative risk assessments (CRA) (*80;81*) would be used to provide estimates of risk factor exposures for each region of the world for selected risk factors. Where available, country-specific information would be used to provide country-specific exposure estimates. Currently observed total incidence and mortality risks would be adjusted using CRA estimates of effect sizes. In the first instance, we would envisage that such an analysis would only be carried out for smoking and perhaps diet and exercise. It would be necessary to model the joint effect on incidence and mortality of the combined current exposure to these risks and to be transparent about the assumptions used in the analysis.

■ Estimation of the overall difference in severity-weighted prevalences for current prevalences and incidence-based prevalences for the GBD-based priors. These factors would be used to adjust health survey-based prevalences as well (as these will reflect current prevalences in the survey countries).

■ Calculation of new life tables for each Member State based on the adjustments to mortality risks described above (to reflect current risk factor exposures and current incidence rates where relevant).

■ Calculation of an incidence-based HALE for each Member State using Sullivan's method with the incidence-based prevalences and the new life tables.

These incidence-based period HALE estimates would provide measures of the healthy life expectancy that could be expected by a cohort exposed to current risk factor levels at each age (for the selected risk factors) and current incidence, remission, and case fatality rates (reflecting current rather than past risks of disease and injury). This would provide a better measure of the health outcome for current health system activities than a measure based on prevalences reflecting past health system activities and past risk factor levels (and other past non-health system determinants).

CONCERNS ABOUT THE USE OF HEALTHY LIFE EXPECTANCY

Several broad concerns about the use of healthy life expectancy as a measure of the health system goal to improve average level of population health have been raised by commentators and in consultations. We discuss these here.

CLAIM 1: HEALTH STATE VALUATIONS DISCRIMINATE AGAINST THE DISABLED

Such claims stem from a misunderstanding of the meaning of health state valuations. As used in summary measures of population health, health state valuations quantify the loss of population health associated with a health state. In other words, they reflect the preferences of societies that people should have better states of health rather than worse ones. The weights do not measure quality of life of people with disabilities and do not measure the value of a person to society (64,66).

Such claims might well emerge from a very narrow view of health which excludes long-term impairments and disabilities. Some groups argue that people with long-term disabilities are as healthy as other people. This clearly relates to the conceptualization of health that is used (64). We believe that the scope of the defi-

nition of health must accord with people's legitimate expectations for their health and their health systems. To exclude long-term disabilities from this scope would mean that populations with a high prevalence of preventable disabilities (such as some African countries where there is a high prevalence of river blindness) would be considered to have the same level of population health as other countries with much lower prevalence of this type of blindness. Such a conceptualization of health would imply that health systems that prevent this type of blindness do no better than those that do not, all else being equal. If improving the level of population health is one of the major goals of health systems, then we must include in the measurement of population health all aspects of health which people expect their health systems to address.

It is important to distinguish the use of SMAPH to measure average level of the health goal from any uses for resource allocation. The inclusion of all five goals in the health systems performance assessment (HSPA) framework means that health system resources should be used broadly to achieve a mix of goals. WHO has never advocated the use of SMAPH by themselves, to set priorities for resource allocation. The level of population health is only one piece of information, though an important one, that decision-makers need to set priorities. *The World Health Report 2000* stated clearly that health policy has objectives in addition to improving the level of population health. It also seeks to reduce health inequalities; increase the responsiveness of the system to the legitimate non-health needs of the population; reduce inequalities in responsiveness; and ensure that financial contribution to the health system is fairly distributed across households. In addition, it is important to ensure that a country uses its scarce resources as efficiently as possible to achieve these goals.

CLAIM 2: METHODS ARE TOO COMPLEX

Some commentators have argued that the data demands and complexity of the calculations make healthy life expectancy an impractical measure for use as a summary measure of population health (82). Although the concept of healthy life expectancy is relatively simple to understand, health encompasses multiple domains and mortality risks, and with the additional requirement to ensure comparability of estimates across countries, any acceptable methods used to compute healthy life expectancy will inevitably be complex.

The analytical and conceptual elements underlying summary measures of population health such as healthy life expectancy are certainly more substantial than for measures of mortality such as life expectancy. However, complexity is not a reason to ignore progress in measuring health in a more appropriate way. Some conceptually simple measures such as income per capita, which are widely used, are in fact extremely complicated to calculate. The intricacies of national income accounts are known only to a few, yet the measure of overall economic performance is widely used. We believe that in order to report on levels of health for WHO Member States, it is important to use a summary measure that is conceptually simple to understand, as well as methods that capture all important aspects of health and result in estimates that are comparable across Member States.

Claim 3: HALE Adds No More Information Than Life Expectancy

Some commentators have argued that HALE correlates highly with life expectancy and hence adds little or no additional information on average levels of population health. While lower life expectancies are generally associated with lower healthy life expectancy—the two indicators are correlated—there are large variations in healthy life expectancy for any given level of life expectancy. For example, for countries with a life expectancy of 70, healthy life expectancy varies from 57 to 61.5, a non-trivial variation. If male and female HALE are considered separately, the range of variation increases to 57 to 65 at total life expectancy of 70.

Claim 4: HALE Is Too Uncertain

Some commentators have argued that HALE estimates are too uncertain or that data are not "available" for some countries. This issue is discussed in detail in (83). Healthy life expectancy estimates for all countries are based on a mix of survey data for some countries (with their own uncertainty due to sampling and systematic biases) and GBD 2000-based estimates, which draw on a wide range of epidemiological and demographic data of varying degrees of uncertainty. Thus, there is no sense in which some HALE estimates are "real" and others "estimates;" rather, HALE is estimated with varying degrees of uncertainty across Member States.

Claim 5: HALE Hides Detailed Health Information

Summary measures of average population health status are constructed from detailed information on incidence rates, prevalence rates, severity distributions, case fatality rates, etc. As such, they complement the detailed health information rather than replace it. They form the apex of a hierarchy of related measures, rather than a piecemeal set of unconnected measures. The macro measures at the apex of the system, such as HALE and DALYs, provide a broad population-based overview of trends and causes. Publication of summary measures such as healthy life expectancy should be accompanied (in background documents perhaps) by more detailed disaggregation of component parts, e.g. incidence rates, prevalence rates, severity distributions, case fatality rates, etc. Thus, WHO plans to publish detailed tabulations from the GBD 2000 project, together with documentation of sources and methods, and also, over the next year, to work towards making available country-level estimates of incidence, prevalence, and mortality by cause, age, and sex.

Claim 6: HALE Is Not Sensitive to Differences or Changes in Population Health

Some commentators have argued that HALE does not distinguish between the average levels of health for countries at a similar level and does not change greatly over time. These comments apply with equal force to most other long established summary measures of population health such as life expectancy at birth or infant mortality. There is clear evidence that all of these indicators, including healthy life expectancy, can change substantially over relatively short periods of time, *if the health of the population changes substantially*. Examples include the dramatic decrease in male life expectancy in Russia during the 1990s. The important issue is to quantify correctly the average level of health of populations. Then the rate of change of the indicator over time, or the difference across populations, will be appropriately captured and will appropriately reflect reality.

Conclusions

We conclude that the SMAPH for the purposes of measuring performance should at least fulfil the following criteria.

- The measure should reflect changes in incidence, remission, health state severity, and mortality such that when these get worse, then the SMAPH would get worse.

- The measure should reflect current, not past risk factor exposures.

- It should be possible to communicate the results of the SMAPH to decision-makers, the media, and the interested public.

- It should be possible to calculate the SMAPH for a wide range of countries with diverse data systems.

For these reasons, WHO used healthy life expectancy as a summary measure of the level of population health for the health system performance analysis in *The World Health Report 2000*. As a summary measure of the average level of health in a population, healthy life expectancy has two advantages over other summary measures. The first is that it is relatively easy to explain the concept of an equivalent "healthy" life expectancy to a non-technical audience. The second is that healthy life expectancy is measured in units (expected years of life) that are meaningful to and within the common experience of non-technical audiences (unlike other indicators such as mortality rates or incidence rates).

We argue that HALE is preferable as a summary measure of population health to indicators such as DFLE which incorporate a dichotomous weighting scheme. Because time spent in any health state categorized as disabled is assigned arbitrarily a weight of zero (equivalent to death), DFLE is not sensitive to differences in the severity distribution of disability in populations. In contrast, HALE adds up expectation of life for different health states with adjustment for severity distribution and thus is sensitive to changes over time or differences between countries in the severity distribution of health states (*12*). Use of a dichotomous measure for health system performance analysis would mean that the analysis could not take any account of health system actions aimed at reducing the severity of health states, as opposed to completely preventing loss of health.

We propose that the calculation of HALE for the health system performance analysis should move from using current health state prevalences to current transition rates (incidence, remission, case fatality), and where current transition rates depend on past risk exposures, to transition rates (including mortality) based on current patterns of risk exposure.

NOTES

1 Figure 27.1 graphically illustrates the magnitude of both health expectancies and health gaps only when a population has a stable distribution with a zero population growth rate. In practice, health expectancies are not sensitive to differences in the age structure of different populations. Health gaps are usually reported in absolute terms so that health gaps are sensitive to variations in the age distribution of different populations, although age independent forms of health gaps can be formulated.

2 This criterion could be weakened to say that if age-specific mortality is lower in any age group, *everything else being the same*, then a summary measure should be the same or better. The weaker version would allow for deaths beyond some critical age to leave a summary measure unchanged. Measures such as potential years of life lost would then fulfil the weak criterion.

REFERENCES

(1) Murray CJL, Frenk J. A framework for assessing the performance of health systems. *Bulletin of the World Health Organization*, 2000, 78(6):717–731.

(2) Gruenberg EM. The failures of success. *Milbank Memorial Fund Quarterly/Health and Society*, 1977, 55: 3–24.

(3) Kramer M. The rising pandemic of mental disorders and associated chronic diseases and disabilities. *Acta Psychiatrica Scandinavica*, 1980, 62(Suppl. 285):282–297.

(4) Manton KG. Changing concepts of morbidity and mortality in the elderly population. *Milbank Memorial Fund Quarterly/Health and Society*, 1982, 60:183–244.

(5) Manton KG. Response to "an introduction to the compression of morbidity." *Gerontologica Perspecta*, 1987, 1:23–30.

(6) Olshansky SJ et al. Trading off longer life for worsening health. *Journal of Aging and Health*, 1991, 3: 194–216.

(7) Robine JM, Mathers CD, Brouard N. Trends and differentials in disability-free life expectancy: concepts, methods and findings. In: Caselli G, Lopez AD, eds. *Health and mortality among elderly populations*. Oxford, Clarendon Press, 1996:182–201.

(8) Robine JM, Romieu I, Cambois E. Health expectancy indicators. *Bulletin of the World Health Organization*, 1999, 77(2):181–185.

(9) van de Water HP, Perenboom RJ, Boshuizen HC. Policy relevance of the health expectancy indicator: an inventory of European Union countries. *Health Policy*, 1996, 36(2):117–129.

(10) Field MJ, Gold GM, eds. *Summarizing population health: directions for the development and application of population metrics.* Institute of Medicine, Washington, DC, National Academy Press, 1998.

(11) Mathers CD, McCallum J, Robine JM, eds. *Advances in health expectancies: proceedings of the 7th meeting of the international network on health expectancy (REVES).* Canberra, Australian Institute of Health and Welfare, 1994.

(12) Murray CJL, Salomon JA, Mathers CD. A critical examination of summary measures of population health. *Bulletin of the World Health Organization,* 2000, 78(8): 981–994.

(13) Murray CJL et al., eds. *Summary measures of population health: concepts, ethics, measurement and applications.* Geneva, World Health Organization, 2002.

(14) Sanders BS. Measuring community health levels. *American Journal of Public Health,* 1964, 54:1063–1070.

(15) Sullivan DF. A single index of mortality and morbidity. *HSMHA Health Reports* 86, 1971:347–354.

(16) Bone MR. International efforts to measure health expectancy. *Journal of Epidemiology and Community Health,* 1992, 46:555–558.

(17) Mathers CD, Robine JM. Health expectancy indicators: a review of the work of REVES to date. In: Robine JM et al., eds. *Calculation of health expectancies, harmonization, consensus achieved and future perspectives.* Colloque INSERM vol. 226. France, John Libbey Eurotext and Les Editions INSERM, 1993.

(18) Robine JM, Blanchet M, Dowd JE, eds. *Health expectancy.* London, OPCS, HMSO, 1992.

(19) Robine JM et al., eds. *Calculation of health expectancies, harmonization, consensus achieved and future perspectives.* Colloque INSERM vol. 226. France, John Libbey Eurotext and Les Editions INSERM, 1994.

(20) Crimmins EM, Saito Y, Ingengneri D. Trends in disability-free life expectancy in the United States, 1970–90. *Population and Development Review,* 1997, 23(3): 555–572.

(21) Robine JM, Jagger C. *Developing consistent disability measures to address public policy needs for older populations.* Background Paper prepared for OECD Meeting on Implications of Disability for Ageing Populations: Monitoring Social Policy Challenges. Paris, 1999.

(22) Saito Y, Crimmins EM, Hayward MD. *Health expectancy: an overview.* NUPRI Research Paper Series No. 67. Tokyo, Nihon University Population Research Institute, 1999.

(23) Organisation for Economic Co-operation and Development. *Eco-santé. OECD Health Database.* Paris, Organisation for Economic Co-operation and Development, 1999.

(24) Romieu I, Robine JM. World atlas of health expectancy calculations. In: Mathers CD, McCallum J, Robine JM, eds. *Advances in health expectancies.* Canberra, Australian Institute of Health and Welfare, 1994.

(25) Wilkins R, Adams OB. Health expectancy in Canada, late 1970's: demographic, regional and social dimensions. *American Journal of Public Health,* 1983, 73(9): 1073–1080.

(26) Murray CJL, Lopez AD. Regional patterns of disability-free life expectancy and disability-adjusted life expectancy: Global Burden of Disease Study. *The Lancet,* 1997, 349(9062):1347–1352.

(27) Murray CJL, Lopez AD, eds. *The global burden of disease: a comprehensive assessment of mortality and disability from diseases, injuries, and risk factors in 1990 and projected to 2020.* Cambridge, Harvard University Press, 1996.

(28) Murray CJL, Lopez AD. *Global health statistics.* Cambridge, Harvard University Press, 1996.

(29) Murray CJL, Lopez AD. Evidence-based health policy —lessons from the Global Burden of Disease Study. *Science,* 1996, 274(5288):740–743.

(30) Murray CJL, Lopez AD. Mortality by cause for eight regions of the world: Global Burden of Disease Study. *The Lancet,* 1997, 349(9061):1269–1276.

(31) Murray CJL, Lopez AD. Global mortality, disability, and the contribution of risk factors: Global Burden of Disease Study. *The Lancet,* 1997, 349(9063):1436–1442.

(32) Mathers CD, Vos T, Stevenson C. *The burden of disease and injury in Australia.* Canberra, Australian Institute of Health and Welfare, 1999.

(33) Wilkins R, Adams OB. Quality-adjusted life expectancy: weighting of expected years in each state of health. In: Robine JM, Blanchet M, Dowd JE, eds. *Health expectancy, OPCS studies on medical and population subjects No. 54.* London, HMSO, 1992.

(34) Wilkins R, Chen J, Ng E. Changes in health expectancy in Canada from 1986 to 1991. In: Mathers CD, McCallum J, Robine JM, eds. *Advances in health expectancies: proceedings of the 7th meeting of the international network on health expectancy (REVES).* Canberra, Australian Institute of Health and Welfare, 1994.

(35) Mathers CD. Gains in health expectancy from the elimination of diseases among older people. *Disability and Rehabilitation,* 1999, 21(5-6):211–221.

(36) Wolfson MC. Health-adjusted life expectancy. *Health Reports,* 1996, 8(1):41–46.

(37) Public Health Service. *Healthy people 2000: national health promotion and disease prevention objectives—full*

report, with commentary. DHHS publication No. (PHS) 91-50212. Washington, DC, US Department of Health and Human Services, Public Health Service, 1991.

(38) Erickson P, Wilson R, Shannon I. *Years of healthy life.* Statistical Notes No. 7. Hyattsville, US Department of Health and Human Services, CDC, National Center for Health Statistics, 1995.

(39) CDC. Years of healthy life—selected states, United States, 1993–1995. *The Journal of the American Medical Association*, 1998, 279(9):649.

(40) U.S. Department of Health and Human Services. *Healthy people 2010. With understanding and improving health and objectives for improving health*, 2nd ed. Washington, DC, U.S. Government Printing Office, 2000.

(41) Murray CJL, Lopez AD. Alternative projections of mortality and disability by cause 1990–2020: Global Burden of Disease Study. *The Lancet*, 1997, 349(9064): 1498–1504.

(42) Lozano R, Frenk J, Gonzalez MA. El peso de la enfermedad en adultos mayores, Mexico 1994. *Salud Publica de Mexico*, 1994, 38:419–429.

(43) Lozano R et al. Burden of disease assessment and health system reform: results of a study in Mexico. *Journal for International Development*, 1995, 7(3):555–564.

(44) Fundación Mexicana Para la Salud. *Health and the economy: proposals for progress in the Mexican health system*. Mexico, Fundación Mexicana para la Salud, 1995.

(45) República de Colombia Ministerio de Salud. *La carga de la enfermedad en Colombia*. Santafé de Bogotá, Editorial Carrera, Séptima, 1994.

(46) Ruwaard D, Kramers PGN. *Public health status and forecasts*. The Hague, National Institute of Public Health and Environmental Protection, 1998.

(47) Bowie C et al. Estimating the burden of disease in an English region. *Journal of Public Health Medicine*, 1997, 19:87–92.

(48) Concha M et al. *Estudio ecarga de enfermedad informe final*. Estudio Prioridades de Inversio en Salud, Minsterio de Salud, 1996.

(49) Murray CJL et al. The *health sector in Mauritius: resource use, intervention cost and options for efficiency enhancement*. Cambridge, Harvard Center for Population and Development Studies, 1997.

(50) Murray CJL et al. *U. S. patterns of mortality by county and race: 1965–1994*. Cambridge, Harvard Center for Population and Development Studies and Centers for Disease Control, 1998.

(51) Murray CJL. Rethinking DALYs. In: Murray CJL, Lopez AD, eds. *The global burden of disease: a comprehensive assessment of mortality and disability from diseases,*

injuries, and risk factors in 1990 and projected to 2020. Cambridge, Harvard University Press, 1996:1–98.

(52) Dempsey M. Decline in tuberculosis: the death rate fails to tell the entire story. *American Review of Tuberculosis*, 1947, 56:143–151.

(53) Romeder JM, McWhinnie JR. Potential years of life lost between ages 1 and 70: an indicator of premature mortality for health planning. *International Journal of Epidemiology*, 1977, 6:143–151.

(54) Ghana Health Assessment Project Team. A quantitative method of assessing the health impact of different diseases in less developed countries. *International Journal of Epidemiology*, 1981, 10(1):72–80.

(55) Hyder AA, Rotllanat G, Morrow RH. Measuring the burden of disease: healthy life-years. *American Journal of Public Health*, 1998, 88(2):196–202.

(56) Murray CJL, Lopez AD. Progress and directions in refining the global burden of disease approach: a response to Williams. *Health Economics*, 2000, 9(1):69–82.

(57) Stouthard et al. *Disability weights for diseases in the Netherlands*. Rotterdam, Department of Public Health, Erasmus University, 1997.

(58) Mathers CD, Murray CJL, Salomon JA. Methods for measuring healthy life expectancy. In: Murray CJL, Evans DB, eds. *Health systems performance assessment: debates, methods and empiricism*. Geneva, World Health Organization, 2003.

(59) Mathers CD, Robine JM, Wilkins R. Health expectancy indicators: recommendations for terminology. In: Mathers CD, McCallum J, Robine JM, eds. *Advances in health expectancies: proceedings of the 7th meeting of the international network on health expectancy (REVES)*. Canberra, Australian Institute of Health and Welfare, 1994.

(60) Mathers CD. Health expectancies: an overview and critical appraisal. In: Murray CJL et al., eds. *Summary measures of population health: concepts, ethics, measurement and applications*. Geneva, World Health Organization, 2002:177–204.

(61) Barendregt J. Incidence- and prevalence-based SMPH: making the twain meet. In: Murray CJL et al., eds. *Summary measures of population health: concepts, ethics, measurement and applications*. Geneva, World Health Organization, 2002:221–231.

(62) Robine JM. Disability-free life expectancy trends in France, international comparison. In: Mathers CD, McCallum J, Robine JM, eds. *Advances in health expectancies*. Canberra, Australian Institute of Health and Welfare, 1994.

(63) Mathers CD. Trends in health expectancies in Australia 1981–1993. *Journal of the Australian Population Association*, 1996, 13(1):1–16.

(64) Salomon JA et al. Quantifying individual levels of health: definitions, concepts, and measurement issues. In: Murray CJL, Evans DB, eds. *Health systems performance assessment: debates, methods and empiricism*. Geneva, World health Organization, 2003.

(65) Sadana R et al. *Describing population health in six domains: comparable results from 66 household surveys*. EIP Discussion Paper No. 43. Geneva, World Health Organization, 2002. URL: http://www3.who.int/whosis/discussion_papers/discussion_papers.cfm#

(66) Salomon JA et al. Health state valuations in summary measures of population health. In: Murray CJL, Evans DB, eds. *Health systems performance assessment: debates, methods and empiricism*. Geneva, World Health Organization, 2003.

(67) Murray CJL et al. Cross-population comparability of evidence for health policy. In: Murray CJL, Evans DB, eds. *Health systems performance assessment: debates, methods and empiricism*. Geneva, World Health Organization, 2003.

(68) Sadana R et al. Comparative analyses of more than 50 household surveys on health status. In: Murray CJL et al, eds. *Summary measures of population health: concepts, ethics, measurement and applications*. Geneva, World Health Organization, 2002.

(69) Tandon A et al. Statistical models for enhancing cross-population comparability. In: Murray CJL, Evans DB, eds. *Health systems performance assessment: debates, methods and empiricism*. Geneva, World Health Organization, 2003.

(70) Üstün TB et al. WHO Multi-country Survey Study on Health and Responsiveness 2000–2001. In: Murray CJL, Evans DB, eds. *Health systems performance assessment: debates, methods and empiricism*. Geneva, World Health Organization, 2003.

(71) World Health Organization. *The World Health Report 2001. Mental Health: New Understanding, New Hope*. Geneva, World Health Organization, 2001.

(72) Murray CJL et al. *The Global Burden of Disease 2000 project: aims, methods and data sources*. EIP Discussion Paper No. 36. Geneva, World Health Organization, 2001. URL: http://www3.who.int/whosis/discussion_papers/discussion_papers.cfm#

(73) Üstün TB et al. The World Health Surveys. In: Murray CJL, Evans DB, eds. *Health systems performance assessment: debates, methods and empiricism*. Geneva, World Health Organization, 2003.

(74) Cutler DM, Richardson E. Measuring the health of the United States population. *Brookings Papers on Economic Activity, Microeconomics*, 1997, 217–272.

(75) Cutler DM, Richardson E. The value of health: 1970–1990. *American Economic Review*, 1998, 88(2): 97–100.

(76) Fleurbaey M. On the measurement of health and health inequalities. In: Murray CJL, Wikler D, eds. *Fairness and goodness: ethical issues in health resource allocation*. Geneva, World Health Organization (forthcoming).

(77) Murray CJL, Salomon JA, Mathers CD. The individual basis for summary measures of population health. In: Murray CJL et al, eds. *Summary measures of population health: concepts, ethics, measurement and applications*. Geneva, World Health Organization, 2002:41–51.

(78) Gakidou E, Murray CJL, Frenk J. A framework for measuring health inequality. In: Murray CJL, Evans DB, eds. *Health systems performance assessment: debates, methods and empiricism*. Geneva, World Health Organization, 2003.

(79) Williams A. Inter-generational equity: an exploration of the 'fair innings' argument. *Health Economics*, 1997, 6(2):117–132.

(80) Ezzati M et al. *CRA Interim guidelines, data collection sheets and toolbox*. Geneva, World Health Organization, 2001. URL: http://www.ctru.auckland.ac.nz/CRA

(81) Murray CJL, Lopez AD. On the comparable quantification of health risks: lessons from the global burden of disease study. *Epidemiology*, 1999, 10(5):594–605.

(82) Almeida C et al. Methodological concerns and recommendations on policy consequences of The World Health Report 2000. *The Lancet*, 2001, 357(9269): 1692–1697.

(83) Murray CJL, Mathers CD, Salomon JA. Towards evidence-based public health. In: Murray CJL, Evans DB, eds. *Health systems performance assessment: debates, methods and empiricism*. Geneva, World Health Organization, 2003.

Chapter 28

LIFE TABLES FOR 191 COUNTRIES FOR 2000: DATA, METHODS, RESULTS

ALAN D. LOPEZ, OMAR B. AHMAD, MICHEL GUILLOT,
BRODIE D. FERGUSON, JOSHUA A. SALOMON,
CHRISTOPHER J.L. MURRAY, KENNETH H. HILL

INTRODUCTION

Basic demographic information on the number of deaths by age and sex in a population is a critical input for the determination and evaluation of health policies and programmes. Beginning with the year 1999, the World Health Organization (WHO) began making annual life tables for all Member States. These life tables have several uses and form the basis of all WHO's estimates about mortality patterns and levels worldwide. A key use of these life tables is in the construction of healthy life expectancy (HALE) which is the basic indicator of average population health levels used by WHO and published each year in *The World Health Report*.

The construction of a life table requires reliable data on a population's mortality rates, by age and sex. The most dependable source of such data is a functioning vital registration system in which all deaths are registered. Deaths at each age are related to the size of the population in that age group, usually estimated from population censuses, or continuous registration of all births, deaths, and migrations. The resulting age/sex-specific death rates are then used to calculate a life table.

Table 28.1 Mortality data sources (number of countries) for WHO subregions, 2000

Subregion*	Category I Complete vital statistics (coverage 95%+)	Category II Incomplete vital statistics	Category III Sample registration and surveillance systems	Category IV Child mortality estimated from surveys and censuses	Category V No recent data on child or adult mortality	Number of countries
AfrD	2	2	0	18	4	26
AfrE	0	2	1	13	4	20
AmrA	3	0	0	0	0	3
AmrB	17	9	0	0	0	26
AmrD	0	4	0	1	1	6
EmrB	4	4	0	5	0	13
EmrD	0	2	0	5	2	9
EurA	26	0	0	0	0	26
EurB	7	9	0	0	0	16
EurC	8	1	0	0	0	9
SearB	1	1	0	1	0	3
SearD	0	2	2	1	2	7
WprA	4	1	0	0	0	5
WprB	3	12	1	6	0	22
Total	75	49	4	50	13	191

*AFR = Africa Region; AMR = Region of the Americas; EMR = Eastern Mediterranean Region; EUR: European Region; SEAR = South-East Asia Region; WPR = Western Pacific Region.

A = subregions have very low rates of adult and child mortality; B = low adult, low child; C = high adult, low child; D = high adult, high child; E = very high adult, high child mortality.

For a complete list of countries by subregion, see Annex 60.1.

Table 28.2 Mortality data sources (% of deaths covered) for WHO subregions, 2000

Subregion	Category I *Complete vital statistics (coverage 95%+) (%)*	Category II *Incomplete vital statistics (%)*	Category III *Sample registration and surveillance systems (%)*	Category IV *Child mortality estimated from surveys and censuses (%)*	Category V *No recent data on child or adult mortality (%)*	*Total deaths 2000 (WHO estimates) (%)*
AfrD	0	4	0	89	7	100
AfrE	0	13	9	54	23	100
AmrA	100	0	0	0	0	100
AmrB	39	61	0	0	0	100
AmrD	0	65	0	14	21	100
EmrB	2	74	0	24	0	100
EmrD	0	18	0	68	14	100
EurA	100	0	0	0	0	100
EurB	51	49	0	0	0	100
EurC	96	4	0	0	0	100
SearB	6	19	0	76	0	100
SearD	0	2	92	4	2	100
WprA	100	0	0	0	0	100
WprB	0	15	84	1	0	100
Total	24	13	36	22	5	100

While the legal requirement for the registration of deaths is virtually universal, the cost of establishing and maintaining a system to record births and deaths implies that reliable data from routine registration are generally only available in the more economically advanced countries. Reasonably complete national data to calculate life tables in the late 1990s were only available for 75 countries, covering about one-quarter of the deaths estimated to have occurred in 2000 (Tables 28.1 and 28.2). In the absence of complete vital registration, sample registration or reliable information on mortality in childhood has been used, together with indirect demographic methods, to estimate life tables. This approach has been greatly facilitated by the availability of reliable estimates of child mortality in many countries of the developing world during the 1980s and 1990s from the Demographic and Health Surveys (DHS) program, and more recently by the Multiple Indicator Child Survey (MICS) Programme led by UNICEF.

Several international agencies and other demographic centres routinely prepare national mortality estimates or life table compilations as part of their focus on sectoral monitoring. Thus, UNICEF has periodically reviewed available data on child mortality to assess progress with child survival targets and to evaluate interventions (*1*). A recent update of trends in child mortality during the 1990s has also been completed (*2*). Three agencies or organizations, the United Nations Population Division, the World Bank, and the United States Census Bureau have all produced

international compilations of life tables, and in the case of the Population Division, at least, tables continue to be updated biennially (*3–5*). These various studies generally rely on the same data sources—censuses, surveys, and vital registration—but can produce quite different results due to differences in the timing of data availability, in judgements about whether or how the basic data should be adjusted, and in estimation techniques and choice of models.

A comparative review of these various exercises highlights the variability in results from different procedures and judgement. For example, in India, adjusting the Sample Registration System (SRS) for under-reporting of adult mortality, estimated at 13–14% in 1999–2000 (*6*), yields an estimate of 9.8 million deaths in 2000, or 1 million more than the 2000 United Nations population assessment (*3*).

Differences such as these are not insignificant and have major implications for the monitoring, evaluation and reorientation of public health programmes in countries as well as at a global level. While it would obviously be desirable to develop a single set of life tables for all countries of the world, technical judgement, data availability, and the timing of periodic assessments will continue to vary. Given WHO's needs for annual life table estimates as part of the continuous assessment of health systems performance, and a preference for a model life table system based on a modification of the Brass logit system rather than other families of model life tables (*7*), WHO has constructed a new set of life tables, the results of which, for 2000, can be found in the full report (*8*).

This chapter provides details on the methods and data sources used to prepare these life tables. We begin with a review of the sources, types and quality of the data available. We examine the different sources of data and the problems and difficulties involved in using them in generating life tables. We also provide a brief review of the two main approaches used by WHO to estimate the parameters of the Brass logit system for each country. For countries with a long series of vital registration data, lagged-time series analysis was used. For all other countries, the parameters were estimated from either shorter time series of vital registration data or from survey or surveillance data on child and adult mortality. This is followed by a discussion of how the basic demographic inputs for the method were estimated for countries, as well as a summary of the major findings.

Data sources and Adjustments

Vital Registration Data

Ideally, life tables should be constructed from a long historical series of mortality data from vital registration where the deaths and population of the *de facto* (or occasionally *de jure*) population-at-risk are entirely covered by the system. In order to compute life tables for a given year for which vital registration of deaths is not yet available for administrative reasons, short-term projections are required from the latest available year. This will require an adequate time series of data, with at least 15–20 years of mortality statistics. Table 28.9 shows the availability of vital registration data on mortality to the World Health Organization that could be used for estimation of life tables for the year 2000.

Firstly, vital registration data since 1980 were systematically evaluated for completeness using an array of demographic techniques including the Brass Growth-Balance method (*9*), the Generalised Growth Balance method (*10*), and the Bennett–Horiuchi technique (*11*). These latter two methods require data on the age–sex distribution of the population from two adjacent censuses, as well as registered intercensal deaths. As a result, the simple Growth-Balance method was more commonly used to evaluate the completeness of death reporting since the basic data requirements (deaths and population by age and sex for a given year or period) were more easily met. On the other hand, the technique assumes that the population of inter-

est is stable, which is unlikely to be the case in many developing countries, and involves a certain degree of arbitrariness in fitting the points used to estimate the extent of under-reporting (*12*).

Application of these methods to each country with vital registration data resulted in selecting 75 countries for which the vital registration data were judged to be sufficiently complete to compute life tables (Table 28.1). These countries are listed under Category I in Table 28.9. For each of these countries, the last year (or last few years for small populations) were used to establish the "standard" pattern of l_x values by age, for each sex separately. Using this standard, time series for α and β, the two parameters of the Brass logit system, were generated. Time series techniques were then used to project the values of α and β to the year 2000, from which the 2000 life table was then obtained. This approach is more fully described in the methods section. For small populations (e.g. Cook Islands) three or four year moving averages were used for time series analysis rather than single-year data.

For Bosnia and Herzegovina, vital registration data were not available after 1991. The 1989–1991 data were judged to be complete and, in the absence of new information, were averaged and assumed to apply in 2000, since any background improvements in mortality were probably counteracted by the effects of the conflict in the 1990s.

For a second group of countries with vital registration (or sample vital registration in the case of Bangladesh, China, India and Tanzania), application of these indirect demographic methods to assess completeness suggested that some correction was required to the vital registration data. These 53 countries are listed under Categories II and III in Table 28.9. The extent of under-reporting varied considerably but was typically on the order of 20–25% in the Central Asian Republics, and somewhat higher (30–40%) in several developing countries. For example, adult mortality was judged to be 84% complete in Egypt, 92% complete in Guatemala, 84–86% in India, 78–84% in Kazakhstan, 82–85% in Republic of Korea, and 73–75% in the Philippines. These completeness ratios were then applied to the vital registration data to correct for under-reporting.

For child mortality, all available data points from child mortality surveys such as the DHS or the MICS were used to correct the vital registration data on child mortality. This analysis benefited greatly from the comprehensive country evaluation of data carried out by Hill et al. (*1*) based on census and survey data available as of 1996. We have updated these country plots with more recent information and adjusted the 2000 predictions of Hill et al. where recent data suggested this was necessary. Where recent survey data were not available, child mortality rates were adjusted, based on the correction factors suggested from the above techniques for adult mortality and on levels estimated for neighbouring countries. To the extent that child deaths are more likely to be under-reported than adult deaths, this will underestimate levels of child mortality.

For those countries with a sufficiently long time series of vital registration or sample registration data, the corrected time series were then analysed (as for Category I countries). For the remainder, levels of child ($_5q_0$) and adult ($_{45}q_{15}$) mortality were projected forward to 2000 using available evidence on the speed of mortality decline, or by assuming a pattern of mortality change in the 1990s consistent with economic growth. These projected values of child and adult mortality were then applied to the modified logit life table system (7) to generate a full life table. In some cases (e.g. South Africa, Tanzania, Cambodia, Dominican Republic, Haiti and Myanmar), death rates were increased by adding on estimated mortality from HIV/AIDS. These methods and data sources for estimating HIV/AIDS mortality are described in a later section.

MULTI-SOURCE APPROACHES FOR SPECIFIC POPULATIONS

In two large developing countries, India and China, several data sources, including vital registration, surveillance systems and surveys are available to estimate mortality rates. None of these systems alone is sufficiently reliable to produce life tables for these countries without adjustments, but all are useful to estimate child and adult mortality. The data sources used and the adjustments made to them are as follows:

China

Three sources of mortality data were used to estimate the life table.

Disease Surveillance Points. The Disease Surveillance Points (DSP) is a nationally representative system of 145 epidemiological surveillance points operated by the Chinese Academy of Preventive Medicine and covering a population of 10 million people throughout China. Data on the age, sex, and cause of 50 000–60 000 deaths are recorded each year. Periodic evaluations of the DSP data by re-surveying households at random suggest a level of under-reporting of deaths of about

15% (*13*), although application of the Growth-Balance method to the data since 1991 suggests an average adjustment factor about twice this level. Annual data for the period 1991–1998 were used, with corrections, to estimate the trend in $_5q_0$ and $_{45}q_{15}$.

Vital Registration. Data on the age, sex and cause of 725 000 deaths are collected annually from the vital registration system operated by the Ministry of Health, covering a population of 121 million (66 million in urban areas, 55 million in rural areas). While the data are not representative of mortality conditions throughout China, they are useful for suggesting trends in mortality, given the number of deaths covered. Trends in $_{45}q_{15}$ for the rural and urban coverage areas separately are shown in Figure 28.1. While under-reporting yields implausibly low levels of $_{45}q_{15}$, these data suggest that there has been only a very modest decline in adult mortality during the 1990s (4–5% for males in both areas and for females in rural areas, and 14% for females in urban areas).

Survey Data. Survey data are obtained from the annual 1 per 1 000 household survey asking about deaths in the past 12 months. For example, the 1997 survey covered a population of 1 243 000 people spread over 864 counties (3 164 townships, 4 438 villages) in 31 provinces, and recorded a total of 7 845 deaths. While this is a nationally representative sample, Growth-Balance methods suggest substantial under-reporting of deaths (27% and 29% for males and females, respectively). Trends in the implied unadjusted $_{45}q_{15}$ from the surveys in the 1990s are shown in Figure 28.2 and

Figure 28.1 Trends in $_{45}q_{15}$ from vital registration data—China, 1990–1998

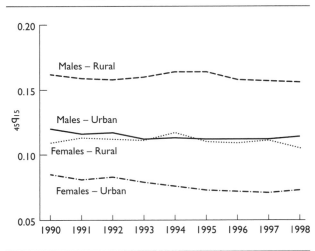

suggest a somewhat more substantial decline, although the much smaller number of deaths compared with vital registration makes trend assessment difficult.

In all three systems, data were available for the period 1991–1998. Since Growth-Balance analyses suggested that under-reporting had remained relatively constant during the 1990s, the average annual decline in $_5q_0$ and $_{45}q_{15}$ suggested by these three data sources was first calculated and applied to the 1990 Chinese life table based on the census to project death rates to 2000. Uncertainty around death rates in 2000 was generated from more optimistic and pessimistic assumptions about the rate of decline during the 1990s.

India

The most representative and reliable data on mortality rates by age and sex in India come from the Sample Registration System which has been in operation for several decades. We used data for the period 1990–1998 (latest year available) to compute annual life tables. Data are collected on vital events in 4 436 rural and 2 235 urban sampling units with a population of about 6 million people covering almost all States and Territories. Comparison of $_5q_0$ from the SRS with the rate reported from the DHS (National Family Health Survey) conducted in 1992–93 yields very similar results, suggesting that under-reporting of child deaths is minimal. On the other hand, under-reporting of adult deaths in the SRS during the 1990s has probably increased to around 15% based on the

Figure 28.2 Trends in $_{45}q_{15}$ (unadjusted) based on estimates from the Sample Survey of Population Change—China, 1991–1998

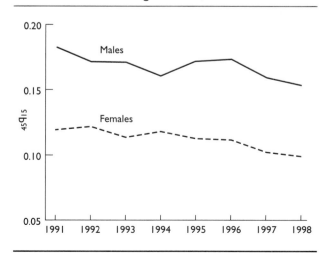

Bennett–Horiuchi variable–r methodology (6). We therefore corrected the SRS death rates at age five and over by 14% for males and 16% for females, and projected these forward to 2000. Uncertainty intervals around age-specific death rates were generated from plausible projections to 2000 of the trend lines in these rates.

Census and Survey Data

For the remaining 63 countries (Table 28.1), no reliable estimates of adult mortality could be obtained. However, extensive direct and indirect estimates of child mortality ($_5q_0$) were available for recent years from various census and survey programmes. These estimates were systematically evaluated and projected to 2000, along with uncertainty intervals (2). These estimates and uncertainty ranges were then applied to the modified logit life table system using the global standard to estimate a corresponding life table. More detail on the procedure is provided in the methods section.

In only a handful of countries in this group (Afghanistan, Angola, Bhutan, Burundi, Democratic People's Republic of Korea, Democratic Republic of the Congo, Djibouti, Equatorial Guinea, Haiti, Liberia, Malawi, Sao Tome and Principe, and Swaziland) was there insufficient evidence in the 1990s to establish estimates of child mortality with reasonable confidence. The life tables for these countries are consequently based on estimated child mortality levels with wide uncertainty. Substantial caution in their use is essential until more recent evidence on child mortality levels becomes available.

For many countries in this category, mortality from HIV/AIDS is likely to be substantial. This would not be captured from the model life table application since the models were built from mortality data in the pre-AIDS era. For these countries, primarily in sub-Saharan Africa, AIDS-free life tables were first estimated by estimating child mortality levels excluding HIV. Age/sex-specific death rates from HIV were then estimated separately (14) and added to the model life table age-specific rates with appropriate adjustment for competing risks.

Methods

Life Table Construction

Standard life table methods were used to construct the time series of life tables for countries in Categories

I and II, where time series data were available. The basic Brass logit system was used to generate the trend in the two parameters (α, β) from these life tables. This system rests on the assumption that two distinct age patterns of mortality can be related to each other by a linear transformation of the logit of their respective survivorship probabilities. Thus, for any two observed series of survivorship values, l_x and l_x^s, where the latter is the standard, it is possible to find constants α and β such that for all ages x greater than zero:

$$\text{logit}\left(l_x\right) = \alpha + \beta \text{logit}\left(l_x^s\right)$$

$$\text{if} \quad \text{logit}\left(l_x\right) = 0.5\ln\left(\frac{(1.0 - l_x)}{l_x}\right)$$

$$\text{then} \quad 0.5\ln\left(\frac{(1.0 - l_x)}{l_x}\right) = \alpha + 0.5\beta\ln\left(\frac{(1.0 - l_x^s)}{l_x^s}\right)$$

If the above equation holds for every pair of life tables, then any life table can be generated from a single standard life table by changing the pairs of (α, β) values used. In reality, the assumption of linearity is only approximately satisfied by pairs of actual life tables. However, the approximation is close enough to warrant the use of the model to study and fit observed mortality schedules. The parameter α varies the mortality *level* of the standard, while β varies the *slope* of the standard, i.e. it governs the relationship between the mortality in children and adults.

In circumstances where a historical sequence of life tables is available, it is possible to generate a time series of α,β pairs using a country-specific standard. Plots of α and β, separately, against time should each produce a trajectory of points (*15*). If the plot of points for each parameter falls along a fairly straight line, that line could theoretically be projected forward to forecast estimates for any time in the future. These α, β estimates can then be substituted into the appropriate logit equations to obtain the corresponding life tables. Where, on the other hand, the trend in the points is erratic, the system cannot provide an adequate forecast. In such situations, suitable techniques must be applied to project mortality, given this pattern. As a result, three models were developed to accommodate different scenarios. In the first model, the parameter at time T is assumed to be a simple linear function of time T:

$$\hat{\alpha}_T = \gamma_1 + \gamma_1 T$$
$$\hat{\beta}_T = \phi_1 + \phi_2 T$$

This model is suited to situations where the trend in α or β is clearly linear. In the second model, the α and β parameters at time T are assumed to be lagged linear functions of the parameters in the preceding periods. Thus, the parameters for time $T + 1$ are based on lag 1 model, those for time $T + 2$ are based on lag 2 model, etc., where T corresponds to the time location of the standard life table. The following equations summarize these relationships:

$$\hat{\alpha}_{T+1} = \gamma_{11} + \gamma_{21}\alpha_T \quad \hat{\beta}_{T+1} = \phi_{11} + \phi_{21}\beta_T \qquad \text{1st forecast point}$$
$$\hat{\alpha}_{T+2} = \gamma_{12} + \gamma_{22}\alpha_T \quad \hat{\beta}_{T+2} = \phi_{12} + \phi_{22}\beta_T \qquad \text{2nd forecast point}$$
$$\hat{\alpha}_{T+3} = \gamma_{13} + \gamma_{23}\alpha_T \quad \hat{\beta}_{T+3} = \phi_{13} + \phi_{23}\beta_T \qquad \text{3rd forecast point}$$
$$\cdots\cdots\cdots\cdots\cdots\cdots \qquad \cdots\cdots\cdots\cdots\cdots\cdots$$
$$\hat{\alpha}_{T+n} = \gamma_{1n} + \gamma_{2n}\alpha_T \quad \hat{\beta}_{T+n} = \phi_{1n} + \phi_{2n}\beta_T \qquad \text{last forecast point}$$

This model is likely to be more suitable in situations where there are clear linear trends, but also regular oscillations in parameter values over time. The third approach combines the above two models:

$$\hat{\alpha}_{T+1} = \gamma_{11} + \gamma_{21}\alpha_T + \gamma_{31}(T+1) \; \hat{\beta}_{T+1} = \phi_{11} + \phi_{21}\beta_T + \phi_{31}(T+1) \; \text{1st forecast point}$$
$$\hat{\alpha}_{T+2} = \gamma_{12} + \gamma_{22}\alpha_T + \gamma_{32}(T+2) \; \hat{\beta}_{T+2} = \phi_{12} + \phi_{22}\beta_T + \phi_{31}(T+2) \; \text{2nd forecast point}$$
$$\hat{\alpha}_{T+3} = \gamma_{13} + \gamma_{23}\alpha_T + \gamma_{33}(T+3) \; \hat{\beta}_{T+3} = \phi_{13} + \phi_{23}\beta_T + \phi_{31}(T+3) \; \text{3rd forecast point}$$
$$\cdots\cdots\cdots\cdots\cdots\cdots\cdots \qquad \cdots\cdots\cdots\cdots\cdots\cdots\cdots$$
$$\hat{\alpha}_{T+n} = \gamma_{1n} + \gamma_{2n}\alpha_T + \gamma_{3n}(T+n) \; \hat{\beta}_{T+n} = \phi_{1n} + \phi_{2n}\beta_T + \phi_{3n}(T+n) \; \text{last forecast point}$$

This model is suitable in situations where there are complex linear trends. In each country, all three models were used to forecast parameter estimates. The model that yielded time series of estimates which best fitted the historical trend was deemed adequate for that country.

To estimate the life table out to age 100+, the Coale-Guo procedure (*16*) was used. It has long been observed that mortality rates at ages over 75 or 80 increase with age at a diminishing rate rather than at the constant Gompertz rate (*17*). Using data from seven populations with relatively reliable mortality data at older ages (Austria, France, Germany, Japan, Netherlands, Norway, and Sweden), Coale and Guo demonstrated that the relative increase from one age group to the next decreases above age 80 or 85. Using these findings, they developed a method of closing out life tables above age 80. Their technique incorporates an assumption of steady rather than Gompertzian constancy in the rate of increase in mortality with age above age 80. More specifically, the logarithm of the ratio of the mortality rate in the interval $(x + 5, x + 10)$ to the ratio from $(x, x + 5)$ is assumed to decline by a constant increment as x rises above 80.

ESTIMATING ADULT MORTALITY

Measuring adult mortality is inherently more difficult than measuring child mortality, in part because of the relative rarity of the former — at younger adult ages death is much less common than in childhood — but more so because recall of deaths via birth histories is undoubtedly more complete than for adult deaths based on household intercensus surveys. Thus, obtaining precise measurement of adult mortality requires large samples of observations covering long reference periods. Also, in contrast to child mortality estimation where information is easily collected from affected mothers, it is often difficult to identify the right informant to provide information on deceased adults. This often results in problems of under-counting and multiple reporting. Often the informant does not know the age of the deceased, and birth certificates often are not available for older people in most developing countries. As a result, errors in the reporting of age can severely limit the ability to obtain good estimates of adult mortality.

The most widely used method of measuring adult mortality from survey data relies on information on the survival of mother and father to estimate adult female and male survivorship, respectively. Other methods use information on a) survival of first husbands to estimate male adult survivorship, b) survival of first wives to estimate female adult survivorship, or c) survival of siblings. These methods, although theoretically sound, have proved difficult to apply in practice, often leading to underestimation of true levels of adult mortality by 15–60% in countries where it has been possible to validate them against registration data (18).

An attempt to systematically review all available direct (primarily from Demographic Surveillance Systems) and indirect estimates on adult mortality levels in Africa concluded that only a relatively small fraction of them yielded plausible estimates, and many of these referred to years well before 2000 (15). As a result, for all countries in Categories IV and V, the modified logit life table system was used. Full details of the rationale and evaluation of the method are given elsewhere (7). Essentially the approach was based on matching the estimated level of child mortality to a plausible range of levels of l_{60} derived from an empirical database of over 1 800 life tables with a wide range of life expectancies. In most cases, the mean value of l_{60} from among those within this plausible range was chosen as a basis for estimating adult mortality levels. In relatively few cases, values other than the mean value were chosen based on an assessment of available evidence about levels of adult mortality.

ESTIMATING MORTALITY FROM HIV/AIDS

For countries with the most extensive HIV/AIDS epidemics and no vital registration data, AIDS mortality was estimated separately and then incorporated into life tables that excluded AIDS. For sub-Saharan African countries, the total number of adult AIDS deaths was derived from sentinel surveillance data on prevalence in pregnant women, with updates of previously published epidemiologic models (14) where more recent data have become available. In order to estimate age and sex-specific mortality, we have analysed registration and surveillance data on AIDS mortality from the following sources: the Adult Morbidity and Mortality Project in three districts of Tanzania; vital registration data from urban and rural South Africa; and Zimbabwe vital registration. These data provided the only reliable sources of population-based information on cause-specific mortality in continental sub-Saharan Africa available to WHO at the time of this analysis. In Figure 28.3 we have plotted the relative age and sex pattern of mortality rates from each of these sources, normalizing on the highest observed rate in each site. There is a remarkable consistency in the pattern across these diverse sources, with the main differences appearing at the youngest and oldest ages. Based on these sources, we have developed a regional standard age pattern by taking the weighted average of the sources. The regional standard appears as a thick line in Figure 28.3. Using this standard, a given estimate of total adult deaths may be translated into age-specific death rates by applying the standard pattern of rates to the population age structure and then rescaling all of the rates such that the total number of deaths matches the specified figure.

Given the dearth of data from which to estimate AIDS mortality directly and the uncertainties introduced through indirect estimation, it is important to try to quantify the level of uncertainty around the mortality estimates that result from these methods. Where enough data were available to undertake a maximum likelihood estimation approach in the epidemiologic models (i.e. about 20 countries), the results included a measure of uncertainty around mortality estimates in each year. For the remaining countries, uncertainty intervals were derived based on an assessment of the coverage and representativeness of sentinel surveillance sites in each country. Probability distributions around the total number of deaths were then trans-

Figure 28.3 Age pattern of HIV mortality

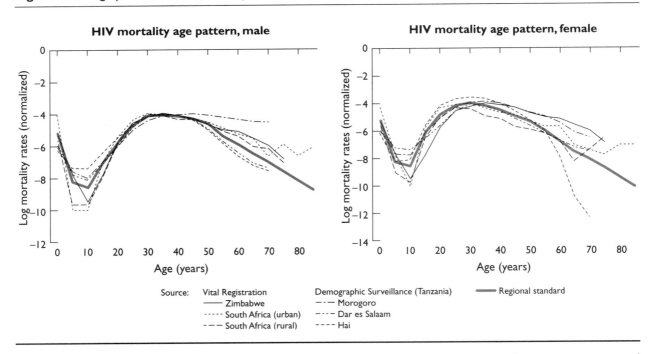

Source:	Vital Registration	Demographic Surveillance (Tanzania)	——— Regional standard
	——— Zimbabwe	–·– Morogoro	
	········· South Africa (urban)	– – – Dar es Salaam	
	– – South Africa (rural)	------ Hai	

lated into distributions around age and sex-specific mortality rates using numerical simulation methods. Monte Carlo methods were used to sample from these distributions in order to incorporate uncertainty around AIDS mortality into the life table uncertainty estimates.

For four countries outside of sub-Saharan Africa (Cambodia, Dominican Republic, Haiti, and Myanmar) where no vital registration data existed or where AIDS was inadequately reflected in registered deaths, we have also merged separate estimates of AIDS mortality into life tables excluding AIDS. The age pattern of AIDS mortality in these cases was based on regional reference patterns from countries with available vital statistics (Argentina, Brazil, Chile, Cuba, Mexico, and Uruguay in the case of Haiti and Dominican Republic; and Thailand in the case of Myanmar and Cambodia).

UNCERTAINTY BOUNDS

There are several sources of uncertainty around the final values of α and β obtained from these models, including model uncertainty as to the correct specification as well as estimation uncertainty in identifying values for the regression coefficients. A detailed discussion of the sources of uncertainty and methods for uncertainty analysis for life tables may be found elsewhere (19). The level of uncertainty around estimates

of α and β depends in part on the uncertainty around the regression coefficients γ_{ij} and ϕ_{ij}, and in turn implies some level of uncertainty around the life tables that are computed from these parameters. Because a complete life table is a complicated nonlinear function of the uncertain parameters, we have used Monte Carlo simulation techniques to develop numerical estimates of the ranges of uncertainty around the life tables. This uncertainty is captured by taking random draws of the regression coefficients γ_{ij} and ϕ_{ij} from normal distributions with means equal to the estimated coefficients and variances derived from the standard errors in the regression. In each of 1 000 iterations, the draws of γ_{ij} and ϕ_{ij} are used to generate α and β estimates, which are then translated into complete life tables. Thus, probability distributions may be defined around life table estimates by analysing the 1 000 different simulated life tables. For example, a range may be defined around the estimate for life expectancy at birth by sorting the 1 000 different estimates of e(0) in the simulated life tables and then identifying the 25th and 975th values as the bounds of an approximate 95% confidence interval.

In the absence of historical data (i.e. for countries in Categories IV and V), the modified logit system was used (7). Like the simple logit system, the new model is anchored on the relationship between two life tables. Unlike the simple logit system, however, the new formulation includes two additional parameters which correct for the nonlinearity in the original Brass method. The main input to the system is an estimated range around $_5q_0$. For any given $_5q_0$ value, this life table system provides a range of plausible values for $_{45}q_{15}$. These ranges have formed the basis for a set of Monte Carlo simulations of different possible life tables consistent with the knowledge and uncertainty regarding adult and child mortality. The range of simulated life tables allow calculation of uncertainty ranges around the various key indicators such as q_x, l_x and e_x.

RESULTS

Overall life expectancy at birth (both sexes combined) in 2000 was estimated to range from 81.1 years in Japan (84.7 females, 77.5 for males) to 37.5 years in Malawi (Table 28.3). For males, the next highest life expectancy was estimated for Sweden (77.3 years), followed by Andorra (77.2), Iceland (77.1), Monaco (76.8), and Switzerland (76.7). Male life expectancy exceeded 75.0 years in 19 countries in 2000 (Table 28.4).

Among females, the second highest life expectancy was estimated for Monaco (84.4 years), followed by San Marino and Andorra (83.8 years), and France (83.1). Twenty-four countries had an estimated life expectancy of 80 years or more for females in 2000 (Table 28.5). Female life expectancy exceeded 75.0 years in 57 countries, or about one-third of WHO's Member States.

Given the extraordinary impact of the HIV/AIDS epidemic in sub-Saharan Africa, it is perhaps not surprising that the countries with the lowest life expectancy in 2000 are all from this Region. Indeed 37 of the 40 countries with the lowest life expectancy are in sub-Saharan Africa. While countries in this Region suffer disproportionately from many of the factors which cause child death and the premature mortality of adults, including acute respiratory infection, diarrhœal diseases, and tuberculosis, the lack of progress in achieving further gains in life expectancy can largely be attributed to the effects of the HIV/AIDS epidemic over the last 15 years or so. If deaths from HIV/AIDS were to be excluded, life expectancy at birth in some countries of the region would be 15 to 20 years higher (Table 28.6). This is particularly true of countries of southern Africa (Botswana, Lesotho, Namibia, South Africa, Swaziland, Zambia, Zimbabwe), but reductions in life expectancy of the order of 5–10 years due to AIDS mortality in 2000 are common in many other

African countries as well. On average, life expectancy at birth in sub-Saharan Africa is 6 years lower for males and slightly more than 7 years lower for females compared to what would have been the case in 2000 in the absence of HIV/AIDS mortality.

Table 28.3 Life expectancy at birth (years), both sexes combined, top 10 and bottom 10 countries, 2000

	Top 10 countries			Bottom 10 countries	
1	Japan	81.1	1	Malawi	37.5
2	Monaco	80.6	2	Sierra Leone	37.9
3	Andorra	80.5	3	Mozambique	38.7
4	San Marino	80.0	4	Zambia	39.4
5	Sweden	79.6	5	Rwanda	39.5
6	Switzerland	79.6	6	Burundi	41.0
7	Iceland	79.5	7	Central African Republic	42.0
8	Australia	79.3	8	Lesotho	42.1
9	Italy	79.2	9	Namibia	42.7
10	France	79.1	10	Dem. Rep. of the Congo	42.8

Table 28.4 Countries with male life expectancy greater than 75.0 years, 2000

Country	e_0 (years)	Country	e_0 (years)
Japan	77.5	Italy	76.0
Sweden	77.3	New Zealand	75.9
Andorra	77.2	Norway	75.7
Iceland	77.1	Netherlands	75.4
Monaco	76.8	Singapore	75.4
Switzerland	76.7	Greece	75.4
Israel	76.6	Malta	75.4
Australia	76.6	Spain	75.4
San Marino	76.1	France	75.2
Canada	76.0		

Table 28.5 Countries with female life expectancy greater than 80.0 years, 2000

Country	e_0 (years)	Country	e_0 (years)
Japan	84.7	Norway	81.4
Monaco	84.4	Austria	81.4
San Marino	83.8	Netherlands	81.0
Andorra	83.8	New Zealand	80.9
France	83.1	Belgium	80.9
Switzerland	82.5	Finland	80.9
Italy	82.4	Luxembourg	80.8
Spain	82.3	Greece	80.8
Australia	82.1	Malta	80.7
Sweden	82.0	Germany	80.6
Iceland	81.8	Israel	80.6
Canada	81.5	Singapore	80.2

Large sex differences in life expectancy persist in the more developed countries. At the beginning of the 20th century, female life expectancy exceeded that of males by 2 to 3 years, on average, at least in Europe, North America, and Australia (20). In 2000, the female advantage had widened to 10 or more years in Kazakhstan (10.4 years), Lithuania (10.4), Ukraine (10.7), Estonia (11.0), Latvia (11.3), and Belarus (12.0), and was highest of all countries in the Russian Federation (12.6). Conversely, the differential was only half a year or less in countries such as Bangladesh, Lesotho, and Zambia, with male life expectancy 0.2 to 0.5 years higher than that of females in a handful of countries including Botswana, Maldives, Namibia, and Nepal. Figure 28.4 shows the distribution of the male–female gap in life expectancy at birth across the 191 Member States of WHO in 2000. The extreme values observed in some Eastern European countries are clear from the tail of the distribution. In about one-third of countries, the male–female differential is between 5 and 6 years in favour of females. Since sex differentials in mortality are typically lower in developing countries, the overall global difference in male–female life expectancy at birth is slightly lower than this (4.5 years).

Useful summary indicators of prevailing mortality risks in a population are the probability of dying between birth and age 5, as an overall measure of health conditions among children, and the probability of dying between ages 15 and 60, as a measure of premature mortality among adults. These are shown for the various WHO Regions, and within them, the various mortality-based subregions, in Figure 28.5.

Differences in levels of child mortality remain vast. Of the 10.9 million deaths below age 5 estimated to have occurred in 2000 (Table 28.7), 99% were in developing regions. The probability of child death ($_5q_0$) is typically less than 1% in industrialized countries (i.e. those classified into the A Regional Strata)

Table 28.6   Difference in life expectancy at birth for all possible causes of death and causes excluding AIDS, by sex, 2000 (years)

Males			
Namibia	18.5	Djibouti	5.9
Botswana	17.3	Haiti	5.4
Zambia	15.2	Eritrea	5.4
Zimbabwe	14.9	Nigeria	4.7
Lesotho	14.8	Somalia	4.7
Swaziland	14.2	Ghana	3.9
South Africa	12.1	Bahamas	3.9
Central African Republic	10.3	Gabon	3.8
Malawi	10.1	Dem. Rep. of the Congo	3.5
Kenya	9.8	Guyana	3.0
Burundi	9.8	Liberia	2.7
Côte d'Ivoire	9.0	Cambodia	2.7
Mozambique	8.3	Myanmar	2.5
Rwanda	7.8	Chad	2.3
Uganda	7.8	Honduras	2.2
United Republic of Tanzania	7.2	Sierra Leone	2.1
Ethiopia	7.2	Dominican Republic	2.1
Burkina Faso	6.6	Benin	2.1
Togo	6.3	Gambia	2.0
Cameroon	6.2	Angola	2.0
Congo	6.0		

Females			
Namibia	21.5	Congo	7.3
Botswana	20.2	Cameroon	7.3
Zambia	18.1	Djibouti	7.0
Zimbabwe	17.6	Eritrea	6.4
Lesotho	17.4	Somalia	5.7
Swaziland	16.8	Nigeria	5.6
South Africa	15.1	Ghana	4.7
Malawi	12.4	Dem. Rep. of the Congo	4.4
Central African Republic	12.2	Gabon	4.4
Burundi	11.7	Liberia	3.3
Kenya	11.6	Chad	2.8
Côte d'Ivoire	10.9	Sierra Leone	2.6
Mozambique	10.3	Angola	2.6
Rwanda	9.9	Gambia	2.4
Uganda	9.2	Benin	2.4
Ethiopia	8.8	Guinea-Bissau	2.1
United Republic of Tanzania	8.6	Haiti	2.1
Burkina Faso	7.8	Senegal	2.1
Togo	7.5		

Figure 28.4   Distribution of male–female difference in life expectancy at birth, WHO Member States, 2000

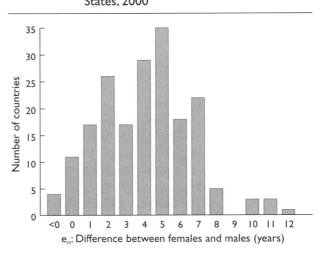

e_o: Difference between females and males (years)

(and 0.4% in Sweden and Singapore), but rises to almost 300 per 1 000 in Sierra Leone. Levels of child mortality well in excess of 10% (100 per 1 000) are still common throughout Africa and in parts of Asia (Afghanistan, Cambodia, Laos, Myanmar, Nepal and Pakistan).

However, perhaps the widest disparities in mortality occur at the adult ages 15–59 years. In some Southern African countries such as Botswana, Malawi, Namibia, and Zambia, where HIV/AIDS is now a major public health problem, 65% or more of adults who survive to age 15 can be expected to die before age 60 on current mortality rates. In several others (e.g. Burundi, Lesotho, Mozambique, Rwanda, Swaziland and Zimbabwe) the risk exceeds 60%. The dramatic increase in $_{45}q_{15}$ in South Africa is also note-

worthy, with estimated levels of 567 per 1 000 and 502 per 1 000 for males and females respectively in 2000, compared with levels around 250 to 350 per 1 000 females and males respectively in 1990 (21). At the other extreme, $_{45}q_{15}$ levels of 90–100 per 1 000 are common in most developed countries for men, with risks as low as half this again for women.

The increasing disparity between levels of child and adult mortality in recent years is apparent from Figure 28.6 which contrasts average levels of $_5q_0$ with levels of $_{45}q_{15}$ for males and females separately based on the estimated country-specific life tables for 2000. Estimates of uncertainty are included for each point. The systematic departure of patterns of mortality in Eastern European countries, particularly males, from expected levels given the traditional relation-

Figure 28.5 Chances of dying in childhood (0–4 years) and adulthood (15–59 years), by subregion, 2000

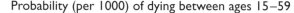

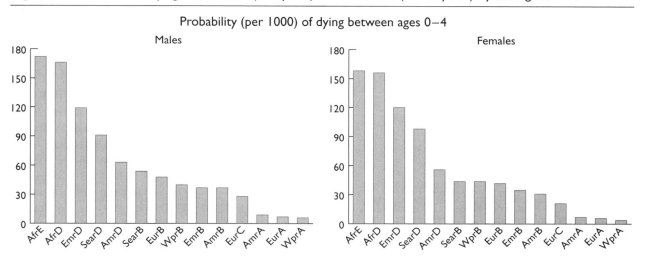

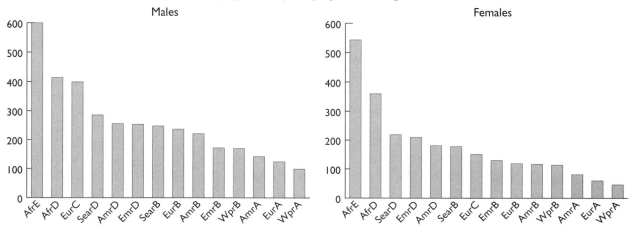

ship between child and adult mortality is clear, as is the vast uncertainty around estimated levels of adult mortality in several, primarily sub-Saharan African countries. By and large, uncertainty around child mortality levels is much less than around adult mortality, reflecting the knowledge gained from the extensive

Table 28.7   Total deaths by sex, age and WHO subregion, 2000

				Age group (years)					
Sex	Total (000)	0–4 (000)	5–14 (000)	15–29 (000)	30–44 (000)	45–59 (000)	60–69 (000)	70–79 (000)	80+ (000)
Both sexes	55 694	10 901	1 444	3 632	5 082	7 007	8 021	10 289	9 317
AFR D	4 245	1 930	187	398	486	379	316	346	203
AFR E	6 327	2 316	250	907	1 198	656	400	391	208
AMR A	2 778	37	9	55	129	308	371	687	1 183
AMR B	2 587	316	36	194	255	387	411	521	467
AMR D	510	119	17	48	55	64	63	76	68
EMR B	690	127	21	50	52	103	112	133	91
EMR D	3 346	1 421	134	208	243	343	357	398	242
EUR A	4 076	27	7	49	120	347	575	1 126	1 824
EUR B	1 952	170	24	67	126	264	370	510	420
EUR C	3 636	57	18	125	295	567	759	967	850
SEAR B	2 142	301	55	191	249	331	370	404	242
SEAR D	12 015	3 012	484	850	1 092	1 714	1 850	1 902	1 110
WPR A	1 152	8	2	16	30	118	179	294	504
WPR B	10 238	1 060	201	475	750	1 427	1 888	2 534	1 903
Males	29 696	5 649	733	1 882	3 026	4 346	4 799	5 504	3 759
AFR D	2 189	1 023	93	165	258	219	169	171	90
AFR E	3 228	1 235	122	357	633	387	216	191	87
AMR A	1 382	21	5	40	84	192	220	371	448
AMR B	1 491	177	21	148	177	240	238	279	212
AMR D	282	65	9	29	34	36	35	41	33
EMR B	387	67	11	32	32	64	65	71	45
EMR D	1 750	723	66	98	134	198	198	209	123
EUR A	2 036	15	4	37	82	233	379	627	659
EUR B	1 053	93	15	46	86	177	224	253	159
EUR C	1 857	33	12	97	229	406	470	409	202
SEAR B	1 185	173	31	122	152	188	203	207	108
SEAR D	6 518	1 489	228	424	646	1 028	1 074	1 052	577
WPR A	626	5	1	11	20	81	124	178	205
WPR B	5 712	529	114	275	459	896	1 184	1 443	812
Females	25 998	5 253	712	1 751	2 056	2 662	3 222	4 786	5 558
AFR D	2 056	907	93	232	228	160	147	175	114
AFR E	3 099	1 081	128	550	566	269	184	200	121
AMR A	1 396	16	4	15	45	116	151	315	735
AMR B	1 096	140	15	46	78	147	173	242	256
AMR D	229	55	8	18	22	28	28	35	36
EMR B	303	60	10	19	21	40	47	61	46
EMR D	1 596	698	68	110	109	145	158	190	119
EUR A	2 040	12	3	12	38	114	197	499	1 165
EUR B	900	77	9	22	40	87	146	257	261
EUR C	1 779	23	6	28	66	160	289	558	648
SEAR B	957	127	23	69	97	142	167	197	134
SEAR D	5 496	1 524	257	427	446	686	776	849	532
WPR A	526	3	1	4	10	37	55	117	299
WPR B	4 526	531	87	200	291	530	704	1 091	1 092

global survey programmes on child mortality levels and determinants over the past decades.

Uncertainty bounds around q_x and l_x tend to widen around young adult ages, particularly in sub-Saharan Africa where reliable direct evidence on adult mortality levels is rare. Indeed, the width of these uncertainty intervals conveys as important a finding as the estimated central value, and argues for urgent investment in measuring adult mortality levels in those countries where the bounds remain unacceptably wide.

An alternative summary index of mortality conditions in a population is the average age of death,

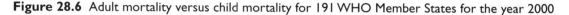

Figure 28.6 Adult mortality versus child mortality for 191 WHO Member States for the year 2000

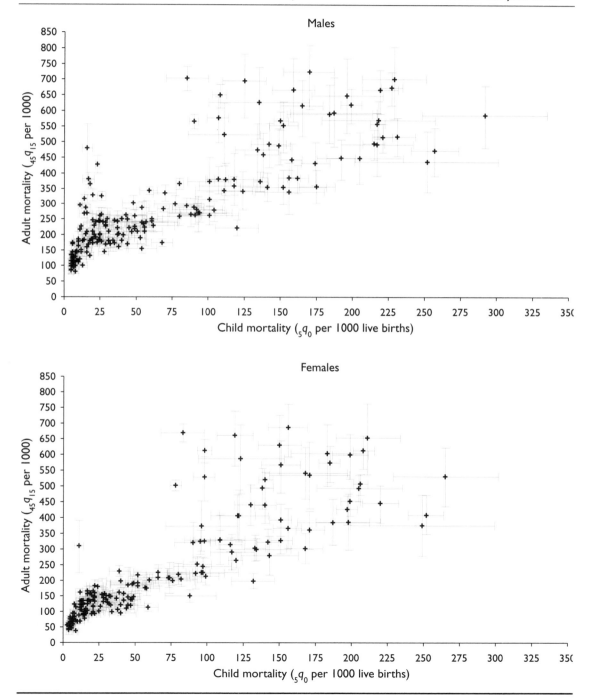

related to the average age of the population. In countries where child mortality is high, both the average age at death and the average age of the population will be comparatively low, and will increase more or less in tandem as health development improves. This is clear from Figure 28.7 which shows the relationship separately for males and females based on the life tables for each country in 2000. Interestingly, beyond an average age of the population of about 30, the average age at death rises somewhat more slowly than at lower average age levels, particularly for females. This no doubt reflects the fact that by the time average age at death reaches 60 years or so, much of the progress in reducing child and adult mortality has been achieved, and hence further reductions will only lead to progressively slower increases in average population age.

Figure 28.7 Average age of death and population, 2000, 191 countries

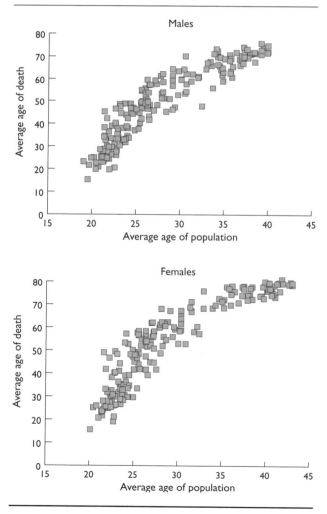

As the Figure also shows, extraordinarily large differences remain in average age at death among WHO Member States in 2000, ranging from as low as 15.5 in Niger (both sexes combined), 19.9 in Afghanistan, 20.3 and 20.5 in Somalia and Sierra Leone, respectively, to almost 80 years in Greece (76.8), Norway (77.1) and Sweden (78.5). This fourfold difference is significantly larger than the range in life expectancy reported earlier.

Just under 56 million people are estimated to have died in 2000, almost 30 million of whom were males (Table 28.7). Worldwide, 10.9 million children below age 5 died in that year, about 3/4 of them in developing regions of Africa and South Asia. Another 10 million or so died in each of the oldest age groups 70–79 and 80+, the vast majority in the lower mortality A, B and C subregions. There were many more deaths in young adults ages 15–59 years (15.6 million), than in children ages 0–14 years (12.3 million), emphasizing the need for a more expansive view of policies to prevent premature death to address leading causes of young adult death as well.

Worldwide, life expectancy at birth in 2000 was estimated at 64.9 years (62.7 for males, 67.2 for females) (Table 28.8). The very substantial differences in age patterns of mortality among subregions evident from Table 28.7 translate into wide variations in average regional life expectancy, with levels ranging from just over 44 years (both sexes) in AfrD where HIV/AIDS is highly prevalent, to an average level almost twice as high (80.9 years) in WprA. Average life expectancies of 70 years or more were obtained

Table 28.8 Life expectancy at birth (years) by WHO subregion, 2000

Subregion	Males	Females	Both sexes
AfrD	50.3	52.4	51.3
AfrE	43.5	45.2	44.3
AmrA	74.1	79.6	76.9
AmrB	67.5	74.5	70.9
AmrD	63.5	68.4	65.9
EmrB	68.6	71.6	70.0
EmrD	59.1	61.0	60.0
EurA	74.8	81.2	78.0
EurB	65.5	72.3	68.8
EurC	60.3	72.1	66.0
SearB	64.1	68.9	66.4
SearD	59.7	62.4	61.0
WprA	77.3	84.2	80.9
WprB	68.2	72.7	70.4
World	62.7	67.2	64.9

in six subregions, but interestingly not in EurB or C. In particular, average male life expectancy at birth in EurC was barely 60 years, among the lowest of any subregion in the world outside of Africa.

DISCUSSION

The life table and its associated parameters are key inputs into the assessment of how well or poorly heath systems are performing. Life tables have numerous other uses in epidemiology, demography, and economics, and the availability of annual, current life tables for all 192 WHO Member States should improve the quality and relevance of the analytical base for such uses. Careful evaluation of the data upon which life tables are to be constructed is essential if the results are to be used with any confidence. This report has tried to set out the countries for which vital registration appears to be working sufficiently well to prepare life tables with no, or very minimal adjustments to data. For countries where this is not the case, we have outlined the procedures used to adjust the data, but the results obtained are very much dependent on a considered judgement of the evidence. This degree of subjectivity is unavoidable given current demographic practices for adjusting data, and further work is required to explore how formal statistical methods might be better applied to reduce this subjectivity in judging the extent of under-enumeration of deaths.

This analysis has also highlighted the vast degree of uncertainty and ignorance that exists with respect to levels and patterns of adult mortality in developing countries. For one-third of WHO's Member States, probably accounting for a similar proportion of deaths, little or nothing is reliably known about levels of adult mortality, particularly among younger adults below age 60. For these countries, there is little alternative but to follow the classical demographic approach of constructing adult mortality levels from child mortality rates on the assumption that the two are linked in some predictable fashion. However, evidence from the past 30 years or so suggests that this is not necessarily the case as new hazards such as HIV have emerged, or old ones, such as alcohol abuse, have become more extreme in some populations. We have attempted to avoid such distortions by using the modified logit life table system to estimate adult death rates, but the results will remain uncertain until verification is eventually possible from systems which reliably capture deaths.

It is unlikely that such systems will be established in the near future in the countries where they are needed. Yet good estimates of adult mortality are required now for planning and monitoring in the health sector. Questions on deaths occurring in households, when asked with sufficient care and rigour, can yield useful, current data on adult mortality levels and patterns, and should be routinely added to censuses and surveys. The ongoing WHO World Health Survey will provide an ideal opportunity to expand our knowledge of adult mortality. At the same time, a focus on collecting data on child survival in the handful of countries (Category V) where no recent data are available will greatly assist programmes concerned with child health promotion.

REFERENCES

(1) Hill K et al. *Trends in child mortality in the developing world: 1960–1996.* New York, Division of Evaluation and Planning, UNICEF, 1999.

(2) Ahmad OB, Lopez AD, Inoue M. The decline in child mortality: a reappraisal. *Bulletin of the World Health Organization,* 2000, 78:1175–1191.

(3) United Nations. *World population prospects: the 2000 revision.* New York, United Nations, 2001.

(4) U.S. Census Bureau. *International data base (IDB).* Washington, DC, U.S. Census Bureau Population Division, International Programs Center (IPC), 2002. URL: http://www.census.gov/ipc/www/ibdnew.html.

(5) World Bank. *World development indicators 2001.* Washington, DC, World Bank, 2001.

(6) Bhat PN. Recent trends in fertility and mortality in India: critical reappraisal of data from sample registration system and national family health surveys. In: Srinivasan K, Vlassoff M, eds. *Population and development nexus in India: challenges for the new millennium.* New Delhi, Tata McGraw-Hill, 2001.

(7) Murray CJL et al. Modified logit life table system: principles, empirical validation, and application. In: Murray CJL, Evans DB, eds. *Health systems performance assessment: debates, methods and empiricism.* Geneva, World Health Organization, 2003.

(8) Lopez AD et al. *World mortality in 2000: life tables for 191 countries.* Geneva, World Health Organization, 2002.

(9) Brass W. On the scale of mortality. In: Brass W, ed. *Biological aspects of mortality.* London, Taylor & Francis, 1971.

(10) Martin LG. A modification for use in destabilized populations of Brass' technique for estimating completeness of registration. *Population Studies*, 1980, 34:381–395.

(11) Bennet NG, Horiuchi S. Mortality estimation from registered deaths in less developed countries. *Demography*, 1984, 21:217–234.

(12) Preston SH. Use of direct and indirect techniques for estimating the completeness of death registration systems. In: United Nations, ed. *Data bases for mortality measurement*. New York, United Nations, 1984:143–153.

(13) Chinese Academy of Preventive Medicine. *Annual report on the disease surveillance system, 1996*. Beijing, 1997.

(14) Salomon JA, Murray CJL. Modelling HIV/AIDS epidemics in sub-Saharan Africa using seroprevalence data from antenatal clinics. *Bulletin of the World Health Organization*, 2001, 79:586–692.

(15) Lopez AD et al. *Life tables for 191 countries: data, methods and results*. EIP Discussion Paper No. 9. Geneva, World Health Organization, 2000. URL: http://www3.who.int/whosis/discussion_papers/discussion_papers.cfm#

(16) Coale A, Guo G. Revised regional model life tables at very low levels of mortality. *Population Index*, 1989, 55:613–643.

(17) Perks W. On some experiments on the graduation of mortality statistics. *Journal of the Institute of Actuaries*, 1932, 63:12–57.

(18) Stanton E, Abderrahim A, Hill K. An assessment of DHS maternal mortality indicators. *Studies in Family Planning*, 2000, 31:111–124.

(19) Salomon JA et al. *Methods for life expectancy and healthy life expectancy uncertainty analysis*. EIP Discussion Paper No. 10. Geneva, World Health Organization, 2001. URL: http://www3.who.int/whosis/discussion_papers/discussion_papers.cfm#

(20) Lopez AD. The sex mortality differential in developed countries. In: Lopez AD, Ruzicka LT, eds. *Sex differentials in mortality: trends, determinants, and consequences*. Canberra, Australian National University Press, 1983.

(21) Timaeus IM. Mortality in sub-Saharan Africa. In: Chamie J, Cliquet RL, eds. *Health and mortality. Issues of global concern*. New York, United Nations Population Division, 1999: 110–131.

Table 28.9 Availability of vital registration data on mortality in the WHO database, 1980–2000 (as of 15 September 2001)

Country	80	81	82	83	84	85	86	87	88	89	90	91	92	93	94	95	96	97	98	99	00
Category I: Complete vital statistics (coverage 95%+)																					
Andorra													x		x	x	x	x	x		x
Antigua and Barbuda				x			x	x			x	x	x	x	x	x					
Argentina	x	x	x	x	x	x	x	x	x	x	x	x	x	x	x	x	x			x	
Australia	x	x	x	x	x	x	x	x	x	x	x	x	x	x	x	x	x	x	x		
Austria	x	x	x	x	x	x	x	x	x	x	x	x	x	x	x	x	x	x	x	x	x
Bahamas	x	x	x	x	x	x	x	x	x	x	x	x	x	x	x	x	x	x			
Bahrain	x	x	x		x	x	x	x	x	x	x	x	x	x	x		x	x	x	x	x
Barbados	x	x	x	x	x	x	x	x	x	x	x	x	x	x	x	x	x				
Belarus		x	x	x	x	x	x	x	x	x	x	x	x	x	x	x	x	x	x	x	
Belgium	x	x	x	x	x	x	x	x	x	x	x	x	x	x	x	x	x	x			
Bosnia and Herzegovina						x	x	x	x	x	x	x									
Bulgaria	x	x	x	x	x	x	x	x	x	x	x	x	x	x	x	x	x	x	x	x	
Canada	x	x	x	x	x	x	x	x	x	x	x	x	x	x	x	x	x	x			
Chile	x	x	x	x	x	x	x	x	x	x	x	x	x	x	x	x	x	x			
Cook Islands	x	x	x	x	x	x	x	x	x	x	x	x	x	x	x	x	x	x	x	x	
Costa Rica	x	x	x	x	x	x	x	x	x	x	x	x	x	x	x	x		x		x	
Croatia		x	x	x	x	x	x	x	x	x	x	x	x	x	x	x	x	x	x		
Cuba	x	x	x	x	x	x	x	x	x	x	x	x	x	x	x	x	x	x	x		
Cyprus	x	x	x	x	x	x	x	x	x	x	x	x	x	x	x	x	x	x			
Czech Republic	x	x	x	x	x	x	x	x	x	x	x	x	x	x	x	x	x	x	x	x	x
Denmark	x	x	x	x	x	x	x	x	x	x	x	x	x	x	x	x	x	x			
Dominica	x	x	x	x	x	x	x	x	x	x	x	x	x	x	x						
Estonia		x	x	x	x	x	x	x	x	x	x	x	x	x	x	x	x	x	x	x	
Fiji	x	x	x	x	x	x	x	x					x	x	x	x	x	x	x	x	
Finland	x	x	x	x	x	x	x	x	x	x	x	x	x	x	x	x	x	x			

continued

Table 28.9 Availability of vital registration data on mortality in the WHO database, 1980–2000 (as of 15 September 2001) *(continued)*

Country	80	81	82	83	84	85	86	87	88	89	90	91	92	93	94	95	96	97	98	99	00
France	x	x	x	x	x	x	x	x	x	x	x	x	x	x	x	x	x	x	x		
Germany	x	x	x	x	x	x	x	x	x	x	x	x	x	x	x	x	x	x	x	x	
Greece	x	x	x	x	x	x	x	x	x	x	x	x	x	x	x	x	x	x	x		
Grenada					x				x							x	x	x			
Hungary	x	x	x	x	x	x	x	x	x	x	x	x	x	x	x	x	x	x	x	x	x
Iceland	x	x	x	x	x	x	x	x	x	x	x	x	x	x	x	x	x	x	x		
Ireland	x	x	x	x	x	x	x	x	x	x	x	x	x	x	x	x	x	x	x		
Israel	x	x	x	x	x	x	x	x	x	x	x	x	x	x	x	x	x	x	x		
Italy	x	x	x	x	x	x	x	x	x	x	x	x	x	x	x	x	x	x	x		
Jamaica	x	x	x	x	x	x	x	x	x	x	x										
Japan	x	x	x	x	x	x	x	x	x	x		x	x	x	x	x	x	x			
Kuwait	x	x	x	x	x	x	x	x	x	x		x	x	x	x	x	x	x	x	x	
Latvia	x	x	x	x	x	x	x	x	x	x	x	x	x	x	x	x	x	x	x	x	
Lithuania		x	x	x	x	x	x	x	x	x	x	x	x	x	x	x	x	x	x	x	
Luxembourg	x	x	x	x	x	x	x	x	x	x	x	x	x	x	x	x	x	x	x	x	x
Malta	x	x	x	x	x	x	x	x	x	x	x	x	x	x	x	x	x	x	x		
Mauritius	x	x	x	x	x	x	x	x	x	x	x	x	x	x	x	x	x	x	x	x	
Mexico	x	x	x	x	x	x	x	x	x	x	x	x	x	x	x	x	x	x			x
Monaco		x	x	x			x	x													
Netherlands	x	x	x	x	x	x	x	x	x	x	x	x	x	x	x	x	x	x	x	x	
New Zealand	x	x	x	x	x	x	x	x	x	x	x	x	x	x	x	x	x	x	x		
Norway	x	x	x	x	x	x	x	x	x	x	x	x	x	x	x	x	x	x	x		
Poland	x	x	x	x	x	x	x	x	x	x	x	x	x	x	x	x	x	x	x	x	
Portugal	x	x	x	x	x	x	x	x	x	x	x	x	x	x	x	x	x	x	x	x	
Qatar		x	x	x		x	x	x	x	x		x	x	x	x	x	x	x			
Republic of Moldova		x	x	x	x	x	x	x	x	x	x	x	x	x	x	x	x	x	x	x	
Romania	x	x	x	x	x	x	x	x	x	x	x	x	x	x	x	x	x	x	x	x	
Russian Federation	x	x	x	x	x	x	x	x	x	x	x	x	x	x	x	x	x	x	x	x	
Saint Kitts and Nevis	x	x	x	x	x	x	x	x	x	x		x	x	x	x						
Saint Lucia	x	x	x	x	x	x	x	x	x	x		x	x	x	x						
Saint Vincent and the Grenadines	x		x	x	x	x	x	x				x				x	x				
San Marino	x	x	x	x	x	x	x	x	x	x	x	x	x	x	x	x	x	x	x		
Serbia and Montenegro		x	x	x	x	x	x	x	x	x	x	x	x	x	x	x	x	x			
Seychelles	x	x	x	x	x	x	x	x	x	x	x	x	x	x	x	x	x	x			
Singapore	x	x	x	x	x	x	x	x	x	x	x	x	x	x	x	x	x	x	x	x	x
Slovakia		x	x	x	x	x	x	x	x	x	x	x	x	x	x	x	x	x	x	x	
Slovenia		x	x	x	x	x	x	x	x	x	x	x	x	x	x	x	x	x	x	x	
Spain	x	x	x	x	x	x	x	x	x	x	x	x	x	x	x	x	x	x	x		
Sri Lanka	x	x	x	x	x	x	x	x	x	x		x	x	x	x	x	x				
Suriname	x	x	x	x	x	x	x	x	x	x	x	x	x	x	x	x	x	x			
Sweden	x	x	x	x	x	x	x	x	x	x	x	x	x	x	x	x	x	x	x		x
Switzerland	x	x	x	x	x	x	x	x	x	x	x	x	x	x	x	x	x	x	x		
TFYR Macedonia		x	x	x	x	x	x	x	x	x	x	x	x	x	x	x	x	x			
Tonga																x	x	x			
Trinidad and Tobago	x	x	x	x	x	x	x	x	x	x	x	x	x	x	x						
Ukraine		x	x	x	x	x	x	x	x	x	x	x	x	x	x	x	x	x	x	x	x
United Kingdom	x	x	x	x	x	x	x	x	x	x	x	x	x	x	x	x	x	x	x	x	
United States of America	x	x	x	x	x	x	x	x	x	x	x	x	x	x	x	x	x	x	x	x	
Uruguay	x	x	x	x	x	x	x	x	x	x	x	x	x			x	x	x	x		
Venezuela	x	x	x	x	x	x	x	x	x	x	x	x	x	x	x						

continued

Table 28.9   Availability of vital registration data on mortality in the WHO database, 1980–2000 (as of 15 September 2001) *(continued)*

Country	80	81	82	83	84	85	86	87	88	89	90	91	92	93	94	95	96	97	98	99	00
Category II: Incomplete vital statistics																					
Albania	x				x	x	x	x	x	x	x	x	x	x	x	x	x	x	x		
Algeria	x	x	x			x	x														
Armenia		x	x			x	x	x	x	x	x	x	x	x	x	x	x	x	x	x	
Azerbaijan		x	x	x	x	x	x	x	x	x	x	x	x	x	x	x	x	x	x	x	x
Belize	x	x	x	x	x	x	x	x	x	x	x	x	x	x	x	x					
Brazil	x	x	x	x	x	x	x	x	x	x	x	x	x	x	x	x					
Brunei Darussalam		x	x	x	x	x	x	x	x	x	x	x	x	x	x	x	x	x	x	x	x
Cape Verde	x	x	x	x	x	x					x	x							x		
Colombia		x	x	x	x	x	x	x	x	x	x	x	x	x	x	x					
Dominican Republic	x	x	x	x	x	x												x	x	x	
Ecuador	x	x	x	x	x	x	x	x	x	x	x	x	x	x	x	x	x	x	x		
Egypt	x	x	x	x	x	x	x	x	x	x	x	x	x	x	x	x				x	
El Salvador	x	x	x	x	x	x	x	x	x	x	x	x	x		x	x	x	x			
Georgia		x	x	x	x	x	x	x	x	x	x	x	x		x	x	x				
Guatemala	x	x	x	x	x	x	x	x	x			x	x	x		x	x	x			
Guyana				x											x	x	x	x			
Honduras	x	x	x	x	x																
Iran (Islamic Republic of)			x	x	x	x	x					x			x	x	x	x	x	x	
Jordan	x													x					x		
Kazakhstan		x	x	x	x	x	x	x	x	x	x	x	x	x	x	x	x	x	x	x	
Kyrgyzstan		x	x	x	x	x	x	x	x	x	x	x	x	x	x	x	x	x	x	x	
Lao People's Dem. Republic															x						
Malaysia											x	x	x	x	x	x	x	x	x		
Maldives					x	x	x	x	x	x	x	x	x	x		x	x	x	x		
Marshall Islands							x	x	x	x	x	x	x	x	x	x	x	x			
Mongolia								x	x	x		x	x	x	x	x	x	x			
Morocco								x	x	x	x	x	x	x	x	x	x	x	x		
Nepal		x										x									
Nicaragua								x	x	x	x	x	x	x		x	x	x			
Niue	x	x	x	x	X	x	x	x	x	x	x	x	x	x	x	x	x	x			
Palau						x		x	x	x	x	x	x	x	x	x	x	x	x		
Panama	x	x	x	x	x	x	x	x	x	x	x	x	x	x	x	x	x	x			
Papua New Guinea	x	x	x	x	x			x	x	x	x	x	x	x	x	x	x	x	x		
Paraguay	x	x	x	x	x	x	x	x	x	x	x	x	x		x						
Peru	x	x	x	x	x	x	x	x	x	x											
Philippines	x	x	x	x	x	x	x	x	x	x	x	x	x	x	x	x	x				
Republic of Korea	x	x	x	x	x	x	x	x	x	x	x	x	x	x	x	x	x	x	x		
Samoa	x												x	x							
South Africa														x	x	x					
Syrian Arab Republic				x	x	x													x		x
Tajikistan		x	x			x	x	x	x	x	x	x	x	x	x		x				
Thailand	x	x	x	x	x	x	x	x	x	x	x	x	x	x	x	x	x	x	x		
Tunisia	x						x	x	x					x	x	x		x	x		
Turkey												x	x	x	x	x	x	x			
Turkmenistan		x	x			x	x	x	x	x	x	x	x	x	x	x	x	x	x		
Tuvalu												x	x	x	x						
Uzbekistan		x	x	x	x	x	x	x	x	x	x	x	x	x	x	x	x	x	x		
Viet Nam										x										x	
Zimbabwe			x								x	x	x	x		x		x			

continued

Table 28.9 Availability of vital registration data on mortality in the WHO database, 1980–2000 (as of 15 September 2001) *(continued)*

Country	80	81	82	83	84	85	86	87	88	89	90	91	92	93	94	95	96	97	98	99	00
Category III: Sample registration and surveillance systems																					
Bangladesh											x	x	x	x	x	x	x	x	x	x	
China								x	x	x	x	x	x	x	x	x	x	x	x	x	
India											x	x	x	x	x	x	x	x	x		
United Rep. of Tanzania													x	x	x	x	x	x	x	x	

Chapter 29

Modified Logit Life Table System: Principles, Empirical Validation, and Application

Christopher J.L. Murray, Brodie D. Ferguson, Alan D. Lopez,
Michel Guillot, Joshua A. Salomon, Omar B. Ahmad

Introduction

Model life table systems (*1–3*) are used extensively in demographic, epidemiological and economic analyses. Probably the most widespread use is to infer age patterns of adult mortality, about which comparatively little is known in developing countries, from levels of child mortality, which are much more reliably documented (*4*). Yet, substantial evidence has accumulated that such model life table systems do not adequately represent the range of age-specific patterns that are empirically observed. The routine use of split-level modifications of the Coale-Demeny and the United Nations model life table systems is one manifestation of the inadequacy of the original models for current estimation purposes. Concomitantly, there has been a major expansion of empirically observed data on age-specific mortality in countries with complete or very nearly complete registration systems over the last 30 years (*5*). These data provide an opportunity to improve the widely used model life table systems through a reappraisal of age patterns of mortality that have been observed in such populations.

In this chapter, we present the development and testing of a new model life table system based on a modification of the Brass logit life table system (*2*). The first section briefly reviews some of the main uses of model life tables and consequently the requirements for a good model life table system. Section two reviews the main two-parameter model life table systems, emphasizing the Coale-Demeny, United Nations and Brass systems. In the third section, we present the logic and mathematical foundation for a modification of the Brass logit life table system. The dataset of high quality life tables which provides the empirical basis for the development of the modified logit system is reviewed in section four. Details of the empirical esti-

mation of the modified logit life table system as well as basic information on the robustness of the model are given in section five. Section six provides a direct empirical assessment of the adequacy and predictive power of the Coale-Demeny, Brass logit and modified logit systems, as well as a discussion of the limitations and implications of this work.

Uses and Required Properties for Model Life Table Systems

Understanding the strengths and weaknesses of model life table systems and thus the direction for an improved system should start with a clear articulation of the multiple uses of model life tables. Model life tables are used extensively for smoothing data, incorporating age-specific mortality patterns in various indirect estimation techniques such as sibling or parental survival, and forecasting age-specific mortality rates (*1;3;6*). One of the most important uses of model life tables is in routine demographic estimation work in settings where complete vital registration is not available. A complete life table often is estimated with information only on child mortality or child mortality and some measure of adult mortality experience derived from censuses or surveys. Another important use of model life tables is in the economic appraisal of health interventions when the benefits of an intervention must be modelled in the context of general levels of mortality.

Model life tables are not models in the usual sense of the word. They are not causal theories or statistical models. Rather, model life tables can be thought of in terms of a representation theorem. The central thesis is that the complex phenomenon of age-specific mortality rates can be adequately represented by two or three parameters such as model family and level. Being able to represent a full schedule of mortality by age with two or three pieces of information simplifies the understanding of mortality patterns and has proven to have multiple analytical uses in many fields. Thinking of model life tables in these terms may help in formulating appropriate empirical tests of the adequacy of a model life table system.

We propose at least three required properties for a model life table system. The first required property is that it be simple and easily used. In practice, this means that a model life table system should use, at most, two parameters to define a unique life table. More complicated systems may perform better on the second and third criteria described below but the fact remains that such systems have not been widely used in applied work. We include in the category of two-parameter systems: the Coale-Demeny family of life tables, the United Nations models, the Brass logit system and the Ledermann system (7). The Coale-Demeny and United Nations systems are *de facto* two-parameter systems, with the choice of family being one parameter and the level being the second parameter. The Brass logit system when a single global standard is used has two parameters, α and β. When multiple standards are used, it becomes a three-parameter system.

Second, any two-parameter model life table system should also adequately capture the true range of age-specific mortality patterns seen in real populations. In other words, model life table systems should not under-represent the extent to which mortality by age can vary across populations. For example, if one looks at child mortality measured using $_5q_0$ plotted against adult mortality measured using $_{45}q_{15}$ in populations with good vital registration data, how much of the diversity of this pattern is captured in the model life table system?

Third, when a model life table system is used to select a life table to represent mortality by age for a population, how close a fit is there between the predicted mortality rates and actual mortality rates? The fit between predicted and actual can be assessed in many ways such as the root mean squared error in the death rates (or log of death rates), the explained variance or the average relative error in age-specific death rates. Formal assessment of the predictive power of a model life table system should be an absolute requirement to judge its adequacy.

There are other uses and therefore other criteria that can be proposed to evaluate a model life table system. For this chapter, however, we focus on two-parameter systems and more formally assess the range

of age-specific mortality patterns they capture and their predictive power.

Two-Parameter Model Life Table Systems

The basic objective in the creation of any model life table is to construct a system that gives mortality rates by sex and age, defined by a small number of parameters that capture the level as well as the age pattern of mortality. If a particular model adequately represents reality, the characteristics of a given population can be summarized by the parameters of that model, thereby facilitating the study of variation among populations or within a population over time. The principles underlying each of the existing model life tables are discussed below.

United Nations

The first set of model life tables was published by the United Nations in 1955 (8). This was a relatively simple one-parameter system indexed on infant mortality levels. Subsequently, the United Nations published a revised set of model life tables in 1981, which included an attempt to construct regional models using data from developing countries judged adequate for inclusion in the empirical dataset. Five families of models were identified, each with a set of tables producing life expectancies ranging from 35 to 75 years for each sex. Although the revision, technically, remains a one-parameter system, it could be argued that the choice of a family constitutes a separate dimension.

The revised UN model life tables for developing countries, while clearly an improvement over the one-parameter system, also have important limitations (9). The relatively small number of empirical life tables (72) limits the applicability of the models to other populations.

Coale and Demeny

Perhaps the most widely used model life table system has been the Coale-Demeny regional model life tables (1). First published in 1966, they were derived from a set of 326 life tables, by sex, from actual populations. Four typical age patterns of mortality were identified, determined largely by the shape of their mortality schedules (corresponding to the geographical location of the population), but also on the basis of their patterns of deviations from previously estimated regression equations. Those patterns were called: North,

South, East and West. As with the revised UN life tables, we consider the Coale-Demeny system to have two parameters, with the second parameter being choice of family. The system was updated in 1989, primarily to include extensions of the model life tables to age 100+ (10).

Strict standards of accuracy imposed in the construction of the Coale-Demeny model life tables limited the number of non-European countries represented. As such, the Coale-Demeny tables may not cover patterns of mortality existing in the contemporary developing world. In fact, there are well-documented examples of mortality patterns that lie outside the range of the Coale-Demeny tables (11). The fact that one of the parameters of the Coale-Demeny system (the "family") is discrete restricts the flexibility of the system, certainly in comparison to other systems where both parameters are continuous.

LEDERMANN

The Ledermann system of model life tables was first published in 1959 and was subsequently revised over the course of the following decade (7). This system is based on a factor analysis of some 157 empirical tables. The method of selection was less rigid than that of the Coale-Demeny tables, and more developing country experiences are represented.

The primary criticism regarding the Ledermann system is its relative complexity, which essentially precludes its use in most developing countries. Even though it does provide some flexibility through a wider variety of entry values, in practice most of these values are not easily estimated for most developing countries. A second major limitation is that the independent variables used in deriving the model refer, with only one exception, to parameters obtained from data on both sexes combined. The user is therefore forced to accept the relationships between male and female mortality embodied in the model even when there is evidence to the contrary. For instance, it is nearly impossible to estimate a Ledermann model life table in which the male expectation of life exceeds that of females.

BRASS

A different approach to constructing life table systems was first proposed by Brass in 1971 (2). The Brass logit life table system belongs to a category of mortality models called relational models. It features a standard life table and two parameters that, through a mathematical transformation, relate any life table to the standard. The general shape of the survivorship

functions is captured through the mortality standard while the parameters help to capture deviations from the standard.

The Brass system rests on the assumption that two distinct age-patterns of mortality can be related to each other by a linear relationship between the logits of their respective survivorship probabilities. Thus, for any two observed survivorship functions, l_x and l_x^s, where the latter is the standard, it is possible to find constants α and β such that

$$\text{Logit}(l_x) = \alpha + \beta \text{Logit}(l_x^s)$$

where
$$\text{Logit}(l_x) = 0.5 \ln\left(\frac{1.0 - l_x}{l_x}\right)$$

for all ages x greater than 0. If the above equation holds for every pair of life tables, then any life table can be generated from a single standard life table by changing the pairs of (α, β) values used.

In reality, the assumption of linearity is only approximately satisfied by pairs of actual life tables. Deviations from linearity appear to be particularly large when the observed mortality of a population is far from that of the standard. Thus, the complexity of variations in levels and age patterns of mortality is not fully captured by the logit system. This observation led authors to modify Brass' original model by including additional parameters that allow for bends in the survivorship function (12;13). These modifications, however, are of limited practical use, because the additional parameters are difficult to estimate empirically and complicate the application of the models.

It is clear, therefore, that there are serious technical considerations in the use of existing empirical models to describe mortality patterns in contemporary developing countries. We are proposing a new modified two-parameter system of model life tables anchored on the logit system. The choice of the logit system was based on a careful comparative evaluation of the logit and the Coale-Demeny systems, presented in a subsequent section.

MODIFICATION OF THE BRASS LOGIT SYSTEM

We can generalize the principle underlying Brass' approach to postulate that there is some transformation of the survivorship function such that all transformed survivorship functions are linear functions of each other. Formally:

$$\Gamma(l_x) = \alpha + \beta \ \Gamma(l_x^s) \qquad [1]$$

If the transformation Γ can be identified, then all survivorship functions can be derived simply from the parameters α and β. Brass's original proposal was that this transformation is a variant of a logit transformation such that:

$$\Gamma(l_x) = 0.5\ln\left(\frac{1-l_x}{l_x}\right) \text{ for all } x > 0 \text{ (and } l_0 = 1.0) \quad [2]$$

The problem is that the logit transformation does not completely linearize the relationship between many survivorship functions. In developing the modified logit model life table system, we sought to identify a transformation that would better linearize the relationships between most survivorship curves without adding the complexity of additional parameters as in previous extensions of the Brass system (*12;13*).

Our modification of Brass' transformation is based upon some simple but powerful empirical observations. The basic observation is that deviations from linearity follow some specific regularities which can be modelled in relation to the amount of mortality change between the standard and the observed life table. These shifts in the structure of mortality can be illustrated by plotting a series of logit life table values against logit values taken from an earlier life table, and examining how the resulting curves depart from linearity. This is shown in Figure 29.1, which presents data for USA males. In this figure, annual logit life table values from 1900 to 1995 are plotted against

Figure 29.1   Annual logit life table values (1900–95) vs. 1900 logit values (US males)

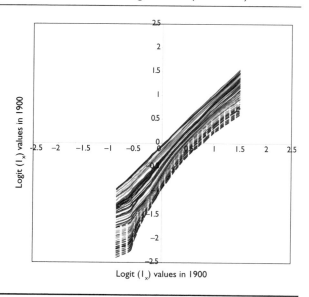

Logit (l_x) values in 1900

logit values for 1900, taken as the standard. It is clear that mortality change over time leads to a change in the age pattern of mortality that is not fully captured by the logit relational model. Indeed, if the logit transformation were fully appropriate, the successive plots in the figure would remain linear over time. Our modification of Brass' transformation is based upon the observation that differences between observed and predicted logit values follow a pattern that is predictable as the mortality level of the observed life table deviates from that of the standard. That is, deviations from linearity in the original Brass model are linked to the relative difference between the mortality rate of the standard and the mortality of the actual life table being estimated.

Empirical investigation of the differences between observed and predicted age-specific mortality rates using the Brass logit transformation with a global standard revealed that this systematic error at each age was related to both the level of child mortality relative to the standard and the level of middle-age adult mortality relative to the standard. Based on this finding, a variety of alternative transformations were investigated. Ultimately, based on multiple tests, the transformation that we have selected is:

$$\Gamma(l_x) = \text{Logit}(l_x) + \gamma_x\left(1 - \left(\frac{\text{Logit}(l_5)}{\text{Logit}(l_5^s)}\right)\right) + \theta_x\left(1 - \left(\frac{\text{Logit}(l_{60})}{\text{Logit}(l_{60}^s)}\right)\right) \quad [3]$$

Thus, the modified transformation includes three standard functions, l_x^s, θ_x and γ_x, which are age- and sex-specific, but invariant across populations. The following sections describe the estimation of these functions.

LIFE TABLE DATASET

Since the 1960's, the World Health Organization has systematically collected vital registration data on causes of death in countries, making every effort to complete the series back to 1950. For most countries, the most recent data refer to the period 1998–2000 (*5*). The data for most countries contain the number of deaths by age, sex and cause, classified according to the Revision of the International Classification of Diseases in use. Data are collected by the conventional 5-year age groups (0, 1–4, 5–9, ..., 85+), although in recent years the terminal age group has been extended to 100+. For each year, mid-year population estimates by age and sex are also provided by reporting countries. These data have been screened for completeness using standard demographic tests, and only those country-years for which mortality was considered complete have been retained for this analysis.

This dataset was supplemented by life tables from two other sources. The historical life tables compiled by Preston, Keyfitz and Schoen (14) were added to the dataset for years not covered by the WHO mortality dataset. The mortality data underlying these life tables had been adjusted, where necessary, for under-reporting. To improve the coverage of developing countries in the dataset, the adjusted national life tables used by the United Nations (3) to produce their model life tables were also added. As more high quality data for developing countries become available, the model life table parameters can be re-estimated. An important initiative to generate age-specific mortality rates for defined populations, primarily in sub-Saharan Africa, is the INDEPTH network (International Network for the continuous Demographic Evaluation of Populations and their Health in developing countries). The first results of this collaboration have recently been published (15) and while the levels of adult mortality in many sites are undoubtedly under-reported, the Network offers considerable promise for rapidly improving knowledge about adult mortality in Africa.

Apart from the criteria of completeness and age- and sex-specific detail, we also applied criteria to exclude life tables of populations during periods of war or those affected by the Spanish influenza pandemic of 1918–19. Data for years prior to 1900 were excluded since the age patterns of mortality tended to be atypical. Small populations with a total size of less than one million people (both sexes combined) were also excluded to minimize the effects of random fluctuations in death rates.

The resulting set of 1 802 life tables used to develop and test the model are shown in Table 29.1. There is, of course, a preponderance of countries from Europe, North America and Australasia, but among the 63 countries represented, about one-third belong to developing regions. For several developed countries, historical datasets back to the beginning of the century have been included. Unfortunately, there is very little empirical data from Africa and most of Asia included in the final life table set used to develop the model. The application of the model to these populations will therefore be more uncertain than elsewhere.

Table 29.2 summarizes the characteristics of the life tables included in the dataset. The mean life expectancies are relatively high (67.5 years for males, 73.4 for females), reflecting the developed country bias, although the range of life expectancies (27 to 77 years for males, 29 to 84 years for females) encom-

pass the experience of all countries (5). Average levels of child and adult mortality are not too dissimilar to what is observed in many developing countries today, and again the range of values more than encompasses estimated levels across all developing countries, with the exception of a few countries in Africa (Namibia, Botswana, Zambia) where female mortality from HIV is extreme.

EMPIRICAL ESTIMATION OF GLOBAL STANDARD, θ_x AND γ_x

ESTIMATING θ_x AND γ_x

By rewriting equations 3 and 1, we can express the age-specific parameters θ_x and γ_x and the country-year-specific parameters α_{ij} and β_{ij} (where i represents country and j year) in a way that allows estimation of the parameter values using OLS regression:

$$\text{Logit}(l_x^{ij}) = \alpha_{ij} + \beta_{ij} \cdot \text{Logit}(l_x^s) + \gamma_x \left(1 - \left(\frac{\text{Logit}(l_5^{ij})}{\text{Logit}(l_5^s)}\right)\right)$$
$$+ \theta_x \left(1 - \left(\frac{\text{Logit}(l_{60}^{ij})}{\text{Logit}(l_{60}^s)}\right)\right) \qquad [4]$$

The last two terms of equation 4 are designed to control for the mortality differential between the standard life table and an observed life table. The first of these captures the effect of differences in child mortality (relative to the standard) while the second captures differences in adult mortality up to age 60. The standard life table used is a sex-specific global standard calculated by taking the average of all sex-specific life tables included in the dataset. As the typical deviation from the standard is neither in the same direction nor of the same magnitude across age groups, θ and γ vary by age but are constant across countries and years.

We have estimated the model parameters by repeated sampling of a randomly selected subset of approximately 70% of the country-years in the full life table dataset (1 261 life tables). The remaining 30% of the empirical observations were reserved for validation purposes, as described below. We ran separate regressions by sex in order to estimate simultaneously the α_{ij} and β_{ij} for each country-year life table and the set of θ_x and γ_x, for all ages except 5 and 60 using OLS regression. After comparing the results of several alternatives, we found it marginally advantageous to set θ_5, γ_5, θ_{60} and γ_{60} to zero in the estimation for identification purposes. The resulting θ_x and γ_x, are

Table 29.1   Life tables comprising the empirical dataset

Country	Year(s)	Total number	Country	Year(s)	Total number
Argentina	1966–70, 77–79, 82–97	48	Latvia	1980–98	38
Australia	1911, 1921, 1950–97	100	Lithuania	1981–98	36
Austria	1955–99	90	Macedonia	1982–97	32
Belarus	1981–98	36	Mauritius	1990–98	18
Belgium	1954–98	90	Mexico	1958–59, 1969–73, 1981–83, 1985–98	48
Bangladesh (Matlab Region)	1975	2	Netherlands	1950–98	98
Bulgaria	1964–98	70	New Zealand	1901, 1911, 1950–98	102
Canada	1921, 1950–97	98	Norway	1910, 1920, 1951–98	100
Chile	1909, 1920, 1930, 1940, 1950, 1955–82, 1984–98	96	Panama	1960	2
			Peru	1970	2
Colombia	1960, 1964	4	Philippines	1964, 1970	4
Costa Rica	1956–83, 1985–98	84	Poland	1959–98	80
Croatia	1982–98	34	Portugal	1920, 1930, 1940, 1955–98	94
Cuba	1970–98	58	Republic of Moldova	1981–98	36
Czech Republic	1934, 1982–99	38	Romania	1963, 1969–98	60
Denmark	1921, 1930, 1952–98	98	Russian Federation	1980–98	38
El Salvador	1950, 1971	4	Serbia and Montenegro	1982–97	32
Estonia	1981–98	36			
Finland	1952–98	94	Singapore	1955–98	88
France	1900–13, 1920–39, 1946–97	172	Slovakia	1982–98	34
Georgia	1981–96	30	Slovenia	1982–98	34
Germany	1969–98	58	South Africa	1941, 1951, 1960	6
Greece	1928, 1956–98	88	Spain	1930, 1940, 1951–69, 1971–98	98
Guatemala	1961, 1964	4	Sri Lanka	1946, 1953	4
Honduras	1961, 1974	4	Sweden	1900–17, 1920–98	194
Hungary	1955–99	90	Switzerland	1951–98	96
India	1971	2	Thailand	1970	2
Iran	1974	2	Trinidad and Tobago	1990–97	14
Ireland	1950–98	98	Tunisia	1968	2
Israel	1975–98	48	Ukraine	1981–98	36
Italy	1901, 1910, 1921, 1931, 1951–97	102	United Kingdom	1901, 1911, 1921, 1931, 1950–98	106
Japan	1950–98	98	United States of America	1900–16, 1920–41, 1945–98	186
Korea, Republic of	1973	2			

Table 29.2   Characteristics of life tables comprising the empirical dataset

Sex	Parameter	Mean	Std. dev.	Minimum	Maximum
Males	e_0	67.46	6.16	26.64	77.29
	$_5q_0$	0.039	0.047	0.005	0.439
	$_{45}q_{15}$	0.208	0.076	0.087	0.762
	$_{20}q_{60}$	0.636	0.078	0.422	0.906
Females	e_0	73.39	6.81	29.20	84.00
	$_5q_0$	0.033	0.043	0.003	0.427
	$_{45}q_{15}$	0.121	0.066	0.049	0.656
	$_{20}q_{60}$	0.478	0.099	0.222	0.833

shown in Table 29.3, along with the global standard l_x values. As Figure 29.2 shows, the values by age for both parameters in males and females follow a consistent pattern.

The effect of this transformation on a set of survivorship functions is shown in Figure 29.3. In the top panel, the deviations (residuals) by age between the logits of the observed l_x and those predicted from the original Brass system using the global standard are plotted for three populations covering a range of mortality experiences. Substantial deviations are evident in the three populations, particularly at ages 0–4 and among older adults. In the bottom panel, the deviations based on this new transformation are shown for the same three populations. Clearly the fit is much better. Because this transformation makes the relation-

Table 29.3   Values of θ_x, γ_x and l_x standard, by sex

Age	Males γ_x	Males θ_x	Males l_x Standard	Females γ_x	Females θ_x	Females l_x Standard
0	0.0000	0.0000	100 000	0.0000	0.0000	100 000
1	0.1607	−0.0097	96 870	0.0855	0.0734	97 455
5	0.0000	0.0000	96 010	0.0000	0.0000	96 651
10	−0.0325	0.0025	95 666	−0.0026	−0.0229	96 370
15	−0.0297	0.0047	95 385	0.0291	−0.0485	96 153
20	0.0427	0.0018	94 782	0.1199	−0.1090	95 795
25	0.1262	−0.0210	93 915	0.1931	−0.1702	95 340
30	0.1877	−0.0518	93 007	0.2352	−0.2117	94 824
35	0.2430	−0.0883	91 949	0.2686	−0.2408	94 197
40	0.2899	−0.1248	90 575	0.3003	−0.2601	93 370
45	0.3148	−0.1482	88 645	0.3203	−0.2594	92 220
50	0.2888	−0.1402	85 834	0.2935	−0.2183	90 569
55	0.1915	−0.0910	81 713	0.1967	−0.1338	88 159
60	0.0000	0.0000	75 792	0.0000	0.0000	84 679
65	−0.2304	0.1170	67 493	−0.2794	0.1859	79 481
70	−0.5523	0.2579	56 546	−0.7066	0.4377	71 763
75	−0.9669	0.4150	42 989	−1.2835	0.7534	60 358
80	−1.5013	0.5936	28 117	−2.0296	1.1360	44 958
85	−2.2126	0.8051	14 364	−2.9576	1.5774	27 123

ship between survivorship functions more linear with respect to age, a two-parameter fit on the transformed standard will perform much better than the original simple logit transformation.

DEVELOPING MODEL LIFE TABLES

Having estimated θ_x and γ_x, we can proceed to developing model life tables using the modified transformation. It is important to note that γ_x and θ_x do not vary across countries or years. Because of this, each life table can still be uniquely defined with this transformation as a linear function of a standard using only two parameters. It is advantageous to use the life table

functions l_5 and l_{60} as parameters to define a unique life table rather than α and β since these values are more readily interpretable. Any pair of l_5 and l_{60} uniquely defines a life table because there is a one-to-one mapping between a pair of α_{ij} and β_{ij} values and a pair of l_5 and l_{60} values. It can be shown that:

$$\alpha_{ij} = \frac{\text{Logit}(l_5^{ij}) \cdot \text{Logit}(l_{60}^s) - \text{Logit}(l_5^s) \cdot \text{Logit}(l_{60}^{ij})}{\text{Logit}(l_{60}^s) - \text{Logit}(l_5^s)} \quad [5]$$

$$\beta_{ij} = \frac{\text{Logit}(l_{60}^{ij}) - \text{Logit}(l_5^{ij})}{\text{Logit}(l_{60}^s) - \text{Logit}(l_5^s)} \quad [6]$$

By sampling systematically from the range of l_5 and l_{60} and discarding combinations that are logically impossible (i.e., $l_5 < l_{60}$), we have generated a large set of model life tables. Using this set, it is possible to visualize various life table functions such as $_nq_x$ and e_x as parameters in the two dimensional space defined by l_5 and l_{60}. Figure 29.4a shows life expectancy at birth isoclines corresponding to given values of l_5 and l_{60}. Each point on the isocline corresponds to a constant level of life expectancy generated by different age patterns of mortality. The same life expectancy is possible with low child mortality and high adult mortality or higher child and lower adult mortality. The isoclines demonstrate that the same life expectancy can occur with widely varying age patterns. This is illustrated more clearly in Figure 29.5, which shows the log of age-specific death rates for four model life tables selected from the isocline of male life expectancy equal to 65 years. The substantial variation in death rates illustrates the heterogeneity of mortality patterns that should be captured by any life table system. Analysis will confirm that the Brass logit and modified logit sys-

Figure 29.2   Values of θ_x, γ_x by age and sex

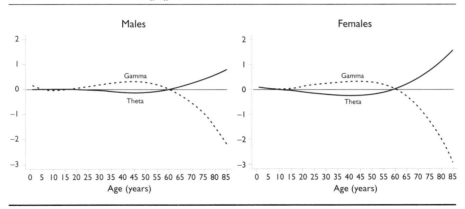

Figure 29.3   Deviations between observed and predicted logits by age, selected countries

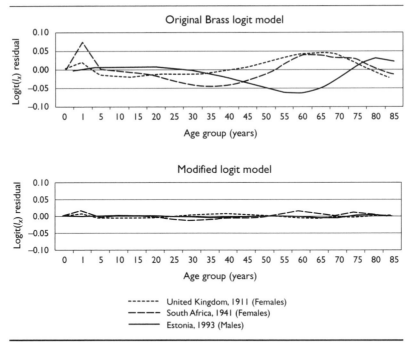

Figure 29.4   Isoclines of e_0, $_{45}q_{15}$ and $_{20}q_{60}$, selected values, males

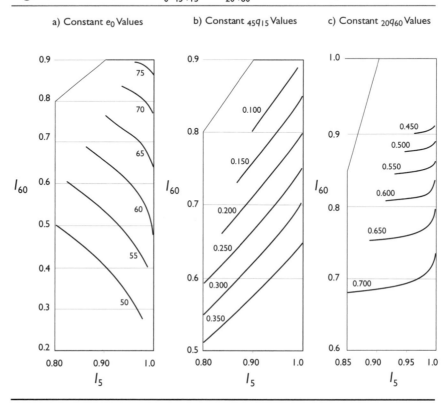

Figure 29.5   Log M_x for four populations with male e_0 = 65 years

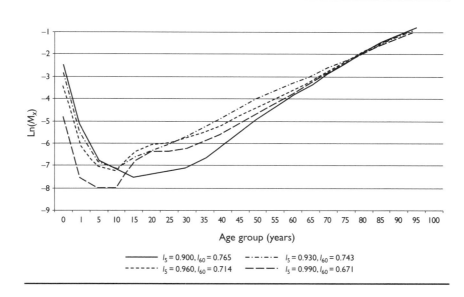

tems exhibit a considerably greater degree of flexibility than the Coale-Demeny system in this regard.

Figures 29.4b and 29.4c show, respectively, how adult mortality $(_{45}q_{15})$ and mortality among the elderly $(_{20}q_{60})$ vary according to the two parameters, l_5 and l_{60} in the set of model life tables. At a given level of child mortality, the slope of successive isoclines remains relatively constant. Figure 29.4c, on the other hand, indicates that the impact on older age mortality of declining levels of child mortality is much less apparent. Levels of $_{20}q_{60}$ are much more strongly determined by levels of adult mortality.

The fact that the isoclines in Figure 29.4 are monotonically increasing or decreasing in the l_5 and l_{60} parameter space implies that it is sufficiently correct to say there is one combination of l_5 and l_{60} that will correspond with any two life table mortality functions. This is not an algebraic relationship but an empirical one that follows from the monotonic isoclines. It means that we can find a matching life table in the modified logit system for most combinations of two life table functions. If two life table indices are known such as $_5q_0$ and e_0, then a unique life table is defined in this system at the point where the different contours intersect. For example, referring to Figure 29.4a, if we know $_5q_0$ is 100 per 1 000 and life expectancy at birth is 60 years, then the unique life table is defined by an l_5 of 0.900 and an l_{60} of 0.652.

The actual contour lines are a function of the global standard survivorship function as well of equation 4 so that they cannot easily be defined analytically. To help in the practical use of this system, we have developed a simple computer program, ModMatch, which identifies a modified logit life table on the basis of any two life table functions as parameters (16). Given the values of two life table functions, such as e_0 and $_5q_0$, the program interactively searches in l_5–l_{60} space to identify a combination of l_5 and l_{60} that yields a life table matching the given input values with a sufficient degree of precision. This program simplifies the matching of model life tables to selected empirical life table functions.

PREDICTIVE VALIDITY OF THE COALE-DEMENY, BRASS LOGIT AND MODIFIED LOGIT LIFE TABLE SYSTEMS

PREDICTIVE VALIDITY OF THE COALE-DEMENY VS. THE MODIFIED LOGIT SYSTEM

A key use of a model life table system is to create a full life table given information on only two life table indices such as life expectancy and child mortality or, more probably, adult mortality and child mortality. A strong test of this predictive use of a model life table system is to take an empirical life table, select a model life table using two aggregates from this empirical life table, and then compare the model life table age-specific death rates to the observed age-specific death rates. We have conducted two such tests: choosing model life tables on the basis of $_5q_0$ and e_0, and choosing on the basis of $_5q_0$ and $_{45}q_{15}$.

How well do these model life table systems capture the observed range of mortality experience? As noted above, one important criterion for a model life table system is that it adequately represents the known range of mortality experience across countries. Figures 29.6–29.8 make three types of comparisons: $_5q_0$ and e_0, $_5q_0$ and $_{45}q_{15}$, and $_{45}q_{15}$ and $_{20}q_{60}$, respectively. In each figure the observed points from the underlying dataset are shown and compared with the Coale-Demeny model life table values. It is clear that the range of mortality experience captured in the Coale-Demeny system is much smaller than the observed range in the empirical life tables, particularly at medium levels of mortality.

The limited range of mortality patterns captured in the Coale-Demeny model life table systems can be explained, in part, by the relatively recent emergence of the high adult mortality and low child mortality pattern now observed in parts of Eastern Europe and the Newly Independent States. The Coale-Demeny system was developed when there was little evidence of this pattern. Even excluding these countries, however, the range captured in this system is much smaller than the real variation seen worldwide. In contrast, the modified logit life table system can capture the entire range of mortality patterns illustrated in Figures 29.6–29.8 as illustrated in the contour figures shown earlier. On this criterion, the modified logit system is clearly better able to capture the diverse array of mortality patterns now seen.

Using the 30% of the original dataset of life tables (541 life tables) reserved for the validation test, we have applied the Coale-Demeny and modified logit systems to select a model life table on the basis of $_5q_0$ and e_0. The Coale-Demeny model has been selected by first matching each e_0 on all families and then selecting the family with the closest $_5q_0$. The life table from the modified logit system has been selected using the iterative matching algorithm described earlier. After repeating this procedure for each of the 541 life tables, the fit between predicted and observed mortality rates has been summarized using the root mean squared error in the logarithm of the death rates, since the logarithm of the death rates allows a more meaningful comparison across age groups.

Table 29.4 summarizes the goodness-of-fit statistics from the two model life table systems. The upper panel gives the results for the first type of test described above where life tables were selected on the basis of $_5q_0$ and e_0. As the table clearly demonstrates, the modified logit system gives much better predictions of age-specific death rates than the Coale-Demeny system on the basis of this set of 541 empirical life tables, particularly for males. Average root mean squared errors from the modified logit system are approximately 60–65% of those from the Coale-Demeny system.

The second test that we have used to assess the predictive power of these systems is to select model life tables on the basis of $_5q_0$ and $_{45}q_{15}$, a situation that is more likely to be encountered. This is a more difficult test as the selection of the model life table is based on indices of mortality that cover a smaller age range than life expectancy at birth. For each observed life table in the test subset of 541 life tables, the Coale-Demeny model life table has been selected by matching on $_{45}q_{15}$ in all families and then choosing the family with the closest match to the $_5q_0$. The matching procedure was repeated by first matching on $_5q_0$ and then choosing the family with the closest match on $_{45}q_{15}$. Using this approach, however, the magnitude of the root mean square error was considerably greater than when matching on $_{45}q_{15}$ first. The life table from the modified logit system has been selected by matching on the $_5q_0$ and $_{45}q_{15}$. The predicted age-specific death rates have again been assessed using the root mean squared error in the log death rates. Again, the modified logit system clearly outperforms the Coale-Demeny system, with average root mean squared errors being about 45% of those from the Coale-Demeny system for males, and about one-third lower for females. This sex differential in relative performance of the two approaches relates to the fact that the variance in adult male mortality is greater than for females.

Figures 29.9 and 29.10 show the relative performance of the two model life table systems in predicting the actual observed probability of adult death ($_{45}q_{15}$) (Figure 29.9) and life expectancy at birth (Figure 29.10) based on the subset of 541 life tables. If a system could exactly predict the true life table values, then all sample points would lie on a straight line. As Figure 29.9 illustrates, the modified logit system more successfully predicts the true probability of adult death (for males) than the closest match from the Coale-Demeny system, selected on the basis of $_5q_0$ and e_0, as described earlier. In particular, the Coale-Demeny system performs relatively poorly for true levels of $_{45}q_{15}$ in excess of about 150 per 1 000, which would include much of the contemporary developing world. A similar pattern is apparent from Figure 29.10 which

Figure 29.6   Comparison of observed patterns of $_5q_0$ and e_0 vs. Coale-Demeny model values, males

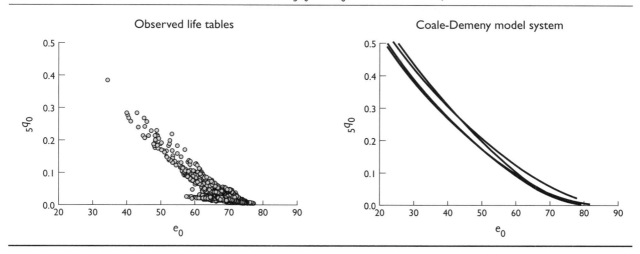

Figure 29.7   Comparison of observed patterns of $_5q_0$ and $_{45}q_{15}$ vs. Coale-Demeny model values, males

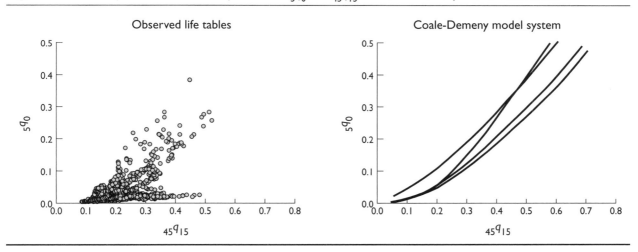

Figure 29.8   Comparison of observed patterns of $_{45}q_{15}$ and $_{20}q_{60}$ vs. Coale-Demeny model values, males

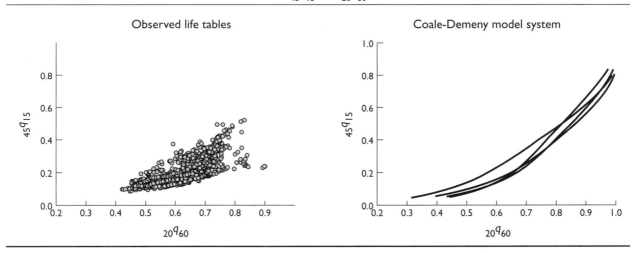

clearly shows the much closer fit between observed and predicted male e_0 for this sample of countries compared with the Coale-Demeny system, selected

Table 29.4 Comparison of root mean square error of $\ln(m_x)$ of the Coale-Demeny, Brass and modified logit systems using the 30% life table subset

Sex/Method	Coale-Demeny	Brass logit	Modified logit
Males (e_0 and $_5q_0$)	0.3412	0.2594	0.2017
Females (e_0 and $_5q_0$)	0.3629	0.2544	0.2146
Males ($_{45}q_{15}$ and $_5q_0$)	0.4285	0.2741	0.1892
Females ($_{45}q_{15}$ and $_5q_0$)	0.2564	0.2820	0.1726

on the basis of $_5q_0$ and $_{45}q_{15}$, irrespective of the level of true life expectancy.

In addition to assessing the overall fit between predicted age-specific death rates and those actually observed, we have tested for any systematic bias in the death rates at different ages. Table 29.5A summarizes the regression results of the observed on predicted values for various life table functions. If the modified logit system were able to perfectly predict the observed life table function (e.g., $_{45}q_{15}$ or $_{20}q_{60}$), then the coefficient of the regression would equal one and the constant would be zero. As is clear from Table 29.5, this is very nearly the case for all tests conducted on the 541 life table subset, with the greatest departure from unity at ages 60–80 years for males. In exploring

Figure 29.9 Predicted vs. observed male $_{45}q_{15}$ using the Coale-Demeny and modified logit systems, selecting on the basis of $_5q_0$ and e_0 ($n=541$)

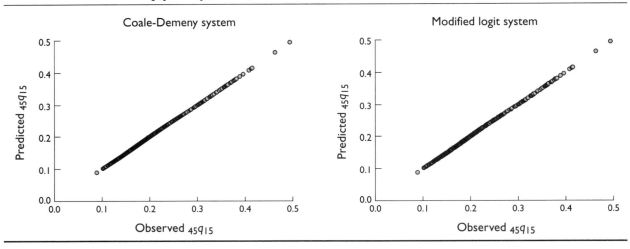

Figure 29.10 Predicted vs. observed male e_0 using the Coale-Demeny and modified logit systems, selecting on the basis of $_5q_0$ and $_{45}q_{15}$ ($n=541$)

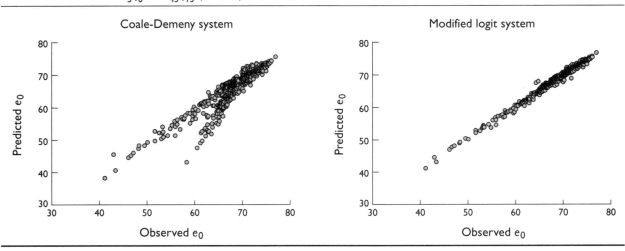

Table 29.5A Results of regression of selected observed life table parameters on those predicted by the modified logit system (*n*=541)

	Males				Females			
	α	β	R^2	RMSE	α	R	R^2	RMSE
e_0	−1.6905	1.0258	0.9882	0.6137	−1.1436	1.0155	0.9845	0.7742
$_{45}q_{15}$	0.0006	0.9972	0.9995	0.0017	0.0008	0.9927	0.9993	0.0016
$_{20}q_{60}$	−0.0360	1.0520	0.6069	0.0474	−0.0002	1.0047	0.7747	0.0438

this bias further, we found that substituting the 25th percentile values for θ_x and γ_x at all ages 65 and over (obtained from their uncertainty distributions) leads to a reduction in the bias of predicted values of probability of death at higher ages while having little effect on the overall R^2 for e_0. As a result, we have used the 50th percentile of the distribution for males at all ages below 65 and the 25th percentile values for θ_x and γ_x at all ages 65 and over, while leaving the estimated values for females unchanged. Table 29.5B shows the effect of this modification on the comparison between observed and fitted life table functions for males.

Table 29.5B Results of regression of selected observed life table parameters on those predicted by the modified logit system, using 25th percentile values for males ages 65+

	Males (25th percentile)[*]			
	α	β	R^2	RMSE
e_0	−0.8250	1.0127	0.9885	0.6068
$_{45}q_{15}$	0.0006	0.9972	0.9995	0.0017
$_{20}q_{60}$	0.0105	0.9799	0.6086	0.0473

[*] 25th percentile values are as follows :
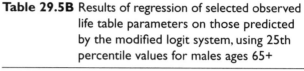
$$\gamma_{65-85+} = (-0.2466, -0.5744, -0.9952, -1.5372, -2.2597)$$
$$\theta_{65-85+} = (0.1148, 0.2544, 0.4099, 0.5862, 0.7939)$$

DISCUSSION

In this chapter, we have demonstrated that the modified logit life table system using a single global standard can represent the full range of mortality patterns seen across the high quality life tables available internationally. The proposed system generates better predictions of age-specific mortality rates than the Coale-Demeny and original Brass systems and is indexed on two life table functions that are relatively easy to understand. While the modified logit system as presented here is indexed on l_5 and l_{60}, for practical use it is approximately possible to identify a unique life table with any two life table functions such as life expectancy at birth and child mortality.

The main limitation of this model life table system and the tests of its predictive validity is that the sample of high quality life tables is heavily weighted towards populations with life expectancies between 60 and 73 (for males) and 66 and 80 (for females). The addition of more high quality and recent life tables for high mortality populations might suggest alternative values of θ_x and γ_x that would minimize prediction error. Such analyses can be undertaken easily if new high-quality life tables become available. Based on the available set of life tables in our empirical dataset, however, the results appear to be quite robust to the selection of even small subsets of life tables. We have re-estimated the θ_x and γ_x for numerous random

samples of 100 life tables selected from the overall database and have found that the parameter estimates are remarkably insensitive to the set of life tables on which they are estimated. This strengthens our view that the addition of new life tables will not alter substantially the estimates of θ_x and γ_x.

There is remaining uncertainty as to how the model system would perform in countries with high levels of HIV. It is quite possible that in high HIV settings the age pattern of mortality projected out of sample by the model may not be accurate, although this cannot be tested due to the lack of high quality life tables for these countries. As a very limited test, we have compared the estimates of age-specific mortality based on selecting a model life table in the absence of HIV with HIV death rates added on *a posteriori* (5) for Zimbabwe, South Africa, and Tanzania with the model life table selected using values of l_5 and l_{60} that reflect the impact of HIV. Predicted life expectancy at birth was within 0.5 years of the value estimated from this two-stage procedure, with an even closer agreement for levels of adult mortality.

The use of the Coale-Demeny and UN systems is so widespread in demographic estimation that there are often circular arguments about levels and patterns of adult mortality. One set of analysts often use the results of other demographic analyses founded on these model life table systems without realizing that they substantially underestimate the variation in age-specific mortality patterns seen in the real world. The use of models is so deeply embedded in available international datasets that it can be difficult to formulate real empirical tests of these models. We have tried to ensure that the observed life tables used in this analysis have not been modified using model life table systems, and hence that the modified system is based exclusively on observed data.

One implication of this analysis is that for sub-Saharan Africa in particular there is much more uncertainty about levels of adult mortality than implied in currently available demographic estimates such as the UN Population Division life tables (*17*). Often, levels of adult mortality have been estimated by selecting a life table on the basis of estimated child mortality and an arbitrary choice of a model life table family (often West by default). This has tended towards a one-to-one mapping of child mortality to adult mortality prior to the HIV epidemic. In reality, even the empirical record of countries outside Africa suggests that there can be much greater variation in levels of adult mortality as compared to child mortality than captured in the Coale-Demeny and UN model life tables. We hope that the convenience of a simple model life table system parameterized using easily recognized aspects of a population's mortality experience and a single global standard will facilitate a wide use of the modified logit system.

A key issue in the application of this new system of model life tables will be the availability of reliable estimates of child and adult mortality which are required to identify a fully specified life table. Decades of demographic interest in the measurement of child mortality have resulted in reasonably reliable estimates for almost all countries (*5*), whereas the measurement of adult mortality has been largely neglected. Estimates of survival from ages 15 to 50 or 60 can be constructed from survey or census data on sibling survival, orphanhood or recent household deaths, but require substantial adjustment for undercounting of deaths. A vast increase in data on adult mortality is urgently required, as is research into methods which can reliably correct the data for systematic underreporting. The World Health Organization, through the World Health Surveys programme, has been at the forefront of international research efforts to address these issues.

REFERENCES

(1) Coale A, Demeny P. *Regional model life tables and stable populations*. Princeton, Princeton University Press, 1966.

(2) Brass W. On the scale of mortality. In: Brass W, ed. *Biological aspects of mortality*. London, Taylor & Francis, 1971.

(3) United Nations. *Model life tables for developing countries*. New York, United Nations, 1981.

(4) Ahmad OB, Lopez AD, Inoue M. The decline in child mortality: a reappraisal. *Bulletin of the World Health Organization*, 2000, 78:1175–1191.

(5) Lopez AD et al. *World mortality in 2000: life tables for 191 countries*. Geneva, World Health Organization, 2002.

(6) United Nations. *Manual X: indirect techniques for demographic estimation*. New York, United Nations, 1983.

(7) Ledermann S. *Nouvelles tables-type de mortalité: travaux et document*. Paris, Institut National d'Etudes Demographiques, 1969.

(8) United Nations. *Age and sex patterns of mortality: model life tables for under-developed countries*. New York, United Nations, 1955.

(9) Menken J. Current status of demographic models. *Population Bulletin of the United Nations*, 1977, 9:22–34.

(10) Coale A, Guo G. Revised regional model life tables at very low levels of mortality. *Population Index*, 1989, 55:613-643.

(11) Demeny P, Shorter F. *Estimating Turkish mortality, fertility and age structure*. Statistics Institute, Istanbul University, 1968.

(12) Zaba B. The four-parameter logit life table system. *Population Studies*, 1979, 33:79–100.

(13) Ewbank D, Gomez de Leon J, Stoto M. A reducible four-parameter life table system. *Population Studies*, 1983, 37:105–127.

(14) Preston SH, Keyfitz N, Schoen R. *Causes of death: life tables for national populations*. New York, Academic Press, 1972.

(15) International Development Research Centre. *Population, health and survival at INDEPTH sites*, vol. 1. Ottawa, International Development Research Centre, 2002.

(16) Ferguson BD. *ModMatch: an algorithm for matching a modified logit system life table to selected life table functions. [v1.1]*. Geneva, World Health Organization, 2002. URL: http://www3.who.int/whosis/life/

(17) United Nations. *The 2000 demographic assessment*. New York, United Nations, 2001.

Chapter 30

Empirical Evaluation of the Anchoring Vignette Approach in Health Surveys

Christopher J.L. Murray, Emre Özaltin, Ajay Tandon, Joshua A. Salomon, Ritu Sadana, Somnath Chatterji

Introduction

Health is more than the absence of disease or the minimization of risks of death. All societies recognize health as a critical component of well-being and as having multiple aspects or domains. The non-fatal aspects of an individual's health state have been the focus of an extensive literature that has grown steadily in the last three decades (*1–12*). Non-fatal dimensions of health have been progressively incorporated into national and international health statistics such as the regular reporting by the World Health Organization (WHO) of Disability-Adjusted Life Years (DALYs) and healthy life expectancy (HALE) (*13*). Both at the individual and at the population level, capturing non-fatal dimensions of health must be seen as central to the challenge of measuring health.

The WHO constitution notes that health is a multidimensional concept (*14*). There are potentially three sets of domains that can be specified in order to describe health and contribute to its operational measurement: 1) core domains of health upon which most people agree; 2) additional domains of health that some people consider core domains; and 3) other domains that are related to health and serve as good proximate measures of the experience of health—health-related domains. The *International Classification of Functioning, Disability and Health* (ICF) (*15*) provides a standardized international framework for understanding these multiple domains of health. While the ICF gives a large number of domains and subdomains, a limited set of core domains capture most people's understanding of the key aspects of a health state. These core domains include affect, mobility, cognition, pain, self-care, and usual activities.

A wide array of measurement instruments has been proposed and used to capture these aspects of health (*16–27*). Some instruments have been designed to focus on specific domains such as mobility, or to have particular sensitivity in measuring reductions in multiple domains due to a given disease process. Other instruments have been designed to capture more general aspects of health states such as the SF-36 (*28*), Quality of Well Being Scale (*29*), Health Utilities Index (*20*), and others. As part of its work on providing coherent tools for individual and population health measurement, WHO has been developing simplified common health status measurement tools that build on the rich experience with multiple instruments in different countries.

The mainstay of health status measurement, regardless of the instrument used, is self-reported responses on health status in survey interviews. Because of issues of cost and feasibility, even if self-reported data are supplemented by measured tests, self-responses will likely remain one of the major data collection methods for population health status assessment. These self-response data typically take the form of ordered categorical (ordinal) responses, such as "excellent"/ "very good"/ "good"/ "poor"/ "bad" or "none"/ "mild"/ "moderate"/ "severe"/ "extreme." One critical issue that has been debated extensively (*8;12;30–32*), is the degree to which self-responses on these items are comparable across individuals, socioeconomic subgroups or populations. The challenge of comparability is central to the future of health status instrument development (*33–35*).

In the past two decades, efforts to enhance comparability have focused on encouraging different investigators and statistical agencies to use identical items that have been carefully translated, back-translated and evaluated for cultural relevance. While these efforts have certainly improved comparability where they have been applied, they have not addressed all, or even the dominant aspects, of response comparability. Even when identical or equivalent items have been used, the results across individuals, groups or populations may not be comparable (8). If the meaning of response categories differs systematically across populations, or even across socio-demographic groups within a population, unrelated to health status, then the observed ordinal responses are not cross-population comparable since they will not imply the same level (36).

WHO, over the last five years, has undertaken an extensive programme of work to develop through empirical testing valid, reliable, and comparable instruments to measure health status in a restricted set of core domains of health. At the heart of this approach is the use of anchoring vignettes, explained in detail below. This chapter reports on the first widespread multi-country experience of using the anchoring vignette approach in household surveys. Data on anchoring vignettes for six health domains and eight responsiveness domains are used to draw some general conclusions about design and implementation issues. A detailed non-parametric and parametric analysis of mobility is used to illustrate some of the lessons learned and the implications of this experience for future instrument development, particularly the World Health Survey.

ANCHORING VIGNETTE APPROACH

The problem of comparability may be conceptualized in terms of response category cut-point shifts across populations, or across subgroups within a population. Figure 30.1 illustrates the primary challenge of using self-reported levels on a health status domain, even when reliability and within-population validity have been well established. For each domain, there is some true latent scale for that domain that is, by definition, unobserved. For instance, imagine that there is a latent mobility scale, depicted in the first column of Figure 30.1. Now imagine a self-reported survey question that asks respondents whether they have difficulty walking up stairs and offers five response categories: "no difficulty," "mild difficulty," "moderate difficulty," "severe difficulty," and "extreme/cannot do." The second column in the figure shows the response category cut-points for population A. These are levels of mobility at which an individual will transition from using one response category to another. The highest cut-point in the figure shows the transition from answering "no difficulty" to "mild difficulty." In population B, the

Figure 30.1   Latent mobility scale and cut-point variation in categorical responses

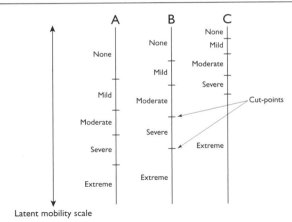

response category cut-points are shifted relative to those in population A so that a higher level of mobility is associated with each of the response categories. Population C shows a third example with even more shift in the cut-points. The implication is dramatic. A response of "mild difficulty" walking up stairs maps to a different level of mobility in populations A, B, and C. In this example, survey results may be reliable and valid within each population, but they cannot be compared across populations without adjustment.

Anchoring vignettes have been developed as a new component of survey instruments that may be used to position self-reported responses on a common, interpersonally comparable scale (37). An anchoring vignette is a description of a concrete level on a given health domain that respondents are asked to evaluate with the same questions and response scales applied to self-assessments on that domain. Vignettes fix the level of ability on a domain so that variation in categorical responses is attributable to variation in response category cut-points. The key objective underlying the anchoring vignette strategy is to elicit responses from subjects for hypothetical levels on a given domain, which reflect individual norms and expectations for health in approximately the same way the self-ratings do for the subjects' own health levels.

The use of vignettes has a long history in social science research, including applications in anthropology, sociology, and psychological research since the 1950s (38–40), as well as numerous applications of the factorial-survey technique pioneered by Rossi and Nock (41). Our anchoring vignette approach departs from previous vignette studies in certain fundamental ways. First, rather than generating random variants of the same vignette (41), our approach depends critically on using vignettes as scale anchors, and therefore requires that a given vignette describe the same domain level to all respondents. Second, our strategy is based on explicit links between vignette ratings and self-ratings through the use of identical questions and response categories.

We have defined two key requirements for the use of anchoring vignettes: *response consistency*, which states that an individual will use the response categories for a particular question in a similar way when evaluating hypothetical scenarios as when providing a self-assessment; and *vignette equivalence*, which states that the underlying domain levels represented in each vignette are understood in approximately the same way by all respondents, irrespective of their age, sex, income, education, country of residence, or other characteristics (37). These two requirements lead to a series of practical considerations in the design and administration of anchoring vignettes.

MULTI-COUNTRY SURVEY STUDY

The WHO Multi-country Survey Study on Health and Responsiveness (MCSS) was carried out in 2000–2001. A total of 61 surveys were completed in 71 countries using face-to-face, postal, and telephone interviewing modes (see Chapter 57 in this book (42)). A 90-minute long version of the interview and a shorter 30-minute version were used. The purpose of this study was to develop a valid, reliable, and comparable instrument to describe individual health and responsiveness, and to test the effects that interviewing mode has on data quality and self-report. The study was also intended to develop a comprehensive methodology for WHO to gather data on important indicators of interest and to assist countries with the fielding of household surveys. The survey was designed to be implemented with careful quality control, appropriate sampling, and data management strategies. Another major goal was to build capacity in countries to analyse data from complex surveys. The MCSS provides the first comprehensive dataset that allows the adjustment of self-reports based on shifts in cut-points using the anchoring vignettes methodology. This large dataset from over 140 000 respondents also allows the investigation of various questions related to this methodology: Can vignettes be used in large household surveys? Can respondents from varying education, income and age levels understand and respond to vignettes? Do responses to vignettes contain the requisite informa-

tion to adjust for biases in self-report? How can we refine the methodology in future iterations?

The MCSS included vignettes for the six core health domains (mobility, self-care, pain, affect, work and household activities, cognition) and vision, and for all the eight domains of responsiveness (prompt attention, dignity, communication, confidentiality, choice of care provider, autonomy, quality of basic amenities, and support).[1] Vignettes were brief, written in simple language presenting precise information and avoiding use of terms used in the self-report question, and written to be applicable in most cultures where the survey was to be implemented. Respondents were instructed to think of the person described in the vignette in terms of the difficulty experienced with a given task, and rate them using the same response categories they used for describing their own health.

Due to the constraints of interview length, each respondent in the survey rated vignettes for only two domains of health and two domains of responsiveness, with a total of 12 to 16 vignettes for the two health domains and 14 vignettes for the two responsiveness domains. These rotations of domains were combined in four sets and randomly allocated to respondents in the survey, such that data on any given vignette were available for at least a quarter of the sample at each site. Since the task required that respondents rate each individual vignette using the five-category response scale rather than merely order them from best to worse, the number of vignettes in every domain exceeded the number of response categories. In each set, the vignettes for the two domains were presented in a non-ordered sequence (i.e. not from best to worst or vice versa) that also mixed the vignettes across both domains.

Table 30.1 provides the breakdown of the number of individuals in the entire MCSS datatset who responded to each vignette. The survey rotations were designed to have approximately twice the number of respondents on mobility as for other domains, to allow for increased power to detect systematic variations in response patterns for at least one domain. In this chapter, data from the Lebanon household and postal surveys have not been included in any of the analyses because the data were not available at the time of writing. Table 30.2 illustrates, as an example, the vignettes that were used for the mobility domain. In this case, the level of mobility represented by Vignette 1, the marathon runner, and the level represented by Vignette 6, the quadriplegic, spans the full range of best to worst imaginable mobility levels.

Table 30.1 Number of respondents for each set of vignettes by domain in 69 MCSS surveys

Domain	N	N responding to vignettes	% responding to vignettes
Affect	141 704	35 187	24.83
Cognition	141 704	34 701	24.49
Mobility	141 704	70 363	49.65
Pain	141 704	35 267	24.89
Self-care	141 704	35 272	24.89
Usual activities	141 704	34 706	24.49

ANALYSIS OF HEALTH AND RESPONSIVENESS VIGNETTES

INTRODUCTION

The anchoring vignette strategy to enhance comparability of individual responses on self-reported items depends on the vignettes invoking the same level of ability for a given domain when presented to different respondents. This requirement of vignette equivalence implies that the set of vignettes for a domain must be generally understood in the same fashion in different languages, cultures, and among respondents of various socioeconomic backgrounds. In this section, we use the large number of ratings of vignettes for six health domains and for eight responsiveness domains to explore the extent to which vignettes have been understood in a similar way. This provides the basis for both analysing the vignette responses and self-reports to assess an individual's level on a domain, and for improving vignettes in subsequent efforts to collect data.

VISUALIZING VIGNETTE RESPONSES

For a sample of respondents, we can summarize the distribution of ratings for a set of vignettes using stacked bars. Figure 30.2 shows, for the household survey in China and the postal survey in the Netherlands, the distribution of responses for each of the six mobility vignettes along with the distribution of self-assessed mobility. On the x-axis, the vignettes are ordered from the best, the marathon runner, to the worst, the quadriplegic, with the self-assessment as the final bar. Each bar is broken down into the percentage of respondents characterizing the overall level of difficulty in moving around described in that vignette as "none," "mild," "moderate," "severe," or "extreme." In both countries, the average responses shift towards the categories "severe" and "extreme" as one moves

Table 30.2 Mobility vignettes as included in the WHO Multi-country Survey Study on Health and Responsiveness 2000–2001

Vignette 1	[Paul] is an active athlete who runs long distance races of 20 kilometres twice a week and engages in soccer with no problems.
Vignette 2	[Mary] has no problems with moving around or using her hands, arms and legs. She jogs 4 kilometres twice a week without any problems.
Vignette 3	[Rob] is able to walk distances of up to 200 metres without any problems but feels breathless after walking one kilometre or climbing up more than one flight of stairs. He has no problems with day-to-day physical activities, such as carrying food from the market.
Vignette 4	[Margaret] feels chest pain and gets breathless after walking distances of up to 200 metres, but is able to do so without assistance. Bending and lifting objects such as groceries produces pain.
Vignette 5	[Louis] is able to move his arms and legs, but requires assistance in standing up from a chair or walking around the house. Any bending is painful and lifting is impossible.
Vignette 6	[David] is paralysed from the neck down. He is confined to bed and must be fed and bathed by somebody else.

from the marathon runner (Vignette 1) to the quadriplegic (Vignette 6). For any vignette, there is a wide range of responses in both countries, such that all five response categories are used by some respondents for all six vignettes. This individual variation in response is likely to be a combination of measurement error and variation in cut-points across individuals in a population. Figure 30.2 also illustrates a substantial difference in response patterns between the Netherlands and China. For Vignette 4 (the individual with difficulties walking 200 metres), in China the most common response is moderate difficulty (47.0%), while in the Netherlands the most frequently used response for this vignette is severe difficulty (60.1%). Clearly, the raw response data on vignettes indicate that response categories are being used differently in these two settings.

CONSISTENCY OF VIGNETTES IN MULTIPLE COUNTRIES

Pooling all the responses for a domain across countries, we can define a global ordering of the vignettes based on the average categorical response. An important requirement of the anchoring vignette approach is that individuals perceive the vignettes at the same level of the domain in the latent variable. One minimal test of this requirement is that an individual's

Figure 30.2 Stacked-bar diagram of vignette responses in China and the Netherlands

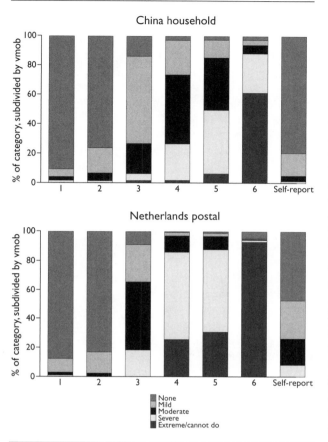

responses are consistent with the global ordering of vignettes on the latent variable. Because test-retest data on self-reported items show that there is considerable stochastic measurement error with any self-reported item, on the basis of stochastic measurement error we would not expect all individuals to order the vignettes in the same way. Examination of the extent to which

individuals do have a consistent ordering of vignettes, however, is one first test of the requirement that the actual domain levels described in the vignettes are perceived in a similar fashion in different cultural and socioeconomic groups.

In examining patterns of vignette ratings, there will be some ambiguity in the exact ordering of vignettes because there are more vignettes than response categories. For the purposes of this analysis, we define a consistent ordering to be a set of categorical vignette ratings that *could be consistent* with the global ordering in the latent variable space, if ambiguities were resolved in favour of the global ordering. For example, consider the case of mobility where there were six vignettes and five response categories on the general question: "How much difficulty do you have in moving around?" One individual might place Vignettes 1, 2, and 3 in the response category "no difficulty," Vignettes 4 and 5 in the category "mild difficulty," and Vignette 6 in the category "extreme difficulty." Another respondent might place Vignette 1 in the category "no difficulty," Vignettes 2, 3, and 4 in "mild difficulty," Vignette 5 in "severe difficulty," and Vignette 6 in "extreme difficulty." Both sets of responses are considered fully consistent with the global ordering of vignettes. The two individuals, however, have different cut-points defining the levels of mobility on the latent variable that map to the five response categories.

For the entire Multi-country Survey Study on Health and Responsiveness dataset, Table 30.3 provides information on the percentage of respondents for each health domain that gave an ordering of vignettes consistent with the global ordering, or had an ordering where only one vignette moved one or two ranks or two vignettes moved one rank each. It is rather remarkable that for two domains, mobility

Table 30.3 Consistent and near consistent orderings of vignettes by domain in 69 MCSS surveys

Domain	# Vignettes	# Raters	Consistent raters		Consistent + near consistent raters	
			#	%	#	%
Mobility	6	68 361	44 834	65.58	62 282	91.11
Affect	6	34 695	19 366	55.82	29 709	85.63
Self Care	7	34 696	9 539	27.49	22 095	63.68
Cognition	8	33 029	5 618	17.01	17 566	53.18
Pain	7	34 435	5 650	16.41	15 941	46.29
Usual Actvities	8	32 251	4 753	14.74	14 625	45.35

Consistent raters: Vignette ordering that is consistent with the global vignette ordering
Near consistent raters: One inversion of one rank, one inversion of two ranks, or two inversions of one rank
Raters is the number responding to all vignettes

and affect, the majority of participants gave responses exactly consistent with the global ordering. Combining the consistent orderings with inversions of ranks involving only one vignette moving one or two ranks or two vignettes moving one rank each, yields a figure of consistent or near consistent orderings of over 90% for mobility, 85% for affect, and 60% for self-care. On the other hand, for cognition, pain, and usual activities, between 40% and 50% were consistent or near consistent. Interpretation of these results must be somewhat tempered by the fact the mobility and affect had six vignettes, self-care and pain had seven, and cognition and usual activities had eight vignettes. Simply on the basis of similar stochastic measurement error, one would expect domains with more vignettes to have a lower percentage with consistent or near consistent orderings.

Table 30.4 shows the percentage of respondents in each survey giving a consistent or near consistent ordering for the six health domains. There is clearly substantial variation across countries. For example, for mobility, the proportion ranges from 51% to more than 99%, with 64 of 69 surveys having more than 80% of respondents giving a consistent or near consistent ordering. For affect, the results are similar, with 62 of 69 surveys reporting over 80% of respondents with consistent or near consistent ordering. Given that affect as a construct might be understood by many as more abstract than mobility, this high degree of consistency across disparate settings is impressive. The table also illustrates five specific cases of less than 35% of respondents in a survey giving consistent or near consistent vignette orderings. These five exceptional cases were self-care in the Korea postal, self-care in the Indonesia postal (in the Indonesia household survey 49% were consistent), usual activities in the Mexico household, pain in the Slovakia household, and usual activities in the Turkey postal (in the Turkey household the figure was 59%). We suspect that these cases were due to specific translation, printing or implementation problems. Nevertheless, it is clear that, overall, the vignettes used for usual activities, pain, and cognition had more variation across countries and performed less well than the vignettes used for mobility, affect, and self-care.

The variation in responses evident in Table 30.4 may be due to a number of factors.

First, despite development efforts in the pilot testing phase, the vignettes may not be written in a way that minimizes ambiguity of interpretation. Test-retest data suggest that some vignettes have lower reliability than others. The variation in test-retest reliability coefficients (kappa values), however, does not seem to account for the consistent differences seen here across domains for the set of vignettes.

Second, despite efforts at quality control in translation, it is possible that there have been unforeseen difficulties in translating certain vignettes into local languages.

Third, a domain may not be unidimensional. For example, one could argue that pain is difficult to present as a unidimensional construct. Duration, intensity and location may be weighted differently in different cultures. In this case, we would expect pain vignettes that include these various aspects to be interpreted differently because of different weights assigned to these different sub-domains.

Fourth, due to interviewer training and other aspects of survey implementation such as questionnaire length, the stochastic measurement error associated with the responses to the vignettes may vary across countries. Increased measurement error will by chance increase the number of inconsistent orderings.

Fifth, measurement error may be a function of the educational status or other socio-demographic characteristics of the respondents. As average levels of education, income and other factors vary across countries, this could account for some cross-national variation in the fraction with consistent orderings.

Finally, there may be systematic variation across cultural groups in the interpretation of the construct of a domain, which could lead to different interpretations of the level associated with a particular vignette on that domain.

EXPLORING CAUSES OF INCONSISTENT ORDERINGS

Quantifying Inconsistent Orderings

For each survey, we have information on the orderings of vignettes for 14 domains—the six health domains and the eight responsiveness domains. The experience on the 14 domains can help in identifying the average effects of domains, surveys, respondent socio-demographic attributes, and survey-domain interactions on vignette ordering. Average domain effects across multiple surveys are likely due to the writing of the vignettes, problems of multidimensionality, or both. Average survey effects that influence all domains in a survey are most likely due to issues of survey implementation including survey mode. Survey-domain interactions would likely discover problems in translation, printing, or interviewer training. Socio-demographic characteristics of the respondents will

Table 30.4 Per cent consistent and near consistent orderings by domain and survey

	Per cent consistent + near consistent vignette ordering					
	Mobility	Affect	Pain	Cognition	Self-care	Usual activities
Australia(p)	98.46	97.93	70.99	86.75	94.23	89.52
Austria(p)	89.00	96.21	62.55	83.11	85.19	72.73
Belgium(b)	94.94	95.91	44.67	91.20	84.03	62.92
Bulgaria(b)	97.64	97.80	61.90	85.25	84.68	70.83
Bahrain(b)	93.16	86.50	52.94	75.13	58.82	57.87
Canada(p)	99.48	97.92	73.33	89.22	95.19	92.16
Canada(t)	95.83	93.62	62.64	73.33	76.92	70.79
Switzerland(p)	96.31	97.30	36.19	79.44	93.46	84.55
Chile(p)	91.63	96.43	78.63	88.60	68.82	82.10
China(h)	90.19	83.92	46.54	79.26	73.53	67.92
China(p)	96.88	96.51	64.02	83.71	76.39	85.90
Colombia(h)	88.80	79.31	48.97	71.58	53.18	52.40
Costa Rica(b)	93.50	86.63	57.75	58.29	51.63	63.78
Cyprus(p)	97.17	98.13	52.38	83.22	84.12	77.93
Czech Republic(b)	98.90	94.07	55.00	90.59	84.90	68.36
Czech Republic(p)	97.57	97.92	63.20	84.74	91.88	83.47
Germany(b)	94.39	92.80	43.01	87.64	80.51	66.00
Denmark(p)	96.24	98.69	57.77	—	94.86	—
Egypt(h)	91.32	80.84	47.91	76.26	66.23	59.23
Egypt(p)	83.53	71.80	45.32	72.22	51.95	50.46
Spain(b)	98.98	95.02	55.10	81.25	88.89	57.08
Estonia(b)	98.96	96.15	51.68	91.89	72.03	69.20
Finland(b)	98.57	95.92	66.27	90.46	80.24	76.38
Finland(p)	98.89	98.71	69.10	80.82	89.23	89.54
France(b)	97.76	92.68	45.12	90.53	89.20	65.40
France(p)	94.10	98.37	62.11	87.39	83.02	81.51
United Kingdom(p)	96.71	97.93	63.36	85.89	95.30	88.07
Georgia(h)	90.85	76.67	46.90	80.41	72.00	67.56
Greece(p)	98.03	98.14	51.10	90.34	88.59	78.82
Croatia(b)	97.12	94.65	53.46	75.65	76.39	79.71
Hungary(p)	96.79	94.92	37.19	80.89	79.12	76.54
Indonesia(h)	86.32	70.36	60.93	73.71	56.70	51.66
Indonesia(p)	68.03	88.61	48.74	68.90	6.54	62.71
India(h)	95.20	90.01	69.82	65.55	57.92	60.43
Ireland(b)	95.77	89.01	52.90	83.71	80.75	75.56
Iran(h)	96.55	92.09	60.08	80.56	75.39	77.37
Iceland(b)	98.74	97.50	59.32	92.50	88.89	78.99
Italy(b)	92.48	86.99	41.81	85.48	90.46	40.65
Jordan(b)	96.47	92.96	59.50	88.56	78.50	71.14
Kyrgyzstan(p)	63.82	80.95	44.67	60.45	68.83	56.70
Korea, Republic of (p)	79.39	83.33	53.33	69.05	11.43	60.00
Lthuania(p)	51.22	96.18	44.27	85.82	88.84	78.59
Luxembourg(t)	93.86	90.12	37.14	83.54	84.83	60.57
Latvia(b)	98.67	91.40	46.60	67.20	78.76	62.77
Morocco(b)	97.35	85.05	54.26	77.01	72.34	52.41
Mexico(h)	84.23	81.20	50.05	65.34	51.41	15.73
Malta(b)	98.78	96.00	42.98	95.87	84.30	79.03
Nigeria(h)	98.28	85.63	59.74	63.14	76.63	86.47
Netherlands(b)	92.51	95.58	44.58	90.11	80.24	72.55
Netherlands(p)	94.70	95.68	67.33	93.50	84.56	86.40
New Zealand(p)	98.43	97.83	52.14	89.33	83.73	82.67

continued

Table 30.4   Per cent consistent and near consistent orderings by domain and survey *(continued)*

	Per cent consistent + near consistent vignette ordering					
	Mobility	*Affect*	*Pain*	*Cognition*	*Self-care*	*Usual activities*
Oman(b)	91.87	89.18	69.87	72.50	59.39	54.00
Poland(p)	97.28	98.49	45.25	87.14	84.09	91.90
Portugal(b)	96.70	95.42	50.82	74.24	74.60	58.64
Romania(b)	94.21	94.09	58.33	77.54	77.29	68.12
Russia(b)	98.22	93.83	66.84	92.33	82.99	50.28
Singapore(h)	87.44	76.75	47.38	76.27	62.80	63.12
Slovakia(h)	96.48	85.92	33.56	81.89	80.94	81.58
Sweden(b)	99.39	98.77	61.54	93.55	94.58	70.73
Syria(h)	91.94	87.01	58.64	79.58	59.98	67.00
Thailand(p)	87.20	88.14	60.80	56.54	62.38	47.06
Trinidad and Tobago(p)	90.74	94.33	69.74	77.99	76.30	77.57
Turkey(h)	91.60	60.75	42.49	70.61	72.12	59.26
Turkey(p)	70.34	78.80	57.34	36.50	42.18	31.98
Ukraine(p)	98.66	96.32	55.68	96.77	82.26	70.97
United Arab Emirates(b)	95.32	92.69	60.00	81.45	68.57	65.16
United States of America(p)	95.28	97.47	62.72	91.61	93.50	83.70
Venezuela(b)	87.26	84.62	57.92	71.81	63.19	58.51
Total	91.11	86.17	54.22	77.24	69.17	66.60

p=Postal, h=Household, t=Telephone, b=Brief face-to-face

help identify the extent to which the cognitive task of responding for anchoring vignettes can work in individuals with different socioeconomic status.

To facilitate this quantitative assessment of the vignette performance, we first calculate a variant of the Spearman's rank order correlation coefficient. Since we want to quantify the extent to which an ordering is *in*consistent with the global ordering of vignettes on the latent variable, we must pay careful attention to ties. For example, Figure 30.3 shows three respondents who all have a consistent ordering with the global ordering. We define a benefit-of-the-doubt rank order correlation coefficient (BDROCC) to be the Spearman's rank order correlation coefficient when all ties have been resolved to be consistent with the global ordering.

Table 30.5 provides the frequency distribution of BDROCC values for all respondents in the entire data-

Figure 30.3   Three examples of consistent vignette orderings

	Respondents		
Response categories	*A*	*B*	*C*
No difficulties	1, 2	1, 2, 3	1
Mild	3		2, 3
Moderate	4, 5	4	
Severe	6	5	4, 5
Extreme		6	6

set on the mobility and the cognition vignettes. In the case of mobility, 66% have a correlation of 1, which is the same as the percentage with a consistent ranking in Table 30.3. 19% have a BDROCC of 0.94, which corresponds to cases of inverting a single vignette with an adjacent vignette. Only three other particular levels of inconsistency occur with a frequency greater than 1%. In contrast, for cognition, 14 different inconsistency levels occur with frequencies greater than 1%, as well as 63 other levels appearing at least once.

This examination of the more common alternative patterns of vignette order inconsistencies in different countries may provide some insight into the relative importance of the various sources of measurement error versus problems of multidimensionality or variation in cultural constructs of a domain. Increased measurement error—whether due to the writing, translation or implementation of the vignettes—should lead to a large number of alternative orderings due to chance, such as what we observe for cognition, pain, and usual activities, even bearing in mind that these domains had seven or eight vignettes as compared to six for mobility and affect. Multidimensionality or cultural variation in the construct would more likely be associated with a predominance of a limited number of alternative orderings, reflecting some other weighting of the components of a multidimensional construct or alternative cultural constructs. For example, some

Table 30.5 Benefit of the doubt rank order correlation coeffcients for mobility and cognition, 69 surveys

Mobility				Cognition			
BODCORR	N	%	Cum. %	BODCORR	N	%	Cum. %
−0.94	2	0.00	0.00	−0.88	2	0.01	0.01
−0.89	16	0.02	0.03	−0.86	1	0.00	0.01
−0.83	15	0.02	0.05	−0.83	1	0.00	0.01
−0.77	27	0.04	0.09	−0.76	2	0.01	0.02
−0.71	48	0.07	0.16	−0.74	3	0.01	0.03
−0.66	16	0.02	0.18	−0.69	5	0.02	0.04
−0.60	35	0.05	0.23	−0.67	4	0.01	0.05
−0.54	36	0.05	0.29	−0.64	4	0.01	0.07
−0.49	36	0.05	0.34	−0.62	6	0.02	0.08
−0.43	54	0.08	0.42	−0.60	7	0.02	0.11
−0.37	71	0.10	0.52	−0.57	8	0.02	0.13
−0.31	63	0.09	0.61	−0.55	4	0.01	0.14
−0.26	54	0.08	0.69	−0.52	4	0.01	0.15
−0.20	58	0.08	0.78	−0.50	10	0.03	0.18
−0.14	56	0.08	0.86	−0.48	4	0.01	0.20
−0.09	107	0.16	1.02	−0.45	11	0.03	0.23
−0.03	185	0.27	1.29	−0.43	13	0.04	0.27
0.03	31	0.05	1.33	−0.40	6	0.02	0.29
0.09	163	0.24	1.57	−0.38	8	0.02	0.31
0.14	360	0.53	2.10	−0.36	10	0.03	0.34
0.20	71	0.10	2.20	−0.33	20	0.06	0.40
0.26	233	0.34	2.54	−0.31	10	0.03	0.43
0.31	161	0.24	2.78	−0.29	14	0.04	0.48
0.37	361	0.53	3.30	−0.26	8	0.02	0.50
0.43	366	0.54	3.84	−0.24	15	0.05	0.54
0.49	178	0.26	4.10	−0.21	19	0.06	0.60
0.54	483	0.71	4.81	−0.19	5	0.02	0.62
0.60	511	0.75	5.55	−0.17	23	0.07	0.69
0.66	1 178	1.72	7.28	−0.14	23	0.07	0.76
0.71	478	0.70	7.98	−0.12	25	0.08	0.83
0.77	626	0.92	8.89	−0.10	32	0.10	0.93
0.83	3 778	5.53	14.42	−0.07	19	0.06	0.99
0.89	706	1.03	15.45	−0.05	19	0.06	1.04
0.94	12 964	18.96	34.42	−0.02	55	0.17	1.21
1.00	44 834	65.58	100.00	0.00	38	0.12	1.33
Total mobility	68 361	100.00		0.02	29	0.09	1.41

continued

groups may view running a marathon not as evidence of increased mobility but of talent, or as an attribute that is not related to health but to sport. Interpretation of Table 30.5 appears to be more consistent with problems of measurement error due to writing of vignettes, translation or implementation for cognition, compared to the results for mobility.

Determinants of Inconsistent Orderings

Using the BDROCC for every individual that responded to each set of vignettes in all surveys, we can examine the variation in these individual coefficients, which is related to a range of factors. Figure 30.4 shows the median BDROCC across the dataset for each domain of health and responsiveness that included vignettes. For four domains—mobility, affect, quality of basic amenities, and dignity—the vignettes as written and implemented in various sites have worked remarkably well with median correlation greater than 0.9. Further five domains—prompt attention, self-care, support, cognition, and confidentiality—have median correlation coefficients between 0.85 and 0.9. The next four domains in terms of the median correlations are

Table 30.5 Benefit of doubt rank order correlation coeffcients for mobility and cognition, 69 surveys *(continued)*

	Cognition		
BODCORR	N	%	Cum. %
0.05	41	0.12	1.54
0.07	37	0.11	1.65
0.10	36	0.11	1.76
0.12	18	0.05	1.81
0.14	109	0.33	2.14
0.17	59	0.18	2.32
0.19	54	0.16	2.49
0.21	45	0.14	2.62
0.24	60	0.18	2.80
0.26	108	0.33	3.13
0.29	59	0.18	3.31
0.31	80	0.24	3.55
0.33	110	0.33	3.88
0.36	129	0.39	4.28
0.38	83	0.25	4.53
0.40	74	0.22	4.75
0.43	230	0.70	5.45
0.45	110	0.33	5.78
0.48	203	0.61	6.39
0.50	172	0.52	6.92
0.52	172	0.52	7.44
0.55	183	0.55	7.99
0.57	274	0.83	8.82
0.60	158	0.48	9.30
0.62	313	0.95	10.25
0.64	715	2.16	12.41
0.67	186	0.56	12.97
0.69	356	1.08	14.05
0.71	423	1.28	15.33
0.74	911	2.76	18.09
0.76	932	2.82	20.91
0.79	609	1.84	22.76
0.81	1 652	5.00	27.76
0.83	885	2.68	30.44
0.86	2 274	6.88	37.32
0.88	1 144	3.46	40.79
0.90	1 992	6.03	46.82
0.93	5 505	16.67	63.48
0.95	1 137	3.44	66.93
0.98	5 306	16.06	82.99
1.00	5 618	17.01	100.00
Total cognition	33 029	100.00	

choice, communication, autonomy, and usual activities. The worst domain, as implemented in the MCSS is pain, with median correlation below 0.8. It is interesting to note that vignettes have been successfully designed and implemented for some domains both for health and responsiveness, while examples of less effective panels of vignettes have also occurred both for health and responsiveness.

From cognitive interviews, reports from implementation teams, and analysis of survey data, it is clear that some surveys have had more implementation difficulties in general than others. Üstün et al. (*42*) in this volume, for example, explore variation in response rates, item missingness, and sample deviation indices across surveys. Figure 30.5 shows the median value of the BDROCC across domains in each survey, which can be considered as a metric of the quality of implementation of the vignettes in a survey. This ranges from a high value of 0.928 in the Sweden brief face-to-face survey, to six surveys having median values below 0.8, including Turkey postal, Mexico household, Egypt postal, Turkey household, Bahrain brief face-to-face, and Indonesia postal. It is unlikely that this variation in the median BDROCC is due to cultural differences in interpretation across countries, as it is unlikely that such cultural variation would exist across the full set of 14 health and responsiveness domains. Rather, this variation seems to be due to increased stochastic measurement error in the implementation of all the panels of vignettes.

Table 30.6 provides the average BDROCC score by survey and domain. This table helps identify cases where specific sets of vignettes in a country appear to have had some major implementation problems. For example, in Bulgaria, three responsiveness domains have very low average correlation coefficients, namely support, choice, and autonomy. On the basis of these results, further investigation demonstrated that by mistake, the printed version of the instrument in Bulgarian used the health response categories "none," "mild," "moderate," "severe," "extreme" instead of the responsiveness response categories of "very good," "good," "moderate," "bad," "very bad" on these three specific domains. Similar implementation difficulties are likely to underline the few cases of exceptionally low correlation coefficients. This table points to an important distinction between cases where there were specific implementation difficulties with particular domains of health or responsiveness in a country, as compared to low correlation coefficients for all domains, which is likely due to some general aspect of survey implementation such as interviewer training.

To explore the effect of educational attainment on responses to the vignettes, Table 30.7 provides the average BDROCC across all surveys for individuals with 0 years of schooling, 1–4 years, 5–11 years, and

Figure 30.4 Median BDROCC across domains*

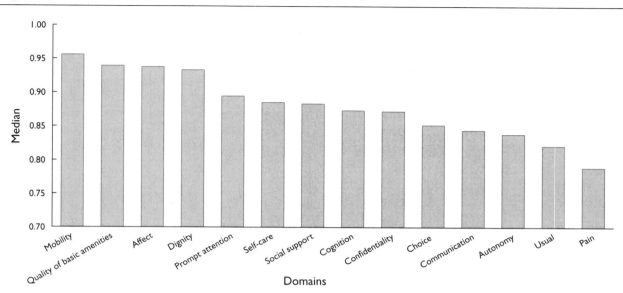

* Benefit of the doubt rank order correlation coefficients

Figure 30.5 Median BDROCC across countries*

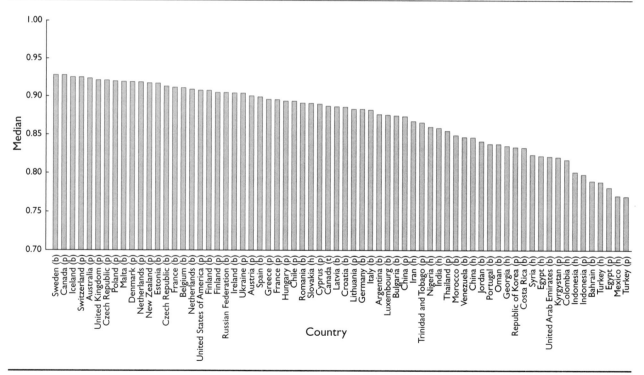

* Benefit of the doubt rank order correlation coefficients

p = Postal, h=Household, t=Telephone, b=Brief face-to-face

12 or more years. For some domains, as expected, the average BDROCC is lower for individuals with no schooling as compared to those with more than 12 years. Overall, however, it is remarkable that individuals with no formal schooling not only understand the vignettes, but also give orderings very close to the

Table 30.6   Average BDROCC (benefit of the doubt rank order correlation coefficient) by domain and survey

Country	Mobility	Affect	Quality of basic amenities	Dignity	Prompt attention	Self-care	Support	Cognition	Confidentiality	Choice	Communication	Autonomy	Usual	Pain	Median
Sweden (b)	0.980	0.977	0.960	0.946	0.933	0.950	0.951	0.923	0.912	0.899	0.863	0.827	0.826	0.831	0.928
Canada (p)	0.986	0.980	0.955	0.978	0.918	0.948	0.928	0.902	0.901	0.899	0.943	0.912	0.928	0.853	0.928
Iceland (b)	0.967	0.970	0.991	0.816	0.706	0.940	0.945	0.929	0.921	0.904	0.864	0.937	0.853	0.799	0.925
Switzerland (p)	0.968	0.965	0.971	0.965	0.938	0.932	0.929	0.871	0.878	0.922	0.865	0.909	0.868	0.729	0.925
Australia (p)	0.979	0.974	0.974	0.957	0.929	0.948	0.956	0.890	0.919	0.906	0.873	0.915	0.916	0.858	0.924
United Kingdom (p)	0.972	0.970	0.954	0.974	0.917	0.960	0.919	0.893	0.909	0.889	0.944	0.924	0.911	0.836	0.921
Czech Republic (p)	0.970	0.972	0.958	0.962	0.931	0.940	0.903	0.894	0.906	0.925	0.917	0.903	0.890	0.817	0.921
Poland (p)	0.958	0.966	0.977	0.960	0.918	0.900	0.946	0.893	0.882	0.933	0.863	0.907	0.922	0.760	0.920
Malta (b)	0.980	0.963	0.969	0.957	0.914	0.901	0.964	0.923	0.916	0.862	0.838	0.924	0.874	0.736	0.919
Denmark (p)	0.967	0.977	0.957	0.959	0.898	0.946	0.878		0.884	0.896	0.929	0.908		0.810	0.919
Netherlands (p)	0.953	0.968	0.950	0.948	0.922	0.909	0.883	0.918	0.894	0.919	0.938	0.911	0.895	0.848	0.919
New Zealand (p)	0.976	0.970	0.977	0.967	0.889	0.905	0.917	0.905	0.922	0.830	0.918	0.926	0.884	0.801	0.917
Estonia (b)	0.987	0.963	0.967	0.962	0.917	0.879	0.944	0.917	0.902	0.934	0.870	0.868	0.820	0.786	0.917
Czech Republic (b)	0.977	0.941	0.961	0.969	0.898	0.914	0.953	0.912	0.896	0.927	0.828	0.907	0.821	0.796	0.913
France (b)	0.964	0.920	0.942	0.939	0.922	0.916	0.924	0.907	0.884	0.869	0.839	0.815	0.803	0.777	0.912
Belgium (b)	0.935	0.948	0.939	0.945	0.928	0.919	0.945	0.903	0.866	0.824	0.826	0.881	0.758	0.728	0.911
Netherlands (b)	0.944	0.956	0.971	0.952	0.925	0.885	0.897	0.904	0.907	0.927	0.874	0.911	0.834	0.757	0.909
United States of America (p)	0.952	0.959	0.937	0.943	0.889	0.950	0.900	0.911	0.876	0.851	0.904	0.932	0.890	0.812	0.908
Finland (b)	0.978	0.963	0.976	0.929	0.909	0.906	0.937	0.903	0.880	0.899	0.858	0.914	0.856	0.842	0.907
Finland (p)	0.980	0.971	0.919	0.885	0.899	0.928	0.931	0.882	0.648	0.868	0.543	0.911	0.917	0.849	0.905
Russian Federation (b)	0.975	0.933	0.959	0.943	0.933	0.896	0.933	0.913	0.836	0.887	0.844	0.834	0.735	0.830	0.905
Ireland (b)	0.956	0.908	0.966	0.952	0.925	0.900	0.949	0.883	0.890	0.843	0.861	0.914	0.847	0.786	0.904
Ukraine (p)	0.979	0.967	0.916	0.934	0.926	0.915	0.877	0.926	0.878	0.826	0.893	0.795	0.844	0.808	0.904
Austria (p)	0.917	0.964	0.948	0.953	0.917	0.906	0.880	0.840	0.915	0.879	0.891	0.895	0.831	0.816	0.901
Spain (b)	0.978	0.953	0.938	0.969	0.892	0.926	0.954	0.881	0.904	0.894	0.883	0.894	0.783	0.811	0.899
Greece (p)	0.974	0.976	0.924	0.934	0.921	0.926	0.818	0.900	0.871	0.852	0.892	0.852	0.866	0.793	0.896
France (p)	0.955	0.967	0.935	0.970	0.911	0.906	0.930	0.883	0.851	0.829	0.844	0.819	0.886	0.827	0.896
Hungary (p)	0.960	0.948	0.938	0.916	0.909	0.885	0.903	0.873	0.882	0.859	0.912	0.857	0.874	0.712	0.894
Chile (p)	0.906	0.953	0.950	0.838	0.936	0.830	0.761	0.908	0.909	0.807	0.903	0.813	0.884	0.858	0.894
Romania (b)	0.933	0.949	0.972	0.954	0.891	0.875	0.943	0.813	0.894	0.892	0.822	0.838	0.779	0.803	0.891
Slovakia (h)	0.959	0.893	0.947	0.934	0.856	0.895	0.924	0.891	0.877	0.891	0.847	0.837	0.875	0.700	0.891
Cyprus (p)	0.970	0.978	0.952	0.967	0.923	0.899	0.842	0.879	0.906	0.804	0.881	0.848	0.873	0.793	0.890
Canada (t)	0.958	0.942	0.951	0.935	0.916	0.886	0.900	0.845	0.887	0.870	0.851	0.888	0.828	0.847	0.887
Latvia (b)	0.979	0.930	0.964	0.948	0.909	0.892	0.882	0.815	0.859	0.922	0.825	0.845	0.804	0.765	0.887
Croatia (b)	0.971	0.942	0.928	0.927	0.930	0.885	0.917	0.859	0.848	0.854	0.887	0.881	0.862	0.785	0.886
Lithuania (p)	0.773	0.957	0.973	0.957	0.909	0.933	0.886	0.894	0.852	0.881	0.843	0.693	0.852	0.763	0.884
Germany (b)	0.941	0.932	0.915	0.930	0.887	0.881	0.901	0.884	0.883	0.855	0.824	0.882	0.815	0.745	0.883

Italy (b)	0.896	0.903	0.962	0.950	0.921	0.933	0.892	0.870	0.873	0.759	0.854	0.846	0.624	0.750	0.882
Argentina (b)	0.953	0.929	0.913	0.915	0.901	0.813	0.844	0.833	0.902	0.877	0.876	0.823	0.848	0.795	0.877
Luxembourg (b)	0.933	0.920	0.924	0.930	0.930	0.911	0.801	0.873	0.868	0.829	0.755	0.878	0.745	0.710	0.876
Bulgaria (b)	0.971	0.954	0.973	0.951	0.239	0.905	0.354	0.893	0.881	0.412	0.869	0.268	0.838	0.830	0.875
China (p)	0.958	0.966	0.918	0.943	0.834	0.874	0.776	0.874	0.886	0.746	0.834	0.791	0.888	0.848	0.874
Iran (h)	0.961	0.926	0.953	0.926	0.845	0.869	0.876	0.875	0.866	0.795	0.799	0.765	0.861	0.805	0.868
Trinidad and Tobago (p)	0.922	0.938	0.910	0.903	0.867	0.866	0.832	0.841	0.866	0.824	0.880	0.832	0.852	0.834	0.866
Nigeria (h)	0.976	0.908	0.932	0.900	0.888	0.881	0.830	0.803	0.770	0.806	0.721	0.839	0.905	0.816	0.860
India (h)	0.954	0.906	0.948	0.920	0.795	0.777	0.916	0.824	0.875	0.867	0.781	0.839	0.781	0.851	0.859
Thailand (p)	0.884	0.904	0.924	0.924	0.745	0.803	0.849	0.630	0.844	0.876	0.861	0.893	0.617	0.801	0.855
Morocco (b)	0.967	0.889	0.909	0.922	0.923	0.845	0.764	0.869	0.827	0.853	0.815	0.772	0.738	0.741	0.849
Venezuela (b)	0.905	0.867	0.848	0.880	0.875	0.793	0.865	0.800	0.846	0.838	0.850	0.760	0.754	0.779	0.847
China (h)	0.919	0.862	0.920	0.902	0.817	0.854	0.897	0.860	0.838	0.819	0.767	0.774	0.806	0.745	0.846
Jordan (b)	0.969	0.922	0.935	0.935	0.863	0.883	0.811	0.909	0.679	0.776	0.808	0.811	0.819	0.817	0.841
Portugal (b)	0.967	0.940	0.936	0.920	0.791	0.868	0.902	0.819	0.810	0.804	0.857	0.817	0.774	0.771	0.838
Oman (b)	0.941	0.908	0.927	0.892	0.868	0.797	0.765	0.815	0.739	0.720	0.829	0.856	0.750	0.846	0.838
Georgia (h)	0.925	0.822	0.894	0.904	0.806	0.840	0.884	0.869	0.830	0.851	0.775	0.748	0.809	0.744	0.835
Republic of Korea (p)	0.801	0.880	0.894	0.933	0.840	0.535	0.848	0.798	0.838	0.874	0.802	0.829	0.786	0.771	0.834
Costa Rica (b)	0.938	0.900	0.930	0.888	0.845	0.778	0.822	0.754	0.867	0.823	0.843	0.802	0.771	0.777	0.833
Syria (h)	0.929	0.886	0.918	0.896	0.826	0.797	0.838	0.859	0.821	0.724	0.750	0.731	0.788	0.776	0.824
Egypt (h)	0.922	0.842	0.909	0.886	0.807	0.800	0.838	0.840	0.843	0.776	0.730	0.673	0.759	0.745	0.822
United Arab Emirates (b)	0.950	0.927	0.914	0.889	0.857	0.834	0.797	0.862	0.804	0.793	0.809	0.770	0.805	0.785	0.821
Kyrgyzstan (p)	0.797	0.873	0.970	0.923	0.886	0.842	0.784	0.768	0.863	0.809	0.756	0.832	0.705	0.745	0.821
Colombia (h)	0.908	0.829	0.913	0.890	0.817	0.737	0.871	0.808	0.843	0.817	0.794	0.782	0.741	0.744	0.817
Indonesia (h)	0.894	0.793	0.896	0.866	0.717	0.758	0.834	0.828	0.801	0.805	0.728	0.695	0.732	0.801	0.801
Indonesia (p)	0.804	0.903	0.913	0.906	0.814	0.335	0.772	0.812	0.789	0.668	0.792	0.818	0.786	0.742	0.798
Bahrain (b)	0.927	0.896	0.875	0.870	0.839	0.774	0.749	0.862	0.744	0.747	0.791	0.752	0.788	0.763	0.789
Turkey (h)	0.927	0.753	0.894	0.828	0.794	0.823	0.857	0.810	0.758	0.782	0.687	0.677	0.761	0.719	0.788
Egypt (p)	0.867	0.801	0.818	0.798	0.765	0.723	0.663	0.800	0.804	0.668	0.797	0.635	0.715	0.685	0.781
Mexico (h)	0.872	0.843	0.856	0.824	0.759	0.730	0.803	0.786	0.782	0.732	0.719	0.702	0.528	0.736	0.771
Turkey (p)	0.751	0.820	0.877	0.895	0.812	0.659	0.539	0.552	0.775	0.620	0.843	0.775	0.574	0.764	0.769
Median	0.956	0.939	0.938	0.933	0.895	0.885	0.883	0.873	0.872	0.852	0.844	0.839	0.821	0.789	

p=Postal, h=Household, t=Telephone, b=Brief face-to-face

global ordering. The gradient by educational attainment in general is rather small. For some domains, including self-care, prompt attention, and communication, there appears to be a stronger gradient. Even in these cases, the difference in the average correlation coefficient between the highest level of educational attainment and the lowest level is 0.05.

We have regressed the individual BDROCC on dummy variables for age group, sex, educational attainment, and type of survey. The results are shown in Table 30.8. In this multivariate analysis, individu-

als with less than 12 years of schooling have lower BDROCC even when age, sex, and survey type are also taken into account. Of note, men have lower correlation coefficients than women, but the magnitude of this effect is quite small. Older respondents have higher correlation coefficients on the vignettes than younger respondents, a result that seems at first to be somewhat counter-intuitive. This could perhaps be explained by the fact that their range of personal experience may be greater, and they are therefore better able to identify with the range of vignettes in a domain. Finally, the survey mode dummy variables explore the impact of standard household surveys, brief household surveys, and postal surveys (only two telephone surveys were conducted). Because the health vignettes in the household surveys come before the responsiveness vignettes, we have interacted health and responsiveness with survey mode to test for ordering or fatigue effects. In this regression analysis, the reference category is responsiveness in the brief face-to-face surveys. These effects suggest that in the longer household surveys, there was a marked reduction in the responsiveness vignette correlation coefficients when these vignettes appeared at the end of a long instrument. This effect is not seen in the comparison of health and responsiveness in the brief face-to-face surveys, which suggests that fatigue may have been an issue in the longer form of the instrument. In general, the best results were obtained in the brief face-to-face instrument, followed by the postal version, with the longer household version producing the worst correlations.

Table 30.7 Average BDROCC (benefit of the doubt rank order correlation coefficient) by education group for all domains

	Years of education			
Domains	*0*	*I to 4*	*5 to II*	*> I2*
Quality of basic amenities	0.927	0.921	0.919	0.931
Autonomy	0.778	0.766	0.783	0.797
Choice	0.801	0.814	0.812	0.817
Communication	0.755	0.778	0.794	0.815
Confidentiality	0.827	0.838	0.834	0.848
Dignity	0.892	0.898	0.901	0.923
Prompt attention	0.803	0.829	0.828	0.849
Support	0.864	0.859	0.859	0.860
Affect	0.876	0.861	0.875	0.906
Cognition	0.836	0.817	0.836	0.865
Mobility	0.933	0.917	0.921	0.934
Pain	0.803	0.774	0.768	0.786
Self-care	0.799	0.792	0.820	0.847
Usual activities	0.793	0.771	0.793	0.817

Table 30.8 Regression analysis of BDROCC (benefit of the doubt rank order correlation coefficient) as a function of age, sex, educational attainment, and survey mode

Variables	*Coef.*	*Std. Err.*	*t*	*P > |t|*	*[95% Conf.*	*Interval]*
Responsiveness and household survey	−0.043	0.001	−34.5	0	−0.045	−0.040
Responsiveness and postal survey	−0.002	0.001	−1.6	0.106	−0.005	0.000
Health and brief face-to-face survey	0.010	0.002	6.6	0	0.007	0.013
Health and household survey	−0.023	0.001	−18.6	0	−0.026	−0.021
Health and postal survey	−0.014	0.001	−9.8	0	−0.017	−0.012
Age (29 to 44 years)	0.005	0.001	6.0	0	0.003	0.007
Age (45 to 59 years)	0.013	0.001	13.8	0	0.012	0.015
Age (60 to 100 years)	0.017	0.001	15.4	0	0.015	0.019
Education (5 to II years)	−0.013	0.001	−17.2	0	−0.014	−0.012
Education (I to 4 years)	−0.020	0.001	−15.1	0	−0.023	−0.017
Education (0 years)	−0.012	0.001	−8.7	0	−0.014	−0.009
Sex (male)	−0.006	0.001	−8.4	0	−0.007	−0.004
Constant	0.875	0.001	699.3	0	0.873	0.878
Number of obs	476 979					
Adj R^2	0.009					

General Assessment of Vignette Implementation

The substantial empirical experience of using anchoring vignettes for health and responsiveness domains in the MCSS demonstrates that vignettes appear to be understood in a similar fashion by individuals with widely varying levels of education and age and diverse cultural backgrounds. This general success of the vignettes is reassuring. Nevertheless, the clear evidence that vignettes were more effectively implemented for some domains than for others, and in some surveys more than in others, highlights the opportunities for improving this approach in future data collection.

Building on the experience of the MCSS, anchoring vignettes have been incorporated in the World Health Survey modules for health, responsiveness, and social capital. Vignettes used in the MCSS were modified based on some of the results shown here and pilot-tested in 12 countries before being included in the final WHS instrument. In general, vignettes have been modified on the basis of both the descriptive results presented in this section and the application of statistical models to the vignette responses, described in later sections. The goal of this development has been to identify vignettes that appear to be widely understood and represent clearly different levels on the domain of concern.

Non-Parametric Analysis of Cut-Point Shift for Mobility

For the majority of respondents that have ordered the vignettes in the same fashion, examination of the categorical rating for each vignette provides evidence of differences in cut-points between individuals and groups. For the domain of mobility, the most common response pattern has been to place Vignettes 1 and 2 in the category "no difficulty," Vignette 3 in the category "moderate difficulty," Vignettes 4 and 5 in the category "severe difficulty," and Vignette 6 in the category "extreme difficulty." 88% of respondents, however, used alternative response patterns, which indicate where individuals have different cut-points.

Overall, 205 different response patterns were used for the six vignettes across all the mobility respondents. Table 30.9 comprises the 18 most common vignette response patterns that account for nearly three-quarters of all responses. In all 18 of these response patterns, the top two vignettes, the marathon runner and the jogger, are placed in the response category "no difficulties." The variation across these

18 is entirely in the pattern of response categories for the other four vignettes. For other domains where the vignettes are more evenly spaced on the latent variable, variation across the position of all vignettes is probably larger. In the case of mobility, the top two vignettes are clearly close to the maximum conceivable level of mobility. The same is not true of the top vignettes for other domains.

Table 30.10 shows the most common response pattern for the vignettes in each country and the percentage of respondents in that country using this response pattern. Across the countries in this sample, 13 different (including all ties) modal response patterns are used. The percentage of respondents giving the modal response pattern, a crude measure of homogeneity of cut-points in a population, ranges from under 10% in Singapore, Indonesia, Mexico, and India, to over 30% in New Zealand, Switzerland, Chile, Czech Republic, and Poland. Given the small number of unique modal patterns across countries (13), compared to the 205 different patterns used by all individual respondents, it appears that there is greater variation in cut-points within countries than across countries for the domain of mobility. The nature of the mobility vignettes and the nature of the domain of mobility may mean that for other domains there is greater cross-country variation in the average or modal cut-points.

Table 30.9 Eighteen most commonly used vignette response patterns in 69 surveys among consistent raters

Pattern	Frequency	Per cent	Cum. per cent
553221	5 404	12.05	100.00
554221	4 905	10.94	90.77
554321	4 298	9.59	79.53
553321	3 110	6.94	57.55
554331	2 247	5.01	41.58
553211	1 497	3.34	27.70
554421	1 271	2.83	23.52
552221	1 203	2.68	22.26
554211	1 096	2.44	20.28
554431	957	2.13	17.71
553331	952	2.12	17.62
555321	925	2.06	17.12
555221	917	2.05	16.97
554311	775	1.73	14.34
554332	745	1.66	13.79
552211	726	1.62	13.43
553311	673	1.50	12.45
554322	673	1.50	12.45

The fact that there are so many different response patterns within a country highlights that cut-point variation is not simply a question of culture or language. Some of this variation may be due to characteristics such as age, sex, or education. It is likely, however, that a considerable fraction of variation in cut-points across individuals may be due to other individual psychological attributes. Individuals of the same age, sex, and education in the same country have a wide range of response patterns and thus, highly variable cut-points. Optimism or pessimism, for example, may influence response categories. It would

be interesting in future analyses to investigate if the modal response pattern is different as a function of responses on questions about general outlook on life or general satisfaction with life experiences.

Non-Parametric Analysis of Self-Reported Mobility

Anchoring vignettes were included in the MCSS so that they could be used with appropriate statistical models to understand how individuals' cut-points vary

Table 30.10 Modal mobility vignette response patterns for consistent raters, pooled and across 69 surveys

Country	Modal pattern	Freq	Per cent	Country	Modal pattern	Freq	Per cent
ALL 69	553221	5 404	12.05	India (h)	554221	97	8.60
Argentina (b)	553221	51	20.90	Ireland (b)	553321	32	12.26
Australia (p)	553221	114	21.23	Iran (h)	554221	394	11.58
Austria (p)	553221	88	24.86	Iceland (b)	553221	40	21.98
Belgium (b)	553221	50	14.41	Italy (b)	554321	42	12.54
Bulgaria (b)	553221	87	24.79	Jordan (b)	554221	32	11.11
Bahrain (b)	554421	30	13.27	Kyrgyzstan (p)	554321	19	13.19
Canada (p)	553221	34	21.52	Korea, Republic of (p)	554211	11	12.79
Canada (t)	554321	16	11.03	Lithuania (p)	553221	79	25.48
Switzerland (p)	553221	49	32.03	Luxembourg (t)	553221	41	17.15
Chile (p)	554221	117	34.31	Latvia (b)	553221	52	17.93
China (h)	554321	377	12.00	Morocco (b)	553221	45	16.85
China (p)	554221	65	15.55	Mexico (h)	554331	76	6.97
Colombia (h)	554431	269	15.13	Malta (b)	554221 / 554331	29	15.76
Costa Rica (b)	553221	22	10.19	Nigeria (h)	554221	369	21.89
Cyprus (p)	554221	35	14.06	Netherlands (b)	553221	64	18.66
Czech Republic (b)	553221	74	17.92	Netherlands (p)	553221	47	23.15
Czech Republic (p)	553221	125	33.24	New Zealand (p)	553221	206	31.94
Germany (b)	553221	69	16.31	Oman (b)	553221	31	10.44
Denmark (p)	553221	135	22.50	Poland (p)	553221	107	36.15
Egypt (h)	554321	169	11.54	Portugal (b)	554321	39	11.44
Egypt (p)	553221	41	11.42	Romania (b)	554321	48	13.91
Spain (b)	554321	48	12.66	Russia (b)	553221	111	17.90
Estonia (b)	553221	62	14.87	Singapore (h)	554321	154	9.34
Finland (b)	554221	68	17.57	Slovakia (h)	554321	55	14.21
Finland (p)	553221	89	18.16	Sweden (b)	554221	69	18.55
France (b)	553221	50	13.66	Syria (h)	554321	333	12.25
France (p)	553221	61	29.33	Thailand (p)	553221	55	14.75
United Kingdom (p)	553221	43	22.63	Trinidad and Tobago (p)	554221	59	16.16
Georgia (h)	553221	487	14.25	Turkey (h)	554321	198	13.14
Greece (p)	553221	90	25.79	Turkey (p)	553221	67	17.82
Croatia (b)	553221	122	21.75	Ukraine (p)	553221	82	27.70
Hungary (p)	554221	89	19.02	United Arab Emirates (b)	54221 / 554321	31	11.27
Indonesia (h)	553221	213	7.48	United States of America (p)	554321	102	22.32
Indonesia (p)	552211 / 553211 / 553221	97	20.00	Venezuela (b)	554321	31	14.09

p=Postal, h=Household, t=Telephone, b=Brief face-to-face

as a function of individual or cultural characteristics. In this section, however, before resorting to the use of statistical models, we use non-parametric approaches (44) to investigate the responses of individuals who gave both self-assessments and vignette ratings for the domain of mobility. Because only a subset of respondents answered the mobility vignettes, the limitation of this approach is that the self-responses of just over half of the respondents are excluded.

SELF-RESPONSE AND VIGNETTE RESPONSE PATTERNS

For individuals who have ranked the six vignettes consistently with the global ordering, Figure 30.6 illustrates that there are 28 possible patterns of self-response and vignette responses. The first 13 patterns are the simple cases where an individual is in a response category better than the first vignette, equal to a given vignette, between two vignettes or worse than the 6th vignette. The remaining 15 patterns are cases of more complex combinations. For example, an individual may give the same categorical rating to Vignette 1 (the marathon runner), Vignette 2 (the jogger) and him/herself. Table 30.11 gives the frequency distribution of response patterns for respondents who ordered the mobility vignettes consistent with the global ordering.

Over half of all consistent respondents used self-response and vignette response pattern 14, where Vignettes 1 and 2, and self are in the same response category. The second most common pattern is 19, where Vignettes 1, 2, and 3, and self are in the same response category. The next most common (over 7.5%) is pattern 6, where the individual is in the same response category as Vignette 3, Vignettes 2 and 1 are in a higher response category, and Vignettes 4, 5, and 6 are in a lower response category. The fourth most common pattern is where the individual places himself or herself in the category lower than the jogger, but higher than the person who can walk 200 meters but feels breathless after walking 1 kilometre or climbing a flight of stairs.

For the 66% of respondents who answered the vignettes consistently with the global ordering, mapping to these categories is not a difficult task. For the remaining 34%, an algorithm is needed to categorize the vignette responses that deviate from the global ordering. There are several equally plausible strategies for dealing with inversions in the non-parametric analysis. We have first identified the largest number of vignettes that are consistent with the global ordering. Next, we have identified the best vignette that the individual is worse than and the worst vignette that the individual is better than. These pairs of vignettes that bound the individual response can be directly mapped into one of the 28 patterns in Figure 30.6. For example, if an individual ordered the vignettes 1, 3, 2, 5, 6, 4, then the consistent ordering includes only 1, 2, 5, 6. If the individual's self-response positions him or her above Vignette 5 but below Vignette 2, he or she is located in pattern 16. Table 30.11 also provides the distribution of respondents in the MCSS without

Figure 30.6 28 self-response and vignette response patterns

	1	2	3	4	5	6	7	8	9	10	11	12	13	14	15	16	17	18	19	20	21	22	23	24	25	26	27	28
Vignette 1																												
Vignette 2																												
Vignette 3																												
Vignette 4																												
Vignette 5																												
Vignette 6																												

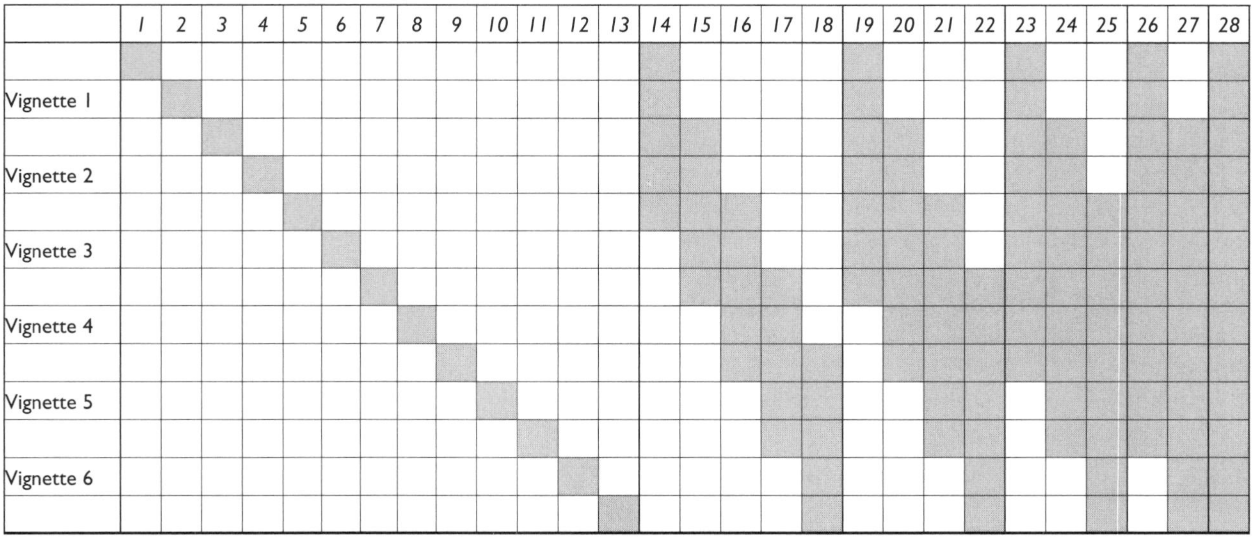

Shading = Self-rating for mobility question, relative to vignette rating

consistent ordering across the 28 patterns. The difference between consistent and inconsistent respondents across the 28 patterns is rather informative. Among consistent raters, over 5% used category 1 or 2, but among inconsistent raters, over 20% used these categories. One is tempted to conclude that in these individuals who rate themselves equal to or better than the marathon runner, we are identifying a group or respondents that either project their levels of mobility above their true levels or are subject to higher levels of measurement error. Pattern 23, where the respondent is in a category better than Vignette 5 but not worse than any vignette between 1 and 4, is also much more common among inconsistent raters.

The 28 self-response and vignette response patterns include a number of overlapping categories, as shown in Figure 30.6. These 28 patterns yield only a partial ordering in terms of the levels of mobility that they represent on the latent scale. In other words, someone with pattern 14 may have higher, equal, or lower levels of mobility than someone with patterns 1, 2, 3, 4, or 5. We can unequivocally say that individuals with pattern 14 have higher levels of mobility than those with pattern 21, but such a definitive statement cannot be made about pattern 14 compared to pattern 20. Assumptions that spread individuals in a broader category such as 14 over patterns 2, 3, and 4, are difficult to justify. This is particularly true in the case of mobility where the majority of respondents in nearly all communities are in response category "no difficulty."

The 28 patterns can, however, be mapped into seven cumulative groups that do have a natural ordering. We may define these cumulative vignette-adjusted response categories (VARS) as follows: VARS 6 includes those individuals who are unequivo-

Table 30.11 Distribution of respondents in 69 multi-country survey studies by 28 self-response and vignette response patterns

Category	Consistent raters		Inconsistent raters		All raters	
	n	%	n	%	n	%
1	690	1.54	2 909	12.37	3 599	5.26
2	1 570	3.50	2 060	8.76	3 630	5.31
3	72	0.16	188	0.80	260	0.38
4	204	0.46	180	0.77	384	0.56
5	2 737	6.10	1 016	4.32	3 753	5.49
6	3 364	7.50	833	3.54	4 197	6.14
7	1 349	3.01	514	2.18	1 863	2.73
8	1 010	2.25	183	0.78	1 193	1.75
9	356	0.79	172	0.73	528	0.77
10	604	1.35	157	0.67	761	1.11
11	273	0.61	299	1.27	572	0.84
12	289	0.64	193	0.82	482	0.71
13	67	0.15	308	1.31	375	0.55
14	24 949	55.65	8 072	34.31	33 021	48.31
15	156	0.35	177	0.75	333	0.49
16	1 075	2.40	597	2.54	1 672	2.45
17	928	2.07	414	1.76	1 342	1.96
18	156	0.35	145	0.62	301	0.44
19	3 848	8.58	2 389	10.15	6 237	9.12
20	47	0.10	102	0.43	149	0.22
21	324	0.72	353	1.50	677	0.99
22	97	0.22	161	0.68	258	0.38
23	381	0.85	1 046	4.45	1 427	2.09
24	23	0.05	74	0.31	97	0.14
25	27	0.06	95	0.4	122	0.18
26	69	0.15	425	1.81	494	0.72
27	10	0.02	64	0.27	74	0.11
28	158	0.35	400	1.70	558	0.82
Total	44 833	65.58	23 526	34.42	68 359	100.00

cally equal to or worse than the 6th vignette, VARS 5 includes those individuals who are equal to or worse than the 6th vignette, and so on. Note that everyone in VARS 6 is by definition included in VARS 5; everyone in VARS 5 is included in VARS 4, and so on. The penultimate category (VARS 1) includes everyone equal to or worse than the best vignette. The difference between this category and the entire sample (VARS 0) is rather small because few individuals in this case have reported themselves in a category better than the marathon runner. In fact, in the specific case of mobility, it could be argued that where individuals have reported themselves as better than the marathon runner, this is likely due to measurement error rather than having a level of mobility better than the marathon runner.

Table 30.12 gives for the entire 68 358 respondents the distribution function for the cumulative VARS categories. 21% of respondents in the entire sample report mobility that is worse than or equal to the individual who becomes breathless after 1 kilometer. 28% are worse than or equal to the jogger, reflecting the large fraction of respondents with levels of mobility that cannot be distinguished from very high levels associated with the best vignettes.

Table 30.12 also shows the cross-tabulation between the raw response categories and the seven VARS categories for the entire set of respondents who answered the mobility vignettes. Of note, nearly all individuals who used the top response category "no difficulty" are included in the vignette-adjusted category equal to or worse than the marathon runner. In fact, individuals in the top response category must logically be included in either VARS 0 (all respondents) and VARS 1 (those respondents equal to or worse than the highest vignette), or in VARS 0 only. For other response categories, the vignette adjustment

identifies individuals with different levels of mobility. For example, individuals whose self-response category was "moderate difficulty" range from some who are included in VARS 1 and VARS 0 only, through others who are included in all seven VARS categories.

Even when one individual is in VARS 6 (and subsequent categories) and another is in VARS 4 (and subsequent), we cannot with certainty (even excluding measurement error) conclude that the first individual has a level of mobility below that of the second individual. Imagine two respondents who give the self-response "extreme difficulty" and have the same latent level of mobility. One places Vignette 6 in the category "extreme difficulty" and Vignette 5 in the category "severe difficulty," and thus falls into VARS 6. The other places Vignettes 4, 5, and 6 in the category "extreme difficulty" because he has different cut-points. The latter falls in VARS 4, but in fact has the same level of mobility as the individual in VARS 6. This illustrates why the VARS distributions should only be examined as cumulative distributions.

Even though in many cases one cannot order individuals, at the population level one can, in certain cases, conclude that one population has a higher level of mobility than another. Based on the principles of first-order stochastic dominance,[2] we can see that if the cumulative distribution of respondents by the vignette-adjusted response categories is always to the left of another, then its mobility is lower. If the cumulative distributions of two populations cross each other, we cannot conclude which population has a lower or higher level of mobility. If stochastic measurement error varies across countries, then the assessment of population levels of mobility using this approach could be biased. In fact, one important advantage of the parametric approach presented below is that it accounts for measurement error more explicitly.

Table 30.12 Distribution of vignette-adjusted raw score (VARS) and self-response categories for mobility in 69 multi-country survey studies

| | | Self-response category | | | | | | | | | | | |
| | Mean | 1 | | 2 | | 3 | | 4 | | 5 | | Total | |
VARS	Self-response	n	cum %	n	cum %	n	cum %	n	cum %	n	cum %	n	cum %
0	4.49	579	100	2 866	100	6 808	100	10 464	100	47 642	100	68 359	100
1	4.47	579	100	2 845	99	6 682	98	10 158	97	44 002	92	64 266	94
2	3.28	568	98	2 811	98	6 461	95	9 293	89			19 133	28
3	3.10	564	97	2 757	96	5 738	84	5 284	50			14 343	21
4	2.71	552	95	2 448	85	3 084	45	1 400	13			7 484	11
5	2.16	513	89	1 214	42	609	9	155	1			2 491	4
6	1.92	390	67	233	8	148	2	86	1			857	1

Figure 30.7 illustrates the distribution across the cumulative VARS categories and, for comparison, the cumulative distribution of the self-response categories for four brief face-to-face surveys in the Czech Republic, Latvia, Romania, and Estonia. According to the self-response data alone, there is a clear ordering of the countries from Latvia with the lowest levels of mobility, to Romania, to the Czech Republic, and finally to Estonia. When differences in cut-points are taken into account through the vignettes, the population level assessment changes. We can conclude that Latvia has lower levels of mobility than Estonia, but we cannot come to conclusions about Romania and the Czech Republic *vis-à-vis* the other two countries. Conclusions about levels of mobility at the individual, or in this case, the population level, using a strictly non-parametric approach, are fairly limited. In addition, even the conclusions drawn using the principles of stochastic dominance may be incorrect in the presence of variation across countries in the extent of measurement error. In the next section, formal parametric models are used to deal more explicitly with measurement error and to increase the range of conclusions possible about the population distributions of health on a given domain.

PARAMETRIC ANALYSIS OF MOBILITY USING THE CHOPIT MODEL

In the previous sections, data collected in the MCSS have been used to demonstrate that individuals, groups, and populations use response categories in different ways. In the language of latent variable models, cut-points between response categories on the latent variable vary across individuals. When individuals respond for themselves and for the vignettes, non-parametric approaches can be used to help distinguish individuals with different levels of mobility. There are major limitations of this approach: first, all individuals in a survey must answer questions not only about themselves, but also about the vignettes; second, non-parametric approaches as illustrated in this chapter provide only a partial ordering across individuals and populations; and third, non-parametric approaches do not explicitly deal with measurement error.

If the evident variation in cut-points across individuals, groups, and populations can be predicted on the basis of individual covariates, then it is possible to increase the efficiency of data collection enormously by gathering anchoring vignette ratings for a given domain on only a subset of respondents. An appro-

priate statistical model can then be used to adjust all individual responses for the expected variation in cut-points. In this section, we apply the CHOPIT model described elsewhere (*36;44*) to analyse the mobility data in the MCSS. For the purposes of developing summary measures of population health such as HALE, the other domains of health in the MCSS have also been analysed using the CHOPIT model. However, in this chapter, we restrict presentation of the results to mobility because of space limitations.

METHODS

Formal details of the basic CHOPIT model are provided elsewhere (*36;44*). In this analysis, however, several aspects of the application of CHOPIT are worth noting.

Figure 30.7 Cumulative mobility distributions in Latvia, Estonia, Romania, and the Czech Republic

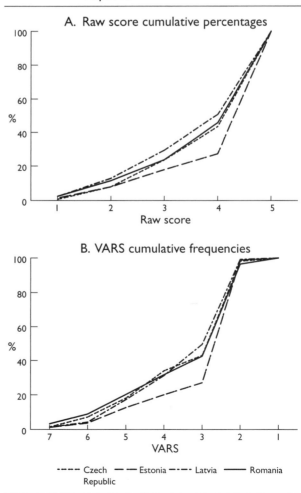

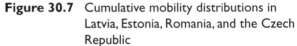

- In the basic CHOPIT model, it is assumed that the stochastic error for each vignette is normally distributed on the latent variable with a constant (and equal) variance for each of the vignettes. This assumption has been relaxed to allow each vignette to have a different variance. Given the variation in the number of inversions in the data for different pairs of vignettes, this elaboration of the model seems appropriate. This modification enables easy identification of those vignettes which are "noisier" than others: i.e. vignettes perceived with more inconsistency by respondents will have larger estimated variances.

- Age, sex, education, country, and interactions of these variables have been included as covariates of latent mobility. Given the strong biological relationship between mobility and age, we have a very strong prior that this variable will predict an important component of mobility. Likewise, educational attainment generally predicts levels of mortality, even in adults (45–49), and we expect will capture some socioeconomic gradients in exposure to health risks and diseases, as well as gradients in access to quality care.

- Age, sex, education, country, and interactions of these variables have also been used as the covariates of the cut-points. Because this is one of the first large-scale systematic explorations of variations in individual cut-points, we do not have strong prior hypotheses that these variables will predict cut-point shift. Given previous observations on some types of morbidity and other functional questions (30;32;34;50–52), we expect that country dummy variables will capture some major cultural variation in cut-points. For mobility particularly, declining health expectations as individuals age may be reflected in cut-point shifts and uncovered through differences in vignette ratings (53). Further research may yield better covariates at the individual level to capture variation due to personality type or outlook.

- In the standard household surveys conducted in 13 countries, more than one mobility item was included. CHOPIT, as opposed to the non-parametric approaches presented earlier, can easily accommodate more than one item on a domain. Inclusion of more than one item is advantageous because it allows more robust estimation of the random effect on the latent variable. The random effect is meant to capture systematic variation in

levels of mobility across an individual, which is otherwise not captured by the covariates of mobility included in the model. Because the postal and brief face-to-face surveys included only one item on mobility, the average fraction of the total variance estimated for the standard household surveys has been applied to the analysis of all the surveys in the estimation of posteriors for each individual. Posteriors are updated estimates of the latent variable taking into account the magnitude of the random effect and the observed categorical response for the individual. The basic idea is that if there is a significant random effect, then there remains information content in the categorical response that is not explained by the measured covariates. In such situations, Bayes' theorem can be invoked in order to exploit this remaining information content (see Tandon et al in this book for more details (36)).

- As with all latent variable models, the underlying scale needs to be identified in CHOPIT. The identification assumptions include the coefficient of Vignette 6 set equal to zero and its variance equal to one.

- For this parametric analysis, we have chosen to include in estimation of the model only those surveys that have met certain explicit criteria reflecting the quality of survey implementation with specific reference to the mobility vignettes. These criteria were a mean Spearman's rank order correlation coefficient greater than 0.8 and a standard deviation of the Spearman's correlation coefficient less than 0.3. The USA postal survey was also excluded because respondents were presented the vignettes in order of severity rather than randomized, as in the case of all other surveys. 55 surveys met these criteria and were included in the model.

- We have repeated the analysis two ways: a) using all the vignette respondents to estimate the model parameters; and b) using only the vignette responses with a BDROCC greater than 0.8. We have included these two analyses to explore the potential impact of non-normal error structures on the CHOPIT model estimation. The CHOPIT model assumes that measurement error on the latent variable is normally distributed. For some surveys, however, some of the inconsistent vignette raters are likely to be not well-represented by a normally distributed error term. By analysing the dataset in both ways and qualitatively comparing the results to some of the non-parametric analyses, we can identify directions for improving instrument design, data collection, and data analysis in the future.

RESULTS

Table 30.13 provides the results of the CHOPIT model for the values of the vignettes on the latent variable and the vignette-specific standard deviations for both the full dataset and the vignette ratings with a BDROCC greater than 0.8. For the full dataset, the worst vignette is set to zero with a variance of one. Vignettes 3, 4, and 5 span from zero to 2.00 on the latent variable, with lower variances than Vignette 6. The marathon runner and the jogger have much higher levels on the latent variable but also much higher variances. This may reflect a lack of consensus among respondents regarding the cut-off on the mobility scale at which further improvements no longer constitute health gains, but rather reflect some other construct (which may be called "fitness" or "talent"). The CHOPIT results for the subset of respondents with a BDROCC > 0.8 are substantively similar, although the scale has expanded to range from 0 to 5.35.

Figure 30.8 allows visualization of the vignettes and expected cut-points for all respondents. On the y-axis, the horizontal lines represent the level on the latent variable of the six vignettes. For each of the four cut-points that define the five response categories on the latent variable, the plot shows the frequency distribution of cut-points across individuals estimated on the basis of age, sex, education, and country, including interactions. It is clear from the figure that many individuals have overlapping cut-points. The cut-point representing the transition from "severe difficulty" to "moderate difficulty" for some individuals overlaps with others' cut-points representing the transition from "moderate difficulty" to "mild difficulty." Figure 30.8 also illustrates how Vignettes 1 and 2 are far from the cut-point between the response categories "mild difficulty" and "no difficulty." Responses to these vignettes are, therefore, less likely to help identify variation in

cut-points across individuals. We have also examined the same relationships for the CHOPIT analysis of the subset of respondents with a BDROCC > 0.8 (Figure 30.8B). Relative to the vignette values on the latent scale, there is not substantive difference in the distribution of the cut-points. This comparison indicates that the estimation of expected cut-points is mostly unaffected by including respondents with large and possibly non-normal measurement error.

While the distribution of predicted cut-points on the basis of age, sex, education, and country is quite wide, Figure 30.8 dramatically underestimates the true variation in cut-points in the populations surveyed. In the figure, no predicted cut-point for the transition between "mild difficulty" and "no difficulty" (cut-point 4) falls below Vignette 3. In the non-parametric analysis, however, more than 14% of respondents have placed Vignette 3 in the same response category as Vignettes 1 and 2, which implies that cut-point 4 is below Vignette 3 (see Table 30.9). Such a large fraction of respondents placing all three vignettes in the top response category is unlikely to be accounted for on the basis of normal measurement error. The most plausible explanation is that the covariates of cut-point shift included in the model fail to capture a substantial component of variation across individuals in cut-points.

Figure 30.9 provides the average predicted cut-points for the set of respondents in each survey, relative to the values of the vignettes. For some countries, cut-point 4 has a lower value than cut-point 3 (which marks the transition between "moderate difficulty" and "mild difficult") in other countries. The figure highlights the values in the Austria postal survey and the Colombia household survey. For each cut-point, Austria is towards the higher end, while the cut-point values in Colombia are at the low end of the distribution across the 55 surveys. In other cases, cut-points are expanded or contracted relative to other countries, i.e. the bottom two cut-points are lower, while the top two cut-points are higher.

Table 30.13 Vignette thetas and sigmas for mobility for full dataset and for BDROCC > 0.8 dataset

	Full dataset				BDROCC > 0.8 dataset			
	Theta	SE Theta	Sigma	SE Sigma	Theta	SE Theta	Sigma	SE Sigma
Vignette 1	4.30	0.04	1.30	0.023	5.35	0.06	1.22	0.028
Vignette 2	3.79	0.03	1.14	0.017	5.03	0.05	1.28	0.023
Vignette 3	2.00	0.01	0.41	0.004	2.68	0.02	0.54	0.006
Vignette 4	1.52	0.01	0.42	0.004	1.96	0.01	0.59	0.006
Vignette 5	1.28	0.01	0.47	0.004	1.60	0.01	0.64	0.007
Vignette 6	0.00	0.00	1.00		0.00	0.00	1.00	

In some countries, we observe strong cut-point gradients by age, sex, and education. Figure 30.10 illustrates that for six surveys (Argentina, Chile, Netherlands, New Zealand, Ukraine, and Portugal), as respondents age, the first cut-points shift to a lower level of mobility. Such an age gradient in the cut-points could be explained by older individuals having lower expectations for mobility as they age; what is considered extreme at a young age is reported as severe at an older age.

Figure 30.11 shows a larger gradient by educational attainment in Austria for all four cut-points. There is a dramatic rise in the top cut-point, a substantial gradient in the two middle cut-points, and little gradient in the bottom cut-point. The rising gradient for mobility in Austria means that in this country, individuals with higher levels of educational attainment have higher

expectations for mobility. This gradient as a function of educational status is present in many but not all countries. Such an educational gradient, as shown in Austria, can mean that gradients in mobility may be larger than revealed by a simple tabulation of self-responses according to educational group.

There is considerable debate about sex gradients in self-responses (30;31;54). Figure 30.12 illustrates for eight countries very different patterns in the variation in cut-points as a function of sex. In Canada and Hungary, cut-points for females are consistently higher than those for males. In Oman and Malta, the reverse is true. More complex patterns unfold in Bahrain, Switzerland, Costa Rica, and Indonesia, where the range of cut-points for males or females is smaller. In Switzerland, for example, males have a lower bottom cut-point but a higher top cut-point. The diversity of

Figure 30.8 Cut-points and vignette ratings for all respondents

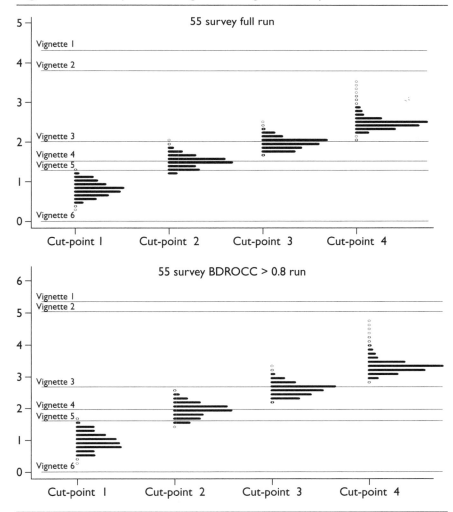

Figure 30.9 Average cut-points for each survey and vignette ratings, 55 survey full run

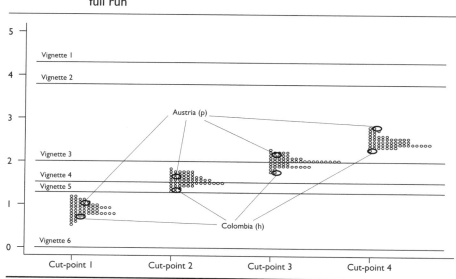

Figure 30.10 Cut-point 1 by age category in six countries, y-axis is normalized to vignette 1 equals 100

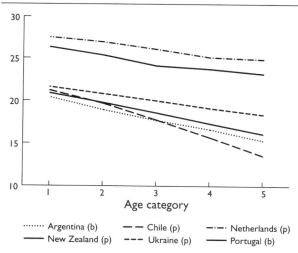

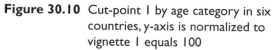

Figure 30.11 Cut-points by educational attainment in Austria Postal Survey, y-axis is normalized to vignette 1 equals 100

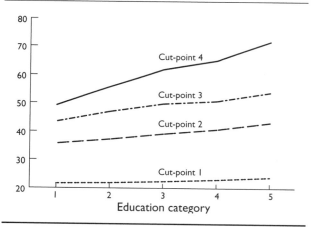

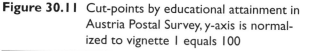

Figure 30.12 Cut-points by sex in eight countries

patterns illustrated by these eight countries indicates that sex differentials in unadjusted self-response data must be interpreted with extreme caution.

A key component of the CHOPIT model is the computation of posterior probability distributions of the latent mobility levels for each individual using his or her covariates (in this case, age, sex, education, and country) and observed self-responses. The self-responses contain additional information beyond what is captured in the covariates because there is, in principle, a random effect across individuals reflecting the impact of unmeasured covariates on mobility. Estimation of the random effect and the width of the

Figure 30.13 Posterior estimates of mobility versus expected values of mobility for the entire dataset

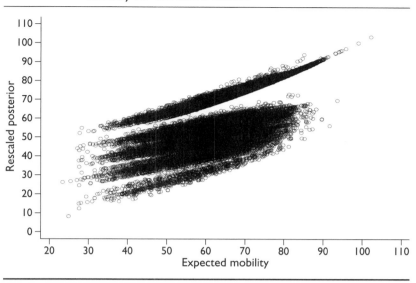

posterior distribution of mobility are improved when more than one item is included for a domain.

Figure 30.13 shows, for the entire dataset, the comparison of the posterior value for mobility for each individual and the expected value based on country and country-specific effects of age, sex, and education. This figure helps visualize how different parts of the model are contributing to the posterior estimate of mobility. Both the y-axis and the x-axis have been transformed so that zero is equal to the worst vignette, the quadriplegic, and 100 is equal to the best vignette, the marathon runner. There are three things to note about this relationship. First, the covariates country, age, sex, and education spread individuals across a wide range in terms of expected mobility. Second, there are five bands representing the effect of each individual's response category on the posterior. In other words, an individual with a value of 50 for mobility, predicted on the basis of covariates, has a very different posterior estimate if he/she responded "no difficulty" or "extreme difficulty." Third, the slopes of each band are different. The steeper slope for the band defined by those responding "no difficulty" is due to the fact that the cut-point for the category "no difficulty" is substantially below the expected value for many individuals. Fourth, the range at any level of expected mobility with a response category band is due to differences in cut-points across individuals. These differences are quite large, even though we know from the non-parametric assessment that it is substantially underestimated in the CHOPIT model,

because we have not identified covariates that predict much of the interindividual variation in cut-points.

When there is more than one item for a domain, the information content of the posterior is greatly increased. If there are two mobility items, Figure 30.13 would have 25 bands representing all the possible answers on the two items, each with five response categories for individuals with a given expected value. Not all of these 25 possibilities are very likely even in the presence of substantial measurement error.

Figure 30.14 compares, for all individuals, the posterior estimate of mobility based on the CHOPIT analysis for the full dataset, including all vignette responders and the CHOPIT analysis using only the vignette responses from those with a BDROCC > 0.8 and all self-responses. Using a dataset that excludes apparently large response errors that were potentially not adequately represented by a normally distributed error term on the latent variable has only a very limited influence on the posterior estimates for individuals. This result suggests that the CHOPIT model is reasonably robust to measurement error in the self-ratings and vignette ratings.

As a final consideration of the impact of taking into account cut-point shift through the use of vignettes and the CHOPIT model, Figure 30.15 presents a comparison of the age-standardized average raw response score with the age-standardized average posterior using the CHOPIT model. The average raw score has been calculated by assigning a value of five to the category "no difficulty," four to "mild difficulty,"

Figure 30.14 Comparison of posterior estimates of mobility for full
run and BDROCC > 0.8 run

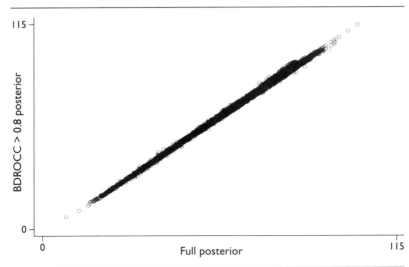

Figure 30.15 Comparison of age-standardized raw score with age-standardized posteriors
in 55 surveys

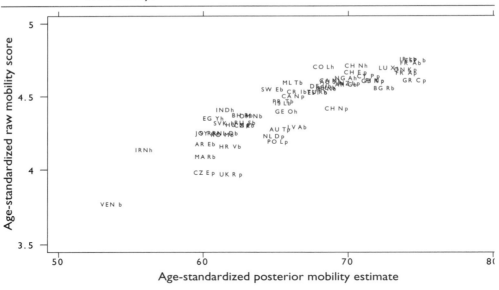

and so on. The figure illustrates that even at the level of comparing national averages, taking into account cut-point shift alters the relative assessment of mobility across countries. Considering, for example, the Netherlands postal survey, a number of countries have the same age-standardized raw score, such as Jordan, Syria, and Romania. After taking into account cut-point differences, the Netherlands has a higher level of mobility. In a similar fashion, there is a wide range of average raw scores associated with the same level

of mobility based on the CHOPIT model. The Netherlands and Sweden have, according to the CHOPIT estimates, similar levels of mobility but substantially different raw scores. The actual levels of mobility from the raw score or from CHOPIT should not be over-interpreted. In many cases, postal surveys appear to have had considerable selection bias in the age of the respondent and potentially the health of the respondent. Likewise, these household surveys do not capture institutionalized populations. Nevertheless, the results demonstrate that cut-point shift, as detected through the use of vignettes, can substantially alter population-level assessments of a domain of health.

DISCUSSION

In this chapter, we explored the use of anchoring vignettes in the MCSS to improve the comparability of self-responses on items measuring some of the core domains of health. While many further investigations have been suggested by this analysis, the overall impression is that in many different societies with individuals of widely disparate socioeconomic status, there is considerable concordance in the understanding of a set of vignettes, which is rather remarkable given that the MCSS was the first large-scale implementation of health vignettes. Against all expectation, individuals with no formal education are able to respond for hypothetical states on a domain in a manner that is consistent with the responses of individuals with more than 12 years of formal education. This result alone suggests that with further work, there are good prospects of using the anchoring vignette approach to develop an in-depth understanding of how individual, group, and population cut-points vary in systematic ways. Such an understanding will help unravel the range of counter-intuitive findings, such as reverse socioeconomic gradients, seen in many health surveys using self-response items (50).

While the health and responsiveness vignettes have been largely understood in similar ways across many societies, this analysis points to a number of design and implementation improvements in future efforts to collect information using anchoring vignettes, such as the World Health Survey. Clearly, some sets of vignettes in the MCSS such as for mobility, affect, quality of basic amenities, and dignity, were better designed and written than others. This is an important warning that developing good panels of vignettes for a domain—whether for health, responsiveness or other areas of investigation—must be seen as an iterative empirical exercise. As with all item design, *a priori* principles or processes cannot yield perfect instruments; these efforts must be supplemented with wide-scale empirical testing.

Our interpretation of the results for different panels of vignettes is that there are several aspects to avoid, or at least that warrant special attention. Where domains are not functionally unidimensional, it is difficult to develop an effective set of vignettes. For example, for pain, it appears that different individuals and groups have different ways of combining duration, location, and intensity of pain into a single pain construct. Improved measurement of pain may require the recognition that pain is not fundamentally unidimensional from a measurement perspective. In some cases, vignettes included in the MCSS were unnecessarily multidimensional; for example, including colour vision deficits in vision vignettes. This type of multidimensionality can be easily addressed in revisions of the vignettes.

Another insight into the design of the vignettes comes from both the non-parametric and parametric analyses: vignettes should not be very close to each other on the latent variable. When two vignettes are very close, in the non-parametric analyses, we would expect a very large number of inversions due to measurement error. Very little information is added by having a second vignette at a similar level on the latent variable. To obtain maximum information, vignettes should be well-spaced across the latent variable.

Salomon et al. (55) have discussed the notion that in the conceptualization of a domain of health, there is a threshold on a domain below which reductions are seen as actual health decrements, but above which improvements are considered by most to be talent and not health. For example, the difference between running a marathon and being able to jog four kilometres may be better characterized as "talent" rather than health. In designing vignettes, the best vignette should not be better than the commonly perceived health-talent threshold. Of course, without broad-based empirical evidence, it is difficult to know precisely where the average health-talent threshold lies. Nevertheless, inclusion of vignettes at exceedingly high levels on a given domain either wastes information or leads to unnecessary confusion on the part of the respondent.

Perhaps the most important design insight from the non-parametric analysis is for the self-response item. Because of the clinical origin of many health domain items, when applied to the general population, the vast majority of respondents often fall in the top response category. Unfortunately, the vignettes yield the least information about differences in the latent variable for individuals who have responded in the top category. In other words, it is important in general population surveys to ask more difficult items. For mobility, rather than asking respondents about general difficulties in moving around, an item referring to vigorous activities such as jogging a kilometre or walking up stairs would be preferable. The target would be to design an item where the most common response category is the middle one. This strategy would maximize the potential of the vignettes to improve comparability of most of the respondents.

The systematic variation across surveys for 14 health and responsiveness domains suggests that issues of survey implementation are also critical to the use of the anchoring vignette approach. Care in the translation and back-translation needs to be supplemented with an increased focus on the training of interviewers to understand why vignette information is important. From this assessment, it is clear that the issue is not the educational attainment of the respondents, but rather some systematic aspect of the survey implementation, probably reflecting the way the interviewer interacts with the respondent in this section of the instrument. Special attention is being given to this challenge in the implementation of the World Health Survey.

Exploration of the data using the CHOPIT model also provides some guidance for future data collection and analysis. Age, sex, education, and country only explain a fraction of the variation in cut-points, evident in the self-response and vignette response patterns across individuals. Future data collection with anchoring vignettes should include additional items that might help predict individual variation in cut-points, for example measures of personality, outlook, or happiness. Finding these covariates of cut-points is essential if the full potential of anchoring vignettes is to be captured in an efficient manner. In the absence of these predictors, one needs to collect vignette information from all respondents, which increases the data collection burden enormously. It is too early to tell if the same set of covariates will predict cut-point variation for all items and domains or whether effective covariates will themselves vary across domains.

The comparison of the parametric analysis using all vignette respondents and only those with a (benefit-of-the-doubt) correlation coefficient greater than 0.8, highlights the importance of understanding and modelling the nature of stochastic error for self-responses and vignettes. One empirical approach that may provide a stronger basis for refining models of stochastic measurement error is high quality test-retest data on self-response and vignettes. The World Health Survey includes a systematic attempt to collect test-retest data on all items in 10% of the sample. Nevertheless, for many interviewers in the field, test-retest is sometimes viewed as an attempt to check on the quality of the interviewer. There are powerful perceived incentives, both in terms of time and supervisor assessment, to not collect a genuine retest. Contamination of the retest with the test results must be carefully avoided if these types of data are to be used to develop a better understanding of the true nature of measurement error.

With a large empirical dataset on test-retest, it will be worthwhile developing and testing modifications of the CHOPIT model that account for the observed nature of measurement error. In the MCSS data, it appears likely that there is both stochastic measurement error well-represented by a normally distributed error term on the latent variable, and in a fraction of respondents, stochastic measurement error related to the observation mechanism itself. For example, a fraction of respondents choose among the five response categories at random. Such errors in response may not be captured well by the parametric assumption of normal errors, as is the case in the current version of the CHOPIT model. Future modifications of CHOPIT are planned in order to examine the sensitivity to differential error structures and to semi-parametric specifications of the model.

A further design implication that has been incorporated into the World Health Survey is including two items per domain, which is important for two reasons. First, it allows an easier and harder item to be included so that the same instrument may be effective in both a general population sample and a clinical sample. Second, for statistical modelling reasons, at least two items are needed to be able to estimate a random effect across individuals. Estimating a random effect can increase the information content of the posterior estimate for an individual dramatically, regardless of the covariates used in the model to predict the latent variable. More than one item per domain also reduces the impact of stochastic measurement error at the individual level. Further work is needed to understand whether the resources required to increase from two items per domain to three would be worthwhile, but the move from one to two items appears essential.

An important agenda item for future research is to provide independent confirmation of the information content of the individual's responses to vignettes. For some domains, it is possible that measured tests could be used to evaluate the extent to which collecting information on vignettes improves the comparability of self-responses. Such validation studies must be undertaken with meticulous attention to test implementation to ensure that the results of the measured test are comparable. In addition, for many domains it is hard to conceive of a measured test that will capture the full range of function that responses to an item or items on a single domain may be capturing. Nevertheless, validation of the vignette strategy using measured tests is an important area for further work.

The World Health Survey (56) represents the next step in large-scale data collection of anchoring vignettes for multiple domains of health and responsiveness. The instrument has been modified from the MCSS instrument to reflect some of the lessons learned from this analysis. The revised instrument was also empirically tested in a 12-country pilot study in 2002. The WHS instrument is being fielded in 2003 in 72 nationally representative household surveys. This further large-scale empirical experience will provide a rich basis for further exploration and development of the anchoring vignette approach to enhancing comparability of self-responses.

NOTES

1   When individuals interact with the health system, it influences their well-being, partly through improvements in health and partly through other aspects of their personal interactions with the system. Aspects related to the way people are treated by the health system and the environment in which they are treated, are defined as responsiveness. Multiple domains characterize responsiveness as well as health, and a common set of domains has been identified for measurement purposes: autonomy, choice, communication, confidentiality, dignity, prompt attention, quality of basic amenities, and access to family and community support (see Chapter 43 of this volume (43)).

2   Three different bases for partial orderings include dominance, first-order stochastic dominance, and second-order stochastic dominance. Dominance describes situations in which all members of a particular population have higher levels (e.g. of mobility) than all members of another population. First-order stochastic dominance occurs when the cumulative distribution of individuals in one population is always to the right of that in another population. Second-order stochastic dominance occurs when the area under the cumulative distribution function for one population is always greater than that of another population. In the example presented here, because the scale on which the cumulative function is described is an ordinal one, it is not possible to make meaningful statements about the area under the c.d.f., and so evaluation of second-order stochastic dominance is not feasible.

REFERENCES

(1)   Chiang CL. *An index of health: mathematical models.* United States Public Health Services Publications Series 1000, Vital and Health Statistics Series 2, No. 5. Washington, DC, National Center for Health Statistics, 1965.

(2)   Cutler DM, Richardson E. Measuring the health of the United States population. *Brookings Papers on Economic Activity, Microeconomics*, 1997, 217–272.

(3)   Fayers PM, Machin D. *Quality of life: assessment, analysis, and interpretation.* Chichester, New York, John Wiley, 2000.

(4)   Fitzpatrick R. A pragmatic defence of health status measures. *Health Care Analysis*, 1996, 4:265–272.

(5)   Katz S et al. Active life expectancy. *The New England Journal of Medicine*, 1983, 309:1218–1224.

(6)   Kramer M. The rising pandemic of mental disorders and associated chronic diseases and disabilities. *Acta Psychiatrica Scandinavica*, 1980, 62(Suppl. 285):282–297.

(7)   McHorney CA. Health status assessment methods for adults: past accomplishments and future challenges. *Annual Review of Public Health*, 1999, 20:309–325.

(8)   Sadana R et al. Comparative analyses of more than 50 household surveys on health status. In: Murray CJL et al., eds. *Summary measures of population health: concepts, ethics, measurement and applications.* Geneva, World Health Organization, 2002:369–386.

(9)   Sullivan DF. A single index of mortality and morbidity. *HSMHA Health Reports*, 1971, 86:347–354.

(10) Chambers LW, Sakett DL, Goldsmith CH. Development and application of an index of social function. *Health Services Research*, 1976, 11:430–441.

(11) Fanshel S, Bush JW. A Health status index and its application to the health services outcomes. *Operations Research*, 1970, 18:1021–1066.

(12) Manderbacka K. Examining what self-rated health question is understood to mean by respondents. *Scandinavian Journal of Social Medicine*, 1998, 26(2):145–153.

(13) World Health Organization. *The World Health Report 2002. Reducing Risks, Promoting Healthy Life.* Geneva, World Health Organization, 2002.

(14) World Health Organization. *Constitution of the World Health Organization.* New York, International Health Conference, 22 July 1946. URL: http://www.who.int/governance/en/.

(15) World Health Organization. *International Classification of Functioning, Disability and Health (ICF).* Geneva, World Health Organization, 2001.

(16) Bergner M. Quality of life, health status, and clinical research. *Medical Care*, 1989, 27(Suppl. 3):S148–S156.

(17) Brazier J et al. Deriving a preference-based single index from the UK SF-36 health survey. *Journal of Clinical Epidemiology*, 1998, 51(11):1115–1128.

(18) Chambers LW et al. The McMaster Health Index Questionnaire as a measure of quality of life for patients with rheumatoid disease. *Journal of Rheumatology*, 1982, 9(5):780–784.

(19) Essink BM et al. An empirical comparison of four generic health status measures. The Nottingham Health Profile, the Medical Outcomes Study 36-item Short-Form Health Survey, the COOP/WONCA charts, and the EuroQol instrument. *Medical Care*, 1997, 35(5):522–537.

(20) Feeny D et al. Multi-attribute health status classification systems: health utilities index. *Pharmaco Economics*, 1995, 7(6):490–502.

(21) Goldberg DP. *The detection of psychiatric illness by questionnaire.* Oxford, Oxford University Press, 1972.

(22) Gudex C, Lafortune G. *An inventory of health and disability-related surveys in OECD countries.* Paris, Directorate for Education, Employment, Labour and Social Affairs, 2000.

(23) Hupkens C. *Coverage of health topics by surveys in the European Union. Population and social conditions.* Eurostat Working Papers 3/1998/E/n.10. Luxembourg, European Commission, 1998.

(24) Hunt SM et al. The Nottingham Health Profile: subjective health and medical consultations. *Social Science & Medicine*, 1981, 15A:221–229.

(25) McDowell I, Newell C. *Measuring health*, 2nd ed. Oxford, Oxford University Press, 1996.

(26) The EuroQol Group. EuroQol—a new facility for the measurement of health-related quality of life. *Health Policy*, 1990, 16(3):199–208.

(27) Ware JE. SF-36 health survey update. *Spine*, 2000, 25(24):3130–3139.

(28) Ware JE. *SF-36 health survey manual and interpretation guide.* The Health Institute, New England Medical Center, Boston, Nimrod Press, 1993.

(29) Kaplan RM, Anderson JP. A general health policy model: update and applications. *Health Services Research*, 1988, 23(2):203–235.

(30) Iburg KM et al. Cross-population comparability of physician-assessed and self-reported measures of health. In: Murray CJL et al., eds. *Summary measures of population health: concepts, ethics, measurement and applications.* Geneva, World Health Organization, 2002:433–448.

(31) Macintyre S, Ford G, Hunt K. Do women 'over-report' morbidity? Men's and women's responses to structured prompting on a standard question on long standing illness. *Social Science & Medicine*, 1999, 48(1):89–98.

(32) Kempen GIJM et al. The assessment of ADL among frail elderly in an interview survey: self-report versus performance-based tests and determinants of discrepancies. *Journal of Gerontology*, 1996, 51B(5):P254–P260.

(33) Sen A. Objectivity and position: assessment of health and well-being. In: Vhen LC, Kleinman A, Ware NC, eds. *Health and social change in international perspective.*

Harvard Series on Population and International Health. Boston, Harvard School of Public Health, 1994.

(34) Sen A. Health: perception versus observation. *British Medical Journal*, 2002, 324(7342):860–861.

(35) Murray CJL et al. New approaches to enhance cross-population comparability of survey results. In: Murray CJL et al., eds. *Summary measures of population health: concepts, ethics, measurement and applications.* Geneva, World Health Organization, 2002:421–431.

(36) Tandon A et al. Statistical models for enhancing cross-population comparability. In: Murray CJL, Evans DB, eds. *Health systems performance assessment: debates, methods and empiricism.* Geneva, World Health Organization, 2003.

(37) Salomon JA, Tandon A, Murray CJL. *Using vignettes to improve cross-population comparability of health surveys: concepts, design, and evaluation techniques.* EIP Discussion Paper No. 41. Geneva, World Health Organization, 2001. URL: http://www3.who.int/whosis/discussion_papers/discussion_papers.cfm#

(38) Anderson HH, Anderson GL. *An introduction to projective techniques and other devices for understanding human behaviour.* Englewood Cliffs, Prentice Hall, 1951.

(39) Herskovits MJ. The hypothetical situation: a technique of field research. *Southwestern Journal of Anthropology*, 1950, 6:32–40.

(40) Walster E. Assignment of responsibility for an accident. *Journal of Personality and Social Psychology*, 1966, 3(1):73–79.

(41) Rossi PH, Nock SL. *Measuring social judgements: the factorial survey approach.* Beverly Hills, Sage Publications, 1982.

(42) Üstün TB et al. WHO Multi-country Survey Study on Health and Responsiveness 2000–2001. In: Murray CJL, Evans DB, eds. *Health systems performance assessment: debates, methods and empiricism.* Geneva, World Health Organization, 2003.

(43) Valentine NB et al. Health system responsiveness: concepts, domains and operationalization. In: Murray CJL, Evans DB, eds. *Health systems performance assessment: debates, methods and empiricism.* Geneva, World Health Organization, 2003.

(44) King G et al. Enhancing the validity and cross-cultural comparability of measurement in survey research. *American Political Science Review*, 2003 (forthcoming).

(45) Mackenbach JP et al. Socioeconomic inequalities in mortality among women and among men: an international study. *American Journal of Public Health*, 1999, 89(12):1800–1806.

(46) Sundquist J, Johansson SE. Self-reported poor health

and low educational level predictors for mortality: a population based follow-up study of 39,156 people in Sweden. *Journal of Epidemiology and Community Health*, 1997, 51:35–40.

(47) Berkman LF, Kawachi I, eds. *Social epidemiology*. Oxford, Oxford University Press, 2000.

(48) Manton KG, Stallard E, Corder L. Education-specific estimates of life expectancy and age-specific disability in the U.S. elderly population: 1982 to 1991. *Journal of Aging and Health*, 1997, 9(4):419–450.

(49) Marmot MG, Shipley MJ. Do socioeconomic differences in mortality persist after retirement? 25 year follow up of civil servants from the first Whitehall study. *British Medical Journal*, 1996, 313(7066):1177–1180.

(50) Murray CJL, Chen LC. Understanding morbidity change. *Population and Development Review*, 1992, 18(3):481–503.

(51) Guralnik JM et al. A short physical performance battery assessing lower extremity function: association with self-reported disability and prediction of mortality and nursing home admission. *Journal of Gerontology*, 1994, 49(2):M85–M94.

(52) Greiner PA, Snowdon DA, Greiner LH. The relationship of self-rated function and self-rated health to concurrent functional ability, functional decline, and mortality: findings from the Nun Study. *Journal of Gerontology*, 1996, 51B(5):S234–S241.

(53) Salomon JA et al. Unpacking health perceptions using anchoring vignettes. In: Murray CJL, Evans DB, eds. *Health systems performance assessment: debates, methods and empiricism*. Geneva, World Health Organization, 2003.

(54) Krieger N. Discrimination and health. In: Berkman LF, Kawachi I, eds. *Social epidemiology*. Oxford, Oxford University Press, 2000:36–75.

(55) Salomon JA et al. Quantifying individual levels of health: definitions, concepts, and measurement issues. In: Murray CJL, Evans DB, eds. *Health systems performance assessment: debates, methods and empiricism*. Geneva, World Health Organization, 2003.

(56) Üstün TB et al. The World Health Surveys. In: Murray CJL, Evans DB, eds. *Health systems performance assessment: debates, methods and empiricism*. Geneva, World Health Organization, 2003.

Chapter 31

Unpacking Health Perceptions Using Anchoring Vignettes

Joshua A. Salomon, Ajay Tandon, Christopher J.L. Murray,
World Health Survey Pilot Study Collaborating Groups[1]

Introduction

Valid, reliable and comparable measures of the health states of individuals are critical components of the evidence base for clinical practice and health policy. Clinical trials and national health surveys rely heavily on self-reported health measures (1–5), but interpretation of these measures is complicated by comparability problems that arise when different persons understand and respond to a given question in different ways. A number of paradoxical findings have been reported in analyses of population health surveys, suggesting that self-reported health measures may give misleading results in the absence of adjustments for these differences (6–9).

A key challenge in the interpretation of self-reported health measures is to distinguish between differences in self-ratings due to actual health differences and those due to varying norms or expectations for health (10;11). If health is understood as consisting of multiple dimensions (for example, mobility, cognition, vision, and affect, among others), then we may conceptualize the level on any given dimension as a continuous but latent (unobserved) scale value, with higher values corresponding to better health levels. Each of the available response choices for a categorical self-report question corresponds to a certain range of values on the latent scale, which may differ across individuals (Figure 31.1). Thus, the influence of varying expectations for health may be expressed in terms of individual differences in the levels on a given dimension at which a person transitions from using one response category to the next, i.e. differences in response category boundaries or cut-points. For example, a 90-year-old person who finds it difficult to walk up a flight of stairs might characterize himself as having only mild difficulties in moving around, while a

40-year-old person at this same level of mobility might describe herself as having moderate difficulties. These responses are not comparable because the two individuals have different response category cut-points for questions regarding mobility.

Strategies for enhancing the comparability of self-reported health measures demand the augmentation of both existing instruments for data collection and existing statistical models for data analysis (12). Standard statistical models for ordinal data, such as the ordered probit model, cannot allow for variation in response category cut-points. Adaptations of these

Figure 31.1 Response category cut-point shift

The problems of interpersonal or cross-population comparability may be conceptualized in terms of response category cut-point shifts. This diagram shows how different individuals, labelled A, B and C, might translate levels on an unobserved, continuous mobility scale into categorical responses in different ways, depending on the location of their cut-points. Cut-points define thresholds on the latent scale at which individuals will transition from using one response category to another.

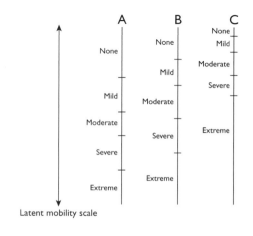

standard models to incorporate systematic cut-point shifts in relation to some defined set of covariates, such as country, age, sex, and education, are described elsewhere (*13,14*). Anchoring vignettes have been developed as a new component of survey instruments used in conjunction with the new statistical models to position self-reported responses on a common, interpersonally comparable scale (*15*). In this chapter, we describe an application of the anchoring vignette strategy from a series of pilot studies for the World Health Survey (*16*). Empirical examples of how anchoring vignettes may be used to understand variation in expectations for health are presented, and implications for interpreting self-ratings of health are discussed.

METHODS

Pilot tests for various components of the World Health Survey were conducted in twelve countries during May and June 2002, including six countries that tested the module on health state measurement: China, Myanmar, Pakistan, Sri Lanka, Turkey, and United Arab Emirates. A non-random sample of the adult population (18 years and older) was selected in each site, with an emphasis on sampling similar numbers of men and women and obtaining sufficient representation at all ages and different levels of income and education. The samples in the six countries that pre-tested the health module included 467 to 605 adults in all sites except Pakistan, which surveyed 234 adults. Face-to-face surveys were conducted using a standardized questionnaire translated into the local language according to defined protocols (*16*).

The health module in the survey included a self-assessment component consisting of one to three questions pertaining to each of twelve domains, along with 15 different anchoring vignettes for each domain. This chapter presents examples of the results for the domain of mobility (Figure 31.2). An anchoring vignette is a description of a concrete level on a given health domain that respondents are asked to evaluate with the same questions and response scales applied to self-assessments on that domain. Vignettes fix the level of ability on a domain so that variation in categorical responses is attributable to variation in response category cut-points. The key objective underlying the anchoring vignette strategy is to elicit responses from subjects for hypothetical levels on a given domain that reflect individual norms and expectations for health in approximately the same way that the self-ratings do for the subjects' own health levels.

Figure 31.2 Mobility items in the World Health Survey Pilot Study

---

Q1. Overall in the last 30 days, how much difficulty did [you/name] have with moving around?

    (a) None (b) Mild (c) Moderate (d) Severe (e) Extreme

Q2. In the last 30 days, how much difficulty did [you/name] have in vigorous activities, such as running 3 kilometres or cycling?

    (a) None (b) Mild (c) Moderate (d) Severe (e) Extreme

Examples of mobility vignettes

- *Paul* is an active athlete who runs long-distance races of 20 kilometres twice a week and plays soccer with no problems.

- *Mary* has no problems with walking, running or using her hands, arms and legs. She jogs 4 kilometres twice a week.

- *Rob* is able to walk distances of up to 200 metres without any problems, but feels tired after walking one kilometre or climbing more than one flight of stairs. He has no problems with day-to-day physical activities, such as carrying food from the market.

- *Anton* does not exercise. He cannot climb stairs or do other physical activities because he is obese. He is able to carry the groceries and do some light household work.

- *Vincent* has a lot of swelling in his legs due to his health condition. He has to make an effort to walk around his home as his legs feel heavy.

- *Louis* is able to move his arms and legs, but requires assistance in standing up from a chair or walking around the house. Any bending is painful, and lifting is impossible.

- *David* is paralysed from the neck down. He is confined to bed and must be fed and bathed by somebody else.

Each survey respondent answered the self-assessment items for all domains and rated 10 different vignettes relating to each of two domains, assigned at random from the universe of 12 domains. The total set of 15 vignettes for a domain included five vignettes that were common to all six study sites and 10 vignettes that were common to three of six sites.

We examined distributions of responses on the two self-assessed mobility questions and ratings for the set of 15 vignettes developed for this domain. Data were analysed using Stata version 7.0. Variation in the categorical ratings of the vignettes was assessed between countries, across age groups, and between the two different domain items pertaining to mobility.

RESULTS

A total of 3 012 respondents participated in the pilot survey on health. Most of the subjects were young adults, and 74 per cent had more than six years of education (Table 31.1). Responses on the self-assessments regarding mobility varied considerably across countries, with the proportion of respondents characterizing themselves as having no difficulty moving

Table 31.1   Distribution of sample used in pilot study of health module for the World Health Survey by country, age, sex, and years of schooling

	Number	%
Age (years)		
18–24	391	13.3
25–34	680	23.2
35–44	724	24.7
45–54	585	20.0
55–64	276	9.4
65+	276	9.4
Sex		
Male	1,296	43.7
Female	1,673	56.3
Years of schooling		
0	228	8.3
1–5	503	18.2
6–12	951	34.5
12+	1,078	39.1
Country		
China	467	15.5
Myanmar	605	20.1
Pakistan	236	7.8
Sri Lanka	594	19.7
Turkey	600	19.9
United Arab Emirates	510	16.9

around ranging from 45 per cent in Sri Lanka to 85 per cent in United Arab Emirates.

Of the total sample completing the health survey, 406 were assigned randomly to complete the version of the questionnaire that included vignettes for mobility. When survey respondents provide ratings for a series of different vignettes on a particular domain, we may visualize the responses in terms of the distribution of categorical ratings for each vignette across different groups of respondents. Figure 31.3 presents an example showing the distribution of responses for five different mobility vignettes in the samples from China and Sri Lanka. In this figure, each stacked bar shows the categorical responses for one vignette, with the sequence of vignettes ordered from higher mobility levels to lower ones, according to average categorical scores.

This type of diagram allows general insights into differences in the use of response categories that may also be examined more formally using the statistical models described elsewhere (*13, 14*). From the distributions of responses, it is evident that respondents in the sample from Sri Lanka tended to give less favor-

able ratings than those in the sample from China, conditional on a fixed level of mobility. Based on insights like these, the differences in self-ratings of mobility in the two samples, shown in the top bars of Figure 31.3, may be understood to arise from a combination of variation in health experiences and variation in expectations. Although the non-probability samples in this study may not allow generalizable inferences regarding the full populations in each country, they provide an illustration of the way that ratings of anchoring vignettes can reveal cut-point differences across populations.

The simple example in Figure 31.3 offers a comparison of the distributions in two countries, but it is important to note that the ratings of anchoring vignettes also allow us to examine differences within countries (e.g., by age, sex, income, education, or other covariates of interest), differences for the same individuals on various questions relating to the same domain, or differences in the same persons over time. For example, Figure 31.4 shows the ratings for an array of 10 different mobility vignettes using the 2 different questions about mobility. This figure demonstrates several key points: a) that the second question is "more difficult" in the sense that it taps a higher level of mobility than the first question; b) that individuals rate themselves favourably on mobility but recognize on average that the top 2 vignettes present higher levels than their own; and c) that there is evidence in favour of respondent consistency in providing self-ratings and vignette ratings, suggested by the similar correspondence between the 2 questions on both the self-assessments and vignette ratings—in both cases, individuals are using the second question in a way that is consistent with tapping a higher level of difficulty.

Figure 31.3 illustrated that there may be significant differences in the use of categorical responses for a given question across countries, but a more basic intuitive understanding of these cut-point differences emerges from an examination of variation relating to individual characteristics of respondents. Figure 31.5 shows the distribution of ratings for one mobility vignette in different age groups for the three countries that included this particular vignette in the pilot study (Myanmar, Pakistan, and Turkey). This figure suggests that older individuals use a more lenient interpretation of the same set of response categories in describing mobility levels, which is consistent with a hypothesis of shifting norms for health during the life cycle.

Figure 31.3 Mobility ratings for self-assessment and selected vignettes, China and Sri Lanka (N=1 061 for self-ratings, N=151 for vignettes)

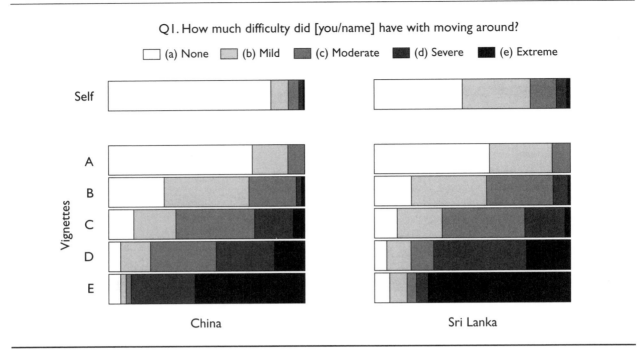

Figure 31.4 Vignette ratings for two mobility questions, pooled results from six countries (China, Myanmar, Pakistan, Sri Lanka, Turkey, United Arab Emirates), N=406

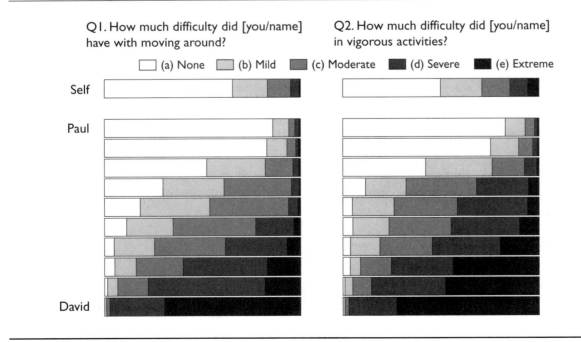

Figure 31.5 Variation in vignette ratings across age groups in three countries, Myanmar, Pakistan and Turkey (N=211)

[Rob] is able to walk distances of up to 200 metres without any problems but feels tired after walking one km or climbing up more than one flight of stairs. He has no problems with day-to-day physical activities, such as carrying food from the market.

Q1. How much difficulty did [Rob] have with moving around?

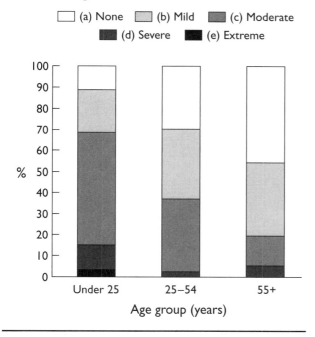

DISCUSSION

Inclusion of anchoring vignettes in health surveys is part of an integrated strategy of instrument design and analytical methods for enhancing the comparability of self-reported health measures across individuals, communities and populations (12). Anchoring vignettes may be applied to many different analytical problems where ordered categorical self-reported responses are observed. This approach provides a means of examining systematic differences in categorical cut-points between populations, within populations across different socio-demographic groups, or within individuals or groups over time. The anchoring vignette method also accommodates comparisons between different questions that relate to a common domain, enabling the interpretation of responses to these related questions on a single underlying scale, and thus providing a bridge between data collected using different health status measurement instruments.

The use of vignettes has a long history in social science research, including applications in anthropology, sociology, and psychological research since the 1950s (17–19), and numerous applications of the factorial-survey technique pioneered by Rossi and colleagues (20). Recent examples of the use of vignettes in health and medicine include applications in nursing research, medical education, and research on clinical practice (21–24). Our anchoring vignette approach departs from previous vignette studies in certain fundamental ways. First, rather than generating random variants of the same vignette (20), our approach depends critically on using vignettes as scale anchors, and therefore requires that a given vignette describe the same domain level to all respondents. Second, our strategy is based on explicit links between vignette ratings and self-ratings through the use of identical questions and response categories.

Two important requirements for the use of anchoring vignettes may be defined as *response consistency*, which states that an individual will use the response categories for a particular question in a similar way when evaluating hypothetical scenarios as when providing a self-assessment; and *vignette equivalence*, which states that the underlying domain levels represented in each vignette are understood in approximately the same way by all respondents, irrespective of their age, sex, income, education, country of residence or other characteristics (15). Empirical investigations regarding these key requirements should be an essential component of the research agenda on anchoring vignettes, and work is underway on developing a range of different evaluative techniques for critical examination and comparison of different candidate vignettes and vignette sets.

In this study, we found that variation in ratings of vignettes for the domain of mobility can shed light on differences in expectations for health across countries, or across subpopulation groups within countries. Although we have developed formal statistical techniques that allow anchoring vignette data to be used in adjusting self-rated health measures (13;14), fundamental insights into differences in the use of particular questions and their associated response categories may be gained through analyses of distributions of vignette ratings, even before any models are applied. Anchoring vignettes have been developed for the World Health Survey for a range of different domains of health, as well as for other areas that share similar methodological challenges, such as health system responsiveness and social capital. While more work is needed to refine individual vignettes and identify those vignettes that perform best, this study demonstrates that the anchoring vignette strategy is feasible in a range of different settings and offers promise for a more widespread application of the approach.

There are a number of important limitations that should be noted. First, the sample size in this pilot study is small, and cannot be assumed to represent the general population in any of the study sites. While this chapter aims to illustrate the types of empirical findings that are available through the use of anchoring vignettes, the wave of data collection that is now underway in the population-representative samples of the World Health Survey will provide a stronger basis with which to examine some of the key questions introduced here. We demonstrate in this chapter how anchoring vignettes can reveal cut-point differences across different groups and questionnaire items, but it will be important to confirm these findings in larger surveys and to cross-validate the anchoring vignette approach, for example, through the use of measured performance tests on selected health domains. There are numerous different possible covariates that could be examined beyond the ones described here, and the current understanding of determinants of cut-point differences remains limited. Research on psychology and decision-making has highlighted a range of different biases and heuristics that shape responses to survey questions (*25*). A similar quantitative understanding of how different health expectations influence self-perceptions of health, and key correlates of these differences, would facilitate interpretation of self-reported health measures.

There has been rising interest recently in the problems of interpretation of self-assessments on health, relating to issues of perception versus observation and experiences versus expectations (*8;10*). We propose that anchoring vignettes can provide a useful tool for unpacking health perceptions and adjusting self-reported health measures to account for variation in norms and expectations of health. As self-ratings of health continue to play an important role in the measurement of health outcomes in clinical trials and the development of summary measures of population health, a strategy of including vignettes in national health surveys and clinical research can contribute to enhancing the utility of these measures by ameliorating important problems of interpersonal comparability.

ACKNOWLEDGEMENTS

We thank David Cutler and Gary King for helpful discussions. This study was supported by the National Institute on Aging (PO1-AG17625).

NOTES

1 World Health Survey Pilot Study Collaborating Groups: *Core survey design, implementation and analysis.* T. Bedirhan Üstün, Somnath Chatterji, Lydia Bendib, Can Çelik, Colin D. Mathers, Abdelhay Mechbal, Christopher J.L. Murray, Emre Özaltin, Alena Petrakova, Ritu Sadana, Joshua A. Salomon, Ajay Tandon, Maria Villanueva, Wan Jun Xie, Cao Yang; *China* Feng Jiang, Keqin Rao; *Myanmar* Kyi Soe, Sanjoy Nandy; *Pakistan* Ashfaq Ahmed; *Sri Lanka* Thushara Fernando; *Turkey* Kutegin Ogel, Adnan Kisa; *United Arab Emirates* Gohar Wajid

REFERENCES

(1) Testa MA, Simonson DC. Assesment of quality-of-life outcomes. *The New England Journal of Medicine*, 1996, 334:835–840.

(2) Kind P et al. Variations in population health status: results from a United Kingdom national questionnaire survey. *British Medical Journal*, 1998, 316:736–741.

(3) Fischer D et al. Capturing the patient's view of change as a clinical outcome measure. *The Journal of the American Medical Association*, 1999, 282:1157–1162.

(4) Shibuya K, Hashimoto H, Yano E. Individual income, income distribution, and self rated health in Japan: cross sectional analysis of nationally representative sample. *British Medical Journal*, 2002, 324:16.

(5) Garratt A et al. Quality of life measurement: bibliographic study of patient assessed health outcome measures. *British Medical Journal*, 2002, 324:1417.

(6) Murray CJL, Chen LC. Understanding morbidity change. *Population and Development Review*, 1992, 18:481–503.

(7) Mathers CD, Douglas RM. Measuring progress in population health and well-being. In: Eckersley R, ed. *Measuring progress: is life getting better.* Collingwood, Victoria, CSIRO Publishing, 1998:125–155.

(8) Sen A. Health: perception versus observation. *British Medical Journal*, 2002, 324:860–861.

(9) Sadana R et al. Comparative analyses of more than 50 household surveys on health status. In: Murray CJL et al, eds. *Summary measures of population health: concepts, ethics, measurement and applications.* Geneva, World Health Organization, 2002:369–386.

(10) Carr AJ, Gibson B, Robinson PG. Measuring quality of life: Is quality of life determined by expectations or experience? *British Medical Journal*, 2001, 322: 1240–1243.

(11) Freedman VA, Martin LG. Understanding trends in functional limitations among older Americans. *American Journal of Public Health*, 1998, 88:1457–1462.

(12) Murray CJL et al. New approaches to enhance cross-population comparability of survey results. In: Murray CJL et al., eds. *Summary measures of population health: concepts, ethics, measurement and applications.* Geneva, World Health Organization, 2002:421–431.

(13) Tandon A et al. Statistical models for enhancing cross-population comparability. In: Murray CJL, Evans DB, eds. *Health systems performance assessment: debates, methods and empiricism.* Geneva, World Health Organization, 2003.

(14) King G et al. Enhancing the validity and cross-cultural comparability of measurement in survey research. *American Political Science Review*, 2003 (forthcoming).

(15) Salomon JA, Tandon A, Murray CJL. *Using vignettes to improve cross-population comparability of health surveys: concepts, design, and evaluation techniques.* EIP Discussion Paper No. 41. Geneva, World Health Organization, 2001. URL: http://www3.who.int/whois/discussion_papers/discussion_papers.cfm#

(16) World Health Organization. *World Health Survey.* Geneva, World Health Organization, 2003. URL: http://www3.who.int/whs/.

(17) Herskovits MJ. The hypothetical situation: a technique of field research. *Southwestern Journal of Anthropology*, 1950, 6:32-40.

(18) Anderson HH, Anderson GL. *An introduction to projective techniques and other devices for understanding human behavior.* Englewood Cliffs, NJ, Prentice Hall, 1951.

(19) Walster E. Assignment of responsibility for an accident. *Journal of Personality and Social Psychology*, 1966, 3: 73–79.

(20) Rossi PH, Nock SL. *Measuring social judgments: the factorial survey approach.* Beverly Hills, Sage Publications, 1982.

(21) Koedoot CG et al. Palliative chemotherapy or watchful waiting? A vignettes study among oncologists. *Journal of Clinical Oncology*, 2002, 20(17):3658–3664.

(22) Goldie J et al. The impact of three years' ethics teaching, in an integrated medical curriculum, on students' proposed behaviour on meeting ethical dilemmas. *Medical Education*, 2002, 36(5):489–497.

(23) Kelly WF et al. Do specialists differ on do-not-resuscitate decisions? *Chest*, 2002, 121:957–963.

(24) Hughes R, Huby M. The application of vignettes in social and nursing research. *Journal of Advanced Nursing*, 2002, 37(4):382–386.

(25) Tversky A, Kahneman D. The framing of decisions and the psychology of choice. *Science*, 1981, 211: 453–458.

Chapter 32

Health State Valuations in Summary Measures of Population Health

Joshua A. Salomon, Christopher J.L. Murray, T. Bedirhan Üstün, Somnath Chatterji

Introduction

The measurement of health, in a way that is comparable across populations and over time within specific populations, is an essential requirement for the evaluation of health policies and assessment of the effectiveness of health interventions. Summary measures of population health, such as healthy life expectancy (1), combine information on mortality and non-fatal health outcomes to provide standardized measures of average health levels in a population (2). An essential input in any summary measure is a set of weights that represent the overall levels of health associated with different states, measured on a meaningful cardinal scale anchored by perfect health and death. These health state valuations constitute the critical link between information on mortality and information on the spectrum of health states experienced by individuals.

To date, there have been limited empirical data on health state valuations collected from representative sample surveys. Most available data have emerged from studies in a small number of industrialized countries among convenience samples of highly educated respondents or patients enrolled in clinical studies. In contrast, the number of valuation surveys in probability samples from the general community has been small. Three widely cited sample surveys on health state valuations in general populations have been completed in the United Kingdom (3), Hamilton, Ontario (4), and Beaver Dam, Wisconsin (5). Important questions have been raised regarding the possibility of variation in health state valuations across different types of respondents (e.g. individuals in a given health state, family members of these individuals, health care providers or the healthy public) (6–8), across countries (9–11) or within countries according to socio-demographic variables such as age, sex, education, or income (12). Although different studies have sought to identify these possible sources of variation, the empirical basis upon which to examine this question has been limited.

A number of key methodological issues relating to health state valuations have been debated extensively in the literature on health economics, psychometrics and health outcomes measurement. One central debate has been over which elicitation technique should be used to obtain valuations. A range of different techniques have been proposed and used widely, including the standard gamble, time trade-off, visual analogue scale, and person trade-off (13;14). Arguments for and against various methods have been based on ethical grounds (15), economic theory (16), and comparisons of psychometric properties (17). For each of the major methods, however, responses depend on the health level of a state, but also capture other values such as risk aversion (dislike of gambling), time preference (discounting of future health), or distributional concerns (14;18). An alternative to selecting a single preferred method is to acknowledge that none of the available methods gives us the exact quantity of interest, but that each of them produces responses from which this quantity may be inferred. New models have been developed to estimate core health values for different states based on responses to multiple measurement methods (19). This approach allows data collected through imperfect instruments to be adjusted to provide better measures of the relative health levels associated with different states.

In order to address some of the fundamental empirical and methodological questions pertaining to health state valuations, the World Health Organization (WHO) has embarked on a series of data collection and analytical efforts on health state valuations as a key component of its research agenda on measuring health. This chapter provides an overview of research at WHO on health state valuations in summary measures of population health. We begin by describing a conceptual and analytical framework for health state valuations, provide a summary of the health state valuation component of the WHO Multi-country Survey Study on Health and Responsiveness 2000–2001 (20), highlight key findings from this effort, and end with a discussion of some of the remaining research questions and directions for future work.

FRAMEWORK FOR HEALTH STATE VALUATIONS

CONCEPTS

The WHO conceptual framework for measuring and reporting on health is elaborated elsewhere in this volume (21). In this framework, health states are described in terms of levels on multiple dimensions such as mobility, pain, hearing, and seeing. Health state valuations, in relation to these multidimensional profiles, constitute scalar index values for the overall health levels associated with different states, measured on a cardinal scale that ranges from zero (for a state equivalent to death) to unity (for a state of ideal health). These valuations formalize the intuitive notions that health levels lie on a continuum and that we may characterize an individual as being more or less healthy than another at a particular moment in time. Health state valuations quantify departures from perfect health, i.e. the reductions in health associated with particular health states. It is important to emphasize that these weights *do not* measure the quality of life of people with disabilities and *do not* measure the value of a person to society.

In fact, there have been various conceptual interpretations of health state valuations that have led to considerable ambiguity in defining the basis for measuring and understanding these valuations. It is useful for us to contrast our conceptual definition of health state valuations with these other concepts.

Utility

Some measurement instruments explicitly define health state valuations in terms of the utility associated with health states (22). Richardson (18) and others have noted, however, that *utility* in this context is defined (somewhat circularly) as the quantity that is maximized when individuals make choices obeying the axioms of expected utility theory, which offer a set of principles relating to preferences under uncertainty. The use of the standard gamble technique for eliciting valuations is linked to the axiomatic foundations of expected utility theory, and as such incorporates both assessments of health levels associated with different states, as well as attitudes towards risk and uncertainty (14;18). The notion of utility applied to health state valuations, therefore, conflates the concept of health with the separate concept of risk aversion, which we do not believe is relevant for characterizations of health levels in summary measures (2). It is reasonable to assume that health state utility, as measured through the standard gamble, is related monotonically to the level of health (19), but responses to the standard gamble may not be interpreted directly as interval-scaled measures of health levels.

Quality of Life, Health-related Quality of Life and Well-being

The term quality of life (QoL) has been used widely in various social science contexts to refer to the overall, subjective appraisals of happiness or satisfaction experienced by individuals (23). In health, the term QoL has been used in a more particular way to refer to a multidimensional construct relating to symptoms, impairments, functional status, emotional states, and what we would label as health domains (24;25). Because this use of QoL diverges from more general uses of the term, health researchers often refer to the distinct construct of "health-related QoL." To the extent that an individual's health-related QoL is conceived of as a vector of levels on "health-related" dimensions of life, it is similar to our conceptual framework for measuring health, albeit with less precisely articulated boundaries. Where health-related QoL is viewed as a summary measure of the contribution of an individual's health to his/her overall well-being, on the other hand, conceptual problems emerge from the fact that well-being is not clearly separable into independent health and non-health components, as Broome argues convincingly (26). In other words, when we compare the well-being or "quality of life" of individuals with different health levels, these relative comparisons may change depending on their levels on non-health dimensions of well-being.

Health Level

We may avoid these difficulties if we seek health state valuations that provide cardinal index values for the overall levels of health associated with multidimensional health states. Unlike the notion of utility, we do not believe that it is necessary to define this construct explicitly in terms of choices or preferences. Almost everybody can agree that a person with one amputated leg is healthier than a person with two amputated legs, all else being equal, without resorting either to the language of choice or to statements about the overall well-being of either person. While this is a simple case of a dominance ordering (because the difference is in the level of only one domain), the same intuitive notion applies to more complicated examples: if we say that somebody with a mild sore throat is, all else being equal, healthier than somebody with two broken arms, perhaps not everybody would agree, but most people could at least interpret this statement in reference to some common-sense understanding of health. Indeed, this common-sense notion extends beyond ordinal comparisons, for example, allowing us to say that going from good health to having a sore throat is a smaller change in health than going from a sore throat to quadriplegia. In all of these cases, we submit that there is an intuitive understanding of the meaning of health that is not based on the concept of choice. People may usually (but not always) prefer to be in a better state of health, but levels of health may be understood as distinct from these individual preferences.

We draw a clear line here between the tools that are used to elicit judgments about health levels and the conceptual definition of the construct itself. One of the common elicitation techniques used in survey research on health state valuations is the *time trade-off*, which asks individuals to indicate preferences between different hypothetical scenarios that involve choices between improved health levels and reduced longevity (27). On the face of it, this technique appears to parallel closely the notion of summary health measures that are based on equivalence between length of life and levels of health. The similarity of the framing, however, does not imply that an individual's *preferences* over different combinations of health levels and longevity are the actual phenomena of interest, which we can illustrate with an example. Imagine that we ask survey respondents whether they would be willing to give up any time at the end of their lives in order to avoid living with a mild hearing impairment. Some respondents may be unwilling to sacrifice any longevity to avoid this minor health problem, even though they acknowledge that the state of having a mild hearing impairment represents a lower level of health than a state with no hearing impairment, *ceteris paribus*. Indeed, empirical research confirms the finding that

there are threshold effects such that respondents are unwilling to trade longevity to avoid minor health problems—see, for example, Robinson et al. (28). In the illustration offered here, it is the judgment that the hearing impairment represents a decrement from perfect health that interests us, not the preferences that result from the combination of this judgment with numerous other considerations. In other words, the preferences that we may infer from techniques such as the time trade-off are likely to depend, at least in part, on assessments of health levels, but they may also reflect a range of other values and considerations that are distinct from evaluations of health levels.

MEASUREMENT

One of the primary objectives in the enterprise of measuring health state valuations is to characterize the relationship between overall valuations and levels on the multiple domains of health (29–31). Estimation of this *valuation function* would ideally be based directly on empirical data on domain levels and corresponding valuations for a wide range of different states, both measured reliably on meaningful, interpersonally comparable scales. In practice, however, neither domain levels nor health state valuations are elicited directly through the current array of available data collection instruments, but rather must be inferred from observations that *are* obtained directly (Figure 32.1). Domain levels are most often characterized in terms of ordered categorical (ordinal) data, while valuations are typically inferred from standard elicitation methods such as the standard gamble, time trade-off, visual analogue scale or person trade-off, which must be interpreted with caution in seeking measures of health levels, for the reasons described above.

Figure 32.1 Measurement framework for health state valuations

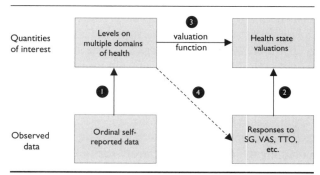

SG=standard gamble; VAS=visual analogue scale; TTO=time trade-off

In Figure 32.1, the key relationships of interest are marked by numbered arrows as follows: 1) mapping function from ordinal self-reported data to unobserved cardinal levels on core domains of health; 2) mapping function between responses to standard elicitation methods and underlying health state valuations; 3) mapping function between multiple domain levels and health state valuations (*valuation function*). The line marked 4) is depicted as a dotted line because this relational function between domain levels and responses on a particular elicitation method may be of interest only as an intermediate step in predicting health state valuations from domain levels. For example, a function relating domain levels to visual analogue scale responses can be used to predict health state valuations if the predicted visual analogue scale responses are then transformed using the estimated function represented as line 2).

Work is underway at WHO on estimating all of the relationships described in Figure 32.1:

- An extensive research agenda on cross-population comparability of health survey data focuses on the mapping from ordinal survey responses into cross-population comparable measurements of health along different domains, using an approach based primarily on anchoring vignettes to adjust for interpersonal differences in the uses of categorical response scales (see (*32*) and Chapters 55, 30, and 31 in this volume (*33–35*)).

- A multi-method data collection protocol and new analytical models for health state valuations have been developed to estimate the relationships between responses on different elicitation techniques (e.g. standard gamble, time trade-off, etc.) and underlying health state levels (*19*).

- New instruments have been developed for the collection of information on individual descriptions of hypothetical health states along a set of core domains, as well as valuations of these health states using the visual analogue scale. This information, combined with the results from the multi-method protocol, allows estimation of the health state valuation function that may be used to predict valuations based on domain levels (adjusted to cross-population comparable scales).

This chapter will focus on the latter two components of this agenda. Readers interested in the first component are referred to relevant background papers (cited above) that present the various aspects of this work in considerable detail.

For the purposes of deriving overall valuations for individuals to be incorporated in summary measures of population health, some have considered whether it would be appropriate simply to elicit individual valuations of their own health states directly (*36*). A focus on estimating and applying a standard valuation function, however, has both pragmatic and normative appeal. Firstly, the measurement of domain levels is more easily achieved in health surveys because it involves more concrete and specific questions, as opposed to the somewhat abstract nature of multi-attribute valuations. It may be particularly challenging to elicit overall self-valuations (i.e. valuations of individuals' own health states rather than hypotheticals) because these valuations may reflect projection of a desired level of health that leads to an upward bias. This possibility is supported empirically by the fact that individuals' direct valuations of their own health states tend to be higher than those of even the mildest hypothetical states. Secondly, it allows for standardized comparisons of overall health levels, such that two individuals with identical levels on all of the core domains of health have the same overall valuations. Individuals' valuations of their own health states will reflect differences in domain levels and differences in the relative weights that people place on various aspects of their health. For comparative purposes, it is useful to apply a global standard valuation function; however, to the extent that variation in the way that individuals aggregate across domains is of substantive interest, estimation of valuation functions at national or subnational levels enables formal analysis of this variation.

DATA COLLECTION STRATEGY

As part of the framework for assessing health systems performance, WHO has embarked on a large-scale effort to collect new data on health state valuations in representative sample surveys from numerous countries through the Multi-country Survey Study on Health and Responsiveness 2000–2001 (*20*) and the ongoing World Health Surveys (*37*). This work is intended to address several key methodological challenges and to fill the empirical gaps on health state valuations across diverse cultural settings.

An important methodological challenge for the measurement of health state valuations is that responses to existing measurement techniques depend not only on assessments of the health levels in different states, but also on other values such as attitudes toward risk and uncertainty, distributional concerns, or preferences for immediate rather than future outcomes (time preference). A related issue is that many of the standard measurement methods for health state valuations are highly abstract and cognitively demanding tasks that may have limited reliability and validity in the general community. In order to address both of these problems, data collection efforts must combine practical and feasible instruments that can be administered in populations with wide ranges of educational attainment levels with analytical strategies for estimating the quantities of interest from responses to these survey questionnaires.

In collaboration with Member States, WHO has pursued a two-tiered data collection strategy that includes a series of general population surveys in representative probability samples, combined with more detailed surveys among respondents with high levels of educational attainment in the same countries. The primary objective of the population-based surveys is to collect information on health state valuations in the general community in order to estimate valuation functions and examine differences in valuations across countries and within countries by age, sex, education, income, and other variables. The more detailed surveys are designed to allow empirical adjustment of the valuation responses obtained in the population surveys to account for the scaling properties of the simple measurement instrument used in these surveys. The present study reports on the household surveys and companion multi-method studies conducted during 2000–2001 as part of the WHO Multi-country Survey Study on Health and Responsiveness.

CONDUCT OF THE HOUSEHOLD SURVEY AND MULTI-METHOD VALUATION STUDY

Household surveys including a valuation module were conducted in fourteen countries: China, Colombia, Egypt, Georgia, India, Iran, Lebanon, Indonesia, Mexico, Nigeria, Singapore, Slovakia, Syria, and Turkey. Sampling plans were developed in each site based on existing national sample frames where possible (20). In three countries (China, India, Nigeria) survey samples were not representative of the whole country because of the size of the countries and language barriers. In China, the study was carried out in the three provinces of Gansu, Henan, and Shandong; in India, the study was carried out in the State of Andhra Pradesh; in Nigeria, it was carried out in the Yoruba speaking regions of Ibadan, Iseyin, Ido, and Ogo of Oyo State.

A workshop was held to train the principal investigators in each household study site on sampling, interviewing techniques, questionnaire review and practice, and general issues related to the survey. Additionally, training manuals and videos were distributed to the sites for ongoing training.

Interviews were conducted face-to-face using paper and pencil questionnaires. In each household, a single adult individual (aged 18 years or older) was selected at random (using the Kish table method (38)) after completing a full household roster. Informed consent was obtained from every respondent in the survey. The survey protocol specified that all interviews should be conducted in privacy. Where other household members, neighbours or friends were present, the interviewers requested privacy, and, where necessary, steps were taken to ensure that interviewers were the same sex as the respondent. Interviewers were supervised on a regular basis during fieldwork to ensure that expectations and production requirements were met, interviewers were performing well, information was kept confidential and professional ethics were followed, questionnaires and other materials were completed accurately and submitted on time, and lastly, that any problems were reported as soon as they arose.

A data entry program was developed by WHO specifically for the survey study and provided to the sites. This program searched for inconsistencies and validated the entries in each field by checking for valid response categories and appropriate ranges. In addition, the data were entered for a second time to capture other data entry errors.

The more detailed multi-method valuation surveys were conducted in eleven of the fourteen countries that implemented the household valuation study: China, Colombia, Egypt, Georgia, India, Indonesia, Mexico, Nigeria, Singapore, Slovakia, and Turkey. The multi-method valuation study in Nigeria, however, was excluded from the analysis reported here because of problems with implementation of the study protocol. Approximately 200 respondents in each site were recruited based on purposive sampling, with an effort to include a range of different ages and a gender balance while recruiting respondents with high levels of educational attainment.

HEALTH STATE VALUATION COMPONENT

In the valuation section of the household survey study, individuals were first presented with a series of 10 different health conditions described by short labels (for example, "Total blindness, acquired as an adult"—see Annex 32.1 for the full set of health condition labels). For a given condition, respondents were asked to imagine a person living in that condition and to describe how they envisioned that person's health along six core dimensions: mobility, self-care, pain, affect, cognition, and usual activities.[1] Using a set of index cards displaying the short labels, each respondent was asked to rank order the 10 conditions, plus his or her own current state of health, and then to assign values to each condition using a thermometer-type (visual analogue) scale (Annex 32.2). There were four different sets of conditions, with overlap between sets, including a total of 34 different conditions across all sets (Annex 32.1). The visual analogue scale (VAS) provides a relatively simple measurement tool for assessing the health levels associated with the hypothetical states. In several previous pilot studies in diverse settings, the VAS was the only existing measurement technique that was consistently comprehensible to respondents, and that had satisfactory levels of reliability in test-retest experiments (39;40). The scaling properties of the VAS have been challenged, however, and there is evidence that the health decrements associated with mild states may be overstated by VAS responses due to scale distortions (41;42). Nevertheless, the general nature of these systematic distortions has been well-defined, which allows for empirical adjustment of valuations obtained using the VAS, once the degree of distortion has been quantified formally (19).

The more detailed surveys among highly educated respondents included more abstract and cognitively demanding valuation tasks, which have potentially limited reliability in general population surveys but have been applied widely in industrialized countries among convenience samples of educated respondents. In the detailed surveys, respondents completed the same tasks as in the household survey (domain descriptions, ordinal ranking and VAS) for a set of 14 conditions, and also provided valuations for the 14 conditions using three other standard elicitation techniques—standard gamble (SG), time trade-off (TTO) and person trade-off (PTO). The objective of these detailed surveys was to use multiple indicators relating to a common set of latent health values in order to impute these underlying health state valuations that inform responses to all different measurement methods, and to adjust the VAS values based on the results (19). Because some sites experienced difficulties in implementing one or more of the valuation methods, as described below, analysis of the multi-method data has focused on the subset of the country-method combinations for which implementation difficulties were minimal.

ANALYSES

The major analytical tasks relating to health state valuations correspond to the estimation of the key relationships defined in the measurement framework outlined above.

MULTI-METHOD ANALYSIS

Analysis of the detailed multi-method surveys focused on estimation of parametric relationships between responses to standard elicitation techniques and latent (unobserved) core values for a range of different conditions. The multi-method analysis was based on the median values for each condition and method in each country. For each elicitation technique, formal models were specified to describe responses on a given technique as a function of the core health values and one auxiliary parameter with direct substantive interpretation (see (19) for an introduction to this approach). For example, standard gamble responses depend on the core health values and a risk aversion parameter; time trade-off responses depend on the health values and a discount rate; person trade-off responses depend on the health values and a parameter reflecting distributional concerns (the so-called "rule of rescue" parameter); and VAS responses depend on the health values and a scale distortion parameter. By formalizing these relationships based on previous theoretical and empirical findings, maximum likelihood methods were used to recover the latent core values for the range of health conditions in the study and simultaneously to characterize the nature of the auxiliary values such as the risk aversion parameter. Of most immediate concern, this analysis produced a function that could be used to adjust for the scale distortion in VAS values, in order to translate the responses obtained in the larger population sample surveys to the appropriate scale for valuations.

The raw data from the multi-method exercise were in units particular to each method, as summarized in Table 32.1.

To facilitate comparisons between responses on the various methods, we first mapped the raw responses on each method onto a scale that ranges between 0 and 1, with 1 representing ideal health, according to the following standard transformations:

$$r_{i,x}^{VAS} = \frac{s_{i,x}}{100} \qquad [1]$$

Table 32.1 Characteristics of responses to different valuation methods

Method	Response	Units and scale	Interpretation
VAS	$s_{i,x}$	0 to 100	Median rating of condition x in country i
TTO	$y_{i,x}$	years 0 to 10	Median number of years of perfect health equivalent to 10 years in condition x in country i
SG	$p_{i,x}$	risk 0 to 100%	Median risk of death at which treatment is equivalent to certainty in condition x in country i
PTO	$n_{i,x}$	persons 100 to ∞	Median number of averted cases of x equivalent to 100 deaths averted in country i

$$r_{i,x}^{TTO} = \frac{y_{i,x}}{10} \quad [2]$$

$$r_{i,x}^{SG} = 1 - p_{i,x} \quad [3]$$

$$r_{i,x}^{PTO} = 1 - \frac{100}{n_{i,x}} \quad [4]$$

where $r_{i,x}^m$ is the median response from country i for condition x using method m.

After mapping responses from each method onto the unit interval, the basic premise behind the multi-method analysis was that the systematic differences between responses to the different methods may be attributed to the extra considerations that each method introduces in addition to the levels of health associated with the hypothetical conditions presented to respondents.

In the analytical model for the multi-method data, it was assumed that a core health value v_x exists for each condition x (but is unobserved), and that observed responses could be related to these latent core values through a series of method-specific, monotonically increasing functions. Each function included one auxiliary parameter to capture the considerations other than the health value that informed responses to each method.

VAS responses were related to the core health values through a power function with parameter θ_1.

$$r_{i,x}^{VAS} = 1 - [1 - v_{i,x}]^{\theta_1} \quad [5]$$

This formulation was based on results from psychophysics experiments (43) and was also used by Torrance (44) in modelling the functional relationship between VAS and SG.

For the time trade-off, we allowed for time preference by translating the two durations referenced in the TTO to their equivalent present values (45), using the formula for discounting a continuous stream of life (with θ_2 representing the discount rate) and then solving for $r_{i,x}^{TTO}$:

$$r_{i,x}^{TTO} = -\frac{1}{10\theta_2} \ln\left[1 - (1 - e^{-10\theta_2})v_{i,x}\right] \quad [6]$$

The standard gamble function had one parameter θ_3 that represented an individual's risk aversion. The formulation was derived from utility theory, as described by Bell and Raiffa (46).

$$r_{i,x}^{SG} = \frac{-e^{-\theta_3 v_{i,x}} + 1}{-e^{-\theta_3} + 1} \quad [7]$$

The person trade-off formulation was parallel to the standard gamble formulation, but in this case the parameter θ_4 represented aversion to decisions resulting in loss of life, the so-called "rule of rescue" (47).

$$r_{i,x}^{PTO} = \frac{-e^{-\theta_4 v_{i,x}} + 1}{-e^{-\theta_4} + 1} \quad [8]$$

It was assumed that the latent core health values giving rise to the different observed values were distributed normally in logit space, with a mean value for each condition that was constant across the different observation mechanisms:

$$\ln\left(\frac{v_{i,x}}{1 - v_{i,x}}\right) \sim N(\beta_x, \sigma) \quad [9]$$

Expressing equations [5]–[8] in the more general form

$$r_{i,x}^m = f_m(v_{i,x}) \quad [10]$$

and substituting in [9] we obtained:

$$\ln\left(\frac{f_m^{-1}(r_{i,x}^m)}{1 - f_m^{-1}(r_{i,x}^m)}\right) \sim N(\beta_x, \sigma) \quad [11]$$

Parameters of the model were estimated by maximizing the likelihood

$$\prod_i \prod_x \prod_m N\left(\ln\left(\frac{f_m^{-1}(r_{i,x}^m)}{1 - f_m^{-1}(r_{i,x}^m)}\right) \middle| \beta, \sigma, \theta\right) \quad [12]$$

where β is a vector of core health values, σ is the variance, and θ is a vector of auxiliary parameters.

ESTIMATION OF VALUATION FUNCTION

The other major analytical task that was undertaken was estimation of the relationships between levels on the different domains of health and the scalar valuations produced for each health state (captured in the *valuation function*). Because it is often easier to collect information on the levels of health domains than it is to elicit valuations directly, it is useful to be able to predict valuations indirectly based on a particular health state profile consisting of specified domain levels.

Approaches to modelling the relationships between domain levels and valuations have differed in terms of the amount of structure that is imposed on the valuation function *a priori* based on theory. For example, derivation of valuation functions for the Health Utilities Index (*48*) is based on multi-attribute utility theory, which outlines a set of alternative assumptions regarding independence between the domains that are aggregated in the valuation function. Stronger independence assumptions lead to simpler functional forms, and the overall structure imposed by multi-attribute utility theory allows for construction of valuation functions based on a limited set of empirical data concentrating on "corner states," for which decrements along one domain are isolated. This approach offers the practical advantage of reducing the burden of data collection, but has the disadvantage of imposing structure on the valuation function that may not be consistent with the way that people actually aggregate across domains in arriving at overall health valuations. Towards the opposite end of the spectrum are approaches that impose minimal *a priori* structure on the valuation function and instead rely more heavily on collecting valuation data for a large enough number of different health states (i.e. different combinations of domain levels) to allow statistical inference regarding empirical regularities in the relationships between domain levels and valuations (see, for example, (*29;30*)). While these statistical approaches may also impose structure on the valuation function through choices regarding the functional form of the models used, the structure is usually not constrained by theoretical assumptions. Without adopting a strictly theoretical approach to defining the structure of valuation functions, it nevertheless may be useful in the latter empirical approach to define a set of criteria for evaluating different valuation functions based on principles of face validity. For example, one reasonable criterion for a valid valuation function would be that the valuations implied by the function should improve when the level on any particular domain improves, all else being equal.

For the analyses presented here, we have elected to impose minimal theoretically-based structure on the valuation function in order to allow flexibility in investigating the empirical regularities in the large number of observations available from our household survey study. The focus of the analysis has been on modelling the relationships between levels on six domains (mobility, affect, cognition, pain, usual activities, and self-care) and visual analogue scale responses, to be combined with the adjustment of VAS responses estimated through the multi-method analysis described above, in order to obtain predictions of overall health levels based on information on multiple domain levels.

In order to estimate the valuation function, we first translated the categorical descriptions of each hypothetical health condition provided by the respondents in the household sample surveys into cross-population comparable estimates on continuous interval scales, using the anchoring vignette approach described elsewhere (*32–34;49*). In brief, the approach was based on an extension to the standard ordered probit model, which postulates the existence of latent values for each health condition distributed normally with condition-specific means and variances (which were also allowed to vary across countries). The standard model was modified to allow for variation in the categorical cut-points according to a set of covariates (country, age, sex, and education), with identification of cut-point values based on ratings for a set of anchoring vignettes describing fixed ability levels on each domain (see Chapter 55 for a full description of the model). Vignette-adjusted scores on each domain were mapped to a censored (0,1) scale bounded by the scores for the best and worst vignettes (and scaled inversely such that lower numbers correspond to better health levels on each domain). The dependent variable in the regression models was (100-VAS), with the exception of the logit model noted below, in order to facilitate comparisons to disease-burden estimates that are based on health gaps rather than positive measures of health. The valuation function regressions were run on data from 10 countries for which vignette analyses were completed and valuation data available at the time of this study (which excluded Iran, Lebanon, Singapore, and Syria from this first round of analysis).

We estimated a range of different regression models that varied in terms of the following methodological choices:

Model Specification

In the process of mapping between the levels on multiple health domains and overall judgments about health levels associated with particular conditions, the impact of incremental changes in one domain may depend on the levels for other domains. Three different formulations were examined to capture different possible degrees of interaction between levels on the different domains: a) six domain levels as main effects only; b) main effects plus all two-way interaction terms; and c) main effects plus all n-way interaction terms (for n = 2,3,4,5,6). Without imposing structure on the functional form of the valuation function according to *a priori* theoretical assumptions, a comparison of models that include different levels of interaction between domains allows empirical evaluation of the descriptive validity of different assumptions about independence between domains.

Error Term

VAS values for any given condition are not normally distributed because 1) the scale is bounded at the top and (aside from states worse than death) the bottom; and 2) distributions are often skewed as a result of these bounds (50). Different possibilities for the error term in the model were considered in order to account for the skewness and bounded nature of the VAS responses: a) normal using ordinary least squares (OLS) regression; b) normal in logit space using OLS regression of $\ln[(1-VAS/100) / (VAS/100)]$; c) censored normal using a tobit model, which related observed responses on the (0,1) interval to values on an unbounded scale under the assumption that (unobserved) values above 1 or below 0 are observed as 1 and 0, respectively; and d) truncated normal, which has a likelihood function based on the *conditional* probability of the observed values given that the values fall within the unit interval.

Covariance Structure

In addition to the non-normality of distributions of VAS values, the data used here also have a complex variance structure that results from having multiple observations per respondent. We therefore considered random effects models for the OLS and tobit models in order to account for variation both within and between respondents (cf. (50)).

Based on the three sets of issues described above, the range of models examined is summarized in Table

32.2. Performance of the different models was evaluated in terms of predictive validity. Each model was estimated using a 75% subset of the observations, selected at random, and model fit was assessed based on the root mean squared error of the model predictions for the remaining 25% compared to observed values.

RESULTS

HOUSEHOLD SURVEY RESULTS

In total, the 14 country household survey on health state valuations included 46 011 respondents, of whom 52% were women, with a mean age of 39 years and an average of approximately 8.6 years of schooling (Table 32.3). The total number of valuations obtained was 488 012.

Median categorical descriptions of the 35 conditions (including "own health state") are reported in Table 32.4, ranked according to the summed scores for each condition (lowest to highest). The health state descriptions spanned a wide range of different severity levels on all domains. Among the 35 conditions, there were 29 different unique combinations of median domain scores.

For any given condition, there was considerable variation in the health state descriptions provided by

Table 32.2 Regression models for visual analogue scale values

Model	Interactions	Error term	Random effect?
1	none	normal	N
2	none	normal	Y
3	none	logit	N
4	none	truncated normal	N
5	none	censored normal	N
6	none	censored normal	Y
7	2-way	normal	N
8	2-way	normal	Y
9	2-way	logit	N
10	2-way	truncated normal	N
11	2-way	censored normal	N
12	2-way	censored normal	Y
13	all n-way	normal	N
14	all n-way	normal	Y
15	all n-way	logit	N
16	all n-way	truncated normal	N
17	all n-way	censored normal	N
18	all n-way	censored normal	Y

Table 32.3   Characteristics of the study population

Country	N	% women	Mean age, years (s.d.)	Mean years of schooling (s.d.)
China	4 706	46.9	40.0 (14.0)	9.2 (4.2)
Colombia	2 955	64.4	39.9 (15.7)	7.5 (4.4)
Egypt	2 192	55.1	39.4 (14.6)	8.1 (6.1)
Georgia	4 949	57.2	46.3 (16.8)	12.2 (3.1)
Indonesia	4 963	56.1	39.6 (14.8)	7.5 (4.5)
India	2 490	53.5	39.7 (14.5)	3.9 (5.1)
Iran	4 776	52.3	37.5 (15.5)	6.6 (5.3)
Lebanon	1 382	54.5	41.8 (16.4)	10.4 (5.7)
Mexico	2 448	40.3	41.9 (16.5)	9.3 (5.0)
Nigeria	2 452	58.4	35.2 (15.3)	8.2 (4.9)
Singapore	2 769	47.3	40.6 (13.3)	10.1 (4.1)
Slovakia	578	56.2	43.6 (16.7)	12.2 (2.9)
Syria	4 254	52.7	37.9 (15.0)	7.3 (5.2)
Turkey	5 097	42.8	33.4 (12.1)	10.1 (4.0)
Total	46 011	52.2	39.4 (15.3)	8.6 (5.1)

Figure 32.2   Distribution of categorical ratings on difficulties performing usual activities for the condition of drug dependence

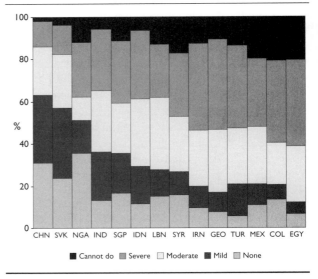

different respondents both within and between countries. Figure 32.2 presents an example of cross-country variation in descriptions for drug dependence along the domain of usual activities. The average categorical rating ranged across countries between 2.2 and 3.6 (if "no difficulty" is coded as 1, "mild difficulty" as 2, and so on), and Figure 32.2 shows a wide variation in the distributions of ratings for this condition in the 14 survey countries. For example, in China fewer than 2% of respondents assessed drug dependence as producing the most severe category of usual activity limitations, while approximately 20% of respondents

in Mexico, Colombia and Egypt chose the most severe category in describing this condition.

Overall, the set of six domains used in this study allowed a total of 15 625 possible combinations of domain levels, of which 11 236 different combinations (72%) were used by respondents. By allowing respondents to provide their own descriptions of each condition, this study has produced valuations for a much larger number of unique states than in studies based on a limited set of generic health state profiles,

Figure 32.3   Average VAS score by condition and country

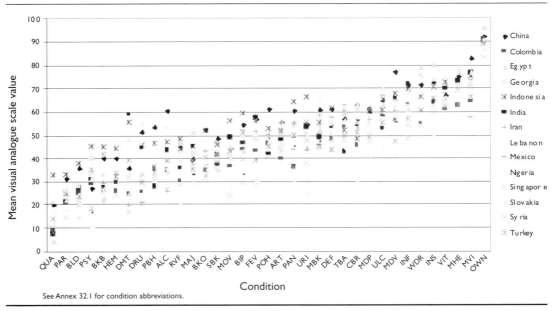

See Annex 32.1 for condition abbreviations.

Table 32.4 Median categorical descriptions of each condition by domain

Condition*	Mobility	Self-care	Usual activities	Pain	Affect	Cognition
Own health state	1	1	1	1	1	1
Mild hearing problems	1	1	1	2	2	1
Skin discolorations on face	1	1	1	2	3	1
Infertility	1	1	1	2	4	1
Mild vision problems	2	1	2	2	2	1
Deafness	1	1	2	2	3	2
Insomnia	1	1	2	2	3	2
Watery diarrhœa	2	1	2	3	2	1
Pain in stomach (as in ulcer)	2	1	2	3	3	1
Chronic bronchitis	2	2	2	3	3	2
Moderate vision problems	3	2	2	2	3	2
Urinary incontinence	2	2	2	3	3	2
Paralysis in one hand	2	3	3	3	3	1
Bipolar disorder	2	2	3	3	3	3
Below the knee amputation, one leg	3	3	3	3	3	1
Moderate depression	2	2	3	3	3	3
Moderate chronic lower back pain	3	3	3	3	3	2
Panic disorder	3	2	3	3	4	3
Recto-vaginal fistula	3	2	3	4	4	2
Alcohol dependence	3	3	3	3	3	4
Arthritis	3	3	4	4	3	2
Drug dependence	3	2	3	3	4	4
Two broken arms in stiff casts	3	4	4	4	3	1
Dementia	3	3	4	3	3	4
Major depression	3	2	3	4	4	4
Severe fevered state	3	3	4	4	4	3
Paralysis in both hands	3	4	4	4	4	2
Psychosis	3	3	4	3	4	4
Severe chronic lower back pain	4	3	4	4	4	2
Below the knee amputation, both legs	4	4	4	4	4	2
Total blindness	4	4	4	4	4	2
Hemiparesis	4	4	4	4	4	2
Paraplegia	4	4	4	4	4	2
Movement disorder	4	4	4	4	4	3
Quadriplegia	5	5	5	4	5	3

* Abbreviated condition labels are presented here. Complete labels are reported in Annex 32.1.

which typically have elicited valuations for 40 to 60 different states (30;51). A large amount of variation is useful in developing mapping functions from domain levels to valuations (29–31).

The average VAS scores in each country for the 35 conditions in this study are plotted in Figure 32.3. While there was substantial variation across countries for each condition, there was nevertheless evidence of a considerable level of agreement overall. Pearson's correlation coefficients for the mean valuations across countries were almost all greater than 0.8 (Table 32.5). The intraclass correlation coefficient for the mean valuations was 0.795. Pearson's correlation

coefficients and the intraclass correlation coefficient for the median valuations (not shown) were similar.

Behind these summary statistics, variation in the valuations within each country was also observed. Figure 32.4 presents an example of the different ranges in values reported for four conditions (own health state, infertility, major depression, and quadriplegia) in each country. In these box-plots, the box indicates the interquartile range (IQR), while the whiskers show the furthest data point that is within 1.5 times IQR beyond either boundary of the IQR. Outliers, defined as data points more than 1.5 times IQR beyond the boundaries of the IQR, appear as circles.

It is worth noting that although respondents were allowed to rate a health state as worse than death (i.e. less than 0 on the visual analogue scale), only 135 (0.02%) responses in total gave values below 0, in contrast to findings in other valuation studies (*51–52*).

Although variation in VAS scores within and across countries may suggest cross-cultural differences in the valuation of health conditions, it is important to recognize that observed variation may be due to several distinct sources. One key feature of our study was that

Table 32.5 Correlation coefficients for mean VAS scores across countries

	China	Colombia	Egypt	Georgia	Indonesia	India	Iran	Lebanon	Mexico	Nigeria	Singapore	Slovakia	Syria	Turkey
China	1.000													
Colombia	0.908	1.000												
Egypt	0.879	0.925	1.000											
Georgia	0.928	0.917	0.904	1.000										
Indonesia	0.869	0.905	0.875	0.855	1.000									
India	0.865	0.882	0.872	0.889	0.932	1.000								
Iran	0.905	0.930	0.938	0.896	0.855	0.823	1.000							
Lebanon	0.911	0.934	0.946	0.918	0.869	0.833	0.972	1.000						
Mexico	0.878	0.960	0.918	0.871	0.872	0.872	0.917	0.922	1.000					
Nigeria	0.845	0.861	0.786	0.855	0.799	0.773	0.819	0.833	0.815	1.000				
Singapore	0.893	0.900	0.905	0.915	0.931	0.951	0.834	0.859	0.878	0.795	1.000			
Slovakia	0.895	0.898	0.913	0.937	0.860	0.868	0.890	0.908	0.870	0.806	0.903	1.000		
Syria	0.856	0.905	0.956	0.858	0.823	0.792	0.967	0.964	0.914	0.747	0.823	0.857	1.000	
Turkey	0.865	0.925	0.910	0.874	0.924	0.870	0.903	0.913	0.896	0.794	0.908	0.887	0.894	1.000

Figure 32.4 Box-and-whisker plots of VAS scores by country for four states: own health state, infertility, major depression, and quadriplegia

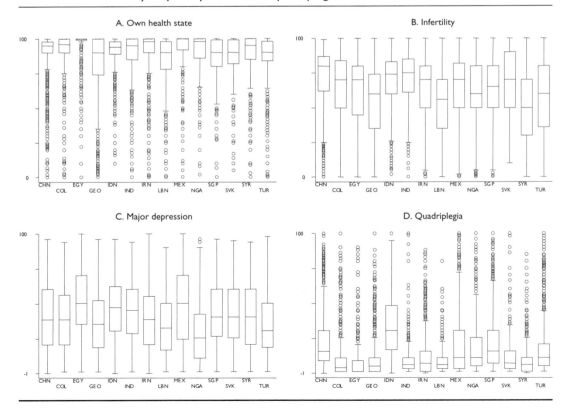

we elicited individual descriptions from respondents for each of the conditions they valued. Thus, individuals were asked to provide their own assessments of how they imagined each condition in terms of the core domains of health, so that in fact, the condition label "deafness" represented not a single defined set of domain levels across all respondents, but a range of different states depending on how each respondent envisioned the domain levels associated with deafness. A significant component of the variation in visual analogue scale values attached to the same disease label may therefore be related to variation in these health state descriptions. Figure 32.5 shows the relationship between the standard deviation (across countries) of the mean summed categorical domain scores for the range of conditions and the standard deviation of the mean VAS scores across countries. This figure shows a strong correlation between the variation in health state descriptions and valuations for the conditions in this study. Thus, some of the differences that have been observed previously (9;53) may be due to differences in the health state descriptions conjured by a particular label in various settings.

Multi-method Results

Characteristics of the study population in 10 sites for the multi-method valuation study appear in Table 32.6. Approximately 200 respondents were included in most sites. The average age of the multi-method study populations was similar to the average age in the

household surveys, but the education levels were significantly higher in the multi-method study, by design.

The analytical model used for the multi-method data was based on the assumption that observed responses on the different methods resulted from a mapping between a set of core underlying health values and method-specific scales. In the model, this mapping was based on a series of increasing functions that captured other values and considerations tapped by each method (such as risk aversion in the standard gamble, time preference in the time trade-off, etc.) (19). The existence of a core set of latent health values was supported in this dataset by high rank order correlations across the different methods. Table 32.7 shows the Spearman's rank correlation coefficients for median valuations on the different methods within and between countries. The within-country correlations indicate the level of correspondence in pairwise comparisons of the rankings for the set of conditions produced by different methods within a particular country. The between-country correlations reported in Table 32.7 are averaged across the set of nine other countries in each case; for example, to compute the VAS-VAS between-country correlation for China in Table 32.7, rank correlations were first computed between the median VAS results in China and the median VAS results in each of the other nine countries, and then these nine coefficients were averaged. This table confirms high levels of correlations both within and between countries, with the exception of the person trade-off in Mexico and Georgia, where the lack of correlations is consistent with implementation difficulties reported by the sites. In Georgia, for example, the median person trade-off values were identical for all 34 states. For the multi-method analysis reported

Figure 32.5 Standard deviation of domain descriptions and VAS scores

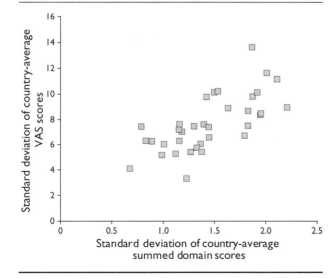

Table 32.6 Characteristics of the multi-method study population

Country	N	% women	Mean age, years (s.d.)	Mean years of schooling (s.d.)
China	201	49.3	40.8 (13.2)	14.5 (2.6)
Colombia	207	52.7	37.0 (14.4)	17.8 (4.0)
Egypt	203	47.8	40.0 (14.0)	16.2 (3.0)
Georgia	200	55.5	43.9 (16.3)	14.3 (2.9)
Indonesia	137	46.0	41.5 (13.1)	15.6 (3.8)
India	200	54.5	35.8 (13.8)	16.3 (2.9)
Mexico	192	49.5	35.5 (12.6)	14.7 (2.9)
Singapore	150	54.0	35.2 (13.0)	14.1 (3.1)
Slovakia	200	65.0	37.6 (14.4)	14.3 (3.1)
Turkey	198	50.0	33.9 (11.2)	15.2 (3.4)
Total	1 888	52.6	38.1 (14.0)	14.7 (2.6)

Table 32.7   Spearman's rank order correlation coefficients for different valuation methods, within and between countries

Methods	China	Colombia	Egypt	Georgia	Indonesia	India	Mexico	Singapore	Slovakia	Turkey
Within countries										
VAS-TTO	0.97	0.93	0.94	0.97	0.78	0.96	0.89	0.96	0.97	0.91
VAS-SG	0.97	0.94	0.92	0.97	0.67	0.94	0.87	0.97	0.97	0.92
VAS-PTO	0.98	0.86	0.92	0.30	0.54	0.83	−0.27	0.84	0.96	0.89
TTO-SG	0.98	0.96	0.97	0.97	0.79	0.97	0.93	0.96	0.94	0.96
TTO-PTO	0.99	0.86	0.86	0.30	0.75	0.77	−0.34	0.84	0.95	0.94
SG-PTO	0.98	0.79	0.84	0.30	0.60	0.75	−0.34	0.84	0.93	0.95
Between countries										
VAS-VAS	0.84	0.90	0.88	0.88	0.84	0.88	0.84	0.85	0.85	0.87
VAS-TTO	0.82	0.87	0.84	0.84	0.83	0.87	0.80	0.81	0.84	0.83
VAS-SG	0.79	0.85	0.83	0.81	0.83	0.85	0.80	0.81	0.82	0.80
VAS-PTO	0.58	0.61	0.64	0.67	0.60	0.60	0.71	0.61	0.61	0.63
TTO-VAS	0.84	0.85	0.86	0.86	0.73	0.84	0.84	0.84	0.84	0.86
TTO-TTO	0.81	0.83	0.83	0.83	0.72	0.84	0.81	0.81	0.82	0.83
TTO-SG	0.80	0.81	0.82	0.80	0.70	0.82	0.80	0.80	0.80	0.81
TTO-PTO	0.56	0.57	0.63	0.67	0.58	0.59	0.69	0.61	0.59	0.59
SG-VAS	0.84	0.85	0.84	0.86	0.62	0.80	0.84	0.84	0.85	0.86
SG-TTO	0.81	0.83	0.81	0.83	0.62	0.80	0.81	0.80	0.83	0.81
SG-SG	0.80	0.82	0.81	0.79	0.60	0.79	0.81	0.80	0.82	0.80
SG-PTO	0.56	0.55	0.61	0.67	0.49	0.54	0.68	0.63	0.58	0.58
PTO-VAS	0.86	0.81	0.79	0.30	0.53	0.78	−0.22	0.74	0.84	0.83
PTO-TTO	0.82	0.77	0.75	0.30	0.50	0.77	−0.18	0.73	0.81	0.80
PTO-SG	0.80	0.75	0.75	0.30	0.48	0.75	−0.23	0.70	0.79	0.78
PTO-PTO	0.59	0.58	0.60	0.22	0.46	0.55	−0.11	0.56	0.60	0.56

here we have excluded the person trade-off results for Mexico and Georgia.

The different elicitation techniques produced substantially different results across the range of conditions in the study. Table 32.8 reports the overall mean, median and standard deviations of the responses by method (after rescaling responses onto the unit interval using equations [1]–[4]) in the pooled dataset, but excluding the person trade-off in Mexico and Georgia. Overall, the lowest mean and median values arose from the visual analogue scale, while the highest values were usually produced by the person trade-off technique. Standard gamble values were close to person trade-off values for many states, while time trade-off values tended to be closer to VAS scores. The skewness of the data is evident by the gap between the mean and median values, which is most pronounced towards the upper and lower ends of the scale.

Within every country, a range of values was observed across respondents on each of the different elicitation techniques. Figure 32.6A presents the results from China, which was the site with the highest degree of correlation across methods. In this figure, results from all methods were rescaled to the (0,1) interval,

as described earlier, in order to facilitate comparisons. The pattern of responses is similar to that reported previously (*19*), with lower values and smaller variances in the VAS scores compared to the other methods. As in previous studies, the size of the variance tended to be larger near the middle of the scale than at the ends. In Figure 32.6B, we have graphed the same results for Indonesia, where the cross-method correlations were lowest (among the set of eight countries with acceptable results on all four methods). Although the data from Indonesia show a substantially greater level of measurement error, similar relationships between the responses on the different methods are broadly discernible even in the presence of considerable error. The remaining sites show results falling between the two extremes of China and Indonesia in terms of levels of measurement error and the degree of correlation between responses on the different methods.

MODELING MULTI-METHOD RESPONSES

The multi-method analysis focused on estimating the series of relationships between responses on the four methods and a set of latent core health values, based

Table 32.8 Mean, median and standard deviation of valuation results by method and condition

Condition*	Visual analogue			Time trade-off			Standard gamble			Person trade-off		
	Mean	Median	S.D.	Mean	Median	S.D.	Mean	Median	S.D.	Mean	Median	S.D.
Mild vision problems	0.786	0.830	0.170	0.873	0.990	0.233	0.926	0.995	0.186	0.911	0.998	0.226
Mild hearing problems	0.744	0.780	0.151	0.857	0.950	0.222	0.913	0.990	0.188	0.916	0.998	0.209
Skin discolorations on face	0.732	0.780	0.189	0.832	0.950	0.254	0.899	0.990	0.200	0.910	0.998	0.232
Insomnia	0.738	0.780	0.170	0.811	0.905	0.254	0.901	0.990	0.203	0.902	0.995	0.225
Moderate vision problems	0.695	0.740	0.191	0.818	0.920	0.240	0.904	0.982	0.188	0.884	0.990	0.234
Infertility	0.699	0.795	0.236	0.766	0.900	0.301	0.831	0.970	0.268	0.874	0.990	0.241
Pain in stomach (as in ulcer)	0.653	0.680	0.192	0.775	0.900	0.247	0.859	0.960	0.216	0.879	0.990	0.233
Watery diarrhœa	0.665	0.700	0.215	0.761	0.900	0.281	0.853	0.960	0.243	0.884	0.990	0.235
Chronic bronchitis	0.630	0.660	0.195	0.754	0.850	0.266	0.854	0.950	0.215	0.869	0.981	0.239
Paralysis in one hand	0.557	0.600	0.221	0.714	0.800	0.271	0.804	0.900	0.239	0.861	0.980	0.238
Deafness	0.556	0.580	0.204	0.700	0.800	0.276	0.819	0.930	0.247	0.854	0.980	0.240
Two broken arms in stiff casts	0.576	0.600	0.205	0.689	0.790	0.283	0.785	0.900	0.267	0.849	0.967	0.243
Moderate depression	0.573	0.600	0.199	0.679	0.750	0.284	0.794	0.900	0.250	0.850	0.960	0.246
Severe chronic lower back pain	0.545	0.590	0.205	0.648	0.700	0.280	0.748	0.850	0.264	0.847	0.975	0.245
Arthritis	0.512	0.500	0.193	0.653	0.700	0.289	0.757	0.880	0.278	0.834	0.950	0.251
Urinary incontinence	0.518	0.520	0.239	0.644	0.700	0.300	0.746	0.850	0.278	0.827	0.960	0.274
Panic disorder	0.482	0.500	0.224	0.583	0.600	0.292	0.729	0.850	0.288	0.827	0.950	0.251
Bipolar disorder	0.471	0.490	0.230	0.583	0.625	0.312	0.746	0.885	0.293	0.806	0.900	0.278
Below the knee amputation, one leg	0.460	0.465	0.221	0.624	0.700	0.289	0.742	0.850	0.291	0.777	0.900	0.285
Alcohol dependence	0.472	0.500	0.237	0.587	0.600	0.311	0.700	0.820	0.316	0.812	0.950	0.289
Severe fevered state	0.471	0.500	0.243	0.557	0.600	0.326	0.693	0.800	0.322	0.756	0.933	0.327
Movement disorder	0.434	0.430	0.207	0.569	0.600	0.290	0.675	0.800	0.311	0.783	0.900	0.289
Paralysis in both hands	0.400	0.400	0.223	0.540	0.550	0.284	0.681	0.800	0.297	0.753	0.872	0.297
Recto-vaginal fistula	0.406	0.400	0.251	0.545	0.600	0.316	0.641	0.750	0.330	0.755	0.900	0.318
Drug dependence	0.396	0.400	0.242	0.501	0.500	0.314	0.630	0.700	0.334	0.767	0.900	0.314
Below the knee amputation, both legs	0.327	0.300	0.212	0.501	0.500	0.307	0.598	0.650	0.331	0.713	0.817	0.315
Psychosis	0.317	0.280	0.220	0.441	0.400	0.305	0.578	0.600	0.330	0.744	0.867	0.308
Major depression	0.338	0.300	0.220	0.452	0.450	0.309	0.576	0.610	0.339	0.692	0.857	0.340
Hemiparesis	0.318	0.300	0.182	0.479	0.500	0.303	0.546	0.600	0.331	0.708	0.800	0.306
Dementia	0.335	0.300	0.231	0.426	0.400	0.323	0.538	0.550	0.355	0.679	0.800	0.339
Total blindness	0.295	0.240	0.222	0.454	0.464	0.314	0.521	0.535	0.344	0.695	0.833	0.332
Paraplegia	0.255	0.210	0.177	0.388	0.400	0.288	0.428	0.400	0.330	0.652	0.800	0.345
Quadriplegia	0.146	0.100	0.168	0.255	0.100	0.284	0.279	0.100	0.321	0.484	0.500	0.381

on the median observed responses for each condition, method and country. The full set of parameters to be estimated included, in this case, 34 latent health values, four auxiliary parameters and a variance term (for the distribution of health values, assumed to be normal in logit space). Because the parametric specifications of the four different functions relating responses on each method to the core health state values are quite similar in terms of their general shapes, the model is only weakly identified without the imposition of additional constraints on the estimation problem. Thus, to simplify the estimation task we have chosen to fix one of the auxiliary parameters (the discount rate) and estimate the remaining auxiliary parameters

(which capture risk aversion, the rule of rescue and VAS scale distortions) and core health state values conditional on this fixed discount rate. Results in the empirical literature on levels of time preference for health outcomes in different populations have varied (54–56), so we have taken a baseline value of 3% per annum for the discount rate, but also examined the results under alternative assumptions of 1% and 5% annual discount rates. Table 32.9 reports the results for the baseline analysis and sensitivity analyses on the discount rate.

The baseline estimate of the risk aversion parameter was 2.54, where 0 indicates risk neutrality and positive numbers indicate risk aversion. The implication

Figure 32.6 Valuation results by method and condition

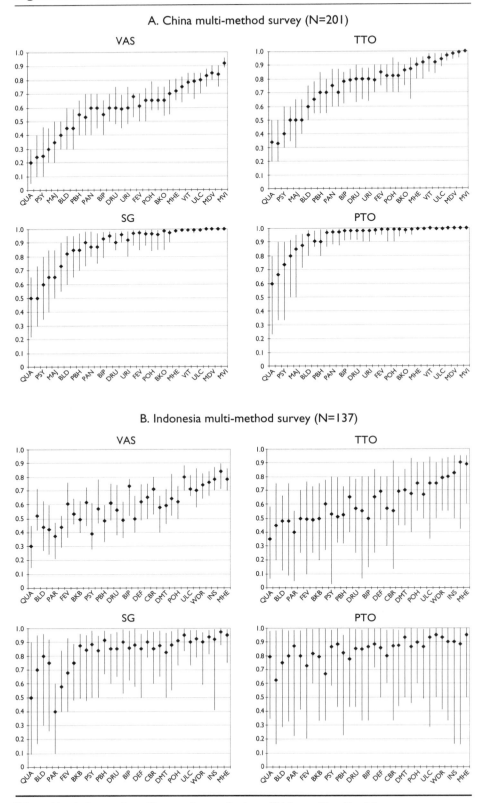

Points and bars indicate median and interquartile range. See Annex 32.1 for condition abbreviations.

Table 32.9   Results from multi-method analyses

	Baseline (discount rate = 3%)			Discount rate = 1%			Discount rate = 5%		
	Estimate	2.5th percentile	97.5th percentile	Estimate	2.5th percentile	97.5th percentile	Estimate	2.5th percentile	97.5th percentile
Auxiliary parameters									
Scale distortion	0.64	0.59	0.69	0.68	0.62	0.73	0.60	0.56	0.65
Risk aversion	2.54	2.22	2.85	2.79	2.47	3.11	2.28	1.97	2.59
Rule of rescue	4.81	4.47	5.15	5.07	4.72	5.41	4.56	4.22	4.89
Time preference	0.03			0.01			0.05		
Core health state values									
Mild vision problems	0.967	0.955	0.976	0.961	0.948	0.972	0.971	0.961	0.979
Mild hearing problems	0.940	0.920	0.956	0.931	0.909	0.949	0.948	0.930	0.962
Vitiligo	0.937	0.916	0.953	0.927	0.904	0.946	0.945	0.926	0.960
Insomnia	0.918	0.892	0.939	0.907	0.879	0.931	0.928	0.905	0.947
Moderate vision problems	0.903	0.873	0.928	0.890	0.858	0.918	0.914	0.887	0.936
Infertility	0.900	0.869	0.925	0.887	0.854	0.915	0.912	0.884	0.935
Watery diarrhoea	0.870	0.832	0.902	0.854	0.813	0.889	0.884	0.849	0.913
Peptic ulcer	0.856	0.815	0.891	0.840	0.795	0.878	0.872	0.834	0.904
Chronic bronchitis	0.810	0.759	0.853	0.790	0.737	0.837	0.828	0.781	0.869
Deafness	0.764	0.706	0.815	0.743	0.683	0.797	0.785	0.729	0.833
Two broken arms	0.751	0.691	0.804	0.729	0.666	0.785	0.772	0.715	0.823
Paralysis, one hand	0.744	0.684	0.799	0.722	0.660	0.779	0.766	0.708	0.818
Moderate depression	0.732	0.669	0.788	0.709	0.645	0.768	0.754	0.694	0.808
Arthritis	0.690	0.623	0.752	0.667	0.598	0.730	0.714	0.648	0.773
Severe back pain	0.687	0.620	0.749	0.663	0.595	0.727	0.711	0.645	0.770
Urinary incontinence	0.684	0.616	0.746	0.660	0.591	0.724	0.707	0.642	0.767
Bipolar disorder	0.635	0.564	0.702	0.610	0.539	0.679	0.659	0.589	0.725
Alcohol dependence	0.631	0.559	0.699	0.607	0.534	0.675	0.656	0.585	0.722
Amputation, one leg	0.631	0.560	0.698	0.607	0.535	0.676	0.655	0.584	0.721
Panic disorder	0.612	0.540	0.682	0.588	0.515	0.658	0.637	0.565	0.705
Severe fever	0.591	0.517	0.661	0.566	0.492	0.637	0.616	0.543	0.685
Movement disorder	0.548	0.474	0.621	0.524	0.450	0.597	0.573	0.498	0.645
Recto-vaginal fistula	0.532	0.458	0.606	0.508	0.435	0.581	0.557	0.482	0.630
Paralysis, both hands	0.518	0.444	0.591	0.494	0.421	0.568	0.542	0.467	0.616
Drug dependence	0.512	0.437	0.586	0.488	0.415	0.561	0.537	0.462	0.611
Amputation, both legs	0.441	0.369	0.514	0.419	0.349	0.491	0.463	0.389	0.538
Major depression	0.427	0.356	0.500	0.405	0.336	0.477	0.449	0.376	0.524
Hemiparesis	0.422	0.352	0.495	0.401	0.332	0.472	0.444	0.372	0.519
Psychosis	0.418	0.347	0.490	0.396	0.328	0.467	0.440	0.368	0.515
Dementia	0.414	0.344	0.487	0.393	0.325	0.464	0.437	0.365	0.512
Total blindness	0.360	0.294	0.430	0.340	0.277	0.408	0.381	0.312	0.453
Paraplegia	0.307	0.247	0.372	0.289	0.232	0.352	0.325	0.263	0.393
Quadriplegia	0.088	0.066	0.113	0.082	0.062	0.106	0.094	0.071	0.122

of a risk aversion parameter of 2.54 is that a person would be willing to accept only an 8% risk of death to avoid living in a state that constitutes a 25% reduction from perfect health, or to accept only a 22% risk of death to avoid living in a state that falls at the mid-point between perfect health and death on a scale of overall healthiness.

The baseline estimate of the rule of rescue parameter implies that respondents tend to have strong preferences for mortality aversion over prevention of non-fatal outcomes. Similarly to the risk aversion parameter, a value of 0 would indicate "rescue-neutrality," while positive values are consistent with the rule of rescue. The estimated baseline value of 4.81 implies that saving the life of one healthy individual would be equivalent to averting 12 cases of a non-fatal condition that falls halfway between perfect health and death (rather than two cases, which would be the "rescue-neutral" point of equivalence).

Of most direct relevance for the present study are the estimates of the scale distortion parameter for the VAS responses. From the baseline estimation, the following transformation is required to adjust for end-aversion bias in the visual analogue scale:

$$VAS_{adjusted} = 1 - (1 - VAS_{raw}/100)^{(1/0.64)} \quad [13]$$

At the estimated level of scale distortion in the baseline, a health state with a true value of 0.95 would result in an observed VAS score of 85 out of 100. Across the full uncertainty range spanning the lower bound of the confidence interval for a 5% discount rate to the higher bound of the confidence interval for a 1% discount rate, the range of observed scores consistent with a true value of 0.95 would be 81 to 89 out of 100.

ESTIMATION OF VALUATION FUNCTION

The 18 different regression models that were estimated, relating VAS scores to vignette-adjusted levels on six domains, varied in terms of the level of interaction between domains that were included in the models, the specification of the error term, and the inclusion or omission of an individual-level random effect. Coefficient estimates for all 18 models are reported in Table 32.10. The first section of the table reports on the six models that incorporated main effects only; the second section reports on models including two-way interaction terms; and the third section reports on the full model including all two-way, three-way, four-way, five-way, and six-way interactions. In each of these models, both the dependent and independent variables have been scaled such that higher numbers correspond to larger health decrements, i.e. lower levels of overall health for the left-hand side variable—(100-VAS) or the corresponding logit transformation of this quantity—and lower levels on specific domains for the right-hand side variables, with each scaled between 0 and 1.

Regression coefficients from the OLS models are similar to those from the tobit models which allow for censoring in the data set. The similarity between OLS and the censored models is due in part to the fact that only a relatively small number of observations are stacked at either 0 or 100 on the visual analogue scale. Coefficients in the truncated normal models tend to be larger overall than those in the other models. In the

range of different models with two-way interactions and those with higher order interactions, a large number of the interaction terms are statistically significant.

To aid in the substantive interpretation of the regression results from the alternative models considered here, Table 32.11 shows the changes in overall health valuations (expressed as decrements from full health) associated with changes in individual domain levels. For models with interactions, the relative changes due to changes in different domain levels will vary depending on the starting point for the evaluation. Table 32.11 therefore provides two different types of examples: (a) reductions in overall health decrements starting from halfway between the best and worst levels on all domains, then raising the individual domain levels, one at a time, from the midpoint to the best level on that domain, while holding all others constant at 50%; and (b) increases in overall health decrements starting from the best levels on all domains and lowering the individual domain levels, one at a time, from the best level to the 50% level, while holding all others constant at 100%. The results in Table 32.11 were computed by first calculating predicted levels for (100-VAS) based on the regression results, and then adjusting these predicted values using the power function estimated through the multi-method analysis (equation [13]).

For the first six models, which include main effects only, changes in overall valuations move in the same direction as changes in individual domain levels, which we propose as a minimal criterion for face validity. The relative importance of changes in different domains varies somewhat across the different models, but there is some consistency in the broad patterns that emerge, with affect, mobility and self-care tending to be the most important domains in all of the main-effects-only models. In models 7 through 12, which include main effects and all two-way interactions between domains, changes in valuations move in the expected direction when starting from the midpoint level on all domains, but in the opposite direction for certain domains when starting from the best levels. Note that this finding occurs because some of the coefficients on the main effects are negative, and when all domains are at their best levels, none of the interaction terms are relevant to changes in only one domain (as the domain scores are scaled such that the best level has a value of 0). For the full models including all *n*-way interaction terms, no inversions with respect to the direction of domain-specific changes appear. It is interesting to note that in the full models the relative importance of decrements in cognition is much greater when the other domains are at favorable levels than when they are all at intermediate levels. In moving from the 50% level on all domains, improvements in cognition produce small benefits in terms of overall health valuations relative to other domains, while in moving from the best levels on all domains, changes in cognition pro-

Table 32.10 Estimation of valuation function

A. Regression results for models with main effects only

	(1) Normal		(2) Normal RE		(3) Logit		(4) Truncated		(5) Censored		(6) Censored RE	
	Coef	|t|	Coef	|t|	Coef	|t|	Coef	|t|	Coef	|t|	Coef	|t|
aff	**15.63**	65.87	**16.59**	75.57	**0.895**	54.20	**26.65**	61.85	**15.75**	64.65	**16.68**	74.32
cog	**7.25**	48.31	**9.92**	71.07	**0.468**	44.82	**12.36**	45.28	**7.48**	48.44	**10.39**	72.41
mob	**10.02**	45.34	**12.07**	59.24	**0.761**	49.49	**15.72**	40.72	**10.57**	46.60	**12.77**	61.23
pain	**5.71**	18.05	**8.10**	27.52	**0.701**	31.83	**9.01**	15.75	**6.69**	20.56	**9.32**	30.84
self	**14.57**	59.30	**12.04**	53.93	**0.935**	54.67	**22.85**	53.16	**15.00**	59.52	**12.40**	54.34
usual	**6.92**	27.91	**8.31**	36.45	**0.221**	12.80	**10.89**	25.39	**6.53**	25.66	**7.83**	33.58
cons	**21.35**	155.73	**17.81**	124.35	**−1.744**	182.77	**2.43**	7.60	**20.75**	147.30	**17.04**	114.43
Adj. R²	0.33		0.33		0.29							

Abbreviations: aff = affect, cog = cognition, mob = mobility, self = self-care, usual = usual activities, cons = constant.
Coefficients in bold are significant at 0.05 level.

B. Regression results for models with main effects and all two-way interactions

	(7) Normal		(8) Normal RE		(9) Logit		(10) Truncated		(11) Censored		(12) Censored RE	
	Coef	|t|	Coef	|t|	Coef	|t|	Coef	|t|	Coef	|t|	Coef	|t|
aff	**15.59**	32.11	**15.55**	36.34	**0.802**	23.89	**30.05**	33.64	**15.28**	30.66	**15.12**	34.65
cog	**19.29**	36.73	**23.32**	50.22	**1.158**	31.88	**32.18**	34.49	**19.59**	36.30	**23.83**	50.23
mob	**−4.98**	6.82	−0.87	1.34	**−0.663**	13.12	**9.00**	6.91	**6.07**	8.10	**1.68**	2.54
pain	**3.76**	4.54	1.42	1.93	**0.648**	11.29	2.53	1.66	**5.27**	6.19	0.22	0.30
self	**4.72**	5.39	0.89	1.14	**0.493**	8.14	**4.11**	2.69	**3.19**	3.55	**2.67**	3.36
usual	**19.37**	25.72	**17.75**	26.47	**1.518**	29.14	**35.73**	26.72	**20.46**	26.47	**18.64**	27.26
X12	**13.09**	18.11	**16.17**	25.11	**1.006**	20.11	**22.07**	17.68	**13.70**	18.45	**16.78**	25.53
X13	**8.96**	8.73	**7.37**	8.16	**0.846**	11.92	**11.67**	6.55	**9.75**	9.24	**8.00**	8.67
X14	**17.53**	16.30	**21.52**	22.49	**1.502**	20.20	**24.13**	12.52	**19.35**	17.51	**23.67**	24.22
X15	**10.87**	9.48	**8.53**	8.47	**0.644**	8.12	**14.94**	7.60	**11.20**	9.53	**8.71**	8.48
X16	**6.30**	5.69	**5.92**	6.07	**0.618**	8.06	**13.61**	7.20	**6.82**	6.00	**6.50**	6.54
X23	**13.57**	21.50	**12.89**	23.22	**0.889**	20.39	**19.23**	17.71	**13.91**	21.46	**13.13**	23.15
X24	1.36	1.48	**2.40**	2.96	**0.290**	4.56	0.09	0.06	1.81	1.92	**2.22**	2.68
X25	**3.57**	4.91	0.04	0.07	**0.135**	2.69	**4.25**	3.45	**3.49**	4.68	0.24	0.37
X26	**7.88**	10.53	**8.00**	12.15	**0.549**	10.60	**9.49**	7.51	**8.09**	10.53	**8.13**	12.12
X34	**26.96**	19.73	**13.88**	11.49	**2.109**	22.32	**45.95**	19.42	**28.96**	20.62	**14.99**	12.14
X35	**20.54**	27.04	**19.79**	29.42	**1.775**	33.78	**34.52**	26.50	**22.02**	28.25	**21.22**	30.92
X36	**14.74**	15.73	**6.82**	8.20	**1.225**	18.91	**24.11**	15.22	**15.68**	16.32	**7.20**	8.50
X45	**4.10**	2.74	**2.68**	2.04	**0.469**	4.54	3.48	1.37	2.31	1.51	0.82	0.61
X46	**22.73**	15.61	**19.80**	15.40	**1.765**	17.53	**38.91**	15.77	**24.10**	16.13	**20.81**	15.87
X56	**15.74**	19.95	**14.11**	20.01	**1.098**	20.13	**23.41**	17.43	**16.28**	20.11	**14.46**	20.11
cons	**22.20**	88.34	**18.68**	80.29	**1.407**	80.96	**1.87**	3.57	**22.46**	87.10	**18.78**	78.64
Adj R²	0.34		0.34		0.32							

Abbreviations: aff = affect, cog = cognition, mob = mobility, self = self-care, usual = usual activities, cons = constant. Interaction terms refer to domains in alphabetical order (1 = affect, 2 = cognition, etc.).
Coefficients in bold are significant at 0.05 level.

continued

Table 32.10 Estimation of valuation function (continued)

| | C. Regression results for models with main effects and all n-way interactions | | | | | | | | | | | |
| | (13) Normal | | (14) Normal RE | | (15) Logit | | (16) Truncated | | (17) Censored | | (18) Censored RE | |
	Coef	|t|	Coef	|t|	Coef	|t|	Coef	|t|	Coef	|t|	Coef	|t|
aff	22.63	28.76	22.53	32.94	1.505	27.77	50.83	32.96	22.93	28.42	22.72	32.64
cog	26.00	12.08	27.66	14.70	1.751	11.81	57.76	15.13	26.45	11.98	28.12	14.68
mob	14.22	5.51	16.23	7.21	1.354	7.63	33.65	6.61	15.18	5.74	17.36	7.58
pain	14.10	7.93	18.26	11.74	1.127	9.21	42.41	12.20	14.37	7.89	18.73	11.83
self	22.18	3.00	13.34	2.06	1.591	3.13	62.98	4.79	23.04	3.04	14.13	2.15
usual	18.44	7.49	20.48	9.50	1.161	6.85	46.54	10.14	18.78	7.44	21.08	9.62
X12	-17.72	5.72	-20.19	7.46	-1.423	6.67	-49.53	9.19	-18.13	5.71	-20.47	7.43
X123	37.38	2.95	39.59	3.59	3.107	3.56	65.91	2.94	38.42	2.96	39.52	3.52
X1234	-54.20	1.75	-69.11	2.56	-5.376	2.52	-96.21	1.75	-56.72	1.78	-71.10	2.59
X12345	-29.05	0.27	11.17	0.12	2.841	0.39	-79.13	0.43	-24.86	0.23	18.82	0.20
X123456	-45.99	0.42	-56.78	0.60	-7.575	1.01	-72.87	0.38	-57.85	0.52	-70.45	0.73
X12346	140.47	3.10	152.74	3.87	9.730	3.12	262.34	3.26	145.02	3.12	156.82	3.90
X1235	-29.47	0.57	-21.70	0.48	-1.506	0.43	-51.72	0.57	-27.00	0.51	-18.23	0.40
X12356	111.13	2.09	70.64	1.52	5.465	1.49	193.39	2.04	111.71	2.04	68.83	1.45
X1236	-101.42	5.12	-88.37	5.11	-5.825	4.27	-181.92	5.16	-102.48	5.04	-88.24	5.01
X124	26.39	2.86	33.34	4.14	1.790	2.81	75.51	4.72	26.29	2.78	33.30	4.06
X1245	25.35	0.45	12.13	0.25	-0.035	0.01	-13.67	0.14	26.17	0.45	11.21	0.22
X12456	-119.41	1.99	-94.82	1.81	-7.045	1.70	-103.77	0.98	-121.20	1.96	-93.02	1.74
X1246	37.42	2.06	4.74	0.30	3.507	2.80	9.23	0.29	40.35	2.16	5.14	0.32
X125	8.63	0.34	-8.44	0.38	0.599	0.34	65.66	1.48	8.13	0.31	-9.00	0.40
X1256	-2.04	0.07	16.05	0.66	0.133	0.07	-66.90	1.34	-3.11	0.11	14.60	0.59
X126	-8.13	1.14	-1.19	0.19	-0.682	1.40	16.24	1.27	-8.67	1.19	-0.82	0.13
X13	-20.44	4.26	-21.45	5.12	-1.928	5.84	-45.62	5.10	-21.96	4.46	-23.00	5.39
X134	69.21	5.60	62.90	5.83	6.260	7.36	129.54	5.67	74.50	5.87	68.06	6.17
X1345	-186.68	3.29	-211.63	4.27	-16.949	4.34	-339.85	3.43	-208.25	3.58	-237.20	4.69
X13456	364.58	6.13	331.75	6.39	33.449	8.17	700.69	6.67	411.58	6.75	378.44	7.15
X1346	-188.06	7.74	-162.61	7.65	-15.515	9.28	-353.84	8.10	-203.68	8.17	-176.87	8.17
X135	85.43	3.06	95.14	3.90	6.094	3.17	162.11	3.31	91.10	3.18	101.64	4.09
X1356	-193.97	6.51	-162.26	6.24	-13.938	6.79	-363.97	6.86	-209.16	6.84	-175.71	6.62
X136	95.90	8.42	78.00	7.83	6.940	8.85	178.28	8.63	101.32	8.68	82.75	8.16
X14	-10.83	3.94	-5.74	2.39	-1.053	5.57	-43.30	8.46	-11.21	3.98	-5.75	2.36
X145	78.67	2.78	62.24	2.52	5.971	3.07	178.91	3.66	83.67	2.89	67.15	2.67
X1456	-104.74	3.25	-73.24	2.61	-8.063	3.64	-251.42	4.48	-116.06	3.51	-83.69	2.92
X146	35.98	3.65	43.45	5.04	2.296	3.38	91.76	5.26	37.77	3.73	46.22	5.27
X15	-51.31	3.94	-39.91	3.50	-3.029	3.38	-120.53	5.27	-52.50	3.93	-40.95	3.53
X156	69.81	4.43	48.68	3.55	4.125	3.81	162.94	5.88	73.56	4.55	51.76	3.70
X16	-22.30	5.29	-23.45	6.37	-1.491	5.14	-53.99	7.18	-23.16	5.36	-24.84	6.63
X23	-32.17	3.65	-28.14	3.66	-2.586	4.26	-61.33	3.91	-33.19	3.67	-28.54	3.65
X234	36.48	1.48	48.89	2.28	4.156	2.45	73.98	1.71	38.96	1.54	51.92	2.38
X2345	180.00	2.17	125.52	1.73	4.414	0.77	275.90	1.90	173.78	2.04	115.17	1.56
X23456	-109.75	1.27	-74.95	1.00	1.686	0.28	-94.30	0.62	-92.89	1.05	-55.50	0.72
X2346	-95.45	2.62	-113.15	3.56	-6.879	2.74	-213.45	3.30	-98.82	2.65	-117.17	3.63
X235	-56.99	1.61	-60.93	1.97	-1.168	0.48	-75.59	1.21	-54.97	1.51	-60.17	1.91
X2356	-11.31	0.30	14.75	0.46	-3.461	1.35	-68.10	1.02	-18.87	0.49	9.45	0.29
X236	59.34	4.31	48.75	4.06	3.299	3.48	132.30	5.33	59.83	4.24	48.87	4.00
X24	-28.77	4.06	-34.34	5.55	-1.976	4.05	-71.81	5.79	-29.09	4.00	-34.77	5.52
X245	-105.34	2.52	-62.02	1.70	-3.752	1.31	-111.64	1.53	-104.69	2.44	-58.53	1.58

continued

Table 32.10 Estimation of valuation function (continued)

X2456	**195.42**	4.34	**137.64**	3.51	**8.954**	2.89	**212.68**	2.65	**193.10**	4.17	**131.17**	3.27
X246	**-38.20**	2.68	-11.93	0.96	**-2.906**	2.97	-15.05	0.59	**-40.09**	2.75	-12.30	0.97
X25	31.01	1.90	**32.22**	2.26	0.678	0.60	5.98	0.21	29.93	1.79	**31.03**	2.14
X256	**-48.19**	2.66	**-42.33**	2.68	-1.066	0.85	-13.95	0.42	**-44.42**	2.38	**-37.82**	2.34
X26	**20.86**	4.43	**14.85**	3.62	1.341	4.14	3.40	0.39	**21.45**	4.44	**14.79**	3.53
X34	-15.41	1.84	**-25.71**	3.52	**-2.352**	4.09	**-42.65**	2.75	-18.15	2.12	**-29.35**	3.95
X345	49.47	1.24	**71.51**	2.05	**6.248**	2.27	115.56	1.67	60.24	1.47	**85.62**	2.42
X3456	**-146.87**	3.40	**-135.59**	3.60	**-15.060**	5.06	**-342.66**	4.51	**-171.87**	3.88	**-161.67**	4.21
X346	**94.69**	5.22	**88.25**	5.56	**7.553**	6.05	**206.79**	6.32	**101.91**	5.48	**95.18**	5.90
X35	-28.75	1.67	**-30.03**	2.00	**-2.876**	2.42	**-66.83**	2.20	-32.46	1.84	**-33.92**	2.22
X356	**112.98**	5.82	**88.45**	5.23	**8.816**	6.60	**231.92**	6.67	**122.77**	6.17	**97.09**	5.63
X36	**-63.63**	8.50	**-46.65**	7.12	**-4.348**	8.43	**-130.75**	9.38	**-66.24**	8.63	**-48.59**	7.29
X45	-9.88	0.53	-8.68	0.53	-1.660	1.28	-56.48	1.73	-12.30	0.64	-11.87	0.71
X456	-12.02	0.53	-14.72	0.75	0.696	0.45	51.00	1.29	-6.35	0.27	-8.07	0.40
X46	**-20.88**	3.01	**-28.92**	4.78	**-1.219**	2.55	**-64.55**	5.16	**-21.44**	3.02	**-29.98**	4.87
X56	-5.83	0.59	-0.09	0.01	-0.902	1.33	**-51.29**	2.93	-8.21	0.81	-2.80	0.32
cons	**17.59**	42.43	**14.52**	39.47	-1.914	67.03	-12.19	13.13	**17.34**	40.77	**14.14**	37.63
Adj R2	0.35		0.35		0.33							

Abbreviations: aff = affect, cog = cognition, mob = mobility, self = self-care, usual = usual activities, cons = constant. Interaction terms refer to domains in alphabetical order (1=affect, 2=cognition, etc.).

Coefficients in bold are significant at 0.05 level.

Table 32.11 Implications of estimated valuation functions: changes in overall health decrements associated with changes in levels on individual domains

	Reduction in overall health decrement from raising domain levels from 50% to 100%							Increase in overall health decrement from lowering domain levels from 100% to 50%						
Model	Base	Affect	Cog	Mob	Pain	Self	Usual	Base	Affect	Cog	Mob	Pain	Self	Usual
1	35.3	8.0	3.8	5.2	3.0	7.5	3.6	9.0	5.6	2.5	3.5	1.9	5.2	2.4
2	35.3	8.5	5.2	6.3	4.3	6.2	4.4	6.7	5.5	3.2	3.9	2.5	3.9	2.6
3	40.6	11.9	6.4	10.2	9.4	12.3	3.0	5.1	3.9	1.8	3.2	2.9	4.2	0.8
4	35.1	13.2	6.4	8.1	4.7	11.4	5.7	0.3	5.3	1.9	2.6	1.2	4.3	1.6
5	35.7	8.1	4.0	5.5	3.5	7.8	3.5	8.6	5.6	2.5	3.6	2.3	5.3	2.2
6	35.7	8.6	5.4	6.6	4.9	6.5	4.1	6.3	5.4	3.2	4.1	2.9	3.9	2.4
7	33.7	6.9	4.5	4.7	3.0	6.9	4.8	9.5	5.7	7.2	−1.6	−1.2	1.6	7.2
8	33.0	7.4	5.9	5.0	3.4	5.3	6.3	7.3	5.3	8.2	−0.3	0.4	−0.3	6.1
9	34.4	10.4	7.1	8.1	8.2	9.8	6.8	7.9	4.9	7.7	−2.7	−2.7	−2.1	10.9
10	33.1	11.1	7.1	7.7	5.8	10.7	7.0	0.2	6.0	6.6	−0.2	−0.2	0.4	7.7
11	33.7	7.1	4.6	4.9	3.4	7.0	4.8	9.7	5.6	7.4	−2.0	−1.7	1.1	7.7
12	33.0	7.5	6.0	5.2	3.9	5.3	6.4	7.3	5.1	8.5	−0.5	0.1	−0.8	6.4
13	33.3	7.2	3.4	2.6	0.9	6.7	4.8	6.6	7.8	9.1	4.6	4.6	7.6	6.2
14	33.1	6.9	5.3	3.2	2.6	5.4	6.0	4.9	7.1	9.0	4.9	5.6	3.9	6.4
15	34.4	9.5	5.3	2.7	0.1	8.6	7.2	4.1	6.6	8.2	5.7	4.4	7.1	4.6
16	32.6	10.2	4.6	3.8	1.8	9.9	6.8	0.0	4.2	6.1	0.8	2.3	7.7	3.2
17	33.4	7.2	3.5	2.6	0.9	6.7	4.9	6.5	7.8	9.2	4.9	4.7	7.9	6.3
18	33.1	6.9	5.4	3.3	2.6	5.4	6.1	4.7	7.1	9.1	5.2	5.7	4.2	6.5

The first section uses as a starting point the health decrement associated with 50% levels on all domains, and shows improvements in overall health resulting from improvements along each domain from 50% to 100%, while holding all other domain levels constant at 50%. The second section uses as a starting point the health decrement associated with the best levels on all domains, and shows declines in overall health resulting from declines along each domain from 100% to 50%, while holding all other domain levels constant at 100%.

duce the largest changes in overall health valuations in five of the six model variants. This type of complex interaction between domains is not captured in the parsimonious model that includes only main effects, but may be important for deriving overall valuations for incorporation in summary measures of population health, particularly at ages when most members of the population are relatively healthy.

Table 32.12 provides a summary of the out-of-sample predictive validity of the different models. Overall, it is notable that only the truncated models allow for predictions that span the full range of the scale, while the other models tend to collapse predictions toward the midpoint of the scale. This result is also apparent in comparisons of the root mean squared errors of the model predictions at different levels of observed VAS scores. While the various models are similar in terms of the overall average errors, the truncated models significantly outperform all other models at values towards the high end of the scale, while performing less well on predictions near the middle of the scale. For the purposes of estimating health state valuations in the general population, the advantage of predictive validity at the upper register where mostly healthy respondents are found may be important.

It is also useful to note from Table 32.12 that models with the full set of interaction terms offer slight improvements in predictive validity in some cases, but perform worse than more parsimonious models in other cases, which points to certain instances of over-fitting. Based on the results reported here, the truncated normal model appears to be most appropriate for use in summary measures of population health because of its ability to produce valuations across the full scale and its better performance at high health levels. While the truncated model including two-way interactions offers a reasonable compromise between parsimony and completeness, the general finding that the models with two-way interactions can in some cases violate the principle that overall valuations should move in the same directions as changes in any specific domain, may point to the need for more elaborate specifications including higher-order interactions. Of the models considered here, the most promising candidate therefore appears to be the truncated normal model including the full set of interactions. However, further work should be pursued to examine whether a more parsimonious model including some but not all of the higher-order interactions may be preferred.

DISCUSSION

As interest rises in summary measures of population health as a major element of health systems performance assessment, continued attention to the various conceptual, methodological and empirical issues relating to health state valuations is critical. This report has described the key components of the WHO research agenda on health state valuations, including new instruments for data collection, empirical results from the first round of the large-scale multi-country valuation survey project that has been launched, and analytical strategies for interpreting responses to standard elicitation techniques and understanding relationships

Table 32.12 Predictive validity of regression models

| | | Range of predicted VAS | | RMSE of predicted compared to observed VAS | | | | |
| | | | | | Range of observed values | | | |
Model	Description	Min	Max	Overall	[0,25)	[25,50)	[50,75)	[75,100]
1	normal, main effects	18.5	78.6	18.65	23.84	12.18	15.03	23.96
2	RE normal, main effects	15.2	82.2	18.36	23.13	12.82	15.41	22.42
3	logit, main effects	9.6	85.1	18.44	17.98	15.74	18.89	21.36
4	truncated normal, main effects	0.1	97.6	18.29	19.00	17.88	19.18	17.14
5	tobit, main effects	17.2	79.2	18.59	23.29	12.36	15.27	23.81
6	RE tobit, main effects	13.6	83.0	18.30	22.58	13.05	15.68	22.23
7	normal, 2-way interactions	15.7	81.6	18.42	23.15	12.40	14.70	23.79
8	RE normal, 2-way interactions	15.4	82.0	18.18	22.51	13.06	15.00	22.46
9	logit, 2-way interactions	5.7	88.6	18.29	18.35	15.89	17.29	21.80
10	truncated normal, 2-way interactions	0	100.0	18.21	18.89	17.80	18.69	17.49
11	tobit, 2-way interactions	13.7	82.8	18.37	22.56	12.65	14.83	23.81
12	RE tobit, 2-way interactions	13.2	83.6	18.14	21.94	13.35	15.15	22.41
13	normal, all interactions	13.4	84.1	18.26	23.07	12.31	14.64	23.39
14	RE normal, all interactions	12.6	85.5	18.05	22.48	12.95	14.90	22.19
15	logit, all interactions	4.4	88.4	18.02	18.86	15.02	17.01	21.40
16	truncated normal, all interactions	0	100.0	18.22	19.51	17.19	18.27	17.99
17	tobit, all interactions	10.4	84.2	18.20	22.50	12.52	14.77	23.35
18	RE tobit, all interactions	9.6	85.9	18.00	21.93	13.21	15.03	22.10

between domain levels and valuations. The data collection enterprise described here represents the largest empirical undertaking to date on valuations of health states in general populations, including more than 46 thousand respondents from 14 countries, providing a total of nearly 500 thousand VAS valuations.

The conceptual basis for health state valuations outlined in this chapter differs from many previous interpretations of health state valuations by focusing on *levels of health* as the key quantity of interest for use in summary measures, rather than on choices under uncertainty (as reflected in health utilities) or on general notions of well-being (as reflected in health-related quality of life measures). This conceptual framework has motivated the development of new methods for recovering the underlying assessments of health levels associated with different states from answers to different types of measurement techniques such as the visual analogue scale, standard gamble, time trade-off, and person trade-off. We found that individuals in the samples examined in this study were, on average, strongly risk averse and even more strongly adherent to the "rule of rescue."

The multi-method analyses described here have been anchored by the choice of a discount rate in order to gain statistical strength; further empirical evidence on levels of time preference for health outcomes may narrow the range of uncertainty around the findings from this study. Nevertheless, very high rank order correlation coefficients between responses on different measurement methods, both within and across countries, lend support to the premise that the various methods can be related to an underlying set of core health values through a series of monotonic functions. Assertions that available techniques somehow tap fundamentally unrelated constructs are seriously undermined by these high rank correlations. Even in the presence of large amounts of measurement error, systematic differences between the valuations produced by the four measurement methods considered here may be discerned, and the patterns are largely consistent across countries.

This study has relied on the visual analogue scale for collecting information on valuations in general population samples, combined with adjustments to VAS responses using the detailed multi-method exercises among highly educated respondents. The use of the VAS is appealing because of its simplicity and its demonstrated reliability in previous studies. However, other investigators have challenged the use of the VAS on the grounds that it lacks a theoretical basis, and an implicit (or sometimes explicit) equating of method-

ological rigor with the use of preference-based questions. Based on the strong evidence of predictable monotonic relationships between the different measurement methods, strategies based on the adjustment of VAS responses seem appropriate. However, further empirical investigations of some of the more demanding elicitation methods such as the time trade-off, or on the other hand more basic methods such as simple ordinal ranking exercises, are worth pursuing.

One implication of defining the quantity of interest in terms of health levels rather than individual preferences concerns the interpretation of states regarded as "worse than death." While it is easy to conceive of the possibility that an individual might *prefer* death to living in the most severe health states imaginable, this preference may be more closely linked to notions of overall well-being than to assessments of health levels, strictly defined. Indeed, it seems inherently problematic to describe a person in any living state, even one characterized by the most severe decrements along the key dimensions of health, as having *less health* than somebody who is dead. In this study, we observed a very low occurrence of states rated as worse than death on the visual analogue scale than what has been reported in some previous studies. The infrequency of this type of response is consistent with a conceptual framework which seeks to disentangle evaluations of health levels from stated or revealed preferences over hypothetical or real life choices.

Another key finding from this study is that cross-country variation in the way respondents weigh different domains of health in producing overall assessments of health levels may be smaller than previously believed. A key innovation of the work presented here is that respondents were allowed to provide both domain descriptions and valuations for hypothetical conditions, rather than simply being presented with generic multidimensional profiles as stimuli for valuation. Overall, valuations for more than 11 thousand unique combinations of levels on six core domains of health were elicited. This new approach presents several different advantages: a) it reduces the cognitive load on respondents, no longer requiring them to juggle a large number of different pieces of information in providing ratings for a set of health states; b) it eliminates the need to assume (implausibly) that a particular condition label or even a defined profile conjures up the same imagined health state across all individuals; and c) it allows estimation of the valuation function based on a vastly larger number of unique health states than in studies based on defined health state profiles. In considering the amount of variation in valuations explained by different valuation functions versus variation in health state descriptions, we found that cross-country differences in descriptions accounted for a large component of the systematic differences in valuations across countries.

The primary focus of this chapter has been to describe the new data and analyses that were used in estimating health state valuations based on the WHO Multi-country Survey Study on Health and Responsiveness 2000–2001. A number of methodological challenges persist, and research is proceeding in several different directions. In terms of the estimation of valuation functions linking domain levels to overall health assessments, it will be important to explore the full array of options for modelling the stochastic component of valuation distributions, to resolve issues of measurement error in the explanatory variables (domain levels), and to examine alternative functional forms for aggregating across domains. In the work we have described here, a range of different statistical models was considered, and various options for including interactions between domains were examined. Based on different criteria for predictive validity of these models, there remains some ambiguity about which model specification is most appropriate. There is some evidence that higher order interactions are statistically significant and potentially substantively important, while other evidence supports more parsimonious formulations. We have also proposed one simple criterion for face validity of valuation functions, requiring that overall valuations should improve if the level on any given domain improves, all else being equal. Based on this criterion alone, it appears that the models including only two-way interaction terms may produce results that lack face validity in some instances. Continuing work on specifying alternative models, and on developing a full set of criteria for evaluating these alternatives, will be useful.

As ongoing data collection efforts bear fruit, we will also seek to examine the generalizability of the results reported in this study of fourteen countries. It will be important to extend the cross-country analyses described here to include additional individual-level socioeconomic variables such as age, sex, education and income, as well as health-related variables including diagnostic categories, comorbidities, interactions with the health system and other factors. Both simple models involving separate estimation for different subgroups and more complicated hierarchical models may be applied in order to quantify these differences.

The development and refinement of data collection instruments for improving comparability of categorical domain responses is a relatively new enterprise that holds promise for enhancing the validity of survey research. Adjustment of categorical ratings of domain levels to continuous, comparable values on a common interval scale is a major area of investigation at WHO, which is considered in detail elsewhere in this volume (33–35), but has critical importance in the estimation of valuation functions. In the work described here, the anchoring vignette approach has been used for adjustment of categorical domain scores for the hypothetical health conditions in the valuation study, as it is with self-reported health levels in the population surveys. As this approach continues to evolve and further modifications are made both to the data collection instruments and analytical models used in conjunction with these data, the models for estimating the relationships between domain levels and overall valuations should be revisited in parallel. Comparisons of valuation functions estimated using raw categorical scores with those estimated using the adjusted, continuously scaled domain values may provide useful insights into the impact of data comparability problems in research on valuation functions.

In the long-term research agenda on health state valuations, the goal of continuing to seek improvements in measurement instruments must remain a priority. Further methodological work on instruments for eliciting health state valuations may eventually ameliorate the difficulties of interpreting responses to the current range of available valuation elicitation techniques in terms of cardinal health measures, and reduce the need for adjustments to these data through statistical models. In the meantime, however, as the refinement of data collection tools proceeds, it seems prudent to apply strategies for making optimal use of the imperfect tools currently available.

Notes

1   Categorical ratings on a seventh dimension, community participation, were also elicited for each of the hypothetical states, but this dimension was considered to be "health-related" rather than a direct component of health. Furthermore, comparable cardinal measurements for community participation were not available because the anchoring vignette strategy was not applied for this dimension.

References

(1) Mathers CD et al. Healthy life expectancy in 191 countries, 1999. *The Lancet*, 2001, 357(9269):1685–1691.

(2) Murray CJL, Salomon JA, Mathers CD. A critical ex-

amination of summary measures of population health. *Bulletin of the World Health Organization*, 2000, 78(8): 981–994.

(3) Kind P et al. Variations in population health status: results from a United Kingdom national questionnaire survey. *British Medical Journal*, 1998, 316(7133):736–741.

(4) Torrance GW et al. Multiattribute utility function for a comprehensive health status classification system. Health Utilities Index Mark 2. *Medical Care*, 1996, 34(7):702–722.

(5) Fryback DG et al. The Beaver Dam Health Outcomes Study: initial catalog of health-state quality factors. *Medical Decision Making*, 1993, 13(2):89–102.

(6) Froberg DG, Kane RL. Methodology for measuring health-state preferences—III: population and context effects. *Journal of Clinical Epidemiology*, 1989, 42(6): 585–592.

(7) Kind P, Dolan P. The effect of past and present illness experience on the valuations of health states. *Medical Care*, 1995, 33(Suppl.4):AS255–AS263.

(8) Ubel PA, Richardson J, Menzel P. Societal value, the person trade-off, and the dilemma of whose values to measure for cost-effectiveness analysis. *Health Economics*, 2000, 9(2):127–136.

(9) Jelsma J et al. The global burden of disease disability weights. *The Lancet*, 2000, 355(9220):2079–2080.

(10) Üstün TB et al. Are disability weights universal? WHO/NIH Joint Project CAR Study Group. *The Lancet*, 1999, 354(9186):1306.

(11) Baltussen RM et al. Obtaining disability weights in rural Burkina Faso using a culturally adapted visual analogue scale. *Health Economics*, 2002, 11(2):155–163.

(12) Dolan P. Effect of age on health state valuations. *Journal of Health Services Research & Policy*, 2000, 5(1): 17–21.

(13) Nord E. Methods for quality adjustment of life years. *Social Science & Medicine*, 1992, 34(5):559–569.

(14) Froberg DG, Kane RL. Methodology for measuring health-state preferences—II: scaling methods. *Journal of Clinical Epidemiology*, 1989, 42(5):459–471.

(15) Arnesen T, Nord E. The value of DALY life: problems with ethics and validity of disability adjusted life years. *Leprosy Review*, 2000, 71(2):123–127.

(16) Torrance GW. Toward a utility theory foundation for health status index models. *Health Services Research*, 1976, 11(4):349–369.

(17) Krabbe PF, Essink-Bot ML, Bonsel GJ. The comparability and reliability of five health-state valuation methods. *Social Science & Medicine*, 1997, 45(11):1641–1652.

(18) Richardson J. Cost utility analysis: what should be measured? *Social Science & Medicine*, 1994, 39(1):7–21.

(19) Salomon JA, Murray CJL. A multi-method approach to measuring health state valuations. *Health Economics*, 2003 (forthcoming).

(20) Üstün TB et al. WHO Multi-country Survey Study on Health and Responsiveness 2000-2001. In: Murray CJL, Evans DB, eds. *Health systems performance assessment: debates, methods and empiricism.* Geneva, World Health Organization, 2003.

(21) Salomon JA et al. Quantifying individual levels of health: definitions, concepts, and measurement issues. In: Murray CJL, Evans DB, eds. *Health systems performance assessment: debates, methods and empiricism.* Geneva, World Health Organization, 2003.

(22) Torrance GW. Utility approach to measuring health-related quality of life. *Journal of Chronic Diseases*, 1987, 40(6):593–603.

(23) Gill TM, Feinstein AR. A critical appraisal of the quality of quality-of-life measurements. *The Journal of the American Medical Association*, 1994, 272(8): 619–626.

(24) Patrick DL, Erickson P. *Health status and health policy: quality of life in health care evaluation and resource allocation.* New York, Oxford University Press, 1993.

(25) McDowell I, Newell C. *Measuring health: a guide to rating scales and questionnaires.* New York, Oxford University Press, 1987.

(26) Broome J. Measuring the burden of disease by aggregating well-being. In: Murray CJL et al., eds. *Summary measures of population health: concepts, ethics, measurement and applications.* Geneva, World Health Organization, 2002: 91–113.

(27) Torrance GW. Measurement of health state utilities for economic appraisal. *Journal of Health Economics*, 1986, 5(1):1–30.

(28) Robinson A, Dolan P, Williams A. Valuing health status using VAS and TTO: what lies behind the numbers? *Social Science & Medicine*, 1997, 45(8):1289–1297.

(29) Dolan P. Modeling valuations for EuroQol health states. *Medical Care*, 1997, 35(11):1095–1108.

(30) Brazier J et al. Deriving a preference-based single index from the UK SF-36 Health Survey. *Journal of Clinical Epidemiology*, 1998, 51(11):1115–1128.

(31) Busschbach JJ et al. Estimating parametric relationships between health description and health valuation with an application to the EuroQol EQ-5D. *Journal of Health Economics*, 1999, 18(5):551–571.

(32) Salomon JA, Tandon A, Murray CJL. *Using vignettes to improve cross-population comparability of health surveys: concepts, design, and evaluation techniques.*

EIP Discussion Paper No. 41. Geneva, World Health Organization, 2001. URL: http://www3.who.int/whosis/discussion_papers/discussion_papers.cfm#

(33) Tandon A et al. Statistical models for enhancing cross-population comparability. In: Murray CJL, Evans DB, eds. *Health systems performance assessment: debates, methods and empiricism.* Geneva, World Health Organization, 2003.

(34) Murray CJL et al. Empirical evaluation of the anchoring vignette approach in health surveys. In: Murray CJL, Evans DB, eds. *Health systems performance assessment: debates, methods and empiricism.* Geneva, World Health Organization, 2003.

(35) Salomon JA et al. Unpacking health perceptions using anchoring vignettes. In: Murray CJL, Evans DB, eds. *Health systems performance assessment: debates, methods and empiricism.* Geneva, World Health Organization, 2003.

(36) Hausman D. Why not just ask? Preferences, "Empirical Ethics" and the role of ethical reflection. In: Wikler D, Murray CJL, eds. *Fairness and goodness: ethical issues in health resource allocation.* Geneva, World Health Organization (forthcoming).

(37) World Health Organization. *World Health Survey.* Geneva, World Health Organization, 2003. URL: http://www3.who.int/whs/

(38) Kish L. *Survey sampling.* New York, John Wiley & Sons, Inc., 1965.

(39) Sadana R. Measurement of variance in health state valuations in Phnom Penh, Cambodia. In: Murray CJL et al., eds. *Summary measures of population health: concepts, ethics, measurement and applications.* Geneva, World Health Organization, 2002:593–618.

(40) Shibuya K. *Quantifying the economic impact and health consequences of disease: implications for the studies on smoking* [Doctoral Thesis]. Boston, Harvard School of Public Health, 1999.

(41) Dolan P, Sutton M. Mapping visual analogue scale health state valuations onto standard gamble and time trade-off values. *Social Science & Medicine,* 1997, 44(10): 1519–1530.

(42) Nord E. The validity of a visual analogue scale in determining social utility weights for health states. *International Journal of Health Planning and Management,* 1991, 6(3):234–242.

(43) Stevens SS. On the psychophysical law. *Psychological Review,* 1957, 64(3):153–181.

(44) Torrance GW. Social preferences for health states: an empirical evaluation of three measurement techniques. *Socio-Economic Planning Sciences,* 1976, 10129–10136.

(45) Johannesson M, Pliskin JS, Weinstein MC. A note on QALYs, time tradeoff, and discounting. *Medical Decision Making,* 1994, 14(2):188–193.

(46) Bell DE, Raiffa H. Marginal value and intrinsic risk aversion. In: Bell DE, Raiffa H, Tversky A, eds. *Decision making: descriptive, normative and prescriptive interactions.* Cambridge, Cambridge University Press, 1998.

(47) Hadorn DC. Setting health care priorities in Oregon. Cost-effectiveness meets the rule of rescue. *The Journal of the American Medical Association,* 1991, 265(17): 2218–2225.

(48) Torrance GW et al. Multi-attribute preference functions. Health Utilities Index. *Pharmacoeconomics,* 1995, 7(6): 503–520.

(49) King G et al. Enhancing the validity and cross-cultural comparability of measurement in survey research. *American Political Science Review,* 2003 (forthcoming).

(50) Brazier J, Rice N, Roberts J. Modelling health state valuation data. In: Murray CJL et al., eds. *Summary measures of population health: concepts, ethics, measurement and applications.* Geneva, World Health Organization, 2002: 529–547.

(51) Dolan P et al. The time trade-off method: results from a general population study. *Health Economics,* 1996, 5(2):141–154.

(52) Patrick DL et al. Measuring preferences for health states worse than death. *Medical Decision Making,* 1994, 14(1):9–18.

(53) Üstün TB et al. Multiple-informant ranking of the disabling effects of different health conditions in 14 countries. WHO/NIH Joint Project CAR Study Group. *The Lancet,* 1999, 354(9173):111–115.

(54) Redelmeier DA, Heller DN. Time preference in medical decision making and cost-effectiveness analysis. *Medical Decision Making,* 1993, 13(3):212–217.

(55) Dolan P, Gudex C. Time preference, duration and health state valuations. *Health Economics,* 1995, 4(4): 289–299.

(56) Ganiats TG et al. Population-based time preferences for future health outcomes. *Medical Decision Making,* 2000, 20(3):263–270.

ANNEX 32.1
HEALTH CONDITIONS AND CARD SETS

Code	Condition label	Set
ALC	Alcohol dependence, marked by excess drinking that cannot be controlled	D
ART	Arthritis, causing major pain, swelling and deformities in hands and wrists	B
BIP	Bipolar disorder, with alternating periods of depression and mania marked by increased energy and activity, sleep loss, extreme talkativeness and irresponsible behaviour	A
BKB	Below the knee amputation in both legs, with no prosthesis but with basic crutches available	A
BKO	Below the knee amputation in one leg, with no prosthesis but with basic crutches available	A
BLD	Total blindness, acquired as an adult	A
CBR	Chronic bronchitis, marked by frequent cough and occasional difficulty breathing	A
DEF	Deafness, acquired as an adult; able to hear shouting at a close distance, but cannot distinguish words or sounds	B
DMT	Dementia, marked by memory loss and difficulties with concentration, language and organization	B
DRU	Drug dependence, marked by excessive and uncontrollable drug use and withdrawal problems upon stopping use	C
FEV	Severe fevered state with continuous hallucinations, as in typhoid fever	D
HEM	Hemiparesis; paralysis of one half of the body, including one arm and one leg, but not affecting sexual function	B
INF	Infertility, in somebody who wants to have a child	C
INS	Insomnia; difficulty falling asleep, waking up earlier than wanted and frequently during the night	A
MAJ	Major depression, with profound sadness, loss of pleasure in activities, slowness and irritability, poor sleep and appetite and suicidal thoughts	C
MBK	Moderate chronic lower back pain, with stiffness in the morning, problems sitting or bending and to a lesser degree, walking; difficulties in all physical activities	D
MDP	Moderate depression, marked by sadness, loss of pleasure in many activities, decreased energy and appetite and some difficulty thinking	A
MDV	Moderate vision problems; cannot distinguish the fingers of a hand across the room and sees poorly after the sun goes down, no glasses available	A
MHE	Mild hearing problems; able to hear and understand loud sounds and speech	B
MOV	Movement disorder with stiffness, trembling and slowness in movements and speech, poor balance and walking problems	D
MVI	Mild vision problems; able to distinguish faces across the room but not across the road, no glasses available	A,B,C,D
PAN	Panic disorder, marked by recurrent and unpredictable attacks of severe anxiety including sweating, tremors, dry mouth, and discomfort in the chest and stomach	C
PAR	Paraplegia, paralysis from the waist down, including loss of sexual function; rudimentary wheelchair available	B
PBH	Paralysis in both hands; unable to move fingers or thumb at all.	C
POH	Paralysis in the one hand that is used most for work, unable to move fingers or thumb	C
PSY	Psychosis, marked by problems in thinking and distortions in reality; individual often hears voices and has strange behaviour and speech	D
QUA	Quadriplegia, paralysis from the neck down, unable to move arms or legs or use hands, but able to breathe independently; basic wheelchair available	A,B,C,D
RVF	Recto-vaginal fistula, abnormal connection between rectum and vagina that allows stool to pass through the vagina, may be a complication of childbirth	C
SBK	Severe chronic lower back pain, making bending and walking painful and strenuous work or exercise impossible	D
TBA	Two broken arms set in stiff casts encasing the elbow and wrist but leaving the fingers free	B
ULC	Pain and burning sensation in stomach, as in peptic ulcer	D
URI	Loss of control over urination	C
VIT	Skin discolorations (vitiligo), covering 10 per cent of the face and visible from a distance	D
WDR	Watery diarrhœa five times per day, without major pain or cramps	B

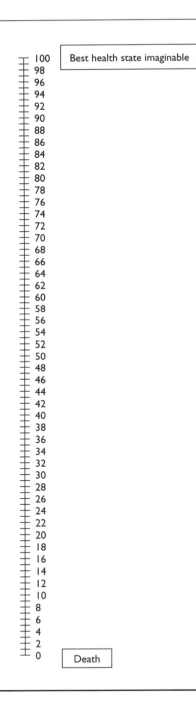

Chapter 33

METHODS FOR MEASURING HEALTHY LIFE EXPECTANCY

COLIN D. MATHERS, CHRISTOPHER J.L. MURRAY, JOSHUA A. SALOMON

INTRODUCTION

In *The World Health Report 2000*, the indicator used to report the average levels of population health for WHO Member States was disability-adjusted life expectancy, or DALE, which measures the equivalent number of years of life expected to be lived in full health (1). Following the feedback from Member States and to better reflect the inclusion of all states of health in the calculation of healthy life expectancy, the name of the indicator used to measure it was changed to health-adjusted life expectancy (HALE). Life expectancy and healthy life expectancy estimates for Member States for the year 2000 were published in *The World Health Report 2001* and *The World Health Report 2002* as part of WHO's regular annual reporting on health in Member States. In addition, healthy life expectancy is the measure used to assess the health system goal to improve average levels of population health in the health systems performance assessment framework (2).

Because substantial resources are devoted to reducing the incidence and the impact on people's lives of conditions that cause ill health but not death, it is important to capture both fatal and non-fatal health outcomes in any measure of population health. For this reason, it is proposed to use healthy life expectancy as a summary measure of the level of population health that captures the full health experience of the population and not just mortality (3). Healthy life expectancy adds up expectation of life for different health states with adjustment for severity distribution and thus is sensitive to changes over time or differences between countries in the severity distribution of health states (4;5). This is an advantage compared to other forms of health expectancy such as disability-free life expectancy (DFLE) which gives zero weight to years lived in less than full health (3).

Health expectancy estimates based on self-reported health status information are not comparable across countries due to differences in survey instruments and cultural variations in reporting of health (6;7). Analyses of over 50 national health surveys for the calculation of healthy life expectancy in *The World Health Report 2000* identified severe limitations in the comparability of self-report health status data from different populations, even when identical survey instruments and methods were used (8). We have demonstrated how these comparability problems relate not only to differences in survey design and methods, but also more fundamentally to unmeasured differences in expectations and norms for health (9). In order to improve the methodological and empirical basis for the measurement of population health, WHO has initiated a data collection strategy with the Member States consisting of household and/or postal or telephone surveys in representative samples of the general populations using a standardized instrument together with new statistical methods for adjusting self-reported health measures to comparable scales (10;11).

In constructing estimates of healthy life expectancy for 191 countries for the year 2000, we sought to address these methodological challenges regarding comparability of health status data across populations and cultures (12). The method involved three inputs. First, life expectancy at each age is calculated in the standard way. Second, estimates of the prevalence of various states of health at each age are required. Finally, a method of weighting time in less than full health relative to full health must be developed.

Because comparable health status prevalence data are not yet available for all countries, a three-stage strategy is proposed to estimate severity-weighted health state prevalences for countries in a way that maximizes cross-country comparability:

■ Firstly, data from the Global Burden of Disease 2000 Study (*13*) will be used to estimate severity-adjusted disability prevalences by age and sex for all 191 countries. Proposed methods are described in the third section of this chapter.

■ Secondly, data on health state prevalences and health state valuations from the World Health Survey will be used to make independent estimates of severity-adjusted disability prevalences by age and sex. Proposed methods are described in section four.

■ Finally, for the survey countries, "posterior" prevalences will be calculated using Bayesian methods and "prior" distributions based on the GBD 2000-based prevalences. The relationship between the GBD 2000-based prevalences and the survey prevalences among the survey countries will then be used to adjust the GBD 2000-based prevalences for the non-survey countries.

Uncertainty intervals for the posterior prevalences will be estimated based on the uncertainty in the survey estimates and the prior distributions.

GLOBAL PATTERNS OF HEALTHY LIFE EXPECTANCY IN 2000

In this section, we give an overview of the estimates of healthy life expectancy for the year 2000 published for WHO Member States in *The World Health Report 2001* (*14*). Methods and data sources used are described by Mathers et al (*12*) and incorporate a number of significant improvements compared to the estimates for 1999 published in *The World Health Report 2000* (*15*). These methods and data sources, together with proposed improvements, are described in sections three to six of this chapter.

HALE FOR WHO REGIONS AND SUBREGIONS IN 2000

We first summarize the results at the regional level. Country-level estimates for mortality and disability were aggregated to estimate life expectancy (LE) and healthy life expectancy (HALE) for each of the six WHO Regions and for the world (Table 33.1). Regional healthy life expectancies at birth in 2000 ranged from a low of 39 years for African males and females to a high of almost 66 years for females in the low mortality countries of Western Europe. Regional healthy life expectancies at age 60 in 2000 ranged from a low of 8.3 years in Africa to a high of around

Table 33.1   Life expectancy (LE), healthy life expectancy (HALE), and lost healthy years as per cent of total LE (LHE%), at birth and at age 60, by sex and total, WHO regions and world, 2000

WHO Region	Persons			Males			Females		
	HALE (years)	LE (years)	LHE% (%)	HALE (years)	LE (years)	LHE% (%)	HALE (years)	LE (years)	LHE% (%)
At birth									
AFRO	38.8	47.3	18.0	39.1	46.4	15.8	38.5	48.2	20.2
AMRO	63.2	73.0	13.4	61.3	69.8	12.2	65.1	76.2	14.5
EMRO	51.2	62.4	17.9	52.0	61.3	15.2	50.4	63.5	20.6
EURO	62.9	71.9	12.6	59.9	67.9	11.7	65.8	76.0	13.4
SEARO	52.7	61.9	15.0	52.6	60.4	12.8	52.7	63.5	17.0
WPRO	63.0	71.6	12.0	61.4	69.2	11.2	64.6	74.0	12.7
World	56.0	65.0	13.8	54.9	62.7	12.5	57.0	67.2	15.1
At age 60									
AFRO	8.3	14.8	43.9	8.3	13.8	40.2	8.3	15.8	47.3
AMRO	15.0	20.5	27.0	13.9	18.7	25.8	16.0	22.3	28.0
EMRO	9.8	16.5	40.9	9.9	15.6	36.7	9.7	17.5	44.7
EURO	14.2	19.2	26.2	12.7	17.1	25.5	15.6	21.3	26.7
SEARO	10.7	16.3	34.3	10.2	14.9	31.6	11.2	17.7	36.6
WPRO	14.1	19.3	26.8	12.7	17.3	26.7	15.6	21.3	26.9
World	13.0	18.4	29.4	11.9	16.7	28.3	14.1	20.2	30.3

16 years for females in Europe, North America, and the Western Pacific.

Overall, global healthy life expectancy at birth in 2000 for males and females combined is 56.0 years, 9.0 years lower than total life expectancy at birth. Global HALE at birth for females is just over 2 years greater than that for males (Table 33.1). In comparison, total life expectancy at birth is almost 4 years higher for females than for males. The difference between HALE and total life expectancy is LHE ("lost" healthy life expectancy). The equivalent "lost" healthy years range from 20% (of total life expectancy at birth) in Africa to 11–12% in the European and the Western Pacific regions. The equivalent "lost" healthy years at age 60 are a higher percentage of the remaining life expectancy, due to the higher prevalence of disability at older ages. These range from around 40–50% in sub-Saharan Africa to around 25% in developed countries.

When HALE is calculated for the 17 epidemiological subregions of the world,[1] the range is even greater (Table 33.2). Subregional healthy life expectancies at birth in 2000 ranged from a low of 36 years for the very high mortality subregion of Africa to a high of 76 years for females in the low mortality countries of the Western Pacific region (these include Japan, Australia, New Zealand, and Singapore). The very low health expectancies of the African countries in both subregions D and E reflect the high burden of HIV/AIDS, tuberculosis, malaria, other communicable, maternal, perinatal and nutritional conditions, and injuries.

Despite the fact that people live longer in the richer, more developed countries, and have greater opportunity to acquire non-fatal disabilities in older age, disability has a greater absolute (and relative) impact on healthy life expectancy in poorer countries. Separating life expectancy into equivalent years of good health and years lost to sub-optimal health thus widens rather than narrows the difference in health status between the rich and the poor countries.

The relative contributions of diseases and injuries to variations in HALE are best summarized in terms of the loss of healthy life measured in DALYs. *The World Health Report 2001* provides detailed estimates of DALYs for over 100 disease and injury categories for the 14 mortality subregions, and contains tables of the leading causes of DALYs worldwide and by region. While the rankings are broadly similar for the two sexes, there are important differences. Thus, while lower respiratory infections, perinatal conditions, and HIV/AIDS are the three leading causes of DALYs, their relative significance differs slightly for

males and females. More importantly, depression is the fourth leading cause of disease burden for females but ranks seventh for males. Maternal conditions constitute the seventh leading cause for females, accounting for almost 4% of their global disease burden in 2000. Road traffic accidents are a leading cause of overall disease and injury burden for males (3.1%) but not for females (1.3%).

HALE ESTIMATES FOR WHO MEMBER STATES, 2000

The annex table of this chapter gives estimates of life expectancy and healthy life expectancy at birth together with 95% uncertainty intervals for 191 WHO Member States. Annex Table 4 of *The World Health Report 2001* also presents healthy life expectancy at age 60.

Japanese women lead the world with an estimated average healthy life expectancy of 76.3 years at birth in the year 2000, which is 8.4 years lower than total life expectancy at birth. HALE at birth for Japanese males is 5.1 years lower than that for females at 71.2 years. This is a narrower gap than that for total life expectancy at birth of 7.2 years. After Japan, in second to sixth places, are Switzerland, San Marino, Andorra, Monaco, and Australia with healthy life expectancies at birth (males and females combined) in the range 71.5 to 72.1 years, followed by a number of other industrialized countries of Western Europe. It should be noted, however, that there is a considerable range of uncertainty in the ranks for countries other than Japan, with typical 95% uncertainty ranges of around 3 years for developed countries. Canada is in the 17th place (70.0 years) and the United States of America in the 28th place (67.2 years).

Other countries with reasonably high healthy life expectancies in the Americas include Chile (65.5 years), Costa Rica (65.3 years), Dominica (64.6 years), Mexico (64.2 years), and Uruguay (64.1 years). Brazil is split, with a high healthy life expectancy in its southern half and a lower one in the north. The total average is a relatively low 57.1 years, with 54.9 for males and 59.2 for females.

China has a healthy life expectancy above the global average, at 62.1 years, 63.3 years for women and 60.9 for men. Other countries in the Asian region generally have lower HALE. Improving health in Viet Nam has resulted in a healthy life expectancy of 58.9 years. Simultaneously, Thailand has not improved significantly over the past decade, though it is still ahead of Viet Nam, at 59.7 years. Healthy life expectancy in

Table 33.2   Life expectancy (LE), healthy life expectancy (HALE), and lost healthy years (LHE) as per cent of total LE (HLE%), at birth and at age 60, by sex and total, by mortality subregion, 2000

WHO Region	Persons			Males			Females		
	HALE (years)	LE (years)	LHE% (%)	HALE (years)	LE (years)	LHE% (%)	HALE (years)	LE (years)	LHE% (%)
At birth									
AFRO D	42.1	51.6	18.5	42.4	50.5	16.2	41.8	52.7	20.6
AFRO E	36.5	44.4	17.8	36.7	43.5	15.6	36.2	45.2	19.9
AMRO A	68.0	77.2	11.8	66.3	74.4	10.9	69.7	79.9	12.8
AMRO B	60.7	71.1	14.7	58.6	67.6	13.2	62.7	74.6	15.9
AMRO D	55.4	65.9	16.0	54.2	63.5	14.6	56.6	68.4	17.3
EMRO B	59.5	69.9	15.0	59.3	68.4	13.3	59.6	71.4	16.5
EMRO D	52.8	65.7	19.5	53.5	63.8	16.3	52.2	67.5	22.6
EURO A	70.2	78.0	10.0	68.2	74.8	8.9	72.2	81.2	11.1
EURO B1	60.5	70.3	14.0	58.4	66.9	12.8	62.6	73.7	15.1
EURO B2	54.3	64.7	16.1	52.5	61.6	14.8	56.0	67.8	17.3
EURO C	56.0	66.2	15.4	51.1	60.3	15.2	61.0	72.1	15.5
SEARO B	58.7	67.1	12.6	57.2	64.6	11.3	60.1	69.7	13.8
SEARO D	51.1	60.5	15.6	51.5	59.3	13.2	50.7	61.7	17.8
WPRO A	73.5	80.8	9.1	70.9	77.4	8.3	76.1	84.3	9.7
WPRO B1	62.2	70.9	12.2	60.9	68.8	11.5	63.6	73.0	13.0
WPRO B2	53.7	62.1	13.4	52.4	59.6	12.1	55.0	64.5	14.6
WPRO B3	50.1	59.5	15.8	49.6	58.0	14.4	50.5	60.9	17.1
World	56.0	65.0	13.8	54.9	62.7	12.5	57.0	67.2	15.1
At age 60									
AFRO D	8.4	15.1	44.3	8.5	14.2	40.2	8.3	16.0	47.9
AFRO E	8.2	14.5	43.6	8.1	13.5	40.1	8.3	15.6	46.7
AMRO A	16.4	21.6	23.8	15.3	19.8	22.6	17.6	23.4	24.9
AMRO B	13.4	19.3	30.8	12.4	17.6	29.6	14.3	21.0	31.8
AMRO D	11.9	18.0	33.9	11.3	16.8	32.4	12.5	19.3	35.2
EMRO B	11.5	17.6	34.8	11.1	16.7	33.1	11.8	18.5	36.3
EMRO D	9.3	16.4	43.4	9.5	15.4	38.2	9.1	17.5	47.9
EURO A	17.0	21.6	21.2	15.6	19.4	19.4	18.4	23.8	22.6
EURO B1	12.8	18.1	29.1	11.6	16.3	28.6	14.0	19.9	29.5
EURO B2	11.1	16.7	33.5	10.1	15.3	33.9	12.1	18.1	33.1
EURO C	10.6	16.1	34.5	8.5	13.7	37.5	12.6	18.6	32.2
SEARO B	12.6	17.4	27.6	12.0	16.3	26.2	13.2	18.6	28.7
SEARO D	10.3	16.1	36.0	9.9	14.7	32.9	10.7	17.5	38.7
WPRO A	19.6	23.9	17.9	17.6	21.2	17.0	21.6	26.5	18.6
WPRO B1	13.2	18.5	28.7	11.9	16.6	28.7	14.5	20.4	28.7
WPRO B2	11.4	16.5	31.1	10.8	15.4	30.0	12.0	17.6	32.0
WPRO B3	10.6	16.5	35.5	9.9	15.2	34.8	11.3	17.7	36.2
World	13.0	18.4	29.4	11.9	16.7	28.3	14.1	20.2	30.3

Myanmar is just 49.1 years, substantially behind its south-east Asian neighbours.

In Russia, healthy life expectancy is 60.6 for females, which is 5 years below the European average, but just 50.3 years for males, 9.6 years below the European average. This is one of the widest sex gaps in the world and reflects the sharp increase in adult male mortality in the early 1990s. The most common explanation is the high incidence of male alcohol abuse, which led to high rates of accidents, violence, and cardiovascular disease. From 1987 to 1994, the risk of premature death increased by 70% for Russian males. Between 1994 and 1998, life expectancy improved for males, but has declined significantly again in the last three years. Similar rates exist for other countries of the former Soviet Union.

The bottom 10 countries for HALE are all in sub-Saharan Africa, where the HIV/AIDS epidemic is rampant. The lowest health expectancy in 2000 was estimated at 29.5 years in Sierra Leone. Life expectancy in several countries in southern Africa has been reduced 15–20 years in comparison to life expectancy without HIV. Other African countries have lost 5–10 years of life expectancy because of HIV (16). AIDS is now the leading cause of death in sub-Saharan Africa, far surpassing the traditional deadly diseases of malaria, tuberculosis, pneumonia, and diarrhœal disease. AIDS killed 2.2 million Africans in 2000, versus 300 000 AIDS deaths 10 years ago.

The worldwide pattern of health expectancies at birth in 2000 is shown in Figure 33.1, highlighting the enormous variation between developing and developed countries, as well as between the lower and higher mortality regions of Europe. Figure 33.2 shows the distribution of healthy life expectancy at age 60 in 2000. Both figures show average HALE for males and females combined.

Figure 33.3 shows average HALE at birth versus total life expectancy at birth for 191 countries. While lower life expectancies are generally associated with lower healthy life expectancy—the two indicators are correlated—there are large variations in healthy life expectancy for any given level of life expectancy. For example, for countries with a life expectancy of 70, healthy life expectancy varies from 57 to 61.5. If male and female HALE are considered separately, the range of variation increases to 57 to 65 at total life expectancy of 70.

Figure 33.4 shows the relationship between healthy life expectancy at birth for males and females for the Member States. In the countries with HALE at birth of 45 years or lower, male and female HALE are about the same. These countries are almost entirely in Africa, but include the Lao People's Republic, Haiti, and Nepal as well. In a number of countries with HALE around 50 years, female HALE at birth is actually lower than male HALE. These countries are mostly in Africa and the Eastern Mediterranean region, but also include Afghanistan, Pakistan, and Bangladesh. For other countries with HALE at birth greater than 50 years, female HALE is generally higher than male HALE, though the gap is lower than the one for total life expectancy. In many countries of Eastern Europe, female HALE at birth is substantially higher than male, reflecting very high levels of adult mortality in men in the 1990s. Similar patterns are apparent for the male-female gap in healthy life expectancy at age 60, although the male-female reversal in the Eastern Mediterranean countries no longer occurs. Figure 33.5

Figure 33.1 Average HALE at birth (males and females combined), 191 Member States, 2000

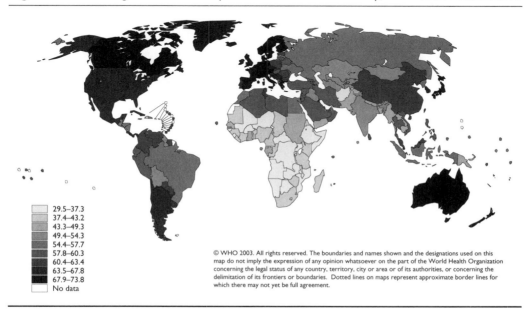

	29.5–37.3
	37.4–43.2
	43.3–49.3
	49.4–54.3
	54.4–57.7
	57.8–60.3
	60.4–63.4
	63.5–67.8
	67.9–73.8
	No data

Figure 33.2 Average HALE at birth (males and females combined), 191 Member States, 2000

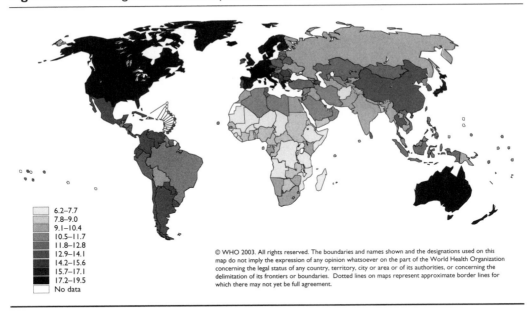

6.2–7.7
7.8–9.0
9.1–10.4
10.5–11.7
11.8–12.8
12.9–14.1
14.2–15.6
15.7–17.1
17.2–19.5
No data

Figure 33.3 Healthy life expectancy at birth versus total life expectancy at birth, by sex, WHO Member States, 2000

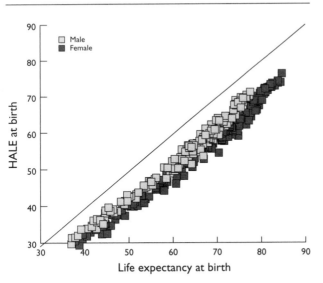

Figure 33.4 Healthy life expectancy at birth: males versus females, WHO Member States, 2000

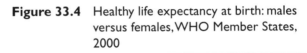
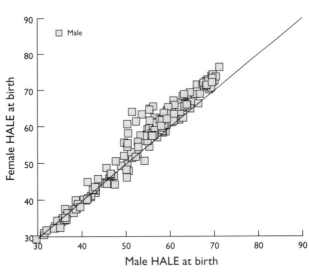

shows the worldwide patterns of female-male differences in healthy life expectancy at birth.

METHODS FOR CONSTRUCTING LIFE TABLES

As a first step towards the estimation of HALE, it is crucial to develop for each WHO Member State the

best possible assessment of overall mortality levels by age and sex for the year 2001 in order to construct a period life table. Since the publication *of The World Health Report 2000*, there has been intensive contact between WHO and Member States in an effort to verify the best sources of recent data on vital registration and cause of death, and new life tables for the year 2000 have been constructed for all 191 WHO Member States (*17*). Complete or incomplete vital

Figure 33.5 Female-male difference in HALE at birth, 191 Member States, 2000

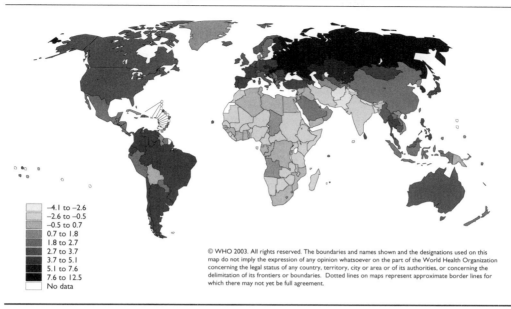

-4.1 to -2.6
-2.6 to -0.5
-0.5 to 0.7
0.7 to 1.8
1.8 to 2.7
2.7 to 3.7
3.7 to 5.1
5.1 to 7.6
7.6 to 12.5
No data

registration data together with sample registration systems cover 76% of global mortality. Survey data and indirect demographic techniques provide information on levels of child and adult mortality for the remaining 24% of estimated global mortality. Details of the methods and data sources used to estimate all cause mortality for WHO Member States are given elsewhere (18;19).

For countries in each of the categories described above, there are several sources of uncertainty that will result in uncertainty around the final life tables. The general approach for describing and estimating uncertainty is described in Salomon et al. (20). For those countries with vital registration data projected using time series regression models on the parameters of the logit life table system, uncertainty around the regression coefficients will be accounted for by taking 1 000 draws of the parameters using the regression estimates and variance covariance matrix. For each of the draws, a new life table will be calculated. For countries that do not have time series data on mortality by age and sex, point estimates and ranges around $_5q_0$ and $_{45}q_{15}$ for males and females will be developed on a country-by-country basis as described in Lopez et al. (18). Monte Carlo simulation will be used with the modified logit life table system described by Murray and colleagues (19), to generate 1 000 random life tables, which will then be used to describe ranges around key indicators such as life expectancy at birth.

There have been substantial improvements in the estimates of life expectancies for WHO Member States for *The World Health Report 2002*, compared to those estimated for 1999 for *The World Health Report 2000*. This results from substantial new and more recent data on mortality rates provided by Member States, and improvements in the model life table system used for Member States with limited data.

METHODS FOR ESTIMATING GBD-BASED PRIORS

REGIONAL HEALTH STATE PREVALENCE ESTIMATES

Burden of disease analysis uses a disease-specific approach to estimate the disability and loss of healthy years of life associated with an exhaustive set of health conditions. In particular, DALYs are calculated as the sum of years of life lost due to mortality (YLL) and years lived with disability (YLD). YLD for a particular health condition (disease or injury) are calculated by estimating the number of new cases (incidence) of the condition occurring in the time period of interest. For each new case, the number of years of healthy life lost is obtained by multiplying the average duration of the condition (from onset to remission or death) by a severity weight that quantifies the equivalent loss of healthy years of life due to living with the health condition (*21*).

The Global Burden of Disease 2000 project is estimating YLD for a comprehensive set of 135 disease and injury categories involving analysis of many more disease stages, severity levels, and sequelae (*13*). These estimates are made by age and sex and for the 17 epidemiological subregions. While Global Burden of Disease 2000 results are reported for the 14 mortality subregions described above, YLDs are estimated for the 17 epidemiological subregions, chosen to maximize epidemiological homogeneity (*13*).

For some conditions, numbers of incident cases are available directly from disease registers or epidemiological studies, but for most conditions only prevalence data are available. In these cases, a software program called DISMOD⌷ is used to model incidence and duration from estimates of prevalence, remission, case fatality, and background mortality. Many different sources of information are used to calculate YLD. An iterative process and extensive consultation with relevant experts are required to ensure consistency of epidemiological estimates. For *The World Health Report 2000*, burden of disease estimates were updated for many of the cause categories based on the wealth of data available on major diseases and injuries available to WHO technical programmes through collaboration with Member States and scientists worldwide. Examples are the extensive datasets on tuberculosis, maternal conditions, injuries, diabetes, cancer, and sexually transmitted infections. This process of updating Global Burden of Disease 2000 estimates will continue and contribute to the improvement of the analytic base for estimation of GBD prior prevalences. Further details of Global Burden of Disease 2000 data and methods are given by Murray et al. (*13*). In particular, the ongoing analysis of cause of death and epidemiological data have been used to estimate mortality, incidence and prevalence, and YLD for the Global Burden of Disease 2000 regions for the year 2001.

As part of the Global Burden of Disease 2000 project, undiscounted and non-age-weighted prevalence YLD have been estimated directly from prevalence estimates for each cause sequela by age and sex as follows:

$$YLD_c^{Prev} = Prev_c DW_c \qquad [1]$$

where $Prev_c$ is the point prevalence of cases, and DW_c is the disability weight (in the range 0–1).

In order to estimate disability prevalence at the population level, it is also necessary to estimate the YLD associated with residual categories of disease and injury such as "other chronic respiratory diseases" or "other malignant neoplasms." We follow the procedure developed by the Global Burden of Disease 1990 (*22*) to estimate YLD for all of these residual categories. Further attention will be paid to refining these estimates and assessing the uncertainty around them.

Summation of prevalence YLD over all causes would result in overestimation of disability prevalence because of comorbidity between conditions. We correct for comorbidity between major cause groups as described below to obtain estimates of all-cause YLD by age and sex for each WHO subregion.

This burden-of-disease-based approach to the calculation of HALE has a number of advantages over the health survey approach:

■ It guarantees consistency with the health gap measure (DALYs) of the burden of disease.

■ It ensures inclusion of all causes of disability (also those resulting in forms of disability poorly reported in health surveys, e.g. substance abuse, intellectual disability).

■ It avoids problems of self-report biases.

However, there are currently two major limitations with this approach:

■ Problems with comorbidities, and

■ The data demands for calculating YLD for a comprehensive set of conditions.

Comorbidity refers to the not uncommon situation where a person has two or more health problems that result in disability (either dependently or independently of each other). It makes little sense simply to add the independently determined disability weights for conditions that are found to coexist as this can lead to the illogical possibility of having a combined weight of more than one (i.e. more disabling than death), particularly in the case of two heavily weighted conditions. Both the Global Burden of Disease 1990 and the Australian Burden of Disease Study made adjustments for comorbidity assuming that conditions occurred independently (i.e. the probability of having two conditions was the product of the average probabilities for having each condition) and adjusted the disability weights for comorbid conditions assuming a multiplicative model. A similar approach is used here, but some dependent comorbidity is also taken into account, as described below in the section on country-specific estimates of health state prevalences.

Figure 33.6 compares the overall age-sex specific prevalence YLD rates (adjusted for comorbidity) for the six WHO regions based on Global Burden of Disease 2000 Version 1 estimates for the year 2000. Table 33.3 gives age-sex specific prevalence YLD rates for the 17 epidemiological subregions for the year 2000.

There have been substantial improvements in the Global Burden of Disease 2000 estimates, compared to those used for *The World Health Report 2000*. Global Burden of Disease 2000 Version 2 results were used in the construction of Global Burden of Disease prior estimates for *The World Health Report 2002* and include much additional data. In 2003, particular effort is being put into improving the assessments of chronic respiratory diseases, cardiovascular diseases, injuries, perinatal and maternal causes, selected infectious diseases, and nutritional deficiencies.

COUNTRY-SPECIFIC CAUSE OF DEATH ESTIMATES

Causes of death for the 17 subregions and the world have been estimated based on data from national vital registration systems that capture about 17 million deaths annually. In addition, information from sample registration systems, population laboratories, and epidemiological analyses of specific conditions has been used to improve estimates of the cause of death patterns (*16;23–25*). WHO is intensifying efforts with Member States to obtain and verify recent vital registration data on causes of death.

Cause of death data are carefully analysed to take into account incomplete coverage of vital registration in countries and the likely differences in cause of death patterns that would be expected in the uncovered and often poorer subpopulations. Techniques to undertake this analysis have been developed based on the Global Burden of Disease Study (*22*), and further refined using a much more extensive database and more robust modelling techniques (*26*).

Special attention has been paid to problems of misattribution or miscoding of causes of death in cardiovascular diseases, cancer, injuries, and general ill-defined categories. A correction algorithm for reclassifying ill-defined cardiovascular codes has been developed (*23*). Cancer mortality by site has been evaluated using both vital registration data and population based cancer incidence registries. The latter have been

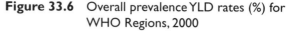

Figure 33.6 Overall prevalence YLD rates (%) for WHO Regions, 2000

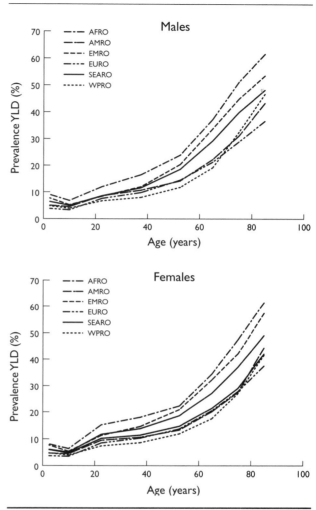

analysed using a complete age-period-cohort model of cancer survival in each region (*24;25*).

As a general rule, vital registration data, suitably corrected for ill-defined coding and probable systematic biases in certifying deaths to non-specific vascular, cancer, and injury codes are used to estimate the cause of death pattern. Such vital registration data were available for about 65 countries. In a further 20 countries or so, cause of death models are used to correct vital registration data by age and sex to yield more plausible patterns across Groups I, II, and III. The distribution of specific causes within groups is then based on the recorded cause of death patterns from vital registration data. The resulting estimates are systematically corrected on the basis of other epidemiological evidence from registries, community studies, and disease surveillance systems.

Table 33.3 Overall prevalence YLD rates (%) for WHO epidemiological subregions for the year 2000

Sex	Subregion	Age group (years)								
		0–4	5–14	15–29	30–44	45–59	60–69	70–79	80–89	Age-std[a]
Males										
	AFRO D	9.0	6.6	11.0	15.0	23.9	37.7	50.6	60.0	15.4
	AFRO E	9.0	6.9	12.8	17.7	23.9	36.9	51.7	63.4	16.5
	AMRO A	2.3	2.8	8.0	8.8	10.3	16.8	26.7	40.5	8.1
	AMRO B	6.1	5.3	8.9	12.0	18.1	28.2	37.4	49.1	11.9
	AMRO D	6.0	5.4	9.3	13.0	19.9	29.3	39.2	49.9	12.6
	EMRO B	5.4	3.8	6.5	9.8	16.5	30.3	40.9	46.7	10.4
	EMRO D	8.4	5.7	9.2	13.0	22.3	35.3	46.6	56.4	13.7
	EURO A	2.0	2.3	6.1	7.4	9.0	13.8	23.1	33.4	6.7
	EURO B1	4.5	3.5	6.7	9.2	13.5	19.2	25.5	35.6	8.7
	EURO B2	7.8	5.3	8.9	12.3	22.5	31.1	41.6	52.6	13.0
	EURO C	4.7	3.8	9.2	12.8	18.7	24.2	32.8	44.9	11.4
	SEARO B	6.0	4.5	7.7	10.2	17.2	26.9	38.6	52.8	10.9
	SEARO D	6.5	5.0	8.8	11.9	19.0	29.9	40.2	47.2	12.1
	WPRO A	2.8	2.9	5.2	6.6	7.8	12.0	18.7	30.3	6.0
	WPRO B1	4.7	3.9	6.7	7.8	11.9	20.0	35.5	52.7	8.7
	WPRO B2	5.5	4.4	7.6	9.9	16.1	25.5	38.1	53.9	10.5
	WPRO B3	6.0	4.6	8.4	12.5	22.6	34.1	41.7	45.1	12.7
	World	6.3	4.7	8.3	10.4	15.1	23.2	33.4	44.0	10.5
Females										
	AFRO D	8.2	6.2	13.9	16.6	22.3	35.1	48.0	61.4	16.8
	AFRO E	8.0	6.5	16.2	19.2	22.3	34.0	47.2	61.3	17.7
	AMRO A	2.2	2.8	8.4	8.6	10.7	16.2	24.5	43.7	8.7
	AMRO B	5.7	5.1	9.8	11.9	15.7	23.9	32.1	46.0	11.9
	AMRO D	5.7	5.3	10.6	13.1	17.5	25.8	34.7	48.3	12.9
	EMRO B	5.5	3.9	8.5	11.5	16.8	27.6	35.3	48.0	11.8
	EMRO D	8.4	6.0	12.6	15.9	22.6	34.0	44.8	61.6	16.1
	EURO A	1.9	2.4	6.9	7.7	9.2	14.2	22.4	36.1	7.4
	EURO B1	4.3	3.8	9.4	10.8	13.4	18.2	23.6	36.5	10.0
	EURO B2	7.7	5.4	11.2	13.2	19.0	25.5	32.3	44.0	13.3
	EURO C	4.4	3.9	8.8	10.9	13.8	18.7	24.4	36.9	10.0
	SEARO B	5.6	4.5	9.9	11.1	15.4	23.5	32.6	45.4	11.6
	SEARO D	6.3	5.2	12.2	14.5	19.4	28.3	38.2	50.0	14.1
	WPRO A	2.5	2.9	6.1	6.8	7.9	11.6	17.4	32.7	6.6
	WPRO B1	4.8	4.0	7.2	8.4	12.3	18.2	29.3	45.1	9.4
	WPRO B2	5.4	4.4	9.6	10.9	14.7	22.9	33.1	48.4	11.4
	WPRO B3	5.8	4.8	10.7	13.5	19.4	28.8	35.1	41.9	13.2
	World	6.0	4.8	10.2	11.4	14.7	21.4	29.1	42.1	11.4

a. Total rate age-standardized to World Standard Population

For China and India, cause patterns of mortality are based on existing mortality registration systems, namely the Disease Surveillance Points System (DSP) and the Vital Registration System of the Ministry of Health in China, the Medical Certificate of Cause of Death (MCCD) for urban India and the Annual Survey of Causes of Death (SCD) for rural areas of India.

For all other countries lacking vital registration data, cause of death models are used first to estimate the distribution of deaths across the broad categories of communicable, non-communicable diseases and injuries, based on estimated total mortality rates and income, and using regional standards of deviation from the cause of death distribution predicted solely from total mortality and income (*26*). A regional model pattern of specific causes of death is then constructed based on local vital registration and verbal autopsy data, and this proportionate distribution is applied within each broad cause group. Finally, the resulting estimates are adjusted based on other epidemiological evidence from specific disease studies.

Global Burden of Disease 2000 Version 1 estimates of death by cause, age, and sex for the 14 mortality subregions are summarized in *The World Health Report 2001* Annex Table 3 and in Murray et al. (*13*).

There have been substantial improvements in the Global Burden of Disease 2000 cause of death estimates for WHO Member States, compared to those used for *The World Health Report 2000*. Most recent data from Member States are used, together with specific analyses of mortality due to certain causes, to improve the accuracy of cause of death estimates.

COUNTRY-SPECIFIC ESTIMATES OF HEALTH STATE PREVALENCES

Where feasible, country-specific prevalence YLD estimates are being made for a number of causes. For the estimates for 2000, these included childhood vaccine preventable diseases, malnutrition, HIV/AIDS, cancers, and diabetes. For other causes, regional YLD estimates are being used, together with country-specific and regional cause of death information, to develop country-specific estimates of severity-weighted prevalence YLD by age and sex. The five methods used are described below. The causes for which each method was used for the year 2000 estimates are listed in Table 33.4. The average per cent of total prevalence YLD (all cause) estimated using each of these methods is shown by region in Table 33.5 for the year 2000 results. For HALE estimates for *The World Health Report 2002* (*27*), a similar strategy has been followed.

Country-specific Prevalence Data

For the causes listed in the first column of Table 33.4, prevalence YLD estimates are being made directly for Member States using available data on the prevalence of each condition. For the Group I conditions, databases of country-level studies developed by WHO programmes and UNAIDS can be used to estimate country-level prevalences. Methods used to estimate the prevalence of malignant neoplasms at the country level, based on national incidence, mortality and survival data, are described by Mathers et al. (*24*). Diabetes prevalence is based on updated country-level prevalence estimates prepared by the WHO Management of Non-communicable Diseases and Mental Health Programme (NMH) according to the revised WHO definition of diabetes cases (this updates previous work published by King et al. (*28*)). Variations in the prevalence of unipolar depressive disorders in some European countries, Australia, New Zealand, and Japan have been estimated directly from relevant population studies for the Global Burden of Disease 2000. For other countries in the A (lowest mortality) regions, country-specific prevalences P_c for males and females aged 15–59 have been estimated using a regression model on suicide rates as follows:

$$P_c = P_R + 0.0919(S_c - S_R) \qquad [2]$$

where P_R is the regional depression prevalence, S_c and S_R are the country and regional suicide rates (ages 15–59 both sexes combined). For other regions, it was assumed that the variation of depression prevalence with suicide rate was half that of A countries, and the range of variation was restricted from a minimum of one half the regional average to a maximum of twice the regional average.

YLD/YLL Ratios—Short Duration Causes

For specific disease and injury causes where mortality is responsible for a significant proportion of the total burden (incidence YLD/YLL ratio less than 5), regional estimates of incidence YLD/YLL ratios by age and sex together with country-level estimates of YLL are used to estimate country-level YLD. This process ensures that country-specific knowledge on the epidemiology of the disease (as reflected in the country-level mortality estimates of that disease) is used to adjust the regional-level patterns of disability due to that cause.

For causes where the sequelae causing most YLD are of short duration (i.e. less than around 10-15 years), prevalence YLD are approximately equal to undiscounted, non-age-weighted incidence YLD within the age bands used in the Global Burden of Disease 2000. For these causes, country-level prevalence YLD are estimated within each age-sex group *a,s* as follows:

$$PREVYLD_{c,a,s} = PREVYLD_{R,a,s} \left(\frac{YLL[0,0]_{c,a,s}}{YLL[0,0]_{R,a,s}} \right) \quad [3]$$

YLD/YLL Ratios—Long Duration Causes

For causes where the sequelae causing most YLD are of longer duration (as is typical for injuries), prevalence

Table 33.4　Cause-specific methods used for estimation of country-level prevalence YLD

Country-specific prevalence data	Inc. YLD/YLL ratios short duration causes	Inc. YLD/YLL ratios long duration causes	Prevalence YLD regression models	Regional prevalence YLD rates
Pertussis	Tuberculosis	Endocrine disorders	Maternal conditions	STDs excluding HIV
Diphtheria	HIV/AIDS	Other respiratory diseases	Perinatal conditions	Poliomyelitis
Measles	Hepatitis B	Other digestive diseases	Unipolar depressive disorders*	Trypanosomiasis
Tetanus	Hepatitis C	Other genitourinary system diseases	Parkinson disease	Chagas disease
Meningitis	Malaria	Road traffic accidents	Ischæmic heart disease	Schistosomiasis
Onchocerciasis	Lower respiratory infections	Poisonings	Cerebrovascular disease	Leishmaniasis
Trachoma	Rheumatic heart disease	Falls	COPD	Lymphatic filariasis
PE Malnutrition	Hypertensive heart disease	Fires	Congenital anomalies	Leprosy
Iodine deficiency	Inflammatory heart disease	Other unintentional injuries		Dengue
Malignant neoplasms	Other cardioavscular	Self-inflicted injuries		Japanese encephalitis
Diabetes mellitus	Peptic ulcer disease	Violence		Intestinal nematode infections
Unipolar depressive disorders*	Cirrhosis of the liver	War		Upper respiratory infections
Alcohol use disorders	Appendicitis	Other intentional injuries		Otitis media
Drug use disorders	Nephritis and nephrosis			Iron-deficiency anaemia
Asthma				Other nutritional causes
				Other neoplasms
				Bipolar disorder
				Schizophrenia
				Epilepsy
				Alzheimer/dementias
				Multiple sclerosis
				PTSD
				Obsessive-compulsive disorder
				Panic disorder
				Insomnia (primary)
				Migraine
				Other neuropsychiatric
				Sense organ diseases
				Benign prostatic hypertrophy
				Skin diseases
				Musculoskeletal diseases
				Oral conditions
				Drownings

Some country data plus regression model based on suicide rates

YLD at a given age derive from incident YLD at that age and at earlier ages. For these causes, country-level prevalence YLD are estimated using a life table method from the undiscounted, non-age-weighted incidence YLD at previous ages, calculated as follows:

$$YLD[0,0]_{c,a,s} = YLD[0,0]_{R,a,s} \left(\frac{YLL[0,0]_{c,a,s}}{YLL[0,0]_{R,a,s}} \right) \quad [4]$$

Prevalence YLD Regression Models

For certain causes, regression models have been developed for prevalence YLD on cause-specific mortality and selected other variables using the dataset provided by estimates for the 17 epidemiological regions of the Global Burden of Disease 2000.

For perinatal causes, regression based on a selected set of developing regions gave a slope of 0.7 PREVYLD per 100 000 against perinatal mortality per 100 000

Table 33.5 Average per cent of total prevalence YLD estimated by every method, for WHO Member States within each epidemiological subregion, GBD 2000 Version I

Subregion	Cause-specific method used for estimation of country-level prevalence YLD				
	Country-specific prevalence data	Incidence YLD/YLL ratios	Prevalence YLD regression models	Regional prevalence YLD rates	All methods
AFRO D	10	52	6	32	100
AFRO E	9	56	6	29	100
AMRO A	18	23	15	44	100
AMRO B	11	39	14	37	100
AMRO D	11	42	10	37	100
EMRO B	8	49	10	33	100
EMRO D	8	49	9	34	100
EURO A	14	20	20	46	100
EURO B1	7	36	18	39	100
EURO B2	5	49	13	33	100
EURO C	12	36	16	36	100
SEARO B	8	40	13	40	100
SEARO D	7	42	14	36	100
WPRO A	16	24	16	43	100
WPRO B1	7	35	23	35	100
WPRO B2	8	39	16	37	100
WPRO B3	6	46	10	38	100

for 0–4 year-olds. To avoid problems resulting from statistical fluctuations in countries with small numbers of perinatal deaths, the perinatal mortality rate for each country is adjusted to the 80% confidence limit (upper or lower) closest to the regional perinatal mortality rate before applying this regression relationship and the final country/regional PREVYLD ratio not allowed to exceed the range (1/3,3). This ratio is be applied to regional perinatal prevalence YLD rates for each age group to estimate the country YLD rates.

For maternal causes, a similar regression procedure gave slopes of 61 and 4.41 PREVYLD per 100 000 for developed and developing regions, respectively, against maternal mortality per 100 000 for 15–44 year old women. To avoid problems resulting from statistical fluctuations in countries with small numbers of maternal deaths, the maternal mortality rate for each country is adjusted to the 80% confidence limit (upper or lower) closest to the regional maternal mortality rate before applying the regression relationship and the final country/regional PREVYLD ratio capped in the range (1/3,3). This ratio is then applied to regional maternal prevalence YLD rates for each age group to estimate the country YLD rates.

For Parkinson disease, ischæmic heart disease, cerebrovascular disease, and chronic obstructive pulmonary disease (COPD), regression models have been fitted for prevalence YLD at a given age, including in the models those variables which are significant out of the following set: age-sex specific mortality rates for the cause at that age and all earlier ages, all-cause mortality for that age and for earlier ages, life expectancy at various ages.

Regional Prevalence YLD Rates

For specific disease and injury causes where mortality is not responsible for a significant proportion of the total burden (incidence YLD/YLL ratio is 5 or higher), or where there is insufficient evidence to predict variations in YLD rates from variations in mortality rates, regional estimates of YLD rates per 1 000 population by age and sex are used together with country-level population distribution estimates to estimate prevalence YLD for each country. Work continues on refining these regional estimates in the Global Burden of Disease 2000 and in analysis of uncertainty in the estimates (see below).

Methods for the estimation of country-level prevalence YLD for specific causes are now based on considerably more country-level prevalence data, and on improved methods for the direct estimation of prevalence YLD compared to the methods based on incidence YLD rates and ratios used for the estimation of DALE for 1999 in *The World Health Report 2000* (29).

Adjustment for Comorbidity

The total prevalent YLD per 100 population can be thought of as a severity-weighted disability prevalence measured as a percentage of the population of that age. However, summation over all conditions of the prevalence YLD for a Member State would result in overestimation of disability prevalence because of comorbidity between conditions. We are correcting for independent comorbidity between the major condition groups listed in Table 33.6 as follows:

$$PREVYLD_{a,s} = 1 - \prod_g \left(1 - PREVYLD_{a,s,g}\right) \quad [5]$$

where $PREVYLD_{a,s,g}$ is the prevalence YLD per 100 population for age a, sex s and cause group g. The resulting PREVYLD per 100 population for age a, sex s gives the severity-weighted prevalence of disability by age and sex.

For the year 2000 and 2001 estimates of HALE published in *The World Health Report 2001* and *The World Health Report 2002*, it was assumed that there is no comorbidity between specific conditions within these groups, with the following exceptions:

■ Vitamin A deficiency: 50% of the absolute prevalence assumed to be comorbid with protein-energy malnutrition,

■ Iron-deficiency anæmia: 25% of the absolute prevalence assumed to be comorbid with protein-energy malnutrition,

■ Diabetes: relative risk of cardiovascular disease assumed to be 4.0,

■ COPD (age < 70): region-specific comorbidity with cardiovascular disease estimated from smoking prevalence data separately for males and females aged > 70 and males and females aged 70+.

For the calculation of HALE for the year 2002, work will continue on refining and improving the estimation of dependent comorbidity, particularly at older ages.

Figures 33.7 and 33.8 illustrate the range of variation across and within regions in the age-standardized YLD prevalence estimates for the 191 WHO Member States for the year 2000.

> Estimation of country-level prevalence YLD for all causes for the year 2001 takes into account some dependent comorbidity, whereas independent comorbidity was assumed between all cause groups in the calculation of Global Burden of Disease priors for DALE for 1999.

UNCERTAINTY IN GBD PRIOR ESTIMATES OF HEALTH STATE PREVALENCES

The degree of uncertainty in the country-level weighted disability prevalences is mainly determined by levels of uncertainty in:

■ epidemiological estimates for prevalence and/or incidence of disability associated with specific causes or cause groups,

■ disability weights arising from uncertainty in health state valuations and, in some cases, also in the disability severity distribution associated with a condition,

■ estimation of prevalence YLD at the country level from the regional prevalence YLD rates,

■ estimation of prevalence YLD from incidence YLD, and

■ the approximate nature of adjustments for comorbidity.

Table 33.6 Major cause groups for which independent comorbidity assumed

Cause groups		
Tuberculosis+HIV	Maternal conditions	Digestive diseases
STDs excluding HIV	Perinatal conditions*	Genito-urinary diseases
Diarrhoeal diseases	Nutritional deficiencies	Skin diseases
Childhood-cluster diseases	Malignant and other neoplasms	Rheumatoid arthritis
Meningitis*	Endocrine disorders	Osteoarthritis
Hepatitis B+C	Mental disorders	Gout
Malaria	Neurological conditions	Back pain
Tropical-cluster diseases and nematodes	Vision disorders	Other musculoskeletal disorders
Trachoma	Hearing loss plus other sense disorders	Congenital anomalies
Other infectious diseases	Cardiovascular diseases/diabetes/COPD	Oral conditions
Respiratory infections	Asthma plus other respiratory	Injuries

For each WHO Member State, uncertainty in the country-level weighted disability prevalences for the year 2000 was estimated for a subset of specific causes as is summarized in Table 33.7. For the remaining specific causes, the overall level of uncertainty was assumed to be greater than that for the causes where detailed uncertainty estimates were made. For specific causes, where the uncertainty in the disability weights reflected uncertainty in health state valuations, this was estimated as well. For some causes where the disability weight also reflects the distribution of health state severity, additional uncertainty in the severity distribution was modelled.

High levels of uncertainty were specified for a number of residual categories, where there is a sub-stantial burden of disease due to mortality. For these categories, provisional YLD estimates were based on the methods used in the 1990 Global Burden of Disease Study (22), and a high level of uncertainty was included (Table 33.7).

A Monte-Carlo simulation (125 iterations) was run for the country-level weighted disability prevalences using @RISK© (30). @RISK© is an add-in software program to commercial spreadsheet packages. It allows the entry of uncertainty distributions instead of point estimates for input variables. It then recalculates the spreadsheet many times over, every time picking a value from each of the specified distributions, and produces an output dataset containing the resulting distribution of values for the output cells of interest.

Figure 33.7 Estimated age-standardized prevalence YLD rate versus life expectancy at birth, by sex, WHO Member States, 2000

Figure 33.8 Estimated age-standardized prevalence YLD: country versus regional rate, by sex, WHO Member States, 2000

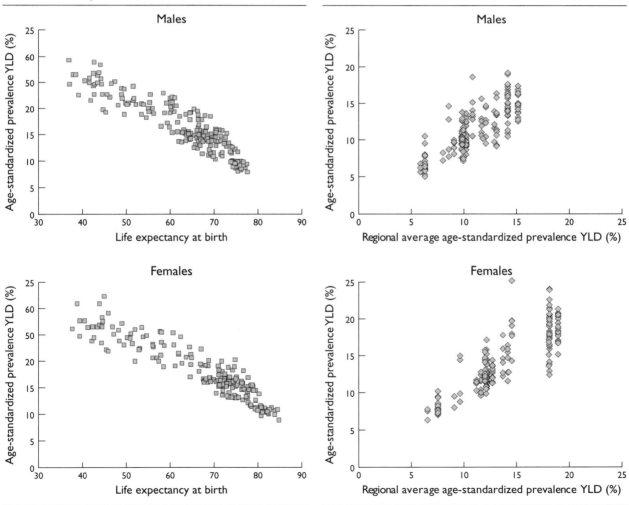

These output datasets were used to estimate 95% uncertainty intervals for the age-sex specific weighted prevalences for the WHO Member States.

The 95% uncertainty intervals are quite wide for any individual age-sex group, reflecting the total uncertainty in epidemiological estimates, health state valuations, and in the adjustments for covariance and for residual cause categories. Since some of these sources of uncertainty are not dependent on age and because uncertainty in age distributions

Table 33.7 Estimation of uncertainty in GBD prior estimates of comorbidity-adjusted prevalences by age and sex for WHO Member States in the year 2000

Category	Cause	Uncertainty estimation
Group I	Chlamydia	Uncertainty in regional prevalence and uncertainty in disability weight
	Gonnorhoea	Uncertainty in regional prevalence and uncertainty in disability weight
	HIV/AIDS	Uncertainty in country prevalence (AFRO D), other regional prevalences and uncertainty in disability weight
	Diarrhœal diseases	Uncertainty in regional prevalence and uncertainty in disability weight
	Malaria	Uncertainty in regional incidence and uncertainty in disability weight
	Maternal causes	Uncertainty estimated from uncertainty in regional prevalence YLD rates together with estimated uncertainty in country/region YLD ratios
	Perinatal conditions	Uncertainty estimated from uncertainty in regional prevalence YLD rates together with estimated uncertainty in country/region YLD ratios
	Protein-energy malnutrition	Estimated from analysis of uncertainty in epidemiological estimates of prevalence of stunting, wasting and developmental disability
	Iron-deficiency anæmia	Uncertainty in regional prevalence and uncertainty in disability weight
Group II	Depressive episodes	Uncertainty in regional prevalence, uncertainty in disability weight, additional uncertainty in prevalences among children and at older ages
	Bipolar disorder	Uncertainty in regional prevalence and uncertainty in disability weight
	Schizophrenia	Uncertainty in regional prevalence and uncertainty in disability weight
	Dementia	Uncertainty in regional prevalence and uncertainty in disability weight
	Migraine	Uncertainty in regional prevalence and uncertainty in disability weight
	Hearing loss, adult onset	Uncertainty in regional prevalence and uncertainty in disability weight
	Ischæmic heart disease	Uncertainty in regional mortality estimates, uncertainty in case fatality rates and uncertainty in disability weights
	Stroke	Uncertainty in regional mortality estimates, uncertainty in case fatality rates and uncertainty in disability weights
	Osteoarthritis	Uncertainty in regional prevalence and uncertainty in disability weight
	Gout	Uncertainty in regional prevalence, severity and duration
	Low back pain	Uncertainty in regional prevalence, severity and duration
Group III	Road traffic accidents	For each of these injury causes, uncertainty estimated from uncertainty in regional YLD/YLL ratios, uncertainty in country mortality estimates and age-specific uncertainty in estimation of prevalence YLD from incidence YLD
	Falls	
	Other unintentional injuries	
	Violence	
Residual categories	Other perinatal causes	Relative uncertainty modelled by triangular distribution 0.9-1-2
	Other neuropsychiatric	Relative uncertainty modelled by triangular distribution 0-1-5
	Other cardiovascular	Relative uncertainty modelled by triangular distribution 0-1-5
	Other respiratory	Relative uncertainty modelled by triangular distribution 0-1-5
	Other digestive	Relative uncertainty modelled by triangular distribution 0-1-5
	Other genitourinary	Relative uncertainty modelled by triangular distribution 0-1-5
	Other musculoskeletal	Relative uncertainty modelled by triangular distribution 0-1-5
Other sources of uncertainty	Causes for which uncertainty not estimated	Aggregate relative uncertainty assumed to be equal to the aggregate relative uncertainty for the causes listed above multiplied by a triangular distribution 0.5-1-4
	Comorbidity adjustment	Uncertainty in level of dependent comorbidity and in adjustment to disability weights for co-morbid conditions
	Adjustment to prior prevalence	Relative uncertainty modelled by triangular distribution 0-1-5

* For a uniform distribution, every value in the specified range has an equal probability of being chosen in each iteration of the simulation. For a triangular distribution, the probability of being chosen rises linearly from zero at the minimum value, to a maximum at the most probable value, then falls linearly to zero at the maximum value.

of epidemiological estimates may be smaller than uncertainty in the overall level for the population, the uncertainty distributions for different age groups will have non-zero correlations. The correlation in age-specific uncertainty distributions was estimated for the age-sex specific prevalence YLD for selected WHO Member States in all regions and average correlation matrices were estimated for Member States in three groups for the year 2000 (an example for one group is presented in Table 33.8). Sensitivity analysis showed that the uncertainty distribution for HALE at birth was not strongly dependent on the level of correlation, so that it was acceptable to use the average correlation matrices.

As part of the ongoing Global Burden of Disease 2000 work programme, estimates of uncertainty in YLD estimates for specific causes will continue to be revised and improved. In addition, the estimation of uncertainty introduced in estimating residual categories, adjusting for comorbidity, and in estimating prevalence YLD at country level will also be reviewed and refined.

> Estimation of uncertainty in country-level prevalence YLD for all causes for the year 2001 has been reviewed and refined, based on continuing revision of the Global Burden of Disease 2000 analyses of epidemiological and other health data for the WHO Member States.

USING HEALTH SURVEY DATA TO IMPROVE ESTIMATION

THE WHO HOUSEHOLD HEALTH SURVEY PROGRAM

Comparability is fundamental to the use of survey results for calculating healthy life expectancy (9). Existing national health surveys do not address this issue. To overcome the problem of cross-population comparability, the WHO survey instrument includes case vignettes and some measured tests on selected domains that are intended to calibrate the description that respondents provide of their own health (10). Data from 63 surveys in 55 Member States were used to estimate the true prevalence of different states of health by age and sex for HALE estimates reported in *The World Health Report 2001* for the year 2000 (Table 33.9). Just over one half (34) of these surveys were household interview surveys, two were telephone

Table 33.8 Estimated correlation matrix for age-specific uncertainty distributions for prevalence YLD estimates for the AFRO and SEARO D regions, year 2000 estimates

Age	Males								Females							
	0–4	5–14	15–29	30–44	45–59	60–69	70–79	80–89	0–4	5–14	15–29	30–44	45–59	60–69	70–79	80–89
0–4	1.00								1.00							
5–14	0.13	1.00							0.09	1.00						
15–29	0.12	0.30	1.00						0.07	0.22	1.00					
30–44	0.15	0.29	0.38	1.00					0.09	0.22	0.29	1.00				
45–59	0.19	0.22	0.25	0.32	1.00				0.13	0.19	0.22	0.26	1.00			
60–69	0.17	0.17	0.18	0.26	0.38	1.00			0.13	0.15	0.16	0.21	0.29	1.00		
70–79	0.11	0.12	0.13	0.21	0.32	0.37	1.00		0.09	0.10	0.11	0.16	0.24	0.28	1.00	
80–89	0.05	0.09	0.10	0.15	0.21	0.28	0.36	1.00	0.04	0.07	0.07	0.11	0.16	0.19	0.25	1.00

surveys, and the remainder postal surveys. Thirty five of the surveys were carried out in 31 European countries, 22 surveys in 19 developing countries, and the remainder in Canada, USA, Australia, and New Zealand. The sampled populations were adults aged 18 years and over. It is proposed to use more extensive data from the World Health Survey (11) together with statistical methods for correcting biases in self-reported health data, based on the hierarchical ordered probit (HOPIT) model (31) for the estimation of HALE in in future years.

Health state valuations will also be derived from the World Health Survey using the methods outlined by Salomon et al. (32). A global average valuation function will be applied to the individual domain levels

estimated using the HOPIT model in order to derive severity-adjusted prevalences of health states by age and sex for each survey country.

The World Health Survey using a standardized health survey module together with statistical methods to improve comparability of self-report data across Member States, will be used to estimate severity-weighted prevalences from health surveys for future years. This differs from the approach used to calculate DALE for 1999, where latent factor analysis methods were used to extract a common health factor from existing non-comparable surveys (1).

Table 33.9 Population surveys conducted using WHO survey instrument 1999–2000

Region	Country	Type of survey	Sample size	Region	Country	Type of survey	Sample size
AFRO	Nigeria	Household	5 108		Ireland	Brief face to face	711
AMRO	Canada	Postal	816		Italy	Brief face to face	1 002
	Canada	Telephone	778		Luxembourg	Telephone	719
	United States of America	Postal	1 792		Malta	Brief face to face	500
	Argentina	Brief face to face	1 555		Netherlands	Brief face to face	1 085
	Chile	Postal	2 078		Netherlands	Postal	3 794
	Colombia	Household	8 158		Portugal	Brief face to face	1 001
	Costa Rica	Brief face to face	1 508		Spain	Brief face to face	1 000
	Mexico	Household	4 813		Sweden	Brief face to face	1 000
	Trinidad and Tobago	Postal	2 583		Switzerland	Postal	962
	Venezuela	Brief face to face	1 495		United Kingdom	Postal	976
EMRO	Bahrain	Brief face to face	1 609		Georgia	Household	9 847
	Cyprus	Postal	1 311		Poland	Postal	1 751
	Jordan	Brief face to face	1 604		Slovakia	Household	1 183
	Oman	Brief face to face	1 719		Turkey	Household	5 207
	United Arab Emirates	Brief face to face	1 686		Turkey	Postal	5 013
	Egypt	Household	4 490		Kyrgyzstan	Postal	2 209
	Egypt	Postal	2 778		Estonia	Brief face to face	1 000
	Morocco	Brief face to face	1 506		Hungary	Postal	2 996
EURO	Austria	Postal	2 773		Latvia	Brief face to face	1 512
	Belgium	Brief face to face	1 100		Lithuania	Postal	3 513
	Croatia	Brief face to face	3 000		Russian Federation	Brief face to face	1 601
	Costa Rica	Brief face to face	1 508		Ukraine	Postal	1 562
	Czech Republic	Postal	2 038	SEARO	Indonesia	Household	9 994
	Denmark	Postal	3 014		Indonesia	Postal	5 074
	Finland	Brief face to face	1 021		Thailand	Postal	2 382
	Finland	Postal	2 692		India	Household	5 196
	France	Brief face to face	1 003	WPRO	Australia	Postal	1 185
	France	Postal	1 525		New Zealand	Postal	3 401
	Germany	Brief face to face	1 123		China	Household	9 486
	Greece	Postal	1 803		China	Postal	2 078
	Iceland	Brief face to face	489		Republic of Korea	Postal	705

Health state valuations used to estimate severity-weighted prevalences from health surveys for the year 2001 are based on valuations derived from representative population samples in WHO Member States using a multi-methods approach.

HEALTH STATE PREVALENCES FOR 55 MEMBER STATES IN 2000

This section reviews the results from the WHO Household Health Survey Program for 63 surveys in 55 countries during 2000–2001 that were used in the estimation of HALE for the year 2000. Figure 33.9 compares the average age-sex specific sever-

Figure 33.9 Comparison of severity-weighted average prevalences from surveys and GBD priors, developed and developing countries

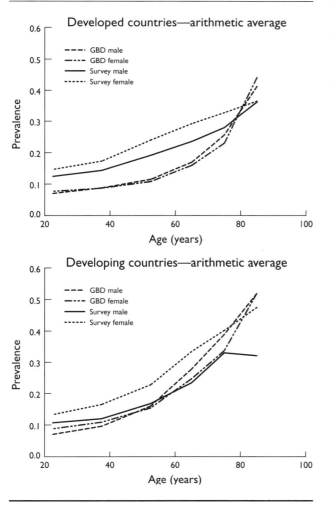

ity-weighted prevalences of health states for the 61 surveys with the corresponding average prevalence YLD from the Global Burden of Disease 2000 based estimates for those countries. Averages are compared for developed and developing countries separately. Figure 33.10 compares the average calibrated severity-weighted prevalences for developed and developing countries and also, for the developed countries, the A regions versus EURO B and C (predominantly the former Soviet countries of Eastern Europe). Survey respondents in the latter countries reported substantially worse health than for the A regions. This is consistent with the high adult mortality rates in many of these countries.

Figure 33.11 shows the age-standardized average severity-weighted prevalences versus per capita GDP (PPP 1998) for the 55 Member States where surveys were conducted. Unlike many cross-national surveys collecting self-report data on health, there is a clear trend to higher levels of average health status with increasing per capita GDP.

Figure 33.12 shows the female versus male age-standardized average severity-weighted prevalences for the 55 Member States where surveys were conducted. There were three surveys where male age-standardized prevalences were significantly higher than those for females: Australia, Venezuela, and Costa Rica. All three of these were postal surveys and two of them, Australia and Venezuela, had low response rates (less than 40%). This raised concerns about non-response bias for these particular surveys and, following consultation, it was decided to base the HALE estimates for these countries on the methods used to estimate posterior prevalences for non-survey countries (see the section on posterior health state prevalences for Member States in this chapter).

Uncertainty intervals for survey-based severity-weighted prevalences were derived to reflect several different sources of uncertainty. First, multiple estimates of individual domain levels were generated during the calibration procedure in order to capture uncertainties that arise in the mapping from categorical self-reported responses into continuous measures of domain levels. Estimation uncertainties in the fitting of the model parameters were propagated by sampling from draws from the joint distribution of the coefficient estimators. The standard errors for the survey means also reflect the sampling uncertainty arising from the development of inferences about the entire population based on a random sample from it.

It is important to include uncertainty arising from systematic error so as not to underestimate total uncertainty in estimates (*20*). In the case of the surveys, the potential average systematic error was estimated by comparing the survey prevalences with the GBD-based prior prevalences for survey countries. Uncertainty arising from non-random causes such as sampling bias, or unknown systematic differences between the GBD disability weights and the health state valuation function, was estimated for postal and other surveys separately using least squares regression to estimate the root mean squared error of the survey estimates around the prior estimates.

Uncertainty in survey prevalences is estimated taking account of sampling uncertainty, uncertainty in HOPIT estimation, and potential systematic biases.

Figure 33.11 Age-standardized average severity-weighted prevalences versus per capita Gross Domestic Product (PPP 1998), 63 surveys in the WHO 2000–2001 household survey study

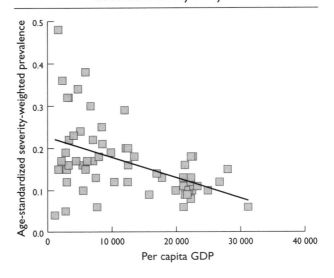

Figure 33.10 Comparison of severity-weighted average prevalences from surveys for developed and developing countries and for A regions versus Euro B and Euro C regions

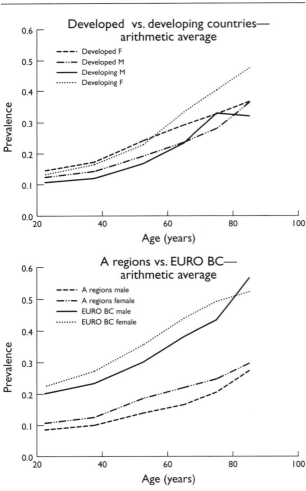

Figure 33.12 Age-standardized average severity-weighted prevalences for females versus males, 63 surveys in the WHO 2000–2001 household survey study

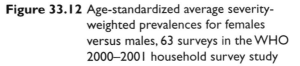
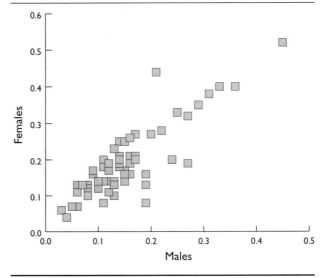

POSTERIOR HEALTH STATE PREVALENCES FOR MEMBER STATES

We have thus far described two sets of evidence on the severity-weighted health state prevalences for WHO Member States:

■ GBD-based estimates for all 191 Member States,

■ Survey-based estimates for a subset of Member States (55 for the year 2000).

In order to make the best use of the survey data to obtain estimates for all WHO Member States, we used Bayesian methods to calculate a posterior prevalence distribution for each Member State based on the prior distributions (GBD-based) updated by the survey evidence.

Bayesian statistics provide a conceptually simple process for updating uncertainty in the light of new evidence (20). If we denote the prior probability distribution for the quantity of interest by $P(H)$, and the new evidence by E, then the posterior probability distribution of H given the evidence, is given by Bayes' theorem as follows:

$$P(H \mid E) = \frac{P(H)P(E \mid H)}{P(E)} \qquad [6]$$

The term $P(E \mid H)$ gives the probability of E given a particular value of H. In this case, we propose to treat the GBD-based estimates of prevalences and their uncertainty distributions as expressing our prior beliefs in the form of probability distributions about the prevalences for WHO Member States. The surveys provide new evidence about the age-sex specific prevalences for specific Member States, and we can calculate the posterior probability distribution for each of these as follows:

$$P(\mu_i \mid y_i) = \frac{P(y_i \mid \mu_i)P(\mu_i)}{\int P(y_i \mid \mu_i)P(\mu_i)d\mu_i} \qquad [7]$$

where μ_i is the mean severity-weighted prevalence (for a given age, sex, and country all denoted by subscript i), $P(\mu_i)$ is the prior probability (the GBD-based prevalence estimates), and y_i is the observed prevalence from the survey.

When the evidence (survey mean severity-weighted prevalences by age and sex) and the prior means are both normally distributed, then the above equation for the posterior mean severity-weighted prevalence reduces to a weighted sum of the survey mean and the prior mean as follows:

$$Prev_{Post} = w_1 Prev_{Survey} + w_2 Prev_{Prior} \qquad [8]$$

where the weights are defined in terms of the standard deviation SD_1 for the average survey prevalence (for a given age and sex) and the standard deviation SD_2 for the prior prevalence (for the given age and sex) as:

$$w_1 = \frac{SD_2^{\,2}}{\left(SD_1^{\,2} + SD_2^{\,2}\right)} \qquad [9]$$

$$w_2 = \frac{SD_1^{\,2}}{\left(SD_1^{\,2} + SD_2^{\,2}\right)} \qquad [10]$$

For the calculation of HALE for the year 2000, the above normal approximation was used. The standard deviations for the prior means were estimated by carrying out an uncertainty analysis of the GBD prevalence YLD estimates at the country level, as described above. The standard deviations for the survey means were derived from the sampling variation together with uncertainty arising from the HOPIT calibration process and uncertainty due to systematic sampling bias (see the section on health state prevalences for 55 Member States in 2000).

The resulting survey weight w_1 varied across survey countries by age and sex, due to variation both in survey standard deviations and in prior standard deviations. The average survey weight across all countries ranged from around 0.2 at younger and older ages to 0.4 for middle age groups for males, and from around 0.15 at younger and older ages to 0.2 for middle age groups for females (Figure 33.13). In estimating the posterior prevalences for the survey countries, survey prevalences for 18–29 year-olds were assumed to apply to the age group 15–29 years. Posterior prevalences for 0–4 and 5–14 year age groups were assumed to be the same as the prior prevalences for those age groups.

Because the survey mean prevalences are on average higher than the GBD priors, the posterior estimates are on average higher than the priors. If GBD priors for non-survey countries are not updated, then the use of posteriors for survey countries only would result in a systematic difference in prevalences between survey and non-survey countries.

To avoid this problem for the year 2000 estimates, the evidence from the surveys was also used to update the non-survey priors. Least squares ordinary regression was used to fit the following model for the survey countries:

$$Prev_{Post} = \alpha + \beta Prev_{Prior} + \delta_1 POSTAL + \delta_2 EUROBC \quad [11]$$

where POSTAL is 1 for postal surveys, 0 otherwise, and EUROBC is 1 for countries in the EURO region in mortality strata B and C (high adult mortality countries), 0 for countries in other regions.

A range of models including factors such as dummies for other survey types and regions, country life expectancy, country-specific risk of death at given ages, and GDP per capita were also examined. None of these models provided significantly better fit to the data. Only the above terms were important in the model and retained. Goodness of fit was taken into account through the uncertainty analysis as outlined below.

The fitted model was used to estimate posterior severity-weighted prevalences for all non-survey countries. The Bayesian posterior for survey countries was adjusted for countries with postal surveys using the regression coefficient for the postal dummy. This adjusts for the systematic and significant differences in prevalences between postal and household surveys, so that the reference standard for all posterior estimates is household survey type. Where a country had a household and postal or telephone survey, the posterior based on the household survey was used. Where a country had a brief face-to-face and postal or telephone survey, the arithmetic average of the two posteriors was used.

Figure 33.14 shows the resulting estimated posterior severity-adjusted prevalence rates (age-standardized to the World Standard Population (33)) versus life expectancy at birth for the year 2000 estimates.

Figure 33.15 shows the range of variation in the age-standardized posterior prevalences within each of the WHO epidemiological subregions.

It is proposed to investigate the use a similar Bayesian estimation technique for HALE estimates for future years, but to explicitly use the likelihood function to compare posterior prevalences rather than make assumptions that priors and survey estimates are normally distributed. Work will continue on uncertainty analyses in the Global Burden of Disease 2000, and the uncertainty distributions will be used directly,

Figure 33.14 Estimated age-standardized posterior prevalence YLD rate versus life expectancy at birth, by sex, WHO Member States, 2000

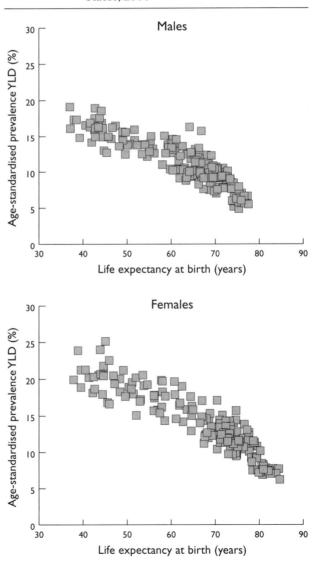

Figure 33.13 Survey weights by age and sex, 63 surveys in 55 countries, 2000–2001

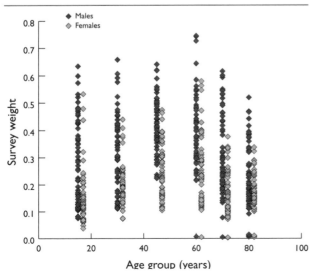

together with the multiple draws (125 were used for year 2000 results) of survey estimates, to compute posterior distributions for prevalences.

Additionally, the more comprehensive dataset of posterior and prior estimates for the World Health Survey countries will be used to find a best-fit regression model for estimation of posterior prevalences for non-survey countries. This regression model may include more or different terms to those included in equation [11], depending on the relationships that exist in the expanded dataset for survey countries in the World Health Survey.

Figure 33.15 Estimated age-standardized posterior prevalence YLD: country versus regional rate, by sex, WHO Member States, 2000

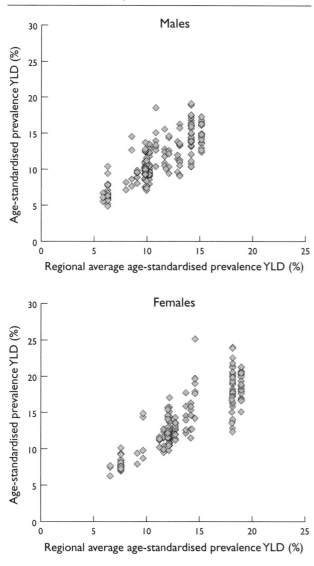

Bayesian estimation techniques will be investigated to calculate posterior prevalences for 191 Member States by utilizing prior prevalence estimates based on the GBD 2000 and country-level data, together with independent evidence from the World Health Survey for as many Member States as possible.

UNCERTAINTY IN POSTERIOR HEALTH STATE PREVALENCES

The variance of the posterior estimate for countries with surveys is given by:

$$SD_{POST}^2 = \frac{SD_1^2 SD_2^2}{\left(SD_1^2 + SD_2^2\right)} \qquad [12]$$

The inter-age correlation for the survey estimates is assumed to be zero. Thus, the inter-age correlation matrix for the posterior estimates is approximately estimated for each country by adjusting the inter-age correlation matrix for the prior estimates (see example given in Table 33.8) by a country-specific factor reflecting the average prior weight across age groups.

A regression model similar to that shown in equation [11] will be used to estimate posterior prevalences for non-survey countries. One of the assumptions of the classic linear regression model is that the independent variables are fixed in repeated measures. Stochastic error around the independent variables included in the regression will produce biased estimates of the regression coefficients, which is known as the "errors-in-variables" problem. Because practical analytical methods are generally lacking, it is almost universal to ignore this layer of uncertainty. We have addressed this problem, however, using a Monte Carlo procedure, described below for the year 2000 estimates. It is proposed to follow a similar procedure for future years.

Consider the regression model above for a specific age-sex group (subscripts are suppressed for ease of the presentation):

$$Y = X\beta + \varepsilon, \qquad [13]$$

where Y is the posterior prevalence, X is the matrix of regressor variables, and β is the coefficient vector.

■ To account for the stochastic error in X (arising from the uncertainty in the priors) and the uncertainty in Y (arising from the combined uncertainties of the priors and the surveys), one observation of the prior value and the survey value was drawn for each survey country from the relevant uncertainty distributions (assumed to be normal). In drawing observations of prior values, it was assumed that one half of the uncertainty arose at the regional level (so all countries in the same region shared the same draw) and the other half was country-specific. For each country, the posterior value Y was calculated and the regression model estimated. This process was repeated 10 times, resulting in 10 estimates of the coefficient vector and the stochastic error term.

■ For each of the 10 regressions, 10 draws of the coefficient vector were then made based on the variance-covariance matrix of the regression estimators, resulting in a set of 100 coefficient vectors.

■ For each of these 100 coefficient vectors, 10 random draws of the prior prevalence for each of the 191 WHO Member States were made and the regression model was used to compute the posterior prevalences. This results in a sample of 1 000 posterior estimates for the age-specific prevalences in each of the 191 WHO Member States. These 1 000 posterior prevalences are sorted and the 2.5th percentile and 97.5th percentile of the distribution are estimated, providing a 95% uncertainty interval for the posterior prevalence for each WHO Member State.

For the non-survey countries, inter-age correlation between posterior estimates was assumed to be the same as that for the prior estimates.

CALCULATION OF HALE

SULLIVAN'S METHOD

Sullivan's method is used to compute HALE for each Member State from the country life table and the severity-weighted prevalence estimates. Sullivan's method involves using the severity-weighted prevalence of health states (adjusted for comorbidity) at each age in the current population (at a given point of time) to divide the hypothetical years of life lived by a period life table cohort at different ages into years of equivalent full health (34). The method is illustrated in detail in Mathers et al. (29).

Using standard notation for the country life table parameters, we calculate HALE at age x as follows:

D_x Severity-weighted prevalence between ages x and $x + 5$

L_x Total years lived by the life table population between ages x and $x + 5$

$YD_x = L_x D_x$ Equivalent lost years of healthy life between ages x and $x + 5$

$YWD_x = L_x (1 - D_x)$ Equivalent years of healthy life lived between ages x and $x+5$

HALE at age x is the sum of YWD_i from $i = x$ to w (the last open-ended age interval in the life table) divided by l_x (survivors at age x):

$$HALE_x = \frac{\sum_{i=x}^{w} YWD_i}{l_x} \qquad [14]$$

$$LHE_x = \frac{\sum_{i=x}^{w} YD_i}{l_x} = LE_x - HALE_x \qquad [15]$$

LHE_x, the equivalent healthy years of life lost, is the sum of YD_i from $i = x$ to w divided by l_x (survivors at age x).

Sullivan's method is applied in abridged life tables using five year age intervals, up to an open-ended interval of 100+ years. The first interval is subdivided into 0 years and 1–4 years. Posterior prevalences are calculated for the GBD age groups (0–4, 5–14, 15–29, 30–44, 45–59, 60–69, 70–79, 80+) and are assumed to be constant for the five-year age groups within each GBD age group. More detailed calculations for the 2000 estimates showed that error in the final estimate of HALE introduced by this approximation is less than 0.1 years.

UNCERTAINTY ANALYSIS FOR HALE

For each of the inputs to the Sullivan calculation, the measurement and estimation efforts generate an uncertainty distribution. This uncertainty must be propagated forward into the computation of the overall healthy life expectancy. The method follows the general principles outlined by Salomon et al. (20).

For each country, the distribution of each component is randomly sampled to generate 1 000 draws. This process results in the compilation of component matrices (191 columns × 1 000 rows), the column values of which represent all available information, for 191 countries, about the uncertainty surrounding each component of the HALE. Each component matrix is sampled a row at a time without replacement, and the overall HALE is computed 1 000 times for each of the 191 countries. The HALE estimates for each Member State are then used to calculate for each age and sex, the median value and 95% uncertainty intervals (2.5th and 97.5th percentiles) of HALE.

In sampling from the component uncertainty distributions, it is important to recognize inter-dependencies between multiple uncertain components. If we fail to model these inter-dependencies, the joint probability will be incorrect. Correlation between uncertainty in prevalences across age groups has been discussed above. These correlations must be built into the prevalence draws by making random draws from a multivariate normal distribution with a correlation matrix appropriately specified for each country.

Because a proportion of the country-specific prior prevalences is derived making use of country-level cause-specific mortality information (see the section on country-specific estimates of health state prevalences), there will be a correlation between uncertainty in life expectancy and the prevalences. This was taken into account for the year 2000 estimates by estimating the country-level prevalences for selected Member States using the complete set of life table draws for each, and computing the correlation between the age-standardized severity-adjusted prevalence and life expectancy at birth for males and females separately. A simple regression model was fitted to this data to estimate the corresponding correlation for other Member States as a function of life expectancy at birth. The correlation estimates ranged from around 0.2 in developed countries to around 0.3 to 0.4 in the African WHO Region. For survey countries, the survey uncertainty was assumed to have zero correlation with life expectancy uncertainty, resulting in lower correlation estimates for these countries (typically around half the prior correlation). A similar method will be used to quantify the mortality-prevalence correlation for future estimates.

The prevalence-mortality correlations are taken into account in selecting draws for input to Sullivan's method as follows. The prevalence draws are ranked in ascending order of age-standardized prevalence and the life table draws in ascending order of life expectancy at birth. We then draw from these two ranked columns to obtain paired prevalence and life table draws with the required rank order correlation using the methods of Vose (35). These pairs of draws are used with Sullivan's method to compute a set of HALE estimates. These distributions are then used to estimate the 95% uncertainty intervals for HALE at birth and at age 60.

Annex Table 4 of *The World Health Report 2001* gives 95% uncertainty ranges for HALE at birth and at age 60 for males and females for all WHO Mem-

ber States.[2] Average uncertainty ranges in estimates of healthy life expectancy at birth (both sexes combined) are shown for the 191 WHO Member States in Figure 33.16, plotted against health expenditure per capita (measured in international dollars for 1998 using purchasing power parity conversion factors). Average 95% uncertainty intervals for Member States in each of the 17 epidemiological regions of the Global Burden of Disease 2000 are shown in Figure 33.17 together with average healthy life expectancy at birth for these regions.

The uncertainty ranges for HALE in 2000 are larger than those estimated for DALE in 1999 as published in *The World Health Report 2000* (15). There are two main reasons for this: a) more detailed analysis of uncertainty in GBD-based priors for 2000, particularly for health state valuation uncertainty, uncertainty in residual categories, and co-morbidity, and b) estimation of non-random uncertainty due to survey data. Additionally, *The World Health Report 2001* reports 95% uncertainty intervals rather than the 80% intervals reported in *The World Health Report 2000*.

Apart from the more detailed uncertainty analyses carried out for the 2000 estimates, which included more sources of uncertainty and improved estimates of its magnitude, the methods used to deal with correlation between components of uncertainty were also more sophisticated. For the 1999 analysis, a more con-

Figure 33.16 Uncertainty in average healthy life expectancy at birth (males and females combined) for the year 2000 versus average health expenditure per capita (1998) for 191 WHO Member States

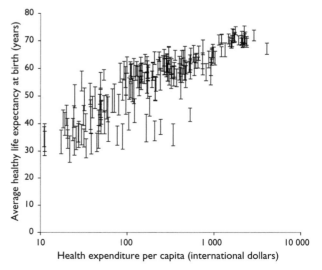

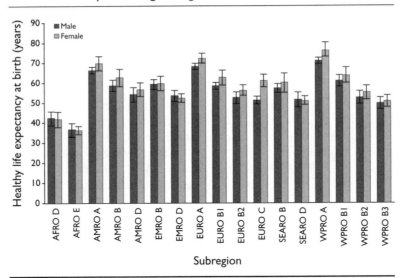

Figure 33.17 HALE at birth with 95% uncertainty intervals, by sex, 17 epidemiological regions, 2000

servative set of approximations was used as follows: we assumed 100% correlation between uncertainty at each age within broad age ranges 0–14, 15–29, 30–44, 45–59, 60–69, and 70+ years (so that for a given sample of the disability prevalence distribution, it is high at all ages or low at all ages within one of these ranges).

The annex table also gives 95% uncertainty intervals for HALE at birth and total LE at birth, by sex, for all Member States. These uncertainty intervals will enable readers to compare HALE estimates for Member States, keeping in mind the uncertainty in these comparisons. This will help readers to avoid giving undue emphasis to small differences in mean ranks for countries.

> The uncertainty estimates for HALE in 2001 are based on a more comprehensive analysis of all sources of uncertainty in the life tables, GBD prior estimates, survey estimates, and Bayesian posterior estimation which takes into account inter-age correlations and correlations between uncertainty in mortality and prevalences.

PROPOSAL TO USE INCIDENCE HALE FOR HSPA

The HALE that has been estimated for the health systems performance analysis published in *The World*

Health Report 2000 and for reporting on average levels of population health (*The World Health Report 2001* and *The World Health Report 2002*), is a prevalence-based HALE that reflects the estimated current prevalence of health states in the population for the reference year.

Elsewhere (3) we discuss a number of possible summary measures of average population health based on capturing current health conditions in a period measure, or on estimating expected current and future HALE for individuals in the population. We argue that using an incidence-based HALE that also takes into account some current risk factor prevalence information for the population may offer advantages for health systems performance analysis.

We propose that for the estimation of HALE for health systems performance analysis, we calculate an incidence-based HALE that also takes into account current exposures for selected risk factors. The proposed analytic approach is as follows:

■ Inclusion in the Global Burden of Disease 2000 of prevalence estimates based on current transition rates (so-called "incidence-based" prevalences) as well as the observed prevalence rates. These two types of prevalence estimates would differ only for causes where there was evidence of a non-equilibrium state for the disease model, due to time trends in incidence, remission or case fatality, e.g. HIV/AIDS in many regions. GBD-based prior estimates would be calculated using prevalences derived from currently estimated incidence rates (rather than the currently observed prevalences). For many diseases, such as HIV/AIDS, use of current incidence rather than prevalence would ensure that current risk factor profiles were taken into account.

■ For selected risk factors where there are long lags to health outcomes, estimation of incidence and mortality for the population would be based on a counterfactual assumption that the population had been exposed to current levels of the risk factor for a long time in the past. The Global Burden of Disease 2000 comparative risk assessments (CRA) (36;37) would be used to provide estimates of risk factor exposures for each region of the world for selected risk factors. Where available, country-specific information would be used to provide country-specific exposure estimates. Currently observed total incidence and mortality risks would be adjusted using CRA estimates of effect sizes. In the first instance, we would envisage that such analysis would only be carried out for smoking, and perhaps diet and exercise. It would be necessary to model the joint effect on incidence and mortality of the combined current exposure to these risks and to be transparent about the assumptions used in the analysis.

■ The country-specific differences between incidence-based and prevalence-based overall comorbidity adjusted prevalence YLD would be used to adjust the survey-based prevalences (so that they also represent an estimate of severity-weighted prevalence of health states if current incidence rates and risk factor exposures were experienced at each age).

■ Posterior prevalences would be derived using Bayesian estimation methods as above.

■ Calculation of new life tables for each Member State based on the adjustments to mortality risk described above (to reflect current risk factor exposures and incidence rates where relevant).

■ Calculation of an incidence-based HALE for each Member State using Sullivan's method with the incidence-based prevalences and the new life tables.

These incidence-based period HALE would provide estimates of the healthy life expectancy that could be expected by a cohort exposed to current risk factor levels at each age (for the selected risk factors) and current incidence, remission, and case fatality rates (reflecting current rather than past risks of disease and injury). This would provide a better measure of the health outcome for current health system activities than a measure based on prevalences reflecting past health system activities and past risk factor levels (and other past non-health system determinants).

DISCUSSION AND CONCLUSIONS

This chapter has described the methods proposed for producing estimates of healthy life expectancy (HALE) for WHO Member States in the next health systems performance analysis. There are considerable improvements in both data and methods over those used for the HALE estimates for 1999 published in *The World Health Report 2000*. These are highlighted in text boxes throughout sections three to seven of this chapter and summarized below.

Healthy life expectancy estimates for Member States for the year 2000 published in *The World Health Report 2001* are not directly comparable with those published in *The World Health Report 2000* for 1999 as they incorporate new epidemiological information, new data from health surveys, and new information on mortality rates, as well as improvements in methods. The new evidence from the WHO Multi-country Household Survey Study has resulted in an overall increase in severity-weighted prevalences, an increase for females relative to males, and hence to a reduction in HALE estimates. This has affected all Member States and at the global level, reduced HALE at birth from the previous estimate of 56.8 years in 1999 to the current estimate of 56.0 years for the year 2000. For some Member States, there have also been changes in HALE estimates due to new information provided on age-specific mortality rates.

Ensuring that healthy life expectancy estimates for Member States are comparable is an overriding consideration for assessing the average level of health of WHO Member States. Because comparable health status prevalence data are not yet available for all Member States, it is recommended to continue to use a three-stage strategy based on use of the Global Burden of Disease 2000, health survey data, and statistical methods to construct maximum likelihood posterior estimates that maximize cross-country comparability. Implemented and proposed data and methodological improvements relative to methods and data used for *The World Health Report 2000* are summarized below.

DATA IMPROVEMENTS

- New and more recent data on mortality (all causes and cause-specific) will be available for many Member States.

- Use of later revisions of the Global Burden of Disease 2000 estimates for constructing GBD-based priors. These will incorporate updated epidemiological assessments for many diseases, including chronic respiratory diseases, cardiovascular diseases, injuries, perinatal and maternal causes, and selected infectious diseases and nutritional deficiencies.

- Increased use of country-specific data for estimation of country-level prevalence YLD for constructing GBD-based priors.

- Improved estimation of uncertainty in country-level prevalence YLD for all causes, based on continuing reviews of epidemiological and other health data.

- Cross-population comparable survey data on health status will be available for more than 70 Member States through the World Health Survey.

- Health state valuations will be derived from representative population samples in the World Health Survey.

METHODOLOGICAL IMPROVEMENTS

- Use of modified logit life table system for countries without time series data on mortality by age and sex.

- Improved methods for direct estimation of prevalence YLD compared to the methods previously based on incidence YLD rates and ratios.

- Improved modelling of uncertainty distributions for age patterns and co-morbidity in the Global Burden of Disease 2000 estimates.

- Allowance for dependent comorbidity for some causes will be made, whereas previously independent co-morbidity was assumed between all causes.

- The World Health Survey, using a standardized health survey module together with statistical methods to improve comparability of self-report data across Member States, will be used to estimate severity-weighted prevalences from health surveys, rather than attempting to utilize information from existing non-comparable surveys as previously.

- Health state valuations will be derived using a multi-method approach that considers the different biases in each of the available valuation methods.

- Uncertainty in survey prevalences will be estimated taking account of sampling uncertainty, uncertainty in HOPIT estimation, and potential systematic biases.

- It is proposed to use Bayesian estimation techniques to calculate posterior prevalences for all 191 Member States utilizing prior prevalence estimates based on the Global Burden of Disease 2000 and country-level data, together with independent evidence from the World Health Survey for as many Member States as possible.

- Uncertainty estimates for HALE will take into account inter-age correlation in uncertainty as well as correlation between prior prevalences and mortality levels.

- For the health systems performance analysis, it is proposed to calculate an incidence-based HALE for each Member State, which also incorporates the mortality risks associated with exposure at each age to the current period levels for selected risk factors.

Some commentators have argued that the data demands and complexity of the calculations make healthy life expectancy an impractical measure for use as a summary measure of population health or as a measure of the attainment of the health system goal for level of health (38). Although the concept of healthy life expectancy is relatively simple to understand, health encompasses multiple domains and mortality risks, and with the additional requirement to ensure comparability of estimates across countries, any acceptable methods used to compute healthy life expectancy will inevitably be complex. Ignoring aspects or domains of health that people value would not, we believe, be acceptable in measuring the health attainment of WHO Member States.

It is our conviction that in order to report on levels of health for WHO Member States, it is important to use a summary measure that is conceptually simple to understand, and methods that capture all important aspects of health and result in estimates that are comparable across Member States.

ACKNOWLEDGEMENTS

Many people have contributed to the data collection and analyses providing inputs to the estimation of healthy life expectancy for 1999 and 2000. We wish to particularly acknowledge the contributions of staff in various WHO programmes and expert groups outside WHO, who have provided advice, collaborated in the reviews of epidemiological data and in the estimation of burden of disease and the conduct of health surveys. Apart from the authors, staff within EIP/GPE who worked directly on the analysis of mortality data for the year 2000 and the Global Burden of Disease 2000 Version 1 up to July 2001 include Alan D. Lopez, Omar B. Ahmad, Jose Ayuso, Cynthia Boschi-Pinto, Marisol Concha, Majid Ezzati, Brodie D. Ferguson, Mie Inoue, Matilde Leonardi, Rafael Lozano, Doris Ma Fat, Eduardo Sabaté, Joshua A. Salomon, Toshi Satoh, Lana Tomaskovic, and T. Bedirhan Üstün. Ajay Tandon, Ritu Sadana, Somnath Chatterji, Maria Villanueva, Lydia Bendib, Nicole B. Valentine, Juan Pablo Ortiz, Yang Cao, Can Çelik, and Wan Jun Xie were also involved with the WHO Multi-country Household Survey Study.

NOTES

1 The Global Burden of Disease 2000 project uses 17 epidemiological subregions of the world for the purposes of epidemiological analyses. The resulting estimates are mapped back into 14 subregions of the 6 WHO regions for the purposes of reporting. Definitions of the regions are given by Murray et al. (*13*).

2 In the Annex Notes of *The World Health Report 2001*, the ranges are erroneously described as 80% intervals.

REFERENCES

(1) Mathers CD et al. Healthy life expectancy in 191 countries, 1999. *The Lancet*, 2001, 357(9269):1685–1691.

(2) Murray CJL, Evans DB. Overview. In: Murray CJL, Evans DB, eds. *Health systems performance assessment: debates, methods and empiricism*. Geneva, World Health Organization, 2003.

(3) Mathers CD et al. Alternative summary measures of average population health. In: Murray CJL, Evans DB, eds. *Health systems performance assessment: debates, methods and empiricism*. Geneva, World Health Organization, 2003.

(4) Murray CJL, Salomon JA, Mathers CD. A critical examination of summary measures of population health.

Bulletin of the World Health Organization, 2000, 78(8):981–994.

(5) Murray CJL et al., eds. *Summary measures of population health: concepts, ethics, measurement and applications*. Geneva, World Health Organization, 2002.

(6) Robine JM, Mathers CD, Brouard N. Trends and differentials in disability-free life expectancy: concepts, methods and findings. In: Caselli G, Lopez AD, eds. *Health and mortality among elderly populations*. Oxford, Clarendon Press, 1996:182–201.

(7) Romieu I, Robine JM. World atlas of health expectancy calculations. In: Mathers CD, McCallum J, Robine JM, eds. *Advances in health expectancies*. Canberra, Australian Institute of Health and Welfare, 1994.

(8) Sadana R et al. *Comparative analyses of more than 50 household surveys on health status*. EIP Discussion Paper No. 15. Geneva, World Health Organization, 2000. URL: http://www3.who.int/whosis/discussion_papers/discussion_papers.cfm#

(9) Murray CJL et al. Cross-population comparability of evidence for health policy. In: Murray CJL, Evans DB, eds. *Health systems performance assessment: debates, methods and empiricism*. Geneva, World Health Organization, 2003.

(10) Üstün TB et al. WHO Multi-country Survey Study on Health and Responsiveness 2000–2001. In: Murray CJL, Evans DB, eds. *Health systems performance assessment: debates, methods and empiricism*. Geneva, World Health Organization, 2003.

(11) Üstün TB et al. The World Health Surveys. In: Murray CJL, Evans DB, eds. *Health systems performance assessment: debates, methods and empiricism*. Geneva, World Health Organization, 2003.

(12) Mathers CD et al. *Estimates of healthy life expectancy for 191 countries in the year 2000: methods and results*. EIP Discussion Paper No. 38. Geneva, World Health Organization, 2001. URL: http://www3.who.int/whosis/discussion_papers/discussion_papers.cfm#

(13) Murray CJL et al. *The Global Burden of Disease 2000 project: aims, methods and data sources*. EIP Discussion Paper No. 36. Geneva, World Health Organization, 2001. URL: http://www3.who.int/whosis/discussion_papers/discussion_papers.cfm#

(14) World Health Organization. *The World Health Report 2001. Mental Health: New Understanding, New Hope*. Geneva, World Health Organization, 2000.

(15) World Health Organization. *The World Health Report 2000. Health Systems: Improving Performance*. Geneva, World Health Organization, 2000.

(16) Salomon JA, Murray CJL. Modelling HIV/AIDS epidemics in sub-Saharan Africa using seroprevalence data

from antenatal clinics. *Bulletin of the World Health Organization*, 2001, 79(7):596–607.

(17) Lopez AD et al. Life tables for 191 countries for 2000: data, methods, results. In: Murray CJL, Evans DB, eds. *Health systems performance assessment: debates, methods and empiricism*. Geneva, World Health Organization, 2003.

(18) Lopez AD et al. *World mortality in 2000: life tables for 191 countries*. Geneva, World Health Organization, 2002.

(19) Murray CJL et al. Modified logit life table system: principles, empirical validation, and application. In: Murray CJL, Evans DB, eds. *Health systems performance assessment: debates, methods and empiricism*. Geneva, World Health Organization, 2003.

(20) Salomon JA et al. *Methods for life expectancy and healthy life expectancy uncertainty analysis*. EIP Discussion Paper No. 10. Geneva, World Health Organization 2001. URL: http://www3.who.int/whosis/discussion_papers/discussion_papers.cfm#

(21) Murray CJL. Rethinking DALYs. In: Murray CJL, Lopez AD, eds. *The global burden of disease: a comprehensive assessment of mortality and disability from diseases, injuries, and risk factors in 1990 and projected to 2020*. Cambridge, Harvard University Press, 1996:1–98.

(22) Murray CJL, Lopez AD, eds. *The global burden of disease: a comprehensive assessment of mortality and disability from diseases, injuries, and risk factors in 1990 and projected to 2020*. Cambridge, Harvard University Press, 1996:211.

(23) Lozano R et al. *Miscoding and misclassification of ischæmic heart disease mortality*. EIP Discussion Paper No. 12. Geneva, World Health Organization, 2001. URL: http://www3.who.int/whosis/discussion_papers/discussion_papers.cfm#

(24) Mathers CD et al. Global and regional estimates of cancer mortality and incidence by site: I. Application of regional cancer survival model to estimate cancer mortality distribution by site. *BMC Cancer*, 2002, 2:36.

(25) Shibuya K et al. Global and regional estimates of cancer mortality and incidence by site: II. results for the global burden of disease 2000. *BMC Cancer*, 2002, 2:37.

(26) Salomon JA, Murray CJL. The epidemiologic transition re-examined: compositional models for causes of death by age and sex. *Population and Development Review*, 2002, 28(2): 205–228.

(27) World Health Organization. *The World Health Report 2002. Reducing Risks, Promoting Healthy Life*. Geneva, World Health Organization, 2002.

(28) King H, Aubert RE, Herman WH. Global burden of diabetes, 1995-2025. *Diabetes Care*, 1998, 21(9): 1414–1431.

(29) Mathers CD et al. *Estimates of DALE for 191 countries: methods and results*. EIP Discussion Paper No. 16. Geneva, World Health Organization, 2000. URL: http://www3.who.int/whosis/discussion_papers/discussion_papers.cfm#

(30) Palisade. *@RISK: advanced risk analysis for spreadsheets*. New York, Palisade Corporation, 1996.

(31) Tandon A et al. Statistical models for enhancing cross-population comparability. In: Murray CJL, Evans DB, eds. *Health systems performance assessment: debates, methods and empiricism*. Geneva, World Health Organization, 2003.

(32) Salomon JA et al. Health state valuations in summary measures of population health. In: Murray CJL, Evans DB, eds. *Health systems performance assessment: debates, methods and empiricism*. Geneva, World Health Organization, 2003.

(33) Ahmad OB et al. *Age standardization of rates: a new WHO standard*. EIP Discussion Paper No. 31. Geneva, World Health Organization, 2001. URL: http://www3.who.int/whosis/discussion_papers/discussion_papers.cfm#

(34) Sullivan DF. A single index of mortality and morbidity. *HSMHA Health Report*, 1971, 86:347–354.

(35) Vose D. *Risk analysis: a quantitative guide*. New York, Wiley, 2000.

(36) Murray CJL, Lopez AD. On the comparable quantification of health risks: lessons from the global burden of disease study. *Epidemiology*, 1999, 10(5):594–605.

(37) Ezzati M et al. *CRA interim guidelines, data collection sheets and toolbox*. Geneva, World Health Organization, 2001. URL: http://www.ctru.auckland.ac.nz/CRA

(38) Almeida C et al. Methodological concerns and recommendations on policy consequences of the World Health Report 2000. The Lancet, 2001, 357(9269): 1692–1697.

Healthy Life Expectancy and Total Life Expectancy at Birth, by Sex, WHO Member States, 2000

Rank	Member State	Persons	Healthy life expectancy (HALE) at birth				Life expectancy at birth			
			Males		Females		Males		Females	
1	Japan	73.8	71.2	(69.9–72.5)	76.3	(74.6–77.8)	77.5	(77.4–77.7)	84.7	(84.4–85.1)
2	Switzerland	72.1	70.4	(68.7–72.1)	73.7	(71.3–75.7)	76.7	(76.3–77.0)	82.5	(82.1–82.9)
3	San Marino	72.0	69.7	(68.0–71.8)	74.3	(72.2–76.4)	76.1	(75.1–77.2)	83.8	(82.8–84.7)
4	Andorra	71.8	69.8	(67.4–73.0)	73.7	(70.7–77.9)	77.2	(74.4–81.7)	83.8	(80.2–89.5)
5	Monaco	71.7	69.4	(67.5–72.1)	73.9	(71.1–76.7)	76.8	(75.2–79.8)	84.4	(81.6–86.4)
6	Australia	71.5	69.6	(67.8–71.5)	73.3	(69.8–75.4)	76.6	(76.3–77.1)	82.1	(81.7–82.5)
7	Sweden	71.4	70.1	(68.7–71.6)	72.7	(70.6–74.6)	77.3	(77.0–77.6)	82.0	(81.7–82.4)
8	Iceland	71.2	69.8	(68.1–71.5)	72.6	(70.3–74.9)	77.1	(75.7–78.6)	81.8	(80.5–83.9)
9	Italy	71.2	69.5	(68.4–70.8)	72.8	(70.5–74.5)	76.0	(75.6–76.3)	82.4	(82.0–82.7)
10	Greece	71.0	69.7	(68.5–70.8)	72.3	(69.9–74.0)	75.4	(75.0–75.7)	80.8	(80.1–81.5)
11	New Zealand	70.8	69.5	(68.0–71.0)	72.1	(69.8–74.0)	75.9	(75.2–76.7)	80.9	(79.8–81.9)
12	France	70.7	68.5	(67.4–69.5)	72.9	(71.4–74.5)	75.2	(74.8–75.5)	83.1	(82.5–83.8)
13	Spain	70.6	68.7	(67.3–70.3)	72.5	(70.3–74.2)	75.4	(74.7–75.8)	82.3	(82.0–82.6)
14	Norway	70.5	68.8	(67.0–70.5)	72.3	(70.2–74.6)	75.7	(75.5–76.0)	81.4	(80.9–82.0)
15	Malta	70.4	68.7	(67.3–70.2)	72.1	(69.7–74.1)	75.4	(74.7–76.2)	80.7	(79.3–82.0)
16	Austria	70.3	68.1	(66.9–69.4)	72.5	(70.3–74.3)	74.9	(74.4–75.4)	81.4	(81.0–81.8)
17	Canada	70.0	68.3	(66.9–69.7)	71.7	(70.0–73.5)	76.0	(75.6–76.5)	81.5	(81.1–81.9)
18	Israel	69.9	69.3	(67.7–71.0)	70.6	(68.3–72.9)	76.6	(76.3–76.9)	80.6	(80.3–81.0)
19	United Kingdom	69.9	68.3	(66.8–69.7)	71.4	(69.2–73.1)	74.8	(74.6–75.0)	79.9	(79.7–80.2)
20	Luxembourg	69.8	67.6	(66.2–69.2)	72.0	(69.5–74.0)	73.9	(73.0–74.8)	80.8	(79.8–82.1)
21	Netherlands	69.7	68.2	(67.1–69.3)	71.2	(69.7–72.7)	75.4	(74.9–76.0)	81.0	(80.4–81.5)
22	Denmark	69.5	68.9	(67.5–70.3)	70.1	(68.2–72.0)	74.2	(73.8–74.5)	78.5	(78.2–79.0)
23	Germany	69.4	67.4	(66.0–68.7)	71.5	(69.4–73.3)	74.3	(74.0–74.8)	80.6	(80.3–80.9)
24	Belgium	69.4	67.7	(66.2–69.2)	71.0	(69.0–73.0)	74.6	(74.2–75.0)	80.9	(80.5–81.3)
25	Ireland	69.3	67.8	(66.3–69.1)	70.9	(68.6–72.7)	74.1	(73.6–74.5)	79.7	(79.3–80.0)
26	Finland	68.8	66.1	(64.9–67.2)	71.5	(69.9–73.0)	73.7	(73.5–74.0)	80.9	(80.5–81.3)
27	Singapore	67.8	66.8	(64.3–69.0)	68.9	(65.8–71.7)	75.4	(74.7–76.0)	80.2	(79.5–81.1)
28	United States of America	67.2	65.7	(63.8–67.5)	68.8	(66.5–71.0)	73.9	(73.7–74.2)	79.5	(79.3–79.6)
29	Slovenia	66.9	64.5	(62.1–66.7)	69.3	(66.5–71.9)	71.9	(71.5–72.3)	79.4	(78.9–80.2)
30	Cyprus	66.3	66.4	(64.6–68.7)	66.2	(63.4–68.8)	74.8	(74.3–75.6)	79.0	(78.3–79.8)
31	Portugal	66.3	63.9	(62.5–65.4)	68.6	(66.2–70.5)	71.7	(71.4–72.0)	79.3	(78.8–79.8)
32	Republic of Korea	66.0	63.2	(60.8–65.3)	68.8	(64.0–71.4)	70.5	(69.1–72.2)	78.3	(76.8–79.8)
33	Cuba	65.9	65.1	(63.0–67.2)	66.7	(64.4–68.8)	73.7	(73.3–74.0)	77.5	(77.1–77.8)
34	Czech Republic	65.6	62.9	(61.3–64.4)	68.3	(65.7–70.5)	71.5	(71.3–71.7)	78.2	(78.0–78.6)
35	Chile	65.5	63.5	(61.5–66.0)	67.4	(64.5–70.3)	72.5	(72.0–73.8)	79.5	(78.8–80.4)
36	Costa Rica	65.3	64.2	(61.9–66.9)	66.4	(63.1–69.2)	73.4	(72.7–74.5)	78.8	(78.1–79.8)
37	TFYR Macedonia[a]	64.9	63.9	(62.0–65.6)	65.9	(64.1–67.6)	70.2	(69.8–70.8)	74.8	(74.5–75.3)
38	Brunei Darussalam	64.9	63.8	(61.5–66.0)	65.9	(62.4–69.6)	73.4	(72.1–74.8)	78.7	(77.3–80.3)
39	Kuwait	64.7	64.6	(62.1–66.8)	64.8	(61.4–68.0)	74.2	(73.5–75.0)	76.8	(76.0–77.6)
40	Dominica	64.6	63.2	(59.7–66.1)	66.1	(63.3–69.3)	72.6	(71.5–73.6)	78.3	(77.0–79.7)
41	Serbia and Montenegro	64.3	63.3	(62.1–64.7)	65.4	(63.2–67.3)	69.8	(69.6–70.1)	74.7	(74.5–75.0)
42	Mexico	64.2	63.1	(60.8–65.2)	65.3	(61.5–68.1)	71.0	(70.4–72.0)	76.2	(75.7–76.8)
43	Uruguay	64.1	61.7	(59.0–64.6)	66.5	(63.5–69.4)	70.0	(69.8–70.3)	77.9	(77.5–78.2)
44	Croatia	64.0	60.8	(59.5–62.0)	67.1	(64.7–69.2)	69.8	(69.5–70.1)	77.7	(77.3–78.1)

continued

			Healthy life expectancy (HALE) at birth				Life expectancy at birth			
			Males		Females		Males		Females	
Rank	Member State	Persons								
45	Jamaica	64.0	62.9	(59.8–65.8)	65.0	(62.1–68.1)	72.8	(72.0–74.7)	76.6	(75.3–78.3)
46	Panama	63.9	62.6	(60.1–65.1)	65.3	(62.6–68.0)	71.5	(70.7–72.2)	76.3	(75.8–76.7)
47	Argentina	63.9	61.8	(59.6–64.0)	65.9	(63.0–68.6)	70.2	(69.8–70.6)	77.8	(77.3–78.3)
48	Bosnia and Herze-govina	63.7	62.1	(60.3–64.3)	65.3	(62.8–67.9)	68.7	(67.4–70.7)	74.7	(73.3–76.0)
49	Bulgaria	63.4	61.0	(59.4–62.6)	65.8	(63.8–67.7)	67.4	(66.8–67.6)	74.9	(74.6–75.4)
50	Barbados	63.3	62.3	(59.7–65.0)	64.3	(60.9–67.7)	71.6	(70.4–72.8)	77.7	(76.6–78.9)
51	United Arab Emirates	63.1	62.3	(60.0–64.5)	63.9	(59.9–66.9)	72.3	(71.2–73.5)	76.4	(75.4–77.7)
52	Bahrain	62.7	63.0	(61.0–65.2)	62.3	(59.1–65.1)	72.7	(71.9–73.9)	74.7	(73.7–75.8)
53	Slovakia	62.4	59.6	(58.1–60.9)	65.2	(62.3–67.5)	69.2	(68.8–69.6)	77.5	(77.2–77.9)
54	Venezuela	62.3	60.4	(57.7–63.2)	64.2	(59.9–67.2)	70.6	(70.0–71.2)	76.5	(75.8–77.0)
55	China	62.1	60.9	(59.5–62.5)	63.3	(59.1–65.8)	68.9	(68.2–69.7)	73.0	(72.0–74.2)
56	Saint Lucia	62.0	60.7	(58.1–63.0)	63.3	(60.0–66.5)	69.2	(68.2–69.9)	74.2	(73.1–75.2)
57	Grenada	61.9	62.1	(59.5–65.1)	61.8	(57.8–65.7)	70.9	(69.5–72.1)	73.2	(72.1–74.6)
58	Antigua and Barbuda	61.9	61.7	(58.4–64.8)	62.1	(59.0–65.2)	71.8	(70.5–73.1)	76.6	(75.4–77.9)
59	Poland	61.8	59.3	(57.9–60.5)	64.3	(61.2–66.7)	69.2	(68.9–69.5)	77.7	(77.2–78.2)
60	Romania	61.7	59.5	(57.4–61.4)	64.0	(61.6–66.8)	66.2	(65.5–67.0)	73.5	(72.7–74.6)
61	Trinidad and Tobago	61.7	60.3	(57.9–63.1)	63.0	(59.0–65.8)	68.5	(67.4–70.5)	73.8	(72.8–74.7)
62	Malaysia	61.6	59.7	(57.3–62.1)	63.4	(60.3–66.6)	68.3	(67.4–69.4)	74.1	(73.1–75.3)
63	Tunisia	61.4	61.0	(59.2–62.9)	61.7	(58.0–65.4)	69.2	(68.3–70.0)	73.4	(71.9–74.3)
64	Niue	61.1	60.8	(57.1–64.2)	61.4	(58.6–65.2)	69.5	(66.7–71.9)	72.8	(71.4–77.3)
65	Sri Lanka	61.1	58.6	(55.7–61.5)	63.6	(61.0–67.0)	67.6	(65.1–68.9)	75.3	(73.8–76.0)
66	Colombia	60.9	58.6	(56.2–61.0)	63.3	(59.8–66.2)	67.2	(66.3–68.1)	75.1	(74.3–75.8)
67	Paraguay	60.9	59.9	(56.7–63.4)	61.9	(58.8–65.5)	70.2	(69.0–71.5)	74.2	(72.4–75.7)
68	Saint Vincent & Grenadines	60.9	59.7	(57.1–62.2)	62.1	(59.1–65.0)	67.7	(66.5–68.7)	73.3	(72.2–74.8)
69	Estonia	60.8	56.2	(54.7–57.6)	65.4	(62.5–67.7)	65.4	(64.8–66.1)	76.5	(75.6–77.8)
70	Cook Islands	60.7	60.4	(58.1–62.8)	61.1	(57.7–64.9)	68.7	(67.8–69.4)	72.1	(71.2–73.0)
71	Lebanon	60.7	60.3	(57.6–63.1)	61.1	(57.4–65.1)	69.1	(67.7–70.7)	73.3	(72.2–74.7)
72	Tonga	60.7	59.3	(57.0–61.9)	62.0	(58.4–65.2)	67.4	(66.8–68.3)	72.9	(72.6–73.9)
73	Suriname	60.6	59.5	(57.0–61.9)	61.7	(58.5–64.6)	68.0	(66.6–69.6)	73.5	(71.8–75.3)
74	Qatar	60.6	59.3	(56.5–62.6)	61.8	(58.4–65.4)	70.4	(70.1–70.7)	75.0	(74.6–75.4)
75	Mauritius	60.5	58.6	(55.6–61.3)	62.5	(58.4–66.3)	67.6	(67.0–68.1)	74.6	(74.1–75.0)
76	Ecuador	60.3	58.4	(55.4–61.3)	62.2	(58.6–66.0)	68.2	(67.5–68.9)	74.2	(73.6–74.8)
77	Belarus	60.1	55.4	(53.4–57.5)	64.8	(62.7–66.9)	62.0	(61.0–62.9)	74.0	(73.2–74.9)
78	Hungary	59.9	55.3	(53.7–56.9)	64.5	(61.8–66.7)	66.3	(66.1–66.5)	75.2	(74.9–75.5)
79	Samoa	59.9	58.2	(55.6–60.6)	61.6	(59.0–64.4)	66.7	(65.5–67.7)	72.9	(71.8–74.0)
80	Thailand	59.7	57.7	(55.7–59.7)	61.8	(57.9–64.9)	66.0	(65.0–67.1)	72.4	(71.1–74.2)
81	Oman	59.7	59.2	(57.2–61.4)	60.3	(56.6–63.1)	69.5	(68.4–70.6)	73.5	(72.6–74.5)
82	Saint Kitts and Nevis	59.6	57.6	(54.7–60.7)	61.5	(57.8–65.6)	66.1	(65.3–67.3)	72.0	(70.8–73.3)
83	Fiji	59.6	58.7	(55.9–61.3)	60.5	(56.9–64.3)	66.9	(65.7–68.1)	71.2	(69.9–72.3)
84	Syrian Arab Republic	59.6	59.6	(55.3–60.9)	59.5	(54.9–62.2)	67.4	(66.5–68.0)	71.2	(70.4–71.8)
85	Saudi Arabia	59.5	58.3	(55.0–61.1)	60.7	(56.5–64.9)	68.1	(67.1–69.1)	73.5	(72.7–74.5)
86	Albania	59.4	56.5	(54.4–59.9)	62.3	(60.2–65.2)	64.3	(62.8–65.7)	72.9	(71.6–74.1)
87	Belize	59.2	58.0	(55.2–61.0)	60.4	(55.6–64.9)	69.1	(68.0–70.3)	74.7	(74.0–75.2)
88	Solomon Islands	59.0	58.0	(55.1–61.5)	60.1	(56.6–63.8)	66.6	(64.4–69.6)	71.4	(68.5–75.3)
89	Armenia	59.0	56.9	(55.0–58.6)	61.1	(58.1–64.1)	64.4	(63.8–65.0)	71.2	(70.2–72.2)
90	Philippines	59.0	57.0	(54.3–59.4)	60.9	(57.7–64.3)	64.6	(63.6–65.5)	71.1	(70.0–72.7)
91	Viet Nam	58.9	58.2	(55.6–60.7)	59.7	(56.5–62.8)	66.7	(65.7–67.8)	71.0	(69.9–72.0)
92	Peru	58.8	57.8	(55.2–60.6)	59.8	(56.2–63.6)	66.7	(65.9–67.6)	71.6	(70.4–72.7)
93	Iran (Islamic Republic of)	58.8	59.0	(56.4–61.6)	58.6	(55.3–61.9)	68.1	(67.4–69.0)	69.9	(69.2–70.8)
94	Seychelles	58.7	57.0	(54.1–59.7)	60.4	(57.1–64.0)	66.5	(65.2–67.9)	74.2	(72.4–76.2)

continued

Rank	Member State	Persons	Healthy life expectancy (HALE) at birth				Life expectancy at birth			
			Males		Females		Males		Females	
95	Turkey	58.7	56.8	(55.4–58.2)	60.5	(57.4–63.2)	66.8	(66.6–68.0)	72.5	(71.9–74.0)
96	Jordan	58.5	58.2	(56.4–60.3)	58.8	(56.0–61.4)	68.5	(67.4–70.0)	72.5	(72.1–73.8)
97	Libyan Arab Jamahiriya	58.5	58.4	(55.7–61.4)	58.6	(55.2–62.5)	67.5	(66.4–68.7)	71.0	(70.0–72.2)
98	Republic of Moldova	58.4	55.4	(52.4–57.9)	61.5	(59.1–64.3)	63.1	(62.4–63.8)	70.5	(69.6–71.4)
99	Cape Verde	58.4	56.9	(53.7–60.2)	60.0	(56.3–63.8)	66.5	(64.4–67.9)	72.3	(71.1–73.3)
100	Lithuania	58.4	53.6	(51.6–55.5)	63.2	(60.2–65.9)	66.9	(66.1–67.8)	77.2	(76.7–78.2)
101	Algeria	58.4	58.4	(55.8–61.9)	58.3	(54.5–62.2)	68.1	(66.9–69.4)	71.2	(69.9–72.4)
102	Georgia	58.2	56.1	(54.1–58.3)	60.2	(57.3–62.8)	65.7	(64.0–67.7)	71.8	(70.3–74.2)
103	Bahamas	58.1	57.2	(54.0–60.5)	59.1	(54.2–64.0)	68.0	(67.1–68.9)	74.8	(73.9–75.6)
104	Palau	57.7	56.5	(54.3–58.6)	58.9	(55.7–62.4)	64.7	(63.6–65.2)	69.3	(68.4–70.3)
105	Latvia	57.7	51.4	(49.0–53.5)	63.9	(60.9–66.5)	64.2	(62.8–64.9)	75.5	(74.5–76.5)
106	Indonesia	57.4	56.5	(55.7–58.2)	58.4	(55.8–61.0)	63.4	(62.4–64.6)	67.4	(66.4–68.5)
107	El Salvador	57.3	55.3	(52.0–58.7)	59.4	(55.3–63.3)	66.3	(65.4–67.1)	73.3	(72.4–74.4)
108	Egypt	57.1	57.1	(55.4–58.8)	57.0	(54.1–59.3)	65.4	(64.8–66.0)	69.1	(68.5–69.7)
109	Brazil	57.1	54.9	(51.4–58.1)	59.2	(54.8–64.1)	64.5	(63.0–65.7)	71.9	(70.2–73.5)
110	Tuvalu	57.0	56.4	(54.0–58.9)	57.6	(54.0–61.0)	63.6	(62.0–64.8)	67.6	(65.7–68.7)
111	Nicaragua	56.9	55.8	(51.8–60.3)	58.0	(54.3–62.4)	66.4	(65.4–67.5)	71.1	(70.2–72.0)
112	Ukraine	56.8	52.3	(51.0–53.7)	61.3	(58.0–63.5)	62.6	(62.0–63.1)	73.3	(72.9–73.8)
113	Honduras	56.8	55.8	(52.5–59.6)	57.8	(53.6–62.0)	66.3	(64.5–67.9)	71.0	(69.2–72.5)
114	Vanuatu	56.7	56.0	(52.6–59.7)	57.4	(53.6–61.8)	64.2	(60.5–69.1)	68.1	(64.2–72.3)
115	Micronesia[b]	56.6	55.8	(52.8–58.8)	57.5	(54.0–61.0)	63.7	(61.6–66.1)	67.7	(65.8–69.9)
116	Dominican Republic	56.2	54.7	(50.9–58.2)	57.7	(53.4–61.9)	65.5	(64.5–66.4)	71.6	(70.5–72.6)
117	Marshall Islands	56.1	54.8	(51.9–57.9)	57.4	(54.3–60.3)	62.8	(61.4–64.3)	67.8	(66.6–69.0)
118	Russian Federation	55.5	50.3	(48.6–52.4)	60.6	(57.0–63.3)	59.4	(58.4–60.8)	72.0	(71.6–73.0)
119	DPR Korea[c]	55.4	54.9	(51.5–58.4)	56.0	(52.2–59.8)	64.5	(62.0–66.3)	67.2	(64.6–69.2)
120	Azerbaijan	55.4	53.3	(50.6–56.3)	57.5	(54.3–60.8)	61.7	(59.2–64.2)	68.9	(66.6–71.3)
121	Morocco	54.9	55.3	(53.4–57.3)	54.5	(51.3–57.2)	66.1	(65.2–67.4)	70.4	(68.7–71.4)
122	Guatemala	54.7	53.5	(49.9–57.2)	56.0	(52.3–59.7)	63.5	(62.2–65.2)	68.6	(67.2–70.6)
123	Kazakhstan	54.3	50.5	(48.0–53.1)	58.1	(55.6–60.6)	58.0	(57.6–58.9)	68.4	(67.2–70.0)
124	Uzbekistan	54.3	52.7	(49.2–56.3)	55.8	(51.5–60.2)	62.1	(61.6–62.9)	68.0	(67.3–68.9)
125	Kiribati	53.6	52.8	(49.6–56.1)	54.4	(50.7–57.9)	60.4	(57.8–64.0)	64.5	(61.2–67.3)
126	Nauru	52.9	50.4	(47.0–54.4)	55.4	(51.0–60.2)	58.8	(55.3–62.9)	66.6	(62.5–71.3)
127	Kyrgyzstan	52.6	49.6	(46.5–53.1)	55.6	(51.2–60.1)	60.0	(58.5–61.7)	68.8	(66.8–70.8)
128	Iraq	52.6	52.6	(48.6–57.0)	52.5	(48.6–57.3)	61.7	(59.7–64.0)	64.7	(62.2–67.0)
129	Mongolia	52.4	50.3	(46.3–54.3)	54.5	(50.8–58.2)	61.2	(59.1–62.6)	66.9	(65.4–68.4)
130	Maldives	52.4	54.2	(50.3–58.2)	50.6	(46.4–55.9)	64.6	(62.9–66.2)	64.4	(62.4–66.7)
131	Turkmenistan	52.1	51.2	(48.3–54.3)	53.0	(50.1–56.7)	60.0	(59.3–60.8)	64.9	(64.3–66.0)
132	Guyana	52.1	51.4	(48.3–54.6)	52.8	(47.7–58.4)	61.5	(59.2–63.2)	67.0	(64.9–69.8)
133	India	52.0	52.2	(50.2–54.2)	51.7	(48.5–54.8)	59.8	(58.5–62.0)	62.7	(60.8–65.6)
134	Bolivia	51.4	51.4	(47.4–55.5)	51.4	(47.1–55.9)	60.9	(59.1–62.4)	63.6	(62.7–65.9)
135	Tajikistan	50.8	49.6	(46.2–53.2)	52.0	(47.8–56.1)	60.4	(59.0–62.3)	64.7	(63.0–66.9)
136	Sao Tome and Principe	50.0	50.3	(46.8–53.6)	49.7	(44.8–54.7)	60.3	(57.8–62.5)	61.9	(60.0–64.2)
137	Bangladesh	49.3	50.6	(47.4–54.1)	47.9	(43.6–52.6)	60.4	(58.6–62.3)	60.8	(59.1–62.6)
138	Bhutan	49.2	50.1	(44.8–55.1)	48.2	(43.5–53.7)	60.4	(57.0–64.4)	62.5	(58.9–66.3)
139	Yemen	49.1	48.9	(45.7–51.9)	49.3	(44.4–53.9)	59.3	(57.6–60.9)	62.0	(60.9–63.5)
140	Myanmar	49.1	47.7	(43.8–51.6)	50.5	(45.7–54.3)	56.2	(53.5–58.0)	61.1	(57.6–62.8)
141	Pakistan	48.1	50.2	(46.6–54.2)	46.1	(41.5–51.1)	60.1	(58.6–62.5)	60.7	(58.6–63.1)
142	Cambodia	47.1	45.6	(43.1–48.0)	48.7	(45.4–52.4)	53.4	(52.7–54.2)	58.5	(57.9–59.5)
143	Gambia	46.9	47.3	(44.1–50.6)	46.6	(42.4–50.8)	55.9	(52.4–59.4)	58.7	(55.2–62.2)
144	Papua New Guinea	46.8	46.6	(42.8–50.5)	47.1	(43.6–50.9)	55.1	(52.8–57.7)	57.5	(54.8–60.0)
145	Ghana	46.7	46.5	(43.4–49.7)	46.9	(43.5–51.1)	55.0	(53.7–56.8)	57.9	(56.0–59.8)
146	Gabon	46.6	46.8	(42.9–50.0)	46.5	(42.6–49.9)	54.6	(50.3–59.0)	56.9	(51.9–60.2)

continued

Rank	Member State	Persons	Healthy life expectancy (HALE) at birth				Life expectancy at birth			
			Males		Females		Males		Females	
147	Comoros	46.0	46.2	(42.8–49.6)	45.8	(41.4–50.3)	55.3	(53.6–57.1)	58.1	(56.3–59.8)
148	Nepal	45.8	47.5	(44.4–51.1)	44.2	(39.1–49.8)	58.5	(56.8–60.5)	58.0	(56.5–59.7)
149	Sudan	45.1	45.7	(42.2–49.3)	44.4	(39.2–50.2)	55.4	(52.9–59.1)	57.8	(55.1–61.5)
150	Senegal	44.9	45.2	(42.1–48.0)	44.5	(40.9–48.4)	54.0	(52.6–56.0)	56.1	(54.7–58.1)
151	Equatorial Guinea	44.8	44.9	(40.6–48.7)	44.8	(40.2–49.4)	53.5	(49.0–57.0)	56.2	(52.4–59.6)
152	Laos[d]	44.7	43.7	(39.1–47.5)	45.7	(40.6–49.6)	52.2	(47.4–54.9)	56.1	(52.0–58.3)
153	South Africa	43.2	43.0	(41.1–45.0)	43.5	(40.5–46.4)	49.6	(48.8–50.6)	52.1	(51.0–53.0)
154	Haiti	43.1	41.3	(37.0–46.2)	44.9	(38.8–51.1)	49.7	(47.0–56.9)	56.1	(52.4–62.2)
155	Madagascar	42.9	43.2	(40.6–46.1)	42.6	(38.0–47.3)	51.7	(50.3–53.7)	54.6	(53.2–56.6)
156	Togo	42.7	42.7	(39.3–46.5)	42.7	(39.3–46.8)	50.5	(48.1–54.0)	53.0	(50.5–56.6)
157	Congo	42.6	42.5	(39.3–47.0)	42.8	(39.1–47.2)	50.1	(46.8–52.7)	52.9	(49.5–56.4)
158	Benin	42.5	43.1	(39.8–46.5)	41.9	(37.5–46.5)	51.7	(50.4–53.0)	53.8	(52.5–55.8)
159	Nigeria	41.6	42.1	(39.2–45.0)	41.1	(37.7–45.0)	49.8	(48.3–51.9)	51.4	(49.8–53.6)
160	Mauritania	41.5	42.1	(37.7–46.3)	40.8	(35.5–46.0)	51.7	(49.2–54.2)	53.5	(51.1–56.2)
161	Eritrea	41.0	41.4	(38.1–45.0)	40.5	(36.5–45.0)	49.1	(46.6–52.6)	51.0	(48.3–54.6)
162	Kenya	40.7	41.2	(38.7–44.4)	40.1	(36.7–43.8)	48.2	(46.2–50.3)	49.6	(47.5–51.8)
163	Cameroon	40.4	40.9	(37.6–44.0)	39.9	(36.7–43.2)	49.0	(47.6–50.4)	50.4	(48.9–51.9)
164	Guinea	40.3	40.4	(36.7–44.0)	40.1	(35.9–45.5)	49.0	(47.4–51.1)	52.0	(50.4–54.1)
165	Chad	39.3	38.6	(35.3–43.7)	39.9	(36.1–44.5)	47.4	(46.1–48.7)	51.1	(49.7–52.6)
166	Cote d'Ivoire	39.0	39.1	(36.7–42.6)	38.9	(35.9–42.1)	46.4	(44.9–48.5)	48.4	(46.8–50.6)
167	Zimbabwe	38.8	39.6	(37.4–41.9)	38.1	(34.7–41.3)	45.4	(44.7–46.5)	46.0	(44.9–47.1)
168	Swaziland	38.2	38.8	(34.1–44.2)	37.6	(32.6–42.7)	44.7	(39.4–50.7)	45.6	(40.8–52.0)
169	Tanzania[e]	38.1	38.6	(35.4–42.7)	37.5	(34.0–41.1)	45.8	(45.1–46.7)	47.2	(46.4–47.9)
170	Liberia	37.8	38.2	(34.0–42.4)	37.4	(33.5–41.5)	46.6	(43.3–51.3)	49.1	(45.7–53.9)
171	Botswana	37.3	38.1	(34.3–42.0)	36.5	(33.2–40.0)	44.6	(42.4–47.1)	44.4	(42.3–46.5)
172	Angola	36.9	36.2	(33.7–42.0)	37.6	(33.3–42.8)	44.3	(40.8–47.9)	48.3	(44.9–52.0)
173	Guinea-Bissau	36.6	36.7	(33.6–39.8)	36.4	(33.0–40.3)	44.5	(43.4–46.0)	46.9	(45.7–48.5)
174	Uganda	35.7	36.2	(33.4–39.8)	35.2	(31.1–39.6)	43.5	(40.8–47.3)	44.6	(41.7–48.7)
175	Namibia	35.6	36.5	(32.5–41.2)	34.7	(31.4–38.8)	42.8	(39.2–48.1)	42.6	(39.2–47.6)
176	Ethiopia	35.4	35.7	(32.2–40.9)	35.1	(30.4–40.9)	42.8	(39.0–48.3)	44.7	(40.5–50.5)
177	Lesotho	35.3	36.1	(33.1–39.7)	34.5	(31.2–38.7)	42.0	(38.8–45.7)	42.2	(38.6–47.3)
178	Djibouti	35.1	35.6	(31.3–40.4)	34.6	(30.1–39.6)	43.5	(39.9–48.2)	44.7	(40.1–49.3)
179	Somalia	35.1	35.5	(32.5–38.9)	34.7	(30.6–38.8)	43.8	(42.6–45.4)	45.9	(44.7–47.6)
180	Burkina Faso	34.8	35.4	(32.5–38.3)	34.1	(30.5–37.9)	42.6	(42.0–43.4)	43.6	(42.9–44.4)
181	Mali	34.5	34.8	(31.5–39.3)	34.1	(29.5–38.9)	42.7	(40.3–45.2)	44.6	(42.2–47.3)
182	DR Congo[f]	34.4	34.4	(31.6–39.4)	34.4	(30.5–39.3)	41.6	(38.6–45.8)	44.0	(41.2–47.5)
183	Central African Republic	34.1	34.7	(31.6–38.2)	33.6	(30.3–37.3)	41.6	(40.3–43.1)	42.5	(41.1–44.4)
184	Afghanistan	33.8	35.1	(30.3–40.4)	32.5	(26.2–39.5)	44.2	(38.5–50.1)	45.1	(39.2–51.7)
185	Burundi	33.4	33.9	(30.4–37.5)	32.9	(29.3–36.9)	40.6	(37.7–43.7)	41.3	(38.2–45.5)
186	Niger	33.1	33.9	(30.9–37.7)	32.4	(27.1–37.6)	42.7	(40.5–46.1)	43.9	(42.1–46.7)
187	Zambia	33.0	33.7	(30.6–37.0)	32.3	(28.9–36.1)	39.2	(36.1–43.8)	39.5	(36.5–43.7)
188	Rwanda	31.9	32.0	(29.6–36.5)	31.8	(28.3–36.2)	38.5	(36.8–41.1)	40.5	(38.6–43.3)
189	Mozambique	31.3	31.5	(28.9–34.9)	31.1	(28.1–34.7)	37.9	(36.7–39.5)	39.5	(38.2–41.2)
190	Malawi	30.9	31.4	(28.2–34.6)	30.5	(26.8–34.4)	37.1	(33.6–41.1)	37.8	(34.0–42.2)
191	Sierra Leone	29.5	29.7	(26.4–36.0)	29.3	(25.2–35.1)	37.0	(32.9–43.3)	38.8	(35.3–44.7)

a. The Former Yugoslav Republic of Macedonia

b. Federated States of Micronesia

c. Democratic People's Republic of Korea

d. Lao People's Democratic Republic

e. United Republic of Tanzania

f. Democratic Republic of the Congo

Chapter 34

A Framework for Measuring Health Inequality

Emmanuela Gakidou, Christopher J.L. Murray, Julio Frenk[1]

Introduction

Health inequalities are prominent in the policy agenda (*1–22*). Average achievement is no longer considered a sufficient indicator of a country's performance on health; rather, the distribution of health in the population is also key and should be measured as a distinct dimension of the performance of health systems (*23*).

Health inequality is defined as variations in health status across individuals in a population (*16*). This approach, which is consistent with the measurement of inequality in other fields, such as economics, allows us to perform cross-country comparisons and study the determinants of health inequality (*24*).

This chapter addresses the question of measuring health inequalities as distinct from measuring the average levels of health. An important policy debate is the trade-off between policies that improve the average level of health and policies that primarily reduce inequalities in health. How this trade-off should be resolved is not, however, the subject of this chapter.

In the first section, we ask what is the quantity that we would fundamentally want to be equally distributed in a population. In other words, we attempt to answer the classic question in the context of health: equality of what (*25*)? We believe it is critical for a clear debate on health inequality to first articulate what the quantity of interest is and why, and then proceed to measure it, depending on the available data. There has to be a clear definition and measurement framework before the applied work can be undertaken. In section two we discuss various ways of summarizing the distribution of the quantity of interest and calculating an index of health inequality, and address the three distinct normative issues that are raised. In section three, we discuss the overall WHO strategy for measurement and we conclude by highlighting the critical relevance to

research and policy formulation of this approach to measuring health inequality.

Equality of What?

In addressing the question "What would we like to be equally distributed in the population," several ethical and technical issues arise. Would we consider that perfect equality exists when all individuals live the same number of years? When they enjoy the same level of health? When they have the exact same health status at all points in their lives? In this section we address some of the normative issues surrounding the choice of the quantity that we would like to have equally distributed in a population.

Equality of Healthy Life Span

Imagine a cohort of individuals born in the year 2000. What would we need to observe in order to say that there was complete equality in health among them? One starting point might be to argue that everyone in the population should have the same healthy life span. In other words, we would like all members of a cohort to live the same number of years and to have on average the same health status during their lives. Later, we will return to further considerations of equality of healthy life span.

Healthy life span is a summary measure of survival and of the non-fatal health outcomes weighted by their preference weights. Figure 34.1 illustrates the healthy life span for an individual i. The horizontal axis is the age of the individual; here the individual is assumed to live to the age of 100 years. On the vertical axis is the per cent of full health the individual enjoyed at each age. If the individual in the diagram lived for 100 years in full health and suddenly died at the age of 100, his

Figure 34.1 Healthy life span for an individual

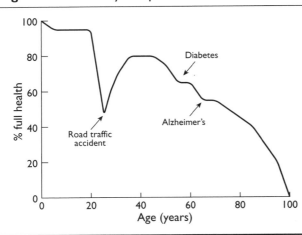

healthy life span would be the whole area of the graph and would be equal to 100. If this individual during his lifetime experienced any sort of decrement from full health, then we would represent his healthy life span by a different curve, such as the one shown in Figure 34.1, which would take into account the time spent in health states less than full health that this individual experienced. The individual shown in Figure 34.1 was born in full health, had a motor vehicle accident at the age of 25, experienced diabetes at the age of 50, and Alzheimer's disease at the age of 65.

The actual calculation of the healthy life span for individual *i* depends on the weights that one assigns to the various health states worse than full health; the methods and debates surrounding the measurement of health state weights are addressed elsewhere (*26–31*).

We need to distinguish between an individual's healthy life span and the set of health risks that he/she is exposed to at each age of his/her life. Health risks are the probabilities of death, and incidence and remission of non-fatal health outcomes of differing severities that individuals face at each age. We are not able to measure health risks at the individual level, but we are developing methods to approximate them. By combining across all ages an individual's risks of being in a state less than full health, we calculate health expectancy, i.e. the expected number of years lived in full health, given a set of health risks. A given level of health expectancy can result from more than one underlying pattern of health risks. Health risks can be seen as underlying healthy life span, or healthy life span may be considered the realization of a set of health risks.

For all individuals in a cohort to have equal healthy life spans, two conditions are necessary and sufficient: a) all individuals have equal health expectancies; and b) individuals' risks of death, and incidence and remission for non-fatal health outcomes are rectangular. Equal health expectancies means that the area under the health survivorship function (Figure 34.2) is equal.[2] A rectangular risk curve means the risks of mortality, incidence and remission are either 0 or 1 at all ages.[3] Because it is essentially impossible for all risks to be rectangular—for example, we will never be able to reduce the risk of injury to zero—the ideal of equal healthy life spans will never be realized.

In addition, some may argue that differences in healthy life spans that are strictly due to chance are not relevant to measuring health inequality. Individuals faced with exactly the same health survival function at each age may have very different healthy life

Figure 34.2A Health survivorship function

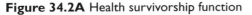
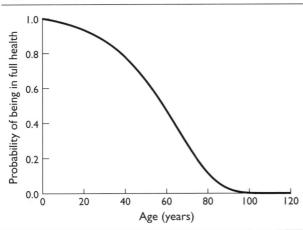

Figure 34.2B Distribution of healthy life span

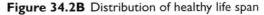
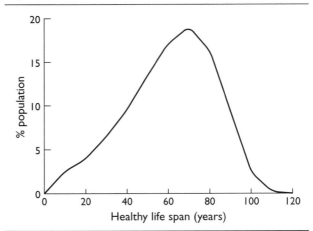

spans due to chance. Healthy life span is the realization of a health survivorship function. Figure 34.2A illustrates a particular health survival function by age which corresponds to a health expectancy of 56.5 years, and Figure 34.2B the distribution of healthy life spans that may be observed in a population of 50 000 in which all individuals were exposed to the distribution of the health risks shown. In Figure 34.2A, the y-axis is the average proportion of full health attained by the population at each age, and the x-axis is age. In Figure 34.2B, the x-axis is healthy life span observed and the y-axis is the per cent of individuals that achieved this value of healthy life span from a cohort of 50 000. At the onset, everyone in this cohort had a healthy life expectancy of 56.5 years, but due solely to chance healthy life spans range from 1 to 110 years. It is impressive that all of the variation in healthy life span that is seen in Figure 34.2B has resulted from complete equality in health risks for the cohort of 50 000 individuals.

If some individuals have a healthy life span of 10 years and others of 90 years simply due to chance, should this be reflected in a measure of health inequality? Clearly, for all populations that are large enough, the chance component of the distribution of healthy life spans would be the same if the underlying set of health risks by age were the same.

Equality of healthy life span is not an achievable goal for a population. It could only be realized if risks of incidence and remission of non-fatal health outcomes, and risks of mortality were either zero or one for the entire population. Given that this is unfeasible and that it is unlikely that differences in the level of health inequality observed across countries are due to distinct levels of luck/chance in those countries, we

are more interested in the distribution of health risks across individuals in a population and comparing these distributions across populations.

EQUALITY OF HEALTH RISKS

Each individual has a profile of health risks by age that can be summarized in a health survivorship function (similar to the one shown for a cohort in Figure 34.2A). This profile of health risks can be characterized by two distinct attributes. First, the area under the curve shown in Figure 34.2A is the health expectancy of the individual: the average healthy life span for an individual faced with a health survivorship function.[4] Different profiles of health risks by age can have equal health expectancies. In other words, health survivorship curves can differ in their shape, while the area under the curve remains constant.

Both differences in the health expectancies across individuals and differences in the shape of health risks across age can contribute to unequal healthy life spans above and beyond those contributed by chance. To help understand the contribution of these two factors to the inequality of healthy life spans, we will take advantage of the often observed linear relationship between the log of age-specific mortality rates and age (32;33).[5] The shape of the health risks which incorporate the probabilities of non-fatal health outcomes will be somewhat different, but as there is a strong relationship between the prevalence of non-fatal health outcomes worse than full health with age (34), these curves will be used to illustrate the general point.

Figure 34.3A shows the log of the risk of an ill-health outcome or death for two different populations. In each of the populations, all individuals have an

Figure 34.3A Health risk by age

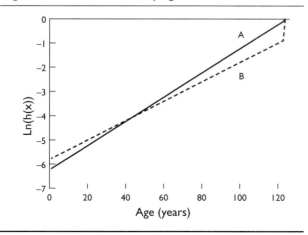

Figure 34.3B Distribution of realized healthy life span

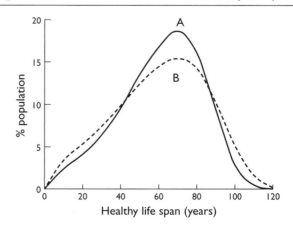

identical set of ill-health risks (or health survivorship functions) by age, as shown, and the health expectancy in each population is 56.5 years. Because the slope of the health risk curve in population A is steeper than the one in population B, the distribution of healthy life span (shown in Figure 34.3B) for population A has a lower variance that the distribution for population B (variance of 437 for population A versus 568 for B), although they have the same mean.

Silber (*35*) and LeGrand (*36;37*) have sought to measure the inequality in the age of death due to variations in the slope of the log death rate. The concept is quite similar to inequality in healthy life span, instead applied solely to risks of death. Figure 34.4 illustrates a generally observed phenomenon for women in the UK: as mortality declines, the slope of the logarithm of the death rate increases. In other words, there is a strong relationship between the level of mortality and the inequality in the age of death (or years of life lived) that is contributed by the slope of the death rate. Not surprisingly, LeGrand and Silber conclude that as mortality declines, inequality measured in this way declines.

If everyone in populations A and B has an identical health expectancy but the age profile of health risks differs only in the slope and intercept of the log of health risks as a function of age, is this contributor to the inequality in healthy life span relevant to measuring health inequality? A number of arguments suggest that variation in the average pattern of health risks between populations may not be of much substantive interest. First, across populations there is a strong relationship between the slope of the mortality risk and age—and presumably the health risk function and age—such that inequality measured in this way decreases as mortality declines. Second, holding health expectancy constant, there are few policies or interventions to alter the slope of this relationship and thus reduce inequality in healthy life span. Third, it is not at all clear that everyone would share a common preference for the age profile of health risks. Consider a choice of health risk profiles both with the same health expectancy of 54 years. In the first, there is a 10% probability of death in the first week of life, followed by 0% risk of death until the age of 60, and then a 100% risk of death. In the second, there is a 0% chance of death until age 20, when the risk of death is 10%, followed by 0% risk until the age of 57.8 years, and then a 100% risk of death. Few would choose the latter as death at 1 day seems preferable to death at age 20, but consideration of the inequality of the

distribution of realized life spans (as in Figure 34.3B) would lead to preferring the second scenario.

Studies of social group differences and small area analyses have shown that within a cohort there is great variation in health expectancy across individuals (*1;15;17;38–40*). Some individuals face higher risks of ill health and mortality at every age and others face much lower risks. This variation in health expectancy across individuals at a given age is not reflected in the average health survivorship curve of the population. The health survivorship function shows the average probabilities, without any additional information on how these probabilities are distributed across the population.

Figure 34.5 illustrates the healthy life span for a population where individual health expectancies vary from 47 to 82 years, but the slope of the log health risk function is the same for all individuals. All individuals' health survivorship functions lie in between the bounds shown, and are parallel to the bounds. The thicker curve in the middle, curve B, represents the average risk of ill-health for the population at each age, which corresponds to a health expectancy of 56.5 years. Figure 34.5B shows that a population in which health risk curves lie anywhere between the two bounds shown in Figure 34.5A, will have almost the same inequality in terms of healthy life spans shown in Figure 34.5B, as a population in which all individuals have the same health risk curve, curve B in Figure 34.5A. So, in terms of healthy life span, the two populations have almost the same amount of health inequality. However, looking at the distribution of expected life span, or health expectancy (Figure 34.5A) most would agree that the population where individuals lie anywhere in the range of 47 to 82 years has much greater health inequality

Figure 34.4   Mortality rates by age, UK females, 1901–1995

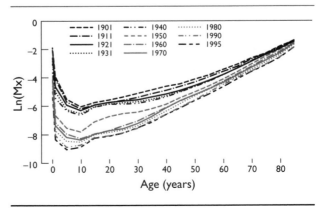

than the population where health expectancy is 56.5 years for all individuals.

For the reasons detailed above, our concern about variation across individuals in health expectancy seems much more important than differences between populations in the slope of the average health risk curve as a function of age.

Figure 34.5 also illustrates an important phenomenon in observing any cohort. The average health expectancy in Figure 34.5A is 56.5 years, but the realized average cohort life span is 58.7 years. The high risk individuals tend to die at younger ages so the realized mortality at older ages reflects the risks of those with better health expectancies. This selection effect which can be substantial in populations with considerable inequality, leads to the paradoxical situation that inequality in health expectancy will increase the average realized cohort life span.

It is notable that the difference between the distributions of health expectancy is very large in the populations in Figure 34.5A, ranging from no variation for population B to a large variation for population A. The difference in the distribution of the outcome, i.e. healthy life span, resulting from these very different distributions of risk, is not that large. A remarkable increase in inequality of health expectancy has a relatively small effect on the distribution of healthy life span. This indicates that the chance component in the realization of the expectation is large.

We believe that the distribution of health expectancy for a cohort is of more interest for studying health inequality than the distribution of healthy life spans. Likewise, we think that the shape of the average health risk curve or variation in the shape of health risk curves holding health expectancy constant may be

of interest. However, for the study of health inequality we find it to be less relevant than simply the distribution of health expectancy.

The Distribution of Health Expectancy Attributable to Unavoidable Factors or Choice

One might argue that we should be uninterested in two components of the distribution of health expectancy for a cohort: the component that is not amenable to change and the component that arises from fully informed choices of individuals to decrease their health expectancy through the pursuit of risky activities.

If there were differences in health expectancy that could never be remedied either with current or with future technology, one could perhaps persuasively argue that we should be uninterested in the above just as we have argued that we are uninterested in the dispersion of healthy life spans strictly due to chance. If such differences were measurable and common, it would be a strong argument to measure inequality in terms of health gaps rather than health expectancies. (Health gaps are the difference between the maximum achievable health expectancy for a given individual and the actual health expectancy.) But which component of the distribution of health expectancy is not amenable to intervention? That due to genes? That due to chance during birth? In both cases, the argument that we cannot intervene to change the effects on the distribution of health expectancy is most likely specious. With current improvements in technology and future progress, it is likely that these components of the distribution of health expectancy will become amenable to change and thus should not be excluded

Figure 34.5A Health risk by age

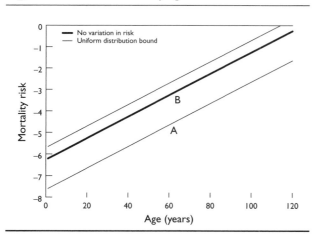

Figure 34.5B Distribution of healthy life span

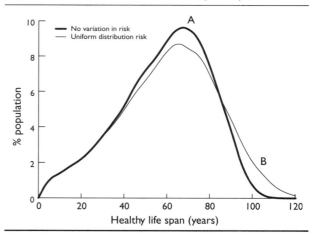

from a measure of health inequality. Perhaps as important is the argument that there is little evidence of significant cross-population variation in the contribution of genes etc. No convincing evidence exists at the health expectancy level that any population group has a lower distribution of health expectancy due to factors which are impossible to change. The component of health expectancy distribution due to unavoidable factors is likely to be small and completely impossible to assess. From here on, we will assume that it is best to not worry about this aspect.

What about volition? How much of the distribution of health expectancy for a population is due to fully informed choices of individuals who have a taste for risky behaviour? This seems like a very slippery slope. What real choices affecting health are fully informed? Would we exclude the effects of tobacco on health expectancy which are likely to be very great because smoking is a choice? In most cases, it is not a well informed choice when a minor takes up the addictive habit. But in the cases where we can claim the choice is informed, should it be excluded? We would argue that it should not. First, in most cases health risks are not adopted because of a love for risky behaviour, but rather for other, less informed reasons. Second, the true volitional component of the distribution of health expectancy is likely to be very small and can well be ignored. This argument is similar to the ones in the field of income inequality, where the variation in the distribution of income due to different leisure income trade-offs in the population is routinely ignored in the measurement of income inequality.

From Cohort to Period Measures of Health Expectancy

If we could directly measure every individual's risks of incidence, remission and mortality at each age, we would be able to construct the distribution of health expectancies for a cohort. To estimate each individual's cohort health expectancy, we would in principle need to know the health risks for individuals who by chance may have died at a young age. In theory, a reasonably good estimate of the distribution of health expectancy for the cohort could be obtained. From a policy perspective, waiting over 100 years to measure health inequality for each birth cohort would not be useful. Since health inequality is a critical component of measuring health systems performance, we need to measure health inequality using only information collected in one period of time. In other words, we have

to conceptualize a period measure of the distribution of health expectancy.

In the estimation of a period measure, however, we only have information on individual i at one age a. To estimate the distribution of health expectancies, we need to relate this measurement to the distribution of risks at another age for a different set of individuals. In order to relate risks for different groups of individuals across time, there has to be a formal principle for linking observed risks of various individuals to estimate the health expectancy of a hypothetical birth cohort, exposed to currently observed risks. In order to estimate the period distribution of health expectancy, we could follow one of two strategies: 1) Use some other variable, such as a socioeconomic status indicator that can link individuals at different ages. This approach would underestimate the distribution of health expectancies in a period because it assumes that all variation in health risks is predicted by the socioeconomic variable selected. 2) Assume an arbitrary correlation of risk between age groups, less than or equal to one.

It is clearly a bigger issue to address the basic challenge of estimating risk distributions since they are largely unobservable, but nevertheless, the development of standardized and comparable health inequality measures will require some explicit method of developing a period distribution of health expectancy from various age-specific distributions of health risks.

In summary, we argue that the most relevant quantity of interest for studying health inequality is the distribution of health expectancy across individuals, constructed for a period, using a clearly defined method for linking the distributions of health risks at different ages.

Summarizing the Distribution of Health Expectancy in a Measure of Health Inequality

Figure 34.6 illustrates the distribution of health expectancies for three populations, A, B, and C. Which distribution of health expectancy is more unequal? If the x-axis in the graph were income, rather than health expectancy, most people would agree that distribution B is less unequal than C and A. This simple conclusion is based on the concept of decreasing marginal utility of income, namely that an extra dollar generates less utility as income rises. Distribution B has the same variance as A, but a higher mean, so that if this were income the variance would have less importance. In terms of a commonly used measure of inequality, the

Figure 34.6   Distribution of healthy life expectancy

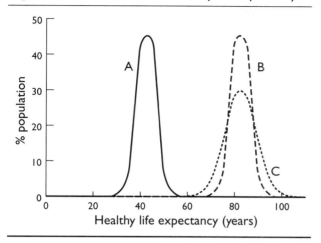

Gini coefficient, distributions A and C have the same amount of inequality, while distribution B has lower inequality than A and C. While for income some people may be in agreement that distributions A and C have equal amounts of inequality, for health, this finding may be met with less accord. The notion of declining marginal utility does not apply as persuasively, as some would claim that an extra year of healthy life generates as much utility at high levels of health expectancy as at low levels. Those who want to measure absolute inequalities in health would say that C is clearly worse than A or B, and that they cannot distinguish between A and B. The vast literature on measuring income inequality (25;41–44) is very helpful in the design of a health inequality measure, but this simple example illustrates that health has some fundamental differences from income that require special consideration. To date in the literature on measuring health inequality, there has been little substantive discussion on summary measures of distributions of health.

TWO FAMILIES OF HEALTH INEQUALITY MEASURES

Based on the wide array of measures used to summarize the distribution of income (44) and taking into account the fact that absolute, and not just relative, differences in health expectancies may matter, we propose two families of measures: individual-mean differences and interindividual differences.

Individual-Mean Differences

Measures of individual-mean differences compare each individual's health to the mean of the population. The general form is:

$$IMD(\alpha, \beta) = \frac{\sum_{i=1}^{n} \left| h_i - \bar{h} \right|^{\alpha}}{n\bar{h}^{\beta}}$$

where h_i is the health of individual i, $\bar{h}$ is the average health of the population, and n is the number of individuals in the population. The parameter α changes the significance attached to differences in health observed at the ends of the distribution, compared to differences observed near the mean of the distribution. The parameter β controls the extent to which the measure is purely relative to the mean or absolute. A common example of individual-mean differences is the variance when $\alpha = 2$ and $\beta = 0$. However, many other individual-mean difference measures are possible. When $\alpha = \beta = 1$ the measure is strictly relative, and when $\beta = 0$ it is measuring absolute deviations from the mean but β could be any value between 0 or 1, reflecting some mix of concern between relative and absolute individual-mean difference.

Interindividual Differences

Another family of measures is based on comparing each individual's health (or income) to every other individual's health, rather than comparing each individual to the mean of the population. We propose the general form of these measures to be:

$$IID(\alpha, \beta) = \frac{\sum_{i=1}^{n} \sum_{j=1}^{n} \left| h_i - h_j \right|^{\alpha}}{2n^2 \bar{h}^{\beta}}$$

where h_i is the health of individual i and h_j is the health of individual j, $\bar{h}$ is the mean health of the population and n is the number of individuals in the population. The parameters α and β are the same as for the individual-mean measures described above. A well-known example of this family is the Gini coefficient (45), a relative measure often used to report income distribution, where $\alpha = 1$ and $\beta = 1$. The Gini is frequently represented as being derived graphically from the Lorenz curve (46) of a population, but in fact it is algebraically equal to the equation above. It is worth noting that when $\alpha = 2$ the individual-mean difference and the interindividual difference for any given population distribution are identical. For any other values of α they are different.

CHOOSING A SINGLE INDEX OF HEALTH INEQUALITY

For standard comparisons we need to choose a single index of health inequality to summarize the distribution of health expectancy for a population. This choice requires the resolution of three fundamentally normative issues: which family of measures, what should be the value of α, and what should be the value of β. These choices are normative and an individual's preferences for these can be elicited through a series of questions that isolate the effect of each on the index of inequality.

We will provide illustrative examples of what these choices entail. For simplicity reasons we will use a population of seven individuals (which can be thought of as seven homogeneous groups of individuals). In each example we will transfer a specified amount of years of health expectancy from an individual who is better off (i.e. has higher health expectancy) to an individual who is worse off. The transfers will be described in the text and are also depicted in Figures 34.7–34.9. There are three types of choices to be made. For each choice we present two populations and ask "Which represents a greater decrease in inequality: the transfer in population A or the transfer in population B?"

β: Relative versus Absolute Inequality

One of the key choices that has to be explicitly made is whether we are more concerned about absolute differences in health, relative differences in health, or a mix of both with some weights, depending on our preferences. Figure 34.7 illustrates reductions of health inequality in two populations brought about by transferring equivalent years of health expectancy from the better off to the worse off. With this question we can attempt to measure the extent to which individuals are concerned about relative inequality, absolute inequality, or some mixture of both. The situation depicted in Figure 34.7 is the following: populations A and B have similar distributions of healthy life expectancy across the seven individuals, but at different levels. In population A the mean is 20 years, while in population B it is 60 years. In population A, 5 years of healthy life expectancy are transferred from an individual whose healthy life expectancy is 35 years to an individual whose healthy life expectancy is 5 years. In population B, 5 years of health expectancy are transferred from an individual with health expectancy of 75 years (highest in the population) to an individual with health expectancy of 45 years (lowest in the population). Which of the two transfers results in a greater decrease of health inequality?

With questions such as this, we can elicit people's preferences for a value of β, between 0 and 1, i.e. for their preferences for an absolute or a relative measure of inequality.

α: Intensity of Health Gain/Loss

The second normative choice has to do with whether gains or losses of health that occur at the ends of the distribution should be treated differently from gains or losses of health that occur near the mean. Consider the two reductions in health inequality depicted in Figure 34.8. Both populations are at the same level of health expectancy, with a mean value of 20 years. In population A, 5 years of health expectancy are transferred from the individual with the highest value (35 years) to the individual with the lowest value (5 years). In population B, 5 years of health expectancy are transferred from the individual with health expectancy of 30 years to the individual with a health expectancy of 10 years. Which of the two transfers represents a greater decrease in health inequality?

If scenario A is chosen, then the measure used would need to weigh more heavily transfers of health occurring at the ends of the distribution. If the respondent

Figure 34.7 Transfer of healthy life expectancy

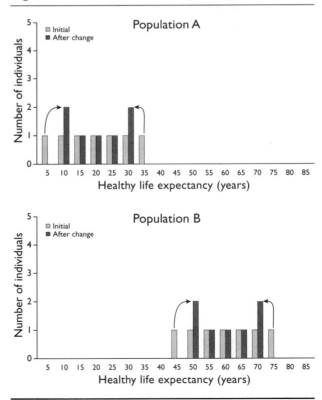

is indifferent, then all transfers of the same amount should be weighed equally, regardless of which part of the distribution they occurred in. If the choice is A, then α will be greater than one; if the respondent is indifferent between the two scenarios, then α = 1. By constructing other questions where the amount of health expectancy that is transferred is different in magnitude, the exact value of α could be elicited.

Interindividual versus Individual-Mean Differences

The third choice refers to the family of measures: individual-mean or interindividual comparisons. In the calculation of inequality in a population all measures include a difference between individual *i* and another entity. In Figure 34.9, the two reductions in health inequality illustrate the choice. Both populations have the same mean value of health expectancy (both before and after the transfer) and the exact same amount of health is transferred in both cases. The initial distribution of health is different in the two populations. In both populations 15 years of health expectancy are transferred from the individual at the upper end of the distribution (35 years) to the individual at the lower

end of the distribution (5 years). The question again is: "Which of the two scenarios represents a greater decrease in inequality?" Those who prefer A are expressing a view that what counts is not only where the individual starts and where he/she ends up, but also where the rest of the population is. Those who are indifferent between A and B believe that what is really important is the absolute change achieved, regardless of where other people are in the distribution. In the first case, we would use a measure of interindividual comparisons, while in the second one we would use a measure of individual-mean differences.

Through a series of such questions, we could elicit an individual's values for the design of a summary index for the distribution of health expectancy. Population surveys or convenience samples could provide information from a wide range of individuals.

OPERATIONALIZING THE MEASUREMENT OF INEQUALITY IN HEALTH EXPECTANCY

While we have argued that the quantity of interest for measuring health inequality is the distribution of

Figure 34.8   Transfer of healthy life expectancy

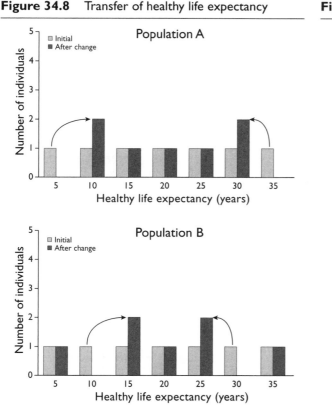

Figure 34.9   Transfer of healthy life expectancy

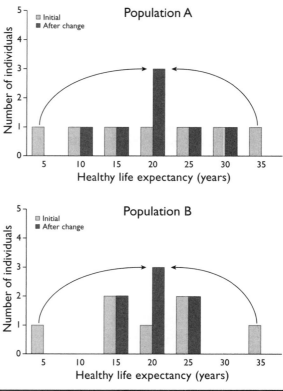

period health expectancy, how can this be measured? Risk is not observed, only outcomes. An individual with a 10% chance of death is either alive or dead at the end of a time period; survival at a given point in time provides us with no information as to the underlying risk of death of an individual. Nevertheless, we believe that the distribution of health risks can be reasonably approximated through a variety of techniques. The combination of the latter lays out a reasonable strategy to estimate the distribution of health expectancy. The strategy can be divided into four distinct approaches: measuring the distribution of child mortality risk, measuring the distribution of adult mortality risk, measuring the distribution of life expectancy and health expectancy directly through small area analyses, and measuring the distribution of non-fatal health outcomes.

Child Mortality Risk

While we cannot observe child mortality risk, we can observe the variation in the proportion of a mother's children who have died, which provides information at a very fine level of aggregation (namely households) on the distribution of child death risk. Using statistical models we can evaluate the difference in the distribution of outcomes from that which would be expected based on a distribution of equal risk. Data on children ever born and children surviving for women of reproductive age are widely available for a large number of developing countries from the Demographic and Health Surveys (DHS) (47) and many censuses and population surveys. A strategy for measuring inequality in child mortality risks has been implemented and is presented in Chapter 35.

Adult Mortality Risk

For children, grouping data by mother provides fine grained information on the distribution of mortality risks in the population. Unfortunately, we have no such handle to measure the distribution of adult mortality. Similar information on the survivorship of siblings, which is available from a number of household surveys, could in principle be used, but it would refer to average mortality experience over decades and the estimates of the distribution of mortality risks would be for older time periods. Chapter 37 proposes some potential strategies for the measurement of inequalities in adult health, based on the experience of measuring child health inequalities.

Distribution of Life Expectancy or Health Expectancy for Groups

One method to approximate the distribution of health expectancy in the population is to divide the population into groups that are expected to have similar health expectancies and measure directly the health expectation for those groups. Inevitably, this will underestimate the distribution of health expectancy in the population even if the groups are perfectly non-overlapping in terms of their individual health expectancies. The more refined the groupings, the more we will approximate the true underlying distribution of health expectancy. Analyses based on data from small geographical areas hold out the promise of being one of the most refined methods for revealing the underlying distribution of health expectancy in a population. For example, a detailed age-sex-race group analysis of counties in the US showed a range in life expectancy across counties of 41.3 years (17).

The Distribution of Non-fatal Health Outcomes

Measurement of non-fatal health outcomes on continuous or polychotomous scales provides more information from which to estimate the distribution of risk across individuals. Numerous surveys contain data on self-reported health status using a variety of instruments. The main problem to date with this information is the comparability of the responses across different cultures, levels of educational attainment, and incomes. For example, the rich often report worse non-fatal health outcomes than the poor (48;49). Problems of comparability must be resolved before such datasets can be used to contribute to estimation of health expectancy in the population. Recent efforts to resolve the problem of cross-population comparability of self-reported health status by the World Health Organization and other agencies are promising to result in better data in the next few years (see Chapter 53).

The ideal would be to simultaneously pursue the development of methods and datasets to measure these different dimensions of the distribution of health expectancy. There is a great need for new methods to integrate these various measurements into one estimation of the distribution of health expectancy in populations. The models developed in subsequent chapters are an attempt to resolve some of these methodological challenges.

CONCLUSIONS

This chapter has proposed an innovative approach to the measurement of health inequality, which is based on four key notions. First, we start with the principle that health is an intrinsic component of well-being and thus we should be concerned with inequality in health, whether or not it is correlated with inequality in other dimensions of well-being. Second, we propose that any measure of health inequality should reflect the complete range of fatal and non-fatal health outcomes in order to capture the rich complexity of health. We operationalize this notion through the concept of healthy life span. Third, we propose health expectancy as an improved measure compared to healthy life span, since it excludes those differences in healthy life span that are simply due to chance. In other words, the quantity of interest for studying health inequality is the distribution of health expectancy across individuals in the population. Fourth, the inequality of the distribution of health expectancy can be summarized by measures of individual-mean differences or inter-individual differences. The exact form of the measure to summarize inequality depends on three normative choices. A firmer understanding of people's views of these choices will provide a basis for deliberating on the final WHO measure of health inequality.

Our approach contrasts with that proposed by LeGrand (36;37) and Silber (35). Their primary concern is not variation in the set of age-specific health risks facing individuals, but the shape of the average population mortality rate as a function of age. This approach concludes that on average health inequality is decreasing worldwide. This finding is entirely attributable to the fact that the shape of average mortality risks across ages changes in a predictable fashion as life expectancy increases. We argue that we should focus on the distribution of health expectancy across individuals. In these terms there is no reason to expect that this distribution steadily narrows as the average health expectancy increases. The enormous variation in life expectancy (17) in the US across small areas is one indication of this.

A focus on the inequality of age-specific health risks (inputs to the distribution of health expectancy) may reinvigorate interest in some health problems. For example, many specific occupational exposures are not major contributors to average levels of population health expectancy, but may result in markedly elevated risks for a small minority. Such increases in risks will add to the inequality of health expectancy. As we quantify better the distribution of health expec-

tancy, the role of occupational and local environmental exposures in contributing to risk inequality may become apparent. Interest in inequality in health risks in developed countries may also draw attention to the impressive inequality in adult male mortality risk. In a country like the US, there is considerably more inequality in adult male mortality risk than in child or adult female mortality risks (17).

The task of measuring the distribution of health expectancy will need to make use of cross-sectional survey data on the prevalence of various non-fatal health outcomes. Measuring health inequality is fundamentally about comparing the distribution of the health status of individuals within populations and comparing distributions of different populations. If self-reported responses from the application of various health status surveys using instruments such as SF-36, EUROQOL, or activities of daily living are to be used in estimating health expectancy, special attention will need to be paid to the comparability of these responses across cultural groups. There is evidence that current instruments for measuring health status in surveys may not be comparable (49–51). Hopefully the work on inequality will improve comparability of health status survey responses across cultural groups.

There is a growing consensus that improvements in average levels of health is not a sufficient indicator of health systems performance. The distribution of such improvement is an equally important dimension of performance. In order to place health inequality at the center of the policy debate, we must develop better methods for measuring it. That will be the only way to ascertain the true magnitude of the problem and of monitoring progress towards its solution.

NOTES

1 An earlier version of this chapter appeared in the *Bulletin of the World Health Organization*, 2000, 78(1):42–54.

2 Some formal notation will be helpful for those familiar with survival analysis. $S(x)$ is the traditional survivorship function defining the probability of being alive at age x given a set of mortality risks, $\mu(x)$ at each age. In addition to mortality risks, individuals face incidence and remission rates from full health into health states less than full health and transition probabilities between these states. This complex set of health risks can be summarized by the health survivorship function. This is the probability of being alive and in equivalent full health at each age. Formally, for an individual it is calculated by weighing the survivorship function (the probability of being alive at each age) by the probability of being in any health state j at each age by the severity weight for that health state:

$$HS(x) = S(x)\sum_{j}\left(P_{jx} \cdot W_{jx}\right)$$

where $HS(x)$ is health survival at age x, $S(x)$ is probability of being alive at age x, P_{jx} is the probability of being in state j at age x (which takes into account both incidence and remission for condition j), and W_{jx} is the severity weight attached to state j at age x, measured on a scale where 0 is like-death and 1 is full health. For heuristic purposes, if we assume that $HS(x)$ monotonically declines with age, we can summarize the combination of health risks and the severity weight for different health states and mortality into one measure, $h(x)$, health risk, which can be thought of as the sole hazard to which an individual would be exposed such that health survivorship would be $HS(x)$.

3   For mortality, rectangular risks means that all individuals have a zero risk of death until some age x, at which the risk becomes one for the entire population (i.e. they all die at the same age). For non-fatal health outcomes, rectangular risks means that at a given age, the risk of incidence of a condition or remission from that condition is either zero or one for the entire population. This would correspond to no variance in the outcomes, as all individuals would be faced with the same set of conditions with certainty. Different individuals may have different rectangular risk curves as long as the health expectancy is the same. For different risk curves to have the same health expectancy, the duration of each condition would have to be the same, and if individuals had more than one condition, they would have to have the same comorbidity profile, despite different risk curves.

4   Formally:

$$HALE = \int_{0}^{L} HS(x)dx$$

where $HALE$ is health expectancy, $HS(x)$ is the probability of being in full health at age x, and L is the limit of human life.

5   Gompertz' Law of Mortality (*32*) applies only to mortality rates above age 20. Risks of death from birth to age 20 decline with age. Recently, careful analyses of mortality rates over age 75 or 80 have shown that they do not increase as fast as the Law of Mortality would predict (*33*).

REFERENCES

(1)   Acheson D. *Independent inquiry into inequalities in health*. London, The Stationery Office, 1998.

(2)   Antonovsky A. Social class, life expectancy and overall mortality. *Milbank Memorial Fund Quarterly*, 1967, 45: 31–73.

(3)   Barker J. Inequalities—whose health for all? *Health Visit*, 1990, 63:232–233.

(4)   Beaglehole R, Bonita R. Public health at crossroads: which way forward? *The Lancet*, 1998, 351:590–592.

(5)   Judge K, Mulligan JA, Benzeval M. Income inequality and population health. *Social Science & Medicine*, 1998, 46:567–579.

(6)   Kaplan G, Lynch J. Whither studies on the socioeconomic foundations of population health? *American Journal of Public Health*, 1997, 87:1409–1411.

(7)   Kawachi I, Kennedy BP. Income inequality and health: pathways and mechanisms. *Health Services Research*, 1999, 34:215–227.

(8)   Krieger N, Fee E. Measuring social inequalities in health in the United States: a historical review, 1900–1950. *International Journal of Health Services*, 1996, 26: 391–418.

(9)   Kunst AE, Geurts JJ, van den Berg J. International variation in socioeconomic inequalities in self reported health. *Journal of Epidemiology and Community Health*, 1995, 49:117–123.

(10) Mackenbach JP. Socioeconomic inequalities in health in The Netherlands: impact of a five year research programme. *British Medical Journal*, 1994, 309: 1487–1491.

(11) Mackenbach JP. Tackling inequalities in health. *British Medical Journal*, 1995, 310:1152–1153.

(12) Mackenbach JP, Gunning-Schepers LJ. How should interventions to reduce inequalities in health be evaluated? *Journal of Epidemiology and Community Health*, 1997, 51:359–364.

(13) Marmot M et al. Social inequalities in health: next questions and converging evidence. *Social Science & Medicine*, 1997, 44:901–910.

(14) Marmot MG, McDowall ME. Mortality decline and widening social inequalities. *The Lancet*, 1986, 2:274–276.

(15) Marmot MG et al. Health inequalities among British civil servants: the Whitehall II study. *The Lancet*, 1991, 337:1387–1393.

(16) Murray CJL, Gakidou E, Frenk J. Health inequalities and social group differences: what should we measure? *Bulletin of the World Health Organization*, 1999, 77: 537–543.

(17) Murray CJL et al. *U.S. patterns of mortality by county and race: 1965–1994*. Cambridge, Harvard School of Public Health and National Center for Disease Prevention and Health Promotion, 1998.

(18) Power C, Matthews S. Origins of health inequalities in a national population sample. *The Lancet*, 1997, 350: 1584–1589.

(19) Townsend P. Widening inequalities of health in Britain: a rejoinder to Rudolph Klein. *International Journal of Health Services*, 1990, 20:363–372.

(20) van Doorslaer E et al. Income-related inequalities in health: some international comparisons. *Journal of Health Economics*, 1997, 16:93–112.

(21) Wagstaff A, Paci P, van Doorslaer E. On the measurement of inequalities in health. *Social Science & Medicine*, 1991, 33:545–557.

(22) Whitehead M, Scott-Samuel A, Dahlgren G. Setting targets to address inequalities in health. *The Lancet*, 1998, 351:1279–1282.

(23) Murray CJL, Frenk J. A framework for assessing the performance of health systems. *Bulletin of the World Health Organization*, 2000, 78(6):717–731.

(24) Murray CJL, Frenk J, Gakidou E. Measuring health inequality: challenges and new directions. In: Leon D, Walt G, eds. *Poverty, inequality and health: an international perspective*. Oxford, Oxford University Press, 2001.

(25) Sen A. *Inequality reexamined*. Cambridge, Harvard University Press, 1992.

(26) Murray CJL. Rethinking DALYs. In: Murray CJL, Lopez AD, eds. *The global burden of disease: a comprehensive assessment of mortality and disability from diseases, injuries, and risk factors in 1990 and projected to 2020*. Cambridge, Harvard University Press, 1996.

(27) Nord E. Methods for quality adjustment of life years. *Social Science & Medicine*, 1992, 34:559–569.

(28) Nord E, Richardson J, Macarounas-Kirchmann K. Social evaluation of health care versus personal evaluation of health states. Evidence on the validity of four health-state scaling instruments using Norwegian and Australian Surveys. *International Journal of Technology Assessment in Health Care*, 1993, 9:463–478.

(29) Richardson J. Cost utility analysis: what should we measure? *Social Science & Medicine*, 1994, 39:7–21.

(30) Torrance GW. Measurement of health-state utilities for economics appraisal: a review. *Journal of Health Economics*, 1976, 5:1–30.

(31) Ware JE. Standards for validating health measures: definition and content. *Journal of Chronic Diseases*, 1987, 40:473–480.

(32) Gompertz B. On the nature of the function expressive of the law of human mortality and on a new mode of determining life contingencies. *Philosophical Transactions of the Royal Society of London*, 1825, 115:513–585.

(33) Olshansky SJ, Carnes BA. Ever since Gompertz. *Demography*, 1997, 34:1–15.

(34) Murray CJL, Lopez AD. Regional patterns of disability-free life expectancy and disability-adjusted life expectancy: Global Burden of Disease Study. *The Lancet*, 1997, 349:1347–1352.

(35) Silber J. Health and inequality. Some applications of uncertainty theory. *Social Science & Medicine*, 1982, 16:1663–1666.

(36) Le Grand J. Inequalities in health and health care: a research agenda. In: Wilkinson RG, ed. *Class and health: research and longitudinal data*. London and New York, Tavistock Publications, 1986.

(37) Le Grand J. An international comparison of measures of distributions of ages-at-death. In: Fox J, ed. *Health inequalities in European countries*. Aldershot and Brookfield, Gower, 1988.

(38) Corchia C et al. Social and geographical inequalities in prenatal care in Italy. *Prenatal Diagnosis*, 1995, 15: 535–540.

(39) Hart CL, Smith GD, Blane D. Inequalities in mortality by social class measured at 3 stages of the lifecourse. *American Journal of Public Health*, 1998, 88:471–474.

(40) Hollingsworth JR. Inequality in levels of health in England and Wales, 1891–1971. *Journal of Health and Social Behavior*, 1981, 22:268–283.

(41) Dagum C, Zenga M, eds. *Income and wealth distribution, inequality and poverty. Proceedings of the Second International Conference on Income Distribution by Size: Generation, Distribution, Measurement and Applications, held at the University of Pavia, Italy, September 23–30, 1989*. New York, Berlin, London, Tokyo, Springer, 1990.

(42) Kakwani NC. On the estimation of income inequality measures from grouped observations. *The Review of Econometrics Studies*, 1976, 43:483–492.

(43) Nygard F, Sandstrom A. Income inequality measures based on sample surveys. *Journal of Econometrics*, 1989, 42:81–95.

(44) Sen A. *On economic inequality*. Oxford, Oxford University Press, 1997.

(45) Gini C. *Variabilita e mutabilita*. Bologna, Tipogr. di P. Cuppini, 1912.

(46) Lorenz MO. Methods for measuring the concentration of wealth. *Journal of the American Statistical Association*, 1905, 9.

(47) Macro International Inc. *Demographic and Health Surveys*. URL: http://www.measuredhs.com/

(48) Australian Institute of Health and Welfare. *Australia's health: the fifth biennial report of the Australian Institute of Health and Welfare*. Canberra, AGPS, 1996.

(49) Murray CJL, Chen LC. Understanding morbidity change. *Population and Development Review*, 1992, 18:481–503.

(50) Johansson SR. The health transition: the cultural inflation of morbidity during the decline of mortality. *Health
Transition Review,* 1991, 1:39–68.

(51) Johansson SR. Measuring the cultural inflation of morbidity during the decline of mortality. *Health Transition
Review*, 1992, 2:78–89.

Chapter 35

MEASURING TOTAL HEALTH INEQUALITY: ADDING INDIVIDUAL VARIATION TO GROUP-LEVEL DIFFERENCES

EMMANUELA GAKIDOU, GARY KING

BACKGROUND

The distribution of health, or health inequality, has become prominent on global policy agendas as researchers have come to regard average health status as an inadequate summary of a country's health performance (*1;2*). Almost all health inequality studies have in fact documented *differences in average health status across groups* of people. Those with an economic focus have measured differences in average health status across income groups (*3;4*). Researchers with a sociological focus have examined inequalities in average health status among social classes (*5;6*), and those with a political focus have looked at how political structure is related to differences in the average level of health (*7*). Other scholars have focused on differences in average health status among racial or ethnic groups or by educational attainment or occupation (*8–10*). Most researchers consider differences across political entities such as countries or local governments. Similarly, demographers have also long studied variations in average health status, particularly in children, across age, sex, education, and racial groups (*11–13*). In low- and middle-income countries, there exists a rich demographic literature on levels and trends in child mortality and causes associated with them (*14–16*).

In this chapter, we define the concept of *total health inequality*, and demonstrate how to measure it by the variation in health status across *individuals* (within a country as a whole or any subgroup within a country). This approach complements the existing group-level approaches, a fact that can even be demonstrated mathematically. That is, the standard analysis of variance identity applies to variations in health status just as it does to all other coherent variables:

"Total" = "Between Group" + "Within Group"

Literature in this area has focused exclusively on the "between group" component. In this chapter, the missing "within group" component is added to the existing measures to arrive at total health inequality. With the latter, no individual variation in health status is ignored. With this measure added to the existing reporting standards, public health policy can be targeted at reducing inequalities across individuals, in addition to its present goal of reducing disparities in average health status across countries and groups in society.

We would like to emphasize that total health inequality complements group-level measures; it does not replace them. After all, if average health attainment is the same across a given set of groups, total health inequality could still be unacceptably high (because of intragroup variation across individuals), whereas if total health inequality is small, then the differences among any set of groups, albeit potentially systematic, must also be small. In our view, between, within, and total levels of health inequality should be reported henceforth.

Preferably, measures of inequality in healthy life expectancy (the number of years in full health an individual born today can expect to live (*17*)) would be computed, but this chapter focuses on a preliminary step for which data are more readily available – developing methods for the measurement of total inequality in the probability of child survival. Survival from birth to two years of age is only one aspect of health, but it is a useful place to start since it is a critical part of health status, particularly in developing countries (*4;18*).

The normative principles involved in choosing a measure of inequality are discussed briefly. Instead of making an arbitrary choice, the inequality measure selected is consistent with the results of a survey of normative preferences of over 1 000 health professionals conducted by WHO and used in *The World Health Report 2000* (*19*). Comparisons with applications of other popular measures of income inequality to health are also presented.

METHODS

The data analysed are from 50 countries where a Demographic and Health Survey (DHS) had been conducted and the data were available. Table 35.1 lists the countries, sample size, and year of the surveys used. The DHS is a 20-year project conducting high quality national sample surveys on population, maternal and child health. Funded primarily by the United States Agency for International Development (USAID), DHS is administered by Macro International Inc. (*20*). Low-income country governments and international organizations have long relied on DHS data to monitor a variety of child and maternal health and family planning indicators (*21*). One of the most significant contributions of the DHS is the collection of internationally comparable data on the demographic and health characteristics of populations in developing countries (*22–25*).

The DHS are conducted through in-person interviews. The samples, which are all above 3 000 households in the countries analysed in this study, are the result of a multistage stratified sampling design (*26*). The DHS sampling weights are used to produce nationally representative estimates.

For each country we used the latest year of available data from a nationally representative DHS, ranging from 1987 to 1997. For each mother surveyed, the number of children born and the number that survived to age two was calculated. A ten-year observation period was used ending two years prior to the interview year, to avoid censoring effects. This period is a compromise between providing recent estimates and ensuring enough births to reduce the effects of sampling error. Measuring survival to (or death by) age five, would involve a longer censoring period, produce older estimates of inequality, and not differ much from the under two mortality because on average, 80% of under five deaths occur in the first two years of life (*26;27*).

To provide a partial but independent validation of the DHS-based results, mortality data by municipality in Mexico (*28*) and Brazil (*29*) from different data sources were analysed. Data on socioeconomic

Table 35.1 DHS survey year and sample size

Country	Year	No. of households interviewed
Bangladesh	1997	9 127
Benin	1996	5 491
Bolivia	1994	8 603
Brazil	1996	12 612
Burkina Faso	1993	6 354
Burundi	1987	3 970
Cameroon	1997	5 501
Central African Republic	1995	5 884
Colombia	1995	11 140
Comoros	1996	3 050
Côte d'Ivoire	1994	8 099
Dominican Republic	1996	8 422
Ecuador	1987	4 713
Egypt	1995	14 779
Ghana	1994	4 562
Guatemala	1995	12 403
Haiti	1995	5 356
India	1993	89 777
Indonesia	1994	28 168
Kazakhstan	1995	3 771
Kenya	1993	7 540
Liberia	1986	5 239
Madagascar	1997	7 060
Malawi	1992	4 849
Mali	1996	9 704
Mexico	1987	9 310
Morocco	1992	9 256
Mozambique	1997	8 779
Namibia	1992	5 421
Nepal	1996	8 429
Nicaragua	1998	13 634
Niger	1995	7 577
Nigeria	1990	8 781
Pakistan	1991	6 611
Paraguay	1990	5 827
Peru	1996	28 951
Philippines	1998	13 983
Rwanda	1992	6 551
Senegal	1997	8 593
Sudan	1990	5 860
Thailand	1987	6 775
Togo	1998	8 569
Trinidad and Tobago	1987	3 806
Tunisia	1988	4 184
Uganda	1995	7 070
United Republic of Tanzania	1996	8 120
Uzbekistan	1996	4 415
Yemen	1992	6 010
Zambia	1996	8 021
Zimbabwe	1994	6 128

variables (30) and on the political system (31) of each country were also collected to help us explore possible causes of differences in inequality. The socioeconomic variables were gathered for the year the survey was conducted in each country.

The population of interest includes all children born alive in a country in a given time period. Ideally, one would measure the length of time each child is *expected* to live from birth to two years and then use a measure of inequality to summarize the distribution of these survival expectations. Making the inference from the dichotomous data on child survival to health inequality requires several methodological steps.

The first one is to estimate the distribution of the probability of death across children in each national sample. The chief methodological difficulty here is that for any one child, only the dichotomous variable of survival to two years is measured, while the probability of dying for each child is not observed. These probabilities are estimated using the extended beta-binomial model (32;34). The latter has been widely applied in biomedical research, most commonly for modelling animal littermate survival probabilities, and in political science to model voting statistics (32; 34–38). In this application, we model the number of child deaths within a family with a binomial distribution with equal risk of dying per child, and then allow the risks to vary across families according to a beta distribution (35). (See Annex 35.1 for more details on the specification of the model.)

Potential confounders, including mother's age, number of children, level of education, and average birth interval, were controlled for (13). This procedure relaxes the assumptions of the model, making it more flexible. However, the basic model fits the data well, and controlling for these variables does not materially affect the estimates of health inequality. When the covariates have no effect, the beta distributed random effect portion of the model ensures that the level of variability is not underestimated.

For Mexico and Brazil, the extended beta-binomial model was also applied to the municipality-level mortality datasets to validate the model. The underlying assumption is that small geographical areas (which are treated analogously to families) include mostly homogeneous populations for which the risk of death is similar. In both countries, the estimates of inequality from the extended beta-binomial model did not materially differ between the two datasets used.

As an example of the results of the analysis, Figure 35.1 shows the estimated distribution of the probabil-

ity of dying before age two in Benin and the Central African Republic, and the corresponding distributions of expected childhood survival time (up to two years) for those countries. These two countries were chosen because they have very similar average probabilities of death (0.13 and 0.12, respectively), and therefore very similar mean survival times (1.86 and 1.87 years, respectively), but markedly different distributions of actual survival time around these means and hence divergent levels of health inequality. For example, in the Central African Republic, about 25% of children born have a probability of death lower than 4%. In contrast, children in Benin have risks of death more closely distributed around its mean, with only 4% of its children having a probability of death lower than 3%. Clearly at the lower end of the distribution Benin does worse than the Central African Republic, but it does much better at the higher extreme. For example, in Benin less than 1% of children born have a probability of death greater than 40%, contrasted with the Central African Republic, where more than 4% of children have that probability of death. This is merely one striking example of why summarizing health status with only mean levels is misleading.

The second step is to transform the estimated probability of death between birth and age two for each child ($_2q_0$ in demographic notation) to the expected survival time in the first two years of life, S. Although the results do not change materially, we opted to measure inequality in survival time, instead of probability of survival, as it is analogous to inequality in health expectancy and is more interpretable. Expected survival time can be calculated as:

$$S = \frac{1}{_2m_0} - \frac{e^{-2\,_2m_0}}{_2m_0},$$

where S is expected survival time, and $_2m_0$ is the mortality rate in the first two years of life (39). $_2m_0$ can, in turn, be calculated from the probability of dying in the first two years of life, $_2q_0$:

$$_2m_0 = \frac{\ln[1-_2q_0]}{2} \quad (39).$$

Finally, since plotting fifty graphs like Figure 35.1 would be unwieldy, we give numerical summaries of health inequality. To do this, several normative criteria have to be addressed. At least three general normative dimensions are relevant (17). First, measures of inequality range from absolute to relative. Absolute measures are independent of mean survival

Figure 35.1   Distribution of probability of death between birth and age two ($_2q_0$) for Benin
and the Central African Republic

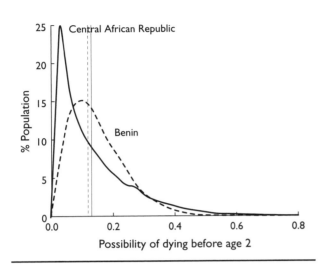

Note: The curves are density estimates and the vertical lines are the average $_2q_0$
for each country.

$$II = \frac{\sum\limits_{i=1}^{n} \sum\limits_{j=1}^{n} |s_i - s_j|^3}{2n^2 \sqrt{s}},$$

where s_i is the expected survival time between birth
and age two of individual i, and s is the average
expected survival time in the first two years of life in
the population. This index of inequality (II) is logically
between a relative and an absolute measure, so the
average survival time is included in the denominator.
The index is based on comparing each child with every
other child in the population (thus the sum of the differences in the numerator), and gives a large weight
to the best and worst off (the differences are raised to
the power of three). Larger values of II indicate more
individual-level inequality in child survival. The health
inequality point estimates and uncertainty bounds are
mean posterior estimates and 95% credible intervals,
respectively, computed from the extended beta-binomial model with flat priors and the traditionally used
asymptotic normal approximations, e.g. (*40*).

time, whereas relative measures adjust for the mean.
If one believes that more variation in health states is
acceptable when average survival time is higher, then
a measure close to the relative end of the continuum
would reflect that choice. On the other hand, if one
believes that a given discrepancy in expected survival
across people should be considered in the same way,
irrespective of the mean survival time in that population, then an absolute measure of inequality would be
appropriate. The second normative dimension is the
weight given to outliers. One might believe that the
majority of children is what measures should be based
on, or one might instead want to focus primarily on
the worst and best off. The final dimension is whether
individuals should be compared to the average of their
communities or to each of the individuals within their
communities separately.

A range of measures of inequality that reflect a lot of
different normative positions were developed, including measures used in quantifying income inequality
(such as the Gini index), variance measures, and
many that have not been previously considered (*17*).
Although it need not have turned out this way, in the
present analysis these measures all gave substantively
consistent empirical results. For empirical analyses,
the inequality index (*II*) used was derived from a survey of the normative preferences of over 1 000 health
professionals and other individuals with an interest in
health systems (*19*). The index is defined as:

RESULTS

Table 35.2 lists estimates of child survival inequality
using *II* for each of the 50 countries, ranked from
most unequal (Liberia) to least unequal (Colombia).
For comparison, estimates of child survival inequality
were calculated for three other commonly used summary measures of distributions—the variance, the Gini
index, and the coefficient of variation. The pairwise
rank order correlations between the four measures
were all higher than 0.93. Table 35.3 presents the
ranking of countries from most to least unequal by
the four measures of inequality used in this analysis.

To get a sense of the uncertainty in estimation,
Figure 35.2 plots the inequality estimates with 95%
confidence intervals for each country (the size of the
confidence intervals is mostly a function of the sample
size in each country). These kinds of basic data could
be used by health professionals as a basis for further
research, particularly into the determinants of total
health inequality, and eventually public policy to
reduce inequalities.

Figure 35.3 presents an exploratory view of the
relationship between our measure of health inequality and five plausible explanatory variables, interacted
with the type of government. The purpose of these
graphs is to understand the measure of inequality
developed and to explore correlations with other relevant variables. Determining what causes changes in

Table 35.2 Child survival inequality index for 50 countries, estimates and 95% confidence intervals

Country	Inequality index	95% CI	Country	Inequality index	95% CI
Liberia	.75	.56 – .91	Comoros	.36	.17 – .53
Mozambique	.73	.59 – .87	Egypt	.35	.29 – .42
Central African Republic	.69	.53 – .85	Uganda	.34	.23 – .48
Nigeria	.66	.55 – .77	Burkina Faso	.34	.21 – .47
Malawi	.62	.44 – .78	Kenya	.34	.24 – .44
Rwanda	.56	.43 – .68	Ecuador	.32	.18 – .44
Niger	.54	.42 – .66	Benin	.31	.19 – .45
Pakistan	.54	.43 – .64	Bangladesh	.30	.20 – .41
Côte d'Ivoire	.52	.40 – .64	Bolivia	.27	.17 – .37
Mali	.51	.41 – .60	Tunisia	.25	.14 – .35
Namibia	.47	.31 – .61	Morocco	.25	.15 – .34
United Republic of Tanzania	.47	.35 – .59	Brazil	.23	.14 – .33
Togo	.46	.35 – .57	Guatemala	.23	.16 – .30
Zambia	.46	.32 – .59	Senegal	.22	.14 – .32
Madagascar	.45	.33 – .58	Peru	.22	.17 – .26
Yemen	.44	.34 – .53	Zimbabwe	.21	.11 – .31
Nepal	.41	.29 – .52	Dominican Republic	.21	.11 – .30
Cameroon	.40	.25 – .54	Nicaragua	.20	.13 – .27
Sudan	.40	.29 – .51	Trinidad and Tobago	.15	.04 – .25
Burundi	.40	.24 – .55	Thailand	.15	.05 – .24
Indonesia	.40	.34 – .45	Mexico	.14	.06 – .21
India	.39	.36 – .43	Paraguay	.12	.05 – .20
Haiti	.39	.22 – .55	Kazakhstan	.11	.01 – .21
Ghana	.39	.23 – .53	Philippines	.10	.05 – .16
Uzbekistan	.36	.21 – .52	Colombia	.08	.03 – .15

inequality is a critical issue, but we do not pursue it in any detail here. Among the variables included, GDP per capita and health expenditures per capita are negatively correlated with health inequality, which lends face validity to the inequality measure. As with average level of mortality, the relationship between health inequality and GDP per capita and health expenditure per capita is very strong at low levels of income and expenditure, and the effect is smaller at higher levels. The relationship between health inequality and absolute poverty (defined as the per cent of the population earning less than one international dollar per day) appears to be more linear, with considerable variation in inequality at each given level of poverty. More surprisingly, health inequality seems entirely uncorrelated with income inequality (r = –0.16), as measured by economists' most commonly used measure, the Gini index calculated for income.

Additionally, inequality in childhood survival is positively related to the mean probability of death ($2q0$), but at a given level of mortality there is significant variation in inequality. This confirms the expected relationship and also reflects the fact that traditionally reported measures of average levels of health are

insufficient for summarizing the health experience of a population. Finally, each point in each graph also codes the type of political system. The graphs seem to indicate that full democracies (represented as diamonds) tend to have lower values of inequality than partial democracies (squares) or autocracies (triangles), as would be expected. (Partial democracies include countries that have adopted some democratic practices, such as popular elections to legislatures with limited powers, but most have not completed the transition from autocratic practices.) However, and perhaps surprisingly, health inequality is otherwise unrelated to the type of political system either directly or in interaction with any of the five potential explanatory variables.

The individual-level approach to conceptualizing and measuring health inequality appears to complement the group-level approaches. To show that the total health inequality measures offered here are at least sometimes distinct from group-level analyses, the results of the present analysis are compared to those of Wagstaff (4) and Brockerhoff and Hewett (16). Wagstaff calculated inequalities among income groups in 7 countries, measured by a concentration

Table 35.3 Relative ranks of child survival inequality by four measures of inequality (Rank 1 refers to the most unequal)

Country	II	Std. deviation	Coefficient of variation	Gini coefficient
Liberia	1	2	1	1
Mozambique	2	1	2	2
Central African Republic	3	3	5	6
Nigeria	4	4	7	7
Malawi	5	5	3	3
Rwanda	6	6	8	9
Nigeria	7	9	4	4
Pakistan	8	7	13	17
Côte d'Ivoire	9	8	10	10
Mali	10	10	6	5
Namibia	11	14	22	26
Tanzania	12	11	12	12
Togo	13	12	16	18
Zambia	14	13	9	8
Madagascar	15	15	11	11
Yemen	16	16	14	13
Nepal	17	17	15	14
Cameroon	18	19	23	23
Sudan	19	18	20	21
Burundi	20	20	17	15
Indonesia	21	24	30	31
India	22	21	26	25
Haiti	23	22	19	19
Ghana	24	23	25	24
Uzbekistan	25	30	35	39
Comoros	26	25	27	27
Egypt	27	26	28	29
Uganda	28	27	24	22
Burkina Faso	29	28	18	16
Kenya	30	29	32	32
Ecuador	31	32	33	33
Benin	32	31	21	20
Bangladesh	33	33	29	28
Bolivia	34	34	31	30
Tunisia	35	36	38	37
Morocco	36	35	36	35
Brazil	37	39	40	40
Guatemala	38	37	37	36
Senegal	39	38	34	34
Peru	40	40	39	38
Zimbabwe	41	41	41	41
Dominican Republic	42	42	42	42
Nicaragua	43	43	43	43
Trinidad & Tobago	44	46	47	48
Thailand	45	45	45	45
Mexico	46	44	44	44
Paraguay	47	47	46	46
Kazakhstan	48	50	50	50
Philippines	49	48	48	47
Colombia	50	49	49	49

index. Brockerhoff and Hewett measured ethnic differences in 11 countries via odds ratios. Brockerhoff and Hewett used subsets of the same DHS datasets as used in this analysis, while Wagstaff used mostly data from the Living Standards Measurement Surveys.

Figure 35.4 plots the ranks of the total health inequality measure (*II*) by each of these group-level measures (with rank 1 assigned to the country with the largest inequalities). Clearly the individual-level measure is tapping into different concepts as the two pairs are not even positively correlated. For example, the Central African Republic and Rwanda have large individual-level inequalities in child survival, but relatively smaller inter-ethnic group inequalities. (These results do not contradict, but rather imply that there is considerable intra-ethnic group inequality that is, by definition, not picked up by the group-level measures.) In contrast, Kenya has less individual-level health inequality relative to other sub-Saharan African countries, but more ethnicity–related inequalities. Similarly, Brazil and Nicaragua have large differences in child mortality levels across income groups, but less individual-level inequality than Pakistan and Cote d'Ivoire. These results establish that measures of total health inequality are indeed measuring different concepts and uncovering different findings than the existing group-level approaches.

CONCLUSIONS

This chapter presents the first measures of total health inequality of a population. Such measures could serve as an important complement to existing group-level approaches in the literature on health inequalities among groups. Including individual-level variation, as done here, produces estimates of inequality that capture the entire distribution of risk of death in the population and that are directly comparable across countries.

At the same average level of health status, countries can achieve widely varying levels of health inequality. Since measuring and communicating this type of information seems essential to making informed public policy, we believe inequality should be measured and reported together with average levels of health status.

Estimating the underlying distribution of risk is useful for understanding the nature and possibly the causes of health inequality using observed dichotomous outcomes such as survival and death. This or a related approach should prove useful for examining

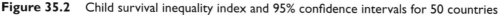

Figure 35.2 Child survival inequality index and 95% confidence intervals for 50 countries

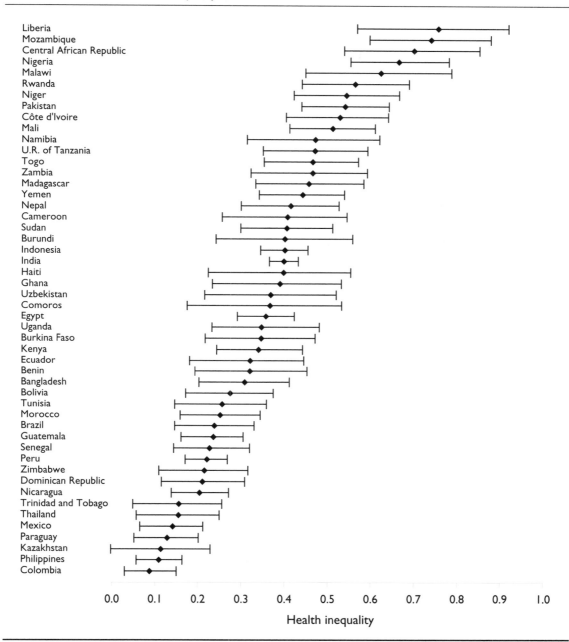

the risk of ill-health for all age groups, such as in measures of inequality in health expectancy.

Considerable future research needs to be conducted into health inequality. For one area, efforts should continue to measure inequalities in child survival outside of the fifty countries analysed here. For another, the normative underpinnings of popular measures of health inequality should be further clarified. Similarly, other measures that formalize richer normative principles should be developed. Further efforts need to be

made to measure what types of people, policy-makers, and democratic electorates prefer one normative position over another. Third, new databases need to be created and statistical methods developed that enable researchers to expand measures of inequality in child survival in the first two years of life to inequality in health expectancy in general. Fourth, we have to seek further external validation of these results, along the lines of the vital registration-based analysis conducted for Mexico and Brazil. Finally, and most importantly

Figure 35.3   Child survival inequality index, plotted against five economic and demographic indicators by type of government

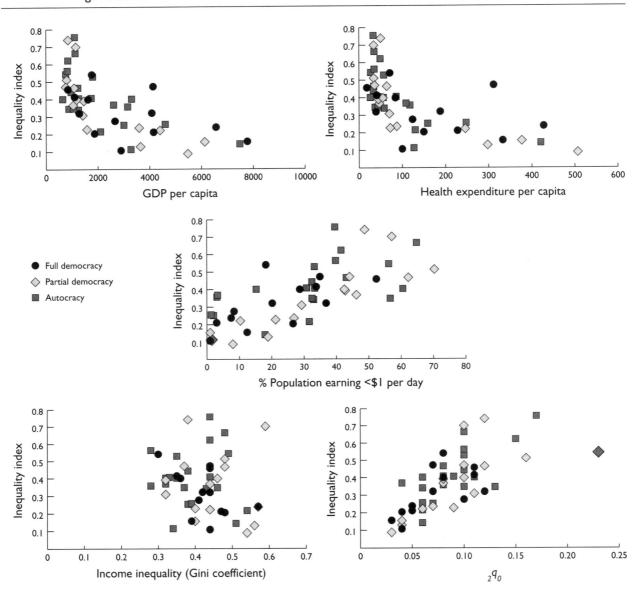

for influencing health policy globally, scholars should pursue an understanding of the determinants of inequality. We need to comprehend not only how average levels of health status of populations can be raised, but also how health inequalities can be reduced.

There are several limitations to this study. The ranking of countries is influenced by the year the data were collected and particularly for those most affected by the HIV/AIDS epidemic, the estimate of the inequality index might change if more recent data were available. Since women of reproductive age are the basic sampling units in these surveys, their premature death (from maternal or other causes) excludes their children from the studies. Such children often have an elevated mortality risk and their exclusion may bias estimates of child mortality (both level and inequality) downward. This bias is likely to be greater in countries with higher maternal mortality and HIV/AIDS epidemics. Our preliminary explorations of this issue indicate that the estimate of the inequality index changes very little, and not enough to result in a change of rankings across countries.

Figure 35.4 Country rankings of child survival inequality: comparing the individual-level inequality index with existing indices of income- and ethnicity-related inequalities in child survival. A rank of I on all scales indicates the highest levels of inequality.

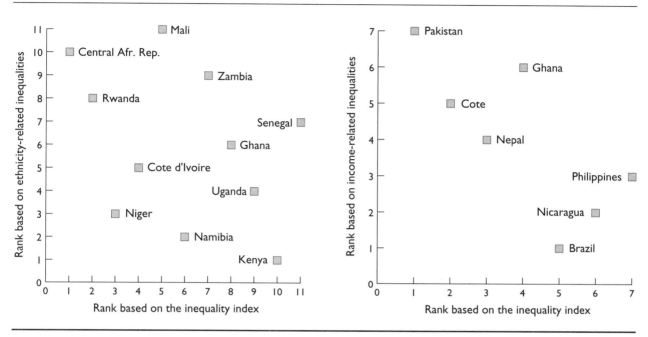

Some of the potential implications of this chapter include a research programme devoted to developing and improving measures of health inequality, a substantial change in data collection efforts by public health authorities internationally, and even ongoing changes in national and international public policy as a result. All this possible activity takes nothing away from the important existing focus on differences in average health levels across groups, but measuring and reporting individual health inequality adds an essential new perspective as well.

ACKNOWLEDGEMENTS

The authors thank Christopher J.L. Murray, Julio Frenk, Alan D. Lopez, Brad Palmquist, Joshua A. Salomon, Lana Tomaskovic, and Brodie D. Ferguson for valuable comments. Our thanks go to the World Health Organization, the U.S. National Science Foundation (SBR-9729884), and the National Institutes on Aging (PO1 AG17625-01) for research support.

REFERENCES

(1) World Health Organization. *The World Health Report 2000. Health Systems: Improving Performance.* Geneva, World Health Organization, 2000.

(2) Acheson D. *Independent inquiry into inequalities in health.* London, The Stationery Office, 1998.

(3) World Bank. *Country reports on health, nutrition, population, and poverty.* Washington, DC, World Bank, 2002. URL: http://www.worldbank.org/poverty/health/data/intro.htm

(4) Wagstaff A. Socioeconomic inequalities in child mortality: comparisons across nine developing countries. *Bulletin of the World Health Organization*, 2000, 78:19–29.

(5) Marmot MG, et al. Health inequalities among British civil servants: the Whitehall II study. *The Lancet*, 1991, 337:1387–1393.

(6) Kawachi I, Marshall S, Pearce N. Social class inequalities in the decline of coronary heart disease among New Zealand men, 1975–1977 to 1985–1987. *International Journal of Epidemiology*, 1991, 20:393–398.

(7) Navarro V. Health and equity in the world in the era of "globalization." *International Journal of Health Services*, 1999, 29:215–225.

(8) Kunst AE, Geurts JJ, van den Berg J. International variation in socioeconomic inequalities in self reported health. *Journal of Epidemiology and Community Health*, 1995, 49:117–123.

(9) Kunst AE, et al. Occupational class and cause specific mortality in middle aged men in 11 European countries: comparison of population based studies. EU Working Group on Socioeconomic Inequalities in Health. *British Medical Journal*, 1998, 316:1636–1642.

(10) Mackenbach JP, Kunst AE. Measuring the magnitude of socio-economic inequalities in health: an overview of available measures illustrated with two examples from Europe. *Social Science & Medicine*, 1997, 44:757–771.

(11) Preston SH, Haines MR. *Fatal years: child mortality in late nineteenth-century America*. Princeton, Princeton University Press, 1991.

(12) Caldwell JC, McDonald P. Influence of maternal education on infant and child mortality: levels and causes. In: *International Population Conference, Manila*, vol. 2, 1981:79–96.

(13) Bicego G, Ahmad O. *Infant and child mortality*. Demographic and Health Surveys Comparative Studies No. 20. Calverton, Macro International Inc., 1996. URL: http://www.measuredhs.com/pubs/

(14) Hill K, Pande R, Mahy M, Jones G. *Trends in child mortality in the developing world: 1960 to 1996*. New York, UNICEF, 1999.

(15) Hill K, Pande R. *The recent evolution of child mortality in the developing world*. Arlington, VA, Partnership for Child Health Care, Basic Support for Institutionalizing Child Survival [BASICS]. Current Issues in Child Survival Series, 1997.

(16) Brockerhoff M, Hewett P. Inequality of child mortality among ethnic groups in sub-Saharan Africa. *Bulletin of the World Health Organization*, 2000, 78(1):30–41.

(17) Gakidou E, Murray CJL, Frenk J. Defining and measuring health inequality: an approach based on the distribution of health expectancy. *Bulletin of the World Health Organization*, 2000, 78(1):42–54.

(18) Zaba B, David P. Fertility and the distribution of child mortality risk among women: an illustrative analysis. *Population Studies*, 1996, 50:263–278.

(19) Gakidou E, Murray CJL, Frenk J. *Measuring preferences on health system performance assessment*. EIP Discussion Paper No. 20. Geneva, World Health Organization, 2000. URL: http://www3.who.int/whosis/discussion_papers/discussion_papers.cfm#

(20) USAID & Macro International. *Demographic and Health Surveys*. 1984. URL: http://www.measuredhs.com

(21) Stanton C, Abderrahim N, Hill K. An assessment of DHS maternal mortality indicators. *Studies in Family Planning*, 2000, 31:111–123.

(22) Sullivan J, Rutstein S, Bicego G. *Infant and child mortality*. Demographic and Health Surveys Comparative Studies No. 15. Calverton, Macro International Inc., 1994. URL: http://www.measuredhs.com/pubs/

(23) Curtis SL. *Assessment of the quality of data used for direct estimation of infant and child mortality in DHS-II surveys*. Calverton, Maryland, Macro International, Inc., Demographic and Health Surveys, 1995.

(24) Boerma JT, Sommerfelt AE. Demographic and Health Surveys (DHS): contributions and limitations. *World Health Statistics Quarterly*, 1993, 46:222–226.

(25) Hill K, et al. *Trends in child mortality in the developing world: 1960–1996*. New York, UNICEF, 1999.

(26) Rutstein S. Factors associated with trends in infant and child mortality in developing countries during the 1990s. *Bulletin of the World Health Organization*, 2000, 78: 1256–1270.

(27) Macro International Inc. *An assessment of the quality of health data in DHS surveys #2*. Calverton, Macro International Inc., 1993.

(28) Fundacion Mexicana para la Salud, Instituto Nacional de Estadística Geografía e Informática. *Deaths and population by municipality in Mexico*. 1998.

(29) Instituto Brasilero de Geografía e Estadística (IBGE). *Sistema de Informacao sobre Mortalidade*. 1994. URL: http://www.datasus.gov.br, http://www.ibge.gov.br.

(30) World Health Organization. *GPE Socio-economic database*. Geneva, World Health Organization, 2000.

(31) Gurr TR, Jaggers K. *Polity III: regime change and political authority, 1800–1994*. Computer file, Inter-university Consortium for Political and Social Research, Ann Arbor, MI, 1996.

(32) Prentice RL. Binary regression using an extended beta-binomial distribution, with discussion of correlation induced by covariate measurement errors. *Journal of the American Statistical Association*, 1986, 81:321–327.

(33) King G. *Unifying political methodology: the likelihood theory of statistical inference*. Cambridge, Cambridge University Press, 1989.

(34) Palmquist B. *Analysis of proportions data*. College Station, Texas, 1999.

(35) Brooks SP, et al. Finite mixture models for proportions. *Biometrics*, 1997, 53:1097–1115.

(36) Yamamoto E, Yanagimoto T. Statistical methods for the beta-binomial model in teratology. *Environmental Health Perspective*, 1994, 102S:25–31.

(37) Liang KY, McCullagh P. Case studies in binary dispersion. *Biometrics*, 1993, 49:623–630.

(38) Griffiths D. Maximum likelihood estimation for the beta-binomial distribution application to the household distribution of the total number of cases of a disease. *Biometrics*, 1973, 29:637–648.

(39) Preston SH, Keyfitz N, Schoen R. *Causes of death: life tables for national populations*. New York and London, Seminar Press, 1972.

(40) King G, Tomz M, Wittenberg J. Making the most of statistical analyses: improving interpretation and presentation. *American Journal of Political Science*, 2000, 44:341–355.

THE EXTENDED BETA-BINOMIAL MODEL

The first step in the analysis is to estimate the distribution of the probability of death across children in each national sample. The chief methodological difficulty here is that for any one child, only the dichotomous variable of death or survival to two years of age is measured, while the probability of dying is not observed. One possibility would be to estimate these probabilities with a child-level logit or probit model, but this would make our estimates heavily dependent on the quality and choice of available covariates, and in some cases would underestimate the true variability.

An alternative is to model children with the same mother as having the same independent probability of survival, with probabilities that vary across families, or in other words as a binomial distribution. (Allowing the probabilities of death among children within a family to vary does not necessarily lead to different observable data on the total number of children who die in a family.)

Thus, we begin by assuming that the probability of death, π, for each child follows independent and identically distributed Bernoulli distributions within families. The total number of dead children in a family, Y, is itself distributed binomially with expectation $n\pi$ and variance $n\pi(1-\pi)$, where n is the number of children in the family.

For each family i the binomial distribution can be parameterized as:

$$\Pr\left(Y_i = y_i \mid \pi, n\right) = \binom{n_i}{y_i}\pi^{y_i}\left(1-\pi\right)^{n-y_i} \quad [\text{A1}]$$

But rather than assuming that the probability of a child dying, π, is constant across families, the variability in these unobserved probabilities across families is modelled with a two-parameter beta density, which allows the probabilities to vary even without covariates (or within categories of the covariates). The beta distribution is a flexible distribution, bounded by 0 and 1, which are the limits of π. Conventionally, the beta distribution is represented as:

$$f(\pi \mid a,b) = \beta^{-1}(a,b)\pi^{a-1}(1-\pi)^{b-1} \quad [\text{A2}]$$

where a and b are the parameters, $\beta(a,b) = \Gamma(a)\Gamma(b)/\Gamma(a+b)$ is the beta function and $\Gamma(a)$ is the Gamma function (which is the same as the factorial function

for integers and interpolations for noninteger arguments).

In this analysis, we use re-parameterization suggested by Palmquist (*34*), where

$$\gamma = (a+b)^{-1}$$
$$\pi = a(a+b)^{-1}$$

The expectation of the beta distribution is π and γ is a dispersion parameter in that the variance is:

$$V(\pi) = \frac{ab}{(a+b)^2}\frac{1}{a+b+1} = \pi(1-\pi)\frac{1}{1+\gamma^{-1}}$$

Thus, a population whose risk distribution followed a beta distribution would have an average risk of mortality of π and a variance of $V(\pi)$. Combining the within-family binomial distribution with the across-family beta distribution produces the beta-binomial model. Mathematically, this is accomplished by integrating [A1] over the re-parameterized version of the density in [A2].

Prentice (*32*) showed that the beta-binomial model can be made into an extended beta-binomial model, allowing both under and over-dispersion, by extending the permissible range of the parameters. This model is often a reasonable approximation even when children within the same family have heterogeneous survival probabilities or dependent outcomes.

The simple extended beta-binomial model without covariates estimates *one* beta distribution for each population, i.e. the most likely beta distribution from which the observed distribution of deaths could have come. The model estimates one π and one γ for each population. Controls can be included in the model by letting π vary over the observations as a logistic function of measured covariates:

$$\pi_i = \frac{1}{1+e^{-X_i\beta}} \; .$$

This procedure allows a different extended beta-binomial distribution to fit each unique combination of values of the covariates, making for a much more flexible overall model. We included covariates for the mother's age, number of children, level of education, and average birth interval, all variables that have been shown to affect childhood survival probabilities. We find in our data that the basic model fits well, and adding covariates does not materially affect the esti- mates of health inequality, even when the covariates themselves have an impact on the risk of death among children.

Chapter 36

DETERMINANTS OF INEQUALITY IN CHILD SURVIVAL: RESULTS FROM 39 COUNTRIES

EMMANUELA GAKIDOU, GARY KING

INTRODUCTION

Few would disagree that health policies and programmes ought to be based on valid, timely and relevant information, focused on those aspects of health development that are in greatest need of improvement. For example, vaccination programmes rely heavily on information on cases and deaths to document needs and to monitor progress on childhood illness and mortality. The same strong information basis is necessary for policies on health inequality. The reduction of health inequality is widely accepted as a key goal for societies, but any policy needs reliable research on the extent and causes of health inequality. Given that child deaths still constitute 19% of all deaths globally and 24% of all deaths in developing countries (1), reducing inequalities in child survival is a good beginning.

Conceptually, the field of health inequalities can be represented by this simple identity:

$$\begin{matrix} Total \\ Health \\ Inequality \end{matrix} = \begin{matrix} Between\text{-} \\ Group \\ Inequality \end{matrix} + \begin{matrix} Within\text{-} \\ Group \\ Inequality \end{matrix} \quad [1]$$

The between-group component of total health inequality has been studied extensively by numerous scholars. They have expertly analysed the causes of differences in health status and mortality across population subgroups, defined by income, education, race/ethnicity, country, region, social class, and other group identifiers (2–9).

Unfortunately, the within-group component of health inequality was not recognized until recently (1;10;11). While no more important than the between-group component, the within-group one may reveal valuable information about policies and interventions to reduce overall inequalities. Indeed, this chapter demonstrates that inequality in child mortality within

groups is considerably larger than inequality between groups in low- and middle-income countries, and this finding is only partially accounted for by differences in average mortality. It therefore seems reasonable to suggest that policy-makers need to take into account both these components of inequality, and that measures of total inequality should appear alongside average health and between-group inequality measures in international comparisons. The analysis presented in this chapter takes a first step towards identifying the policy changes necessary to reduce total health inequality in child mortality by examining the effects of two major sources of inequality—income and health services access.

METHODS

DATA

The data used in this analysis come from 39 countries where a Demographic and Health Survey (DHS) was conducted and comparable data are available on all the determinants of interest, namely child survival, indicators of permanent income, maternal education, and household access to health services (12). For each country the latest year of available data was used from a nationally representative DHS, ranging from 1992 to 1997. Table 36.1 displays the countries in this analysis, along with the survey year, sample size, and three-letter acronym used in figures later in the chapter.

The DHS collects complete birth histories for women of reproductive age (usually defined as 15–49 years), as well as health histories for all children born in the last five years, through in-person interviews. Birth histories include information on the date of birth and current status (alive/dead) of each child that each woman has had. This information is used to construct the dependent variable: whether each child survived to the age of two years.

Health histories collect information on immunization of the children, the type of attendant present at the birth of the child (skilled or unskilled), and the type and number, if any, of antenatal care visits that the mother received for each pregnancy. With this information a proxy variable was constructed for the

Table 36.1   Demographic and Health Surveys used in this analysis: country name, three-letter acronym, survey year, and sample size

Country	Code	Survey year	Sample size
Bangladesh	BGD	1997	9 127
Benin	BEN	1996	5 491
Bolivia	BOL	1994	8 603
Brazil	BRA	1996	12 612
Burkina Faso	BFA	1993	6 354
Cameroon	CAM	1998	5 501
Central African Republic	CAR	1995	5 884
Colombia	COL	1995	11 140
Comoros	COM	1996	3 050
Cote d'Ivoire	CIV	1994	8 099
Dominican Republic	DOR	1996	8 422
Egypt	EGY	1995	14 779
Eritrea	ERI	1995	5 054
Ghana	GHA	1994	4 562
Guatemala	GUA	1995	12 403
Haiti	HAI	1995	5 356
Indonesia	IDN	1994	28 168
Kenya	KEN	1993	7 540
Madagascar	MDG	1997	7 060
Malawi	MWI	1992	4 849
Mali	MAL	1996	9 704
Morocco	MOR	1992	9 256
Mozambique	MOZ	1997	8 779
Namibia	NAM	1992	5 421
Nepal	NEP	1996	8 429
Niger	NER	1998	7 577
Nigeria	NIG	1990	8 781
Pakistan	PAK	1991	6 611
Paraguay	PAR	1990	5 827
Peru	PER	1996	28 951
Philippines	PHI	1998	13 983
Rwanda	RWA	1992	6 551
Togo	TOG	1998	8 569
Uganda	UGA	1995	7 070
United Republic of Tanzania	TZA	1996	8 120
Uzbekistan	UZB	1996	4 415
Yemen	YEM	1992	6 010
Zambia	ZAM	1996	8 021
Zimbabwe	ZWE	1994	6 128

household's access to health services. This variable is derived from a factor analysis based on the proportion of children of each mother that received a measles vaccine, the proportion that received a DTP vaccine, the proportion of pregnancies for which the mother received at least four antenatal care visits, and the proportion of deliveries that were attended by skilled personnel. This proxy variable is referred to as "health services access."

The DHS also collect information on indicators of permanent income for each household. The indicators used in this analysis were: ownership of a radio, television, bicycle, motorbike, car, and fridge; whether the household has electricity and running water; the type of material that the floor, walls and roof of the house are made of; and the type of toilet that the household has. These indicators were used in a hierarchical ordered probit model to arrive at an estimate of permanent income for each household. This method of estimating permanent income from indicator variables is similar to methods developed to construct an asset index from the DHS (*13;14*). Details of the estimation of permanent income and a validation of the model are presented in Ferguson et al. (*15*).

STATISTICAL MODEL

A previous study measuring total health inequality used the extended beta-binomial model to estimate the distribution of mortality risk (*10*). This chapter presents a conceptually similar approach using a modified logit model. In the standard logit model, all variation in the probability of child survival depends on the quality of available covariates, and so any measure of inequality derived from such a model would underestimate total inequality. For this analysis, the usual logit model is modified to include an additional term that captures systematic variability not picked up by the measured covariates. This hierarchical logit model can be estimated with commonly used statistical software such as Stata.

To define the model, let Y_i be 1 for death and 0 for survival to age two, and X_i denote a vector of covariates measured shortly after birth, for child i. Then under the hierarchical logit model, the probability of survival is:

$$\Pr(Y_i \mid \eta_i) = [1 + \exp(-X_i\beta - \eta_i)]^{-1} \qquad [2]$$

where η_i is an extra, but unmeasured, explanatory variable. Since η_i is unmeasured but assumed independent normal, it can be integrated out during estimation:

$$\Pr(Y_i) = \int [1+\exp(-X_i \beta - \eta_i)]^{-1} N(\eta_i | 0, \omega^2) d\eta_i \quad [3]$$

where ω is the standard deviation of η_i and is estimated along with β. When X_i predicts well, ω is small and η_i is superfluous. When X_i omits information and predicts poorly, ω is larger and so η_i corrects the estimated probability by adding the appropriate amount of variability. This model therefore corrects for some, but obviously not all, sources of omitted information in the covariates. It is especially useful for situations where interest lies in measuring variability (or inequality).

The hierarchical logit model is fit to the data for each country separately and the *ex ante* probability that each child will die before age two is estimated. Then the sample variance of these probabilities is computed, which is decomposable according to equation [1] and which correlates with the other measures of inequality, such as the Gini coefficient, presented in Gakidou and King (10), at better than 0.95. The variance is the measure of inequality used in this analysis because it can be additively decomposed into between- and within-group components: i.e. equation [1] holds exactly, not merely as a conceptual framework.

Between-group inequality is measured here by computing the variance across income quintiles of the average probability of child mortality. Obviously, this only includes income-group inequalities and excludes between-group inequalities for other types of groups. However, most research on between-group inequality in child mortality has focused on disparities between income groups or groups highly correlated with income. We have also computed between-group inequality on the basis of several other definitions of groups, such as educational attainment, and the results are similar.

DECOMPOSITION ANALYSIS

We now decompose total health inequality by studying the effects of income inequality and inequality in access to health services. We first explore what portions of total inequality can be accounted for by inequality in permanent income and inequality in access to health services. Then we estimate the reduction in total inequality that would result if all households with incomes or levels of health services access below the mean were raised to the mean.

To compute an estimate of these effects, the analysis is performed sequentially, studying the effect of one variable at a time. To estimate the full effect of permanent income, a hierarchical logistic regression model is run where the only covariate is permanent income and the hierarchical error term picks up all systematic variation across mothers not correlated with income. This model is an estimate of the total effect of income on mortality. Maternal education, health system access, birth interval and age of the mother at birth are excluded, as some of the effects of income are mediated through these (post-treatment) covariates. The hierarchical error term picks up the remainder effect of these covariates, i.e. the effect that is independent of income.

The goal is to estimate the effect of permanent income inequality on inequality in total child mortality. To do that, the value of the permanent income index for each mother is replaced with the average value of all mothers in her country, and the regression model is used to recalculate the probability of mortality for each child. The new sample variance for this counterfactual scenario is then computed. This procedure simulates what would happen to the total variance if income were equally distributed in each country.

A similar procedure is employed to estimate the effect of health services access. The proxy for health services access is introduced in the hierarchical logit model. The effect of health services access inequality is estimated by replacing the value of this proxy variable for each mother with the average level for the country. The additional reduction in total variance, after removing variation due to permanent income inequality, is then considered as the effect of health services access inequality on total child mortality inequality.

From a policy perspective, it is also interesting to explore the effect of improving the situation of the worst off. This analysis is conducted in two steps as well. First, we simulate the reduction in total inequality that would occur if we raised to the mean the level of income for households with incomes lower than the mean. Second, we estimate the additional reduction in total inequality that would occur if the level of health services access were raised to the mean for households with access below the mean.

RESULTS

BETWEEN-GROUP, WITHIN-GROUP, AND TOTAL HEALTH INEQUALITY

Figure 36.1 plots, by country, total inequality by the average risk of death for the 39 countries in this analysis. The horizontal axis is the average probability of

Figure 36.1 Relationship of total child survival inequality with average level of child mortality

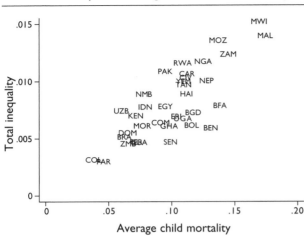

Figure 36.2 Within- vs. between-group inequality for 39 countries

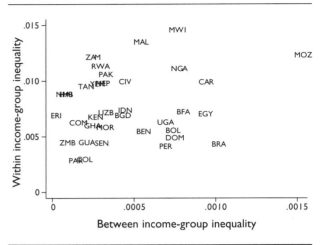

death for all children in the country. The vertical axis is the total variance in risk of death. The figure highlights that as average probability of dying increases, so does total inequality. Even though the relationship is strong, it is far from perfect, as demonstrated by countries such as Benin and Mozambique, which are at approximately the same average level of child mortality (about 135 per 1 000) but have very different levels of total inequality. Benin has a total inequality of 0.006, which is moderate for this sample, while Mozambique has one of the highest levels measured at 0.013.

Figure 36.2 plots between-income-group inequality (horizontally) by within-group inequality (vertically). Mozambique stands out with a high level of both between- and within-group inequality, while Paraguay has low levels of both. The figure indicates that there exists a small relationship between the two, but highlights that knowing one does not help much in predicting the other. Figure 36.2 also demonstrates that between-group inequality is a relatively small fraction of total health inequality. Indeed, within-group inequality is larger than between-group inequality in all 39 countries.

QUANTIFYING THE SOURCES OF HEALTH INEQUALITY

We now present the results of the decomposition analysis of total inequality into the effects of permanent income and access to health services. The reduction in total health inequality that would result if there were no inequality in permanent income is indicated in the horizontal axis of Figure 36.3. Brazil, Peru, and the

Dominican Republic are three of the countries which would benefit the most from a reduction in economic inequality. As was indicated in Figure 36.2, the contribution of economic inequality does not appear to be consistently greater in countries with higher inequality in child mortality. There is large variation in the contribution of economic inequality to total inequality in child mortality, ranging from very small (close to no effect, as in Namibia), up to almost 40% in Brazil. This implies that the sources of total inequality vary significantly across countries and economic inequality may not be a large source of inequality in health for several countries. As mentioned earlier, this counter-

Figure 36.3 Per cent reduction in total inequality resulting from removing income inequality versus removing health services access inequality

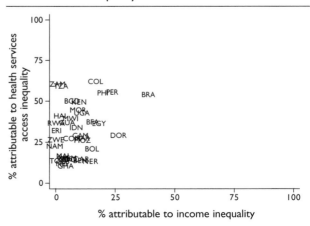

factual scenario attempts to capture the full effect of economic status on child mortality.

The vertical axis of Figure 36.3 shows the per cent reduction in total inequality that would result if there were no inequality in access to health services in each country. In most countries, the effect of inequality in health services access is larger than that of income inequality. The magnitude of the effect varies significantly across countries; in Colombia, Zambia, the United Republic of Tanzania, Peru, Philippines, and Brazil, more than 50% of the inequality in child mortality would be eliminated if access to health services were equal within each country. The effect of access to health services is larger than the effect of income inequalities in all included countries except Niger, which suggests that a good start for policies to reduce inequalities in child survival might be addressing inequalities in, and increasing the level of access to, health services in most countries.

Figure 36.4 presents the results of the second set of counterfactual analyses, examining the effect of potential policies to increase the income and health system access for the worst off. The horizontal axis displays the per cent reduction in total inequality that would result if the income of households currently below the mean were raised to the average level for their country. The figure shows that the countries that would benefit most from such a policy would be Brazil, Peru, and the Dominican Republic, with Brazil showing a decrease in total inequality of 50%. The vertical axis depicts the reduction in total child mortality inequality after raising the level of health system access for

those households below the average for their country. Colombia, Zambia, and the United Republic of Tanzania appear to be the countries where increasing health services access would have the greatest effect. It is interesting to note that there are a few countries which would benefit greatly from both an increase in income of the poorest and in level of access for those lacking access. In countries such as Colombia, Peru, Egypt, Brazil, Dominican Republic, and the Philippines, most inequality in child mortality would be eliminated by policies to reduce economic and health services access inequalities.

DISCUSSION

This chapter presents a decomposition of total inequality in two ways. First, it divides total inequality into between-income-group and within-income-group components and shows that most of the variation occurs within groups. Second, it examines the effect of two major policy-relevant determinants of total health inequality. Under the analytical assumptions presented, areas of intervention for public policy are identified that would seem most likely to be successful in producing large reductions in total inequality. In the vast majority of countries, a variable approximating access to health services accounts for a significant proportion of inequality, although the results indicate that public policy needs to be formulated on a country by country basis, as there are significant differences across the set of countries in this analysis.

Income-related inequalities, while important in their own right, appear to be a major component of total inequality in child survival in only a handful of countries. In most countries, they explain less than $\frac{1}{5}$ of total inequality. In some countries, particularly in Brazil, Peru, and the Dominican Republic, income-related inequalities account for more than a quarter of total health inequality. It is worth highlighting that the analytical approach followed here attempts to capture the full effect of permanent income on child survival.

The surprising and encouraging finding of this chapter is the size of the effect of health services access on total inequality. In all countries in this analysis except for Niger, the effect of health services access is larger than the effect of permanent income. The types of services that constitute the health services access proxy are amenable to interventions within the health sector, whether they are health education or family planning programmes, or programmes to improve accessibility

Figure 36.4 Per cent reduction in total inequality resulting from raising income to the mean versus raising health services access to the mean for those below the mean

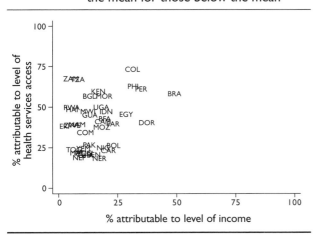

to health services in particular areas. In terms of policy implications, the present findings suggest that the most effective ways to reduce inequalities in child survival would be by reducing inequalities in health services access and increasing coverage of health services.

In this analysis, health services access has been approximated by four related variables which were available in the dataset. It is likely that jointly these four variables are a good proxy for access to health services; however, it is also possible that they are capturing different effects in different countries. These variables and their significance depend on the structure of a country's health system and a more in-depth analysis is required to arrive at concrete policy recommendations to reduce total health inequality for each country. With the variables currently available in the data, it is not possible to distinguish whether financial or physical access is of greater importance, as these cannot be differentiated in the present analysis.

As in all counterfactual analyses, the results of the procedures in this chapter can be sensitive to assumptions. In the present analysis in particular, the order in which terms are introduced and hypothetical scenarios are implemented influences the estimate of the effect of each component of total inequality. Some, but not all, of these effects can be studied by reordering the manipulations. When the scenarios are reordered so that the health system access variables are introduced first, the size of the effect of permanent income inequality drops. As such, the results here should be considered conservative estimates of the effects of health interventions on total health inequality.

The results also suggest that the causes of inequality in child mortality are related to, but are quite distinct from, the causes of average level of childhood mortality, and that they vary significantly across countries. Therefore, variables which predict inequality need to be further researched, even if they do not predict average levels of health attainment.

References

(1) World Health Organization. *The World Health Report 2000. Health Systems: Improving Performance*. Geneva, World Health Organization, 2000.

(2) Preston SH, Haines MR. *Fatal years: child mortality in late nineteenth-century America*. Princeton, Princeton University Press, 1991.

(3) Caldwell JC, McDonald P. Influence of maternal education on infant and child mortality: levels and causes. In: *International Population Conference, Manila*, vol. 2, 1981:79–96.

(4) Bicego G, Ahmad O. *Infant and child mortality*. Demographic and Health Surveys Comparative Studies No. 20. Calverton, Macro International, Inc., 1996. URL: http://www.measuredhs.com/pubs/

(5) Kunst AE, Geurts JJ, van den Berg J. International variation in socioeconomic inequalities in self reported health. *Journal of Epidemiology and Community Health*, 1995, 49:117–123.

(6) Wagstaff A. Socioeconomic inequalities in child mortality: comparisons across nine developing countries. *Bulletin of the World Health Organization*, 2000, 78: 19–29.

(7) Marmot MG, et al. Health inequalities among British civil servants: the Whitehall II study. *The Lancet*, 1991, 337:1387–1393.

(8) Kawachi I, Marshall S, Pearce N. Social class inequalities in the decline of coronary heart disease among New Zealand men, 1975–1977 to 1985–1987. *International Journal of Epidemiology*, 1991, 20:393–398.

(9) Mackenbach JP, Kunst AE. Measuring the magnitude of socio-economic inequalities in health: an overview of available measures illustrated with two examples from Europe. *Social Science & Medicine*, 1997, 44:757–771.

(10) Gakidou E, King G. Measuring total health inequality: adding individual variation to group-level differences. *International Journal for Equity in Health*, 2002, 1.

(11) Braveman P, Starfield B, Geiger HJ. World Health Report 2000: how it removes equity from the agenda for public health monitoring and policy. *British Medical Journal*, 2001, 323:678–681.

(12) Macro International Inc. *Demographic and Health Surveys*. 2001. URL: http://www.measuredhs.com/

(13) Filmer D, Pritchett L. Estimating wealth effects without expenditure data—or tears: an application to educational enrolments in states of India. *Demography*, 2001, 38: 115–132.

(14) World Bank. *Country reports on health, nutrition, population and poverty*. 2001. URL: http://www.worldbank.org/poverty/health/data/index.htm

(15) Ferguson BD et al. Estimating permanent income using indicator variables. In: Murray CJL, Evans DB, eds. *Health systems performance assessment: debates, methods and empiricism*. Geneva, World Health Organization, 2003.

Chapter 37

MEASUREMENT METHODS FOR INEQUALITY IN THE RISK OF ADULT MORTALITY

EMMANUELA GAKIDOU, AJAY TANDON

INTRODUCTION

Unlike with children, many fewer datasets are readily available for the estimation of inequality in adult risk of dying. Particularly in low- and middle-income countries, information on average levels of mortality is often unreliable, let alone data on the distribution of mortality risk within countries. Intensive efforts have been made to identify datasets that are well suited for the analysis of inequality in mortality risk in adults, and models have been modified to fit this analysis.

This chapter presents an overview of data available, proposes a model to estimate the distribution of mortality risk in adults and an alternative process of approximating that distribution in countries where data are not readily available.

INDIVIDUAL-LEVEL DATA

To estimate the distribution of hazard in each age-sex group in a population, individual-level data are needed. The ideal dataset would be records of individuals from health surveys or censuses linked to death registration records. This type of dataset would provide multiple years of observation for each individual and a survival outcome at the end of the observation period. The longer the observation period, the better for the model. In some countries, it is possible to directly link records from health surveys to death registration; in others, techniques have been developed to find probabilistic matches.

DIRECT RECORD LINKAGE

Directly linked death registration and census/health survey datasets exist for a few countries. A direct record linkage can happen when an individual record

has a unique identifier for each person which is the same in the census/health survey and in the death registration index.

An example of a dataset that is directly linked are the data from the National Health Interview Survey in the United States from 1987 to 1994 that have been linked to the National Death Index from 1987 to 1997. So, for example, for individuals in the 1987 National Health Interview Survey the follow-up period is eleven years. Survival analysis can be performed on these individuals some of whom died during the eleven year period, and the majority of whom would be considered "censored" observations, as they were alive at the end of the observation period and we have no further information on them.

Similar datasets exist for a few countries around the world; however, there are strict confidentiality agreements that do not allow their dissemination. WHO is arranging with the Statistical Offices of these countries to gain access to the data only for the purposes of this analysis, and without disclosing any of the individual-level information. We are hoping that in collaboration with the Statistical Offices, we will be able to perform the analysis of inequality in adult mortality risk. Some of the countries with identified linked data are listed in Table 37.1.

PROBABILISTIC RECORD LINKAGE

In some countries, direct record linkage is not feasible because unique identifiers that could link records from the census or surveys to death registration do not exist. Since the 1960s, techniques on probabilistic record linkage have been developed that allow for matches to be made between records from different datasets within certain constraints and probability structures.

Table 37.1 Some existing individual-level datasets

Country	Data available
USA	NHIS 1987–1994–NDI 1987–1997
UK	1970, 80 & 90 census linked to death registry—1% sample
UK	since 1993, linked birth and death certificates for children who die < 5yrs
Sweden	1960 to 1985 censuses, linked to between census data and mortality data for 5 or 10 years
Finland	5 yearly censuses since 1970, linkage between censuses and to mortality data for the following 5 years
Denmark	1970–86 census, linkage to mortality and cancer registry data
Norway	1970 and 1980 censuses, linkage between censuses, linkage to 1980–90 mortality data
Italy	1981 census linked to mortality data for the following 6 months
Italy	for Turin: linked to 1981–89 mortality data
Canada	Manitoba county census
France	2–3% sample of 1975 census, linked to 1975–1989 mortality data

Probabilistic record linkage involves assigning agreement and disagreement weights (or odds) for each value of each matching variable. The matching variables commonly used as they are often present in both mortality and census data include geocodes (codes for area of residence—county, municipality, etc.), sex, age, ethnic/racial group, country of birth, date of birth, education, and occupation. A larger number of variables common to both records leads to a better overall matching of records between the two datasources.

When records are probabilistically matched, a balance has to be found between maximizing the number of links obtained and minimizing the estimated percentage of false-links. Commercial software packages are available that conduct probabilistic record linkage. Statistics Canada has developed a software named *Generalized Record Linkage Software* (GRLS) and another commonly used commercially available package is *Automatch*.[1]

MODELS FOR ESTIMATING RISK OF DEATH DISTRIBUTION IN ADULTS

Survival analysis models are a good starting point for the estimation of probability of death in age groups other than children. For the most part, data available refer to observations of individuals over the course of several years and dichotomizing this information into survival or death like we do in children would discard valuable data on length of survival.

For adults we want to model survival time in order to estimate baseline hazard (or risk) at time t. This baseline hazard is the component of the hazard that is solely a function of time. The second component of the hazard is a function of covariates. For each adult we have a number of covariates available such as income, education, age, occupation, race/ethnicity, etc. These covariates can help us estimate the risk of death for individual i. However there are still many unmeasured covariates and community-level variables that are not captured by individual i's covariates. Therefore, we would like to add a term to capture systematic variation across individuals that is not explained by the available covariates and operates at the level of the residence/geographic variable.

Therefore, for individual i, conditional on his/her having survived to time t, his/her hazard (or instantaneous probability) of dying in time t is:

$$h(t_i) = e^{\gamma t_i} e^{\beta x_i}$$

The parameter γ is usually positive with mortality data and indicates that the hazard increases with time and as time goes to infinity, the hazard goes to 1.

The probability of having survived to time t is given by $S(t)$ and is equal to:

$$S(t) = e^{\frac{-e^{\beta x_i}}{\gamma}\left(e^{\gamma t} - 1\right)}$$

The probability density function $f(t)$ is:

$$f(t) = e^{\left(\beta x_i + \gamma t\right) - \frac{e^{\beta x_i}}{\lambda}\left(e^{\lambda t} - 1\right)}$$

The simple Gompertz regression model assumes that the hazard of an individual can be entirely determined by his or her covariates and the baseline hazard function, based on the γ parameter of the distribution. This parametric specification with the available covariates can only explain part of the variability in observed time to death. Excess systematic variability is known as over-dispersion. Over-dispersion is caused by misspecification or omitted covariates. "Frailty" models attempt to measure this over-dispersion by modelling it as a multiplicative effect on the hazard function. In adult survival data we do not have measures of community-level variables. To capture this unmeasured effect at the community level, we include a group-level effect on the hazard, i.e. the hazard for individual i of group j becomes:

$$h(t_{ij} \mid \alpha_j) = \alpha_j h(t_{ij}) = \alpha_j e^{\gamma t} e^{\beta x_{ij}}$$

The hazard of each individual i includes his/her vector of covariates βx_i and the unmeasured variables which are shared within the group j and are estimated by α_j. α_j is a random positive quantity, and for purposes of model identifiability it is assumed to have mean one and variance θ. The Gamma distribution is often used to parameterize this deterministic variability, as it is very flexible and can easily be parameterized to have mean one and variance q. The probability density function of the $\text{Gamma}(1/\theta, \theta)$ is:

$$g(x) = \frac{x^{\frac{1}{\theta}-1} e^{-\frac{x}{\theta}}}{\Gamma\left(\frac{1}{\theta}\right) \theta^{\frac{1}{\theta}}}$$

Performing the integrations shows that specifying the unmeasured variability as Gamma will result in the survival model where probability of survival to time t, $S(t)$ will be equal to:

$$S_\theta(t) = \left[1 - \theta \ln\left\{S(t)\right\}\right]^{-\frac{1}{\theta}}$$

This specification of the model is used in the example of the United States presented below. This model may need to be modified to fit the needs of specific datasets.

AN APPLICATION OF THE ADULT SURVIVAL MODEL TO DATA FROM THE USA

DATA

The data used in this example come from the National Health Interview Survey from 1987 to 1994. The records of the interviewed individuals have been linked using a unique person identifier to the National Death Index for the years 1987 to 1995. There are 415 158 records in the dataset. Individuals interviewed by the NHIS are a nationally representative sample of the non-institutionalized population of the US aged over 18. The questionnaire includes questions on their socio-demographic characteristics, such as age, sex, occupation, education, income, race, as well as questions on how individuals rate their own health and whether they are limited in their usual activities. The questionnaire also has information on the geocode of the place of residence of the respondents. For confidentiality reasons the public files include randomized geocodes, i.e. the users of the data know which individuals lived in the same area, but do not have information on where this area is.

MODEL USED

The model used in this analysis was a survival analysis model with a Gompertz distribution on the baseline hazard and a gamma distribution on the random effect. The Gompertz distribution on the baseline hazard means that the risk of death rises monotonically with age; the parameter of the Gompertz distribution γ has been set equal to 0.09 for males and 0.08 for females. The value of this parameter was taken from the life table for the US and it reflects the rate of increase of the mortality risk with age.

Based on the parameterization described above, the hazard of individual i living in area j at time t is being estimated as:

$$h(t_{ij} \mid \alpha_j) = \alpha_j h(t_{ij}) = \alpha_j e^{\gamma t} e^{\beta x_{ij}}$$

where aj is the "over-dispersion" or excess systematic variability (called random effect in our child survival model) for area j in which individual i lives, γ is set to the value of 0.09 for males and 0.08 for females, and βx_{ij} is the vector of covariates for individual i which include: age, education, race, income, whether he/she is above or below the poverty line, whether he/she lives alone or not, whether he/she was employed or not, if he/she has any difficulties in performing major daily activities, and his/her rating of his/her own health status.

PRELIMINARY RESULTS

A preliminary analysis of variation in predicted risk of death was done using the model described above. The model was run separately for each age-sex group. There are not enough observations in the data to group the population in five year age groups, as would be ideal; the groupings used in this analysis were: 25–34 years, 35–44, 45–54, 55–64, and over 65 years.

Figure 37.1 shows one example of the output of the survival analysis model. From the model a predicted probability of death for each individual can be estimated, based on the individual's set of covariates and the geographic area in which he/she resides. Figure 37.1 shows the predicted distribution of risk of death for males and females aged 45–54 years. The distribution of risk of death seems to be less unequal for females than for males. This finding is consistent with results from small area analyses (1) which report much greater inequality in adult males than females. Patterns

Figure 37.1   Predicted distributions of risk of death for males and females aged 45–54 years, USA

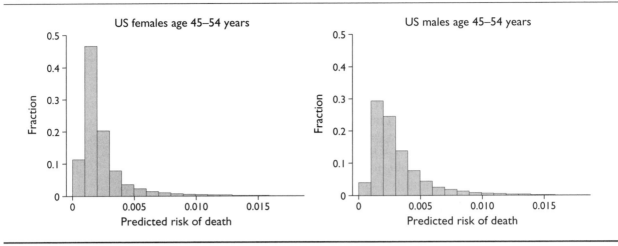

of inequality in risk of death across ages and the causes of these inequalities need to be explored further.

Table 37.2 presents the main results of the model for five age groups. It shows the predicted average hazard rate at the onset of observation, as well as the median (since these distributions are very skewed, it is also interesting to look at the median). The table also lists three measures of the variation in the distributions, the interquartile range, the standard deviation, and the coefficient of variation. The results confirm the patterns seen in age-specific mortality rates by sex from the US life tables. Males have a higher mortality rate than females in the age groups studied here. In terms of the distribution of that mortality rate, according to absolute measures of inequality such as the interquartile range or the standard deviation, there is more variation in males than females, at all ages. According to the coefficient of variation, a relative measure of inequality, there is more variation in females than males in the age group 25–34, but more inequality in males in all other age groups.

This type of analysis should also be performed on individual-level datasets from other countries. A cross-national comparison of inequalities in risk of death at different ages is likely to yield very interesting results.

HOUSEHOLD SURVEY DATA

WHO has engaged in a World Health Survey programme conducting household, postal, and telephone surveys in nationally representative samples of the population. Primarily the World Health Survey has

been used to collect information on current health of the interviewees along with their socio-demographic characteristics.

WHO is considering adding questions to collect information on household deaths in the 12 months preceding the interview. Such questions would increase the data available on adult mortality, particularly in low-income countries. Information on the socio-demographic characteristics of the deceased household members could also be collected. If the sample size were large enough, this would result in an individual-level dataset that could be used to estimate inequality in adult mortality.

In addition to enquiring about deaths in household members, a more ambitious project would entail linking individuals from the World Health Survey probabilistically to census records and to future death registration records. This would result in a dataset of individuals with baseline information on health state and follow-up for mortality.

USING SMALL-AREA ANALYSIS TO ESTIMATE THE DISTRIBUTION OF MORTALITY RISK ACROSS INDIVIDUALS

Where sufficiently large linked individual record datasets are available, it is possible to estimate the distribution of mortality risk across individuals in an age group. Unfortunately, for many countries such linked datasets are not currently available. The computerization of the latest round of decennial censuses in many countries holds out the prospect that these datasets

Table 37.2 Predicted mean and median hazard rate, interquartile range, standard deviation, and coefficient of variation, by age and sex, USA

Age group	Mean			Median		
	Both sexes	Males	Females	Both sexes	Males	Females
25–34	0.001	0.001	0.000	0.000	0.001	0.000
35–44	0.001	0.002	0.001	0.001	0.001	0.001
45–54	0.003	0.004	0.003	0.002	0.003	0.002
55–64	0.008	0.010	0.006	0.005	0.007	0.004
65–74	0.026	0.031	0.022	0.019	0.024	0.016

Age group	Interquartile range			Standard deviation			Coefficient of variation		
	Both sexes	Males	Females	Both sexes	Males	Females	Both sexes	Males	Females
25–34	0.0006	0.0006	0.0002	0.0008	0.0010	0.0005	1.22	0.98	1.32
35–44	0.0008	0.0009	0.0006	0.0017	0.0020	0.0013	1.33	1.30	1.26
45–54	0.0020	0.0024	0.0015	0.0035	0.0041	0.0028	1.11	1.10	1.05
55–64	0.0055	0.0071	0.0039	0.0075	0.0092	0.0051	0.96	0.93	0.83
65–74	0.0192	0.0231	0.0158	0.0219	0.0255	0.0181	0.85	0.83	0.82

may become more common in the near future. Nevertheless, for the vast majority of countries alternative methods are needed to quantify the extent of inequalities in mortality risks. For nearly 80 countries in the world with complete vital registration systems and another 40 countries with partial vital registration data, the analysis of mortality rates for small areas is feasible. In this section, we explore the extent to which the analysis of the distribution of mortality rates across small areas can be used as an estimator of the distribution of mortality risks across individuals.

The well-known large variation in mortality risks across small areas (1–4) suggests that the distribution of mortality risks across small areas does reveal a considerable fraction of the variance in mortality risks across individuals. For example, within the United States, the variation in life expectancy across counties is 61 to 77.5 for males and 70.5 to 83.5 for females. To use small-area variation in mortality risk as a valid and reliable indicator of the variation of mortality risk across individuals would require a number of assumptions. In this section, we explore these more carefully and use the United States as an empirical illustration of the strengths and weaknesses of this proxy approach.

PRINCIPLES

If the probability of living in a given small area is independent of mortality risk for any individual, then we would observe the same expected value of average mortality risk across all small areas (5). The only observed variation across small areas would be due to chance or measurement error. As the unit for small-area analysis was decreased in size, the observed stochastic variation in death rates would increase. Given random association with appropriate statistical methods (see below), however, no systematic variation in expected average mortality rate would be detected. It is clear, nevertheless, in all countries studied that people with similar socioeconomic status and other health-related covariates are more likely to live together than at random. In addition, community-level factors such as environmental quality, quality of health services, and community health interventions can also determine mortality risks. For both of these reasons, we anticipate that there is considerable deterministic variation in expected average death rates across small areas. The survival analysis models that include a random effect by location developed in the previous section, show the potential significance of location and also the relatively high covariance between important predictors of individual mortality risk and location.

For deterministic variation in average mortality risk across small areas to be used as a proxy for the variation in mortality risk across individuals, we must address three key questions. First, what fraction of the variance in individual mortality risks is captured by the deterministic variance in average death rates across small areas? Second, in order to make meaningful comparisons across countries, we would also need to know how the measured deterministic variance across small areas is affected by the size of the small areas included in the analysis? Third, is the relationship between deterministic variance in death rates across small areas and the variance in mortality risks across individuals consistent across populations and over time? If it is consistent, then the observed variation across small areas can be used to make comparable estimates of the variation in mortality risks across individuals.

In the following subsections, we first explore models that can be used to decompose the observed distribution of mortality rates for an age-sex group across small areas into the stochastic and deterministic components. The next section compares small-area assessments for the United States with the linked individual record data analysis presented earlier for the US. The influence of the size of small areas on the results is explored next. Finally, further extensions of small-area studies requiring supplementary data are discussed.

MODELS TO DECOMPOSE OBSERVED VARIATION IN DEATH RATES ACROSS SMALL AREAS INTO STOCHASTIC AND DETERMINISTIC COMPONENTS

The observed variation in death rates across small areas is due to a combination of stochastic variance which is in proportion to the number of individuals in an age-sex group in each small area and deterministic variation in the average death rate across small areas. Two strategies have been traditionally used to deal with this problem in small-area studies. First, small-area data have been combined over time or across adjacent locations to achieve a threshold population size that provides "acceptable" confidence intervals for the mortality parameter being estimated. The main advantage of this approach is that it allows for estimates with a known uncertainty interval for each particular small area or grouping of small areas. The distribution across small areas is, nevertheless, still a function of both stochastic and deterministic variation in the average death rate across small areas. If we are not concerned about obtaining estimates of the expected mortality risk for each small area but only about the distribution of mortality risks across small areas, then a variety of statistical models can be used to decompose the observed variation in death rates across small areas into stochastic and deterministic components.

The Beta-Binomial Model

The beta-binomial model presented earlier to estimate the distribution of mortality risk across mothers,

given data on the survival of their children, can also be applied to small-area data for an age-sex group. Each small area has a certain number of individuals observed in an age-sex group and a certain number of deaths. Assuming that each individual in the small area experiences the same mortality risk, then the number of deaths observed will be distributed binomial. If we assume that mortality risks across small areas are distributed beta, then the beta-binomial model presented earlier can be used to estimate the deterministic variation in mortality risk across small areas. The main limitation of this model is that the computational time for each age-sex group is very long and depends on the number of individuals in each small area. Given available computing power, it may not be feasible to run this model on datasets that include multiple small areas with large populations until an alternative algorithm for its estimation has been developed.

Compound Normal Model

A much more efficient model can be used to estimate the distribution of mortality risk across small areas if some simplifying assumptions are made. First, we assume that for each small area, the observed death rate y_i is distributed normally with mean μ_i and standard deviation σ_i:

$$y_i \sim N(\mu_i, \sigma_i^2)$$

σ_i is assumed to be the normal approximation of the binomial and is equal to:

$$\sigma_i = \sqrt{\frac{pq}{N}}$$

where p is the observed death rate, q is one minus the death rate, and N is population size in the age-sex group.

Second, we assume that μ_i is distributed normally across small areas with mean μ and standard deviation θ:

$$\mu_i \sim N(\mu_i, \theta^2)$$

It follows that the distribution of observed death rates is:

$$y_i \sim N(\mu, \sigma_i^2 + \theta^2)$$

Although the assumption that expected mortality risk across small areas is distributed normally cannot be true as mortality risks cannot be less than zero or greater than one, it appears that the approximation gives reasonable answers. Estimates of μ and θ can be obtained using maximum likelihood methods. In other terms, for every age and sex group, the observed death rate has a small area-specific deterministic component—which is the same as saying there is fundamental variability or a small area-specific random effect with a mean μ and standard deviation θ, and a stochastic component with mean 0 and (known) standard deviation σ_i.

Using data from the US Burden of Disease study for 2 077 counties or country clusters, this model has been estimated for each age-sex group. Table 37.3 shows the mean death rate across small areas, the observed standard deviation of the death rates, and the estimated θ or the standard deviation of the expected death rate.

Figure 37.2 illustrates for males and for females for the US the coefficient of variation in the expected death rate as a function of age. As can be seen in the graph, the largest coefficient of variation is age group 35–39 for males and 30–34 for females.

For comparison, the same model has been estimated for district-level data for the UK, 1997. Data from the UK (illustrated in Figure 37.3) were available for 403 districts. One notable distinction is that in the UK data, there appears not to be a big difference in the coefficient of variation of the expected death rate for males versus females. In the data from the US, on the other hand, males tended to have a higher expected death rate for almost all age groups.

Comparing age group 65–69, it appears that the normal-normal model gives a similar standard devia-

tion of mortality risk across small areas as did the more computationally intensive beta-binomial model. One advantage of the beta-binomial model is that it can handle when there are zero deaths in an age-sex group in a small area. Zero deaths in an age-sex group present some problems for the normal-normal model. In this analysis for districts with zero deaths, the average death rate for that age group across all districts was used in place of a zero death rate.

Table 37.3 Expected death rates and estimated standard deviation of the expected death rate across small areas in the USA

Age group	Expected death rate		Std deviation of expected death rate	
	Females	Males	Females	Males
0–4	0.00189	0.00242	0.00028	0.00035
15–19	0.00041	0.00112	1.99E-07	0.00017
20–24	0.00046	0.00155	5.87E-05	0.00040
25–29	0.00055	0.00158	6.84E-05	0.00034
30–34	0.00071	0.00181	0.00013	0.00052
35–39	0.00101	0.00222	0.00018	0.00069
40–44	0.00148	0.00289	0.00021	0.00079
45–49	0.00252	0.00454	0.00028	0.00096
50–54	0.00424	0.00742	0.00039	0.00121
55–59	0.00684	0.01228	0.00056	0.00162
60–64	0.01049	0.01896	0.00090	0.00205
65–69	0.01553	0.02842	0.00132	0.00289
70–74	0.02473	0.04468	0.00188	0.00409
75–79	0.03803	0.06616	0.00220	0.00473
80–84	0.06319	0.10154	0.00305	0.00565
85+	0.10682	0.15262	0.00353	0.00590

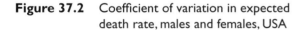

Figure 37.2 Coefficient of variation in expected death rate, males and females, USA

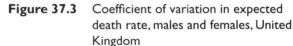

Figure 37.3 Coefficient of variation in expected death rate, males and females, United Kingdom

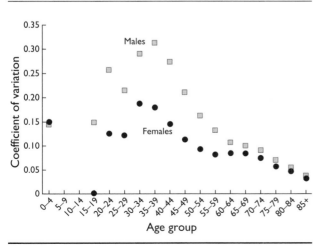

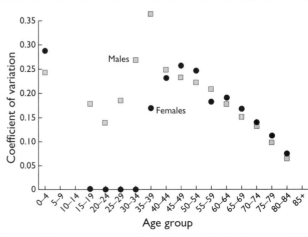

What Fraction of the Total Variation in Mortality Risk across Individuals Is Captured by the Variation in Mortality Risk across Small Areas?

There is clearly no theoretical answer to the question what is the fraction of total variance in mortality risk across individuals captured by the variance in mortality risk across small areas. If small-area analysis captures a predictable fraction of the variance, this must be established empirically. If generalizable statements on this relationship are to be made, they will need to be based on careful empirical assessments in a wide range of settings. Here, we present only one comparison based on the individual analysis for adult mortality in the US and small-area analysis for the US.

Table 37.4 shows the standard deviation of the estimated mortality risk across individuals in the US by age and sex, using the full survival model and the standard deviation estimated across small areas.[2]

The standard deviation increases with age in both analyses, and is larger in the individual-level analysis than in the small-area analysis. Figure 37.4 presents for males and for females the coefficient of variation of risk of death with age. The same age pattern is observed from the survival analysis model and the small-area analysis in both males and females. As demonstrated in Table 37.4 above, the survival analysis model is showing more inequality in risk of death than the small-area analysis one.

Further empirical studies in settings where linked individual datasets and small-area data are available

Table 37.4   Standard deviation of estimated risk of death across individuals from two analyses: full survival analysis model with random effect and small-area analysis

	Full model	*Small-area analysis*
Males		
25–34	0.0010	0.0005
35–44	0.0020	0.0008
45–54	0.0041	0.0012
55–64	0.0092	0.0021
65+	0.0255	0.0050
Females		
25–34	0.0005	0.0001
35–44	0.0013	0.0002
45–54	0.0028	0.0004
55–64	0.0051	0.0009
65+	0.0181	0.0027

will help establish if there is a consistent relationship between the variation in mortality risk across small areas and the variation across individuals. If such a relationship does exist, it implies that there is some common process that underlies patterns of human aggregation. If true, patterns of human aggregation where individuals with similar mortality risk tend to live close to each other is an interesting and important phenomenon in its own right. Perhaps the stability over time of small-area deviations in mortality rates observed in the US and the UK over decades is related to this process. Alternatively, community-level factors may be more important determinants of mortality risk than has generally been appreciated.

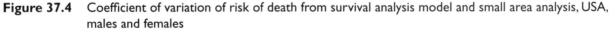

Figure 37.4   Coefficient of variation of risk of death from survival analysis model and small area analysis, USA, males and females

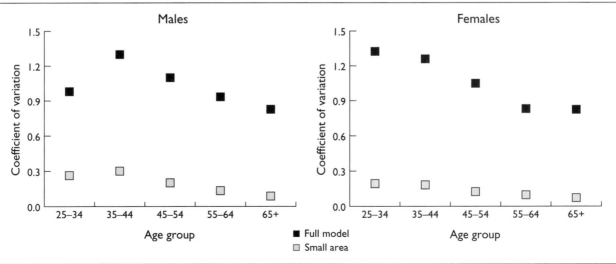

SIZE OF SMALL AREAS AND VARIATION IN MORTALITY RISK

The magnitude of the variation in expected mortality risk across small areas depends on the size of the small areas being analysed. In other words, the systematic variation in mortality risks across states in the USA is much smaller than across counties. Further research needs to be conducted into the ideal size of small areas that is best suited for this type of analysis, so that there are enough person-years in the data to estimate the distribution of risk of death, but the small areas are still homogeneous enough to capture the effect of unmeasured covariates on risk.

SUPPLEMENTING SMALL-AREA ANALYSIS

Small-area analysis will always underestimate the total variance in mortality rates across individuals. The key problem lies in the fact that individuals within a small area experience different mortality risks. This inter-individual variation is not captured in the small-area data. In some countries, such as the Russian Federation, linked individual data are available for a few small areas. This type of data can provide a direct assessment of within small area variance in risk. Individual-level data from a few small areas can be used to improve estimates of the variation in risk achieved with small-area data only. Another possible way to capture some of the variation within small areas is to include in the estimation model indices of heterogeneity for each small area. These could be indices of income inequality or education inequality, which are often available at the small-area level or can be computed from census data.

NOTES

1 Generalized Record Linkage System (GRLS) Software was developed by Statistics Canada. Automatch Generalised Record Linkage System was developed by MatchWare Technologies, Inc.

2 Note that the age groups are different from those in the previous section because there are not enough observations in the individual-level data to group individuals in smaller age groups.

REFERENCES

(1) Murray CJL et al. *U.S. patterns of mortality by county and race: 1965–1994.* Cambridge, Harvard School of Public Health and National Center for Disease Prevention and Health Promotion, 1998.

(2) Benach J et al. Material deprivation and leading causes of death by gender: evidence from a nationwide small area study. *Journal of Epidemiology & Community Health*, 2001, 55(4):239–245.

(3) Reading R et al. Do interventions that improve immunisation uptake also reduce social inequalities in uptake? *British Medical Journal*, 1994, 308(6937): 1142–1144.

(4) Galal OM, Qureshi AK. Dispersion Index: measuring trend assessment of geographical inequality in health—the example of under-five mortality in the Middle East/north African region, 1980–1994. *Social Science & Medicine*, 1997, 44(12):1893–1902.

(5) Wolfson M, Rowe J. On measuring inequalities in health. *Bulletin of the World Health Organization*, 2001, 79(6): 553–560.

Assessing the Distribution of Household Financial Contributions to the Health System: Concepts and Empirical Application

Christopher J.L. Murray, Ke Xu, Jan Klavus, Kei Kawabata, Piya Hanvoravongchai, Riadh Zeramdini, Ana Mylena Aguilar-Rivera, David B. Evans

INTRODUCTION

In the past decade, there has been considerable interest in analysing and understanding the distribution of health system contributions across households (1–11). The fairness in financial contribution measure presented in *The World Health Report 2000* (12) contributed to this heightened attention towards health system financing arrangements (9;13–19). Protecting households from excessively large or catastrophic health payments has also played a prominent role recently in national policy debates in a number of countries (20–23).

The analysis of the consequences of household health system contributions can be divided into two broad approaches: the income approach and the burden approach. The former examines the effect of health system payments in the space of income. The key concern is the marginal effect of health systems financing arrangements on the broader construct of total household income. The effects in the space of income have been measured in terms of changes in its distribution (5–7;18) and more recently on changes in levels of poverty (10). The latter examines health system payments in terms of the impact or disutility experienced by households because of these payments.

The WHO measures of the fairness in financial contribution (2;11) and studies of catastrophic health payments (24) are examples of the burden approach.

To further clarify the conceptual distinction between the income and the burden approaches, Table 38.1 summarizes the main approaches and types of measurements that are possible. The effects of health system payments on households in the space of income can be assessed in terms of changes in the full distribution of income, most commonly reported using the redistributive effect (RE), or in terms of differences in the number of households falling below the poverty line (DH) before and after health system payments.

In the burden space, the complete distribution of disutility or impact of financial payment on households requires a distributional measure analogous to the ones used in the income space; the WHO fairness in financial contribution index (FFC) was developed for this purpose. The fraction of households facing a burden above a fixed threshold (%CAT), considered to involve catastrophic payments, is analogous to the DH in the income space and focuses attention on one tail of the distribution of household financial burden.

The purpose of this chapter is to use household survey data from 59 countries to illustrate the two different approaches to analysing the consequences

Table 38.1 Main indicators used in the income and burden approaches to analysing the consequences of household health system payments

Approach	Complete distribution	Threshold
Income	Change in the distibution of income due to health system payments (redistributive effect or RE)	Change in the number of households falling below the poverty line due to health system payments (DH)
Burden	Distribution of disutility or burden due to health system payments (fairness in financial contribution index or FFC)	Households above a threshold level of disutility or burden due to health system payments (Percentage of households with catastrophic payments or %CAT)

of household health system contributions. This empirical assessment helps to illustrate how changes in income distribution, changes in the percentage of households below the poverty line, the FFC, and the fraction of households facing catastrophic health payments all capture different dimensions of health financing arrangements. Through this analysis, it is argued that the different approaches for analysing the distribution of health system payments can be seen as complementary and useful in different ways for policy review and formulation.

The chapter is organized as follows. The next section reviews some core principles that underlie both the income and burden approaches. Section three reviews the income approach and gives an overview of the statistical indices that are used in this context to summarize the distribution. It also proposes an important modification of the standard methods used in this work that we believe will enhance the conceptual clarity of the measurements. The following section examines the burden approach towards health system contributions with a presentation of the respective summary distributional measures. Sections three and four also present the threshold measures of poverty or catastrophic payments associated with these two measurement approaches. Section five shows the empirical results based on an extensive database comprising household survey data from 59 countries. The last section concludes and discusses the findings.

COMMON CONCEPTUAL UNDERPINNINGS OF THE INCOME AND BURDEN APPROACHES

Analysis of the consequences of household health system contributions whether using the income or burden approach, examines the distribution of contributions to the financing of the health system in isolation from the distribution of the benefits of the health system. This is in keeping with a long tradition of analyses of the equity of public finance systems (25–30). The underlying principle is that any given distribution of benefits delivered by health systems could be financed in many different ways with various households contributing more or less to the overall resources that are raised. Because the distribution of household contributions can be considered as an independent policy choice to the distribution of benefits, it is interesting and important from a social policy perspective to investigate the consequences of this component by itself. Of course, analysing the distribution of the

benefits in terms of the coverage of interventions or their impact on health outcomes is also a critical issue which is addressed in detail elsewhere (31–33).

In both approaches health payments comprise four main sources: taxation, social security contributions, private health insurance premiums, and out-of-pocket payments. The methods and assumptions used in the context of estimating tax and social security contributions are the same. The differences between the approaches presented in the empirical section of this paper, therefore, do not reflect differences in the practical methods used to attribute financial contributions to particular households.

As a result of the distinction between health payments and health benefits, it is possible that in a situation where poorer households do not purchase health care because they cannot afford it, health payments appear relatively progressive in the income approach and relatively fair in the burden approach. Such an outcome could emerge if, for example, out-of-pocket payments for health services were concentrated in the upper income groups because the lower income groups chose not to use the services even though they needed them. The lack of available health services for the poor because of inadequate resources or because of a lack of financial protection mechanisms are important determinants of non-use and access to health services. It is important to identify non-users and the reasons for non-use, but for policy relevance they merit separate analysis.

MEASUREMENT OF THE IMPACT OF HEALTH SYSTEM PAYMENTS IN THE SPACE OF INCOME

PUBLIC FINANCE ORIGINS OF MEASURING TAX DISTRIBUTION

The literature on the distribution of government revenue collection has developed a standard set of measurement tools. These tools are built on one important approach to analysing the distribution of income, namely the Lorenz curve $L_x(p)$. It can be defined as the proportion of total income, x, received by the lowest pth fraction of the population, arranged in ascending order of income. It is shown in Figure 38.1. Perfect equality—each successive percentile of the population receiving 1% of the income—is denoted by the 45-degree line from the origin (the diagonal).

The Gini coefficient G_x is the proportion between the diagonal and the Lorenz curve (the observed devia-

Figure 38.1 Illustration of the progressivity index

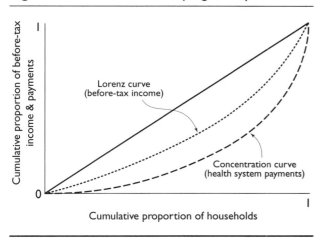

tion from perfect equality) divided by the total area under the diagonal (the maximum possible deviation from perfect equality). Because of the symmetry between the areas above and below the diagonal, it can be defined as one minus twice the area under the Lorenz curve:

$$G_x = 1 - 2 \int_0^1 L_x(p)dp \qquad [1]$$

Here the subscript x is used to refer to before-tax income. The Gini coefficient can have values in the range [0,1], with the degree of inequality increasing as the coefficient approaches unity—as the area between the Lorenz curve and the diagonal gets closer to the total area below the diagonal.

The concentration curve of a tax $C_t(p)$ is defined similarly to the Lorenz curve, replacing the cumulative proportion of income received by each fraction p, by the cumulative proportion of taxes or other payments contributed by each fraction of the population ordered by income (Figure 38.1). The concentration curve can be above or below the diagonal—when payments are progressive (e.g. the bottom 1% of income earners pay less than 1% of tax) it lies below, and when they are regressive it is above.

The tax concentration index C_t corresponds to the Gini coefficient—the area between the diagonal and the concentration curve divided by the area under the diagonal. Because the curve can lie above or below the diagonal, it can have values between –1 and 1. It is important to note that the concentration index of a tax is a bivariate function of both tax payments and household income. As it is not uniquely related to either distribution, the underlying income distribution could change substantially with no effect on

the concentration index, as long as the income ranks are preserved.[1] Clearly then, the distribution of tax payments needs to be related more concretely to the income distribution and the degree of income inequality that prevails in different countries or at different periods of time than is possible using the concentration index alone.

In a progressive tax system the average tax rate increases with income, while the opposite defines a regressive system. Progressive tax payments reduce income inequality while regressive taxes increase it. The Kakwani index of tax progressivity is given by the difference between the concentration index of taxes and the Gini coefficient of income:

$$K_t = C_t - G_x = 2 \int_0^1 \left[L_x(p) - C_t(p) \right] dp \qquad [2]$$

The subscript t refers to taxes and the subscript x refers to before-tax income. Graphically the Kakwani index is represented as twice the area between the concentration curve of taxes and the Lorenz curve of before-tax income. If the tax system is progressive and $C_t(p)$ lies below $L_x(p)$, (i.e. C_t has a higher value than G_x), K_t is positive. Where taxes are regressive or $C_t(p)$ lies above $L_x(p)$, the index is negative. The value of K_t ranges from –2 to 1. It approaches the lower limit when the income distribution is extremely unequal ($G_x \to 1$) and the tax burden falls on the poorest population groups ($C_t \to -1$). It approaches the upper limit with the converse: there is almost no income inequality and the tax burden falls on the richest groups.

Unlike the Kakwani index which measures departures from proportionality, the Reynolds-Smolensky index (29), often called the redistributive effect (RE), measures the extent to which the tax system redistributes income. Denoting the after-tax Gini coefficient by G_{x-t}, the redistributive effect is:

$$RE = G_x - G_{x-t} = 2 \int_0^1 \left[L_{x-t}(p) - L_x(p) \right] dp \qquad [3]$$

The index is defined in the range [–1,1], a negative value indicating regressivity and redistribution towards the better-off, and positive values pointing to the opposite. This is depicted in Figure 38.2.

Aronson et al. (34) have suggested a decomposition where the redistributive effect is partitioned into three components: indicating vertical equity, horizontal equity, and a reranking component in turn. It can be formalized as follows:

Figure 38.2 The redistributive effect (RE)

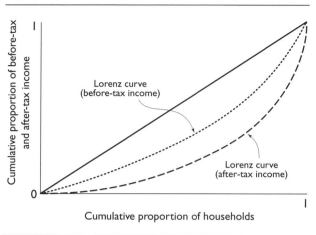

$$RE = \left(\frac{g}{1-g}\right)K_t - \sum \alpha_x G_{F(x)} - \left[G_{x-t} - C_{x-t}\right]$$
$$= V - H - R \qquad [4]$$

K_t is the Kakwani progressivity index and g is the average tax rate. The first component reflects vertical equity (V) of tax payments. The second term, corresponding to horizontal inequity, H, is obtained as a weighted sum of after-tax Gini coefficients, $G_{F(x)}$, computed within each group of before-tax equals. Non-zero values of H are associated with situations where households with the same before-tax income end up with different after-tax income due to differential tax treatment. Reranking, R, measures the extent to which households move up or down the order of households ranked by income in the process of moving from the before-tax income distribution to the after-tax income distribution. The value of V indicates the extent of redistribution that could have been attained in the absence of differential treatment of equals and rank reversals (i.e. when $H = R = 0$). The H and R terms are by definition non-negative and they reduce the redistributive effect below its potential maximum.

EXTENDING INCOME REDISTRIBUTION ANALYSIS TO HEALTH SYSTEM PAYMENTS

The policy interest in the impact of health payments on income has focused on the marginal impact of health system payments. It starts with the question: given the redistributive effect of non-health public financing, what further redistributive effect is produced by health financing (6)? Health payments influence income distribution through general taxation, social security contributions used on health, and direct private pay-

ments for health services. To see the distinct effect of health payments on the amount of money that is left for the household after all health payments, the redistributive effect should be addressed with respect to the distribution of after-tax income before any health payments (public and private) and after-tax income after all health payments.

Figure 38.3 shows total gross income (before any taxes) as the area A + B + C + D. Area A is after-tax income after all health payments, social security contributions and taxes, B represents private health payments, C is health payments through general taxation and social security contributions, and D shows tax payments used for purposes other than health. Total health payments are area B + C, and total tax and social security contributions are area C + D. Without health payments total after-tax income would equal the area A + B + C; with health payments after-tax income becomes area A.

In their analysis of OECD countries Wagstaff, van Doorslaer et al. (*18*) defined RE as the difference between the Gini coefficient of gross income (A + B + C + D) and the Gini coefficient of gross income after health payments (A + D). It can be argued that this does not measure what is intended, namely income distribution changes resulting from health payments taking as the starting point society's efforts to redistribute income through non-health public finance. To measure the true marginal redistributive effect of health payments alone, the income distribution changes created by health payments are better captured by measuring the difference between the Gini of after-tax income before health payments (A + B + C) and the Gini of after-tax income after health payments (A). The two methods will give different results. In the following

Figure 38.3 Conceptual framework for the calculation of redistributive effect (RE)

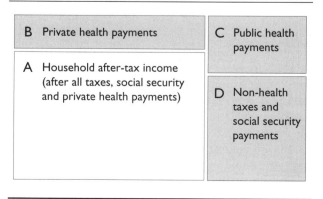

empirical work, we have adopted the approach of examining (A + B + C) compared with (A).

As was shown above, RE can be decomposed as:

$$RE = V - H - R = \frac{g}{1-g} K_t - (H+R)$$

$$= \frac{g}{1-g} (C_t - G_x) - (H+R) \quad [5]$$

In this context, g is the average share of household after-tax or before-tax income spent on health depending on the method used. Decomposition of RE helps to understand the difference between the methods. In the Wagstaff and van Doorslaer approach, the health payment share of income, g, is smaller because health payments (B + C) are divided by total income (A + B + C + D), while in the latter approach the same health payments are divided by the area (A + B + C). Where general non-health taxation is progressive overall, the before-payment Gini, G_x, becomes smaller in the method proposed here because it is based on after-tax income and tax payments used exclusively on health, while in the former method the Gini coefficient is based on total gross income. Although the directions of changes in the average contribution rate (g) and the before-payment income Gini can be identified, other terms in the formula, such as the concentration index (C_t) horizontal inequity (H) and reranking (R) could become either bigger or smaller because they depend on both the distribution of health payments and the income rank order.

EXTENDING THE ANALYSIS TO THE IMPACT ON POVERTY

Wagstaff and van Doorslaer (10) extended recently the analysis of health system contributions on overall income distributions to include changes in the number of households falling below the poverty line. The poverty impact is illustrated in Figure 38.4 by a hypothetical distribution of income, where the horizontal axis measures cumulative income and the vertical axis shows the cumulative percentage of the population.

The vertical line is the poverty line. Before health payments, about 30% of the population is under the poverty line. The poverty gap can be defined as area A, which equals total income required to push these households above the poverty line. After health payments, about 50% of the population is under the poverty line and the poverty gap has increased to A + B. Besides their impact on the number of households falling below the poverty line, health payments can also influence the extent of poverty for households already below the poverty line, sometimes called the depth of poverty.

A simple measure quantifying the impact of health system contributions on poverty is given by the difference in the percentage of households under the poverty line before and after health payments. Denoting the percentage of households under the poverty line after health payments as H_a and before health payments as H_b, the headcount difference DH is given as:

$$DH = H_a - H_b \quad [6]$$

Wagstaff and van Doorslaer (10) also propose measures that reflect changes in the depth of poverty in addition to the simple headcount measures. In this paper, for simplicity we focus on changes in the fraction of households falling beneath the poverty line.

HEALTH PAYMENTS IN THE SPACE OF BURDEN

EQUAL BURDEN OF HEALTH PAYMENTS

Murray et al. (2) and WHO (12) proposed that the impact of health system payments should be examined in the space of burden on households. Although the extension of public finance analysis to health payments has yielded interesting information on progressivity and income redistribution, it can be argued that a society does not seek to finance the health system for the purpose of redistributing income. Instead, societies expect health payments to be arranged in a fair way. Consistent with public financing studies that follow the capacity to pay principle, health payments should be viewed as a distinct entity, independent of income determination (27). We argue that the appropriate

Figure 38.4 Distribution of income and the poverty line

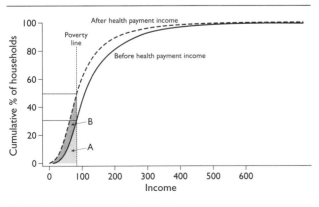

principle for this purpose is one where the burden created by health payments is equalized across all households.

The equal burden principle is different from the progressivity principle developed and used in the public finance context. Analysis of tax progressivity defines a tax function without reference to the total amount of revenue to be raised. Under the principle of equal burden, a given amount of total revenue is needed and each individual is requested to contribute according to his/her capacity to pay (35). The equal sacrifice principle advanced by Mills (36) proposed that everyone should suffer the same absolute loss of utility. Under a particular form of utility function, this proposition is equivalent to each individual paying the same proportion of income in taxes (37). The equal burden principle could also imply progressive payments when capacity to pay is defined as income net of basic needs spending instead of total income. Other definitions of the capacity to pay follow from alternative forms of the household's utility function.

WHO has argued that health system payments should be organized in such a way that the burden of payments is equalized across households. The concern about equal burden or sacrifice among households is explicitly not a matter in the space of income or the marginal contribution of the health system to an overall social goal of redistributing income. Rather, this concern is expressed in terms of raising revenue for the health system in such a way that the burden of payments on households is distributed fairly. As the term "equity" is associated with the distribution of income, WHO introduced the term "fairness" in financial contribution to describe the distribution of the burden of health payments. Equalizing burden is a proposition about what is fair for health system contributions not about what is the overall social policy regarding the distribution of income.

How can equal burden be defined? We argue that equal burden is equivalent to an equal fraction of households' capacities to pay. The debate on what is a fair contribution in this construct is in fact a debate on what is capacity to pay.

Adopting a utility function commonly used in the poverty literature (38), the utility of household i before (U_i) and after health payments (U_i') can be expressed as:

$$U_i = \ln(C_i - S_i) \qquad [7]$$

$$U_i' = \ln(C_i - S_i - HE_i) \qquad [8]$$

where C_i is household consumption, S_i is the minimum

consumption required for subsistence and HE_i is the total household contribution to the health system. The reduction in utility for household i (ΔU_i) due to a household's contribution of the health system is given by:

$$\Delta U_i = U_i - U_i' = \ln(C_i - S_i) - \ln(C_i - S_i - HE_i) \qquad [9]$$

If we define a household's consumption net of subsistence requirements as household capacity to pay (CTP_i), total household health contribution (HE_i) can be written as household capacity to pay multiplied by household financial contribution (HFC_i). So equation [9] becomes:

$$\Delta U_i = \ln(CTP_i) - \ln(CTP_i - CTP_i HFC_i) \qquad [10]$$

$$= \ln\left[\frac{CTP_i}{CTP_i(1 - HFC_i)}\right] = \ln\left[\frac{1}{1 - HFC_i}\right]$$

Then according to the equal burden principle we have:

$$\ln\left[\frac{1}{1 - HFC_i}\right] = \ln\left[\frac{1}{1 - HFC_j}\right] = \dots = \ln\left[\frac{1}{1 - HFC_n}\right] \qquad [11]$$

From equation [11], we get:

$$HFC_i = HFC_j = \dots = HFC_n = HFC_o \qquad [12]$$

where HFC_o is the total health expenditure share of total capacity to pay. It can be written as:

$$HFC_o = \frac{\sum HE_i}{\sum CTP_i} \qquad [13]$$

In other words, equalizing HFC across households can be justified as the basis for assessing the fairness in financial contribution from the premise that the disutility due to financing the health system should be equalized across households. Capacity to pay for a household follows from the form of the utility function. In the case of the utility function in equation [7], capacity to pay is household consumption minus subsistence expenditure.

The above formulation for determining the distribution of the health financial contribution may also have implications for determining a measure to summarize the distribution of HFC. Figure 38.5 shows the distribution of HFC in four countries. The x-axis shows the household financial contribution, HFC, while the y-axis shows fractions of households. The HFC-norm (HFC_o) is represented by the vertical line. The more

Figure 38.5 Distribution of household financial contribution (HFC)

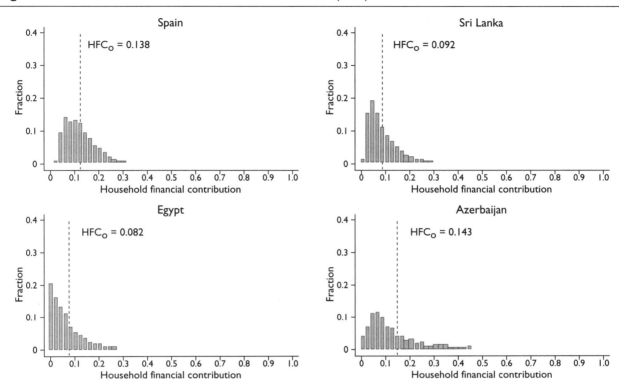

tightly the distribution is concentrated around HFC_o, the fairer the system.

The HFC distributions of Spain and Sri Lanka are narrower than those of Egypt and Azerbaijan. On these grounds, Spain is the fairest, followed by Sri Lanka, Egypt, and Azerbaijan.

A summary index of the distribution should permit a comparison of fairness across countries. A discussion of various summary measures and their properties is found in Xu et al. (11) and based on a variety of considerations, they propose the fairness in financial contribution index (FFC) as the most appropriate summary measure, defined as:

$$FFC = 1 - \sqrt[3]{\frac{\sum_{i=1}^{n}\left|HFC_i - HFC_o\right|^3}{n}} \qquad [14]$$

More details on the derivation of this summary index are provided elsewhere including a discussion of the difference between it and the index used in *The World Health Report 2000* (11). The FFC index can vary between 0 and 1, with 1 representing perfect fairness and 0 representing maximal unfairness.[2]

Catastrophic Financial Burden on Households

In the income space analysis, the effect of health system contributions was examined with respect to changes in the overall distribution and changes in the share of households below the poverty line. The same logic applies when considering the impact of health payments in the burden space, where interest lies not only with the distribution of payments, but also with the households at the right-hand tail of the distribution facing particularly high financing burdens.

Accessing the services that can improve people's health can lead to households having to pay catastrophic shares of their available income, and may subsequently push them into poverty. The desire to protect people from such payments has influenced the design of health systems and insurance mechanisms in many different settings including the USA, Australia, India, and Indonesia and is now widely accepted as a desirable objective of health policy (12;21;22;39–50).

In designing health systems, policy-makers need to know what system characteristics are associated with the incidence of catastrophically high health payments.

Catastrophic payments need not be synonymous with high health care costs (*51*). A large bill for surgery, for example, may not be catastrophic if households do not bear the full costs because the service is provided at a subsidized price or covered by a third party insurance. On the other hand, even relatively small expenditures for common illnesses can be financially disastrous for poorer households lacking insurance coverage.

Capacity to pay was defined earlier as total household consumption net of subsistence requirements, adjusted for equivalent household size. Health expenditures consist of out-of-pocket payments in addition to direct and indirect tax payments and social security contributions. As with the poverty line, defining what level of HFC is catastrophic calls for an arbitrary choice of threshold. The incidence of catastrophic payments in a country is calculated here as the percentage of households with health payments equaling or exceeding a 40% threshold of capacity to pay. For a full rationale behind these choices, see Xu et al. (*24*).

EMPIRICAL ILLUSTRATION

DATA SOURCES AND DEFINITION OF VARIABLES

The empirical results reported in this chapter are based on nationally representative household surveys from 59 countries conducted between 1991 and 2000. The sample size ranges from 1 103 households in Sweden to 62 946 households in the Republic of Korea (see the Table 42.1 for more details).

Household consumption expenditure was used to estimate household capacity to pay. The choice of consumption expenditure instead of current income was based on two considerations. First, the variance of current expenditure is smaller than the variance of current income over time. Income data reflect random shocks while expenditure data conform better to the notion of effective income and consumption smoothing. Second, in most of the household surveys available for this study, expenditure data are more reliable than income data. This is particularly true in developing countries, where the informal sector is typically quite large and survey respondents may not wish to reveal their true income for various reasons (*52–53*).

All out-of-pocket payments and private health insurance premium information were taken directly from the surveys. The general tax and social security contributions used for health were estimated from salary income (for income tax and social security contributions) and expenditure data (for expenditure taxes such as value added taxes or VAT) when the infor-

mation was not directly available from the survey. In order to distinguish the part of government spending that is used on health, each household's tax payments were multiplied by the proportion of total government spending that goes to finance the health system. These ratios were available from National Health Accounts estimates.

For determining poverty, as well as for measuring household subsistence expenditure, a food share based poverty line was used. Subsistence needs and the poverty line were defined for each country separately to allow for different consumption patterns and prices. This is based on the observation that the share of food expenditure to income falls as household income rises, and that the poor have higher shares of food in total income or consumption than the rich (*54*). The food expenditure of the household with the median share of food expenditure in total expenditure, adjusted for household size, was taken to reflect subsistence requirements and the poverty line, although because of variation across households, the average food expenditures of households with food shares from the 45th to 55th percentile was used. An equivalence scale of *eqsize* = *hhsize*$^\beta$ was used to adjust for household size. The value of β was estimated from the data from the 59 countries using the following fixed-effects regression:

$$\ln food = \ln k + \beta \ln hhsize + \sum_{i=1}^{N-1} \gamma_i country_i \quad [15]$$

The value of the coefficient β was estimated as 0.564 with a confidence interval of 0.556–0.572 (see (*55*) for more details).

RESULTS

The Income Approach

The augmented methodology proposed in the present chapter was used to calculate the redistributive effect (RE) and its constituent parts—the vertical, horizontal, and reranking components. The RE and headcount difference (DH) for each country is presented in Table 38.2. The largest positive value of the overall RE, indicating the largest decrease in income inequality after health payments, is 0.019 for Nicaragua. The other extreme is Switzerland where health system payments increased income inequality as measured by the Gini coefficient by 0.021. While there is considerable variation within this set of 59 countries in the RE, overall health system payments appear to have only a small impact on the distribution

Table 38.2 Redistributive effect (RE) and poverty headcount difference (DH)

Country	Distribution			Threshold		
	RE	V	H+R	Before health pay-ments $(H_b)^a$ (%)	After health pay-ments $(H_a)^a$ (%)	Difference^a DH=H_a−H_b (%)
Argentina	0.008	0.020	0.012	19.54	26.28	6.74
Azerbaijan	0.006	0.010	0.004	39.35	43.67	4.32
Bangladesh	0.006	0.008	0.001	31.69	35.12	3.43
Belgium	0.011	0.016	0.005	0.00	0.00	0.00
Brazil	0.007	0.014	0.006	25.13	30.23	5.10
Bulgaria	0.007	0.009	0.003	7.16	10.44	3.28
Cambodia	0.005	0.016	0.011	22.10	24.97	2.87
Canada	0.004	0.010	0.005	0.02	0.04	0.02
Colombia	0.010	0.014	0.004	18.45	21.77	3.32
Costa Rica	0.008	0.010	0.003	13.90	16.92	3.02
Croatia	0.012	0.019	0.008	3.30	4.48	1.18
Czech Republic	0.011	0.023	0.011	0.05	0.05	0.00
Denmark	−0.003	0.001	0.004	0.03	0.07	0.03
Djibouti	−0.002	0.000	0.001	18.90	20.69	1.79
Egypt	0.003	0.004	0.001	19.45	22.23	2.78
Estonia	0.009	0.012	0.004	17.42	21.09	3.67
Finland	−0.001	0.005	0.006	0.08	0.15	0.08
France	0.002	0.008	0.006	0.34	0.47	0.13
Germany	−0.007	−0.002	0.004	0.00	0.01	0.01
Ghana	0.003	0.004	0.002	30.54	34.13	3.58
Greece	0.003	0.010	0.007	0.72	1.28	0.56
Guyana	0.009	0.010	0.001	23.48	28.55	5.07
Hungary	0.012	0.017	0.005	0.86	1.31	0.45
Iceland	−0.008	−0.003	0.006	0.00	0.00	0.00
Indonesia	0.007	0.008	0.002	20.47	22.14	1.68
Israel	0.009	0.013	0.004	0.31	0.74	0.43
Jamaica	−0.006	−0.005	0.001	28.73	33.72	4.99
Korea, Republic of	−0.008	−0.002	0.006	0.36	0.75	0.38
Kyrgyzstan	0.000	0.002	0.002	30.96	34.34	3.38
Latvia	0.002	0.005	0.002	9.34	12.45	3.12
Lebanon	−0.011	−0.005	0.006	1.94	4.07	2.13
Lithuania	0.009	0.011	0.001	6.21	7.66	1.45
Mauritius	0.006	0.008	0.002	8.84	10.19	1.35
Mexico	0.007	0.008	0.002	15.33	17.08	1.75
Morocco	0.010	0.011	0.001	20.41	21.59	1.19
Namibia	0.001	0.003	0.002	31.13	34.71	3.58
Nicaragua	0.019	0.023	0.004	28.02	30.91	2.90
Norway	−0.013	−0.006	0.008	0.09	0.09	0.00
Panama	0.013	0.018	0.004	17.51	19.97	2.47
Paraguay	0.001	0.005	0.003	16.71	20.39	3.68
Peru	0.007	0.011	0.004	22.49	25.17	2.68
Philippines	0.005	0.005	0.001	27.35	29.17	1.82
Portugal	0.002	0.004	0.002	5.40	7.20	1.79
Romania	0.002	0.002	0.000	29.94	32.26	2.31
Senegal	0.007	0.009	0.001	20.28	22.33	2.05
Slovakia	0.010	0.011	0.001	0.33	0.42	0.09
Slovenia	−0.006	0.001	0.008	2.03	3.66	1.63
South Africa	0.006	0.008	0.002	29.50	30.82	1.32
Spain	0.005	0.009	0.004	0.89	1.33	0.44

continued

Table 38.2   Redistributive effect (RE) and poverty headcount difference (DH) *(continued)*

Country	Distribution			Threshold		
	RE	V	H+R	Before health pay-ments $(H_b)^a$ (%)	After health pay-ments $(H_a)^a$ (%)	Difference^a $DH=H_a-H_b$ (%)
Sri Lanka	0.005	0.007	0.002	21.74	25.19	3.45
Sweden	−0.001	0.002	0.003	0.00	0.31	0.31
Switzerland	−0.021	−0.016	0.005	0.00	0.08	0.08
Thailand	0.005	0.008	0.002	6.79	8.28	1.50
UK	0.006	0.007	0.002	0.53	0.71	0.18
Ukraine	0.006	0.010	0.004	21.79	25.79	4.01
USA	−0.003	0.002	0.005	1.19	1.62	0.42
Viet Nam	0.000	0.006	0.007	28.35	36.09	7.75
Yemen	0.006	0.009	0.002	27.16	29.82	2.66
Zambia	0.004	0.006	0.002	52.95	54.86	1.91

^{a} Households under the poverty line

V=Vertical effect; H+R=Horizontal and reranking effects-

of income. In percentage terms, the largest impact of health system payments was to increase the Gini coefficient by 7% in Switzerland and to decrease it by 5% in Slovakia. Given that health system contributions range from 1.3% to 13% of GDP in the world, their relatively minor impact on the distribution of income is not surprising.

While the overall impact on the distribution of income as measured by the Gini coefficient is relatively small, the pattern across countries is interesting. A group of Scandanavian countries, Denmark, Finland, Iceland, Norway, and Sweden all have negative REs, indicating that health contributions in those countries make the after-payment distribution of income less equal than the before-payment distribution, i.e. health payments are regressive despite the existence of public prepayment mechanisms.

The values of the horizontal inequity and reranking components are relatively low but for some countries the H and R components outweigh the pro-poor redistributive impact deriving from vertical redistribution, with the consequence that the total effect becomes negative. This is the explanation for the results in Denmark, Finland, and Sweden but not in Norway where the vertical effect is also regressive. Other countries where health system payments worsen the distribution of income include Germany, Djibouti, the Republic of Korea, Jamaica, Lebanon, Slovenia, Switzerland, and the USA. In nine countries, the RE is greater than 0.01: Belgium, Colombia, Croatia, Czech Republic, Hungary, Morocco, Nicaragua, Panama, and Slovakia. The cluster of Eastern European countries with health systems that contribute to greater income equality is notable.

In fact, in most of the countries where RE is negative the principal reason seems to be vertical redistribution. This illustrates that it is important to identify the reasons behind a negative RE—whether it is due to vertical or horizontal inequalities—because the appropriate policy response could well differ depending on the source of the negative RE. The RE is, however, relatively insensitive to the horizontal and reranking effects. In Figure 38.6 the x-axis depicts the redistributive effect, while the y-axis shows the vertical (V), horizontal and reranking effects (H + R). The horizontal and reranking components are relatively constant regardless of the level of RE, whereas the vertical effect explains much of the variation in RE.

Results from a variance decomposition analysis of RE strengthen the above argument that RE is not sensitive to horizontal inequity and reranking. The RE index can be written as:

$$RE = V - (H + R) \qquad [16]$$

and the variance of RE can be expressed as:

$$\mathrm{var}(RE) = \mathrm{var}(V) + \mathrm{var}(H+R) - 2\,\mathrm{cov}(V, H+R) \quad [17]$$

Since the horizontal and reranking effects reduce the impact of the vertical effect on RE, the covariance of the vertical effect and the horizontal and reranking effects must be subtracted from the variance of RE. If both sides of the equation are divided by the variance of RE, we obtain the percentage effect of each component on the total variance of RE as:

$$\frac{\mathrm{var}(RE)}{\mathrm{var}(RE)} = \frac{\mathrm{var}(V)}{\mathrm{var}(RE)} + \frac{\mathrm{var}(H+R)}{\mathrm{var}(RE)} - \frac{2\,\mathrm{cov}(V, H+R)}{\mathrm{var}(RE)} \quad [18]$$

Figure 38.6 Redistributive effect (RE) and its components (V, H and R)

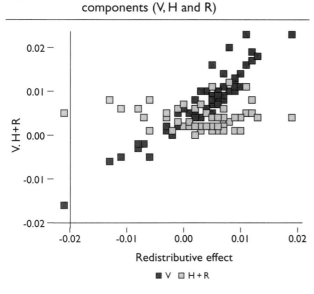

Figure 38.7 Redistributive effect (RE) and out-of-pocket (OOP) share

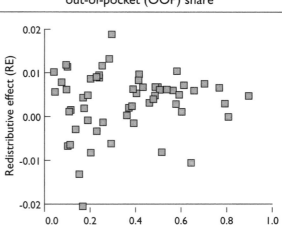

The results show that the variances of the horizontal and reranking effects contributed for only 16% of the total variance. This suggests that the variance of RE is determined predominantly by the variance of the vertical effect.

In an effort to identify health system characteristics associated with different types of redistributive effects, some studies have suggested a negative relationship between RE (or progressivity) and the proportion of total health expenditures met by out-of-pocket payments (OOP) (7;18). Figure 38.7 does not support this hypothesis for the 59 countries. In countries with a low proportion of health expenditure met by OOP in particular, there is very substantial variation in the RE, and no obvious trend in RE as OOP increases in importance.[3]

Turning next to the poverty impact of health payments, the way the health system is financed can have a significant effect. Table 38.2, in the last three columns, shows the proportion of people living in poverty before and after health contributions, and the difference between the two. Across this sample of countries, the percentage of households driven below the absolute poverty line by health system contributions ranged from near 0 in Belgium, Canada, Czech Republic, Denmark, Germany, Iceland, and Norway to 7.7% in Viet Nam. Argentina, Brazil, Guyana, and Jamaica also have more than 5% of households impoverished through health system contributions. Substantial effects can be noted as well in some of the former socialist countries, such as Azerbaijan, Esto-

nia, Kyrgyzstan, and Ukraine. It is important to note that the marginal impact of health system payments on the levels of poverty appears to be substantially larger than the impact of health system payments on the overall distribution of income.

The weak relationship between the impact of health system payments on the distribution of income and their impact on the levels of poverty is exemplified by Brazil. Overall in that country, the RE was 0.007 indicating progressive health system payments, yet these same payments increased the poverty rate by 5.1 percentage points. In contrast, Norway with a RE of –0.013 had no change in the poverty rate due to health payments. Clearly, the RE does not capture the impact of health system contributions on poor households very well. Health payments can still force people living close to the poverty line into poverty even if these payments are progressive in the system, which indicates the importance of focusing not only on the distribution as a whole through the RE, but also on the tail of the distribution using the DH.

As a general rule, health payments have a greater impact on poverty in countries with a higher proportion of the population already living in poverty. However, Figure 38.8 shows that there is substantial variation in the levels of impoverishment at any given level of overall poverty, suggesting that some countries have been more effective in protecting the poor from impoverishing health payments than others. Notable examples include South Africa and Zambia where health payments caused little additional poverty despite high levels of the population living in poverty. On the other hand, substantial impoverishment took

Figure 38.8 Level of poverty and impoverishment due to health payments

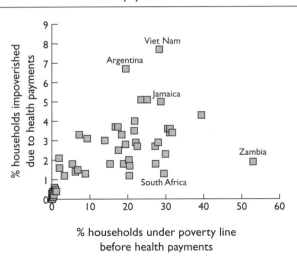

Figure 38.9 The fairness in financial contribution index (FFC) and the prepayment share of total health expenditure (%)

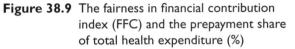
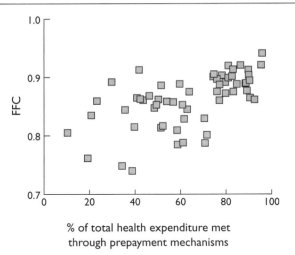

place in Jamaica and Viet Nam, although these countries were at the same level of poverty as South Africa before health payments. Argentina stands out as a country with lower than average poverty before health payments, but with a large fraction of the population pushed into poverty due to health system payments.

The Burden Approach

The summary measure of the distribution of household financial contributions in the burden space, the FFC, is reported in Table 38.3. It ranges between 0.740 in Brazil to 0.941 in Slovakia. In this sample of countries, the high levels of fairness are also seen in a number of high-income OECD countries including the United Kingdom, Sweden, Denmark, Germany, and Canada. Nevertheless, there is considerable variation within the OECD, with the United States of America, Switzerland, and Norway having substantially lower levels of fairness. In the case of the USA and Switzerland, the role of private insurance with regressive premiums is important, while in Norway general taxation is regressive. The lowest scores (less than 0.800) were found in a group of countries in transition from socialist economies (Azerbaijan, Ukraine, and Viet Nam) and a group in Latin America and the Caribbean (Argentina, Brazil, and Jamaica).

The crudest measure of the extent of financial risk protection mechanisms in a society is the share of health expenditure channelled through prepayment mechanisms including taxes, social insurance, and private insurance. Not surprisingly, Figure 38.9 shows that there is a moderately strong relationship between

the FFC and the share of expenditure through prepayment. At any given level of prepaid health financing, however, there is considerable variation in the FFC suggesting that the progressivity of taxes, social insurance, and private insurance matter as well as the types of out-of-pocket expenditures that households incur.

Table 38.3 also reports the threshold measure in the burden space, the proportion of households with catastrophic health contributions. The overall proportion is reported in addition to the proportion facing catastrophic expenditures solely because of out-of-pocket payments. The impact of health system contributions is notably high in many Latin American countries—in Argentina and Brazil more than 10% of households had payments that exceeded 40% of their capacities to pay, while in Colombia, Nicaragua, Panama, and Paraguay the share was more than 5%. Similarly, more than 5% of households faced catastrophic expenditure in the same group of countries in transition from socialist economics listed above, and in Cambodia. The fact that the countries with the lowest scores on the FFC also had a high proportion of households with catastrophic spending reflects the general finding that there is a strong negative correlation between these two measures (–0.903)—the fairer the distribution of financial burden across households, the lower the proportion of households facing catastrophic payments.

Although the proportion of households with catastrophic payments was high in some countries in transition, others have been better at protecting households against catastrophic payments, including

Table 38.3 Fairness in financial contribution and catastrophic payments

Country	Distribution Fairness in financial contribution (FFC)	Threshold Households with catastrophic payments (Total health expenditure) (%)	Households with catastrophic payments (Out-of-pocket expenditure) (%)
Argentina	0.785	11.84	5.77
Azerbaijan	0.748	11.27	7.15
Bangladesh	0.868	1.73	1.21
Belgium	0.903	0.23	0.09
Brazil	0.740	13.27	10.27
Bulgaria	0.862	2.79	2.00
Cambodia	0.805	5.54	5.02
Canada	0.913	0.48	0.09
Colombia	0.809	7.82	6.26
Costa Rica	0.861	3.06	0.12
Croatia	0.865	2.45	0.20
Czech Republic	0.904	0.01	0.00
Denmark	0.920	0.38	0.07
Djibouti	0.853	0.82	0.32
Egypt	0.835	3.24	2.80
Estonia	0.872	2.47	0.31
Finland	0.901	1.36	0.44
France	0.889	0.68	0.01
Germany	0.913	0.54	0.03
Ghana	0.862	2.47	1.30
Greece	0.858	3.29	2.17
Guyana	0.887	1.73	0.60
Hungary	0.905	0.96	0.20
Iceland	0.891	1.30	0.30
Indonesia	0.859	1.34	1.26
Israel	0.897	1.09	0.35
Jamaica	0.787	5.39	1.86
Korea, Republic of	0.847	2.57	1.73
Kyrgyzstan	0.875	1.32	0.62
Latvia	0.828	4.05	2.75
Lebanon	0.844	8.50	5.17
Lithuania	0.875	1.68	1.34
Mauritius	0.861	1.59	1.28
Mexico	0.857	1.93	1.54
Morocco	0.913	0.27	0.17
Namibia	0.877	1.65	0.11
Nicaragua	0.829	5.02	2.05
Norway	0.888	1.22	0.28
Panama	0.801	5.53	2.35
Paraguay	0.815	5.07	3.51
Peru	0.813	4.01	3.21
Philippines	0.886	0.99	0.78
Portugal	0.845	4.01	2.71
Romania	0.901	0.31	0.09
Senegal	0.892	0.86	0.55
Slovakia	0.941	0.00	0.00
Slovenia	0.890	1.88	0.06
South Africa	0.894	1.12	0.03

continued

Table 38.3 Fairness in financial contribution and catastrophic payments *(continued)*

Country	Distribution	Threshold	
	Fairness in financial contribution (FFC)	Households with catastrophic payments (Total health expenditure) (%)	Households with catastrophic payments (Out-of-pocket expenditure) (%)
Spain	0.899	0.89	0.48
Sri Lanka	0.865	1.75	1.25
Sweden	0.920	0.39	0.18
Switzerland	0.875	3.03	0.57
Thailand	0.888	0.99	0.80
UK	0.921	0.33	0.04
Ukraine	0.788	6.82	3.87
USA	0.860	3.23	0.55
Viet Nam	0.762	11.46	10.45
Yemen	0.853	2.29	1.66
Zambia	0.816	4.02	2.29

the Czech Republic, Romania, Slovakia, and Slovenia. While catastrophic payments were relatively low in most OECD countries, they were relatively high, effecting more than 3% of households, in the USA, Switzerland, Portugal, and Greece, and more than 1% in Korea, Mexico, Finland, and Norway.

In most cases, the principal source of catastrophic payments was direct payments made by the users of services. This can be seen by comparing the proportion of households facing catastrophic financial burdens due to out-of-pocket payments with the proportion facing catastrophic expenditure from all causes in Table 38.3. In some countries, however, public prepayment mechanisms played a significant role, causing over 2% of households to face catastrophic health spending in Argentina, Brazil, Costa Rica, Jamaica, and Panama in the Americas; Azerbaijan, Croatia, and Estonia among the transition economies; Switzerland and the USA among the OECD countries; and Lebanon. In the Latin American countries it is likely to be due to social insurance payments that can constitute a relatively high share of salaries, and people with low incomes are not usually exempt as they are in the case of income taxes. In the USA and Switzerland, it is more related to the nature of the health insurance system where payments are not levied in proportion to incomes.

The chapter by Xu et al. *(24)* in this volume explores further the factors related to the variation in the proportion of households facing catastrophic expenditures due to out-of-pocket payments. The triad of poverty or low capacity to pay, the ready availability of health services, and the absence of risk pooling

mechanisms, are closely associated with increases in catastrophic payments on a cross-country basis.

WHAT IS THE EMPIRICAL RELATIONSHIP BETWEEN THE INCOME AND BURDEN APPROACHES?

Comparison of the results of Table 38.2 with those in Table 38.3 shows that health payments in the income space improve the after-payment distribution of income over the prepayment distribution (i.e. the RE was positive) in all of the countries shown to perform at the low end of the FFC scale in the burden space (e.g. Argentina, Azerbaijan, Brazil, Jamaica, Ukraine, and Viet Nam). At the other extreme, health payments in Denmark and Sweden resulted in an increase in income inequality (RE was negative) but the distribution of household financial contributions in the burden space was relatively fair with FFC scores in excess of 0.9. There appears to be little correlation between the RE and the FFC across countries.

On the other hand, a comparison of the threshold measures shows more consistency—countries where health payments resulted in a relatively high proportion of households falling below the poverty line were also those where a relatively high percentage of households faced catastrophic payments. These correlations are explored formally in Table 38.4.

The two measures used in the burden space (FFC and %CAT) are highly correlated, negatively. This means that the fairer the distribution of household financial payments, the lower is the proportion of households facing catastrophic expenditure. The FFC also has a strong negative correlation with DH, the

Table 38.4 Correlation coefficients between measures in the income and burden space

		Burden space		Income space	
		FFC	%CAT	RE	DH
Burden space	FFC	1.000			
	%CAT	−0.903	1.000		
Income space	RE	−0.071	0.028	1.000	
	DH	−0.740	0.708	0.251	1.000

threshold measure in the income space. Not surprisingly, the two threshold measures, DH and %CAT, show a high, positive correlation. By contrast, the income space summary measure of the distribution of payments, RE, shows only a weak relationship with the threshold measure in the income space (DH), and almost no relationship with the threshold (%CAT) and the distribution (FFC) measures in the burden space. In fact, the correlation between RE and the FFC is negative, suggesting that the fairer the distribution of household financial contributions in the burden space, the worse is the measured impact of health payments on the distribution of incomes.

Why is the FFC closely correlated with %CAT and with DH while the RE is not? Part of the answer lies in the fact that contributions by household in the middle and upper parts of the income distribution can have an important influence on the Gini coefficient and thus the RE. All three measures, the FFC, %CAT, and DH are highly sensitive to payments of poor households. In the burden space, health system contributions are analysed as a fraction of household capacity to pay so that contributions by middle and upper income house-

holds have relatively little effect. While the three are empirically correlated, they do capture distinct aspects of the experience of poorer households.

Wagstaff and van Doorslaer (*10*) have argued that the main concern of the FFC, a concern with equalizing the burden of payments across households, can be captured by the income space measure (RE). Their logic was that subsistence expenditure which is deducted from total expenditures to estimate capacity to pay for the FFC, is highly regressive. A fairly financed system with equal financial burdens implies, therefore, a particular level of progressivity (or redistributive effect) and deviations from financial fairness can be mapped into the RE.

This is not necessarily the case as two populations with the same RE can have different levels of the FFC index and vice versa. Comparison of Tables 38.2 and 38.3 shows that in Azerbaijan and Bangladesh, for example, the RE was 0.006 but the FFC was 0.748 in the former and 0.868 in the latter. The fact that the two approaches capture different features of the health payment distribution and that the same level of progressivity or redistributive effect of health payments can lead to different levels of fairness as measured by the FFC index can be illustrated using simulated data. Let us assume two populations, A and B, with the same redistributive effect (RE = −0.0011). In order to demonstrate the sensitivity to horizontal inequity of the two approaches, we make the variance of the health financing contributions (HFC) within income deciles in population A smaller than in population B.

Figure 38.10 shows the distribution of HFC across income deciles for both populations. The y-axis shows HFC and the x-axis income deciles ranked from the lowest to the highest. The horizontal line in the middle of the box represents the median of the HFC. The

Figure 38.10 The distribution of household financial contribution by income deciles

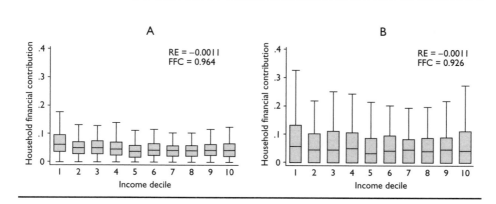

box extends from the lower 25th percentile to the upper 25th percentile. The upper value is equal to $HFC_{[75]} + 1.5(HFC_{[75]} - HFC_{[25]})$, and the lower one is $HFC_{[25]} - 1.5(HFC_{[75]} - HFC_{[25]})$. The mean HFC in each decile is the same, but there are larger variances within each decile in population B than in population A.

The redistributive effect of health payments is the same in both populations. However, the FFC is lower in population B than in population A. This is because the income space measure is not sensitive to horizontal inequity (as shown earlier) and it does not give great weight to households in the tails of the distribution, e.g. those with catastrophic health expenditures. FFC and RE, therefore, capture different concerns. Fairness in financial contribution is measured in the burden space, a concern with the equal burden of health system payments. It is not a concern with progressivity of health payments with respect to income, the focus of the income space approach.

One implication is that countries with a high degree of out-of-pocket financing of their health systems can be shown to be progressive in the income space (a relatively high RE), yet they also have high catastrophic payments in the burden space. A health financing system with a relatively large share of expenditure provided by out-of-pocket payments can be progressive because the rich spend more on health than the poor, both in absolute terms and as a share of their total capacity to pay. At the same time, the smaller payments of the poor can be catastrophic, putting them into poverty. If health policy focuses exclusively on the progressivity of payments, this consequence of out-of-pocket payments—and the converse, the benefits of the prepayment mechanism—will be ignored.

In conclusion, an in-depth analysis in the burden space provides additional insights into the impact of different insurance coverage arrangements than those indicated by the RE index alone.

CONCLUSIONS

This paper described two approaches for measuring the distributional consequences of financial contributions to the health system. The first is derived in the income space while the second is derived in the burden space. The income space distributional measure is based on the progressivity principle, while the burden space approach is based on capacity to pay or the equal burden principle. Each approach has its own distribution and threshold measures.

The income space approach focuses on the changes in income distribution due to health payments. The most common distribution measure used in this context is the redistributive effect, which compares income Gini coefficients before and after health payments. Progressive health payments will reduce the income Gini and make the resulting distribution of income more equal while regressive health payments will have an opposite impact. The threshold measure explores how many households fall into poverty because of health payments.

The burden space approach focuses on the proportion of capacity to pay contributed to health. The summary measure, FFC, captures three common concerns: protecting households against extreme financial loss due to ill health (preventing catastrophic health expenditure); equal payments by households with equal capacity to pay (horizontal equity); and an element of progressivity (richer households should contribute more of their total income than poorer households). The threshold measure indicates the proportion of households with catastrophic health expenditures.

While the two approaches explore different aspects of the impact of health payments, they both provide useful information for policy-makers. The income space approach is sensitive to progressivity and gives feedback on this aspect of the health financing system, but it gives little information on risk protection and catastrophic outcomes leading to impoverishment. The burden space approach is sensitive to horizontal inequity, and particularly to catastrophic health payments. It allows policy-makers to identify shortcomings associated with risk pooling and other financial protection mechanisms in the health financing system.

We believe that the purpose of health policy is not to redistribute income, although its impact on the distribution of income is of obvious interest. Accordingly, it was shown in the present paper that an analysis based on the examination of financing burdens offers an important new insight to the development of health financing policies. Analyses using both approaches will provide more comprehensive information for policy-makers who wish to improve the performance of their health financing systems and who may be operating under rather different circumstances.

ACKNOWLEDGEMENTS

The authors would like to thank Guy Carrin and William D. Savedoff for their helpful comments on earlier versions of the manuscript and Felicia Knaul for her contribution to the early stage of the development of the methodology. We are also grateful to Nathalie Etomba and Anna Moore for data and reference searches.

NOTES

1 Anand (56) showed that it is a measure of the covariance between the income ranks and the tax payments of households.

2 The FFC index approaches zero when households with lower financial contributions to health have substantially larger capacities to pay than households that contribute a higher proportion of their capacities to pay. Consider a hypothetical example of 10 households where 1 household contributes 0% and the remaining 9 households contribute 100% of their capacities to pay. The larger the share of the summed capacity to pay belonging to the household with zero contributions, the smaller the FFC index becomes, approaching its lowest value of zero when virtually all capacity to pay belongs to the one household that pays nothing to health, and all contributions are made by the rest. Of course, in practice such an outcome is not feasible, as health system contributions can only be made from positive capacity to pay, but at the limit the condition applies. This result of the FFC being bounded by 0 and 1 is specific to the formulation in which the sum-mean formulation of HFC_o is used. If the arithmetic mean of household financial contributes was used instead, the FFC would be bounded by 0.5 and 1.

3 This is confirmed in regression analysis where the coefficient of OOP/THE was never significant in explaining RE regardless of the functional form used.

REFERENCES

(1) Kakwani N, Wagstaff A, Van Doorslaer E. Socio-economic inequalities in health: measurement, computation and statistical inference. *Journal of Econometrics*, 1997, 1997:87–103.

(2) Murray CJL et al. *Defining and measuring fairness in financial contribution to the health system*. EIP Discussion Paper No. 24. Geneva, World Health Organization, 2000. URL: http://www3.who.int/whosis/discussion_papers/discussion_papers.cfm#

(3) Pannarunothai S, Mills A. The poor pay more: health-related inequality in Thailand. *Social Science & Medicine*, 1997, 44:1781–1790.

(4) Rasell E, Bernstein J, Tang K. The impact of health care financing on family budgets. *International Journal of Health Services*, 1994, 24:691–714.

(5) van Doorslaer E, Wagstaff A, Rutten F. *Equity in the finance and delivery of health care: an international perspective*. Oxford, Oxford Medical Publications, 1993.

(6) Wagstaff A, van Doorslaer E. Progressivity, horizontal equity and reranking in health care finance: a decomposition analysis for the Netherlands. *Journal of Health Economics*, 1997, 16(5):499–516.

(7) Wagstaff A et al. Equity in the finance of health care: some further international comparisons. *Journal of Health Economics*, 1999, 18:263–290.

(8) Wagstaff A, van Doorslaer E. Equity in health finance and delivery. In: Culyer AJ, Newhouse JP, eds. *Handbook of health economics*. Amsterdam, New York, Elsevier, 2000.

(9) Wagstaff A. *Measuring equity in health care financing: reflections and alternatives to the World Health Organization's fairness of financial contribution index*. Washington, DC, World Bank, 2001. URL: http://www.healthsystemsrc.org/.

(10) Wagstaff A, van Doorslaer E. *Paying for health care: quantifying fairness, catastrophe, and impoverishment, with applications to Vietnam 1993–1998*. World Bank Working Paper, No. 2715. Washington, DC, World Bank, 2001.

(11) Xu K et al. Summary measures of the distribution of household financial contributions to health. In: Murray CJL, Evans DB, eds. *Health systems performance assessment: debates, methods and empiricism*. Geneva, World Health Organization, 2003.

(12) World Health Organization. *The World Health Report 2000. Health Systems: Improving Performance*. Geneva, World Health Organization, 2000.

(13) Almeida C, Braveman P, Gold MR. Methodological concerns and recommendations on policy consequences of the World Health Report 2000. *The Lancet*, 2001, 357:1692–1696.

(14) Klavus J. The measure of fair financing in the World Health Report 2000. *STAKES Themes*. Helsinki, 2000.

(15) Ministry of Health, Viet Nam. *Comments and suggestions of Viet Nam Ministry of Health/Health Policy Unit as regards the World Health Report 2000*. Hanoi, Viet Nam, 2001.

(16) Navarro V. World Health Report 2000: responses to Murray and Frenk. *The Lancet*, 2001, 357:1701–1702.

(17) Shaw RP. Financial fairness indicator: useful compass or crystal ball? *International Journal of Health Services*, 2002, 32(1):195–203.

(18) van Doorslaer E et al. The redistributive effect of health care finance in twelve OECD countries. *Journal of Health Economics*, 1999, 18:291–313.

(19) Williams A. Science or marketing at WHO? A com-

(20) Merlis M. Family out-of-pocket spending for health services: a continuing source of financial insecurity. *The Commonwealth Fund*, 2002.

mentary on 'World Health 2000'. *Health Economics*, 2001, 10(2):93–100.

(21) Pradhan M, Prescott N. Social risk management options for medical care in Indonesia. *Health Economics*, 2002, 11:431–446.

(22) Ranson K. Reduction of catastrophic health care expenditures by a community-based health insurance scheme in Gujarat, India: current experiences and challenges. *Bulletin of the World Health Organization*, 2002, 80: 613–621.

(23) Sesma S, Merino MF, Martinez R. *Hogares con gastos catastróficos por motivos de salud*. México DF, SSA, 2002.

(24) Xu K et al. Understanding household catastrophic health expenditures: a multi-country analysis. In: Murray CJL, Evans DB, eds. *Health systems performance assessment: debates, methods and empiricism*. Geneva, World Health Organization, 2003.

(25) Kakwani NC. Measurement of tax progressivity: an international comparison. *The Economic Journal*, 1977, 87:71–80.

(26) Kakwani NC. On the measurement of tax progressivity and redistributive effect of taxes with applications to horizontal and vertical equity. *Advances in Econometrics*, 1984, 3:149–168.

(27) Musgrave RA. *Public finance in theory and practice* . New York, McGraw-Hill, 1973.

(28) Pfäheler W. Redistributive effects of tax progressivity: evaluating a general class of aggregate measures. *Public Finance*, 1987, 37:1–31.

(29) Reynolds M, Smolensky E. *Public expenditures, taxes, and the distribution of income: the United States, 1950, 1961, 1970*. New York, New York Academic Press, 1977.

(30) Suits D. Measurement of tax progressivity. *American Economic Review*, 1977, 67:747–752.

(31) Gakidou E, King G. Measuring total health inequality: adding individual variation to group-level differences. In: Murray CJL, Evans DB, eds. *Health systems performance assessment: debates, methods and empiricism*. Geneva, World Health Organization, 2003.

(32) Moussavi S et al. Inequalities in coverage: valid DTP3 and measles vaccination in 40 countries. In: Murray CJL, Evans DB, eds. *Health systems performance assessment: debates, methods and empiricism*. Geneva, World Health Organization, 2003.

(33) Shengelia B, Murray CJL, Adams OB. Beyond access and utilization: defining and measuring health system coverage. In: Murray CJL, Evans DB, eds. *Health systems*

performance assessment: debates, methods and empiricism*. Geneva, World Health Organization, 2003.

(34) Aronson JR, Johnson P, Lambert PJ. Redistributive effect and unequal income tax treatment in the U.K. *The Economic Journal*, 1994, 104:262–270.

(35) Ok EA. A note on the existence of progressive tax structures. *Social Choice and Welfare*, 1997, 14:527–543.

(36) Mills JS. *Principles of political economy*. London, Penguin, 1970.

(37) Young P. Equal sacrifice and progressive taxation. *American Economic Review*, 1990, 80:253–266.

(38) Malinvaud E. *Lectures on microeconomic theory*. Amsterdam, New York, Elsevier, 1985.

(39) Bovbjerg RR. *Covering catastrophic health care and containing costs: preliminary lessons for policy from the U.S. experience*. LCSHD Paper Series No. 66. Washington, DC, World Bank, 2001.

(40) Evans RG et al. Controlling health expenditures - the Canadian reality. *The New England Journal of Medicine*, 1989, 320(9):571–607.

(41) Filmer D, Hammer J, Prichett L. Weak links in the chain II: a prescription for health policy in poor countries. *World Bank Research Observer*, 2002, 17:47–66.

(42) Havighurst et al. Strategies in underwriting the cost of catastrophic disease. *Law and Contemporary Problems*, 1976, 40:195.

(43) Kawabata K, Xu K, Carrin G. Preventing impoverishment through protection against catastrophic health expenditure. *Bulletin of the World Health Organization*, 2002, 80:612.

(44) Musgrove P. Public spending on health care: how are different criteria related? *Health Policy*, 2000, 53:61–67.

(45) Najman JM, Western JS. A comparative analysis of Australian health policy in the 1970s. *Social Science & Medicine*, 1984, 18:949–958.

(46) Rice T, Desmond K, Gabel J. The Medicare Catastrophic Coverage Act: a post mortem. *Health Affairs*, 1990, 9: 75–87.

(47) Russel S, Gilson L. User fee policies to promote health service access for poor: a wolf in sheep's clothing? *International Journal of Health Services*, 1997, 27:359–379.

(48) Trapnell GR, et al. *Strategies for insuring catastrophic illness: financial burden, prototype plans, and cost estimates*. Report to DHHS, printed under grant from Hoffmann-La Roche Inc., 1983.

(49) World Health Organization. *The World Health Report 2001. Mental Health: New Understanding, New Hope*. Geneva, World Health Organization, 2001.

(50) World Health Organization. *The World Health Report*

2002. *Reducing Risks, Promoting Healthy Life.* Geneva, World Health Organization, 2002.

(51) Wyszewianski L. Financially catastrophic and high-cost cases: definitions, distinctions, and their implication for policy formulation. *Inquiry*, 1986, 23(4):382–394.

(52) Deaton A. *Understanding consumption.* Oxford, Oxford University Press, 1992.

(53) Bouis HE. The effect of income on demand for food in poor countries: are our food consumption database giving us reliable estimates? *Journal of Development Economics*, 1994, 44:199–226.

(54) Deaton A, Muellbauer J. *Economics and consumer behavior.* Cambridge, Cambridge University Press, 1980.

(55) Xu K et al. Household health system contributions and capacity to pay: definitional, empirical, and technical challenges. In: Murray CJL, Evans DB, eds. *Health systems performance assessment: debates, methods and empiricism.* Geneva, World Health Organization, 2003.

(56) Anand S. *Inequality and poverty in Malaysia: measurement and decomposition.* New York, Oxford University Press, 1983.

Chapter 39

Household Health System Contributions and Capacity to Pay: Definitional, Empirical, and Technical Challenges

Ke Xu, Jan Klavus, Kei Kawabata, David B. Evans,
Piya Hanvoravongchai, Juan Pablo Ortiz, Riadh Zeramdini,
Christopher J.L. Murray

Introduction

In addition to improving population health, an important goal of health systems is to ensure that the financial burden of paying for health is distributed fairly across households (1). Exploring fairness in financial contribution requires the ability to measure each household's financial contribution (HFC), defined as the ratio of a household's health system contributions to its capacity to pay. This chapter, organized into five sections, introduces a method for estimating the HFC from household survey data. Section two presents the framework for analysis and the definition of the numerator and denominator of HFC. The third and fourth sections describe in detail the calculation of households' health system payments through different payment mechanisms and the measurement of capacity to pay. In this context, the data required for estimation are also presented. The last section describes some remaining challenges concerning the measurement of capacity to pay, which are related to the quality of survey data.

Defining a Household's Financial Contribution

The household financial contribution (HFC) represents the household's financial burden due to health system payments. It is a ratio that relates total household expenditure for health (HE) through general taxes, social health insurance contributions, private health insurance premiums, and out-of-pocket payments, to the household's capacity to pay (CTP). The capacity to pay of household i is essentially its effective income minus subsistence expenditure requirements (SE):

$$HFC_i = \frac{HE_i}{CTP_i} \qquad [1]$$

Ideally HFC is defined over a period of one year, a unit of time that encompasses many predictable fluctuations in income and expenditure. The period of evaluation of health expenditure and effective non-subsistence income is of theoretical importance. Depending on the availability of various formal and informal mechanisms to borrow and save, households may behave as if they smoothed their income over longer periods of time. In the extreme, the life cycle consumption hypothesis claims that households smooth consumption over the stream of all future income (2). It is possible that in different countries the period over which permanent income is defined will vary, being generally longer in high-income countries (3). In practice, HFC must be estimated using data covering a shorter period, typically one month, because surveys seldom include questions about expenditures over an entire year, let alone over a longer period.

Household Expenditures for Health

The numerator (HE_i) includes all financial contributions to the health system attributable to the household through taxes, social security contributions, private insurance, and out-of-pocket payments. These include financial outlays that the household itself is not necessarily aware of paying, such as the share of sales or value-added taxes that governments then devote to health. As taxes and social security contributions are rarely earmarked for their ultimate financing purpose, total household payments must be multiplied by the share of these revenues that goes to finance the health system.

THE CONCEPT OF EFFECTIVE INCOME

To operationalize the denominator of HFC, capacity to pay, it is necessary to define effective income and subsistence expenditure. The notion of effective income is meant to reflect household tendencies to smooth consumption over time, taking into account expected variations in income, the household's assets (allowing for saving or non-saving), and future earnings potential.

There is a rich economic literature on different theories of how households make consumption decisions. For example, in the life cycle income hypothesis (4), households are assumed to smooth their consumption over the life cycle, so that expected consumption is equal in all subsequent time periods. One formulization of this theory of consumption behavior adapted to the circumstances of health financing is:

$$C_0 = \frac{Y_0 + A_0 + \sum_{t=1}^{l} Y_t P_t \delta^t}{1 + \sum_{t=1}^{l} P_t \delta^t} \qquad [2]$$

where C_0 is the consumption of a household at time $t = 0$, given complete access to consumption smoothing mechanisms and the ability to consume assets, Y_t is income at time $t > 0$, P_t is the probability of being alive in each future year, A_0 is the annualized value of assets (savings or debts) at time $t = 0$, and δ is $1/(1+r)$, where r is the market interest or discount rate.

The life cycle hypothesis is particularly important under three sets of circumstances: when households face predictable fluctuations in income during the course of the year; when their income in future years is expected to change; and when they have positive assets (savings) or negative assets (debts). In these circumstances the household's consumption over the period of time that is usually incorporated into income and expenditure surveys—e.g. a month—could be lower or higher than its observed earnings over that period.

In order for a household to be able to smooth its consumption over long periods of time effective capital markets must be available. This involves access to formal or informal mechanisms that allows households to borrow on the basis of the present value of their future earnings, or to convert savings that are in the form of assets into monetary value. If the household possesses assets, these can be sold and converted into income although temporary problems that impede the sale and create liquidity problems for the household may exist. A more serious constraint is posed by the fact that in many countries mechanisms that allow households to adjust their consumption by borrowing may not be readily available.

Because of imperfections associated with formal and informal consumption smoothing mechanisms, the income that a household is able to consume and would seek to consume given its current income, assets and access to future earnings, could differ from that predicted by the life cycle hypothesis. Where no mechanisms exist to borrow or save, effective income equals income at that time; where imperfect mechanisms exist, effective income would be somewhere between current income and the expression given in equation [2] (5). The effects of limited access to a borrowing mechanism can be formulated as:

$$C_0 = Min\left[\frac{Y_0 + A_0 + \sum_{t=1}^{L} Y_t P_t \delta^t}{1 + \sum_{t=1}^{L} P_t \delta^t}, Y_o + A_0 F_0 + \sum_{t=1}^{L} Y_t P_t F_t \delta^t \right] \qquad [3]$$

The expression means that a household would like to consume at the level suggested by the life cycle hypothesis, but when its access to borrowing is less than required, it is forced to consume less. F_t is a measure of the access a household has to future earnings at time t. When F_t is zero, but $F_0 > 0$, the household cannot draw on future income, but is limited in its consumption to its current income and assets.

At first glance, the notion of consumption smoothing may seem confusing. Figure 39.1 shows an example of the movements of current income (Y), permanent income (PY), and effective income (EY) over time. Current income for the hypothetical household is expected to increase irregularly for the next 15 years and then steadily decrease. If the household has access to perfect consumption smoothing mecha-

Figure 39.1 Current income, permanent income, and effective income

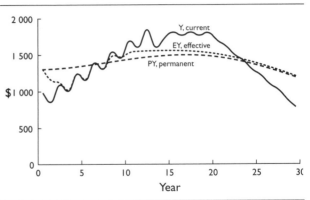

nisms (and perfect foresight), it would be expected to consume along the dashed line (PY). During the first 8–10 years the household borrows money (or uses its savings), as indicated by the fact that the PY line lies above the Y line. Between the 10 and 25-year period, the household makes savings, as its current income is higher than its expenditure expressed by the permanent income line, PY. From the 25th year onwards, the household uses its savings (or borrows) to achieve a higher expenditure level than that allowed by its current income. With access to partial consumption smoothing mechanisms, the household's effective consumption may follow the dotted line (EY). In the first third of the consumption cycle, the household does not take full advantage of the consumption smoothing mechanism, and its expenditure follows in part the current income trend. In the middle part of the cycle, the household saves but not at a rate that corresponds to the level that would be required by complete consumption smoothing. In the last years, the household dissaves and takes almost full advantage of the available consumption smoothing devices.

Because considerations of fairness in financial contribution are normative, the denominator in HFC needs to be defined in terms of some meaningful and comparable standard across households. In order to reflect the desire of households to smooth consumption over time and the limitations to consumption smoothing existing in many circumstances, we define effective income as the level of consumption that a household is able to achieve, based on a life cycle perspective, and assuming that all households share a standard discount rate. To avoid any ambiguity, it is assumed that effective income is as defined in equation [3] with the added constraint that all households face the market interest rate as the discount rate.

Because we define capacity to pay in terms of effective income, it leads naturally to certain conclusions about what should be included in the denominator. For example, subsidies raise a household's net income and, therefore, its effective income. Likewise, tax payments lower the income the household receives. Because F_t cannot be easily observed, estimating effective income presents a number of challenges. These are addressed in more detail in section five that discusses implementation and issues associated with data collection and quality.

SUBSISTENCE EXPENDITURE

The second step in defining capacity to pay is to determine expenditure required for subsistence. There is an

extensive literature on basic needs which addresses this question (6–9). Subsistence is often defined to include basic expenditures on food, shelter, and clothing. This expenditure is subtracted from household total expenditure in order to better capture the household's economic resources available for health and other spending. Therefore, HFC can be considered as a ratio of health expenditure to the income left after expenditure necessary to keep the household alive has been subtracted. The choice of a measure of subsistence expenditure should also be based on definitions that are comparable across populations. Ways of estimating subsistence expenditure from survey data are discussed in the next section.

MEASURING HOUSEHOLD HEALTH EXPENDITURES

As mentioned earlier, household contributions (10–11) to the health system include all direct and indirect payment sources: general taxes, social security contributions, private insurance premiums, and out-of-pocket payments (12). This section describes how these components can be captured from a household survey.

GOVERNMENT SPENDING ON HEALTH

Household contributions to health that are channelled through government spending comprise income tax, property tax, value-added taxes (VAT), sales tax, excise duty, corporate income tax, and other tax sources. In order to distinguish the part of government spending that is used on health (GHE), each household's tax payments are multiplied by the proportion of total government spending allocated to finance the health system (including any government subsidies or transfers to social health insurance):

$$GHE_i = \left(\frac{GHE}{GC}\right)_N \left[(inctax + vat + excise + other)_i (scalar(x))\right] \quad [4]$$

The first bracketed term is simply the fraction of total government consumption (GC) that is allocated to health on a nationwide basis. The second bracket includes terms used for estimating the government revenue originating from the household. Usually only income tax ($inctax_i$), value-added tax (vat_i), and excise duties ($excise_i$) can be captured from a household survey. These constitute only a part of total taxes paid by the household. The remaining tax (such as corporate income, import duties or property taxes) and non-tax revenues (fees, fines, etc.) must be estimated indirectly. Even for income tax, it may be difficult to obtain accurate figures from a household survey because: (a) people may under- or over-report their income and correspondingly the income tax will be underestimated or overestimated; (b) sometimes the tax treatment of an income source cannot be clearly identified for particular countries; (c) even when income subject to tax can be clearly identified, there may be various deductions that may be difficult to capture from the information provided in the survey, despite knowledge of a country's tax laws.

The estimation on VAT/sales tax is more straightforward than the estimation of income tax because the official rates in a country can simply be applied to the reported purchases in the surveys. However, inconsistencies may still exist because of: (a) memory bias associated with certain expenditure items in the survey; (b) a complicated structure of applicable tax rates; (c) the fact that excise duties are sometimes levied on quantity purchased instead of price, but the household survey may only record the money value of that item.

Because of the likely under- and over-reporting in surveys, an adjustment scalar is used to approximate the total government revenue received from households. In doing so it is assumed that the distribution of the non-observed tax and non-tax revenue across households is identical to the distribution of the observed tax revenue from the survey.

The scalar is defined as the ratio of expected government revenue (GC_e) to the government revenue (GC_s) estimated from the survey:

$$scalar(x) = \frac{GC_e}{GC_s} \qquad [5]$$

Expected government revenue shows how much government revenue would be generated by the tax payments of all households included in the survey, if the ratio of government revenue to GDP reported in National Account estimates applied. For the estimation of GC_e, the GDP implied by the expenditure reported in the survey (gdp_s) must be calculated. It is calculated combining survey and National Accounts information as follows:

$$gdp_s = \frac{pc_s}{(PC/GDP)_N} = \frac{\sum w_i(\exp_i)}{(PC/GDP)_N} \qquad [6]$$

pc_s is private consumption from the survey, PC/GDP_N is private consumption share of GDP at the national level, $\exp_i$ is household consumption expenditure, and w_i is the household weight from the survey. Survey weights are applied to account for estimation bias aris-

ing from sampling design and systematic non-response in the sample.

Once the survey GDP has been calculated, GC_e can be derived from:

$$GC_e = gdp_s(GC/GDP)_N \qquad [7]$$

where $(GC/GDP)_N$ is the government consumption share of GDP at the national level. Government tax revenue from the survey is calculated as:

$$GC_s = \sum w_i\left(inctax_i + vat_i + excise_i + other_i\right) \qquad [8]$$

When formulae [7] and [8] are substituted into formula [5], we have:

$$scalar(x) = \frac{(GC/GDP)_N \, gdp_s}{\sum w_i\left(inctax_i + vat_i + excise_i + other_i\right)} \qquad [9]$$

As mentioned earlier, the scalar x is designed to capture the part of government tax revenue that cannot be estimated from the survey data. However, it also includes any measurement error from the survey. In order to separate these effects, scalar x could be decomposed into two parts—one comprising the survey measurement error (scalar x_1) and another comprising the missing tax information part from the survey (scalar x_2). In equations [10] to [12] national level data are denoted by uppercase letters and survey data by lowercase letters:

$$scalar(x_1) = \frac{\left[(INCTAX + VAT + EXCISE + OTHER)/GDP\right]_N \, gdp_s}{\sum w_i\left(inctax_i + vat_i + excise_i + other_i\right)} \qquad [10]$$

This equation represents the extent to which the household tax contributions derived from the survey reflect total national receipts from those sources alone, and

$$scalar(x_2) = \frac{(GC/GDP)_N \, gdp_s}{scalar(x_1)\sum w_i\left(inctax_i + vat_i + excise_i + other_i\right)} \qquad [11]$$

Substituting for scalar x_1 in equation [11] gives:

$$scalar(x_2) = \frac{GC_N}{(VAT + INCTAX + EXCISE + OTHER)_N} \qquad [12]$$

that is the extent to which total government tax revenue is provided by the forms of taxes to which the households contribute directly and which were captured from the analysis of the surveys.

Scalar x_2 equals 1 if the government collects taxes only from households, while it is less than 1 if it collects revenue from other sources. It should be noted that scalar $x = (scalar(x_1))(scalar(x_2))$. The advantage of decomposing the scalar is that the two sources of under- or overestimation could be more clearly identified.

In the analysis, total household consumption is assumed to equal total private consumption. Strictly speaking, this is not the case since private consumption is the market value of all goods and services purchased, or received in kind, by households and non-profit institutions. If the non-profit component is large, the scalar will be underestimated as a result of underestimation of survey GDP.

Whenever income tax ($inctax_i$) is not available directly from a survey, it is estimated from reported income and the country's tax schedule information. Reported income includes salaries and non-salary earnings from all employment activities. Non-salary earnings include in kind benefits. Employment includes self-employment as well as a second job when relevant. The income tax paid by each individual in the household is then aggregated to a monthly value at the household level. The question arises as to which individuals are subject to income tax. In many countries, particularly the poorer ones, only formal sector employees pay income taxes. The way to identify formal sector workers varies by country. Usually answers to the job classification questions in the surveys will indicate whether an individual works in the private, public or informal sector. Other methods of identification can be used in more difficult cases.

Sales tax or value-added tax (vat_i) and excise duties can be imputed from household expenditures on various categories of goods and services. This involves applying the tax rates derived from official tax documents to household expenditures on the corresponding commodities reported in the survey.

The information on other taxes ($other_i$), such as those paid on real estate, can often be obtained directly from the household survey. Otherwise, the value of property owned by the household can be estimated from the questionnaire. Tax rates obtained from the tax schedule of each country are then applied for the calculation.

SOCIAL HEALTH INSURANCE CONTRIBUTIONS

The second component of HE that needs to be estimated is the total social health insurance contribution of the household (SSH_i), which can be formulated as follows:

$$SSH_i = soc_i(scalar(y)) \qquad [13]$$

Household social security contributions (soc_i) are computed similarly to income tax. If social security contributions are provided directly by the survey in the form of a specific question on payments or contributions, this information is used. When this is not the case, the official contribution rate is applied to the salary from the primary job of the individual (after determining whether the earnings are pre-tax or post-tax). The assumption is that only formal sector employees, or full-time permanent workers, contribute to social security.

Although contribution rates may vary with respect to level of income, and sometimes the sector of the economy in which the individual works, it is assumed that the employer's contribution share is borne by the employee in the form of reduced net salaries. For the computation, this implies that employers' contributions should be added to those of the employee. This assumption is generally applied in the tax incidence literature and it simplifies the analysis and comparison across countries (13). As with income tax, the social security contributions by individuals are summed to obtain the contributions at the household level.

Because only a share of social security payments are used in the health sector, the scalar y is introduced. It can be formalized as:

$$scalar(y) = \frac{gdp_s(SSH/GDP)_N}{\sum w_i(soc_i)} \qquad [14]$$

The numerator reflects the expected social security contributions to health for the GDP observed in the survey—the survey GDP (gdp_s) multiplied by the share of health social security payments in GDP at the national level. The denominator is the weighted sum of the household contributions to social insurance of all forms.

This scalar also can be decomposed into two parts. The first is due to measurement error of social security contributions in the survey—in some household surveys, social security contributions reported at the household level can, in sum, differ from the value stated in the National Accounts. These discrepancies are essentially the result of under- or over-reporting social security contributions in the household survey. This can be expressed as:

$$scalar(y_1) = \frac{gdp_s(SOC/GDP)_N}{\sum w_i(soc_i)} \qquad [15]$$

or the extent to which reported household contributions sum to the contributions expected from national aggregates. This scalar could be higher or lower than unity.

The second part of scalar y is related to the fact that only part of social security payments go to health. This component of the scalar y can be expressed as:

$$scalar(y_2) = \frac{gdp_s(SSH/GDP)_N}{scalar(y_1)\sum w_i(soc_i)}. \quad [16]$$

After substituting for scalar y_1 in equation [16], scalar y_2 can be expressed as SSH/SOC, or the proportion of social security payments going to health. Note that, as in the case of the x scalar, scalar y = (scalar (y_1)) (scalar (y_2)).

PRIVATE HEALTH INSURANCE

The third component of HE is the private health insurance premiums paid by households (PRV_i). In most cases, data are available directly from the household survey. In some countries, employers contribute to private health insurance on behalf of their employees (we continue to assume that the employer's contribution to private health insurance is *de facto* part of the employee's income). Hence the employers' contributions should also be included in the analysis. It is likely that excluding the employers' part will lead to underestimation of this component of prepayment in countries where private health insurance plays a dominant role in health system financing, and employers subsidize employees' private health insurance premiums. In the case of social health insurance and tax contributions, a scalar was used to adjust the level of household spending to nationally reported figures. This procedure, however, cannot be undertaken in the case of private insurance premiums since reliable sources of the employers' contribution share at the national level are usually not available. The same applies to out-of-pocket payments.

To avoid an upward bias in the estimation of private health insurance contributions, premium refunds or credits granted from the private insurance company, for example for not using the services in a previous period, must be deducted from the declared level of household private health insurance premiums.

OUT-OF-POCKET PAYMENTS

Out-of-pocket payments (OOP_i) include all categories of health-related expenses paid directly by the household at the time the household receives the health service. Typically these include doctor's consultation fees, purchases of medication, and hospital bills. Spending on alternative and/or traditional medicine is included

in out-of-pocket spending, whereas expenditure on health-related transportation is excluded.

It is important to note that some people may be paying out-of-pocket for health care, but receiving a reimbursement later from social and/or private health insurance schemes. To avoid introducing an upward bias in health expenditures, reimbursements are deducted from household "gross" out-of-pocket payments. Details of these reimbursements are usually given in the surveys.

TOTAL HOUSEHOLD HEALTH EXPENDITURES

Putting the components together, household i's health expenditure comprises its payments to government that are channelled to health, as well as its health-related social insurance contributions, private health insurance contributions, and out-of-pocket payments:

$$HE_i = GHE_i + SSH_i + PRV_i + OOP_i \quad [17]$$

MEASURING HOUSEHOLD CAPACITY TO PAY

As mentioned in section two, household capacity to pay is defined as effective income net of subsistence expenditure. This section describes how to estimate effective income and subsistence expenditure from survey data.

EFFECTIVE INCOME

It is not possible to try to estimate permanent income over the life cycle in a multi-country context with the surveys available, which would require information on likely future income, assets, and the potential to borrow or lend. To reduce the short-term fluctuations observed in income data as reported in surveys, however, household consumption expenditure is used as the proxy for effective income. This choice is based on two considerations. First, the variance of current expenditure is smaller than the variance of current income over time. Income data reflect random shocks while expenditure data conform better to the notion of effective income. In defining capacity to pay, it is important to try to eliminate the effect of random shocks on income to the greatest extent possible. Second, in most of the household surveys expenditure data are more reliable than income data. This is particularly true in developing countries where the informal sector is typically relatively large and survey respondents may not wish to reveal their true income for various reasons (14–15).

SUBSISTENCE EXPENDITURE

It was argued earlier that household capacity to pay for health services should not be determined with respect to its total effective income. The reason is that unless households first meet basic subsistence needs, they will not be in a position to finance health services. In *The World Health Report 2000*, actual food expenditure was used as a proxy for household subsistence expenditure (1).

However, food expenditure may not capture the actual subsistence expenditure of the household, even though effort was made to limit this expenditure to basic food only. A rich family may spend a greater absolute amount on food than a poor family although the food expenditure share of total household consumption expenditure still follows Engel's law—i.e. the share of food to total income falls with increases in income (16). For this reason, the approach has been modified.

In order to eliminate spending on non-essential food and to improve international comparability, one possibility would be to use the international poverty line as a measure of subsistence expenditure. This poverty line is set at one international dollar per day per person in 1985 currency terms, first used by the World Bank in the *World Development Report 1990* (17). The one international dollar subsistence level is based on a study of absolute poverty lines in 33 countries (18).

This alternative was explored by adjusting the 1985 level to nominal units corresponding to the year of the household survey using an appropriate price deflator. To account for differences in consumption patterns and prices, food PPPs (Purchasing Power Parities) rather than general GDP PPPs, were used to convert the international poverty line expressed in international dollars into local currency units. This conversion was made to express subsistence expenditures in the same units as data collected in the surveys. Finally, an adjustment for household size was made to bring the poverty line, defined at the individual level, to the household level.

The introduction of the food poverty line eliminates the problem that actual food expenditure includes spending on non-essential food for many households. It also improves international comparability. Since the food poverty line stays the same as income increases, more progressivity is built into the distribution of HFC

compared to the situation where actual food expenditure is used. Figure 39.2 shows the share of actual food expenditure and the share of the food poverty line in total household consumption expenditure across expenditure deciles. The food poverty level share of total expenditure declines more rapidly with increases in expenditure (income) than does actual food expenditure. This indicates that the capacity to pay of richer households would be underestimated by using actual food expenditure.

The problem with the international poverty line is that several causes of uncertainty are unavoidably built into estimation. These include various problems associated with the construction of food PPP conversion factors. For this reason, we explored an approach that partly resembles the assessment of national poverty lines. Using the observation that food expenditure as a proportion of total expenditure increases with increasing poverty, a food share based poverty line for each country was estimated. The poverty line for a given survey was set equal to the average food expenditure of households whose food share of total expenditure was in the 45 to 55 percentile range (used in preference to the single household at the 50th percentile). This was adjusted for household size using an equivalence scale of *eqsize* = *hhsize*$^\beta$. The adjustment factor β was obtained from household survey data from all 59 countries using the following fixed-effects regression:

$$\ln food = \ln k + \beta \ln hhsize + \sum_{i=1}^{n-1} \gamma_i country_i + \varepsilon \qquad [18]$$

Figure 39.2 Subsistence expenditure as a share of total consumption expenditure, Bangladesh

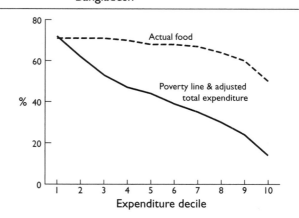

The estimated value of β was 0.564 with confidence interval 0.564–0.572. The estimation of food poverty line is explained further in Xu et al. (*19*).

This approach has the advantage that it does not require the estimation of PPPs for countries where price observations have not been made, nor does it require as many intermediate calculation steps that can introduce uncertainty in the analysis. In addition, it is an indicator estimated directly from the survey data. The food share based measure still eliminates luxurious food spending and introduces more progressivity to the underlying expenditure distribution than the original measure based on actual food expenditure.

Household Capacity to Pay

The numerator of the HFC comprises all health expenditures by the household, including those deducted at source (e.g. tax and social security payments). The denominator of HFC, household's capacity to pay (CTP_i), is a measure of the non-subsistence effective income of the household (effective income minus subsistence expenditure). Total household expenditure is used as the proxy for effective income. However, the expenditure reported in household surveys does not include the health expenditures deducted from income at source, which are included in the numerator. In order, then, to maintain consistency between the numerator and the denominator, tax and social security contributions deducted at source must be added to the denominator which becomes:

$$CTP_i = EXP_i - SE_i + GHE_i - indtax_i(GHE/GC)_N + SSH_i \ [19]$$

The expression $GHE_i - indtax_i(GHE/GC)_N$ represents that part of household tax contributions which is deducted at source—indirect taxes ($indtax_i$) are included in EXP_i and are not deducted at source.

Household expenditure information is available directly from the household survey and converted into a monthly value. Total household consumption expenditure (EXP_i) includes both monetary and in kind payments on all goods and services, as well as the money value of the consumption of household-made products. Household consumption expenditure includes indirect taxes such as the VAT/sales tax, excise duties, as these taxes are viewed as part of the household's capacity to pay.

As a means of quality control, responses from households reporting zero expenditure or zero food expenditure were considered to be reporting errors and were excluded from the analysis.

Additional Data Requirements and the Reference Period

The way the household financial contribution (HFC) can be calculated using information from national household income and expenditure surveys was the focus of the last two sections. It was shown, however, that additional information was required including detailed government taxation documents, and national health accounts figures.

The main sources of this additional information are:

■ Government taxation documents, including information on the systems of income tax, sales tax, value-added tax, excise tax, and property tax.

■ National Health Accounts (NHA) figures. WHO provides yearly estimates of various components of health expenditure from private and public sources for all its Member States, and these were used to give a reference for checking the reliability of the survey data (*1*).

■ Social security and health insurance laws that provide information on premiums and other contributions to the health system.

Ideally the HFC would be measured over a long enough period to allow smoothing of consumption. In practice, this is not possible where data must be taken from existing surveys, which ask about short recall periods, usually less than a year. For this reason, all the variables needed for computing HFC are converted into monthly figures regardless of the recall periods used in the individual surveys. If the recall period in any survey was greater than one month and the inflation rate differed between the months for which information was sought, expenditures were deflated to a common month using the local consumer price index.

Summary and Conclusions

In summary, the household financial contribution, or HFC, is defined as a ratio of health payments made by the household to its capacity to pay. Household health payments consist of four sources: general taxation, social security contributions, private health insurance premiums, and out-of-pocket payments. Household capacity to pay is measured as non-subsistence effective income, which is in practice calculated as total household expenditure net of the food poverty line. Most of the required information can be obtained from household survey data combined with knowledge of the tax and social security systems in the different countries. However, a number of challenges associated with improving the quality of the data and comparability across countries remain.

Measurement error in the context of income or expenditure data derived from surveys is a well known problem (20–21). Measurement error could be introduced at any stage of the survey: design of the survey instrument, data collection or data entry. The typical problem with income survey data is underestimation. This is due to the design of the questions and the tendency of respondents to understate their true earnings. The more detailed the income question, for example the more income categories used, the more accurate the figures generated. Another problem associated with the construction of income questionnaires is whether the respondents understand the desired income concept correctly and in the same way. If the questions and the implementation of the survey are not carefully controlled, situations may arise where some of the respondents report their income gross of taxes while others are reporting their income net of taxes. These problems also complicate comparison of income-based measures between countries.

While expenditure may be reported more accurately by household book-keeping, certain expenditure items may be difficult to capture, or they may be only partly captured by the survey. It may, for example, be difficult to record and impute correctly the value of home production that is consumed in the home rather than sold. If consumption from own-production is substantial, it is possible to produce per capita expenditure figures that are higher than the corresponding GDP figures derived from national accounts. To the extent that these differences are real and they are due to the fact that home-production is not adequately imputed in the calculation of the country GDP, this discrepancy is acceptable. However, in some cases the value of own-production is clearly overestimated in surveys and it is then difficult to know how to treat the survey data.

The time period over which households are asked to recall their expenditures is not identical across surveys or countries. This has been a concern in the analysis of catastrophic expenditures. A short recall period will have a smaller memory bias than a long recall period, while the latter may capture catastrophic expenditures better than the former. The direction of biases generated by different recall periods is not self-evident.

In estimating government spending on health, it is assumed that government revenue comes from general taxes, which is true for the majority of countries.

When revenue from other sources, however, such as the sale of oil or other national assets is substantial, the question arises as how or whether to assign such revenue to households. As there are no common guidelines on how best to deal with revenue accruing from nationally owned assets, it was decided in this context to exclude it from the calculation of HFC. This decision was based on the consideration that revenues arising from the sales of national assets do not represent either a financing burden to the household or an increase in capacity to pay that is freely at its disposal. The effect of this kind of government revenue will be reflected in the HFC since it will reduce health service prices in public facilities or increase health funds in public insurance, thereby reducing the out-of-pocket payments of households.

The application of scalars to adjust for the unobserved part of government (or social health insurance) revenue is necessary for obtaining estimates that are consistent with macro-level information. If, for some reason, the households' tax outlays are overestimated or underestimated, this will have a corresponding impact on HFC and any summary measure of the distribution calculated on the basis of these ratios. Discrepancies between survey and national data can occur if substantial parts of government revenue accrue from state-owned enterprises, non-tax revenue, or external donations rather than from households. Bias may also be generated if the income data that are used for estimating income taxes, and in some cases the social health insurance contributions, are of poor quality. The adjustment scalar is critical to ensure that the level of the revenues is correct, although the distribution of this revenue is not known. The fact that the unobserved revenue is being contributed to households in the same proportions as the observed revenue, could in some cases lead to misleading estimates of the true distribution of the HFCs.

As explained above, the household financial contribution to the health system should include all the components paid directly or indirectly by the household. In principal, private health insurance premiums paid by both employer and employee should be included in the calculation. Information on employer's contribution to private health insurance is very difficult to obtain from household surveys. In countries where private insurance is substantial and employers participate in its funding, like in the United States, household health expenditures and consequently HFC could be underestimated.

Because of the time lag between the recorded out-of-pocket payment and the insurance reimbursement received at a later date, negative out-of-pocket payments could be estimated for some households. For the same reason, negative direct taxes might occur from income register data. Two possible solutions have been suggested: one is to delete the observations with negative values and the other is to set the negative value at zero. The currently followed practice in HFC calculation conforms to the latter approach.

Household surveys are a rich source of data that allows for a detailed micro-level analysis on a relatively comparative basis across countries. Nevertheless, differences in survey design and quality exist. In addition, some of the available surveys are not very recent and may not be suitable for analysing health system fairness if substantial health financing reforms have taken place since they were undertaken. It is important, therefore, to continually try to improve survey design and conduct so that the problems associated with data quality and comparability are reduced.

ACKNOWLEDGEMENTS

The authors are grateful to Guy Carrin and William D. Savedoff for comments on an earlier draft, to Felicia Knaul for her contribution to the early stage of the development of the methodology, to Ana Mylena Aguilar-Rivera for formatting the tables and graphs, and to Nathalie Etomba and Anna Moore for data and reference searches.

REFERENCES

(1) World Health Organization. *The World Health Report 2000. Health Systems: Improving Performance.* Geneva, World Health Organization, 2000.

(2) Ando A, Modgliani F. The life cycle hypothesis of saving: aggregate implication and tests. *American Economic Review,* 1963, 53:55–84.

(3) Friedman M. *A theory of the consumption function.* Princeton, Princeton University Press, 1957.

(4) Romer DH. *Advanced macroeconomics.* New York, McGraw-Hill, 2000.

(5) Behrman P. *Health sector reform in developing countries: making health development sustainable.* Boston, Harvard University Press, 1995.

(6) Sen A. *Poverty and famines: an essay on entitlement and deprivation.* Oxford, Clarendon Press, 1981.

(7) Sen A. *Resources, values and development.* Oxford, Blackwell, 1984.

(8) Sen A. *The standard of living.* New York, Cambridge University Press, 1987.

(9) Streeten P et al. *First things first: meeting basic human needs in the developing countries,* New York, Oxford University Press, 1981.

(10) Fuchs VR. *Who shall live? Health, economics and social choice.* Stanford, Stanford University, 1982.

(11) Iglehart JK. The American health care system - expenditures. *The New England Journal of Medicine,* 1999, 340:70–76.

(12) Murray CJL et al. *Defining and measuring fairness in financial contribution to the health system.* EIP Discussion Paper No. 24. Geneva, World Health Organization, 2000. URL: http://www3.who.int/whosis/discussion_papers/discussion_papers.cfm#

(13) Wagstaff A et al. Equity in the finance of health care: some further international comparisons. *Journal of Health Economics,* 1999, 18:263–290.

(14) Deaton A. *Understanding consumption.* Oxford, Oxford University Press, 1992.

(15) Bouis HE. The effect of income on demand for food in poor countries: are our food consumption databases giving us reliable estimates? *Journal of Development Economics,* 1994, 44(1):199–226.

(16) Mas-Colell A, Whinston MD, Green JR. *Microeconomic theory.* New York, Oxford University Press, 1995.

(17) World Bank. *World development report: poverty.* New York, Oxford University Press, 1990.

(18) Ravillion M et al. *Quantifying the magnitude and severity of absolute poverty in the developing world in the mid-1980s.* Pre Working Paper Series No. 587. Washington, DC, World Bank, 1991.

(19) Xu K et al. Understanding household catastrophic health expenditures: a multi-country analysis. In: Murray CJL, Evans DB, eds. *Health systems performance assessment: debates, methods and empiricism.* Geneva, World Health Organization, 2003.

(20) Paulin GD, Ferraro DL. Imputing income in the consumer expenditure survey. *Monthly Labor Review,* 1994, 117(12):23–31.

(21) McGregor P, Nachane D. Identifying the poor: a comparison of income and expenditure indicators using the 1985 Family Expenditure Survey. *Oxford Bulletin of Economics & Statistics,* 1995, 57(1):119–128.

Chapter 40

Summary Measures of the Distribution of Household Financial Contributions to Health

Ke Xu, Jan Klavus, Ana Mylena Aguilar-Rivera, Guy Carrin, Riadh Zeramdini, Christopher J.L. Murray

Introduction

Considerable attention has recently been focused on the conceptual and empirical issues of measuring the fairness of household financial contributions to the health system (1–4). WHO has argued that fairness requires that health system payments are organized in such a way that the burden of payments is equalized across households. Equal burden is defined as an equal fraction of each household's capacity to pay (CTP). The ratio of a household's health payments to its capacity to pay is called the household financial contribution (HFC). If all households contribute the same share of their CTP, the HFC of each household will equal the ratio of a country's total health expenditure (HE) to its total capacity to pay (2).

The distribution of HFC across households varies across countries. Figure 40.1 shows the HFC distributions for Spain and Azerbaijan.[1] The x-axis depicts the HFC and the y-axis measures proportion of households at various levels of HFC. The HFC distribution of Azerbaijan is clearly more dispersed than that of Spain. In Spain, only a very small proportion of households have high health payments relative to capacity to pay, whereas in Azerbaijan the proportion of the population with a relatively high HFC is considerably greater. Visually, a long right-hand tail indicates more unequal distributions and potentially catastrophic payments for households.

For many purposes, however, visual comparisons are insufficient. To allow comparisons of the relative fairness of financial contributions across countries or over time, the information provided by the HFC distribution needs to be captured in a summary measure. The purpose of this chapter is to explore various summary measures and to develop a justification for the choice of a summary measure for the HFC distribu-

tion. Section two discusses various desirable properties that the measure should possess. The subsequent section contains an overview of the survey data used in the analysis. Some common measures of income inequality are presented in the fourth section and a new measure, called the fairness in financial contribution index (FFC), is proposed. Section five undertakes a comparative analysis of the properties of different

Figure 40.1 Distribution of household financial contributions (HFC), Spain and Azerbaijan

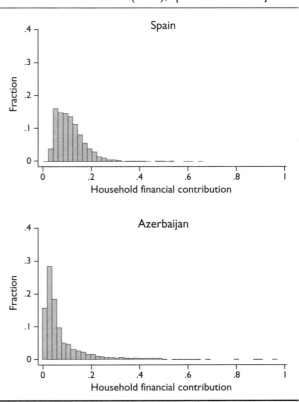

measures and highlights some important advantages of the FFC measure.

CRITERIA FOR A SUMMARY MEASURE OF HFC

There is a vast literature on indices to summarize income distributions (5–8) and their application to the measurement of inequality in the context of health care (9–13). Ideally, a summary measure of any distribution should reflect the normative views of the society by displaying various properties that are consistent with those normative expectations. This could be achieved, for example, by choosing a measure that is more sensitive to relative than to absolute differences between households, or by emphasizing various parts of the distribution more heavily than others.

Before turning to an overview of different indices, a number of criteria that a summary measure of HFC should possess are explored. These include a concern for catastrophic expenditure, the preference for individual-mean rather than interpersonal differences, the property of constant invariance, and the requirement that the index can be displayed in interpretable units.

CONCERN FOR CATASTROPHIC EXPENDITURE

A good summary measure should reflect the normative view of the general public and policy-makers about the importance of different parts of the HFC distribution. In particular, there is a strong preference in most societies for protecting individual households from potentially catastrophic expenditures and for sharing the burden of health financing across households. For example, the possible impact of various health system financing mechanisms on the well-being of poor people has influenced the design of health systems and health insurance mechanisms in many different settings, and protecting people from catastrophic payments is now widely accepted as an important objective of health policy (14–21). These concerns were tested on the general public in a WHO survey about preferences for financing arrangements in the health system. The 1 007 respondents comprised health professionals and people with a special interest in health from over 100 countries, people with knowledge of the health system and how it is financed. Respondents were asked the question in Box 40.1. More than 70% of respondents favoured the option of ensuring that two households paid an equal proportion of their disposable income (capacity to pay), rather than one household risking

catastrophic expenditure. Two variations were asked subsequently: in the first the choice was between one household contributing 200% of its capacity to pay (by borrowing) versus two contributing 100%; in the second the choice was between a single household contributing 50% versus two contributing 25%. In both variations all other households contributed 5% of their capacity to pay. Again, a substantial majority of respondents thought it was more fair to avoid the risk of catastrophic payments by ensuring equal proportional contributions of capacity to pay, the majority increasing as the payments became more catastrophic. These findings are consistent with a strong preference for protecting households from catastrophic expenditures (22). We believe, therefore, that these concerns should be captured by the summary index of HFC.

INDIVIDUAL-MEAN DIFFERENCE

Many commonly used summary measures of inequality can be classified into two main groups: those measuring interindividual differences and those measuring individual-mean differences. An interindividual measure is concerned with differences between every pair of individuals or households in the sample. This type of measure would be preferable in settings where people care more about the difference between their own contribution relative to contributions of all other individuals in the population than the difference between their own contribution relative to the average contribution in the population. The Gini coefficient, widely used to summarize the distribution of income, belongs to this group of measures.

The preference for an individual-mean measure in the context of HFC assessment arises from the normative considerations underlying the equal burden principle. The concern with individual-mean differences is consistent with measuring the extent to which the

---

Box 40.1   Fairness in Financial Contribution Survey

Question 1. In Population A all households contribute 5% of their disposable income towards the health system, except for one household that must contribute 100% of its disposable income. Disposable income is income left after food expenditures are deducted. In population B all households contribute 5% of their disposable income towards the health system, except for two households that each must contribute 50% of their disposable income.

Which one of the two scenarios do you think is more fair?

■ The scenario in Population A

■ The scenario in Population B

■ The two scenarios are equally fair

■ I don't know

distribution of HFC deviates from the norm of equal burden.

Constant Invariance Property

The general formula for an individual-mean difference (IMD) measure of inequality in the distribution of variable y (in this case the HFC) is:

$$IMD(\alpha,\beta) = \frac{\sum_{i=1}^{n}|y_i - \mu|^\alpha}{n\mu^\beta} \qquad [1]$$

where y_i is the household financial contribution (HFC) of household i, μ is the mean financial contribution (i.e. mean HFC), and n is the number of households in the sample. The choice of the parameter α is related to the significance attached to differences in financial contributions observed at the tails of the distribution compared to those observed closer to the mean. For the distribution of HFC, the higher α becomes, the more importance is attached to the tails of the distribution, namely catastrophic spending.

The β coefficient determines the extent to which the inequality measure is relative to the mean, or absolute. A value of $\beta = 1$ reflects an interest in a relative measure. The measure is strictly relative when $\beta = \alpha = 1$. It is invariant to proportionate changes in all observations. This property is called scalar invariance, or mean-independence, under which the inequality index remains unchanged if each individual's HFC is multiplied by the same positive scalar. In contrast, when $\beta = 0$ concern lies exclusively with absolute deviations from the mean and the measure is invariant to the addition of a positive constant to each individual's observed HFC. This property is known as constant invariance. A value of β between zero and one reflects a mix of concern between relative and absolute differences.

Constant invariance is consistent with the equal burden principle. Consider a hypothetical HFC distribution A = {0.1, 0.2, 0.4, 0.5} with a mean HFC of 0.3. Adding a constant of 0.1 to each contribution share yields a distribution of A_1 = {0.2, 0.3, 0.5, 0.6}. Now the mean contribution share has increased to 0.4, relative differences have decreased, but according to the constant invariance property with $\beta = 0$, the fairness of these two distributions is equal. This is implied by the equal burden principle, where fairness is assessed with respect to deviations from the ideal state of all households paying equal shares of their capacity to pay, which would be the mean HFC.

It can also be shown that the equal burden principle is inconsistent with the scalar invariance property. Multiplying the HFC in distribution A by a scalar of, say, 1.5 gives rise to a distribution A_2 = {0.15, 0.3, 0.6, 0.75}. The mean of this distribution is 0.45. While the relative differences with respect to the mean have remained unchanged in the two distributions, the differences between each observation and the mean have increased. There is greater absolute divergence from the ideal of equal burden (mean HFC) in A_2.

It is also true that multiplying the distribution A by a scalar increases the higher contribution shares relatively more than the addition of a constant to each observation. In the above example the relative increase in A_1 due to adding a constant of 0.1 is smaller the higher the contribution share. In contrast, in distribution A_2 the HFC shares of all observations increase by the same relative amount. If the chosen inequality measure attaches more weight to the highest contribution shares, there is likely to be an elevated potential for catastrophic payments, but the measure will be totally insensitive to these changes under scalar invariance. The same applies, of course, to a measure that is constant invariant, but the unobserved welfare implications will be smaller as the relative effect becomes smaller at higher contribution shares.

In the context of income inequality, scalar invariance is usually considered desirable (8). One reason for this is its robustness to linear transformations. For example, the welfare implications of the measure remain the same whether a country's income distribution is expressed in domestic or foreign currency units (e.g. all observations in domestic currency units are multiplied by a constant). This property is especially important for cross-country comparisons or comparisons over time. In addition, even if income is measured in common currency units, mean incomes are likely to differ substantially between countries so reference to the mean level of income is important. In this sense, the invariance property (whether constant or scale) does not have a great impact in the context of summarizing the HFC distribution, which is bounded by zero and unity. The variation of mean HFC is relatively small, the lowest value being 0.062 and the highest value being 0.206 (see below for a description of data).

Interpretable Units

A somewhat related property concerns the scaling properties of the measure. The strictest type of measure is determinable on a ratio scale, where the ratio of two observations remains the same regardless of the units of measurement that are being used. It is, therefore, possible to say that the second poorest household earns twice as much as the poorest household whether incomes are measured in dollars or rupees. A looser type of measure is one that is expressed on an interval scale, where ratios themselves have no meaning, but the ratios of differences do. For example, the difference between the third and first observation in two distributions might be twice that of the difference between the third and the second observations. Measures with ratio or interval scale properties are called cardinal measures. In contrast, an ordinal measure is one that is concerned only with the orderings or rankings of the observations and the ratios of differences have no meaning. An ordinal measure is invariant to any positive monotonic transformation. For example, an income ranking of 1, 2, 3, 4 can be replaced by 100, 106, 120, 399 without any loss of consistency.

In the context of an inequality measure defined in the range 0 to 1, a measure with interval scale properties implies that the difference between 0.9 and 0.8 means the same thing as the difference between 0.7 and 0.6. This property allows the measure to be interpreted more easily, but to formally establish the interval-scale properties of an index of the fairness of the distribution of the HFC would require some type of preference measurement. For example, this would enable it to be established if society regarded a reduction of the index from 0.9 to 0.8 to be equally as valuable as a reduction from 0.5 to 0.4. Such an attempt to measure preferences has not been undertaken.

In the absence of knowing the preferences underlying such choices, an inequality index that has a straightforward interpretation and is expressible in natural units is preferable to an index that involves some arbitrary transformation of functional form. This means that indices such as the standard deviation or the coefficient of variation, both of which are interpretable in natural units, would be more desirable measures than some of the entropy measures that have been proposed in the literature, which do not have readily interpretable units (7–8) (a more detailed description of these measures will be given below).

CRITERIA FOR A SUMMARY MEASURE: SUMMARY

In summary, it would be desirable for an index of the fairness of household financial contributions to give more weight to households with potentially catastrophic contributions; to be based on comparison of individual-mean differences; to have the property of

constant invariance; and to be interpretable in terms of some natural unit.

DATA SOURCES

The empirical analysis is based on household surveys conducted by various statistical agencies in 59 countries, between 1991 and 2000. The sample size ranges from 1 103 households in Sweden to 62 946 households in the Republic of Korea. They include Living Standards Measurement Studies (LSMS), Household Budget Surveys (HSB), Household Income and Expenditure Surveys (HIES), and selected other surveys with adequate information on household income and expenditure.

There are several limitations of these data. Firstly, some of the surveys undertaken in the early 1990s might not reflect the impact of more recent reforms in health system financing. Secondly, there is variation in the recall periods used to ask questions related to health service utilization and associated expenditure. Some surveys use a one month recall period, some use three months, some use one year, and some use combinations such as one month for outpatient services and three months or a year for inpatient services. Thirdly, some survey data are of lower quality than others. Efforts are continually being made to identify high quality and most recent household surveys.

AN OVERVIEW OF INEQUALITY MEASURES

GENERAL CLASS OF INEQUALITY MEASURES

As mentioned above, there are two general types of inequality measures: one measuring interindividual differences and another measuring individual-mean differences.

The standard deviation, a commonly used statistical dispersion measure, is of the IMD class where $\alpha = 2$ and $\beta = 0$. The standard deviation for the HFC can be expressed as:

$$\sigma = \sqrt{\frac{\sum (HFC_i - \mu)^2}{n}} \quad [2]$$

where HFC_i is the household financial contribution of household i and μ is the mean HFC. Based on the concept of equal burden, an alternative summary measure closely related to the standard deviation can be proposed. If it is agreed that health expenditures should be pooled and the burden should be shared equally among households, it can be argued that the distribution of HFC should not be compared to the mean HFC, but rather to a reference level that is equal to the ratio of total health spending to total capacity to pay.

Let us assume that a health system raises a certain amount of health revenue (THE)

$$THE = HFC_1 CTP_1 + HFC_2 CTP_2 ... + HFC_n CTP_n \quad [3]$$

where HE_i is the total health financial contribution of household i and CTP_i is its capacity to pay. Following the definition of fairness stating that every household should contribute the same share of its capacity to pay, we have:

$$HFC_1 = HFC_2 ... = HFC_n = \kappa \quad [4]$$

Making use of equation [4] in equation [3] gives:

$$\sum HE_i = \kappa * \sum CTP_i \quad [5]$$

so that

$$\kappa = \frac{\sum HE_i}{\sum CTP_i} = HFC_o \quad [6]$$

HFC_o is the health financing contribution all households would pay under the principle of equal burden.

The standard deviation of HFC, calculated using the mean of the individual observations (labeled $\sigma_{\overline{HFC}}$) and an "augmented standard deviation" using the equal burden HFC (σ_{HFC_o}) are shown in Table 40.1. The five countries with the most dispersion of the HFC (standard deviations in excess of 0.150) are Ukraine, Argentina, Vietnam, Azerbaijan, and Brazil. At the other extreme, the 10 countries with the lowest levels of inequality (0.050–0.071) included six OECD countries as well as Morocco, Philippines, Romania, and Thailand. There are no substantial differences between the standard $\sigma_{\overline{HFC}}$ and the augmented version σ_{HFC_o}.

The standard deviation gives some weight to the tail of the distribution (i.e. the parameter $\alpha = 2$), so it is sensitive to potentially catastrophic payments. It also satisfies the other desirable properties; it is an individual-mean difference measure, it conforms to the constant invariance property, and it is displayed in readily interpretable units because of the square root retransformation.

THE FFC INDEX

The FFC index was proposed recently by WHO to be the appropriate measure to summarize the HFC distribution (14). It is similar in construct to the standard deviation.[2] However, instead of setting α at 2, it is set at 3 to give more weight to the right-hand tail of the distribution, households with potentially catastrophic payments. In addition, the summed dispersions are subtracted from a reference level of 1. Consequently, the range of the index is from 0 to 1, the degree of fairness increasing as the index approaches unity. The FFC index is defined as:

$$FFC = 1 - \sqrt[3]{\frac{\sum_{i=1}^{n} |HFC_i - \mu|^3}{n}} \quad [7]$$

In order to transform the sum of the cubed dispersions from the mean back into natural or original units, the cube root is taken.

Table 40.2 reports the estimates of the FFC using again the two definitions of μ. Again, there is very little difference in the FFC between the two definitions of μ with scores ranging from 0.740 to 0.942. Brazil, Viet Nam, Azerbaijan, and Argentina are still among the five countries with the least fair distributions of HFC, with Jamaica now entering the picture. Ukraine improves one rank. At the other end of the scale, Thailand and the Philippines drop out of the 10 countries with the fairest distributions. The switch in ranks becomes greater the fairer the two measures are.

Figure 40.2 plots FFC using the mean HFC (vertical axis) against the FFC calculated using the equal burden HFC (HFC_o). The rank order of countries is the same under the two approaches, although the absolute values can be slightly higher or slightly lower—evidenced by the fact that some points are just above the imaginary 45-degree line, and others just below. Because the FFC based on the equal burden HFC is consistent with the definition of fairness of financial contributions used in this chapter, it will be used in all subsequent estimations.

FAMILY OF ENTROPY MEASURES

Theil's Inequality Index

Theil's index derives from the notion of entropy in information theory. It is a measure that assesses the value of different events with respect to their likelihood of occurrence. Suppose there are n independent events and each occurs with the probability p_i, $0 \le p_i \le 1$, and $\sum p_i = 1$. If the information content of the more unlikely events is more valuable than that of events that are more likely to occur, the function $h(p_i)$, reflecting the information content, must be decreasing in p_i.

Table 40.1 Standard deviation of HFC and "augmented standard deviation" based on equal burden HFC (HFC$_o$)

Country	σ_{HFC_o}	$\sigma_{\overline{HFC}}$	Country	σ_{HFC_o}	$\sigma_{\overline{HFC}}$
Argentina	0.167	0.167	Lithuania	0.094	0.094
Azerbaijan	0.184	0.180	Mauritius	0.091	0.091
Bangladesh	0.085	0.084	Mexico	0.098	0.098
Belgium	0.086	0.084	Morocco	0.068	0.066
Brazil	0.199	0.198	Namibia	0.099	0.095
Bulgaria	0.102	0.101	Nicaragua	0.137	0.134
Cambodia	0.143	0.143	Norway	0.081	0.081
Canada	0.065	0.065	Panama	0.143	0.142
Colombia	0.145	0.145	Paraguay	0.131	0.128
Costa Rica	0.113	0.113	Peru	0.126	0.126
Croatia	0.115	0.113	Philippines	0.068	0.068
Czech Republic	0.087	0.085	Portugal	0.110	0.110
Denmark	0.059	0.059	Republic of Korea	0.103	0.102
Djibouti	0.076	0.076	Romania	0.069	0.068
Egypt	0.113	0.113	Senegal	0.075	0.075
Estonia	0.104	0.104	Slovakia	0.050	0.050
Finland	0.075	0.075	Slovenia	0.093	0.093
France	0.099	0.098	South Africa	0.080	0.079
Germany	0.071	0.071	Spain	0.073	0.073
Ghana	0.098	0.097	Sri Lanka	0.092	0.091
Greece	0.102	0.102	Sweden	0.061	0.061
Guyana	0.078	0.076	Switzerland	0.090	0.089
Hungary	0.081	0.080	Thailand	0.071	0.071
Iceland	0.083	0.082	United Kingdom	0.058	0.057
Indonesia	0.086	0.086	Ukraine	0.153	0.153
Israel	0.078	0.078	USA	0.108	0.108
Jamaica	0.142	0.132	Viet Nam	0.178	0.171
Kyrgyzstan	0.081	0.077	Yemen	0.100	0.100
Latvia	0.120	0.120	Zambia	0.124	0.122
Lebanon	0.126	0.125			

Figure 40.2 The FFC index based on equal burden HFC (HFC$_o$) and HFC mean ($\overline{HFC}$)

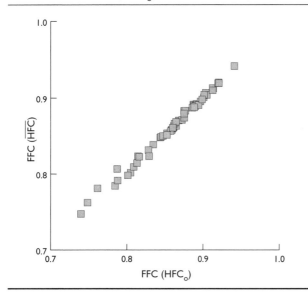

It is assumed that two events i and j are statistically independent and meet the condition

$$h\left(p_i \cdot p_j\right) = h(p_i) + h(p_j) \qquad [8]$$

One function satisfying the decreasing information content property of p_i is:

$$h(p_i) = \ln\left(\frac{1}{p_i}\right) \qquad [9]$$

The expected information content, or entropy, of a situation $H(p)$ is the weighted sum of the individual events $h(.)$, the weights being the respective probabilities:

$$H(p) = \sum p_i h(p_i) = \sum p_i \ln\left(\frac{1}{p_i}\right) \qquad [10]$$

The expression is a measure of the degree to which the probabilities of the various events are equal. It is obvious from equation [10] that the closer the p_i are

Table 40.2   The FFC index based on equal burden HFC (HFC_o) and HFC mean ($\overline{HFC}$)

Country	FFC		Country	FFC	
	HFC_o	$\overline{HFC}$		HFC_o	$\overline{HFC}$
Argentina	0.785	0.784	Lithuania	0.875	0.874
Azerbaijan	0.748	0.762	Mauritius	0.861	0.861
Bangladesh	0.868	0.871	Mexico	0.857	0.857
Belgium	0.903	0.904	Morocco	0.913	0.910
Brazil	0.740	0.747	Namibia	0.877	0.883
Bulgaria	0.862	0.864	Nicaragua	0.829	0.823
Cambodia	0.805	0.802	Norway	0.888	0.890
Canada	0.913	0.913	Panama	0.801	0.798
Colombia	0.809	0.809	Paraguay	0.815	0.823
Costa Rica	0.861	0.862	Peru	0.813	0.814
Croatia	0.865	0.864	Philippines	0.886	0.887
Czech Republic	0.904	0.907	Portugal	0.845	0.849
Denmark	0.920	0.921	Republic of Korea	0.847	0.850
Djibouti	0.853	0.854	Romania	0.901	0.904
Egypt	0.835	0.839	Senegal	0.892	0.891
Estonia	0.872	0.871	Slovakia	0.941	0.942
Finland	0.901	0.901	Slovenia	0.890	0.890
France	0.889	0.889	South Africa	0.894	0.891
Germany	0.913	0.913	Spain	0.899	0.898
Ghana	0.862	0.867	Sri Lanka	0.865	0.869
Greece	0.858	0.858	Sweden	0.920	0.920
Guyana	0.887	0.891	Switzerland	0.875	0.880
Hungary	0.905	0.904	Thailand	0.888	0.888
Iceland	0.891	0.892	United Kingdom	0.921	0.920
Indonesia	0.859	0.858	Ukraine	0.788	0.791
Israel	0.897	0.895	USA	0.860	0.861
Jamaica	0.787	0.807	Viet Nam	0.762	0.781
Kyrgyzstan	0.875	0.883	Yemen	0.853	0.852
Latvia	0.828	0.832	Zambia	0.816	0.823
Lebanon	0.844	0.848			

to $1/n$, the smaller the differences in probabilities, and the greater the entropy. A maximum is obtained when the probability of all events is equal; in that case equation [10] becomes $\ln(n)$, as $p_i = 1/n$.

Theil's index (T) measures the difference between the maximum and the expected information content of a situation, namely:

$$T = \ln(n) - H(p) \qquad [11]$$

Equation [11] can be written as:

$$T = \sum p_i \left[\ln(n) - \ln(\frac{1}{p_i}) \right] \qquad [12]$$

When Theil's entropy index is applied to income inequality measurement, p_i can be interpreted as:

$$p_i = \frac{y_i}{\sum y_i} \qquad [13]$$

where y_i is the income of household i and $\sum y_i$ is total income. Equation [12] can be rewritten as:

$$T = \frac{1}{n} \sum \frac{y_i}{\mu} \ln(\frac{y_i}{\mu}) \qquad [14]$$

where μ is the mean income. Theil's index can have any non-negative value. It equals zero when there is no inequality and increases with more inequality.

The Mean Logarithmic Deviation

Another index belonging to the entropy family of inequality measures is the mean logarithmic deviation (MLD). It is defined as:

$$MLD = \frac{1}{n} \sum \ln\left(\frac{\mu}{y_i} \right) \qquad [15]$$

where y_i is the income of household i and μ is the mean income across all households. *MLD* equals zero in the case of perfect equality and higher values indicate more inequality. Like the Theil index, the *MLD* has no upper limit.

Entropy Measures Applied to the HFC

As the definition of fairness used here requires more weight to be placed on those households that are burdened with potentially catastrophic health payments, we define $y_i = 1 - HFC_i$. In doing so, it can be verified that in the case of Theil's entropy measure, the information content $h(\cdot)$ will be larger, the larger the value of HFC or the financial burden of households. Equation [14] can be rewritten as:

$$T = \frac{1}{n}\sum \frac{1-HFC_i}{1-\overline{HFC_o}} \ln\left(\frac{1-HFC_i}{1-\overline{HFC_o}}\right) \quad [16]$$

The same adjustment can be applied to the *MLD*

$$MLD = \frac{1}{n}\sum \ln\left(\frac{1-\overline{HFC_o}}{1-HFC_i}\right) \quad [17]$$

Inequality results for the 59 countries using Theil's measure and the MLD are presented in Table 40.3. There is very little variation in the level of the indices across countries, although the results are not wholly consistent with the ordering given earlier by the standard deviation or the FFC. For example, some of the countries classified then as relatively unfair are now included among countries with a relatively high degree of fairness (e.g. Egypt, Paraguay), and vice versa (e.g. Sweden, Thailand).

Both the Theil and MLD measures belong to the individual-mean family of inequality measures in the sense that they are comparing individual contributions to the mean (as a ratio). They also attach specific concern to potentially catastrophic health payments, as larger weight is attached to households with very high contribution shares. However, they do not satisfy the constant invariance property. In addition, the units of the indices do not have a straightforward interpretation because of their rather complex structure and the logarithmic transformation.

ATKINSON'S INDEX

Atkinson's index is derived by making additional assumptions about the functional form of the underlying social welfare function, welfare weights, and the relationship between transfers and changes in inequality.

Suppose the utility function for each household is the same and takes the form:

$$U(y_i) = a + b\frac{y_i^{(1-e)}}{1-e} \quad [18]$$

for e not equal to 1, and

$$U(y) = \ln(y) \quad [19]$$

when $e = 1$. The parameter e in the formula, normally bounded by the limits of 0 and 1, determines the level of inequality aversion. The larger the value of e, the greater society's concern about inequality. It is assumed that e is non-negative which implies a concave utility function. It follows that the higher the value of e, the more concave the utility function—when e equals zero, it becomes a straight line.

Under a social welfare function that is an additive function of individual utilities, social welfare will be maximized when everyone's income is equal to the mean income. Atkinson's measure indicates the degree of inequality by taking deviations from this maximum. The measure can be derived as follows.

First, it is necessary to determine the equalized level of income, y_e, that, if given to each individual in the population, would lead to the same level of social welfare (W^*) which is obtained from the observed income distribution

$$W^* = a + b\sum\left(\frac{y_i^{(1-e)}}{1-e}\right) = \frac{1}{n}\sum U(y_e) = U(y_e) \quad [20]$$

which after insertion to equation [18] gives:

$$y_e = \left(\frac{1}{n}\sum y_i^{1-e}\right)^{1/1-e} \quad [21]$$

The second step is to compare the equally distributed income (y_e) and the mean income (μ).

Atkinson's index (A) can now be written as:

$$A = 1 - \frac{y_e}{\mu} = 1 - \left[\frac{1}{n}\sum\left(\frac{y_i}{\mu}\right)^{1-e}\right]^{\frac{1}{1-e}} \quad [22]$$

Atkinson's index lies between zero (complete equality) and one (maximum inequality). A distinguishing feature of this index is its ability to capture movements in different segments of the distribution by changes in the value of the parameter e.

In order for Atkinson's index to reflect the characteristic that people's utility is inversely related to the burden of health payments, set $y_i = 1 - HFC_i$ in the formula, namely:

Table 40.3 Theil's index and the mean logarithmic deviation (MLD)

Country	Theil	MLD	Country	Theil	MLD
Argentina	0.027	0.036	Lithuania	0.015	0.011
Azerbaijan	0.031	0.039	Mauritius	0.014	0.017
Bangladesh	0.005	0.006	Mexico	0.034	0.046
Belgium	0.005	0.005	Morocco	0.003	0.003
Brazil	0.007	0.007	Namibia	0.019	0.011
Bulgaria	0.036	0.053	Nicaragua	0.013	0.017
Cambodia	0.015	0.020	Norway	0.005	0.006
Canada	0.003	0.003	Panama	0.009	0.010
Colombia	0.008	0.009	Paraguay	0.003	0.003
Costa Rica	0.018	0.022	Peru	0.047	0.028
Croatia	0.010	0.016	Philippines	0.002	0.002
Czech Republic	0.009	0.010	Portugal	0.010	0.012
Denmark	0.005	0.005	Republic of Korea	0.012	0.014
Djibouti	0.005	0.007	Romania	0.004	0.004
Egypt	0.003	0.003	Senegal	0.004	0.004
Estonia	0.009	0.011	Slovakia	0.003	0.003
Finland	0.008	0.009	Slovenia	0.015	0.021
France	0.004	0.004	South Africa	0.006	0.007
Germany	0.004	0.004	Spain	0.003	0.004
Ghana	0.007	0.008	Sri Lanka	0.002	0.002
Greece	0.005	0.005	Sweden	0.020	0.026
Guyana	0.005	0.005	Switzerland	0.006	0.007
Hungary	0.005	0.006	Thailand	0.011	0.015
Iceland	0.007	0.008	United Kingdom	0.006	0.007
Indonesia	0.011	0.013	Ukraine	0.018	0.018
Israel	0.004	0.005	USA	0.006	0.007
Jamaica	0.008	0.010	Viet Nam	0.005	0.007
Kyrgyzstan	0.006	0.008	Yemen	0.007	0.009
Latvia	0.007	0.009	Zambia	0.013	0.015
Lebanon	0.007	0.007			

$$A = 1 - \left[\frac{1}{n} \sum \left(\frac{1 - HFC_i}{1 - HFC_o} \right)^{1-e} \right]^{\frac{1}{1-e}} \qquad [23]$$

Not surprisingly, the greater the value of e, the more inequality in health system contributions is observed in all countries (Table 40.4). However, the relative differences between countries vary as e increases. For example, when e increases from 0.30 to 0.35, Atkinson's index increases by 0.0020 in Azerbaijan and only by 0.0003 in Bangladesh. Similarly, the increase is 0.0012 in Ukraine compared to an increase of 0.0001 in the United Kingdom. In countries where the increase is greater there is more unfairness in the HFC at the tail of the distribution.

Atkinson's index satisfies the criteria of individual-mean difference and a concern about potentially catastrophic health payments. An increased concern would be expressed by higher values of the coefficient

e. Atkinson's index is also expressed in interpretable units. However, it does not satisfy the constant invariance property.

COMPARISON OF DIFFERENT MEASURES

This comparison focuses on the rank order differences between the various possible summary measures of the distribution of HFC. Countries are ordered from those with the highest equality (1) to the lowest equality ones (59) in Table 40.5. The ranking of FFC differs substantially from the ranking given by some of the other inequality measures in several cases. For example, the Czech Republic is ranked 9th using the FFC measure, but 24th using the standard deviation, and between 19th and 21st using other indices. Belgium is ranked at 10 by the FFC, 23 by the standard deviation, and between 17 and 19 by the other indices. The rankings given by the standard deviation, Atkinson, Theil,

Table 40.4　Inequality in HFC implied by Atkinson's index

Country	e = 0.2	e = 0.25	e = 0.30	e = 0.35	Country	e = 0.2	e = 0.25	e = 0.30	e = 0.35
Argentina	0.0056	0.0071	0.0087	0.0103	Lithuania	0.0012	0.0016	0.0019	0.0022
Azerbaijan	0.0066	0.0084	0.0103	0.0122	Mauritius	0.0012	0.0015	0.0019	0.0022
Bangladesh	0.0010	0.0013	0.0016	0.0019	Mexico	0.0014	0.0018	0.0021	0.0025
Belgium	0.0010	0.0012	0.0015	0.0017	Morocco	0.0005	0.0007	0.0008	0.0009
Brazil	0.0077	0.0098	0.0119	0.0142	Namibia	0.0013	0.0017	0.0020	0.0024
Bulgaria	0.0016	0.0020	0.0024	0.0029	Nicaragua	0.0028	0.0036	0.0043	0.0051
Cambodia	0.0032	0.0041	0.0049	0.0058	Norway	0.0010	0.0013	0.0015	0.0018
Canada	0.0006	0.0008	0.0009	0.0011	Panama	0.0041	0.0053	0.0065	0.0079
Colombia	0.0036	0.0046	0.0056	0.0066	Paraguay	0.0028	0.0036	0.0043	0.0051
Costa Rica	0.0019	0.0024	0.0029	0.0034	Peru	0.0027	0.0034	0.0041	0.0048
Croatia	0.0020	0.0025	0.0030	0.0035	Philippines	0.0006	0.0008	0.0010	0.0011
Czech Republic	0.0010	0.0012	0.0015	0.0017	Portugal	0.0020	0.0025	0.0030	0.0036
Denmark	0.0005	0.0007	0.0008	0.0009	Republic of Korea	0.0016	0.0020	0.0024	0.0029
Djibouti	0.0011	0.0014	0.0018	0.0022	Romania	0.0006	0.0007	0.0009	0.0010
Egypt	0.0019	0.0024	0.0028	0.0034	Senegal	0.0007	0.0009	0.0011	0.0013
Estonia	0.0016	0.0021	0.0025	0.0029	Slovakia	0.0003	0.0004	0.0005	0.0006
Finland	0.0008	0.0011	0.0013	0.0015	Slovenia	0.0014	0.0017	0.0020	0.0024
France	0.0014	0.0017	0.0021	0.0024	South Africa	0.0008	0.0010	0.0012	0.0014
Germany	0.0008	0.0010	0.0012	0.0013	Spain	0.0008	0.0010	0.0012	0.0014
Ghana	0.0014	0.0018	0.0022	0.0026	Sri Lanka	0.0012	0.0015	0.0018	0.0022
Greece	0.0016	0.0021	0.0025	0.0029	Sweden	0.0005	0.0006	0.0008	0.0009
Guyana	0.0010	0.0012	0.0015	0.0017	Switzerland	0.0013	0.0017	0.0020	0.0024
Hungary	0.0010	0.0012	0.0014	0.0017	Thailand	0.0007	0.0009	0.0011	0.0013
Iceland	0.0011	0.0013	0.0016	0.0019	United Kingdom	0.0004	0.0005	0.0007	0.0008
Indonesia	0.0011	0.0013	0.0016	0.0019	Ukraine	0.0042	0.0053	0.0065	0.0077
Israel	0.0009	0.0011	0.0014	0.0016	USA	0.0018	0.0023	0.0028	0.0033
Jamaica	0.0035	0.0045	0.0055	0.0066	Viet Nam	0.0024	0.0030	0.0036	0.0043
Kyrgyzstan	0.0009	0.0011	0.0014	0.0016	Yemen	0.0015	0.0019	0.0023	0.0027
Latvia	0.0024	0.0031	0.0037	0.0044	Zambia	0.0024	0.0030	0.0036	0.0043
Lebanon	0.0027	0.0035	0.0042	0.0049					

and MLD measures are closer to each other than the ranks given by the FFC. It also seems that the differences in rankings are more pronounced the higher the degree of fairness.

These differences stem from the diverse theoretical approaches and the degree of inequality aversion included in each measure. To illustrate, Figure 40.3 presents the distributions of HFC in Viet Nam and Zambia. The x-axis measures the HFC, and the y-axis shows the density function or the proportion of households observed to have any given HFC.

Visual observation indicates that Viet Nam has a thicker tail to the distribution than Zambia. Correspondingly Zambia has a higher concentration of low HFC shares at the left-hand side of the distribution. Because the FFC index is highly sensitive to the right-hand tail of the distribution, Viet Nam ranks lower than Zambia according to it. Except for the standard deviation, this is not the case for the other inequality measures, which rank the two countries equally (Table 40.5).

Despite the variation in ranks, the rank correlation coefficients of the different indices are high (Table 40.6). The correlation between each index and the FFC is systematically lower than that between the other indices because of the greater weight given to the tail of the distribution by the cubic function used in the FFC. In addition to the rank correlation coefficients, regular Pearson's correlation coefficients were calculated. They confirmed the very high correlation between the different measures.

CONCLUDING REMARKS

A good summary measure for the distribution of HFC should meet the following criteria. It should:

Table 40.5   Rank order using different inequality measures

Country	FFC	σ_{HFC_0}	Atkinson's index				Theil	MLD	Country	FFC	σ_{HFC_0}	Atkinson's index				Theil	MLD
			e= 0.2	e= 0.25	e= 0.30	e= 0.35						e= 0.2	e= 0.25	e= 0.30	e= 0.35		
Slovakia	1	1	1	1	1	1	1	1	Croatia	30	44	43	43	43	43	43	49
United Kingdom	2	2	2	2	2	2	2	2	Sri Lanka	31	28	26	26	26	25	27	26
Denmark	3	3	4	4	4	4	4	4	Ghana	32	32	34	34	34	34	34	33
Sweden	4	4	3	3	3	3	3	3	Bulgaria	33	36	37	37	36	36	37	37
Canada	5	5	7	7	7	7	7	7	Costa Rica	34	42	42	42	42	42	42	41
Morocco	6	6	5	5	5	5	5	5	Mauritius	35	27	27	27	28	28	26	32
Germany	7	10	11	11	11	11	11	9	USA	36	40	40	40	40	40	40	40
Hungary	8	19	18	17	17	17	18	18	Indonesia	37	25	24	24	24	24	24	25
Czech Republic	9	24	20	20	20	20	21	19	Greece	38	37	38	38	39	39	38	38
Belgium	10	23	19	19	19	18	19	17	Mexico	39	33	32	33	33	33	32	34
Romania	11	8	6	6	6	6	6	6	Djibouti	40	14	25	25	25	27	20	30
Finland	12	12	14	14	14	14	14	14	Yemen	41	35	35	35	35	35	35	36
Spain	13	11	12	12	12	12	12	12	Republic of Korea	42	38	36	36	37	37	36	39
Israel	14	17	16	16	16	15	16	16	Portugal	43	41	44	44	44	44	44	44
South Africa	15	18	13	13	13	13	13	13	Lebanon	44	47	49	49	49	49	49	48
Senegal	16	13	10	10	10	10	10	11	Egypt	45	43	41	41	41	41	41	43
Icelend	17	21	23	23	23	22	25	22	Nicaragua	46	51	50	50	50	50	51	52
Slovenia	18	29	31	31	31	31	31	27	Latvia	47	45	47	47	47	47	47	45
France	19	34	33	32	32	32	33	29	Zambia	48	46	45.5	45.5	45.5	45.5	45.5	46.5
Thailand	20	9	9	9	9	9	9	10	Paraguay	49	49	51	51	51	51	50	50
Norway	21	20	21	21	21	21	22	21	Peru	50	48	48	48	48	48	48	53
Guyana	22	15	17	18	18	19	17	20	Colombia	51	54	54	54	54	53	54	55
Philippines	23	7	8	8	8	8	8	8	Cambodia	52	53	52	52	52	52	52	54
Namibia	24	31	30	30	30	30	30	28	Panama	53	52	55	55	56	56	55	42
Lithuania	25	30	28	28	27	26	28	24	Ukraine	54	55	56	56	55	55	56	56
Switzerland	26	26	29	29	29	29	29	31	Jamaica	55	50	53	53	53	54	53	51
Kyrgyzstan	27	16	15	15	15	16	15	15	Argentina	56	56	57	57	57	57	57	57
Estonia	28	39	39	39	38	38	39	35	Viet Nam	57	57	45.5	45.5	45.5	45.5	45.5	46.5
Bangladesh	29	22	22	22	22	23	23	23	Azerbaijan	58	58	58	58	58	58	58	58
Croatia	30	44	43	43	43	43	43	49	Brazil	59	59	59	59	59	59	59	59

give greater weight to the tail of the distribution, particularly households with potentially catastrophic health payments; be based on comparisons of individual-mean differences rather than interindividual differences; have the constant-invariance property; and be interpretable in natural units on the interval scale. Table 40.7 summarizes the properties of the various inequality measures considered. The plus and minus signs indicate whether the criteria are fulfilled or not. If both a + and – are shown, it means that the criterion is not fully satisfied.

The FFC and standard deviation met all four criteria although the standard deviation does not attach as much weight to households with potentially catastrophic health payments as the FFC. Theil's measure and the MLD do not satisfy the constant invariance property, and are less concerned with potentially catastrophic health contributions than the FFC. In addi-

Figure 40.3   HFC distributions, Viet Nam and Zambia

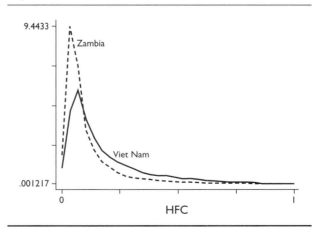

Table 40.6 The rank correlation coefficient of different inequality measures

	FFC	Standard deviation	Atkinson (e=.20)	Atkinson (e=.25)	Atkinson (e=.30)	Atkinson (e=.35)	Theil	MLD
FFC	1							
Standard deviation	0.9101	1						
Atkinson (e=.20)	0.9229	0.9874	1					
Atkinson (e=.25)	0.9249	0.9871	0.9999	1				
Atkinson (e=.30)	0.9265	0.9867	0.9996	0.9998	1			
Atkinson (e=.35)	0.9303	0.9843	0.9991	0.9993	0.9996	1		
Theil	0.9162	0.9898	0.9989	0.9988	0.9985	0.9973	1	
MLD	0.9341	0.9759	0.9878	0.9883	0.9882	0.9887	0.9851	1

Table 40.7 Comparison of different summary measures

Measure	Concern about catastrophic expenditure	Individual-mean difference	Constant invariance	Interpretable units
FFC	+	+	+	+
σHFC_o	+/–	+	+	+
Theil	+/–	+	–	–
MLD	+/–	+	–	–
Atkinson	+	+	–	+

tion, they are not expressed in easily interpretable units. Atkinson's index has considerable flexibility in weighing the different parts of the distribution differently: a higher *e* makes this index more sensitive to the changes at the tail of the HFC distribution. It is also expressed in interpretable units, but it violates the constant invariance property.

No single indicator can explain all features of the unfairness of household financial contributions to the health system. The FFC measure proposed in this chapter satisfies the criteria established for a summary index of the distribution of household financial contributions. As such, it provides a tool for policy-makers to assess how household contributions to health deviate from the concept of equal burden, when the burden of payments is assessed against households' capacity to pay. It also incorporates concern for the burden resulting from potentially catastrophic health payments. As such it is a useful tool for policy analysis.

Acknowledgements

The authors would like to thank David B. Evans and William D. Savedoff for their comments on the manuscript. We are also grateful to Nathalie Etomba and Anna Moore for data and reference searches.

Notes

1 Data for Spain are from the Encuesta Continua de Hogares 1996 with a sample size of 3 104. The Azerbaijian data are the Survey of Living Conditions 1995 with 2 015 households.

2 The FFC index defined here is different from the one used in *The World Health Report 2000* where it was defined as:

$$FFC_{WHR} = 1 - 4\left(\frac{\sum_{i=1}^{n}\left|HFC_i - \overline{HFC}\right|^3}{0.125n}\right)$$

Compared to this version of the FFC index, the new FFC has the additional property of being defined in readily interpretable units because of the cubic root retransformation.

References

(1) Murray CJL et al. Assessing the distribution of household financial contributions to the health system: concepts and empirical application. In: Murray CJL, Evans DB, eds. *Health systems performance assessment: debates, methods and empiricism.* Geneva, World Health Organization, 2003.

(2) Xu K et al. Household health system contributions and capacity to pay: definitional, empirical, and technical challenges. In: Murray CJL, Evans DB, eds. *Health systems performance assessment: debates, methods and empiricism.* Geneva, World Health Organization, 2003.

(3) Xu K et al. The impact of vertical and horizontal inequality on the fairness in financial contribution index. In: Murray CJL, Evans DB, eds. *Health systems performance*

assessment: debates, methods and empiricism. Geneva, World Health Organization, 2003.

(4) Xu K et al. Understanding household catastrophic health expenditures: a multi-country analysis. In: Murray CJL, Evans DB, eds. *Health systems performance assessment: debates, methods and empiricism*. Geneva, World Health Organization, 2003.

(5) Aronson JR, Johnson P, Lambert P. Redistributive effect and unequal income tax treatment in the U.K. *The Economic Journal*, 1994, 104:262–270.

(6) Kakwani N. Measurement of tax progressivity: an international comparison. *The Economic Journal*, 1977, 87:71–80.

(7) Kolm SC. The rational foundations of income inequality measurement. In: Silber J, ed. *Handbook on income inequality measurement*. London, Kluwer Academic Publishers, 1999:19–100.

(8) Jenkins S. The measurement of income inequality. In: Osberg L, ed. *Economic inequality and poverty international perspectives*. London, Sharpe ME, 1991: 3–38.

(9) Wagstaff A et al. Equity in the finance of health care: some further international comparisons. *Journal of Health Economics*, 1999, 18:263–290.

(10) Wagstaff A, van Doorslaer E. *Paying for health care: quantifying fairness, catastrophe, and impoverishment, with applications to Viet Nam, 1993–1998*. World Bank Working Paper No. 2715. Washington, DC, World Bank, 2001.

(11) Kakwani N, Wagstaff A, van Doorslaer E. Socioeconomic inequalities in health: measurement, computation, and statistical inference. *Journal of Econometrics*, 1997, 77(1):87–103.

(12) van Doorslaer E et al. Equity in the delivery of health care: some international comparisons. *Journal of Health Economics*, 1992, 11:389–411.

(13) Wagstaff A, van Doorslaer E. Equity in the finance and delivery of health care: concepts and definitions. In: van Doorslaer E, Wagstaff A, Rutten F, eds. *Equity in the finance and delivery of health care: an international perspective*. Oxford, Oxford Medical Publications, 1993: 2–19.

(14) World Health Organization. *The World Health Report 2000. Health Systems: Improving Performance*. Geneva, World Health Organization, 2000.

(15) World Health Organization. *The World Health Report 2001. Mental Health: New Understanding, New Hope*. Geneva, World Health Organization, 2001.

(16) World Health Organization. *The World Health Report 2002. Reducing Risks, Promoting Healthy Life*. Geneva, World Health Organization, 2002.

(17) Kawabata K, Xu K, Carrin G. Preventing impoverishment through protection against catastrophic health expenditure. *Bulletin of the World Health Organization*, 2002, 80:612.

(18) Filmer D, Hammer J, Prichett L. Weak links in the chain II: a prescription for health policy in poor countries. *World Bank Research Observer*, 2002, 17:47–66.

(19) Musgrove P. Public spending on health care: how are different criteria related? *Health Policy*, 2000, 53: 61–67.

(20) Evans RG et al. Controlling health expenditures—the Canadian reality. *The New England Journal of Medicine*, 1989, 320:571–607.

(21) Russel S, Gilson L. User fee policies to promote health service access for poor: a wolf in sheep's clothing? *International Journal of Health Services*, 1997, 27: 359–379.

(22) Murray CJL et al. *Defining and measuring fairness in financial contribution to the health system*. EIP Discussion Paper No. 24. Geneva, World Health Organization, 2000. URL: http:// http://www3.who.int/whosis/ discussion_papers/discussion_papers.cfm#

Chapter 41

The Impact of Vertical and Horizontal Inequality on the Fairness in Financial Contribution Index

KE XU, JAN KLAVUS, DAVID B. EVANS, PIYA HANVORAVONGCHAI, RIADH ZERAMDINI, CHRISTOPHER J.L. MURRAY

INTRODUCTION

The concept of fairness in household financial contribution to the health system was introduced by WHO in *The World Health Report 2000* (1). In this context, fairness was defined as an equal burden where every household would pay an equal share of its capacity to pay to the health system. The ratio of a household's health payments to its capacity to pay is called the household financial contribution (HFC). If all households contribute the same share of their capacity to pay, the HFC of each household will equal the ratio of a country's total health expenditure to its total capacity to pay (2). An index of fairness in financial contribution (FFC) was defined to measure dispersions from the equal burden criterion. It was constructed to vary from 0 to 1, with 1 representing perfect fairness.

The deviations from perfect fairness can be separated into two distinct effects: a vertical effect and a horizontal effect. The vertical effect refers to the situation where households with different incomes contribute different proportions of their incomes. Horizontal inequality refers to the situation where households facing similar economic conditions pay different proportions of their incomes. Extreme horizontal inequality occurs when households face catastrophically high health expenditures, here defined as 40% or more of their capacities to pay. Moderate horizontal inequality is associated with smaller differences across households faced with similar financial conditions.

The publication of an index of fairness in financial contribution for 191 countries in *The World Health Report 2000* generated considerable debate among policy-makers, international organizations, and the academic world (3–8). It was argued that the FFC index treats progressive and regressive contributions to the health system equally (4;6). In a progressive system, the rich pay a higher share of their incomes than the poor. In contrast, in a regressive system, it is the poor that pay a higher share. According to the critics, the FFC framework ignores the fact that most societies seek to ensure progressive financial contributions because it treats any deviations from equal burden equally; both progressive and regressive contributions are considered unfair. In theory, they argued, the FFC index could penalize a country for being "too progressive" in health financing contributions.

The purpose of this chapter is to investigate empirically the sources of inequality underlying the FFC index. In this analysis it will be possible to test if any countries are penalized for having health financing systems that are "too progressive." The analysis is based on micro-level household survey data from 59 countries. The next section of the chapter introduces the approach used to decompose the observed unfairness into vertical, extreme horizontal, and moderate horizontal inequality. Section three presents the survey data. Section four reports the empirical results on the effects of removing the various inequality components from total unfairness. This is accomplished by a counterfactual analysis that illustrates how much more fair (or less unfair) the health financing system would have been without the various inequality effects. The last section discusses the findings.

METHODS

The household financial contribution (HFC) represents the household's financial burden due to health system payments. It is a ratio that relates total household expenditure for health (HE) through general taxes, social health insurance contributions, private health insurance premiums, and out-of-pocket payments, to the household capacity to pay (CTP).

$$HFC_i = \frac{HE_i}{CTP_i} \qquad [1]$$

Household capacity to pay for health services CTP_i is not defined as its total effective income but as effective income minus subsistence needs (SE) (2). This is because households must first meet certain basic needs before health system payments become relevant and economically feasible. In *The World Health Report 2000*, the actual food expenditure of households was used as a measure of subsistence needs. However, a certain amount of food spending is on non-essential items. For this reason, a food poverty line estimated from the survey data for each country is now used to approximate subsistence needs. Details on the derivation of this poverty line are provided in Xu et al. (9).

This food poverty line is fixed in any country and is equal for all households regardless of their income levels. Because a constant (the food poverty line) is deducted from each household's income, the ratio of health expenditure to total effective income will be lower than the ratio of HE to CTP for all households. The deduction of subsistence expenditures changes this proportion a lot more for poor households, where subsistence needs are a much higher proportion of their total incomes, than for rich households. It means that if all households pay the same proportion of their capacities to pay, the richer pay higher proportions of their total income than the poor—the system is progressive. It also means that after the subsistence deduction, any departure from equal proportional contribution of CTP is considered unfair—the concern for progressivity has already been accounted for in the deduction.

The FFC index is defined as:

$$FFC = 1 - \sqrt[3]{\frac{\sum_{i=1}^{n}\left|HFC_i - HFC_o\right|^3}{n}} \qquad [2]$$

where

$$HFC_o = \frac{\sum HE_i}{\sum CTP_i} \qquad [3]$$

which denotes the equal burden contribution share. It varies between 0 and 1, with 1 representing perfect fairness. A cubic functional form is used to give more weight to households at the tail of the distribution. Because of the cubic transformation, the FFC index cannot be linearly decomposed and the breakdown of the observed unfairness into its components is carried out by a series of counterfactual comparisons.

According to the definition of fairness in equation [2], in the absence of any inequality (vertical, extreme horizontal or moderate horizontal) the FFC index equals 1. Departures from this objective generated by any of the three inequality effects are measured by the extent to which the index departs from 1. The difference between the perfectly fair FFC and the one that is observed ($\Delta FFC = 1 - FFC$) can be partitioned into a vertical effect (ΔFFC_v), a catastrophic spending effect (ΔFFC_c), and a moderate horizontal effect (ΔFFC_h) as:

$$\Delta FFC = 1 - FFC = \Delta FFC_v + \Delta FFC_c + \Delta FFC_h \qquad [4]$$

If the summary measure of the HFC distribution where there is no vertical effect is denoted by FFC_v, and the original distribution incorporating all the effects (the starting point) by FFC, the vertical effect can be written as:

$$\Delta FFC_v = FFC_v - FFC \qquad [5]$$

Now, if FFC_c is the distribution where there is no vertical and no catastrophic effect, the catastrophic effect (net of the vertical effect) can be written as:

$$\Delta FFC_c = FFC_c - FFC_v \qquad [6]$$

The moderate horizontal effect can be obtained from the residual as:

$$\Delta FFC_h = 1 - FFC_c \qquad [7]$$

SEPARATION OF VERTICAL EFFECTS

Observed HFC in any country can be written as a function of household expenditures:

$$HFC_i = f(\exp_i) + \varepsilon_i \qquad [8]$$

The relationship is not linear, and piecewise linear regression can be used to approximate non-linear relationships with the advantage that the parameters are determined by the underlying data and no parametric assumptions about functional form are needed (10). In a fairly financed system, each household would contribute an equal share of its capacity to pay to the health system. This equal burden contribution was defined as HFC_o in equation [3]. Without vertical inequality, households would be observed to pay:

$$HFCv_i = HFC_o + \varepsilon_i \qquad [9]$$

where $HFCv_i$ denotes household i's health financing contribution after dropping the vertical effect. The residual ε_i is the horizontal effect that would still exist and is estimated from the piecewise regression of equation [8]. The counterfactual FFC in the absence of the vertical effect (FFC_v) can be estimated using the $HFCv_i$ from equation [9], and the contribution of the vertical effect to the observed FFC is then estimated as:

$$FFC_c = 1 - \sqrt[3]{\frac{\sum_{i=1}^{n}\left|HFCv_i - HFCv_o\right|^3}{n}} \quad [10]$$

where $HFCv_o$ represents HFC_o re-estimated for the counterfactual distribution of health expenditures in the absence of the vertical effect using equation [3].

SEPARATION OF THE EFFECT OF CATASTROPHIC SPENDING AND MODERATE HORIZONTAL EFFECTS

After eliminating the impact of the vertical effect on the index, the next step is to remove the effect of catastrophic expenditure. This is done by estimating the counterfactual distribution of HFC in the absence of catastrophic health spending. The threshold used for defining catastrophic health expenditure is somewhat arbitrary and in order to facilitate cross-country comparison, it has been set at 40% of the household capacity to pay (9).

Using this threshold, observed household financial contributions (HFC) were truncated at 40% for the households who paid catastrophic shares of their capacities to pay. In order to pool the risk of catastrophic health expenditure, the payments that exceeded 40% of capacity to pay were reallocated to households paying less than 40%. The ratio (α) describes the average additional contribution that would need to be made by all households without catastrophic health expenditures (assuming no vertical effect):

$$\alpha = \frac{\sum\left[(HFCv_i - 0.4)CTP_i \mid HFCv_i \geq 40\%\right]}{\sum\left(CTP_i \mid HFCv_i < 40\%\right)} \quad [11]$$

The new HFC for each household i excluding catastrophic payments ($HFCc$) would then be:

$$HFCc_i = HFCv_i + \alpha \quad \text{if } HFCv_i < 40\% \quad [12]$$
$$HFCc_i = 0.4 \quad \text{if } HFCv_i \geq 40\%$$

The corresponding FFC index that excludes the effect of catastrophic spending (FFC_c) is computed as:

$$FFC_c = 1 - \sqrt[3]{\frac{\sum_{i=1}^{n}\left|HFCc_i - HFCc_o\right|^3}{n}} \quad [13]$$

$HFCc_o$ is HFC_o in the absence of the vertical effect and the effect of catastrophic expenditures (see equation [3]).

Moderate horizontal effects are estimated using equation [7] as described above.

DATA SOURCES

The analysis is based on national representative household surveys from 59 countries. The surveys were conducted between 1991 and 2000, sample sizes ranging from 1 103 households in Sweden to 62 946 in the Republic of Korea. Most of the surveys from developing countries were Living Standards Measurement Studies while Household Budget surveys or Income and Expenditure surveys were used for other countries. Details on the type of survey, survey years, and sample sizes are given in Chapter 42.

RESULTS

REMOVING THE VERTICAL EFFECT

A comparison of the estimates of the FFC_v index with the original FFC for the 59 countries indicates that the vertical effect had a very small impact on total inequality (Figure 41.1). The counterfactual FFC in

Figure 41.1 Decomposing the FFC index: removing the vertical effect

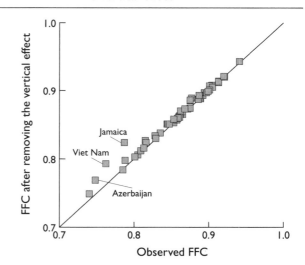

the absence of the vertical effect would have been no more than 1.5% greater than the observed FFC in all but three countries, and the difference is never more than 5%. The rank order correlation coefficient of FFC and FFC_v is also very high at 0.996, with 88% of countries staying at the same rank or changing rank by a maximum of two places after the removal of the vertical effect. The three countries where the impact of the vertical effect was the greatest were Azerbaijan, Viet Nam, and Jamaica. In Jamaica, for example, the FFC index improves from 0.787 to 0.823 as a result of removing the vertical effect, an increase of 4.5%.

To explore the relationship between the progressivity and regressivity of health payments and the impact of the vertical effect on the FFC described above, Figure 41.2 plots the impact of the vertical effect on FFC (shown as the percentage change in the FFC as a result of eliminating the vertical effect) against the concentration index of HFC for all countries. This concentration index shows the progressivity of the household financial contribution to health and is bounded at the lower extreme by –1 (when the entire burden of paying for health falls on the group with the lowest capacity to pay) and 1 at the upper extreme (when the entire burden falls on the group with the greatest capacity to pay). A negative concentration index indicates that the poor contribute a larger share of their capacity to pay than the rich, or regressivity. A positive index indicates progressivity in contributions with respect to capacity to pay.[1]

The results show that the distribution of observed HFC was progressive, i.e. the concentration index was positive, in 19 countries and regressive in the remaining 40. The three countries in which the impact of removing the vertical effect on the FFC was earlier shown to be the greatest (Azerbaijan, Viet Nam, and Jamaica) also had the most regressive HFC distributions using the concentration index. Removing the vertical effect in these countries would improve the FFC by up to 4.5%. On the other hand, progressivity in the HFC distribution is associated with a positive vertical effect in 19 countries. However, in no cases does removal of this vertical effect improve the FFC by more than 0.5%. This indicates that, as Wagstaff (4) and Shaw (6) suggest, an index of fairness based on deviations from equal burden can penalize countries whose health financing contributions are highly progressive, but the resulting impact on the FFC is negligible.

REMOVING THE EFFECT OF CATASTROPHIC SPENDING

Catastrophic spending was defined to occur when households contribute 40% or more of their capacity to pay to the health system. Figure 41.3 depicts the observed FFC for each country on the horizontal axis. The triangles show the relationship between FFC and FFC_v, or the FFC after the vertical effect has been removed, on the vertical axis. This part of Figure 41.3

Figure 41.2 Concentration index of HFC (CI_HFC) vs. percentage increase in FFC after removing the vertical effect

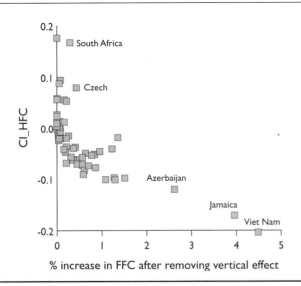

% increase in FFC after removing vertical effect

Figure 41.3 Decomposing the FFC index: removing both vertical and extreme horizontal effect

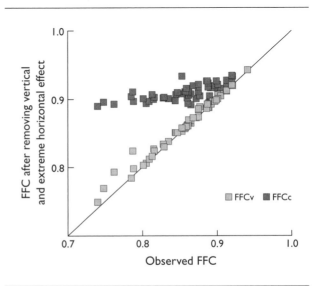

reproduces Figure 41.1 showing that removal of the vertical effect makes very little difference to the FFC.

The vertical axis also shows the relationship between FFC and FFC_c. After removing the effect of catastrophic payments on top of the vertical effect in the manner described above, the FFC improves considerably and is much fairer in most countries (FFC_c is closer to 1 than the original FFC and FFC_v). This is especially noticeable in countries where the initial FFC was less than 0.875, i.e. those countries where financial contributions were distributed across households least fairly. After the removal of catastrophic payments, the FFC for most countries would be concentrated around 0.9, suggesting that policies such as the introduction of health insurance have the potential to dramatically improve the fairness of the health financing system in many settings. With such actions, the resulting degree of fairness would be relatively similar across countries.

REMOVING THE MODERATE HORIZONTAL EFFECT

The moderate horizontal effect refers to the remaining effect that is not due to the vertical effect or to catastrophic payments. This is shown to contribute a relatively high proportion of total unfairness in

Figure 41.4—the FFC would be between 0.05 and 0.1 units higher in its absence. It is comparatively more important, not surprisingly, in countries where the vertical and extreme horizontal effects are low so that in the OECD countries, for example, the main cause of inequality is related to the moderate horizontal effect. This contrasts with findings from earlier research on inequality in health care financing in the OECD countries which highlighted the importance of regressivity in financial contributions to health (e.g. the vertical effect) (11–13).

The importance of the horizontal rather than the vertical effect in determining the fairness in the distribution of HFC is also reinforced by the lack of any relationship between the redistributive effect (RE) and the FFC index. The RE is a measure describing the extent to which income distribution becomes more or less equal after health contributions by households are subtracted from household income. The RE is bordered by −1 at the lower end, negative values indicating that health payments make the after-health payment income distribution more regressive. Positive values (the maximum value is 1) are obtained when the impact of payments on the after-payment distribution is progressive. Figure 41.5 plots the FFC index against RE. There is no clear relationship between the two indices in the survey data for these 59 countries. The

Figure 41.4 Sources of unfairness (1-FFC)

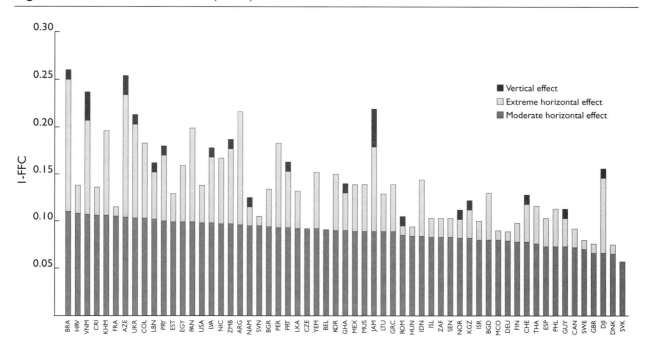

Figure 41.5   Redistributive effect (RE) vs. FFC

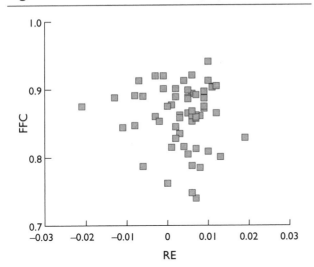

FFC and RE capture different concerns, the former focusing on the fairness of burden that financial contributions impose on households, and the latter focusing on the impact of financial contributions on progressivity in the income space (*14*). The FFC also uses a cubic function, giving more weight to households at the tail of the distribution, e.g. households with catastrophic expenditures. In contrast, RE is not especially sensitive to the tail of the distribution, but is influenced more by households located in the middle part of the distribution. Murray et al. (*14*) show that the RE is also relatively insensitive to horizontal inequality, whereas the FFC index captures horizontal inequalities more systematically, as illustrated above.

CONCLUSIONS AND DISCUSSION

This decomposition analysis of the FFC in 59 countries has showed that vertical inequality played a minor role in the total inequality in household financial contributions captured by the FFC index. Instead, the FFC was sensitive to horizontal inequality. Moderate horizontal inequality is important in all countries while in some, extreme horizontal inequality associated with catastrophic health expenditure is significant as well.

These findings differ from those of earlier studies suggesting the importance of vertical inequality in household contributions to health using the RE as an indicator. There are two ways to think about inequality or fairness in this context: one is defined in the income space addressing the impact of payments on household income, while the other considers the financial burden on households in what has termed

the burden space (*14*). The redistributive effect (RE) belongs to the first class of measures and it is concerned mainly with the progressivity of payments in terms of income. The FFC index conforms to the second approach where concern lies with departures from the equal burden principle.

It should be noted, however, that while the overall health financing system may display vertical fairness, individual financing sources can still include a substantial degree of vertical unfairness. Though the effects may be balanced out when all payments, public and private, are considered simultaneously, certain payments may affect various households differently. For example, out-of-pocket payments are often unexpected and their impact on poor households might be different from the impact of taxation or insurance premiums, which are more predictable.

Certain limitations of the data used in the analysis need to be considered when drawing conclusions for policy. Firstly, some of the surveys undertaken in the early 1990s might not reflect the impact of more recent reforms in health system financing. Some countries may, therefore, have fairer or more unfair systems than implied by the numbers reported in this paper. Secondly, some survey data are of lower quality than others. Efforts are continually being made to identify high quality and more recent household surveys. Thirdly, there is variation in the recall periods used to ask questions related to health service utilization and the associated expenditure. Some surveys use a one month recall period, some use three months, some use one year, and some use combinations such as one month for outpatient services and three months or a year for inpatient services. This has been a concern in the analysis of catastrophic expenditures. A short recall period will have a smaller memory bias than a long recall period, while the latter may capture catastrophic expenditures better than the former. The direction of biases generated by different recall periods is not self-evident. Preliminary regression results indicate that no systematic relationship exists between recall period and catastrophic payments. However, this is an issue that needs to be investigated more in the future.

Despite this, the policy implications of the findings are straightforward. In countries with a relatively high degree of unfairness, the principal means to improve fairness in the health financing system is to introduce risk-sharing mechanisms that help to avoid catastrophically high health payments and reduce the likelihood that people with similar capacities to pay contribute different proportions of their non-subsistence income. One probable reason for the differences in the degree and type of horizontal inequality observed between countries lies in the variations in the share of public financing in overall health system financing. Public financing sources usually incorporate a concern for horizontal equality through the design of the tax system, so the bulk of horizontal inequality is likely to arise from differences in out-of-pocket payments and in differences in access to various private insurance plans and social insurance schemes. Again, this has important implications for policy.

ACKNOWLEDGEMENTS

The authors would like to thank Guy Carrin and William D. Savedoff for their comments on the manuscript. We are also grateful to Ana Mylena Aguilar-Rivera for formatting the tables and graphs, and to Nathalie Etomba and Anna Moore for data and reference searches.

NOTES

1 It should be emphasized that the concentration index is estimated here with respect to HFC, which is a ratio that already incorporates capacity to pay, and consequently an element of progressivity accruing through the subsistence deduction. The other alternative would be to estimate the concentration index with respect to health expenditures, the numerator of HFC. This would not be consistent with the estimation of FFC and would make the comparison of the concentration index and the vertical component of the FFC less appropriate. Because the HFC has progressivity built in through the deduction of the subsistence component, even a neutral concentration index (one that equals 0) indicates a progressive distribution with respect to income from which no subsistence expenditure deduction has been made. Similarly, a progressive HFC distribution indicates an even more progressive distribution with respect to the pre-deduction total income distribution.

REFERENCES

(1) World Health Organization. *The World Health Report 2000. Health Systems: Improving Performance*. Geneva, World Health Organization, 2000.

(2) Xu K et al. Household health system contributions and capacity to pay: definitional, empirical, and technical challenges. In: Murray CJL, Evans DB, eds. *Health systems performance assessment: debates, methods and empiricism*. Geneva, World Health Organization, 2003.

(3) Williams A. Science or marketing at WHO? A commentary on 'World Health 2000.' *Health Economics*, 2001, 10(2):93–100.

(4) Wagstaff A. *Measuring equity in health care financing: reflections and alternatives to the World Health Organization's fairness of financial contribution index*. Washington, DC, World Bank, 2001. URL: http://www.healthsystemsrc.org/

(5) Almeida C, Braveman P, Gold MR. Methodological concerns and recommendations on policy consequences of the World Health Report 2000. *The Lancet*, 2001, 357:1692–1696.

(6) Shaw RP. Financial fairness indicator: useful compass or crystal ball? *International Journal of Health Services*, 2002, 32(1):195–203.

(7) Ministry of Health, Viet Nam. *Comments and suggestions of Vietnam Ministry of Health/Health Policy Unit as regards the World Health Report 2000*. Hanoi, Viet Nam, 2001.

(8) Klavus J. The measure of fair financing in the World Health Report 2000. *STAKES Themes*. Helsinki, 2000.

(9) Xu K et al. Understanding household catastrophic health expenditures: a multi-country analysis. In: Murray CJL, Evans DB, eds. *Health systems performance assessment: debates, methods and empiricism*. Geneva, World Health Organization, 2003.

(10) Greene WH. *Econometric analysis*. New Jersey, Prentice Hall, 2000.

(11) van Doorslaer E, Wagstaff A, Rutten F. *Equity in the finance and delivery of health care: an international perspective*. Oxford, New York, Oxford University Press, 1993.

(12) Wagstaff A et al. Equity in the finance of health care: some further international comparisons. *Journal of Health Economics*, 1999, 18:263–290.

(13) van Doorslaer E et al. The redistributive effect of health care finance in twelve OECD countries. *Journal of Health Economics*, 1999, 18:291–313.

(14) Murray CJL et al. Assessing the distribution of household financial contributions to the health system: concepts and empirical application. In: Murray CJL, Evans DB, eds. *Health systems performance assessment: debates, methods and empiricism*. Geneva, World Health Organization, 2003.

Chapter 42

Understanding Household Catastrophic Health Expenditures: a Multi-country Analysis

Ke Xu, David B. Evans, Kei Kawabata, Riadh Zeramdini, Jan Klavus, Christopher J.L. Murray

Introduction

Health systems can deliver health services, whether preventive or curative, that can make a difference to peoples' health. But accessing these services can lead to individuals having to pay catastrophic shares of their available income and push many into poverty. The potential impact of how health systems are financed on the well-being of households, particularly the poor, has influenced the design of health systems and insurance mechanisms in settings as diverse as the USA, Australia, India, and Indonesia (1–7). Protecting people from catastrophic payments has come to be widely accepted as a desirable objective of health policy (8–15). Catastrophic health expenditure is not always synonymous with high health care costs (16). A large bill for surgery, for example, might not be catastrophic if households do not bear the full costs because the service is provided free or at a subsidized price, or covered by third-party insurance. On the other hand, even relatively small expenditures for common illnesses can be financially disastrous for poor households lacking insurance coverage.

Little, however, is known about either the health system characteristics more likely to protect households from catastrophic payments, or the factors that lead some households within a country to face such payments while others are protected. Most of the limited evidence comes from case studies in individual countries. For example, two US studies showed that households headed by older people, people with disabilities, unemployed or poor, and those with lower access to health insurance were more likely to be affected than other households (17;18).

In Georgia, a survey undertaken after the transition to a decentralized, market-driven system reported that 19% of households seeking care had to borrow money or sell personal items to pay for their care, and that 16% were unable to afford the medications prescribed on seeking care (19). The characteristics of these households were not reported. In Thailand (20), the poor have been reported as more likely to have to pay for health services out-of-pocket than richer people, which, when combined with their lower incomes, places them more at risk of catastrophic health payments (21).

In designing their health systems, policy-makers need to understand if there are characteristics of the system that make people more vulnerable to catastrophic payments. They also need to know which households are more vulnerable for any set of system characteristics. The aim of this chapter, therefore, is to explore the conditions under which catastrophic health expenditures occur more frequently taking advantage of the increasing number of household income and expenditure surveys that are now available.

Methods

Catastrophic health expenditure is defined in relation to a households' capacity to pay (16). The threshold at which health spending has been defined as catastrophic in past studies has varied from 5% to 20% of total family income (16;22). In this chapter, a higher threshold is used to identify the people facing the most extreme difficulties, with health expenditure defined as catastrophic when a household's out-of-pocket payments are greater than or equal to 40% of its capacity to pay.

Household capacity to pay is defined as effective income remaining after basic subsistence needs have been met. Effective income is taken to be the level of total consumption expenditure of the household, considered in many countries to be a more accurate reflection of purchasing power than income reported in household surveys (*23*). Subsistence needs were defined for each country separately to account for different consumption patterns and prices. Building on the fact that the poorer the household, the higher the shares of total income or consumption devoted to food (*24*), the food expenditure of the household with the median share of food expenditure in total expenditure, adjusted for household size, was taken to reflect subsistence requirements. To allow for variation across households, the average food expenditures of households with food shares in total expenditure from the 45th to 55th percentile was used in preference to the expenditure of the single household at the 50th percentile. Similarly, a household was defined as poor if total household expenditure, adjusted for household size, was less than the basic subsistence requirement defined above. This has the advantage of defining poverty in a way that takes into account different consumption patterns in each country, and does not require arbitrary assumptions about purchasing power parities across countries(*25;26*).

Health expenditures requiring out-of-pocket payments include all categories of health-related expenses incurred at the time the household received the service. Typically these include consultation fees, purchases of medication, and hospital bills. Any reimbursements from health insurance schemes are deducted.

Multiple regression was used for the cross-country analysis. The percentage of households with catastrophic expenditures reported in the surveys was regressed on the share of out-of-pocket payments in total health expenditure, the share of total health expenditure in Gross Domestic Product (GDP) and the percentage of households below the poverty line. All variables were transformed into logarithms for the regression, so the estimated coefficients are elasticities—e.g. the proportional change in the dependent variable subsequent to a 1% change in the independent variable.

WHO has systematically tried to identify household income and expenditure surveys that provide enough detail to analyse whether households are facing catastrophic spending. For this analysis, 59 surveys have been included that met the following criterion for quality: national aggregates obtained by scaling-up the survey data to the national level approximated those reported in national accounts. Particular attention was paid to tax revenues and private consumption expenditure. Table 42.1 provides a summary of the years, type, sample size, and key attributes of the surveys. In a number of cases, national surveys have

been part of international survey initiatives or of ongoing national survey programmes including the Living Standards Measurement Studies (LSMS), Household Budget Surveys (HBS), and Household Income and Expenditure Surveys (HES). All surveys provided some basic socioeconomic information about the household including education, place of residence, household size, and age and sex composition.

The household's financial contribution, the share of out-of-pocket payments in total health expenditure and the percentage of households under the poverty line are estimated from the results of these surveys scaled to the national level. The share of total health expenditure in GDP is estimated from the survey data, and GDP per capita figures are obtained from the data used in published National Health Accounts (*10*).

Uncertainty intervals around the reported proportion of households with catastrophic expenditure in each country were calculated using bootstrap methods (*27*). In each country 1 000 subsamples from the sampled population were made, with replacement, and the proportion with catastrophic expenditure recalculated for each of them. The highest and lowest 10% of estimates were eliminated to define the 80% uncertainty interval.

RESULTS

This analysis of household surveys from 59 countries demonstrates an enormous range in the proportion of households facing catastrophic payments from out-of-pocket health expenses, from less than 0.01% in France to 10.5% in Viet Nam (Table 42.2). Not surprisingly, most developed countries have developed social institutions such as social insurance or tax-funded health systems that protect households from catastrophic spending. Among developed countries only Portugal (2.71%), Greece (2.17%), Switzerland (0.57%), and the United States (0.55%) had more than 0.5% of households facing catastrophic health spending. Among developing countries, the range was from below 0.5% in Namibia and Djibouti to ten countries where over 3% of households faced catastrophic health expenditures.

It is notable that there are two clusters of countries that have relatively high rates of catastrophic spending. The first cluster includes a set of selected countries in transition such as Azerbaijan (7.5%), Ukraine (3.87%), Viet Nam (10.45%), and Cambodia (5.02%), although in a number of other countries in transition in the studied set of 59 catastrophic

Table 42.1   Data sources and country codes

Country	Code	Year	Survey name	Sample size
Argentina	ARG	1996/97	Encuesta Nacional de Gasto de los Hogares	27 108
Azerbaijan	AZE	1995	The Azerbaijan Survey of Living Condition	2 015
Bangladesh	BGD	1995/96	Household Expenditure Survey	7 420
Belgium	BEL	1997/98	Household Budget Survey	2 212
Brazil	BRA	1996	LSMS	4 850
Bulgaria	BGR	2000	Bulgarian Integrated Household Survey	5 701
Cambodia	KHM	1999	Cambodia Socioeconomic Survey	6 000
Canada	CAN	1997	Survey of Household Spending	16 495
Colombia	COL	1997	National Quality of Life Survey	9 042
Costa Rica	CRI	1992	Encuesta Nacional de los Hogares	2 472
Croatia	HRV	1999	Housheold Budget Survey	2 935
Czech Republic	CZE	1999	Household Budget Survey	2 675
Denmark	DNK	1997	Danish Household Budget Survey	2 862
Djibouti	DJI	1996	Enquête Djiboutienne auprès des Ménages	2 378
Egypt	EGY	1997	Egypt Integrated Household Survey	2 733
Estonia	EST	1995	Household Budget Survey	2 816
Finland	FIN	1998	Consumption Expenditure Survey	4 348
France	FRA	1995	Household Budget Survey	9 607
Germany	DEU	1993	Income and Consumption Survey	48 270
Ghana	GHA	1998/99	Ghana Living Standards Survey	5 998
Greece	GRC	1998	Household Expenditure Survey	6 235
Guyana	GUY	1992	LSMS	1 499
Hungary	HUN	1993	Household Budget Survey	8 094
Iceland	ISL	1995	Household Budget Survey	1 352
Indonesia	IDN	1999	National Socioeconomic Survey	61 328
Israel	ISR	1999	Household Expenditure Survey	5 904
Jamaica	JAM	1997	Survey of Living Condition	1 984
Kyrgyzstan	KGZ	1998	Poverty Monitory Survey	1 891
Latvia	LVA	1997/98	Household Budget Survey	7 684
Lebanon	LBN	1999	National Household Health Expenditure and Use of Services	6 540
Lithuania	LTU	1999	National Household Budget Survey	8 250
Mauritius	MUS	1996/97	Household Budget Survey	6 233
Mexico	MEX	1996	National Income Expenditure Survey	13 661
Morocco	MCO	1991	LSMS	5 131
Namibia	NAM	1994	Household Income and Expenditure Survey	4 384
Nicaragua	NIC	1993	LSMS	4 144
Norway	NOR	1998	Consumer Expenditure Survey	1 180
Panama	PAN	1997	Encuesta Nacional de Niveles de Vida	4 904
Paraguay	PRY	1996	Household Income and Expenditure Survey	2 588
Peru	PER	1994	Encuesta Nacional de Niveles de Vida	3 615
Philippines	PHL	1997	Family Income and Expenditures Survey	39 520
Portugal	PRT	1994/95	Income and Expenditure Survey	10 450
Republic of Korea	KOR	1999	Household Income and Expenditure Survey	62 946
Romania	ROM	1994	Integrated Household Survey	2 291
Senegal	SEN	1994	Enquête Sénégalaise auprès des Ménages	3 274
Slovakia	SVK	1993	Family Expenditure Survey	2 129
Slovenia	SVN	1997	Annual Household Budget Survey	2 577
South Africa	ZAF	1995	South Africa Income Expenditure Survey	29 594

continued

Table 42.1 Data sources and country codes *(continued)*

Country	Code	Year	Survey name	Sample size
Spain	ESP	1996	Encuesta Continua de Hogares	3 104
Sri Lanka	LKA	1995/6	Household Income and Expenditure Survey	19 631
Sweden	SWE	1996	Household Expenditure Survey	1 103
Switzerland	CHE	1998	Swiss Survey on Income and Expenditure	9 295
Thailand	THA	1998	Thailand Socio-Economic Survey	24 977
UK	GBR	1999/2000	Family Expenditure Survey	7 074
Ukraine	UKR	1996	Income Expendituer Survey	2 272
USA	USA	1997	Consumer Expenditure Survey	7 083
Viet Nam	VNM	1997	Vietnam Living Standard Survey	5 966
Yemen	YEM	1998	Household Budget Survey	13 638
Zambia	ZMB	1996	Living Conditions Monitory Survey	10 921

Table 42.2 Percentage of households with catastrophic health expenditures due to out-of-pocket payments, 59 countries

Country	Percentage of households with catastrophic expenditures	Uncertainty interval (80%)		Country	Percentage of households with catastrophic expenditures	Uncertainty interval (80%)	
		Lower (%)	Upper (%)			Lower (%)	Upper (%)
Argentina	5.77%	5.51%	6.02%	Lithuania	1.34%	1.15%	1.54%
Azerbaijan	7.15%	6.43%	7.86%	Mauritius	1.28%	1.10%	1.46%
Bangladesh	1.21%	1.01%	1.41%	Mexico	1.54%	1.36%	1.71%
Belgium	0.09%	0.01%	0.18%	Morocco	0.17%	0.01%	0.25%
Brazil	10.27%	9.49%	11.04%	Namibia	0.11%	0.04%	0.18%
Bulgaria	2.00%	1.77%	2.23%	Nicaragua	2.05%	1.76%	2.34%
Cambodia	5.02%	4.57%	5.47%	Norway	0.28%	0.08%	0.49%
Canada	0.09%	0.06%	0.13%	Panama	2.35%	2.07%	2.62%
Colombia	6.26%	5.88%	6.64%	Paraguay	3.51%	3.04%	3.98%
Costa Rica	0.12%	0.01%	0.23%	Peru	3.21%	2.84%	3.58%
Croatia	0.20%	0.01%	0.30%	Philippines	0.78%	0.71%	0.85%
Czech	0.00%	0.00%	0.00%	Portugal	2.71%	2.42%	3.01%
Denmark	0.07%	0.01%	0.14%	Republic of Korea	1.73%	1.65%	1.80%
Djibouti	0.32%	0.17%	0.47%	Romania	0.09%	0.01%	0.17%
Egypt	2.80%	2.40%	3.21%	Senegal	0.55%	0.38%	0.72%
Estonia	0.31%	0.13%	0.49%	Slovakia	0.00%	0.00%	0.00%
Finland	0.44%	0.25%	0.63%	Slovenia	0.06%	0.01%	0.12%
France	0.00%	0.00%	0.02%	South Africa	0.03%	0.02%	0.04%
Germany	0.03%	0.02%	0.04%	Spain	0.48%	0.31%	0.64%
Ghana	1.30%	1.11%	1.49%	Sri Lanka	1.25%	1.13%	1.37%
Greece	2.17%	1.93%	2.40%	Sweden	0.18%	0.06%	0.42%
Guyana	0.60%	0.33%	0.87%	Switzerland	0.57%	0.47%	0.68%
Hungary	0.20%	0.11%	0.29%	Thailand	0.80%	0.70%	0.89%
Iceland	0.30%	0.01%	0.50%	UK	0.04%	0.01%	0.07%
Indonesia	1.26%	1.20%	1.32%	Ukraine	3.87%	3.36%	4.39%
Israel	0.35%	0.23%	0.46%	USA	0.55%	0.42%	0.69%
Jamaica	1.87%	1.45%	2.28%	Viet Nam	10.45%	9.90%	11.00%
Kyrgyzstan	0.62%	0.38%	0.86%	Yemen	1.66%	1.46%	1.86%
Latvia	2.75%	2.47%	3.04%	Zambia	2.29%	2.03%	2.54%
Lebanon	5.17%	4.81%	5.53%				

health spending is not as large a problem. The second cluster is in Latin America: Argentina (5.77%), Brazil (10.27%), Colombia (6.26%), Paraguay (3.51%), and Peru (3.21%). As with the first cluster, not all countries in Latin America suffer from these high levels of catastrophic spending. Finally, one country, Lebanon, does not fall into either of these groups but, nevertheless, has high levels of catastrophic spending.

Overall, we would expect that the key factor explaining cross-national variation in the extent of catastrophic payments would be the fraction of total health spending that is through out-of-pocket payments as opposed to the fraction through social insurance, taxation or private insurance. The latter types of health payments are not made at the point of service and are not usually related to an individual's health status or service utilization. Prepayments through social insurance, taxation or private insurance are often labelled as mechanisms to achieve financial risk pooling. Figure 42.1 shows the overall positive relationship between the percentage of households with catastrophic health expenditures and the share of out-of-pocket payments in total health expenditure. (The key to the country codes is found in Table 42.1). Figure 42.1 is shown using a log-log plot because the relationship is notably non-linear. The strong relationship confirms the expectation that in general prepay-

ment and risk pooling protect households from facing catastrophic financial consequences of illness.

At any level of the share of out-of-pocket payments in total health expenditure, the proportion of households facing catastrophic health expenditure varies substantially. For example, in Belgium, Hungary, Israel, USA, Guyana, and Lithuania, out-of-pocket payments range from 20 to 25% of total health expenditure. At the same time, in these countries catastrophic payments range from 0.09% in Belgium to 1.34% in Lithuania. Clearly, a relatively small volume of health payments through out-of-pocket expenditures can nevertheless have very adverse consequences on selected households. As the volume of total health expenditure that is through out-of-pocket payments increases, the range of catastrophic payments also increases. Argentina, Colombia, Mexico, and Thailand have between 40 and 45% of total health expenditure through out-of-pocket payments, while catastrophic expenditures range from 6.26% in Colombia to 0.8% in Thailand. The wide range of the proportion of households with catastrophic payments at the same level of out-of-pocket share demonstrates that other factors are also important determinants of catastrophic payment.

Catastrophic payments occur when households access health services and pay large shares of their

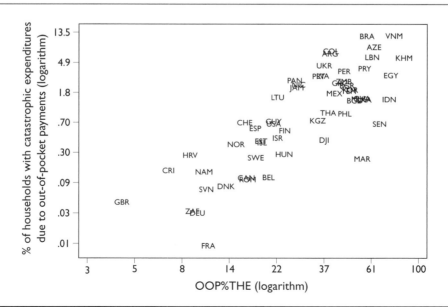

Figure 42.1 Proportion of households with catastrophic expenditures vs. share of out-of-pocket payment in total health expenditures (OOP%THE)

capacity to pay for these services. We would expect, therefore, holding everything else constant, that the probability of catastrophic payments would increase where levels of poverty are higher and where utilization of health care is higher. In all of the household surveys included in this analysis, measures of the proportion of households in poverty are estimated. However, many of these surveys did not include measures of health care utilization. We have used total health expenditure as a share of GDP as an indirect measure of the relative degree of health service delivery. The results of an ordinary least squares (OLS) multivariate regression with these variables is shown in Table 42.3.

The results confirm that countries with a higher share of out-of-pocket payments in total health expenditures are more likely to have a higher proportion of households facing catastrophic expenditure after controlling for other possible determinants. A 1% increase in the proportion of total health expenditure provided by out-of-pocket payments is associated with an average increase in the proportion of households facing catastrophic payments of 2.2%. The coefficients of the percentage of the population living under the poverty line and the share of total health expenditure in GDP are significant, and positively correlated with the percentage of households with catastrophic expenditure as postulated. A 1% increase in poverty will increase catastrophic payments by 0.2%, and a 1% increase in the share of GDP spent on health will increase catastrophic payment by 1.6%. These results are consistent with earlier studies showing that poor households were less able to cope with any given level of health expenditure than richer households (*28–30*). The overall fit of the equation is good, with 77.2% of the variation in the share of households facing catastrophic payments across countries explained by variation in the independent variables. Approximately 23% of variation is not, however, explained by the chosen explanatory variables and it is important for policy purposes to identify other possible determinants.

DISCUSSION

This analysis of household out-of-pocket health spending in 59 countries demonstrates that catastrophic payments are, unfortunately, not rare. They are a common problem in middle-income countries, countries in transition, and a number of low-income countries as well. This negative impact of health systems on households that can lead to impoverishment has long been ignored on the health policy agenda. Once the problem has been identified, however, it is possible for catastrophic payments to quickly become priorities in national health policy debates. Mexico is a recent example.

There is no mystery in understanding the presence of catastrophic health payments. The triad of poverty, health service access and utilization, and the failure of social mechanisms to pool financial risks accounts for most of the variation across countries. Catastrophic payments are the biggest problem when all three of these factors are strong. In other words, we would expect to see high rates of catastrophic spending in countries with high rates of poverty, groups excluded from financial risk protection mechanisms such as social insurance, and moderate to high levels of health care physical access and utilization. Notably a group of countries in Latin America fulfill these criteria as do selected countries in transition.

Catastrophic spending is not a new problem although it may be getting worse in some regions because of the collapse of risk pooling mechanisms. Why has it not been more firmly on national health policy agendas? In developed countries, health systems and financial risk pooling mechanisms evolved in parallel over more than a century. But in many middle-income countries, health service utilization has expanded rapidly and there has been a disconnection with the development of social institutions such as social insurance or tax-financed health services. It appears that the problem of catastrophic health payments is not one that will simply go away with rising

Table 42.3   The determinants of catastrophic health expenditure from cross-country analysis (*n* = 59)

Variable	Coefficient	Standard deviation	t	P > t
Out-of-pocket payment share of total health expenditure (log)	2.161	0.199	10.87	0.00
Total health expenditure share of GDP (log)	1.645	0.362	4.54	0.00
Percentage of households below poverty line (log)	0.173	0.045	3.80	0.00
Constant	2.733	1.141	2.40	0.02
Adjusted *R*-squared	0.7722			
Prob > *F*	0.000			

income; rather, the complex process of developing social institutions to effectively pool financial risk must be placed on the agenda.

It is important to recognize that the impact of out-of-pocket payments is not fully captured by examining catastrophic spending. Many poor households will choose to not seek care rather than become impoverished (*31;32*). Making the users of health services pay out-of-pocket for the services they receive has a potential dual effect at the population level: impoverishing some households that choose to seek services and excluding other individuals from seeking health improving care. Both are important reasons for arguing that health systems are better financed through prepayment mechanisms such as social insurance and general taxation than through user fees.

This analysis uses household survey data on expenditures by category. Measurement error for expenditures is a well recognized problem (*33;34*). If the stochastic component of expenditure recall varies across countries, this could complicate comparisons of the proportion of households facing catastrophic health spending. The strong cross-country relationship found using simple aggregate data, however, suggests that across this set of countries, this problem may not be a dominant issue. As issues of health financing become more central to health policy, public health researchers need to understand and develop improved household survey instruments that capture household health spending for inclusion in various national health surveys.

While the majority of the variation in catastrophic spending can be explained by the triad of poverty, health service utilization, and the absence of risk pooling mechanisms, important unexplained variation remains. Analysis of which households within a country are at a particular risk of catastrophic spending using logistic regression can provide insights into other national determinants of catastrophic spending. Such detailed national assessments can also provide direct input into the design of national policies to increase financial risk protection.

National health systems can be financed in ways that protect households from catastrophic spending and provide access to needed services. The most straightforward approach is to reduce out-of-pocket spending through the development of social insurance or funding through general taxes. Figure 42.1 suggests that if out-of-pocket spending could be reduced to levels lower than 15% of total health spending, few households would be effected by catastrophic payments. The cross-country variation seen in this study, however, demonstrates that there are other more complex strategies that can protect households against catastrophic spending. These may include progressive fee schedules, highly subsidized or free hospital services, or the provision of certain health services to the poor. Regardless of the strategy used, catastrophic health spending is a neglected problem in many parts of the world.

ACKNOWLEDGEMENTS

The authors are grateful to Abdelhay Mechbal and Guy Carrin for their comments, to Piya Hanvoravongchai for the contributions to the previous version, to Ana Mylena Aguilar-Rivera for formatting the tables and graph, and to Nathalie Etomba, and Anna Moore for data and reference searches.

REFERENCES

(1) Bovbjerg RR. *Covering catastrophic health care and containing costs: preliminary lessons for policy from the U.S.experience.* LCSHD Paper Series No. 66. Washington, DC, World Bank, 2001.

(2) Rice T, Desmond K, Gabel J. The Medicare Catastrophic Coverage Act: a post mortem. *Health Affairs*, 1990, 9:75–87.

(3) Trapnell GR et al. *Strategies for insuring catastrophic illness: financial burden, prototype plans, and cost estimates.* Report to DHHS, printed under grant from Hoffmann-La Roche Inc., 1983.

(4) Havighurst CC et al. Strategies in underwriting the cost of catastrophic disease. *Law and Contemporary Problems*, 1976, 40:195.

(5) Najman JM, Western JS. A comparative analysis of Australian health policy in the 1970s. *Social Science & Medicine*, 1984, 18:949–958.

(6) Ranson K. Reduction of catastrophic health care expenditures by a community-based health insurance scheme in Gujarat, India: current experiences and challenges. *Bulletin of the World Health Organization*, 2002, 80: 613–621.

(7) Pradhan M, Prescott N. Social risk management options for medical care in Indonesia. *Health Economics*, 2002, 11:431–446.

(8) World Health Organization. *The World Health Report 2000.Health Systems: Improving Performance.* Geneva, World Health Organization, 2000.

(9) World Health Organization. *The World Health Report 2001. Mental Health: New Understanding, New Hope.* Geneva, World Health Organization, 2001.

(10) World Health Organization. *The World Health Report 2002.Reducing Risks, Promoting Healthy Life*. Geneva, World Health Organization, 2002.

(11) Kawabata K, Xu K, Carrin G. Preventing impoverishment through protection against catastrophic health expenditure. *Bulletin of the World Health Organization*, 2002, 80:612.

(12) Filmer D, Hammer J, Prichett L. Weak links in the chain II: a prescription for health policy in poor countries. *World Bank Research Observer*, 2002, 17:47–66.

(13) Musgrove P. Public spending on health care: how are different criteria related? *Health Policy*, 2000, 53:61–67.

(14) Evans RG et al. Controlling health expenditures—the Canadian reality. *New English Journal of Medicine*, 1989, 320:571–607.

(15) Russel S, Gilson L. User fee policies to promote health service access for poor: a wolf in sheep's clothing ? *International Journal of Health Services*, 1997, 27:359–379.

(16) Wyszewianski L. Financially catastrophic and high-cost cases: definitions, distinctions, and their implication for policy formulation. *Inquiry*, 1986, 23(4):382–394.

(17) Merlis M. Family out-of-pocket spending for health services: a continuing source of financial insecurity. *The Commonwealth Fund*, 2002.

(18) Wyszewianski L. Families with catastrophic health care expenditures. *Health Services Research*, 1986, 21(5): 617–634.

(19) Skarbinski J et al. The burden of out-of-pocket payments for health care in Tbilisi, Republic of Georgia. *The Journal of the American Medical Association*, 2002, 287:1043–1049.

(20) Pannarunothai S, Mills A. The poor pay more: health-related inequality in Thailand. *Social Science & Medicine*, 1997, 44(12):1781–1790.

(21) Frenk J, Knaul F. Health and the economy: empowerment through evidence. *Bulletin of the World Health Organization*, 2002, 80(2):88.

(22) Berki SE. A look at catastrophic medical expenses and the poor. *Health Affairs*, Winter 1986 (DataWatch):139–145.

(23) Xu K et al. Household health system contributions and capacity to pay: definitional, empirical, and technical challenges. In: Murray CJL, Evans DB, eds. *Health systems performance assessment: debates, methods and empiricism*. Geneva, World Health Organization, 2003.

(24) Deaton A, Muellbauer J. *Economics and consumer behavior*. Cambridge, Cambridge University Press, 1980.

(25) Marris R. Comparing the incomes of nations: a critique of the International Comparison Project. *Journal of Economic Literature*, 1984, 22:40–57.

(26) Hill RJ. Measuring substitution bias in international comparisons based on additive purchasing power parity methods. *European Economic Review*, 2000, 44: 145–162.

(27) Davison AC, Hinkley DV. *Bootstrap methods and their application*. Cambridge, Cambridge University Press, 1997.

(28) Wagstaff A. Poverty and health sector inequalities. *Bulletin of the World Health Organization*, 2002, 80(2): 97–105.

(29) Arhin-Tenkorang D. *Mobilizing resources for health: the case for user fees revisited*. CID Working Paper No. 81. Cambridge Center for International Development, 2001.

(30) Bidani B et al. Decomposing social indicators using distributional data. *Journal of Econometrics*, 1997, 77: 125–139.

(31) Creese A, Kuznets J. *Lessons from cost-recovery in health*. Forum on Health Sector Reform. Document No. WHO/SHS/NHP/95.5. Geneva, World Health Organization, 1997. URL: http://mosquito.who.int/docs/hs95_5.htm

(32) Gilson L. *The lessons of user free experience in Africa*. The World Bank Group, Health Reform. Online/Library, 1997. URL: http://www.worldbank.org/healthreform/library/sa/shaw3.pdf

(33) Visaria P. *Poverty and living standards in Asia: an overview of the main results and lessons of selected household surveys*. Living Standards Measurement Working Paper, Washington, DC, World Bank, 1980.

(34) Anand S, Harris C. Choosing a welfare indicator. *American Economic Review*, 1994, 84:226–231.

Chapter 43

Health System Responsiveness: Concepts, Domains and Operationalization

Nicole B. Valentine, Amala de Silva, Kei Kawabata, Charles Darby, Christopher J.L. Murray, David B. Evans

Background

On the creation of WHO in 1948, its constitution defined health as "a state of complete physical, mental and social well-being and not merely the absence of disease or infirmity." It was recognized that the health system must address the medical needs of individuals, but that it must also focus on other factors affecting their well-being, a tradition which has continued since that time. Decades later, Donabedian's (1) pioneering work on the quality of medical care reflected the sentiment of the WHO constitution by defining quality as much broader than simply the ability to enhance health. He named three components: technical quality (the ability to improve health outcomes), process quality (the management of the interpersonal process), and structure quality (related to the quality of amenities). Client satisfaction was of fundamental importance to the management of the interpersonal process because it gave information on the provider's success at meeting the client's values and expectations. These values encompassed health outcomes, the nature of the intervention provided (at home, at the hospital), and an array of factors deemed essential for health care provision, including being served in due time and having access to care when needed. In addition, patient satisfaction was important because it was linked to health outcomes—a dissatisfied patient may fail to follow provider recommendations on treatment or to seek care in the event of future illness.

Since the 1980s, the interest in patient satisfaction as a separate outcome measure has grown and there is now an extensive history of attempts to measure it using questionnaires, particularly in the United States (2–5). With increasing knowledge, however, the need to capture the actual patient experience, in addition to patient satisfaction with the care received, has

also been recognized, since it provides a direct link to actions to improve quality. By 1997, for example, the Agency for Health Research and Quality (AHRQ) in the USA had developed and funded the Consumer Assessment of Health Plans survey and reporting kit (CAHPS) (6) to capture patient experiences through patient reports rather than their satisfaction with these experiences. In 2000, WHO refined and broadened the concept of patient experience to cover not only the interpersonal process between practitioner and patient or client, but also the interaction between the health system and the population it serves. This concept was called responsiveness (7;8).

Although most surveys exploring patient experience have taken place in the high-income countries in North America and Western Europe, there is a growing interest in evaluating the population's experience with health services in other regions, including low-income countries. Haddad et al. identified 16 such studies in 1998 and we have been able to identify another 12 (9–21). The present chapter builds on that body of work.

Section two defines the concept of responsiveness, and describes in more detail its evolution and how it relates to and differs from the concepts of patient satisfaction and quality of care. The third section describes several domains which together capture the notion of the responsiveness of the health system. The related areas of human and patient rights are the focus of section four, while a description of the operationalization process for the measurement of responsiveness is presented in the fifth section. The chapter concludes with a discussion on some of the continued challenges to capturing and measuring responsiveness and the possible strategies for its further development.

The Evolution of the Concept of Responsiveness

Defining Responsiveness

When individuals interact with the health system it influences their well-being. One pathway to achieve well-being is through improvements in health, but well-being is also influenced by other aspects of people's personal interactions with the health system. We define aspects related to the way individuals are treated and the environment in which they are treated as responsiveness. Multiple domains characterize both health and responsiveness. The operationalization of health involves selecting a common set of domains including, for example, mobility and pain. Similarly, for responsiveness, a common set of domains can be identified for measurement purposes.

By convention, only certain levels of functioning in the health domains define whether an individual is considered healthy or unhealthy. There is a threshold above which further increments in functioning are viewed as talent rather than health improvements (22). For example, someone who can run 10 kilometres is regarded as healthier than someone who cannot walk 100 meters. However, someone who can run a marathon is not regarded as healthier than the person who can run 10 kilometres. Similarly, only certain levels on each responsiveness domain define whether the system is responsive or not responsive. Above these thresholds, further improvements are defined as luxury, or the equivalent of talent in health. Improvements in cleanliness and basic ventilation in facilities increase the level of responsiveness, whereas adding luxury items to waiting rooms or hospital wards would not be regarded as part of the responsiveness expected of a health system. The measurement of responsiveness focuses on improvements up to a commonly defined domain threshold.

The well-being of individuals is influenced by their interaction with the health system through its impact on their health and through its responsiveness. The WHO framework for assessing the performance of health systems includes both health and responsiveness as key outcomes on which health systems should be judged, along with the fairness in the way the health system is financed (7). Societies are concerned with the average levels of health and responsiveness, as well as with the distribution, or inequalities in, health and responsiveness across the population. Accordingly, five outcome indicators were defined in the framework: the level and distribution of health, the level and distribution of responsiveness, and fairness in household financial contribution.

The conceptual independence of responsiveness from the health-enhancing aspects of people's encounters with the health system in no way suggests that responsiveness does not impinge on health. Individuals who are treated with concern and cared for in pleasant surroundings are likely to respond better to the counsel offered by health providers in the course of diagnosis and treatment. This could improve treatment outcomes. A responsive health system, therefore, contributes to health enhancement by being more conducive for individuals to seek care earlier, to be more open in their interactions with health care providers, and to better assimilate health information (23). It can also contribute to increased utilization in settings where people might choose not to use available services because of their low responsiveness (9).

Responsiveness and Quality of Care

Responsiveness draws on the quality of care literature, but is distinct from it in many ways. The quality of care literature is diffuse and a number of different frameworks for assessing quality have been proposed. Many draw on the Donabedian framework of technical, process, and structural quality (24). Technical quality has been defined as including dimensions such as appropriateness, effectiveness, and technical competence. Process quality involves dimensions such as courtesy, information provision or communication, respect, choice, and autonomy (25). It has also been called service quality (26) or the interpersonal component of quality (27). Structural quality has included dimensions such as continuity of care, affordability, accommodation, and accessibility. A feature common to the majority of quality of care conceptual frameworks is the rather loose relationship between the concept and its measurement, including the elaboration of an anchored and calibrated scoring system.

By its construct, responsiveness is related more to some of the interpersonal dimensions of quality of care rather than to technical quality. To the extent that technical quality improves health, it is captured in the WHO performance assessment framework through impact on health outcomes. Financial affordability, sometimes considered part of structural quality, is included in the WHO framework partly in the fairness in financial contribution goal and partly through its impact on health outcomes (28). It does not form part of responsiveness. Some of the interpersonal dimensions of quality of care have, therefore, been useful in defining the dimensions of responsiveness, but no single quality of care framework incorporates all the domains that are considered important to responsiveness, nor do any clearly distinguish between health enhancement domains and those that enhance well-being through other mechanisms (24).

RESPONSIVENESS AND PATIENT SATISFACTION

Patient satisfaction tries to capture consumer perceptions of the quality of services delivered by a health provider or the system as a whole (5;6;25;29–39). It is a complex concept that is influenced by a mixture of perceived need, individual expectations, and the experience of care (40). Patient satisfaction surveys have sometimes been used as one component in judging the quality of care (25).

With growing experience in its use, some difficulties have emerged (41). First, the concept becomes ambiguous if it refers to multiple health care events and multiple interactions over long periods. Patient ratings may capture general attitudes or satisfaction rather than recall actual events. Second, respondents may not think along a continuum of dissatisfaction to satisfaction, even if provided with these anchors, making calibration of satisfaction responses difficult. Third, expectations strongly influence satisfaction ratings and paradoxical results may arise. A downturn in the economy, for example, might lower people's expectations of what the system can provide so that they report higher levels of satisfaction. At the same time, system quality might not have improved or might even have fallen. Accordingly, patient satisfaction surveys may not capture what actually happens when people come in contact with the health system, and the responses are strongly influenced by prior expectations of what will or should happen (42).

In addition, satisfaction has been shown to vary with selected socio-demographic characteristics, including income, possibly due to differences in expectations (43;44). The WHO Multi-country Survey Study on Health and Responsiveness 2000–2001 confirmed on a global scale the results of earlier studies that expectations do vary across individuals and populations both between and within countries (45;46).

Partly for these reasons, CAHPS, intended to capture the responsiveness of managed care compared to other forms of service provision, has moved from relying on patient satisfaction surveys to developing means of allowing patients to report on their actual experiences. WHO's approach to responsiveness builds on this idea, the need to capture people's actual experiences with the health system.

Two additional differences between the concepts of responsiveness and patient satisfaction can be highlighted:

- The type of interaction (e.g. at a health service, health insurance, public health campaign): patient satisfaction focuses on interactions in medical facilities, whereas responsiveness includes the scope to evaluate the health system as a whole by concentrating on the different types of interactions people have with the system.

- Components of the interaction: patient satisfaction generally covers both clinical and non-clinical components of an interaction, while responsiveness focuses only on the latter. Responsiveness does not seek to determine whether health is improved by an encounter with the health system; this is captured in the WHO framework on health systems performance assessment by measuring health.

RESPONSIVENESS DOMAINS

The development of the domains of responsiveness and the methodology for their measurement drew on a broad literature review of the areas of quality of care and patient satisfaction. This included the examination of different survey instruments. Details of the studies reviewed are presented in de Silva (47).

FRAMEWORK FOR DEVELOPMENT OF DOMAINS AND ITEMS

Although responsiveness is characterized by multiple domains, its operationalization for comparative purposes across countries requires the selection of a common set of domains that are applicable to all health systems. An extensive literature review was undertaken to answer the question of what, apart from improving health, was valued by people in their interactions with health systems. The review focused on research from the disciplines of sociology, anthropology, health economics, health services and management, ethics, human rights, and patient rights. The precise meaning of the terms developed to describe the domains was tested in a number of pilot surveys. From this process, a common set of eight domains that most comprehensively captured responsiveness was identified. They comprise autonomy, choice, communication, confidentiality, dignity, prompt attention, quality of basic amenities, and support (access to family and community support).

Table 43.1 shows the elements of the proposed WHO measure of responsiveness cross-tabulated with well-known patient satisfaction surveys and studies. As suggested above, none of the existing instruments capture all of the dimensions considered to form part of responsiveness.

CRITERIA FOR SELECTING DOMAINS

The criteria applied in the selection of domains was that the list be exhaustive and widely accepted as an appropriate way to characterize the qualities sought in a responsive health system by the individuals it serves. Although domains may overlap, this should be avoided as far as possible. The following guiding principals were applied. Domains must be:

- validated in related fields as important attributes that individuals seek in their interaction with the health system, in addition to the goal of improving health;

- amenable to self report;

- comprehensive enough, when taken together, to capture all important aspects of responsiveness which people value;

- able to be measured in a way that is comparable within and across populations.

THE COMMON SET OF DOMAINS

In addition to the literature review, WHO undertook an extensive consultative process from 1999 to 2002 that included two expert meetings and three meetings of a Scientific Peer Review Group (48;49). An instrument was developed and tested in a 35-country key informant survey. This was followed by the development of a household survey instrument tested in a 12-country pilot survey, with cognitive testing in seven countries.[1] The full instrument was then fielded in 71 countries as part of the WHO Multi-country Survey Study on Health and Responsiveness 2000–2001 (50). Further cognitive testing was carried out as well as an extensive analysis on the validity and reliability of the data using psychometric testing. With each step of this process, WHO has refined its concepts, methodology, and instruments for measurement. As a culmination of these efforts, the World Health Survey, with a revised instrument for responsiveness, is being implemented in 73 countries in 2002–2003 (51). The next sections describe each of the domains in alphabetical order.

Autonomy

Autonomy is derived from the Greek words *autos* (self) and *nomos* (law). It has two components: decision-making (*autos* or self-directing) and the value system by which decisions are made (*nomos* or natural law). It is also defined as "the freedom of the will" (52). In philosophy, this concept relates to being self-determined instead of being determined from outside. In ethics, autonomy is the notion that ethical rules must be linked to reason, rather than imposed on someone (53). Autonomy in a medical context demands "physicians having a standing duty to respect and at times, an obligation to help promote the free choice of competent patients" (54).

Table 43.1 Existing questionnaires that incorporate domains of responsiveness

Responsiveness dimensions	Patient Survey Quest (5)	Adult Core Quest (30)	Comm. Tracking Study (31)	20 Item Scale (9)	Evaluation Ranking Scale (32)	Picker Patient Experience Quest. (33;34)	Quote-Rheumatic-Patients Instrument (25)
Respect for *autonomy*			X			X	X
Choice of care provider	X	X	X		X		X
Respect for *confidentiality*			X			X	
Communication	X	X	X	X	X	X	X
Respect for *dignity*	X	X	X	X	X	X	X
Access to *prompt attention*	X	X	X		X	X	X
Quality of basic amenities				X	X		X
Access to family and community *support*						X	X

In this context, competency implies being an adult of sound mind, possessing the cognitive and emotional capability of exercising deliberate and meaningful choices consistent with an individual's values (54). Autonomy involves the right to receive medical information, the right of patients to make informed choices, and the right to refuse medical treatment (55).

The principle of autonomy implies that providers must treat people in ways that respect the patients' views of what is appropriate (25;54). This means that the rights of patients who wish to have less autonomy are also respected. The right to autonomy does not force patients to be autonomous.

Autonomy incorporates the concept of empowerment. Judges in some settings have characterized the right to refuse medical treatment as a necessary element of an individual's right to self-determination and, in some instances, they have also recognized a right to privacy as a basis for treatment refusal (56). The right of refusal is not absolute and must be considered alongside other factors such as public well-being and the competence of a patient to make the decision.

Charles, Gafni and Whelan identify four models of autonomy (57). The first is the paternalistic model where the provider makes all decisions on behalf of the patient because the provider is considered to be better informed. The second model, termed the informed decision-making model, imposes the need for information dissemination on the provider and the responsibility for decision-making on the patient. The professional agent model, the third, has the patient willingly forego the right to decision-making by voluntarily and explicitly transferring the decision-making task to the provider. The final model, shared decision-making, focuses on the sharing of both information and decision-making between the patient and the provider. While these models are clearly demarcated in theory, in reality many provider-patient relationships are a combination of these different approaches, varying by disease, patient profile, and interpersonal dynamics.

In certain cultures, family opinions must also be added to the equation and there are various roles that family or friends may play during the decision-making process: information gatherer, recorder or interpreter; coaching the patient to ask certain questions; adviser; or negotiator on the patient's behalf regarding timing, place or treatment option (57). Where an individual voluntarily rescinds a right to sole determination of their own health care, health providers would be expected to consult with family members either in the presence or absence of the patient, the choice being made for the individual. In the case of minors or those who are mentally unstable, patient autonomy would automatically devolve to the family.

This can be further complicated in some cultures where adverse diagnoses, such as cancer, are not traditionally shared with the patient. Anecdotal evidence for this can be found from countries such as Japan, Sri Lanka, and India. The family would make all the decisions in this case, under the conviction that the patient is best left unaware of the actual diagnosis of terminal illness. Health personnel aware of such traditions leave the decision of breaking the news of the diagnosis to the family. In this case, the definition of autonomy includes interaction between providers and the family, as well as the patient. This concept is increasingly being challenged even in these countries, as family wishes may conflict with those of the patient.

The definition of autonomy provided by respondents in the WHO cognitive testing described earlier converged particularly on the desire of patients to be given a choice with regard to treatment. This implies that a system would be judged as more responsive if providers discussed with patients all relevant treatment protocols with an explanation of their relative merits, than if they simply recommended the provider's preferred option. This would give patients the opportunity to make any necessary trade-offs if they wished to do so. Taking this into account, as well as the extensive literature on the topic, autonomy is defined here to focus on four issues:

- the need to provide information to individuals (and their families where appropriate) about their health status and risks, and about alternative treatment options;

- the need to involve the individuals (and their families where appropriate) in the decision-making process to the extent that they wish this to occur;

- the need to obtain informed consent in the context of testing and treatment; and

- the right of patients of sound mind to refuse treatment for themselves.

Choice

The domain of choice relates to health care institutions and health providers. Choice is defined as the power or opportunity to select, which requires more than one option (52). Choice also incorporates the ability of an individual to gain a second opinion (possibly limited to cases of severe or chronic illness or surgery) and access to specialist care when needed (25).

Debate with regard to this domain has centred on the burden imposed on health systems with shortages of human or financial resources. Providing the population with choice could lead to limited resources that could otherwise have been used to improve health and other dimensions of responsiveness. Geographical barriers might also make it very difficult for poor countries to ensure that all people have similar levels of choice.

In many societies, however, the barriers can be procedural. They include lack of flexibility in referral practices and insurance procedures or legislative obstacles to the setting up of health care units. Choice of personal primary health care provider was the most important predictor of high consumer satisfaction in an evaluation of the impact of the Slovenian health reform (58). In the US, where choice is almost infinite, patient satisfaction surveys have become an important planning tool for ensuring the retention of "clients." A survey comparing health maintenance organizations (HMO) and preferred provider organizations (PPO) found lower scores in HMOs because of perceived lack of choice and need for referral approval. Subsequently, HMOs found that the costs of reviewing and approving (or, in some cases, denying) referrals exceeded the savings resulting from the few denials, so it was decided to eliminate referral review (59).

Individuals often seek to consult the same health provider on subsequent occasions, particularly if they are returning for the same complaint. In societies where there is a tradition of confidence and trust in health providers, the option to consult the same person each time is very important and can be a source of comfort even for minor ailments (60). Choice of care provider, therefore, includes the choice of consulting the same provider if desired as much as consulting a different doctor in the event of dissatisfaction with previous encounters. Patient preferences, however, can differ. A study in Sweden found that older patients appreciated retaining the same family physician compared to younger, more educated patients who appreciated more the availability of free choice of physicians (61). There might also be gender differences in these preferences (43). In all of these cases, the ability to consult a specific provider inspires confidence, and the ability to consult someone else if desired increases well-being.

Choice of health care provider can also improve quality and health outcomes indirectly. Providers who know that patients have an option are more likely to treat them with respect and to ensure that they are up-to-date with the latest practices. The debate rests more on how the burden of the demand for choice imposes on resource-constrained health systems. This question can be answered empirically by determining the relative weight people give to choice compared to the other responsiveness domains, and the relative weight to responsiveness compared to health, in different settings.

Clarity of Communication

Clarity of communication is defined as the clarity in conveying information and evoking understanding (52). As a domain of responsiveness, it includes the notion that providers explain clearly to the patient and family the nature of the illness, and details of the required treatment and options (62). It also includes providing time for patients to understand their symptoms and to ask questions.

Individuals in the WHO cognitive testing exercise interpreted the question on communication consistently, referring both to receiving information in simple, non-technical terms and to having the provider listen to their problems and answer their questions. There was some overlap with dignity, in that they would like a provider to treat them with respect and to talk to them in a pleasant and attentive manner. This is consistent with the results of the EUROPEP study where patients valued being well-informed about their illness and feeling free to talk about it with their providers (63).

Clarity of communication implies that the provider listens carefully to the concerns of the patient, and explains about the symptoms and any related illness, its treatment, and implications. This should be done in a manner that is understandable and permits the patient to ask follow-up questions (25).[2] Maintaining such a dialogue is a demonstration of the respect a provider is showing the patient, but remains important in its own right. This combination of attributes of communication and partnership has also been identified as an important aspect contributing to patient satisfaction (64;65).

Different types of communication can occur between health providers and patients: social, non-problem focused talk; positive/partnership talk that involves partnership statements, reiteration, approval and agreement; psychosocial problem talk involving concern, reassurance, psychosocial questions and counselling; disagreements; and medical questions and medical information (43). It may be that all types are important. For example, Gross et al. concluded that there was a positive relationship between longer visits and patient satisfaction (66), suggesting that casual conversation creates a warmer atmosphere for a clearer exchange of medical information subsequently.

Communication involves allowing the time and opportunity for the patient to ask questions and providing answers to them. Fostering a continuing dialogue can help overcome social, psychological, and structural impediments to communication (67). A survey undertaken in the USA identified that 45% of the respondents felt that providers did not communicate adequately (34). Communication was particularly of concern for inpatients at the discharge stage, in terms of providing advice on follow-up and care requirements (34). Another survey of care provided by general practitioners in one city in each of four different high-income countries found that a common source of dissatisfaction was that the practitioner did not communicate enough information (68).

Factors that can improve communication include the use of non-technical language, the frequency of smiles and nods, the degree of eye contact, and voice quality. The use of a person's mother tongue in the dissemination of health information is also important in facilitating better patient-provider relationships. This need, however, imposes a burden on the health system in multi-ethnic societies and may necessitate the use of interpreters in contexts where multilingual health care providers are not available. It has also been suggested that, in addition to being bilingual, there is a need for providers to be bicultural in order to facilitate the provider-patient communication in multi-ethnic societies (69).

The communication domain applies to all types of contacts between the population and the health system, not just to the clinical interactions between a patient and a provider. For example, people need to understand what type of services they can obtain, and where, as well as how to complete any paperwork required for health insurance reimbursements (49).

As with the other domains, communication can improve health outcomes as people are more likely to absorb information if the system communicates well. However, good communication is also valued for its own sake and it is for that reason that communication is included as a domain of responsiveness.

Confidentiality of Personal Information

Confidentiality is defined as being entrusted with secrets (52). It is equated with privacy, which was defined in the U.S. National Information Infrastructure Task Force in 1995 as "an individual's claim to control the terms under which personal information—information identifiable to an individual—is acquired, disclosed, and used" (70).

As a domain of responsiveness, it is related to three specific areas:

- the privacy of the environment in which consultations are conducted by health providers,

- the concept of "privileged communication,"

- the confidentiality of medical records and information about individuals.

The WHO cognitive testing results revealed that there was consistency in the interpretation of the term. The respondents identified confidentiality as requiring health personnel to keep the nature of their illness "secret" from others who are not concerned with its treatment. The notion of not allowing others to overhear conversations during consultations was also mentioned, as was the concern that medical records be kept confidential.

An eight European country study conducted by the European Task Force on Patient Evaluations of General Practice (EUROPEP) also showed that confidentiality of patient information was among the aspects most valued by patients (63). Although this type of confidentiality is a well-established principle in medical practice, its importance is sometimes under-appreciated by medical personnel (71).

Privileged communication relates to the fact that individuals are able to divulge information about themselves to health personnel with the conviction that this information will be kept confidential. The confidentiality of medical records is dependent on proper guidelines and training of health personnel, regardless of whether the records are kept electronically or in paper form. It also requires that members of the health personnel do not discuss cases in a way that permits confidential information to be transmitted to the wider community. An important corollary of this aspect is that individuals may also require access to their own records. Rules for data security have been developed and found to be feasible, at least in countries where the health system is well funded (72;73). Training of health personnel and the existence of physical infrastructure that protects privacy during consultations are prerequisites for the safeguarding of confidentiality (63;71).

Health professionals sometimes face a dilemma between safeguarding patient confidentiality and the need to inform other people, particularly in transmissible conditions where it is important to trace the source of infection and treat others who might require it, as well as to protect other people from becoming infected (73). In the latter case, the emphasis has been on educating individuals of the risks involved in particular types of interactions, and on encouraging them to share the information voluntarily with others at risk. The onus of disclosure in such cases would be on the patient, but health care providers could play a role in inspiring such moves. In cases where ensuring individual autonomy endangers others (such as in the case of major public health threats), there is recourse to established principles developed in international human rights law for deciding about the disclosure of personal information. These principles are examined in more detail in section four of the present chapter.

Dignity

Dignity is derived from the Latin word *dignus,* meaning worthy, defined as the "state of being worthy of honour or respect"(52). The domain of dignity refers to receiving care in a respectful, caring, non-discriminatory setting (47).

The cognitive testing at the seven sites referred to above revealed that "respect" was the term that best defined dignity. The respondents were further probed with another open-ended question requesting asking them to provide the meaning of respect. There was a strong degree of consistency in the individual responses, and the terms politeness, greeting, attention, listening, care, and not being scolded or shouted at, recurred frequently.

Hall and Dornan's review of studies on patient priorities for general practice care finds that many priority lists contain the desire for "'humaneness'" in health sector interactions (74). Privacy during medical examinations has been found to be important in encouraging individuals to utilize health services. The right to privacy in situations such as childbirth is stressed in Gilson, Alilio and Heggenhougen (75). Privacy of the body, defined as preventing undue exposure of the body, is listed as a characteristic of dignity by both the nurses and patients surveyed by Walsh and Kowanko. Nurses also relate privacy to the space provided for patients to express emotions and to share their feelings with family members (76).

Dignity as a notion of respect for persons does not necessarily correlate with the amount of resources spent on health. However, under-paid and over-worked nurses in under-equipped primary health care centres could find themselves too demoralized to treat their patients humanely (77)

There is a close relationship between dignity and the domains of communication, prompt attention, and confidentiality. The way the health provider communicates with an individual, attends to his/her needs promptly, and maintains the confidentiality of any resulting medical information supports individual dignity. Conversely, lack of respect is associated with being shouted at or scolded, being ordered around, and made to wait unreasonably. Morris, in her study on respectful treatment of patients in the US, underlines the critical importance of this domain to patient satisfaction (78). Her definition includes the notions of short waiting times at the facility and convenience, both of which are parts of the domain of prompt attention in the categorization proposed here.

Dignity in the area of public health is as relevant as in curative interactions between a patient and a provider. There is growing evidence on the positive health impact of negative imagery (79). However, public campaigns, for example those aimed at preventing unsafe sex and HIV/AIDS, could, while achieving positive health impact on those who do not have HIV/AIDS, further stigmatize those with it by using insensitive wording. Health care providers are responsible for treating individuals with dignity, while at the system level, appropriate legislation helps to enforce this type of treatment. In addition to laws, patient charters and guidelines developed in consultation with health providers help to ensure that all individuals are treated with dignity in their health encounters. The health educational system can play a major role in training both the provider in the way he/she should treat patients and the consumer regarding his/her rights. Positive incentives also have an impact on provider behaviour towards patients.

Prompt Attention

Prompt attention is defined as care provided readily or as soon as necessary (52). This domain includes people's knowledge that they can have access to rapid care in emergencies, short waiting periods for treatment and surgery even in the case of non-emergencies, convenient times and modes for accessing curative and public health interventions, services within easy travelling distance, and follow-up services (5;25;29;68;77).

Responses during the cognitive testing covered the range of situations described above, but all included the notion of being treated in a timely manner. In addition to this idea of being treated quickly during an emergency, they included the ability to reach a facility, to make an appointment, to be attended once at a facility, to obtain medication to alleviate pain, and to receive test results and diagnosis without delay. Respondents from Nigeria and Slovakia also included the concept of respect in prompt attention, i.e. receiving answers to questions promptly, having their arrival at a facility acknowledged, and being attended in order of arrival or appointment time. Respondents in Slovakia indicated that the latter is not respected due to bribes, a custom that favours the wealthy.

This dimension is not limited only to personal medical services. The lack of prompt attention in terms of the administrative process surrounding an encounter can also affect people's well-being. For example, delays in settling insurance claims or in issuing birth and death certificates can be a source of anxiety (59). It is important in the context of non-personal services as well. Public health issues need to be communicated in a prompt manner, particularly in areas such as outbreaks of diseases (80). Information on preventive measures that can be taken to avoid disease should be accessible and within convenient distance of households. Health education messages should also be provided in a timely manner (81).

These results are consistent with a number of strands of work in the existing literature. For example, in the context of emergency care, patient satisfaction studies have focused on the knowledge of easy access to care if an emergency arises. Such knowledge creates a sense of well-being in addition to the benefit gained by actually obtaining the care (63). Although conceptually this aspect of prompt attention is important, its operationalization is difficult because it relies on an impression rather than the reporting of a person's actual experience.

In preparing his Patient Satisfaction Questionnaire (PSQ), Ware identified seven dimensions of satisfaction that had been included most frequently in previous patient satisfaction studies (5;82). Two were related to our concept of prompt attention—accessibility/convenience and availability of services. In Singapore, a review of complaint cases lodged with the Family Health Service over a two-year period identified excessive waiting time among the top five complaint areas. The study suggested that although this was related to inadequate staff, waiting times could be reduced by improving work flows (83). Similar results have been found in other settings (17). The perception of unreasonable waiting lists for non-emergency operations became a major political issue in the UK in

2001, where the proportion of the population waiting four months or more for elective surgery was 38% compared to 5% in the USA (84).

Achievement of prompt attention can be constrained by at least two factors: a shortage of resources such as personnel, and the lack of an efficient mechanism to smooth work flows over time. Geographical accessibility is important, as is the knowledge that it is possible to access health care quickly in case of emergencies (5). The use of mobile clinics to provide health services could be a way to give more prompt attention for more remote rural communities (85;86).

Quality of Basic Amenities

The domain of quality of basic amenities is related to the extent to which the physical infrastructure of a health facility is welcoming and pleasant (52). It includes clean surroundings, regular maintenance, adequate furniture, sufficient ventilation, enough space in waiting rooms, and clean water, toilets and linen at the institutional level (9;29;32;87). These are sometimes termed "hotel facilities" (88). Drugs, testing facilities, and medical equipment are amenities included in the quality of care literature and are essential to the outcomes of medical care. They are captured in the health part of the WHO performance framework, and therefore are not included in responsiveness (89). The quality of basic amenities domain is linked to health facilities, whether they be inpatient or outpatient, and whether they provide services relating to promotion, prevention, treatment, or rehabilitation.

Respondents at the cognitive testing in all the countries considered cleanliness and comfort as essential elements of this domain. Cleanliness included clean waiting rooms, wards, equipment, toilet facilities, and beds. Comfort included good ventilation, heating in cold climates, roominess, and good quality water.

The question of what level represents "talent" in the sense discussed earlier, and what level is a legitimate part of responsiveness, is particularly difficult to establish with this domain. Although the responses to the cognitive testing focused on cleanliness and space, individuals may associate more amenities as being better, regardless of the current level. A patient satisfaction survey in Bangkok, for example, found that private, for-profit hospitals received lower ratings than either public or non-profit hospitals, except in certain dimensions of amenities where they provided more than the other hospitals (90).

Access to Family and Community Support

Patient welfare is best served if individuals have access to their families and other community support networks during care (91).[3] People who support the patient will help carry some of the weight of illness and its consequences, and give strength to and encourage the patient (92;93). This domain is currently operationalized in the context of inpatient care only. It builds on the work of authors such as Friedland et al. who argued that social support helps people cope better with the stress of illness and its consequences (94). Changes in roles and relationships in a family, income, and employment status due to illness add to this stress. They defined "social support" as the feeling of being cared for and loved, valued, esteemed, and able to count on others should the need arise. This type of support can reduce stress, and health systems that facilitate this support will improve well-being independently of any subsequent health improvement.

This being said, the domain is not entirely separable from health improvements. Freidland et al. also argued that the reduction of stress in this way is correlated with improved health outcomes, and Fadiman claimed that allowing the family access to the patient influenced compliance among the Hmong communities found in Thailand and Laos (69).

While health systems cannot be held responsible for the types of bonds that exist between family members and the extent of support patients receive from the people close to them, health systems can ensure that they provide an encouraging environment within which these beneficial interactions may occur.

Responses for this domain in the cognitive testing exercises indicated that the possibility of having regular visits by relatives and friends was the most important issue. Similar sentiments were expressed in a survey of Czech hospital patients using open-ended questions, where the possibility of having visitors by the bedside was identified as one of the positive changes in the health system since the transition from a communist state (21). In two countries during the cognitive testing, the ability of family and friends to provide food to inpatients was also considered important.

For all these reasons, the domain of access to family and community support has been defined to include visiting rights of family and friends to inpatients, as well as the right to receive food and other consumables from family members if desired. It also comprises the opportunity to carry out religious and cultural practices that are not contrary to the sensitivities of other patients or health care providers, and the right to prac-

tice alternative therapies (such as traditional medicine) which are not contrary to the hospital health care regime. At a broader system level, this domain also captures whether family members of someone who is ill received support and were kept informed by medical personnel (33).

Access to NGOs and community-based organizations has helped resource constrained systems to improve responsiveness, particularly where patients have no family networks to sustain them. In some cases, such organizations interact with health care facilities to improve the well-being of patients at the institution, whereas in other instances, they focus on providing company and comfort to patients in their home environments (95). Health system responsiveness is not determined solely by public sector health providers. It is also influenced by providers in the private and non-government sectors (96). Responsibility for ensuring the entire system is responsive does, however, lie with the government, which needs to be able to encourage and influence the non-government sector to be responsive as well (7).

RESPONSIVENESS AND RELATED SPHERES

RESPONSIVENESS AND HUMAN RIGHTS

Human rights are guaranteed by international agreements and a "rights-based approach" to health heeds the content of these agreements when implementing health policies. The major international treaties documenting human rights are the International Covenant on Economic, Social and Cultural Rights (ICESCR, 1966) and the International Covenant on Civil and Political Rights (ICCPR, 1966). In the human rights approach, limiting the exercise or enjoyment of a right in the name of public health is a last resort and is considered legitimate only if each of the provisions reflected in the Siracusa principles is met.[4] In the responsiveness space, this means that some ways of improving health at the expense of reduced responsiveness are not legitimate. A concern with responsiveness, therefore, is consistent with a concern about human rights in health.

Being treated with dignity whether one is suffering from HIV/AIDS, leprosy, or mental illness, is an important element of human rights. Likewise, discriminating against the physically, mentally, educationally, socially, economically, and politically disadvantaged, in their encounters with the health system, is considered a violation of the human rights of these individuals.

In practice, human rights in the health area are often concerned with the times where responsiveness and health might work in opposite directions. For example, compulsory testing for HIV/AIDS, incarcerating individuals with certain communicable diseases, and enforced sterilization are possible ways of improving population health, but they would reduce system responsiveness on the domains of dignity and autonomy. Such actions are also widely considered as violations of human rights. The domains of responsiveness map well with the principles of a rights-based approach to health (97). For example, autonomy and communication involve seeking, receiving and imparting information, and correspond to freedom of association in human rights. Likewise, confidentiality involves privacy, and autonomy reflects people's right to participate in decisions affecting their health and well-being. The key issue of discrimination in the human rights field is reflected in a concern with inequalities in responsiveness as described in the health systems performance framework (7).

RESPONSIVENESS AND PATIENT RIGHTS

Concern with patient rights has gained prominence over the past few decades (35;36;55). In particular, obtaining patient consent for any invasive procedure has assumed additional importance because law courts have increasingly awarded damages for actions taken without the patient's permission. In 2000, an internal WHO review of legal and regulatory support for patient rights showed that there were entitlements to patient rights under various laws in a diverse range of countries including Algeria, Argentina, Australia, Belgium, Bulgaria, Canada, China, Costa Rica, Denmark, Dominican Republic, Finland, France, Georgia, Greece, Hungary, Iceland, Israel, Kyrgyzstan, Lithuania, Luxembourg, Netherlands, New Zealand, Norway, Peru, Russia, San Marino, Spain, Sweden, Switzerland, Turkey, UK, Uruguay, USA, Venezuela, and Viet Nam.

In some of these countries, the UK for example, patient charters have been developed. The adoption of patient rights in legislation by no means guarantees its effectiveness in delivering responsive health services, but it is an indicator of the official acceptance of the patient's perspective as an important component of the quality of health systems. At the same time, there has been recent growth in the development of non-governmental and consumer organizations advocating for patient or consumer rights.[5]

The responsiveness domains map well into patient rights laws and charters, as is the case with human rights. The right to self-determination about care connects with autonomy; the right to information about the patient's health status and treatment options is similar to communication; the rights to confidentiality and being treated with dignity are both domains of responsiveness; the right of a patient to enjoy family and spiritual support corresponds to the domain of access to family and community support; and the right to humane terminal care is part of dignity.

OPERATIONALIZATION OF THE MEASUREMENT OF RESPONSIVENESS

Once the common set of domains of responsiveness has been selected, there are challenges for measurement. Two are discussed in this section. The first concerns how to define population responsiveness formally taking into account the experiences of individuals across varying numbers of contacts with different parts of the health system. The second is how to the measure population responsiveness based on this construct, in a reliable, valid, and comparable manner. The section concludes by discussing the challenges for the future development of measurement strategies.

It would theoretically be possible to observe people's interactions with a health system in some way, perhaps with direct observation or with cameras. This is not practical and, in any case, someone would need to decide whether the system was responsive to the individual during that encounter. A further problem is that while most domains of responsiveness can be observed, dignity is more related to individual perception. This mirrors the domains of health where some domains can be observed, e.g. mobility, and some cannot, e.g. pain. Accordingly, a more appropriate approach to measuring responsiveness is to ask individuals to report on their experiences using some form of questionnaire, including more than one question (item) on each domain, each of which permits an answer (response) with an unequivocal interpretation (increasing or decreasing responsiveness).

Overall responsiveness is then a multidimensional construct measured at the level of the individual, where scores on each domain are retrieved from individuals and combined into a composite number. This assumes there is some continuum of combined scores which has directionality—the higher the combined score, the higher (or lower) the responsiveness, where "higher" or "lower" refer to a technical choice of the anchors at either side of the scale. This approach builds on a long tradition of "latent constructs" in the social sciences (*98–100*).

FORMALIZING THE MEASUREMENT OF RESPONSIVENESS

In any time period, people can be classified as having the following types of experiences with the health system which serves them:

- inpatient care (hospitals and other long-term care institutions);

- outpatient or ambulatory care;

- interactions with the system that do not involve delivery of personal care, such as public health interventions, health insurance claims, etc.;

- some combination of these experiences;

- none of the above.

An important question is how to treat people who have no interactions with the health system in a given time period. These people can be classified as those who needed care but did not receive it for some reason, and those who did not need care in the time period. Expert meetings on the concept of responsiveness concluded that non-users of the health system who should have received care should be included, on the grounds that their omission would produce an overall responsiveness index without face validity (*49*). It would allow, for example, the average responsiveness of a system that excludes a large proportion of its population from obtaining care, but which is very responsive to the minority of the population who receives care, to be higher than that of a system which does not exclude anyone, but which is not able to be as responsive to each person.

This implies that *health system responsiveness is defined for the counterfactual scenario in which all people who needed to interact with the system in any time period did so.* People who needed care, but did not receive it—here called "denied users"—would be included in the analysis. This requires some way of measuring a responsiveness score for them.

One possibility is to rate responsiveness on each domain as zero for these people. Another is to try to determine the level of responsiveness considered so bad that people would prefer to avoid seeking care, and to use this as the score for patients who did not

use health services because of their poor responsiveness. This would require the ability to separate the different causes of non-use in people requiring care and is the subject of continuing work, but at this stage, zero is used as the responsiveness score for these people on each domain. Methods for estimating the coverage of care in the counterfactual case of people not being excluded for reasons of cost, distance, or cultural acceptability, are discussed in Shengelia et al. (*101*).

THE LEVEL OF HEALTH SYSTEM RESPONSIVENESS

Responsiveness to an Individual

Having defined the different groups of people whose experiences should be represented in any measure of population responsiveness, the first step to measuring responsiveness encompasses the aggregation of responses to question items on a particular domain for a given interaction or contact c:

$$d_{icj} = f(x_{icj1}, x_{icj2}, \ldots, x_{icjn}), \qquad [1]$$

where x_{icjk} refers to respondent i's response to encounter c, on the jth domain and for the kth item (where there are n items). Hence d_{icj} is the domain result for individual i for encounter c on domain j. The f function includes a process of adjustment for the differential use of cut-points or response options, within and across countries, described subsequently. On this basis, d_{icj} is interval-scaled. Next, the responsiveness score for individual i during interaction $c - r_{ic}$ can be expressed as:

$$r_{ic} = g(d_{ic1}, d_{ic2}, \ldots, d_{icm}) \qquad [2]$$

where g is an aggregation function of domain scores 1 to m. This function could be a global, country-specific, or individual-specific aggregation function, or it could be specific to a particular type of encounter, e.g. the relative weights of the various domains might differ for outpatient and inpatient encounters. However, for the purposes of exposition, we retain a single aggregation function g. Conventionally the g function comprises some weighted or unweighted summation procedure, but it may also include some transformation function of item scores, or of the resulting domain scores (e.g. normalizing). We argue that the weights should be determined by the preferences expressed by the population, and a description of how this has been operationalized using nationally representative sample surveys is found in Valentine and Salomon (*102*).

The experience of each individual across q different encounters (c), or the individual's overall responsiveness score, r_i, can be denoted as:

$$r_i = h(r_{i1}, r_{i2}, \ldots, r_{iq}) \qquad [3]$$

where h is the aggregation function across all the individual's contacts during a given time period.

There are many possible ways to aggregate responses over these contacts described in function h. The guiding principles are:

- that weights used in the aggregation process should be a function of the importance of each event to the individuals;

- the importance of each contact or interaction (as opposed to domain importance described by function g in equation [2]) is some monotonic function of the duration of the contact with the system—the longer the interaction, the greater the weight given to the responsiveness score for that interaction. Importance might also be influenced by factors such as perceived severity or the nature of the event.

One strategy would be to treat all contacts or interactions equally, but this would give equal weight to encounters lasting five minutes and those lasting five days. It would also give equal weight to an inpatient stay of 30 days and an application for health insurance lasting 20 minutes. It would violate the principles described above. An alternative would be to base the aggregation function on the time spent in each encounter. In that case, r_{ic} would be multiplied by the proportion of the individual's total contact time in period t contributed by contact c.

Yet another approach would be to base weights on expressed preferences of the population as suggested for weighting function g in equation [2]. This might involve asking individuals to weight the importance of their different interactions with the health system in any given period.

The responsiveness scores would be zero for the group of individuals who needed to interact with the system but were not able to do so. However, some people might have received some care, but been "denied" other types of interactions, raising the question of how to develop time-based weights for the different types of interactions in those cases. For the denied interactions, the average time per encounter for that type of interaction in the population who received it, could be used as the weight.

Health System Responsiveness

The population responsiveness score, R, would be the combination of the individual responsiveness scores for the p individuals in the system and can be expressed as:

$$R = y(r_1, r_2, \ldots, r_p) \qquad [4]$$

where y is an aggregation function.

If the system responsiveness to all individuals counted equally, the aggregation would be:

$$R = \sum_i^p r_i / p \qquad [5]$$

where p is the number of people with at least one contact with the system during the period, plus the denied users. As shown earlier, this would give equal weight to the system's responsiveness to someone who had used the system for five minutes during period t, and to someone who was hospitalized for a large part of the time. On the other hand, a purely time-based weighting system, analogous to that described for function h in equation [3], could be defined. The weight attached to each individual's responsiveness score r_i would be the proportion of total population contact time contributed by that individual during period t. (Population contact time would include the contact time that should have been attributed to denied users.)

The disadvantage of this approach when aggregating across individuals is that the length of a particular interaction in some countries is correlated with insurance status, income, or social standing, independent of severity. It would mean that system responsiveness to the insured or the rich, for example, would count more in the overall responsiveness index than that of the poor, whose interactions for identical conditions have shorter duration. A modified time-based approach in which the weights were based on the time for each encounter under the counterfactual that all people receive standard, good quality attention for that encounter would overcome this problem. Ways of applying this approach to aggregation functions h (equation [3]) and y (equation [4]) are being explored.

In addition to being defined at the population level (equation [4]), responsiveness can be defined for each individual (equation [3]). It could also be defined for a particular type of institution (e.g. hospitals) by limiting the analysis of equation [3] to people who had contact with that institution. Or it could be analysed for particular types of contacts with the system, e.g. outpatient contacts, or contacts with the administrative system, by restricting the focus of c in the equations to those contacts. This gives responsiveness major practical value in the eyes of policy-makers at all levels of the system.

INEQUALITY IN RESPONSIVENESS

The WHO performance assessment framework focuses attention not only on the average level, but also on inequalities in health system responsiveness. Inequalities can be assessed by considering the distribution of responsiveness scores across individuals (r_i). Total inequalities in responsiveness can be measured using one of the available summary measures of the dispersion of the distribution, such as the coefficient of variation (103). In addition, the characteristics of the individuals in the lower tail can help to identify vulnerable or marginalized groups, as well as allow the analysis of responsiveness to particular groups, such as the poor, women, or ethnic minorities.

PRACTICAL LIMITATIONS AND SOLUTIONS

For the World Health Survey, it was not possible to ask respondents about all their interactions with the health system in the past year. Neither has a method been devised to examine the responsiveness of non-personal interactions, such as public health interventions delivered through the media. Attention was focused on inpatient and outpatient encounters. Respondents were asked if they 1) had inpatient care in the previous five years, and 2) had ambulatory care in the the previous year. Respondents reporting care in both settings were asked to report on inpatient care only.

All respondents reporting encounters were asked about the most recent experience. The assumption is that the responsiveness derived for each individual and for each encounter represents the responsiveness to that person for all similar encounters during the time period. The survey contains information on effective coverage and whether respondents were not able to access services for some reason. The responses to those questions will be used to assess if it is possible to identify denied users. With this information, the final weighting function for the three types of experiences will be decided, taking into account the utilization patterns in the different settings.

MEASUREMENT VALIDITY, COMPARABILITY AND RELIABILITY

Household surveys are the most feasible means of collecting information on patient experiences. In order to do this, each domain of responsiveness needs to be a sufficiently coherent construct that can be measured using a cardinal or ordinal scale. The questionnaire approach in which respondents are asked to categorize their experiences into specific response categories,

assumes that there is a true or latent scale for each domain. The measurement and analytical approach for transforming the categorical responses to a continuous scale are discussed in detail elsewhere (104).

Validity can only be established in an indirect way. In the context of measurement of a latent variable at the individual level, specific questions have been shown to ensure greater validity than general ones (55). For example, in the question on choice, the general version of the question would be to ask if the respondent feels free to choose his/her provider, whereas the specific form is to ask whether the respondent was free to choose the desired health provider the last time he/she sought care. The specific form of asking about the most recent encounter has been used in the instruments developed by WHO to measure responsiveness. In addition, observation studies are currently being conducted using the facility surveys described in Annex 43.2. These studies have been designed to test for validity.

The measurement approach used in the two recent WHO population survey studies (WHO Multi-country Survey Study on Health and Responsiveness 2000–2001 and the World Health Survey) requires respondents to rate their interaction with the system into different categories. Other questions called "vignettes" also make respondents characterize a standard set of hypothetical stories into categories. These two pieces of information help to determine the individual's cut-points. A cut-point is a technical term describing the quality of the experience that causes a respondent to change his/her evaluation of the experience from one category to another. The implicit cut-points used by people in their responses might differ; i.e. for the same experience of being greeted with respect, one respondent might rate the experience "good," while another rates it "very good" on a five category scale ("very good," "good," "moderate," "bad," "very bad"). It is necessary to take this variability into account when aggregating responsiveness across individuals, and comparing it across populations and systems.

Expectations have been defined as an individual's beliefs regarding desired outcomes, which are related to a spectrum of personal experiences (89). While for some people a wait of six months for non-emergency surgery is normal, for others, waiting one month would be unacceptable. WHO has introduced the use of vignettes that describe the hypothetical encounter of an individual with the health system, to determine if groups of individuals (for example living in different countries, or those with different levels of education) systematically rate the same scenario differently (*104*). This technique has been also applied by Campbell to identify whether a patient's perception of medical urgency was influenced by his/her socio-economic condition (*105*). A systematic difference in the use of cut-points across individuals or groups can be captured and used to adjust the responses on the individual's own experience to make them comparable with the responses of others. These vignettes also assist in identifying cultural differences in how people rate experiences using categorical scales, and ensure that the final measure of responsiveness can be compared across populations.

Reliability has several faces: the repeatability of scores for the same individual at different points in time, between the individual and an observer, and between two ways of data collection for the same individual. The stability of the concept or its components can also give clues to reliability: for example, do the responses to all questions relating to one domain show the same pattern?

In order to maximize reliability, an extensive process of instrument development was undertaken, involving field-testing as well as consultations with experts (*106*). Item selection took place over a period of three years and included testing in more than 60 countries as part of the WHO Multi-country Survey Study on Health and Responsiveness. The psychometric properties of the responsiveness items used in that study (*107*) were evaluated with additional help from outside experts. Ten of the fifteen items used in the Multi-country Survey Study were found to need only minor changes in wording. Five new items were added and a revised responsiveness module incorporating them was tested in a six-country pilot study. The module was then finalized using a combination of information on psychometric properties and qualitative information from cognitive interviews in the six countries. The wording of some items was changed slightly based on an assessment of face validity of the responses, and some of the items that duplicated common themes but used different response options were dropped (a list of the Multi-country Survey Study questions is given in Annex 43.1). Table 43.2 shows the items covered in the World Health Survey.

There are other challenges in designing any questionnaire, particularly one that will be used in different cultural settings. For example, it is important to establish partially overlapping questions (items) for any domain which permit an answer (response) with an unequivocal interpretation (increasing or decreasing responsiveness). To do this in a way that will have an unequivocal interpretation across cultures is a particular challenge.

A full description of the domain items and a comparison with the Multi-country Survey Study and the World Health Survey is contained in Annex 43.1. Materials related to the World Health Survey are also available (*51*). Domain validity checks inserted in the responsiveness module are available for the domains of choice, dignity, prompt attention, and quality of basic amenities (see Annex 43.1 for details). Further studies of validity also form part of the facility survey exercise described in Annex 43.2.

A final question relates to how system responsiveness to children should be evaluated. On the basis of expert advice (*108*), it was considered acceptable to allow parents to respond for the experience of their children up to the age of 12 years. Accordingly, in the WHO survey instruments, the parent who was present at a child's last encounter with a health provider is asked to report on the child's experience. These responses might be biased if the adult reports on his/her own experiences rather than the ones of the child, but as yet no better way of understanding the system's responsiveness to children is available.

FUTURE DEVELOPMENTS IN MEASURING RESPONSIVENESS

Responsiveness is a new concept. Although it builds on the work of the patient satisfaction and quality of care literature, its measurement within and across countries is in its infancy. Work is continuing, for example, to determine how best to measure responsiveness for individuals who have had multiple contacts with the health system in a given time period, and for denied users. Some additional questions and qualifications are also important.

First, individuals can have a limited vision of domain performance for some domains so their self-reports might not fully reflect system responsiveness. For example, on the domain of confidentiality, patients might know that their conversations with a provider took place in private, but are less likely to know who has access to their medical records.

Second, limited interactions with the system that did not require an inpatient or outpatient visit have not been included in the analysis of responsiveness in the two WHO survey studies. Work is continuing to determine how to evaluate interactions such as applications or claims for health insurance, and population responses to public health interventions such as a media campaign to reduce tobacco con-

Table 43.2 Operationalization of the domains in the World Health Survey 2002

Responsiveness domains		World Health Survey 2002 *
Domain label	Short description	Items for patients and close others (as parents)
Autonomy	Involvement in decisions	* How would you rate your experience of being involved in making decisions about your health care or treatment
		How would you rate your experience of getting information about other types of treatments or tests [I]
Choice	Choice of health care provider	How would you rate the freedom you had to choose the health care providers that attended to you
Communication	Clarity of communication	* How would you rate the experience of how clearly health care providers explained things to you
		* How would you rate your experience of getting enough time to ask questions about your health problem or treatment [I]
Confidentiality	Confidentiality of personal information	* How would you rate the way the health services ensured you could talk privately to health care providers
		* How would you rate the way your personal information was kept confidential [I]
Dignity	Respectful treatment and communication	* How would you rate your experience of being greeted and talked to respectfully
		* How would you rate the way your privacy was respected during physical examinations and treatments [I]
Quality of basic amenities	Surroundings	* How would you rate the cleanliness of the rooms inside the facility, including toilets
		* How would you rate the amount of space you had [I]
Prompt attention	Convenient travel and short waiting times	How would you rate the travelling time to the hospital
		How would you rate the amount of time you waited before being attended to [I]
Access to family and community support	Contact with outside world and maintenance of regular activities	How would you rate the ease of having family and friends visit you
		* How would rate your [child's] experience of staying in contact with the outside world when you [your child] were in hospital [I]

* Similar items appear in the Multi-country Survey Study.

I Item dropped for the short version of the World Health Survey.

sumption or spraying of mosquitoes in city streets or swamps. Finally, responsiveness is valued for its own sake as one of the three intrinsic social goals to which health systems contribute. This section has described a method of measuring this key outcome of health systems. Responsiveness is, however, also instrumental to the achievement of the health goal—people are more likely to seek care and to follow instructions of health providers in a responsive system. The dimensions of prompt attention, dignity and communication may be particularly important in this respect, and interestingly, the respondents to the Multi-country Survey Study questions on the relative importance of responsiveness domains consistently rated these as the most important domains (*102*). Further work is continuing to explore if it can be demonstrated that more responsive systems result in higher levels of population health, holding other determinants constant.

Policy Uses and Challenges

This section is concerned with how information on responsiveness can be used to improve health systems. The first part focuses on the use of the nationally representative information that is currently being collected through the World Health Survey. The second considers the trade-off between undertaking nationally representative population surveys and obtaining information at the facility level. The third outlines several remaining policy challenges.

Uses of National Responsiveness Information

The first use for this type of information is at the political level. The Multi-country Survey Study asked respondents in 61 countries to rate the relative importance of responsiveness, health, and the fairness in household financial contribution. Responsiveness was rated as being only slightly less important than health and more important than fairness in financial contribution (*108*). Intermittent surveys provide people with the opportunity to outline their experiences with the system, and policy-makers and politicians are then in a position to improve health systems performance. The surveys would show which domains were most critical to improve, allowing policy to be developed that is specific to a particular country, region, or population group.

Second, information on inequalities in responsiveness can be used to direct system resources to worse-served populations. Because responsiveness may be instrumental to health, this would improve not only responsiveness, but also health.

Source of Information: National Population Surveys versus Facility Level Surveys

These two sources of information are not mutually exclusive, having different uses, costs, and implications for ensuring validity. Household surveys have three main advantages over facility surveys. First, confidentiality of information can be more difficult to assure in facility-based surveys because facility users might be hesitant to describe their true experiences for fear of being recognized with adverse consequences. Second, facility surveys cannot provide information on non-users and reasons for non-use. Finally, they do not allow interactions between the population and aspects of the health system which are not based at curative facilities to be explored, such as public health interventions.

On the other hand, a facility survey allows a more in-depth exploration of interactions between patients and provider, and can be less expensive. There can also be a much closer link between the measurement of performance and changing the behaviour of providers in a way that will improve responsiveness. Because of the usefulness of both approaches, WHO has developed two types of instruments: a household survey module and a facility survey module. The latter is still in the early testing phases. More details on both types of survey instruments, as well as on the key informant survey instrument are found in Annex 43.2.

Challenges

In spite of the vast body of literature on patient satisfaction and quality of care, there remain a number of challenges for the quantification of the population's experiences with the health system and the introduction of policies to improve responsiveness. Questions relating to measurement were discussed earlier.

On the policy side, improving responsiveness will require understanding the linkages between training, provider payment incentives, and working environments. The role of incentives versus more coercive arrangements to improve responsiveness, such as legislation and professional guidelines, also requires exploration. One option might be the establishment of a responsiveness Ombudsperson to compile information on the state of health system responsiveness and to receive and investigate complaints. The Ombudsperson could make national, subnational, or even disease-specific information available to decision-makers and to the general population.

WHO has recently embarked on a project to develop analytical guidelines for empowering governments to undertake independent policy-relevant analyses of the responsiveness of their health systems. Other approaches for institutionalizing the measurement and use of responsiveness information, and translating them into actions to improve health systems performance, will emerge as research in this field deepens.

Acknowledgements

The authors would like to acknowledge the contributions of Gouke J. Bonsel, Juan Pablo Ortiz, René Lavallée, Ritu Sadana, Geneviève Pinet, Richard Poe, Helena Nygren-Krug, and Daniel Wikler (Harvard School of Public Health), and the panel of ethicists he assembled to discuss the ethics perspective on the domains.

Notes

1 An important step to refining the choice and meaning of domains was the use of cognitive testing at survey sites in seven countries in July–August 2000, as a follow-up to pilot household surveys undertaken in these countries. They included a total of 171 respondents from China, Egypt, Georgia, India, Indonesia, Nigeria, and Slovakia. Individuals were asked open-ended questions to give their definition of the domains used in the survey.

2 The original selection of responsiveness domains based on the review of literature and questionnaires (*47*) did not include communication as a separate domain, but included elements of communication under both the domains of dignity and autonomy. The expert meeting in December 1999 recommended that it be considered as a separate domain and after further review, this was

done in mid-2000 and incorporated into the WHO Multi-country Survey Study questionnaire.

3 This domain was previously titled "access to social support networks."

4 The Siracusa principles on the limitation and derogation provisions in the international covenant on civil and political rights comprise: (Reference: UN Doc. E/CN.4/1985/4)

- The restriction is provided for and carried out in accordance with the law;
- The restriction is in the interest of a legitimate objective of general interest;
- The restriction is strictly necessary to achieve the objective;
- There are no less intrusive and restrictive means available to reach the same objective;
- The restriction is provided for and carried out in accordance with the law;
- The restriction is not drafted or imposed arbitrarily, i.e. in an unreasonable or otherwise discriminatory manner.

5 See, for example URL: http://www.patientconcern.org.uk.

REFERENCES

(1) Donabedian A. *Explorations in quality assessment and monitoring: the definition of quality and approaches to assessment.* Ann Arbor, Health Administration Press, 1980.

(2) Hulka BS et al. Scale for the measurement of attitudes toward physicians and primary medical care. *Medical Care*, 1970, 8:429–436.

(3) Hulka BS et al. Satisfaction with medical care in a low income population. *Journal of Chronic Diseases*, 1971, 24:661–673.

(4) Tessler R, Mechanic D. Consumer satisfaction with prepaid group practice: a comparative study. *Journal of Health and Social Behavior*, 1975, 16:95–113.

(5) Ware Jr JE et al. Defining and measuring patient satisfaction with medical care. *Evaluation and Program Planning*, 1983, 6:247–263.

(6) Agency for Healthcare Research and Quality (AHRQ). *CAHPS 2.0 survey and reporting kit.* Rockville, Agency for Healthcare Research and Quality, 1999.

(7) Murray CJL, Frenk J. A framework for assessing the performance of health systems. *Bulletin of the World Health Organization*, 2000, 78:717–731.

(8) World Health Organization. *The World Health Report 2000. Health Systems: Improving Performance.* Geneva, World Health Organization, 2000.

(9) Haddad S, Fournier P, Potvin P. Measuring lay perceptions of the quality of primary health care services in developing countries. Validation of a 20 item scale. *International Journal for Quality in Health Care*, 1998, 10:93–104.

(10) Applied Research Corporation. *Patient feedback survey (executive summary) prepared for Casemix task force, Ministry of Health, Singapore & Health Corporation of Singapore.* Applied Research Corporation, 1999.

(11) Lim HC et al. Why do patients complain? A primary health care study. *Singapore Medical Journal*, 1998, 39(9):390–395.

(12) Palmer N et al. A new face for private providers in developing countries: what implications for public health? *Bulletin of the World Health Organization*, 2003, 81(4): 292–297.

(13) Kelley E, Boucar M. *Helping district teams measure and act on client satisfaction data in Niger.* Operations Research Results 1(1). Published for the U.S. Agency for International Development (USAID) by the Quality Assurance Project (QAP), Bethesda, 1998. URL: http://www.qaproject.org/

(14) Monawar HGM, Chattterjee N. Health-care utilization by disabled persons: A survey in rural Bangladesh. *Disability and Rehabilitation*, 1998, 20:337–345.

(15) Chimere-Dan GC. Public views on community involvement in local health services in South Africa. *Public Health*, 1997, 111:399–404.

(16) Paul S. *Making voice work: the report card on Bangalore's public services.* Bangalore, Public Affairs Centre, 1998.

(17) Singh H, Mustapha N, Haqq ED. Patient satisfaction at health centres in Trinidad and Tobago. *Public Health*, 1996, 110:251–255.

(18) Scarpaci JL. Help-seeking behavior, use, and satisfaction among frequent primary care users in Santiago de Chile. *Journal of Health and Social Behavior*, 1988, 29: 199–213.

(19) Newman RD et al. Satisfaction with outpatient health care services in Manica Province, Mozambique. *Health Policy and Planning*, 1998, 13(2):174–180.

(20) El Shabrawy A, Eisa AM. A study of patient satisfaction with primary health care services in Saudi Arabia. *Journal of Community Health*, 1993, 18(3):49–54.

(21) Kasalova H et al. Development of patient satisfaction surveys in the Czech Republic: a new approach to an old theme. *International Journal for Quality in Health Care*, 1994, 6:383–388.

(22) Salomon JA et al. Quantifying individual levels of health: definitions, concepts, and measurement issues. In: Murray CJL, Evans DB, eds. *Health systems performance*

assessment: debates, methods and empiricism. Geneva, World Health Organization, 2003.

(23) Williams B. Patient satisfaction: a valid concept? *Social Science & Medicine*, 1994, 38:509–516.

(24) Blumenthal D. Part 1: Quality of care—what is it? *The New England Journal of Medicine*, 1996, 335: 891–893.

(25) Van Campen C et al. Assessing patients priorities and perceptions of the quality of health care. The development of the QUOTE-Rheumatic patients instrument. *British Journal of Rheumatology*, 1998, 37:362–368.

(26) Kenagy JW, Berwick DM, Shore MF. Service quality in health care. *The Journal of the American Medical Association*, 1999, 281:661–665.

(27) Haas-Wilson D. The relationships between the dimensions of health care quality and price: the case of eye care. *Medical Care*, 1994, 32:175–183.

(28) Evans DB et al. Measuring quality: from the system to the provider. *International Journal for Quality in Health Care*, 2001, 13(6):439–446.

(29) Mansour AA, Muneera H, Al-Osimy RN. A study of satisfaction among primary health care patients in Saudi Arabia. *Journal of Community Health*, 1993, 18: 163–173.

(30) Ottosson B et al. Patients' satisfaction with surgical care impaired by cuts in expenditure and after interventions to improve nursing care at a surgical clinic. *International Journal for Quality Health Care*, 1997, 9(1): 43–53.

(31) Center for Studying Health System Change. *Design and methods for the community tracking study.* Washington, DC, Center for Studying Health System change, 2003. URL: http://www.hschange.com/index.cgi?data=01

(32) Pascoe GC, Attkisson CC. The evaluation ranking scale: a new methodology for assessing satisfaction. *Evaluation and Program Planning*, 1983, 6:335–347.

(33) Jenkinson C, Coulter A, Bruster S. The Picker Patient Experience Questionnaire: development and validation using data from in-patient surveys in five countries. *International Journal for Quality in Health Care*, 2002, 14:353–358.

(34) Cleary PD et al. Patients evaluate their hospital care: a national survey. *Health Affairs*, 1991, 10:254–267.

(35) Coulter A, Cleary PD. Patients' experiences with hospital care in five countries. *Health Affairs*, 2001, 20: 244–252.

(36) Crofton C, Lubalin JS, Darby C. Consumer Assessment of Health Plans Study CAHPS. *Medical Care*, 1999, 37.

(37) McKinley RK et al. Reliability and validity of a new measure of patient satisfaction with out of hours primary medical care in the United Kingdom: development of a patient questionnaire. *British Medical Journal*, 1997, 314:193.

(38) Blendon RJ et al. Satisfaction with health systems in ten nations. *Health Affairs*, 1990,185–192.

(39) Wilkin D, Hallam L, Doggett MA. *Measures of need and outcome for primary health care.* Oxford, New York, Oxford University Press, 1992.

(40) Smith C. Validation of a patient satisfaction system in the United Kingdom. *Quality Assurance in Health Care*, 1992, 4:171–177.

(41) Harris-Kojetin LD. The use of cognitive testing to develop and evaluate CAHPS 1.0 core survey items. *Medical Care*, 1999, 37:MS10–MS21.

(42) Avis M, Bond M, Arthur A. Questioning patient satisfaction: an empirical investigation in two outpatient clinics. *Social Science & Medicine*, 1997, 44:85–92.

(43) Hall JA et al. Satisfaction, gender, and communication in medical visits. *Medical Care*, 1994, 32:1216–1223.

(44) Murphy-Cullen CL, Larsen LC. Interaction between the socio-demographic variables of physicians and their patients: its impact upon patient satisfaction. *Social Science & Medicine*, 1984, 19:163–166.

(45) Blendon RJ, Kim M, Benson JM. The public versus the World Health Organization on health system performance. Who is better qualified to judge health care systems: public health experts or the people who use the healthcare? *Health Affairs*, 2001, 20:10–20.

(46) Murray CJL, Kawabata K, Valentine NB. People's experience versus people's expectations. Satisfaction measures are profoundly influenced by people's expectations, say these WHO researchers. *Health Affairs*, 2001, 20:21–24.

(47) de Silva A. *A framework for measuring responsiveness.* EIP Discussion Paper No. 32. Geneva, World Health Organization, 2000. URL: http://www3.who.int/whosis/discussion_papers/discussion_papers.cfm#

(48) World Health Organization. Technical Consultation on Concepts and Methods for Measuring the Responsiveness of Health Systems. In: Murray CJL, Evans DB, eds. *Health systems performance assessment: debates, methods and empiricism.* Geneva, World Health Organization, 2003.

(49) Anand S et al. Report of the Scientific Peer Review Group on Health Systems Performance Assessment. In: Murray CJL, Evans DB, eds. *Health systems performance assessment: debates, methods and empiricism.* Geneva, World Health Organization, 2003.

(50) Üstün TB et al. WHO Multi-country Survey Study on Health and Responsiveness 2000–2001. In: Murray CJL, Evans DB, eds. *Health systems performance assessment:*

debates, methods and empiricism. Geneva, World Health Organization, 2003.

(51) World Health Organization. *World Health Survey.* Geneva, World Health Organization, 2003. URL: http://www3.who.int/whs/

(52) Allen RE, ed. *The Concise Oxford Dictionary of Current English.* New York, Oxford University Press, 1990.

(53) Vesey G, Foulkes P. *Unwin Hyman Dictionary of Philosophy.* Glasgow, Harper Collins, 1999.

(54) Hebert PC. *Doing right—a practical guide to ethics for medical trainees and physicians.* Oxford, Oxford University Press, 1996.

(55) Sitzia J, Wood N. Patient satisfaction: a review of issues and concepts. *Social Science & Medicine,* 1997, 45: 1829–1843.

(56) Darvall L. *Medicine, law and social change: the impact of bioethics, feminism and rights movements on medical decision-making.* Aldershot, Brookfield, Dartmouth Publishing Company, 1993.

(57) Charles C, Gafni A, Whelen T. Shared decision making in the medical encounter: what does it mean? (or it takes at least two to tango). *Social Science & Medicine,* 1997, 44:681–692.

(58) Kersnik J. Determinants of customer satisfaction with the health care system, with the possibility to choose a personal physician and with a family doctor in a transition country. *Health Policy,* 2001, 57:155–164.

(59) Collins H. Patient satisfaction surveys. *Hospital Practice* (15 November 1996):39–45.

(60) Ezeji PN, Sarvela PD. Health-care behavior of the Ibo tribe of Nigeria. *Health Values,* 1992, 16(6):31–35.

(61) Anell A, Rosén P, Hjortsberg C. Choice and participation in the health services: a survey of preferences among Swedish residents. *Health Policy,* 1997, 40:157–168.

(62) Bruster S et al. National survey of hospital patients. *British Medical Journal,* 2002, 309:1542–1546.

(63) Grol R, Wensing M, Mainz J. Patients priorities with respect to general practice care: an international comparison. *Family Practice,* 1999, 16:4–11.

(64) Little P et al. Observational study of effect of patient centredness and positive approach on outcomes of general practice consultations. *British Medical Journal,* 2001, 323:908–911.

(65) Coulter A, Entwistle V, Gilbert D. Sharing decisions with patients: is the information good enough? *British Medical Journal,* 1999, 318:318–322.

(66) Gross DA et al. Patient satisfaction with time spent with their physician. *Journal of Family Practice,* 1998, 47: 133–137.

(67) Coulter A. After Bristol: putting patients at the centre. *British Medical Journal,* 2002, 324:648–651.

(68) Calnan M et al. Major determinants of consumer satisfaction with primary care in different health systems. *Family Practice,* 1994, 11:468–478.

(69) Fadiman A. *The spirit catches you and you fall down: a Hmong child, her American doctors and the collusion of two cultures.* New York, The Noonday Press, 1997.

(70) Lowe M, Hardy Havens DM. Privacy and confidentiality of health information. *Journal of Pediatric Health Care,* 1998, 12:42–46.

(71) Rylance G. Privacy, dignity and confidentiality: interview study with structured questionnaire. *British Medical Journal,* 1999, 318:301.

(72) Anderson RJ. *Security in clinical information systems.* Cambridge, University of Cambridge, 1996. URL: http://www.cl.cam.ac.uk

(73) Denley I, Smith SW. Privacy in clinical information systems in secondary care. *British Medical Journal,* 1999, 318:1328–1330.

(74) Hall JA, Dornan MC. What patients like about their medical care and how often they are asked: a meta-analysis of the satisfaction literature. *Social Science & Medicine,* 1998, 27:935–939.

(75) Gilson L, Alilio M, Heggenhougen K. Community satisfaction with primary health care services: an evaluation undertaken in the Morogoro region of Tanzania. *Social Science & Medicine,* 1994, 39:767–780.

(76) Walsh K, Kowanko I. Nurses' and patients' perceptions of dignity. *International Journal of Nursing Practice,* 2002, 8(3):143–151.

(77) Bassett MT, Bijlmakers L, Sanders DM. Professionalism, patient satisfaction and quality of health care: experience during Zimbabwe's structural adjustment programme. *Social Science & Medicine,* 1997, 45:1845–1852.

(78) Morris NM. Respect: its meaning and measurement as an element of health care. *Journal of Public Health Policy,* 1997, 18:133–154.

(79) Health Canada. *The District of Montreal's Quebec Superior Court Ruling Upholding the Tobacco Act of 1997.* Health Canada, 2003.

(80) Okware SI et al. An outbreak of Ebola in Uganda. *Tropical Medicine & International Health,* 2002, 7: 1068–1075.

(81) Awasthi S, Nichter M, Pande VK. Developing an interactive STD-prevention program for youth: lessons from a north Indian slum. *Studies in Family Planning,* 2000, 31:138–150.

(82) Ware Jr JE, Hays RD. Methods for measuring patient satisfaction with specific medical encounters. *Medical Care,* 1988, 26:393–402.

(83) Lim HC et al. Why do patients complain ? A primary health care study. *Singapore Medical Journal*, 1998, 39: 390–395.

(84) Blendon RJ et al. Inequalities in health care: a five-country study. *Health Affairs*, 2002, 21:182–191.

(85) Ariff KM, Teng CL. Rural health care in Malaysia. *Rural Health*, 2002, 10:99–103.

(86) Mendoza Aldana J, Piechulek H, Al-Sabir A. Client satisfaction and quality of health care in rural Bangladesh. *Bulletin of the World Health Organization*, 2001, 79: 512–517.

(87) Minnick AF et al. What influences patients' reports of three aspects of hospital services? *Medical Care*, 2003, 35:399–409.

(88) Draper M, Hill S. Feasibility of national benchmarking of patient satisfaction with Australian hospitals. *International Journal for Quality in Health Care*, 1996, 8: 457–466.

(89) de Silva A, Valentine NB. *Measuring responsiveness: results of a key informants survey in 35 countries*. EIP Discussion Paper No. 21. Geneva, World Health Organization, 2000. URL: http://www3.who.int/whosis/discussion_papers/discussion_papers.cfm#

(90) Tangcharoensathien V et al. Patient satisfaction in Bangkok: the impact of hospital ownership and patient payment status. *International Journal for Quality in Health Care*, 1999, 11(4):309–317.

(91) Kruse GR, Rohland BM, Wu X. Factors associated with missed first appointments at a psychiatric clinic. *Psychiatric Services*, 2002, 53:1173–1176.

(92) Tekle B, Mariam DH, Ali A. Defaulting from DOTS and its determinants in three districts of Arsi Zone in Ethiopia. *International Journal of Tuberculosis & Lung Disease*, 2002, 6:573–579.

(93) Tomaszewska W et al. Antecedent life events, social supports and response to antidepressants in depressed patients. *Acta Psychiatrica Scandinavica*, 1996, 94: 352–357.

(94) Friedland J, Renwick R, McColl M. Coping and social support as determinants of quality of life in HIV/AIDS. *AIDS Care*, 1996, 8(1):15–31.

(95) Leach E. Our mutual friends. *Nursing Times*, 1999, 95.

(96) Jareg P, Kaseje DCO. World health: growth of civil society in developing countries: implications for health. *The Lancet*, 1998, 351:819–822.

(97) Gostin L, et al. *The domains of health responsiveness: a human rights assessment*. Geneva, World Health Organization, 2002. URL: http://snow.who.int/whosis_stage/menu.cfm?path=hsr

(98) Campbell A, Converse PE, Rodgers WL. *The quality of American life: perceptions, evaluations, and satisfactions*. New York, Russell Sage Foundation, 1976.

(99) Salomon JA et al. *Methods for life expectancy and healthy life expectancy uncertainty analysis*. EIP Discussion Paper No.10. Geneva, World Health Organization, 2001. URL: http://www3.who.int/whosis/discussion_papers/discussion_papers.cfm#

(100) World Health Organization. WHO Meetings of Experts on Measuring and Summarizing Health. In: Murray CJL, Evans DB, eds. *Health systems performance assessment: debates, methods and empiricism*. Geneva, World Health Organization, 2003.

(101) Shengelia B, Murray CJL, Adams OB. Beyond access and utilization: defining and measuring health system coverage. In: Murray CJL, Evans DB, eds. *Health systems performance assessment: debates, methods and empiricism*. Geneva, World Health Organization, 2003.

(102) Valentine NB, Salomon JA. Weights for responsiveness domains: analysis of country variation in 65 national sample surveys. In: Murray CJL, Evans DB, eds. *Health systems performance assessment: debates, methods and empiricism*. Geneva, World Health Organization, 2003.

(103) Ortiz JP et al. Inequality in responsiveness: population surveys from 16 OECD countries. In: Murray CJL, Evans DB, eds. *Health systems performance assessment: debates, methods and empiricism*. Geneva, World Health Organization, 2003.

(104) Tandon A et al. Statistical models for enhancing cross-population comparability. In: Murray CJL, Evans DB, eds. *Health systems performance assessment: debates, methods and empiricism*. Geneva, World Health Organization, 2003.

(105) Campbell JL. General practitioner appointment systems, patient satisfaction and use of accident and emergency services—a study in one geographical area. *Family Practice*, 2000, 11:438–445.

(106) Valentine NB et al. Classical psychometric assessment of the responsiveness instrument in the WHO Multi-country Survey Study on Health and Responsiveness 2000–2001. In: Murray CJL, Evans DB, eds. *Health systems performance assessment: debates, methods and empiricism*. Geneva, World Health Organization, 2003.

(107) World Health Organization. *Background Paper for the Technical Consultation on Responsiveness Concepts and Measurement*. Geneva, World Health Organization, 2001. URL: http://snow.who.int/whosis_stage/hsr/hsr_consultation/hsr_consultation_paper.pdf

(108) Gakidou E, Murray CJL, Evans DB. Quality and equity: preferences for health system outcomes. In: Murray CJL, Evans DB, eds. *Health systems performance assessment: debates, methods and empiricism*. Geneva, World Health Organization, 2003.

COMPARISON OF RESPONSIVENESS DOMAIN QUESTIONS TO RESPONDENTS ABOUT THEIR OWN EXPERIENCES IN THE MCSS AND THE WHS

Responsiveness domains		World Health Survey 2002*		Multi-country Survey Study
Domain label	Short description	Items for patients and close others (as parents)	Items used for internal validity checks	Items for patients
Autonomy	Involvement in decisions	*How would you rate your experience of being involved in making decisions about your health care or treatment? How would you rate your experience of getting information about other types of treatments or tests?	How would you rate the way health care in your country involves you in deciding what services it provides and where it provides them?	How often did doctors, nurses or other health care providers involve you in deciding about the care, treatment or tests? How often did doctors, nurses or other health care providers ask your permission before starting the treatment or tests? Rate your experience of getting involved in making decisions about your care or treatment.
Choice	Choice of health care provider	How would you rate the freedom you had to choose the health care providers that attended to you?	Thinking of the last time you needed to see a health care provider who could treat your condition, how many were there around who you could chose from?	Health care providers available to you, how big a problem, if any, was it to get a health care provider you were happy with? How big a problem, if any, was it to get to use other health services other than the one you usually went to? How would you rate your experience of being able to use a health care provider or service of your choice?
Communication	Clarity of communication	*How would you rate the experience of how clearly health care providers explained things to you? *How would you rate your experience of getting enough time to ask questions about your health problem or treatment?		How often did doctors, nurses or other health care providers listen carefully to you? *How often did doctors, nurses or other health care providers, explain things in a way you could understand? *How often did doctors, nurses or other health care providers give you time to ask questions about your health problem or treatment? Rate your experience of how well health care providers communicated with you in the last 12 months.
Confidentiality	Confidentiality of personal information	*How would you rate the way the health services ensured you could talk privately to health care providers? *How would you rate the way your personal information was kept confidential?		How often were talks with your doctor, nurse or other health care provider done privately so other people who you did not want to hear could not overhear what was said? How often did your doctor, nurse or other health care provider keep your personal information confidential? This means that anyone whom you did not want informed could not find out about your medical conditions.

Responsiveness domains		World Health Survey 2002*		Multi-country Survey Study
Domain label	Short description	Items for patients and close others (as parents)	Items used for internal validity checks	Items for patients
Dignity	Respectful treatment and communica-tion	*How would you rate your experience of being greeted and talked to respectfully? *How would you rate the way your privacy was respected during physical examinations and treatments?	Discrimination (were you treated worse because of….sex, religion, etc.?)	How often did doctors, nurses or other health care providers treat you with respect? How often did the office staff, such as receptionists or clerks there, treat you with respect? How often were your physical exami-nations and treatments done in a way that your privacy was respected? How would you rate your experience of being treated with dignity?
Quality of basic amenities	Surroundings	*How would you rate the cleanliness of the rooms inside the facility, including toilets? *How would you rate the amount of space you had?	How many people slept in the same room as you (inpatient only)?	How would you rate the basic quality of the waiting room, for example, space, seating and fresh air? How would you rate the cleanliness of the place? How would you rate the quality of the surroundings, for example, space, seating, fresh air and cleanliness of the health services?
Prompt attention	Convenient travel and short waiting times	How would you rate the travelling time? How would you rate the amount of time you waited before being attended to?	Did you not seek health care because... you were denied health care?.. How long did it take you to get there (in minutes)? How did you get there?..	How often did you get care as soon as you wanted? How would you rate your experience of getting prompt attention at the health services?
Access to family and community support	Contact with outside world and maintenance of regular activities	How would you rate the ease of having family and friends visit you? *How would you rate your [child's] experience of staying in contact with the outside world when you [your child] were in hospital?		How big a problem, if any, was it to get the hospital to allow your family and friends to take care of your personal needs, such as bringing you your favou-rite food, soap etc..? How big a problem, if any, was it to have the hospital allow you to practice religious or traditional observances if you wanted to? How would you rate your experi-ence of how the hospital allowed you to interact with family, friends and to continue your social and/or religious customs?

* Similar items to those in the Multi-country Survey Study

There are four main types of surveys currently being used or tested by WHO to measure responsiveness. They are:

- facility surveys,
- population-based surveys,
- interviewer-administered (face-to-face or by telephone) questionnaires,
- postal/self-administered questionnaires, and
- key informant surveys.

FACILITY SURVEYS

The main purpose of the responsiveness facility survey instrument currently being tested is to compare the respondent's report of care with what is observed or reported on at the facility itself. A secondary purpose of the facility surveys is to assess the correlation of certain aspects of the functions (e.g. stewardship) with responsiveness.

The facility survey consists of four components:

- interview with management,
- interview with staff,
- observation and collection of documentation on patient complaints, and
- exit interviews with patients.

POPULATION-BASED HOUSEHOLD SURVEYS

INTERVIEWER-ADMINISTERED

As responsiveness is best measured by the reporting by individuals of the well-being gained from an interaction with the health system, the household survey instrument is the best mode of capturing this experience. Household surveys usually sample respondents in a probabilistic manner and are nationally representative.

Telephone surveys are also a form of population-based surveys that have been used in the Multi-country Survey Study (50). Like postal surveys, this type of administration is not an option in many middle- and low-income countries where the poorer segments of society do not live in locations with fixed addresses and postal service remains very unreliable. In some countries (middle and high-income countries) telephone surveys are more efficient.

POSTAL/SELF-ADMINISTERED

The postal survey is also designed with the goal of selecting a representative population sample. The main difference between interviewer-administered and self (respondent)-administered surveys is the need to create a visually striking instrument in order to make people answer and hence increase the response rate. This instrument is not an option in many middle- and low-income countries where the poorer segments of society do not live in locations with fixed addresses and postal service remains very unreliable.

KEY INFORMANT SURVEYS

"Key informant" surveys represent a low-cost means of obtaining information on responsiveness. While this information only reflects "expert opinion," work is currently under way to assess the extent to which this opinion may provide a useful prior on health system responsiveness. In addition, key informants may provide information on aspects of responsiveness that are more difficult for the general population to evaluate (e.g. confidentiality of medical records—knowledge of this would require knowledge of the laws of a country and the workings of the health system, information few ordinary citizens have).

Key informant survey respondents can be sampled in a variety of ways (e.g. snowballing, a process whereby the key informant contacted generates a list of other key informants; an air pollution specialist would then give names of other air pollution specialists), but it usually involves non-probabilistic sampling methods. This makes it difficult to analyse with the usual statistical tests for significance.

Chapter 44

Classical Psychometric Assessment of the Responsiveness Instrument in the WHO Multi-country Survey Study on Health and Responsiveness 2000–2001

Nicole B. Valentine, René Lavallée, Bao Liu, Gouke J. Bonsel, Christopher J.L. Murray

Introduction

The purpose of this chapter is to present the psychometric properties of the responsiveness module used in the WHO Multi-country Survey Study 2000–2001. The responsiveness module measured the quality of aspects of the interaction between individuals and the health system that have the potential to improve well-being, focusing on those aspects which are additional to the improvement in health. The concept was developed out of a review of the previous work relating to quality of care, quality of life, and patient satisfaction (1–3). Eight domains of responsiveness were identified, and a questionnaire was developed to explore people's interactions with the health system on these domains: dignity, autonomy, confidentiality of information, communication (of information), prompt attention, quality of basic amenities, access to family and community support,[1] and choice (of health care provider). A full description of the domains is found in de Silva A et al. (4).

Between 2000 and 2001, the responsiveness module (or instrument or questionnaire; these terms are used interchangeably in this chapter) was implemented in a comprehensive household survey in 60 countries (70 surveys[2]). Data collection involved face-to-face and telephone interviews, as well as self-administered interviews. This chapter starts with a brief introduction to the framework adopted to develop the responsiveness instrument. The rest of it focuses on the psychometrics of the questionnaire from the perspective of operational contents (items) and countries, refraining at this stage from an analysis from the perspective of characteristics of individuals (1;5).

The Framework for Instrument Development

The various issues, criteria, and approaches to constructing such an instrument, in particular in the case of health measures, have been well documented (6;7). These issues are presented in Table 44.1. The key assumption of the concept of responsiveness is that the same domains are relevant to everyone, regardless of nation, culture, and stage of economic development. Beyond this assumption, operationalization meets the traditional difficulties associated with translation of value-laden and context-dependent words or language.

The first part of instrument development involves the description and theoretical foundation of the concept, and the item selection for the questionnaire. The theoretical development of the responsiveness concept is described elsewhere and not repeated here (4). To operationalize the concept in a questionnaire, it is necessary to select items and appropriate response categories. Starting with a pilot set of items and a global structure of the questionnaire, the instrument's feasibility, reliability, and validity are established, whereupon the questionnaire may be further improved. This procedure is reiterated until quality is thought to be sufficient. Finally, distributional characteristics of response patterns are established. In questionnaires pertaining to health and health care with intended multinational or cross-cultural use, particular attention should be paid to general applicability and transferability. The word "psychometrics" is used to describe the ultimate quality of the instrument.

The second phase relates to *feasibility*—the ease of administering the instrument in the field and the

Table 44.1   Criteria and approaches for constructing an instrument

Issue	Discriminative criteria	Approaches
Item and response scale selection	1. Tap important components of each domain of responsiveness	1. Theoretical basis/philosophy, literature review, focus group technique
	2. Selection of operationalization theory	2. Check context
	3. Universal applicability to respondents; includes transferability/translatability	3. Specific translation and transcultural comparison protocol
	4. Initial measurement level; absolute versus relative response mode (e.g. trade-off)	4. Qualitative scale, semi-quantitative scale (grading), numerical scales
	5. Source of information	5. Population (sample), representatives, direct observation

Feasibility	1. Technical performance	1. Technical analysis
		  – Time to respond
		  – Missings, skip patterns

	2. Flexibility	2. Suitable for different types of response modes, dependence on external support
Reliability	Stable results across time ("test-retest"), observers, and mode of asking, etc.	All types of analysis of variance, of which standard test-retest kappa metrics are one
Validity	Note: depends on operationalization theory	Two approaches are prevailing, depending on the degree to which the concept is thought to be unidimensional and ranked [classical psychometric analysis vs. item response theory (IRT)]
	1. Construct validity (parallel measures, [dis]similarity in known groups)	1.,2. Testing differences in measures among groups expected to differ, based on hypotheses; this includes convergent and discriminant validity; relevance of size
	2. Criterion (predictive) validity	
	3. Sensitivity of measure (in psychometrical terms we use this word to avoid any confusion with the term "responsiveness" normally used in psychometric literature) to allow interpretation of scale for improvement	3. Self-reported with other measures/indicators of health when available

Adapted from Sadana et al. (2000), Table 1.

instrument's flexibility. Instrument flexibility refers to its suitability to different types of response modes, and the extent to which administering the instrument depends on external features. Using health instruments as an example, the measurement of vision using Snellen-E chart would be affected by the size of the room in which the respondent is interviewed, and these difficulties cannot always be avoided by standardizing procedures. For example, the distance between the respondent and the chart might be too short in some settings where rooms are small. Techniques such as analyses of missing rates, time to administer the questionnaire, and skip patterns, are examples of approaches for assessing technical performance.

The third phase relates to *reliability*. It is desirable for there to be stable and minimal variation in the responses across time and interviewers. Between individuals and between raters, measurement correlation can be estimated using Kappa reliability statistics, K, calculated as:

$$K = \frac{p_o - p_e}{1 - p_e}, \text{ where } p_o = \sum_{i=1}^{k}\sum_{j=1}^{k} w_{ij}p_{ij}, \dots p_e = \sum_{i=1}^{k}\sum_{j=1}^{k} w_{ij}p_{i\cdot}p_{\cdot j}$$

$$\text{and } p_{i\cdot} = \sum_{j} p_{ij}, \dots p_{\cdot j} = \sum_{j} p_{ij}$$

where i is the rating by the first rater and j is the rating by the second rater, p_o the observed proportion of agreement, p_e the expected proportion of agreement, and k is the number of response categories.

$$w = 1 - \left[\frac{(i-j)}{(k-1)}\right]^2$$

is the weight associated with the degree of deviation from a perfect repetition of the rating.

Another type of reliability, also related to construct validity, is the homogeneity of items within the assumed construct or domain. Correlations of scores for items within a domain and between domains provide some information on the extent to which items form part of the same construct. These results should be reviewed in conjunction with other information from qualitative tests including item-concept mapping and cognitive interviews.

The fourth phase relates to *validity*. Several features of validity can be defined. Construct validity refers to the validity of the measure with respect to the original construct. Is the instrument measuring what it is intended to measure? Testing theories of association between the measurement and other known variables can assess this. For example, measured tests of waiting times and distances travelled can be contrasted with reports on prompt attention. Confirmatory factor analysis can also be used to verify whether assumed item-construct models are valid in different populations. Criterion validity refers to the ability of establishing a causal linkage between the measured construct and other variables as hypothesized. As an example, in a laboratory style case-control study, one group of patients could be assigned to health care providers who do not greet them. The differences in the patient's response to questions on how well they were greeted should be causally related to whether or not they were greeted. The final area of validity assessment is the instrument sensitivity (traditionally referred to as "responsiveness" in classical psychometrics) and linkages of the measure to actions for its improvement. The generic approach to conceptualizing, developing, and applying a measurement instrument is discussed here with respect to the responsiveness instrument.

This chapter mainly draws on a conventional approach in matters of feasibility and reliability, and on classical test theory as a general validity approach (6). In the next section, the development of the module contents is briefly summarized. Then the question of feasibility is addressed. In assessing feasibility, criteria established prior to review of the data are tested. Items where the average rate of missing responses across countries exceeded 20%, and countries where the average rate of missing responses across all items exceeded 20% (taking care of the difference between real missing data and blanks due to incorrectly applied skip patterns), were identified as having problems of feasibility.

Reliability is addressed with a straightforward Kappa analysis of test-retest data. Kappa statistics for eight household surveys[3] were summarized and reviewed on an item-by-item basis. This detailed analysis is particularly important and relevant to the process of questionnaire revision. For validity, we reviewed internal domain-item consistency using confirmatory factor analysis. The final section of this paper draws preliminary conclusions and recommends improvements and further psychometric testing that would be useful.

MODULE: CONTENT, ITEMS, AND STRUCTURE

CONTENT

The responsiveness module contained questions on the eight domains of responsiveness. The questions focused on people's encounters with health providers on two levels: encounters with providers occurring at outpatient health services (broadly defined to include any place outside the home where people sought information, advice, or interventions with respect to improving their health), encounters with health providers at home, and encounters with inpatient services (broadly defined to include all places where the respondent stayed overnight for health care). Table 44.2 documents how the domains were operationalized in the self-report sections of the responsiveness instrument.

Non-personal health actions, such as health promotion campaigns (e.g. anti-smoking or HIV awareness campaigns), were not evaluated. Other aspects of health system activities excluded for practical reasons include specific questions on health in the work place, environmental health, the general health administration system, and information about how to access the health system.

ITEMS

The items in the module were developed using two main sources: reviews of existing instruments and field tests of new and adapted items. Part of the work preceding the development of the module used in the WHO Multi-country Survey Study is described elsewhere (3;5;8).

The Agency for Health Research and Quality (AHRQ), a United States Government policy research agency, provided expert advice on item development. As a result, the WHO instrument built on work that had been undertaken by AHRQ since 1995, in collaboration with researchers from the Harvard Medical School, the Research Triangle Institute, and RAND, to develop questionnaires for reporting consumer's assessments of health plans. The instrument they developed became known as the Consumer Assessment of Health PlanS (CAHPS) survey. WHO used and adapted a number of items relevant to the domains of responsiveness that had been identified as reliable

Table 44.2 The operationalization of responsiveness domains in the WHO Multi-country Survey Study

Domain label	Domain operationalization: description of items for measurement of responsiveness at the individual level
Dignity	being shown respect
	having physical examinations conducted in privacy
Autonomy	being involved in deciding on your care or treatment if you want to
	having providers ask your permission before starting treatment or tests
Confidentiality	having your medical history kept confidential
	having conversations with health care providers where other people cannot overhear
Communication	having health care providers listen to you carefully
	having health care providers explain things so you can understand
	giving patients and family time to ask health care providers questions
Prompt attention	having short waiting times for consultations, appointments, and hospital admissions
	having nurses available when needed during hospital stay
	having short waiting times for having tests done
Support	being able to have family and friends bring personally preferred foods, soaps and other things to the hospital during the patient's hospital stay
	being able to observe religious practices during hospital stay
	interacting with family and friends during hospital stay
Quality of basic amenities	having enough space, seating and fresh air in the waiting room or wards
	having a clean facility
Choice	being able to get to see a health care provider you are happy with
	being able to choose the institution to provide your health care

and valid in the development of the CAHPS survey (Annex 44.1).

Table 44.3 summarizes the sections in the responsiveness module according to their main purpose and to whom they were addressed. The wording of the individual items is contained in Annex 44.3 and Annex 44.4. The largest section of the module was on the level of responsiveness reported by respondents using outpatient/ambulatory medical services (30% in the short form of the module and 21% in the extended form). Table 44.3 also shows the difference in items between the short form (SF) and the extended form (EF) of the responsiveness module. There were differences in the number of items on the utilization of services but the items on the domains of responsiveness were the same. Utilization questions comprised 14% of all items in the short version and 20% in the extended one. The extra utilization questions covered the main reason for the most recent visit to a health provider (needed a check-up for an ongoing chronic problem, not sick, went for a general examination or preventive care, etc.), and the service received (examined, received tests, etc.).

The layout of the questionnaire used in the postal survey was different to the other modes, as it was self-administered. Items in the postal survey were formatted to be attractive and easy for respondents to read and answer. Some other factors, like instructions to interviewers and respondents, were also different.

The items in the home care and outpatient sections were identical, except domain items for quality of basic amenities were excluded from the former due to non-relevance. If respondents had experiences of care at home and outpatient care, answers were elicited only on the outpatient section.

Vignettes are short descriptions of people's experiences with health systems as they relate to the different domains of responsiveness. The respondent was asked to report the level of dignity, for example, with which the person in the vignette is being treated, answering on a scale of "very good," "good," "moderate," "bad," "very bad." This information provides a record of differences in the way people use verbal categories to evaluate a common stimulus. For example, one person might categorize the scenario described in the vignette as "good," while another might consider that the same scenario is "very good." In the analysis of the results, responses to vignettes can be used to adjust all respondents' responses onto a common scale. Full details on this method can be

Table 44.3 The number of items in the responsiveness module of the Multi-country Survey Study with a short description of the sections and the targeted respondents

Description of all sections in the responsiveness module	Targeted respondents	Items in short form of instrument (brief, postal and telephone)		Extra items in EF	Items in extended form of instrument (long)	
		number	%	number	number	%
User filter/skips and name of facility last used	All respondents for the first question, then filtering respondents	8	9		8	6
Outpatient domains (7 domains—excludes support)	Respondents who had used outpatient/ambulatory services in the previous 12 months	26	30		26	21
Inpatient domains (8 domains)	Respondents who had used inpatient/hospital services in the previous 12 months	12	14		12	10
Discrimination for reasons of race, sex, etc.	One question with 12 multiple causes of discrimination asked to users; another question asked only to women in the extended form	12	14	1	13	10
Utilization of different types of providers	Three questions with multiple types of providers, reasons for visit and services provided — users only	12	14	13	25	20
Financial barriers to care	One question users only, one question all respondents	1	1	1	2	2
Section for people receiving care in their homes	Users only		0	23	23	18
Importance	All respondents	2	2	1	3	2
Vignettes (56 vignettes in total rotated through 4 sets)	All respondents	14	16		14	11
Total		87	100	39	126	100

found in Tandon et al. (9). Due to the length of these descriptions and the number needed for each domain (there were seven per domain), it was necessary to divide them between respondents to minimize the module length. Four rotations of vignette sets were used. Each set covered two domains (for wording see Annex 44.4).

STRUCTURE

It is useful to describe the structure of the responsiveness module in detail. The focus of responsiveness measurement is to ask people questions about their actual experiences. In the case of health, everyone can be asked questions on their health as everyone experiences some departure from complete health at some point in time. In responsiveness, not everyone has experiences of outpatient and inpatient interactions with the health system in a defined period of time. As these personal interactions were used as the basis for reporting on the health system's responsiveness, the sample of respondents to questions on experiences

was limited by the extent of these contacts over the recall period (12 months). This approach to the measurement of responsiveness differs from many of the population satisfaction or public/patient opinion surveys which ask about the respondent's satisfaction with the system in general, whether or not they were in contact with it recently, and without referring to specific experiences (10). In contrast, in the responsiveness questionnaire, all respondents were asked a series of questions about the relative importance of different domains regardless of their use of the system.

IMPLEMENTATION

In 2000, the WHO Multi-country Survey Study started with a household survey instrument containing the extended responsiveness module in nine countries. The Study was expanded in 2000–2001 with the launch of a further 61 surveys in different modes: long face-to-face (extended form), brief face-to-face (short form), postal (short form), and telephone surveys (short form). The short form had 87 items and the expanded form (EF) had 126. By 2002, all surveys were concluded. A total of 70 surveys containing the responsiveness module were completed, with data available for 65 for this analysis.

RESPONSE RATES AND MISSING ANALYSIS

RESPONSE ACCORDING TO UTILIZATION PROFILE (INPATIENT, OUTPATIENT, AND NO USE)

Data were provided by 119 991 respondents in the 65 surveys at hand, of which 2 442 (2.1%) were considered incomplete, leaving a total of 117 549 completed responses. For a questionnaire to be regarded as complete, at least one of the following questions had to be answered: sex, age, health status, or one of the filter questions (q6000, q6001, q6300). Figure 44.1 shows the breakdown of completed responses by use of services in the previous 12 months: 49.1% had not used any type of service, 41.1% reported using only outpatient services,[4] 8.6% had used both inpatient and outpatient services, and only 1.1% reported using only inpatient services. Non-users did not complete the questions on the domains of responsiveness, but did respond to the sections on the importance of domains and vignettes. The numbers of respondents per country are shown in Annex 44.2.

FEASIBILITY: MISSING RATE ANALYSIS

The item missing rate is defined as the percentage of non-responses to an item, with refusals to answer and responses of "not applicable" and "don't know" included as missing values. In several items in the long and the brief face-to-face surveys, respondents were given these response options, whereas these options did not exist in the self-administered surveys. As a form of sensitivity analysis, missing rates were calculated with and without this recoding, and the rates did not differ substantively. Country missing rates are the average of their item missing rates, excluding those items which already appeared problematic in the item missing analysis (item missing rates greater than 20% across all countries).

Table 44.4 shows the item missing rates averaged across sections of the questionnaire and across countries (equal weight for each country). Table 44.4 is a compressed version of the full table in Annex 44.5, which shows the average rates, by item, for all items. Three questions had missing rates over 20%. The first concerned the number of times the respondents used different types of providers in the last 30 days (general practitioner, specialist, etc.). This question and its corresponding items had an average missing rate of 29%. The second, asked to women, was whether they felt they were treated badly by the health service because of their sex ("yes" or "no"), which had a missing rate

Figure 44.1 Grouping of respondents (completed questionnaires) to responsiveness module

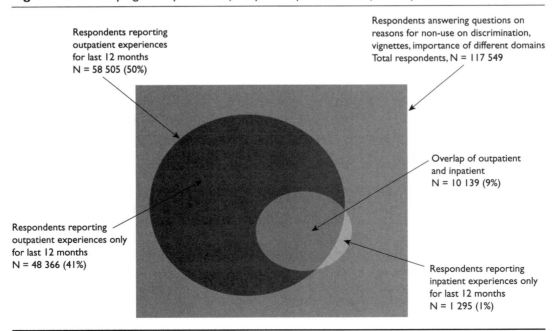

of 41%. Finally, the questions on the services given by the health care provider had an average missing rate of 22%. Excluding these items, the average unweighted missing rate across the others was 4%.

The first two problematic questions seemed to have failed for technical reasons. In the case of the utilization question, if respondents had not visited any of the listed health care providers, there was no clear instruction that they should mark zero. This problem is amenable to technical improvements. In the second case, one problem was that the question had been completed by men as well as women, despite the objective to seek responses from women only. Although the insertion of instructions into the questionnaire and procedural checks might cure this problem, it is not clear why there was such a high missingness for that question. The third problematic question was only asked in the long version of the questionnaire (10 countries). For two thirds of the missings, the respondents answered "not applicable" even if they had used the services. In subsequent analyses of country missing rates, these items are not included.

In the vignette section, the missing rates were surprisingly low. It was anticipated that respondents would have difficulty listening to the stories and drop out, but the missing rate was lower than average at only 3%, with similar performance across domains. This is a promising indication of the feasibility of using vignettes in household surveys, even when questionnaires are self-administered, or when they are administered to people with different cultural and educational backgrounds.

Table 44.5 shows the ranked average item missing rates per country. No country exceeded the arbitrary cut-off that was pre-established at the level of 20%. Three countries had missing rates of more than 10%: Turkey postal (19%), Switzerland postal (18%), and Trinidad and Tobago postal (18%).

A number of general lessons about the feasibility of the responsiveness module emerges from this analysis of missing rates. First, all but three questions meet the pre-set criteria for feasibility, of less than 20% missingness. None of these items was crucial to the measurement of system responsiveness, being included for broader cross-checks on the questionnaire or to enable different types of analysis subsequently. Second, the responsiveness module is a feasible instrument to be used in a variety of settings. None of the 65 country surveys had missing rates higher than the 20% criterion. Third, the face-to-face surveys had lower missing rates (3%) on average than the postal surveys (6%). Another indicator of the relative difficulty associated

Table 44.4 Average item missing rates for the responsiveness module across 65 surveys

Section	Item Missing Rate (%)
Filter	6
Outpatient care	3
Prompt attention	3
Dignity	1
Communication	1
Autonomy	3
Confidentiality	7
Choice	9
Quality of basic amenities	1
Home care	6
Prompt attention	5
Dignity	6
Communication	6
Autonomy	5
Confidentiality	7
Choice	5
Inpatient care	5
Prompt attention	3
Dignity	3
Communication	3
Autonomy	4
Confidentiality	9
Choice	8
Quality of basic amenities	4
Support	8
Discrimination	5
Non-utilization	5
Importance (most and least items)	12
Vignettes	3
Set A	
Dignity	3
Communication	3
Set B	
Confidentiality	3
Quality of basic amenities	3
Set C	
Support	4
Choice	4
Set D	
Autonomy	3
Prompt attention	3
Total	4

with postal surveys is illustrated by the fact that three of them, compared to zero face-to-face surveys, had average missing rates greater than 10%. Fourth, the items focusing on responsiveness domains were mostly unproblematic.

Table 44.5   Average item missing rates by survey for 65 surveys

Survey	Average item missing rates (%)	Survey	Average item missing rates (%)
Turkey—postal	19	Chile—postal	4
Switzerland—postal	18	Russia—brief	3
Trinidad and Tobago—postal	18	Sweden—brief	3
Kyrgyzstan—postal	10	Hungary—postal	3
USA—postal	8	Croatia—brief	3
Bulgaria—brief	8	Ireland—brief	3
Finland—postal	8	Iran—long	3
Austria—postal	7	Belgium—brief	3
Great Britain—postal	7	Italy—brief	3
Iceland—brief	7	Jordan—brief	3
Denmark—postal	6	United Arab Emirates—brief	3
Ukraine—postal	6	Oman—brief	3
Greece—postal	6	Spain—brief	2
Mexico—long	6	Indonesia—postal	2
Estonia—brief	6	Luxembourg—telephone	2
Czech Republic—postal	6	France—brief	2
Netherlands—postal	5	Syria—long	2
Thailand—postal	5	Latvia—brief	2
Egypt—long	5	Egypt—postal	2
Romania—brief	5	China—postal	2
Turkey—long	5	Argentina—brief	2
Colombia—long	5	Canada—postal	2
Slovakia—long	5	Nigeria—long	1
Lebanon—postal	4	India (Andhra Pradesh)—long	1
New Zealand—postal	4	Indonesia—long	1
Cyprus—brief	4	Venezuela—postal	1
Portugal—brief	4	Canada—telephone	1
Australia—postal	4	Republic of Korea—postal	1
Poland—brief	4	Malta—brief	1
France—postal	4	China—long	1
Czech Republic—brief	4	Bahrain—brief	1
Finland—brief	4	Costa Rica—brief	1
Netherlands—brief	4	Georgia—long	1
Germany—postal	4	Morocco—brief	1
Lithuania—postal	4	Average	4

RELIABILITY

GENERAL

The concept of reliability refers to the amount of error, both random and systematic, inherent in any measurement. One form of reliability, called "test-retest" reliability, estimates the error component in case of repetition of a measurement keeping everything else the same. Many other types of reliability are also relevant to questionnaires, such as the source of information (person or interviewer) and mode of administration of the questionnaire. Such a multi-dimensional approach to reliability requires a more complex analysis (*11*).

The focus of this chapter, however, is on test-retest reliability of items with the analysis undertaken for each country separately. No attempt was made to identify which individuals were more likely to provide more stable answers on remeasurement. Following convention, the accordance between the responses to the original and readministered questions is measured with the weighted Kappa statistics (*12*). A score of one indicates perfect concordance between the two sets of responses, and zero indicates that the observed concordance was not better than expected by chance. A negative score suggests that responses are correlated less highly than would be expected by chance. For questions on fact (e.g. "Did you visit the doctor?"),

Table 44.6 Size of samples for retests in eight countries

Survey site	Number of respondents in retest interviews for different sections			
	Not requiring use of health services in previous 12 months	Users of outpatient health services	Users of care at home	Users of inpatient/ hospital services
China	858	412	65	64
Colombia	606	412	0	50
Egypt	452	268	14	32
Georgia	940	254	56	46
India	437	288	9	36
Nigeria	353	58	3	12
Slovakia	96	74	2	16
Turkey	195	127	0	6
Total	3 937	1 893	149	262

Kappas are expected to be higher than for reports on experiences (*13*). It should be kept in mind that a very low prevalence of any item substantially lowers even chance-corrected Kappas. Generally, comparisons within individuals are expected to show higher reliability than comparisons across groups, which is the focus of these surveys (*14*).

In order to establish the test-retest reliability of the responsiveness module, the extended version was readministered in its entirety. This is likely to have resulted in a lower estimate of the reliability of the questionnaire than if only parts of the module had been readministered to different respondents, because length may affect reliability. Respondents in eight countries were selected randomly and approached within one month after the first questionnaire had been administered. A total of 3 937 retests were collected. In the retest data 1 893 individuals reported outpatient or ambulatory care experiences in the previous 12 months; 149 respondents had received home care; 262 had received inpatient or hospital care; and 1 633 individuals had received no care. Table 44.6 presents the sample size of the retest sampling. Data of resamples with n < 30 were omitted from the analysis.

Table 44.7 shows the weighted Kappas for the eight countries separately, with results aggregated for the various sections of the questionnaire described in Table 44.4. The following guidelines are provided to help interpret the table—Kappa or κ > 0.75 denotes excellent reproducibility, 0.4 ≤ κ ≤ 0.75 denotes good reproducibility, and 0 ≤ κ ≤ 0.4 denotes marginal reproducibility (*13*).

ITEM PERSPECTIVE

As it would be expected of filter questions given their factual nature, average Kappas are very high (0.83) for these items. All other items have good or excellent reproducibility. Discrimination items perform the worst, which can partially be explained by the very skewed distribution of responses that is known to reduce the Kappa (rare affirmative responses).[5]

COUNTRY PERSPECTIVE

A strong country effect is visible. Reproducibility was excellent on average in China, Egypt, Slovakia and Turkey, and good in India. It was low in Georgia, Colombia, and Nigeria. The reasons are unclear. Given the consistency of Kappa rates across items within the same country, it is likely that the low rates reflect more on the systematic implementation of the survey, or problems with translation into the local language, rather than on the understandability of the items themselves.

INTERNAL CONSISTENCY METHOD

The analysis in Table 44.8 shows the item-test correlation coefficients (the correlation of the item score with the average of items within a domain), the item-rest correlation coefficients (the correlation of the item score with the domain average that excludes the item in question), the inter-item correlation coefficients (correlation between items), and the alpha coefficients for all countries listed in Table 44.4. The alpha coefficient is formulated as follows:

$$a = \frac{k\bar{r}}{1 + (k-1)\bar{r}}$$

Table 44.7 Kappa rates for sections of the responsiveness module, calculated from retests in eight countries

Section	China	Colombia	Egypt	Georgia	India	Nigeria	Slovakia	Turkey	Average
Filter	0.87	0.41	0.78	0.64	0.80	0.36	0.92	0.89	**0.83**
Outpatients									**0.72**
Prompt attention	0.82	0.43	0.89	0.50	0.71	0.51	0.87	0.87	0.76
Dignity	0.74	0.36	0.84	0.33	0.60	0.43	0.82	0.73	0.70
Communication	0.74	0.34	0.81	0.41	0.60	−0.03	0.82	0.80	0.72
Autonomy	0.81	0.38	0.79	0.43	0.66	0.38	0.90	0.88	0.72
Confidentiality	0.80	0.28	0.79	0.41	0.69	0.04	0.91	0.83	0.75
Choice	0.81	0.27	0.81	0.42	0.68	0.37	0.91	0.87	0.67
Quality of basic amenities	0.79	0.38	0.91	0.45	0.63	0.39	0.88	0.83	0.73
Home care									**0.74**
Prompt attention	0.86			0.42					0.78
Dignity	0.72			0.11					0.64
Communication	0.80			0.09					0.71
Autonomy	0.83			0.32					0.75
Confidentiality	0.91			0.35					0.80
Choice	0.83			0.46					0.77
Inpatients									**0.72**
Prompt attention	0.78	0.64	0.87	0.65	0.69				0.76
Dignity	0.77	0.52	0.96	0.56	0.81				0.74
Communication	0.79	0.34	0.76	0.70	0.65				0.71
Autonomy	0.79	0.47	0.86	0.43	0.65				0.71
Confidentiality	0.76	0.45	0.87	0.45	0.69				0.69
Choice	0.80	0.26	0.97	0.56	0.66				0.66
Quality of basic amenities	0.86	0.60	0.91	0.68	0.75				0.77
Support	0.84	0.37	0.90	0.41	0.66				**0.68**
Discrimination	0.72	0.41	0.58	0.57	0.87	0.36	0.66	0.69	**0.52**
Reasons and service	0.79	0.25	0.67	0.53	0.66	0.34	0.67	0.66	**0.71**
Reasons for non-use	0.78	0.39	0.77	0.52	0.76	0.19	0.65	0.65	**0.72**
Importance	0.79	0.25	0.84	0.34	0.59	0.25	0.71	0.55	**0.61**
Vignettes									**0.56**
Dignity	0.64	0.22	0.90	0.36	0.60	0.12	0.78	0.91	0.57
Autonomy	0.65	0.23	0.89	0.35	0.58	0.11	0.76	0.92	0.56
Confidentiality	0.66	0.21	0.90	0.36	0.61	0.10	0.78	0.91	0.57
Communication	0.66	0.21	0.89	0.36	0.59	0.10	0.77	0.91	0.56
Prompt attention	0.65	0.22	0.90	0.36	0.60	0.11	0.78	0.91	0.57
Support	0.65	0.22	0.90	0.36	0.60	0.11	0.77	0.91	0.56
Quality of basic amenities	0.65	0.22	0.90	0.36	0.60	0.11	0.77	0.91	0.56
Choice	0.65	0.22	0.90	0.36	0.60	0.11	0.77	0.91	0.56
Average Kappa's by country	**0.80**	**0.37**	**0.79**	**0.45**	**0.68**	**0.31**	**0.81**	**0.76**	**0.62**

Blanks mean too few observations to calculate Kappas

where $\bar{r}$ is the average inter-item correlation coefficient, and k is the number of items.

The alpha coefficient ranges from 0 (lowest reliability) to 1 (highest reliability). The coefficient is positively related to the number of items in the scale and the inter-item correlation coefficients. Nunnally and Bernstien (15) suggest that modest values of 0.70 are acceptable in the earlier stages of research. However, where measurements on individuals are of interest (e.g. the results of the test determine whether the individual is at risk for a particular condition), alpha's higher than 0.95 are a desirable standard.

Table 44.8   Item correlations and alpha coefficients for domain questions on the level of responsiveness

Item	Sign	Item-test corr.	Item-rest corr.	Inter-item corr.	Alpha	Short item description
Prompt attention						
q6101	+	0.808	0.456	0.264	0.418	how often did you get care as soon as you wanted
q6103	+	0.633	0.226	0.512	0.677	how long did you have to wait for laboratory tests or examinations
q6104	+	0.834	0.506	0.127	0.226	rate prompt attention
Test scale				0.346	0.614	mean(standardized items)
Dignity						
q6110	+	0.871	0.755	0.560	0.793	how often did health care providers treat you with respect
q6111	+	0.855	0.730	0.577	0.804	how often did office staff treat you with respect
q6112	+	0.797	0.633	0.643	0.844	privacy was respected
q6113	+	0.825	0.678	0.612	0.826	rate dignity
Test scale				0.598	0.856	mean(standardized items)
Communication						
q6120	+	0.859	0.742	0.661	0.854	how often did health care providers listen carefully to you
q6121	+	0.878	0.773	0.639	0.842	explain things in a way you could understand
q6122	+	0.873	0.766	0.644	0.845	give you time to ask questions
q6123	+	0.839	0.709	0.684	0.867	rate communication
Test scale				0.657	0.885	mean(standardized items)
Autonomy						
q6131	+	0.861	0.669	0.587	0.740	did health providers involve you in deciding about the care
q6132	+	0.861	0.629	0.614	0.761	ask your permission
q6133	+	0.868	0.642	0.589	0.741	rate getting involved in making decisions
Test scale				0.596	0.816	mean(standardized items)
Confidentiality						
q6140	+	0.849	0.620	0.614	0.761	how often were talks done privately
q6141	+	0.885	0.718	0.507	0.672	how often did your doctor keep your personal information confidential
q6142	+	0.837	0.603	0.637	0.779	rate confidentiality
Test scale				0.585	0.809	mean(standardized items)
Choice						
q6150	+	0.874	0.672	0.547	0.707	how big a problem to get to a health care provider you were happy with
q6151	+	0.861	0.674	0.569	0.725	to get to use other health services
q6152	+	0.838	0.604	0.652	0.789	rate health care provider or service of your choice
Test scale				0.589	0.811	mean(standardized items)
Quality of basic amenities						
q6160	+	0.916	0.809	0.816	0.898	basic quality of the waiting room
q6161	+	0.922	0.823	0.798	0.887	cleanliness of the place
q6162	+	0.941	0.863	0.746	0.854	rate space, seating, fresh air and cleanliness
Test scale				0.786	0.917	mean(standardized items)
Support						
q6311	+	0.795	0.503	0.489	0.656	get the hospital to allow your family to take care of your personal needs
q6312	+	0.805	0.536	0.445	0.616	have the hospital allow you to practice religious observances
q6313	+	0.814	0.547	0.431	0.602	rate how the hospital allowed you to interact with family, friends
Test scale				0.454	0.714	mean(standardized items)

Overall, the results in Table 44.8 are in the desirable range given that the aim of these surveys is to establish a population estimate. Prompt attention ($\alpha = 0.614$) and support ($\alpha = 0.714$) are the worse performing domains, while the alpha coefficients of the remain-ing domains are greater than 0.8. Within the domain of prompt attention, the item on how long the person waited to have tests or examinations undertaken performed the worst (item-rest correlation of 0.226). Perhaps this question leads people to consider the overall situation in their country rather than to report on their actual experience. The high alpha coefficient for quality of basic amenities might indicate that the items are too similar and are not measuring different aspects of the domain—reviewing the wording of the items, two of the four questions refer to cleanliness.

CONSTRUCT VALIDITY

Construct validity refers to the validity of the measure with respect to the original construct. For establishing the validity of the relevant sections of the questionnaire, the classical psychometric approach was adopted because of the lack of any external reference for responsiveness or other similar instruments to make a more direct comparison with "truth." Thus, the focus here is on the internal structure of the questionnaire, in particular the dimensionality and the homogeneity of items (questions) thought to represent one domain. As the factor structure of the instrument had already been established, confirmatory factor analysis of the seven outpatient domains and two inpatient domains was used (other domains were represented by only one item in the inpatient section of the module, so factor analysis at the item-to-domain level was not possible).

Factor analysis is a statistical technique that can be used to uncover and establish common dimensionality between different observed variables. Exploratory factor analysis is used when the researcher has no *a priori* assumption about the underlying dimensionality of the construct. Confirmatory factor analysis is used when the researcher has a hypothesis about the underlying dimensionality of the construct, and wishes to confirm or refute this hypothesis. The latter type is more restrictive (less arbitrary). The program M-Plus was used because it has a number of technical advantages over other programs, including the ability to have polytomous ordinal categorical variables and continuous variables in the same model (*16*).

Tables 44.9 and 44.10 present the results of the factor analysis on the responses of outpatients and inpatients from the survey countries. The numbers are the factor loadings on the latent variables. The factor loadings range from −1 to +1 and represent the amount of variance that responses to an item have in common with the underlaying latent variable. While there is no strict cut-off to describe strong and weak associations of variance, the closer to +1 or −1, the stronger the unidimensionality of the construct.

From the 65 surveys, the number of respondents for outpatients and inpatients was 58 505 and 11 434 respectively. Data from different countries were pooled and each domain was treated in a separate model. The results generally confirmed the assumed structure of the responsiveness domains. Two items, however, did not perform well: the item on the time elapsing from wanting care to receiving care, and the one on the length of time waited for tests and examinations. In some ways, these are items to be used to test the validity of responses to questions dealing with the promptness of attention, rather than items linked directly to the domains. They seek numerical rather than categorical responses. Accordingly, they might indicate that there is relatively low correlation between people's categorical responses on the promptness of attention and the times they actually waited for care. In addition, question q6100 included travel time to the health care facility, which might not be what respondents were thinking about when asked about prompt attention.

CONCLUSIONS AND RECOMMENDATIONS

This chapter has reported on the feasibility, reliability, and validity of the instrument used to assess responsiveness in the Multi-country Survey Study of 2000–2001. The analyses conducted for this chapter have provided certain insights into the reliability of specific items in the instrument and the validity of the responsiveness construct. The following key conclusions emerge.

The low country missing rates indicated that it is feasible to apply this instrument in different country settings. All but three items met the pre-established 20% threshold of acceptability for missingness. In particular, the responsiveness domain items and vignettes, together forming the core of the module, had missing rates of 9% or less. The Kappa rates varied substantially between different survey sites. Given the consistency across items within a particular country, it seems reasonable to recommend closer quality controls in future surveys. These practices would reduce site variability in Kappas.

A number of lessons were learned about particular items, some of which have already been incorporated into the World Health Survey, the successor to the WHO Multi-country Survey Study. For example, on certain occasions the pattern of missings suggested that either the item or the offered response categories could be adjusted (e.g. by adding "not applicable" to the response categories) to accommodate an apparent reluctance to respond. The reliability and internal consistency of some items was also lower than others, and particular attention focused on the domains of prompt attention and support. Some of these problems could be solved by technical changes to wording, but the domain of support would benefit from an increased conceptual development. It currently refers only to inpatient services relating to the provision of personal comforts (e.g. soap, special food) by family members and friends, the ability to observe religion practices during inpatient stays, and contact with family members and friends during inpatient stays. Other aspects relating to home care in particular have to be explored, including the extent to which family life is affected by the need to care for sick family members in the household. Clearly, any valid measure of health system responsiveness should also include non-personal health actions, such as health promotion campaigns

Table 44.9 Confirmatory factor analysis standardized coefficients—outpatients

Variable description	Prompt attention	Dignity	Commu- nication	Autonomy	Confiden- tiality	Choice	Quality of basic amenities
In the last 12 months, how long did you usually have to wait from the time that you wanted care to the time that you received care?	0.302						
In the last 12 months, when you wanted care, how often did you get care as soon as you wanted?	0.636						
Generally, how long did you have to wait before you could get the laboratory tests or examinations done?	0.336						
Now, overall, how would you rate your experience of getting prompt attention at the health services in the last 12 months?	0.922						
In the last 12 months, when you sought care, how often did doctors, nurses or other health care providers treat you with respect?		0.922					
In the last 12 months, when you sought care, how often did the office staff, such as receptionists or clerks there, treat you with respect?		0.884					
In the last 12 months, how often were your physical examinations and treatments done in a way that your privacy was respected?		0.786					
Now, overall, how would you rate your experience of getting treated with dignity at the health services in the last 12 months?		0.814					
In the last 12 months, how often did doctors, nurses or other health care providers listen carefully to you?			0.869				
In the last 12 months, how often did doctors, nurses or other health care providers there, explain things in a way you could understand?			0.903				
In the last 6 months, how often did doctors, nurses or other health care providers give you time to ask questions about your health problem or treatment?			0.891				
Now, overall, how would you rate your experience of how well health care providers communicated with you in the last 12 months?			0.828				
In the last 12 months, how often did doctors, nurses or other health care providers there involve you as much as you wanted to be in deciding about the care, treatment or tests?				0.841			

continued

Table 44.9 Confirmatory factor analysis standardized coefficients—outpatients *(continued)*

Variable description	Prompt attention	Dignity	Commu-nication	Autonomy	Confiden-tiality	Choice	Quality of basic amenities
In the last 12 months, how often did doctors, nurses or other health care providers there ask your permission before starting tests or treatment?				0.825			
Now, overall, how would you rate your experience of getting involved in making decisions about your care or treatment as much as you wanted in the last 12 months?				0.842			
In the last 12 months, how often were talks with your doctor, nurse or other health care provider done privately so other people who you did not want to hear could not overhear what was said?					0.806		
In the last 12 months, how often did your doctor, nurse or other health care provider keep your personal information confidential? This means that anyone whom you did not want informed could not find out about your medical conditions.					0.954		
Now, overall, how would you rate your experience of the way the health services kept information about you confidential in the last 12 months?					0.786		
In the last 12 months, with the doctors, nurses and other health care providers available to you, how big a problem, if any, was it to get to a health care provider you were happy with?						0.895	
Over the last 12 months, how big a problem, if any, was it to get to use other health care services other than the one you usually went to?						0.866	
Now, overall, how would you rate your experience of being able to use a health care provider or service of your choice over the last 12 months?						0.753	
Thinking about the places you visited for health care in the last 12 months, how would you rate the basic quality of the waiting room, for example, space, seating and fresh air?							0.905
Thinking about the places you visited for health care over the last 12 months, how would you rate the cleanliness of the place?							0.908
Now, overall, how would you rate the overall quality of the surroundings, for example, space, seating, fresh air, and cleanliness of the health services you visited in the last 12 months?							0.943

(e.g. anti-smoking or HIV awareness campaigns), and other aspects of the health system such as the responsiveness of administrative structures. These issues were not evaluated in the Multi-country Survey Study but attempts have been made to include several of them in the World Health Survey.

For the analyses in this chapter, validity investigations could be carried out only to a limited degree. It would be useful if additional items linked to variables associated with better responsiveness could be added to the survey in future iterations to facilitate more analysis of validity. On balance, however, the Survey Study suggests that it is feasible to ask questions on responsiveness with their associated vignettes in different cultural settings. The items proved generally to be reliable and valid, and to elicit consistent responses.

Table 44.10 Confirmatory factor analysis standardized coefficients—inpatients

Variable description	Prompt attention	Support
Did you get your hospital care as soon as you wanted?	0.745	
When you were in the hospital, how often did you get attention from doctors and nurses as quickly as you wanted?	0.892	
Now, overall, how would you rate your experience of getting prompt attention at the hospital in the last 12 months?	0.897	
In the last 12 months, when you stayed in hospital, how big a problem, if any, was it to get the hospital to allow your family and friends to take care of your personal needs, such as bringing you your favourite food, soap, etc.?		0.747
During your stay in hospital, how big a problem, if any, was it to have the hospital allow you to practice religious or traditional observances if you wanted to?		0.826
Now, overall, how would you rate your experience of how the hospital allowed you to interact with family, friends and to continue your social and or religious customs during your stay over the last 12 months?		0.792

ACKNOWLEDGEMENTS

This chapter has benefited from the comments of Ritu Sadana and David B. Evans, both of the World Health Organization.

NOTES

1   This label of "access to social support networks" was applied to this domain during the WHO Multi-country Survey Study. For discussion of subsequent change to the domain label, please refer to the responsiveness concepts chapter in this book (3).

2   This chapter presents analyses from 65 of the 70 surveys containing the responsiveness module (one survey, Singapore, in the 71 Multi-country Survey Study did not contain the responsiveness module).

3   While the WHO Multi-country Survey Study countries covered here included long face-to-face surveys in 10 countries, only 8 of these retested a proportion of their respondents.

4   Outpatient services statistics include services received at home.

5   Rare positive response implies an unfavourable balance of error to valid information, which in turn lowers Kappa statistics that account for chance agreement assuming true response only.

REFERENCES

(1)   Campbell A, Converse PE, Rodgers WL. *The quality of American life: perceptions, evaluations, and satisfactions.* New York, Russell Sage Foundation, 1976.

(2)   Andrews FM, Withey SB. *Social indicators of well-being: Americans' perceptions of life quality.* New York, Plenum Press, 1976.

(3)   de Silva A. *A framework for measuring responsiveness.* EIP Discussion Paper No. 32. Geneva, World Health Organization, 2000. URL: http://www3.who.int/whosis/discussion_papers/discussion_papers.cfm#

(4)   Valentine NB et al. Health system responsiveness: concepts, domains and operationalization. In: Murray CJL, Evans DB, eds. *Health systems performance assessment: debates, methods and empiricism.* Geneva, World Health Organization, 2003.

(5)   World Health Organization. Technical Consultation on Concepts and Methods for Measuring the Responsiveness of Health Systems. In: Murray CJL, Evans DB, eds. *Health systems performance assessment: debates, methods and empiricism.* Geneva, World Health Organization, 2003.

(6)   Sadana R et al. Comparative analyses of more than 50 household surveys on health status. In: Murray CJL et al., eds. *Summary measures of population health: concepts, ethics, measurement and applications.* Geneva, World Health Organization, 2002:369–386.

(7)   Salomon JA et al. Quanitfying individual levels of health: definitions, concepts, and measurement issues. In: Murray CJL, Evans DB, eds. *Health systems performance assessment: debates, methods and empiricism.* Geneva, World health Organization, 2003.

(8)   World Health Organization. *The World Health Report 2000. Health Systems: Improving Performance.* Geneva, World Health Organization, 2000.

(9)   Tandon A et al. Statistical models for enhancing cross-population comparability. In: Murray CJL, Evans DB, eds. *Health systems performance assessment: debates, methods and empiricism.* Geneva, World Health Organization, 2003.

(10) Bernhard HR. *Research methods in anthropology: qualitative and quantitative approaches,* 2nd ed. Thousand Oaks, Sage Publications, 1995.

(11) Gandek B, Ware JE. Methods for validating and norming translations of health status questionnaires: the IQOLA project approach. *Journal of Clinical Epidemiology,* 1998, 51:953–959.

(12) Streiner DL, Norman GR. *Health measurement scales : a practical guide to their development and use.* Oxford, New York, Oxford University Press, 1989.

(13) Rosner B. *Fundamentals of biostatistics*, 4th ed. Belmont, Duxbury Press, 1995.

(14) Sadana R. *Quantifying reproductive health and illness* [Dissertation]. Boston, Harvard School of Public Health, 2001.

(15) Nunnally JC, Bernstein IH. *Psychometric theory*, 3 ed. New York, McGraw-Hill, 1994.

(16) de Silva A, Valentine NB. *Measuring responsiveness: results of a key informants survey in 35 countries*. EIP Discussion Paper No. 21. Geneva, World Health Organization, 2000. URL: http://www3.who.int/whosis/discussion_papers/discussion_papers.cfm#

Annex 44.1

Items from the Consumer Assessment of Health Plans (CAHPS), a USA-based Survey, Included in the Responsiveness Module with Little or No Change

Domain		Question	Response scale
Prompt attention	1	In the last 12 months, when you wanted care, how often did you get care as soon as you wanted?	always(1), usually(2), sometimes(3), never(4)
	2	In the last 12 months, how long did you usually have to wait from the time that you wanted care to the time you received care?	units of time
Dignity	3	In the last 12 months, when you sought care, how often did doctors, nurses or other health care providers treat you with respect?	always(1), usually(2), sometimes(3), never(4)
	4	In the last 12 months, when you sought care, how often did the office staff, such as receptionists or clerks there, treat you with respect?	always(1), usually(2), sometimes(3), never(4)
Communication	5	In the last 12 months, how often did doctors, nurses or other health care providers listen carefully to you?	always(1), usually(2), sometimes(3), never(4)
	6	In the last 12 months, how often did doctors, nurses or other health care providers there, explain things in a way you could understand?	always(1), usually(2), sometimes(3), never(4)
	7	In the last 6 months, how often did doctors, nurses or other health care providers give you time to ask questions about your health problem or treatment?	always(1), usually(2), sometimes(3), never(4)
Autonomy	8	In the last 12 months, how often did doctors, nurses or other health care providers there involve you as much as you wanted to be in deciding about the care, treatment or tests?	always(1), usually(2), sometimes(3), never(4)
Choice	9	In the last 12 months, with the doctors, nurses and other health care providers available to you, how big a problem, if any, was it to get to a health care provider you were happy with?	no problem(1), mild problem(2), moderate problem(3), severe problem(4), extreme problem(5)

ANNEX 44.2
SURVEY COUNTRIES AND NUMBER OF COMPLETED RESPONSES FROM RESPONDENTS WHO USED HOSPITAL SERVICES, OUTPATIENT OR AMBULATORY SERVICES, OR NEITHER (NON-USERS) IN THE LAST 12 MONTHS

	Country	Survey type[a]	Inpatient only	Outpatient only	Both	Neither	Total questionnaires completed	Questionnaires not completed	Total
				Extended form (long face-to-face)					
1	China	1	124	3 782	659	4 877	9 442	44	9 486
2	Colombia	1	14	3 322	518	2 165	6 019	2139	8 158
3	Egypt	1	37	2 399	211	1 839	4 486	4	4 490
4	Georgia	1	85	1 900	272	7 590	9 847	0	9 847
5	India	1	108	2 846	326	1 916	5 196	0	5 196
6	Indonesia	1	85	3 743	228	5 896	9 952	42	9 994
7	Mexico	1	46	1 547	286	2 933	4 812	1	4 813
8	Nigeria	1	44	879	126	3 998	5 047	61	5 108
9	Slovakia	1	3	659	137	384	1 183	0	1 183
10	Turkey	1	28	1 279	102	3 788	5 197	10	5 207
				Short form (postal)					
11	Austria	2	8	581	216	241	1 046	0	1 046
12	Canada	2	2	209	41	155	407	0	407
13	Chile	2	18	322	100	606	1 046	0	1 046
14	China	2	13	350	45	698	1 106	0	1 106
15	Cyprus	2	11	337	121	183	652	0	652
16	Czech Republic	2	4	712	177	128	1 021	0	1 021
17	Denmark	2	11	851	159	490	1 511	0	1 511
18	Egypt	2	12	345	256	770	1 383	0	1 383
19	Finland	2	16	850	204	287	1 357	0	1 357
20	France	2	5	489	181	258	933	0	933
21	Great Britain	2	4	586	123	305	1 018	0	1 018
22	Greece	2	8	439	196	266	909	17	926
23	Hungary	2	35	476	226	763	1 500	0	1 500
24	Indonesia	2	46	956	318	1 150	2 470	1	2 471
25	Kyrgyzstan	2	14	377	180	509	1 080	1	1 081
26	Lebanon	2	30	93	93	896	1 112	0	1 112
27	Lithuania	2	22	796	392	536	1 746	0	1 746
28	New Zealand	2	7	1 198	254	342	1 801	1	1 802
29	Poland	2	3	539	192	148	882	0	882
30	Republic of Korea	2	2	212	51	83	348	0	348
31	Switzerland	2	9	234	58	520	821	2	823
32	Thailand	2	38	484	139	525	1 186	1	1 187
33	The Netherlands	2	5	324	51	230	610	2	612
34	Trinidad and Tobago	2	23	399	174	649	1 245	5	1 250
35	Turkey	2	24	793	528	1 024	2 369	111	2 480
36	Ukraine	2	8	386	203	191	788	0	788
37	USA	2	10	375	71	132	588	0	588

	Country	Survey type[a]	Inpatient only	Outpatient only	Both	Neither	Total questionnaires completed	Questionnaires not completed	Total
				Short form (brief face-to-face)					
38	Argentina	3	3	394	84	300	781	0	781
39	Bahrain	3	9	320	73	407	809	0	809
40	Belgium	3	18	502	116	464	1 100	0	1 100
41	Costa Rica	3	1	421	77	257	756	0	756
42	Croatia	3	10	694	151	645	1 500	0	1 500
43	Czech Republic	3	9	578	139	346	1 072	0	1 072
44	Estonia	3	8	581	144	267	1 000	0	1 000
45	Finland	3	8	576	146	291	1 021	0	1 021
46	France	3	5	526	126	346	1 003	0	1 003
47	Germany	3	4	606	92	421	1 123	0	1 123
48	Iceland	3	6	266	36	181	489	0	489
49	Ireland	3	2	250	87	372	711	0	711
50	Italy	3	12	394	57	539	1 002	0	1 002
51	Jordan	3	28	304	69	402	803	0	803
52	Latvia	3	16	342	103	291	752	0	752
53	Malta	3	2	273	49	176	500	0	500
54	Morocco	3	2	381	53	318	754	0	754
55	Oman	3	8	441	78	308	835	0	835
56	Portugal	3	95	534		372	1 001	0	1 001
57	Romania	3	9	377	161	504	1 051	0	1 051
58	Russian Federation	3	14	753	194	640	1 601	0	1 601
59	Spain	3		534	85	381	1 000	0	1 000
60	Sweden	3	14	471	93	422	1 000	0	1 000
61	Netherlands	3	1	603	83	398	1 085	0	1 085
62	United Arab Emirates	3	15	393	72	338	818	0	818
63	Venezuela	3	11	219	45	479	754	0	754
				Short form (telephone)					
64	Canada	4	10	135	29	219	393	0	393
65	Luxembourg	4	13	429	83	194	719	0	719
	Total		1 295	48 366	10 139	57 749	117 549	2 442	119 991
	Percentage		1.1%	41.1%	8.6%	49.1%	100%		

Item variable name	Item wording in extended form of questionnaire (A stroke before the item variable name indicates the item branched off from a main item)
Q6000	Have you received any health care in the last 12 months? (1) yes, (5) no
Q6001	In the last 12 months, did you get any health care at an outpatient health facility or did a health care provider visit you at home? (An outpatient health facility is a doctor's consulting room, a clinic or a hospital outpatient unit—any place outside your home where you did not stay overnight). (1) yes, (5) no
Q6002	In the last 12 months, did you get most of your health care at a health facility or most of it from a health provider who visited you in your home? mostly at a health facility (1), mostly from a health provider in my home (2), equally from both (3)
Q6003	When was your last visit to a health facility or provider? Was it: last 30 days (1), last 3 months (2), last 6 months (3), between 6 and 12 months (4), don`t remember (5)
Q6004	What was the name of the health care facility? (Please fill in the name of facility, e.g., Oxford Clinic. Only fill in the name of the provider if the facility does not have another name.) enter facility name
Q6005	Was (name of provider) your usual place of care? (1) yes, (5) no
Q6100	In the last 12 months, how long did you usually have to wait from the time that you wanted care to the time that you received care? enter time minutes hours days weeks months
Q6101	In the last 12 months, when you wanted care, how often did you get care as soon as you wanted? always (1), usually (2), sometimes (3), never (4)
Q6102	In the last 12 months, have you needed any laboratory tests or examinations? Some examples of tests or special examinations are blood tests, scans or X-rays. (1) yes, (5) no
Q6103	Generally, how long did you have to wait before you could get the laboratory tests or examinations done? same day (1), 1–2days (2), 3–5days (3), 6–10days (4), specify time if greater than ten days
Q6104	Now, overall, how would you rate your experience of getting prompt attention at the health services in the last 12 months? Prompt attention means…** very good (1), good (2), moderate (3), bad (4), very bad (5)
Q6110	In the last 12 months, when you sought care, how often did doctors, nurses or other health care providers treat you with respect? always (1), usually (2), sometimes (3), never (4)
Q6111	In the last 12 months, when you sought care, how often did the office staff, such as receptionists or clerks there, treat you with respect? always (1), usually (2), sometimes (3), never (4)

continued

Item variable name	Item wording in extended form of questionnaire (A stroke before the item variable name indicates the item branched off from a main item)
Q6112	In the last 12 months, how often were your physical examinations and treatments done in a way that your privacy was respected?
	always (1), usually (2), sometimes (3), never (4)
Q6113	Now, overall, how would you rate your experience of getting treated with dignity at the health services in the last 12 months? Dignity means…**
	very good (1), good (2), moderate (3), bad (4), very bad (5)
Q6120	In the last 12 months, how often did doctors, nurses or other health care providers listen carefully to you?
	always (1), usually (2), sometimes (3), never (4)
Q6121	In the last 12 months, how often did doctors, nurses or other health care providers there, explain things in a way you could understand?
	always (1), usually (2), sometimes (3), never (4)
Q6122	In the last 6 months, how often did doctors, nurses or other health care providers give you time to ask questions about your health problem or treatment?
	always (1), usually (2), sometimes (3), never (4)
Q6123	Now, overall, how would you rate your experience of how well health care providers communicated with you in the last 12 months? Communication means…**
	very good (1), good (2), moderate (3), bad (4), very bad (5)
Q6130	In the last 12 months, when you went for care, were any decisions made about your care, treatment (drugs for example) or tests?
	(1) yes, (5) no
Q6131	In the last 12 months, how often did doctors, nurses or other health care providers there involve you as much as you wanted to be in deciding about the care, treatment or tests?
	always (1), usually (2), sometimes (3), never (4)
Q6132	In the last 12 months, how often did doctors, nurses or other health care porviders there ask your permission before starting tests or treatment?
	always (1), usually (2), sometimes (3), never (4)
Q6133	Now, overall, how would you rate your experience of getting involved in making decisions about your care or treatment as much as you wanted in the last 12 months? Being involved in decision-making means…**
	very good (1), good (2), moderate (3), bad (4), very bad (5)
Q6140	In the last 12 months, how often were talks with your doctor, nurse or other health care provider done privately so other people who you did not want to hear could not overhear what was said?
	always (1), usually (2), sometimes (3), never (4)
Q6141	In the last 12 months, how often did your doctor, nurse or other health care provider keep your personal information confidential? This means that anyone whom you did not want informed could not find out about your medical conditions.
	always (1), usually (2), sometimes (3), never (4)
Q6142	Now, overall, how would you rate your experience of the way the health services kept information about you confidential in the last 12 months? Confidentiality means…**
	very good (1), good (2), moderate (3), bad (4), very bad (5)
Q6150	In the last 12 months, with the doctors, nurses and other health care providers available to you how big a problem, if any, was it to get to a health care provider you were happy with?
	no problem (1), mild problem (2), moderate problem (3), severe problem (4), extreme problem (5)
Q6151	Over the last 12 months, how big a problem if any was it to get to use other health care services other than the one you usually went to.
	no problem (1), mild problem (2), moderate problem (3), severe problem (4), extreme problem (5), never tried (6)
Q6152	Now, overall, how would you rate your experience of being able to use a health care provider or service of your choice over the last 12 months? Choice means…**
	very good (1), good (2), moderate (3), bad (4), very bad (5)
Q6160	Thinking about the places you visited for health care in the last 12 months, how would you rate the basic quality of the waiting room, for example, space, seating and fresh air?
	very good (1), good (2), moderate (3), bad (4), very bad (5)

continued

Item variable name	Item wording in extended form of questionnaire *(A stroke before the item variable name indicates the item branched off from a main item)*
Q6161	Thinking about the places you visited for health care over the last 12 months, how would you rate the cleanliness of the place? very good (1), good (2), moderate (3), bad (4), very bad (5)
Q6162	Now, overall, how would you rate the overall quality of the surroundings, for example, space, seating, fresh air and cleanliness of the health services you visited in the last 12 months? Quality of surroundings means…** very good (1), good (2), moderate (3), bad (4), very bad (5)
Q6300	Have you stayed overnight in a hospital in last 12 months? (1) yes, (5) no
Q6301	What was the name of the hospital you stayed in most recently? enter facility name
Q6302	Did you get your hospital care as soon as you wanted? (1) yes, (5) no
Q6303	When you were in the hospital, how often did you get attention from doctors and nurses as quickly as you wanted? always (1), usually (2), sometimes (3), never (4)
Q6304	Now, overall, how would you rate your experience of getting prompt attention at the hospital in the last 12 months? Prompt attention means…** very good (1), good (2), moderate (3), bad (4), very bad (5)
Q6305	Overall, how would you rate your experience of getting treated with dignity at the hospital in the last 12 months? Dignity means… very good (1), good (2), moderate (3), bad (4), very bad (5)
Q6306	Overall, how would you rate your experience of how well health care providers communicated with you during your stay in the hospital in the last 12 months? Communication means…** very good (1), good (2), moderate (3), bad (4), very bad (5)
Q6307	Overall, how would you rate your experience of getting involved in making decisions about your care or treatment as much as you wanted when you were in hospital in the 12 months? Being involved in decision-making means…** very good (1), good (2), moderate (3), bad (4), very bad (5)
Q6308	Overall, how would you rate your experience of the way the hospital kept personal information about you confidential in the last 12 months? Confidentiality means…** very good (1), good (2), moderate (3), bad (4), very bad (5)
Q6309	Overall, how would you rate your experience of being able to use a hopsital of your choice over the last 12 months? Choice means… very good (1), good (2), moderate (3), bad (4), very bad (5)
Q6310	Overall, how would you rate the overall quality of the surroundings, for example, space, seating, fresh air, and cleanliness of the health services you visited in the last 12 months? Quality of surroundings means…** very good (1), good (2), moderate (3), bad (4), very bad (5)
Q6311	In the last 12 months, when you stayed in hospital, how big a problem, if any, was it to get the hospital to allow your family and friends to take care of your personal needs, such as bringing you your favourite food, soap etc.? no problem (1), mild problem (2), moderate problem (3), severe problem (4), extreme problem (5)
Q6312	During your stay in hospital, how big a problem, if any, was it to have the hospital allow you to practice religious or traditional observances if you wanted to? Would you say it was.. no problem (1), mild problem (2), moderate problem (3), severe problem (4), extreme problem (5)
Q6313	Now, overall, how would you rate your experience of how the hospital allowed you to interact with family, friends and to continue your social and or religious customs during your stay over the last 12 months. Social support means…** very good (1), good (2), moderate (3), bad (4), very bad (5)
Q6400	In the last 12 months, were you treated badly by the health system or services in your country because of your…? (1) yes, (5) no, (7) refuse
/Q64001	nationality
/Q64002	social class
/Q64003	lack of private insurance

continued

Item variable name	Item wording in extended form of questionnaire (A stroke before the item variable name indicates the item branched off from a main item)
/Q64004	ethnicity
/Q64005	colour
/Q64006	sex
/Q64007	language
/Q64008	religion
/Q64009	political/other beliefs
/Q640010	health status
/Q640011	lack of wealth
/Q640012	other
/Q6400113	specify
Q6401*	In the last 12 months, when you used health services in this country, did you feel that you were treated worse because you were a woman?
	(1) yes, (5) no, (7) refuse
Q6500	I will read you a list of different types of places you can get health services. Please can you indicate the number of times you went to each of them in the last 30 days.
/Q6500	general practicioners
/Q6501	dentists
/Q6502	specialists
/Q6503	chiropractors
/Q6504	traditional healers
/Q6505	clinics
/Q6506	hospital outpatient unit
/Q6507	hospital inpatient unit
/Q6508	pharmacy
/Q6509	home health care services
/Q6510	other
/Q6510S	specify
Q6511*	What was the main reason that you went to the health care provider for your most recent visit? Please indicate all that apply.
	yes (1), no (5), DK (8), NA (9)
/Q65111	you needed a check up for a chronic, ongoing problem
/Q65112	you needed care because your chronic, ongoing problem flared up
/Q65113	you needed care because of an injury or illness that had just happened
/Q65114	you needed to follow up with the provider after having an operation or treatment for an injury
/Q65115	you were not sick, you went for a general exam or preventive care
/Q65116	other
/Q65116S	other, specify
Q6512*	What services were provided at your most recent visit? Again, I will read through a list. Please indicate all that apply
	yes (1), no (5), DK (8), NA (9)
/Q65121	you were examined
/Q65122	you received tests
/Q65123	the health care provider gave you treatment
/Q65124	the health care provider talked with you about your health problem
/Q65125	the health care provider talked to you about your health in general
/Q65126	you picked up medicine or a prescription
/Q65127	other
/Q65127S	other, specify
Q6600*	In the last 12 months, were you ever refused health care because you could not afford it?
	(1) yes, (5) no
Q6601	In the last 12 months, did you not seek health care because you could not afford it?
	(1) yes, (5) no

continued

Item variable name	*Item wording in extended form of questionnaire* *(A stroke before the item variable name indicates the item branched off from a main item)*
	Preamble: Ask the respondent to read the cards below or read the cards to the respondent if he/she would prefer. These are descriptions of some different ways the health care services in your country show respect for people and make them the centre of care. Please write the code in the space provided.
Q6602	Most important (1) most important: dignity (DIG), confidentiality of information (CI), choice (CH), prompt attention (PA), autonomy (AUT), surroundings or environment (ENV), social support (SS), communication (COM)
Q6603	Least important (8) least important: dignity (DIG), confidentiality of information (CI), choice (CH), prompt attention (PA), autonomy (AUT), surroundings or environment (ENV), social support (SS), communication (COM)
Q6604	Did the respondent read the cards him/herself? (1) yes, (5) no
Q6701–6714	Vignettes very good (1), good (2), moderate (3), bad (4), very bad (5)
	See Annex 44.4 for wording of vignettes

* Only included in the extended form of the responsiveness module.

** These introductory phrases were used to remind interviewers to describe the domains to the respondents, using the "cards" from Q6602 and Q6603 of the questionnaire.

ANNEX 44.4
WORDING OF RESPONSIVENESS VIGNETTES

Note that the response categories for all vignettes are "very good," "good," "moderate," "bad," "very bad."

SET A

6701. Vignette 1

[Rose] is an elderly woman who is illiterate. Lately, she has been feeling dizzy and has problems sleeping. The doctor did not seem very interested in what she was telling him. He told her it was nothing and wrote something on a piece of paper, telling her to get the medication at the pharmacy.

How would you rate Rose's experience of how well health care providers communicated with her?

6702. Vignette 2

[Conrad] is suffering from AIDS. When he enters the health care unit the doctor shakes his hand. He asks him to sit down and inquires what his problems are. The nurses are concerned about Conrad. They give him advice about improving his health.

How would you rate Conrad's experience of getting treated with dignity?

6703. Vignette 3

[Anya] took her three-month old infant for her vaccination. The nurse asked her why she had not been to the clinic before, and was sympathetic to hear that Anya had a problem finding transport. She advised her about the importance of regularly monitoring the growth of her baby.

How would you rate Anya's experience of getting treated with dignity?

6704. Vignette 4

[Carmen] has gone for a blood test and the doctor has told her that she has diabetes mellitus and that her pancreatic activity is faulty. He has also told her she needs insulin injections three times a day and that she should watch for hypoglycemia. If she does not control her blood sugar she may also go blind. Carmen feels very bad because she does not understand what the doctor is talking about, but she has to leave because he has already called the next patient.

How would you rate Carmen's experience of how well health care providers communicated with her?

6705. Vignette 5

[Julia] visits the health care centre for treatment at a time when the centre is very crowded. The patients are all impatient to get their treatment and are reluctant to queue and wait for their turn. The nurses are very patient most of the time about asking patients to wait their turn, but occasionally they get angry and shout at her for breaking the queue.

How would you rate Julia's experience of getting treated with dignity?

6706. Vignette 6

[Deborah] is a young woman who has been brought to the clinic by her family because she feels very anxious and distressed. She is also afraid that she may die although she is in good health. The doctor has taken time to listen and reassure her and has invited Deborah to come to the clinic whenever she needs to.

How would you rate Deborah's experience of how well health care providers communicated with her?

6707. Vignette 7

[Patricia] goes to a health care unit close to her home regularly. The nurses there are very busy, but they always speak pleasantly to her. The receptionist however is often in a bad mood, and when she is in a bad mood she shouts at Patricia, and at other patients. All appointments to meet doctors and nurses have to be made through this receptionist so the patients put up with her rudeness.

How would you rate Patricia's experience of getting treated with dignity?

6708. Vignette 8

[Sonia] has arrived at the clinic with her three-month-old baby girl. The mother says that the baby has lost a lot of weight, has had fever for two days and will not take her milk. The nurse has listened to the mother without interrupting. She has asked her for additional information and has encouraged the mother to ask her questions if she did not understand.

How would you rate Sonia's experience of how well health care providers communicated with her?

6709. Vignette 9

[Kim] took her six month old infant to the health centre for her regular check-up. The nurse was very annoyed when she found that Kim had

continued

forgotten to bring the baby's growth chart with her. She scolded her loudly in the hearing of all the other mothers who had come to the clinic, and kept grumbling about inconsiderate forgetful mothers who caused extra work as she weighed the baby.

How would you rate Kim's experience of getting treated with dignity?

6710. Vignette 10

[Mario] has been told that he has epilepsy and needs to take medication. The doctor has very briefly explained what the condition is. He is very busy and there is a queue of patients waiting to see him. Mario would like to know more about what he has, but feels that there is no time to ask questions and that the doctor will not be very helpful.

How would you rate Mario's experience of how well health care providers communicated with him?

6711. Vignette 11

[Said] has AIDS. When he goes to his health centre he feels that all the doctors and nurses are unfriendly towards him. They do not talk to him freely. Often they deliberately ignore him. He often has to beg them to answer his questions.

How would you rate Said's experience of getting treated with dignity?

6712. Vignette 12

[Florence] goes to the hospital as she has a pain in her stomach. The nurse shouts at her for not bringing her health card. Two other nurses who are standing by make rude comments about Florence's family and those from her village. Though Florence is in pain and moaning she is not asked to sit down while her personal details are entered in the register.

How would you rate Florence's experience of getting treated with dignity?

6713. Vignette 13

[Thomas] has been told that he has cataracts and that he needs an operation. He has never had his eyes checked and does not understand why he cannot see well. The doctor has explained to Thomas what he has, but he has not understood a word and is afraid to ask again. The doctor has not checked whether or not he has understood.

How would you rate Thomas's experience of how well health care providers communicated with him?

6714. Vignette 14

[Jiang] has been having pain in his chest for a while. Whenever he coughs or exercises his chest is painful. He has been smoking for 30 years. After examining him, the doctor has told him that he will get cancer if he does not stop smoking. The doctor is not very sympathetic and has not even suggested what Jiang could do to give up smoking.

How would you rate Jiang's experience of how well health care providers communicated with him?

SET B

6701. Vignette 1

Dr Johnson is treating [Mark]. Mark seems to be suffering from a rare disease. The press is pressurising Dr Johnson to divulge information regarding this patient. Dr Johnson however is adamant that he will not reveal the personal details regarding his patient.

How would you rate Mark's experience of how well the health services kept information about him confidential?

6702. Vignette 2

[Shedra] had to be hospitalised last year for a hip operation. The hospital had a separate room for her with an attached bathroom. The room was cleaned twice a day by the hospital staff and the sheets changed daily. The bed was comfortable. She could move around in the gardens of the hospital.

How would you rate Shedra's experience of the overall quality of the surroundings, for example space, seating, fresh air and cleanliness, of the health services?

6703. Vignette 3

[Alioune] went to hospital to consult the doctor about some worrying symptoms he was having. He was worried because he had recently visited a commercial sex worker. The waiting room was very crowded. Alioune met some of his friends there. The doctor's consultation room was a little way away from the waiting room. One had to go down the corridor to this room when it was one's turn to consult the doctor. Alioune went in and spoke to the doctor who ordered some tests and advised him about safe sex.

How would you rate Alioune's experience of how well the health services kept information about him confidential?

6704. Vignette 4

[José] was admitted to a local hospital for a week as he developed high fever. The room was clean but small and the toilet was a few metres away down the corridor. It was summer and he felt hot and had to get a table fan from home.

How would you rate José's experience of the overall quality of the surroundings, for example space, seating, fresh air and cleanliness, of the health services?

continued

6705. Vignette 5

[Hans] had an eye operation in a local polyclinic last month. He was in a room that he had to share with four others with no partitions between beds. He had a small locker to keep his things and shared a toilet which was cleaned only every other day.

How would you rate Hans's experience of the overall quality of the surroundings, for example space, seating, fresh air and cleanliness, of the health services?

6706. Vignette 6

As [Ben] has high fever over a long period, his doctor orders a number of tests. The test reports are sent over to the ward from the laboratory. The nurse who is busy attending to some other patients leaves these reports on the counter where they are seen by Ben's neighbour.

How would you rate Ben's experience of how well the health services kept information about him confidential?

6707. Vignette 7

[Albert] sees his general practitioner in his office every month for his diabetes. The office has comfortable chairs in the waiting room and clean toilets. It is well lit and there are magazines and booklets to read while waiting.

How would you rate Albert's experience of the overall quality of the surroundings, for example space, seating, fresh air and cleanliness, of the health services?

6708. Vignette 8

[Simon] went to the hospital to consult the doctor about some worrying symptoms he was having. He wondered if they were connected with his recent heavy drinking. The waiting room was very crowded. Simon met a friend and a couple of his neighbours there. The doctor was sitting in a curtained off area at the end of the waiting room. Due to the noise in the room, the doctor and Simon had to speak very loudly to hear each other. The doctor ordered some tests and advised Simon to reduce his drinking.

How would you rate Simon's experience of how well the health services kept information about him confidential?

6709. Vignette 9

[Paul] goes to visit Dr Jonathan because he is worried about his drinking problem and the effect it is having on his health. Dr Jonathan finds that Paul is suffering from severe stress. Dr Jonathan mentions Paul's visit to a mutual friend Robert, and asks him to advise Paul as well.

How would you rate Paul's experience of how well the health services kept information about him confidential?

6710. Vignette 10

[Fouad] goes to the local public hospital whenever he needs to. The hospital is large but crowded. The waiting rooms are noisy and poorly ventilated. The hospital is generally kept clean though the toilets in the outpatient department tend to smell by the end of the day.

How would you rate Fouad's experience of the overall quality of the surroundings, for example space, seating, fresh air and cleanliness, of the health services?

6711. Vignette 11

[Roger] is suffering from AIDS. He is being treated on a general medical ward. The nurse who knows Roger's HIV status and is worried about her colleagues accidentally becoming infected tells the other nurses in the ward, as well as the orderlies but tells them they must keep this information confidential.

How would you rate Roger's experience of how well the health services kept information about him confidential?

6712. Vignette 12

[Malika] is not keeping in good health and has to go to the dispensary regularly. The place is very crowded, there are not enough chairs for people to sit on as they wait for the doctor. The place is not cleaned regularly and tends to be littered. The corridors are dark and the lights and fans often do not work.

How would you rate Malika's experience of the overall quality of the surroundings, for example space, seating, fresh air and cleanliness, of the health services?

6713. Vignette 13

[Kamal] has a nervous breakdown and had to spend 3 months in the past year in the local hospital. He had to sleep on an uncomfortable mattress with no sheets. There were 30 other patients in the same dormitory style ward and the toilets would smell as they were not cleaned. He came back with a skin infection as he couldn't wash regularly and there were bugs in the bed.

How would you rate Kamal's experience of the overall quality of the surroundings, for example space, seating, fresh air and cleanliness, of the health services?

6714. Vignette 14

[Alma] goes to the hospital to take an HIV test. Though only a number is used to identify the sample, one of the lab technicians recognizes Alma. The test turns out to be positive. The lab technician begins to tell everyone in the village about Alma being HIV positive.

How would you rate Alma's experience of how well the health services kept information about her confidential?

continued

SET C

6701. Vignette 1

[Carol] had to be in hospital over a long period, as her illness was difficult to diagnose. The hospital staff was very considerate in allowing her family to see her and be with her as much as possible. Whenever Carol wanted to contact her family they would allow her to use the phone. Knowing that Carol was worried, the hospital staff arranged for her to visit regularly a place of worship.

How would you rate Carol's experience of how the hospital allowed her to interact with family and friends and to continue social and/or religious customs during her stay?

6702. Vignette 2

[Polly] had to be in hospital for a long time after being involved in a car accident. The hospital staff encouraged her family to visit her daily at any time they could. Her mother often brought her sweets and cakes. Her family would take her to visit a place of worship once a week and spend time praying together.

How would you rate Polly's experience of how the hospital allowed her to interact with family and friends and to continue social and/or religious customs during her stay?

6703. Vignette 3

[Simon] has joint pains and breathlessness. He sees two specialists for these problems once every 2 months. Recently as his breathlessness was worsening, he asked to see a heart specialist and his medicines were adjusted. He sees his general physician regularly to get his prescriptions.

How would you rate Simon's experience of being able to use a health care provider or service of his choice?

6704. Vignette 4

[Alfredo] has a family physician who he consults regularly. Recently friends advised him to consult an alternative medicine provider [substitute appropriate name] for a skin problem. When he asked for a referral, his doctor told him this was not possible and sent him to a skin specialist instead.

How would you rate Alfredo's experience of being able to use a health care provider or service of his choice?

6705. Vignette 5

[Tamara] had to recuperate in hospital for two weeks after a bad fall. Her family visited her regularly during the visiting hours, but she was bored during the rest of the day. The hospital had no common room and patients were not encouraged to go to each other's rooms to chat. There was, however, a little library in the hospital which she visited and the nurses sometimes brought her the daily newspaper.

How would you rate Tamara's experience of how the hospital allowed her to interact with family and friends and to continue social and/or religious customs during her stay?

6706. Vignette 6

[Nathan] has been having headaches for the past year. Initially his general practitioner gave medicines but that did not help. He asked to be referred to a specialist. He has been investigated and detected to have a brain tumour that will require surgery. He knows a famous surgeon and has been able to fix up a date for the surgery by him this month.

How would you rate Nathan's experience of being able to use a health care provider or service of his choice?

6707. Vignette 7

[Dora] had to stay in hospital for two weeks when she broke her leg. Her husband and children were all working far from the hospital and they found it difficult to come and visit her, particularly as the visiting time allowed was very short. Her mother could not visit her at all as the visiting hours did not suit her.

How would you rate Dora's experience of how the hospital allowed her to interact with family and friends and to continue social and/or religious customs during her stay?

6708. Vignette 8

[Ibrahim] has stomach problems for several years. He has been referred to many doctors but has only had to follow the suggestions made by his family doctor. His requests to see a particularly well-known stomach specialist have been turned down by his insurance system.

How would you rate Ibrahim's experience of being able to use a health care provider or service of his choice?

6709. Vignette 9

[Asefa] had to be in hospital for a long time undergoing tests in preparation for his by-pass surgery. His family came to see him during the visiting hours but for the rest of the day he only saw the hospital staff when they came to attend to him. He was told not to listen to his little radio even though he was not disturbing anybody, and his request to have the local spiritual leader visit him was also discouraged on the grounds that other patients would be disturbed.

How would you rate Asefa's experience of how the hospital allowed him to interact with family and friends and to continue social and/or religious customs during his stay?

6710. Vignette 10

[Penelope] had to stay in hospital for two weeks after undergoing surgery. Her family hated coming to see her, because even during visiting time the hospital staff made them feel very unwelcome. Whenever her family brought her some sweets or cakes from home, the nurses would

continued

grumble saying that Penelope was being fussy about the hospital food. Penelope would have liked to have to her closest friends visit her but the nurses did not encourage this.

How would you rate Penelope's experience of how the hospital allowed her to interact with family and friends and to continue social and/or religious customs during her stay?

6711. Vignette 11

[Pascal] needs to go to the local hospital for his blood pressure. Each time that he goes, he is seen by a different doctor. When he asked to see his previous doctor, he was told that it was not possible. Once when he was very sick and had been feeling dizzy he asked to see another doctor or specialist but was told that he could not decide who he should see.

How would you rate Pascal's experience of being able to use a health care provider or service of his choice?

6712. Vignette 12

[Mamadou] goes to the community health centre for his epilepsy. He has to go on a certain day of the week as the unit/team that sees him is available only on those days. Of the four members in the team, though he sees a neurologist each time, he cannot decide who he will see as he gets sent to whoever is free at the time.

How would you rate Mamadou's experience of being able to use a health care provider or service of his choice?

6713. Vignette 13

[Joseph] had to stay in hospital for ten days after a road traffic accident. The nurses asked his family not to visit him as the hospital was crowded with patients, and visitors, they said, added to our workload. Though regular meals were provided in the hospital, Joseph's family thought they would treat him to some of his favourite dishes. Both Joseph and his brother were soundly scolded that day and told to mind the rules of the hospital. When Joseph asked if he could visit a place of worship the nurse in charge said that he could not leave the hospital.

How would you rate Joseph's experience of how the hospital allowed her to interact with family and friends and to continue social and/or religious customs during her stay?

6714. Vignette 14

[Andhaka] goes to the local general hospital. The hospital is large and has several specialities. Depending on his complaints he can decide which department to go to. Once he is registered in a department he must see only the person assigned to him that day.

How would you rate Andhaka's experience of being able to use a health care provider or service of his choice?

SET D

6701. Vignette 1

[Mary] has a serious health problem and knows that she will soon die. Every time she visits her doctor she asks him about her treatment and how much her condition is deteriorating. She wants to be able to plan for the future and make arrangements for her family once she dies. The doctor always tells her not to worry, that things are under control, and that he knows what he is doing.

How would you rate Mary's experience of getting involved in making decisions about her care or treatment as much as she wanted?

6702. Vignette 2

[Xavier] has a stomach ulcer and was advised surgery. His doctor told him it could be arranged only after 3 months as there were other patients in the queue. He now sees the doctor only when he has some discomfort and needs to arrange about 2 weeks in advance a time to meet him.

How would you rate Xavier's experience of getting prompt attention?

6703. Vignette 3

[Romero] has tuberculosis and needs to see his doctor in the primary care centre every month for renewing his prescription. He lives in a village 5 miles (8 km) away and must walk each time to see the doctor. Some days when he gets to the hospital he learns that the doctor is away on leave and must come back without medicines and make the trip again the next day. Once when he coughed blood at night and became very breathless, his relatives had to borrow a neighbour's cart to take him to the hospital.

How would you rate Romero's experience of getting prompt attention?

6704. Vignette 4

[Sarah] visits her doctor regularly because of back pain. She has discussed alternative treatment with her doctor such as special back exercises, acupuncture, yoga, and change in lifestyle, but he only believes in medication. Whenever the pain has got worse, he has adjusted the medication by prescribing higher doses. Despite the side effects that Sue is having, drowsiness, nausea and migraines, he will not consider other options.

How would you rate Sarah's experience of getting involved in making decisions about her care or treatment as much as she wanted?

6705. Vignette 5

[Henry] has recently been diagnosed as having diabetes. The first time he went to the clinic he had to have blood tests, eye check ups and other routine tests. The nurse explained every procedure in detail and asked him for his consent before doing any tests.

How would you rate Henry's experience of getting involved in making decisions about his care or treatment as much as he wanted?

continued

6706. Vignette 6

[Bob] broke his arm a few months ago and had to have a series of X-rays. Initially, the doctors told him about his fractures and explained what they were going to do. After that, they sent him for some other tests all over the hospital without explaining why. Although Bob asked what was happening, the doctors ignored him saying they were busy.

How would you rate Bob's experience of getting involved in making decisions about his care or treatment as much as he wanted?

6707. Vignette 7

[Kofi] has had a heart operation last year. He is now doing well and is on regular medication. He lives outside the city and has to drive once every 3 months to see his doctor. One night he had chest pain and called an ambulance and managed to get to the hospital in 30 minutes.

How would you rate Kofi's experience of getting prompt attention?

6708. Vignette 8

[Dilek] suffers from difficulty breathing and has wheezing attacks almost every week. She lives across the street from the city hospital and can get to the emergency room within 5 minutes of an attack. Within 10 minutes of getting to the emergency room she is given an injection that relieves her distress.

How would you rate Dilek's experience of getting prompt attention?

6709. Vignette 9

[John] has been diagnosed as having HIV. The doctor has been very supportive at the health centre he usually goes to. He has spent time discussing the different drug therapies, the psychological support that is available, and the medical care that he may need. Although he has advised John to start taking medication, he has asked John to decide what he wants to do.

How would you rate John's experience of getting involved in making decisions about his care or treatment as much as he wanted?

6710. Vignette 10

[Gabriel] has a history of chest pain. He usually goes to the local public hospital for his check-ups. One day he had severe pain in his chest and had to have emergency care. As soon as he got there, the doctors had to quickly run tests and take a blood sample. They did not ask for his permission as there was no time and they were concerned about his condition.

How would you rate Gabriel's experience of getting involved in making decisions about his care or treatment as much as he wanted?

6711. Vignette 11

[Aitor] has had backache for several years. The local hospital is always busy and he has to wait about 3 hours each time he has to see a doctor. At times he has to come away without seeing the doctor. He has been advised a special test and will have to wait for 6 weeks before he can get it done as the machine in the hospital is booked.

How would you rate Aitor's experience of getting prompt attention?

6712. Vignette 12

[Stan] fell down from a ladder and broke his leg one evening. He had to be taken to the district hospital, about 10 miles away (15 km), in a private car. He had to wait for an hour in the hospital for the surgeon to arrive and could be operated only the next day.

How would you rate Stan's experience of getting prompt attention?

6713. Vignette 13

[Tara] is always tired and has no energy to do anything. She gave birth to a baby girl two months ago. The doctor has told her that she may be suffering from post-natal depression. After discussing her condition with her, he has suggested that she could either try some anti-depressants or, if she prefers, go to a counsellor.

How would you rate Tara's experience of getting involved in making decisions about her care or treatment as much as she wanted.

6714. Vignette 14

[Niels] has a kidney disease and has to go to the hospital every month for a check up. He sees his regular physician at a pre-arranged time and can reach the hospital on a local bus within 15 minutes. In the past six months he has had to phone his doctor twice for urgent advice about his medication and has received the information he required right away.

How would you rate Niels's experience of getting prompt attention?

Variables	Brief Description of Item	Item missing rates	
		All Sections	Home care section in extended version only
	Filter	**5.7%**	
Q6000	Visit in last 12 months	1.5%	
Q6001	Outpatient visit	1.8%	
Q6002	At facility or at home	4.1%	
Q6003	Time of last visit	2.6%	
Q6004	Name of place	17.3%	
Q6005	Was it your usual place	6.6%	
	Outpatient and home care	**3.3%**	**5.6%**
Q6100	How long waited to get care	5.2%	4.1%
Q6101	How often care as soon as wanted	1.4%	5.9%
Q6102	Laboratory tests or examinations	1.1%	5.7%
Q6103	How long did you wait to get results	5.0%	2.1%
Q6104	Overall rating of prompt attention	1.1%	6.1%
Q6110	How often did health providers treat you with respect	0.6%	5.9%
Q6111	How often did office staff treat you with respect	1.8%	6.2%
Q6112	How often was privacy respected in physical exams	2.0%	6.2%
Q6113	Overall rating of dignity	0.9%	
Q6120	How often did providers listen carefully to you	2.3%	6.3%
Q6121	How often did providers explain things understandably	0.8%	6.2%
Q6122	How often did providers give you time to ask questions	1.1%	6.2%
Q6123	Overall rating of communication	0.9%	6.0%
Q6130	Were any decisions made about your care	1.9%	6.2%
Q6131	How often were you involved as much as you wanted	2.1%	2.0%
Q6132	How often did health providers ask your permission	4.5%	6.3%
Q6133	Overall rating of involvement in decision making as much as wanted	3.2%	6.1%
Q6140	How often were talks done privately	2.3%	6.5%
Q6141	How often did providers keep personal information confidential	12.2%	6.4%
Q6142	Overall rating of confidentiality	6.4%	7.1%
Q6150	How big a problem was it to get a provider of your choice	3.1%	6.5%
Q6151	How big a problem was it to use a health service other than the usual one	18.2%	3.1%
Q6152	Overall rating of choice	4.1%	6.7%
Q6160	How would you rate the quality of the waiting room	1.2%	
Q6161	How would you rate the overall cleanliness	1.2%	
Q6162	Overall rating of space, seating, fresh air and cleanliness	1.3%	

continued

Variables	Brief Description of Item	Item missings
	Inpatient care	**5.3%**
Q6300	Have you stayed in hospital overnight in the last 12 months	1.9%*
Q6301	Name of hospital	17.4%*
Q6302	Did you get hospital care as soon as you wanted	3.3%
Q6303	In hospital, how often could you get a nurse or doctor's attention as quickly as you wanted	3.0%
Q6304	Overall rating of prompt attention	2.9%
Q6305	Overall rating of dignity	2.8%
Q6306	Overall rating of communication	3.0%
Q6307	Overall rating of involvement in decision making as much as wanted	4.4%
Q6308	Overall rating of confidentiality	8.9%
Q6309	Overall rating of choice	7.7%
Q6310	Overall rating of space, seating, fresh air and cleanliness	3.7%
Q6311	How big a problem was it to have family and friends take care of personal needs	5.5%
Q6312	How big a problem was it to practice religious observances	13.6%
Q6313	Overall rating of how hospital allowed you to interact with family, friends and to continue social or religious customs	5.0%
	Discrimination	
	Were you treated badly by the health system because of your (nationality, social class, lack of private insurance, ethnicity, colour, sex, language, religion, political/other beliefs, health status, lack of wealth, other, specify)	
Average		**4.8%**
Q64001	nationality	3.0%
Q64002	social class	3.9%
Q64003	lack of private insurance	4.0%
Q64004	ethnicity	6.1%
Q64005	colour	6.7%
Q64006	sex	4.8%
Q64007	language	3.9%
Q64008	religion	4.2%
Q64009	political/other beliefs	4.4%
Q640010	health status	6.9%
Q640011	lack of wealth	4.4%
Q6401	Did you feel you were treated worse because you were a woman	40.9%
	Types of providers and services	
All types of providers (average)	I will read you a list of different types of places you can get health services. Please can you indiciate the number of times you went to each of them in the last 30 days.	**28.8%**
Q6500	general practitioners (doctors)	27.0%
Q6501	dentists	24.5%
Q6502	specialists	24.1%
Q6503	chiropracters	30.4%
Q6504	traditional healers	29.6%
Q6505	clinics (staffed mainly by nurses, run separately from hospitals)	27.9%
Q6506	hospital outpatient units	25.7%
Q6507	hospital inpatient units	29.0%
Q6508	pharmacy (where you talked to someone about your care and did not only purchase medicine)	22.4%
Q6509	home health care services	29.5%
Q6510	other, specify	46.7%
All reasons for visit (average)	What was the main reason you went for your most recent visit	**18.6%**

continued

Variables	Brief Description of Item	Item missings
All reasons for visit (average)	What services were provided at your most recent visit	**21.7%**
	Non-utilization	**5.4%**
Q6600	In the last 12 months, were you ever refused health care because you could not afford it	5.1%
Q6601	In the last 12 months, did you not seek health care because you could not afford it	5.7%
	Importance	**12.3%**
Q6602	most important domain(s)	9.2%
Q6603	least important domain(s)	15.3%

* Not included in the calculation of the missing percentage of this section; included in the filter section of Table 44.4.

Variables	Item missings	Variables	Item missings
Set A	**3%**	**Set B**	**3%**
vdig1	5%	vcon1	3%
vdig2	4%	vcon2	3%
vdig3	3%	vcon3	4%
vdig4	4%	vcon4	3%
vdig5	4%	vcon5	3%
vdig6	3%	vcon6	4%
vdig7	4%	vcon7	3%
vcom1	2%	vqba1	3%
vcom2	3%	vqba2	2%
vcom3	2%	vqba3	3%
vcom4	2%	vqba4	3%
vcom5	2%	vqba5	3%
vcom6	2%	vqba6	3%
vcom7	2%	vqba7	2%
Set C	**4%**	**Set D**	**3%**
vss1	4%	vaut1	3%
vss2	4%	vaut2	3%
vss3	4%	vaut3	3%
vss4	4%	vaut4	4%
vss5	4%	vaut5	4%
vss6	4%	vaut6	3%
vss7	3%	vaut7	4%
vch1	4%	vpa1	3%
vch2	4%	vpa2	3%
vch3	4%	vpa3	4%
vch4	5%	vpa4	3%
vch5	5%	vpa5	3%
vch6	4%	vpa6	3%
vch7	4%	vpa7	3%

Weights for Responsiveness Domains: Analysis of Country Variation in 65 National Sample Surveys

Nicole B. Valentine, Joshua A. Salomon

Introduction

Improving the responsiveness of health systems is an intrinsic goal of health policy (1). Responsiveness focuses on the interpersonal and contextual aspects of people's interaction with the health system. For measurement purposes, responsiveness has been defined on eight domains: dignity, autonomy, confidentiality of information, communication (of information), prompt attention, quality of basic amenities, access to support, and choice (of health care provider). An overall individual-based measure of health system responsiveness requires aggregation across different interactions of the individual with the system and, for any particular interaction, aggregation across the multiple domains of responsiveness. If a given interaction is described in terms of levels on a set of domains, a composite responsiveness score for this interaction may be computed by applying weights to each domain that reflect the relative importance of different components of responsiveness. The derivation of these weights for the first published assessment of the comparative performance of health systems by the World Health Organization in 2000 has been the subject of technical debate following the publication of *The World Health Report 2000* (2).

One key issue that was raised is the possibility that responsiveness domains might be weighted differently in different countries due to a variety of factors (e.g. culture, history, level of resources, political priorities) (3;4). Domain weights may also vary across different subgroups within a country defined by socio-demographic characteristics (e.g. the elderly compared with the young, males versus females, the employed versus the unemployed, the sick versus the healthy). For purposes of comparison, it is useful to apply a common set of weights in all countries and subpopulations so that interactions with the system characterized by identical levels on all domains receive the same composite responsiveness scores. In addition, within-country or subnational differences in weights may be of interest for local analyses, so a better understanding of the extent of variation in these weights would be valuable as well.

This chapter presents an empirical analysis of the country weights for the responsiveness domains based on a multi-country sample survey study. The goals of the analysis were to estimate the relative country weights for eight different domains of responsiveness using a simple survey instrument, and to examine cross-national variation in these weights.

Methodology

Data

The analyses described in the present chapter are based on the responses to 65 household surveys conducted in 56 different countries as part of the WHO Multi-country Survey Study on Health and Responsiveness 2000-2001 (5).[1] Surveys in the Multi-country Study were administered through four different modes and nine countries included multiple surveys conducted using various modes. The modes are specified in Table 45.1 and are described in more detail elsewhere (5;6). In all of the surveys, respondents selected from the general population were asked to read short descriptions of the eight responsiveness domains and to indicate the most important and the least important of them. Respondents were allowed to include more than one domain in each category. In face-to-face interviews, the interviewers read the domain descriptions to illit-

Table 45.1   List of 65 surveys analysed, survey modes, and respondent numbers

Countries	Mode	Respondents	Countries	Mode	Respondents
Argentina	Brief face-to-face	781	Jordan	Brief face-to-face	803
Austria	Postal	1 046	Kyrgyzstan	Postal	1 080
Bahrain	Brief face-to-face	809	Latvia	Brief face-to-face	752
Belgium	Brief face-to-face	1 100	Lebanon	Postal	1 112
Canada	Postal	407	Lithuania	Postal	1 746
Canada	Telephone	393	Luxembourg	Telephone	719
Chile	Postal	1 046	Malta	Brief face-to-face	500
China *	Postal	1 106	Mexico	Long face-to-face	4 812
China*	Long face-to-face	9 442	Morocco	Brief face-to-face	754
Colombia	Long face-to-face	6 019	Netherlands	Postal	610
Costa Rica	Brief face-to-face	756	Netherlands	Brief face-to-face	1 085
Croatia	Brief face-to-face	1 500	New Zealand	Postal	1 801
Cyprus	Postal	652	Nigeria	Long face-to-face	5 047
Czech Republic	Postal	1 021	Oman	Brief face-to-face	835
Czech Republic	Brief face-to-face	1 072	Poland	Postal	882
Denmark	Postal	1 511	Portugal	Brief face-to-face	1 001
Egypt	Long face-to-face	4 486	Republic of Korea	Postal	348
Egypt	Postal	1 383	Romania	Brief face-to-face	1 051
Estonia	Brief face-to-face	1 000	Russian Federation	Brief face-to-face	1 601
Finland	Postal	1 357	Slovakia	Long face-to-face	1 183
Finland	Brief face-to-face	1 021	Spain	Brief face-to-face	1 000
France	Postal	933	Sweden	Brief face-to-face	1 000
France	Brief face-to-face	1 003	Switzerland	Postal	821
Georgia	Long face-to-face	9 847	Thailand	Postal	1 186
Germany	Brief face-to-face	1 123	Trinidad and Tobago	Postal	1 245
Greece	Postal	909	Turkey	Long face-to-face	5 197
Hungary	Postal	1 500	Turkey	Postal	2 369
Iceland	Brief face-to-face	489	Ukraine	Postal	788
India*	Long face-to-face	5 196	United Arab Emirates	Brief face-to-face	818
Indonesia	Long face-to-face	9 952	United Kingdom	Postal	1 018
Indonesia	Postal	2 470	USA	Postal	588
Ireland	Brief face-to-face	711	Venezuela	Brief face-to-face	754
Italy	Brief face-to-face	1 002	Total respondents	All surveys	117 549

*   The survey covered three provinces in China, Shandong, Henan and Gansu, and one state in India, Andhra Pradesh.

erate respondents. Previously, pilot studies conducted in eight countries in 2000 had included a longer question asking respondents to rank all the domains. This single exercise took at least 15 minutes to perform in several sites, so the question was revised to have the respondents simply indicate the most important and the least important domains (Figure 45.1). 117 549 responses to the surveys were received in total. The average missing rate across all surveys was 9.2% for the most important question and 15.3% for the least important one. Missing rates were fairly constant across surveys. Missing rates for these two questions were higher than the average missing rate of 4% for all questions in all surveys (6).

ANALYSIS

Ordered Probit Model

The statistical model used for the analysis of the data was the ordered probit model, a standard econometric model for ordinal response data (7). Using individual responses on the most important and least important domains, an artificial series of categorical ratings by individuals for the full set of domains was generated on a three category scale, where 1 = least important, 2 = neither least important nor most important, and 3 = most important. In cases where more than one domain was mentioned as being the least or most important, all were given values of 1 or 3, respectively. The data were reshaped to include eight observations

Figure 45.1 Question on the importance of responsiveness domains asked to respondents in the responsiveness module of the Multi-country Survey Study

Read the cards below. These provide descriptions of some different ways the health care services in your country show respect for people and make them the centre of care. Thinking about what is on these cards and about the whole health system, which is the most important and the least important to you?

DIGNITY	AUTONOMY
■ being shown respect ■ having physical examinations conducted in privacy	■ being involved in deciding on your care or treatment if you want to ■ having the provider ask your permission before starting treatments or tests

CONFIDENTIALITY OF INFORMATION	SURROUNDINGS OR ENVIRONMENT
■ having your medical history kept confidential ■ having talks with health providers done so that other people who you don't want to have hear you can't overhear you	■ having enough space, seating and fresh air in the waiting room ■ having a clean facility (including clean toilets) ■ having healthy and edible food

CHOICE	SUPPORT
■ being able to choose your doctor or nurse or other person usually providing your health care ■ being able to go to another place for health care if you want to	■ being allowed the provision of food and other gifts by relatives ■ being allowed freedom of religious practices

PROMPT ATTENTION	COMMUNICATION
■ having a reasonable distance and travel time from your home to the health care provider ■ getting fast care in emergencies ■ having short waiting times for appointments and consultations, and getting tests done quickly ■ having short waiting lists for non-emergency surgery	■ having the provider listen to you carefully ■ having the provider explain things so you can understand ■ having time to ask questions

MOST IMPORTANT_____

LEAST IMPORTANT_____

per person, with each observation consisting of a vector of dummy variables (one for each country-domain combination) as the independent variables, and the score for a particular domain as the dependent variable. No individual explanatory variables were used as the analysis was undertaken at the country level.

The ordered probit model assumes that the categorical response scores arise from an unobserved, continuous latent variable representing the level of importance for a particular domain, normally distributed with variance 1:

$$Y_{i,j}^* \sim N(\mu_{i,j}, 1)$$

where $Y_{i,j}^*$ is the latent weight placed by person i on domain j.

The expected value of the latent variable $\mu_{i,j}$ is expressed as a linear function of a series of indicator variables for the different domains, specific to each country, so that the model coefficients represent the average relative value on the latent scale associated with each domain in each country.

The observed responses $y_{i,j}$ are related to a series of cut-points that represent thresholds on the latent variable at which individuals transition from one response category to another, so that:

$$y_{i,j} = 1 \ \text{if} \ -\infty \le Y_{i,j}^* < \tau_1$$
$$y_{i,j} = 2 \ \text{if} \ \tau_1 \le Y_{i,j}^* < \tau_2$$
$$y_{i,j} = 3 \ \text{if} \ \tau_2 \le Y_{i,j}^* < +\infty$$

Estimation of the model is based on the probabilities of answering in each category, given the distribution of the latent variable for that country and domain, and the set of cut-points (τ_1 and τ_2).

By convention, the model is identified by setting the variance of the normal distribution to 1 and the intercept term in the linear function (an arbitrary reference domain in one country) to 0, which produces a scale that is arbitrary but has interval properties. An interval scale allows us to make meaningful comparisons of the differences between any two domain values, but interpretation of the results in units corresponding to weights (i.e. numbers that lie between 0 and 1 and sum to unity across the set of domains for a given unit of comparison) requires a rescaling of the results, as described below.

Transformation of Parameters to Weights

The results of the ordered probit model reflect an unknown positive affine transformation of the true scale of domain weights. This relationship can be formalized as follows:

$$w_{i,j} = \alpha + \beta X_{i,j}$$

where $w_{i,j}$ is the coefficient for domain i in country j from the regression, $X_{i,j}$ is the properly scaled domain weight for domain i in country j, and α and β are unknown parameters.

In order to transform these results into weights (i.e. determine the values of α and β in order to rescale the coefficients), two additional pieces of information are used. The first is the requirement that the weights, by definition, must sum to unity for any given unit of observation (in this case, a country). The second piece of information that is needed is one known weight that can serve to anchor the scale. The latter was obtained by choosing a value for the lowest estimated weight across all domains and countries, corresponding to the lowest coefficient in the ordered probit regression.

Given the choice of the lowest weight across all domains and countries as the anchor point, there are natural constraints on the possible values for this weight. At the low end, the weight must be greater than or equal to 0, since negative weights have no meaning in this case. At the high end, the minimum weight must be less than or equal to 12.5%, as this represents the value obtained when all eight domains have equal weight (a weight higher than 12.5% would imply that at least one other domain has a weight lower than 12.5%, which is not possible since the chosen anchor has the lowest value across all domains). For any given value of this anchor weight, the coefficients of the linear transformation function are fully determined as follows:

$$\alpha = \frac{X_{D,C} \sum_{i=1}^{8} w_{i,C} - w_{D,C}}{X_{D,C} * 8 - 1}$$

$$\beta = \sum_{i=1}^{8} w_{i,C} - \alpha * 8$$

where the indices D and C indicate the reference domain and country, respectively, and $X_{D,C}$ therefore represents the choice of value for the anchor weight.

The rescaling parameters are computed based only on the reference country's coefficients (i.e. in the equations above, only C appears out of all possible values of j). Once they are applied to all of the regression coefficients, there will be some minor deviations from 1 in the sum of the weights in different countries, since the regression coefficients are estimated without constraint. The weights are therefore normalized to sum to 1 in each country following the application of the transformation function.

Results that would be obtained using anchor values between 0% and 10%, at 0.5% intervals were examined for this chapter. An anchor value of 0% results in the greatest amount of variation within and between countries, while an anchor weight of 10% produces near equality in all weights across domains and countries.

Results

Figure 45.2 shows the frequency with which domains were categorized as most important, least important, or neither most nor least important in each of the 65 surveys. Prompt attention (Figure 45.2f) was most commonly rated as the most important domain, with dignity and communication the next domains most likely to be considered most important (Figures 45.2c & 45.2e). Access to family and community support and quality of basic amenities were selected most often as the least important domains (Figures 45.2h & 45.2g). On average, across respondents from all countries, 42% of respondents selected prompt attention as the most important domain, while 41% selected support as the least important one.

Table 45.2 provides the estimated coefficients from the probit regression. The base country and domain in the probit regression was the United Arab Emirates, which was assigned a coefficient of 0. The country was chosen for convenience as it fell in first position in the alphabetical listing of countries when listed by country label (ARE). Consistent with Figure 45.2,

Figure 45.2 Frequency of respondents in a country rating a domain as least important or most important

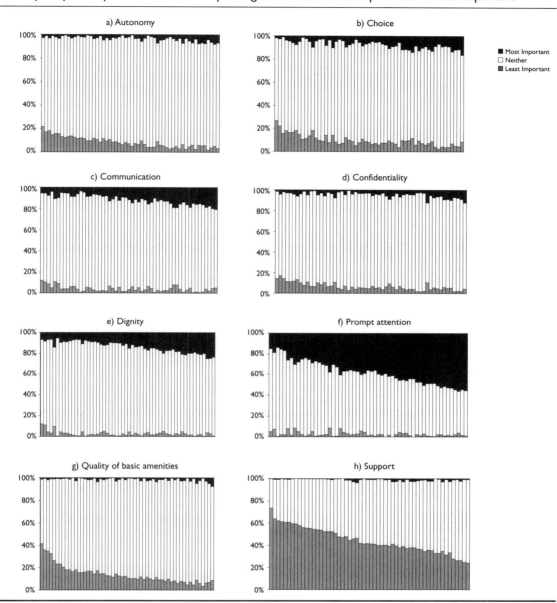

Domains not rated were assigned the label "neither least or most important." The large area of grey shading in (h) shows that across countries, a large proportion of respondents rated the access to family and community support domain as least important.

the coefficients on support are lowest in nearly every survey relative to other domains. The negative sign in front of many of the support domain coefficients indicates that the support domain in that particular country has a lower ranking relative to the base country (United Arab Emirates).

The regression coefficients were converted into weights using the approach described above, which depends on the choice of a particular anchoring value (for the lowest weight across all countries and

domains). Figure 45.3 provides results for a range of different choices for this anchoring value. For the main results in this chapter, the base case has been defined using an anchor weight of 2%. This choice reflects the notion that the *mean* weight in any particular country is unlikely to be zero even for the domain with the lowest relative importance. However, a low non-zero value has been chosen for the anchor because lower values for the minimum imply greater variation across domains and countries. Given the interest in

Table 45.2 Domain coefficients from the ordered probit model for 65 surveys[a]

Country	Autonomy	Choice	Communi-cation	Confiden-tiality	Dignity	Prompt attention	Quality of basic amenities	Support
Argentina	0.749	1.153	1.201	0.867	1.677	2.398	0.807	−0.023
Austria	1.398	1.249	1.620	1.270	1.425	1.901	0.758	−0.471
Bahrain	0.727	0.736	1.440	1.150	1.967	1.799	0.717	0.039
Belgium	1.141	1.183	1.369	1.433	1.584	2.082	0.119	0.137
Canada*	1.171	1.148	1.586	0.982	1.312	2.511	0.673	−0.625
Canada	0.963	1.089	1.429	1.139	1.217	2.419	−0.096	0.634
Chile	1.107	1.146	1.187	0.998	2.176	1.997	0.925	−0.588
China (3 provinces)[b]	1.025	0.949	1.400	0.841	1.682	2.113	0.702	−0.036
China* (3 provinces)[b]	1.305	1.153	1.313	0.902	2.072	1.574	1.151	−0.440
Colombia	1.043	1.008	1.364	1.041	1.693	2.279	0.652	−0.372
Costa Rica	0.898	0.816	1.533	1.071	1.514	2.080	0.770	0.120
Croatia	0.893	1.125	1.370	0.839	1.540	2.446	0.534	−0.062
Cyprus	0.994	1.474	1.293	0.981	1.481	1.961	0.956	−0.270
Czech Republic	0.853	1.176	1.041	1.156	1.351	2.506	0.802	−0.125
Czech Republic*	1.016	1.408	1.741	1.017	1.354	2.055	0.925	−0.591
Denmark	1.230	0.942	1.590	1.101	1.709	2.432	0.746	−0.914
Egypt	0.800	1.002	1.113	1.199	2.394	1.449	0.614	−0.072
Egypt*	0.465	0.988	1.071	1.360	2.247	1.417	1.005	0.076
Estonia	0.779	1.768	1.041	1.080	1.427	2.191	0.555	0.036
Finland	1.080	1.012	1.192	1.291	1.548	2.624	0.549	−0.467
Finland*	1.107	0.919	1.678	1.322	1.305	2.340	0.547	−0.414
France	1.028	1.218	1.450	1.442	1.463	2.236	0.016	0.059
France*	1.097	1.191	1.643	1.051	1.346	2.134	0.704	−0.101
Georgia	0.594	1.294	1.609	0.666	1.750	1.631	0.957	0.156
Germany	1.137	1.371	1.136	1.555	1.320	2.028	0.589	−0.113
Greece	0.839	1.324	1.305	0.886	1.500	2.319	1.059	−0.377
Hungary	1.115	1.243	1.468	1.005	1.529	2.374	0.818	−0.598
Iceland	1.125	1.000	1.392	1.624	1.816	1.772	0.367	−0.100
India (1 province)[b]	0.782	0.464	1.699	0.871	1.238	2.499	0.914	0.032
Indonesia	0.785	0.703	1.387	0.681	1.510	2.716	0.851	−0.132
Indonesia*	0.693	0.592	1.799	1.012	1.173	2.117	1.148	0.340
Ireland	0.964	1.326	1.211	1.245	1.592	2.272	0.509	−0.107
Italy	0.896	1.186	1.142	1.003	1.286	2.759	0.589	−0.008
Jordan	0.887	0.838	1.171	1.087	2.042	2.006	0.833	−0.287
Kyrgyzstan	0.929	1.018	1.180	0.885	1.382	1.817	1.106	0.538
Latvia	0.623	1.535	1.305	0.890	1.613	2.091	0.361	0.380
Lebanon	0.907	0.953	1.520	0.975	2.328	1.538	0.813	−0.150
Lithuania	0.884	1.253	1.356	0.642	1.597	2.241	0.745	0.088
Luxembourg	1.090	1.309	1.439	1.427	1.439	1.732	0.097	0.326
Malta	1.229	1.120	1.530	1.477	1.378	2.095	0.696	−0.251
Mexico	0.875	0.744	1.379	1.147	1.690	2.244	0.572	0.007
Morocco	0.724	0.841	1.310	1.000	2.134	1.924	0.774	0.271
Netherlands	1.212	1.006	1.368	1.514	1.543	2.175	0.431	−0.105
Netherlands*	1.370	0.968	1.576	1.117	1.430	2.281	0.753	−0.569
New Zealand	1.225	0.992	1.570	1.067	1.429	2.504	0.659	−0.569
Nigeria	0.678	0.304	1.582	0.967	0.920	2.555	1.068	0.367
Oman	0.679	0.743	1.581	1.223	1.772	1.953	0.929	−0.170
Poland	1.042	1.374	1.145	1.013	1.343	2.452	0.870	−0.396
Portugal	0.853	1.157	0.865	1.040	1.272	2.592	0.577	0.500

continued

Table 45.2 Domain coefficients from the ordered probit model for 65 surveys *(continued)*

Country	Autonomy	Choice	Communi-cation	Confiden-tiality	Dignity	Prompt attention	Quality of basic amenities	Support
Republic of Korea	1.183	1.231	2.069	1.021	1.293	1.778	1.082	−0.677
Romania	0.560	1.048	1.194	0.791	1.445	2.569	0.970	0.255
Russia	0.643	1.156	1.167	0.918	1.346	2.522	0.632	0.381
Slovakia	0.960	0.993	1.564	1.380	1.344	2.066	0.291	0.091
Spain	0.940	1.047	1.447	1.136	1.401	2.625	0.787	−0.368
Sweden	1.284	0.775	1.430	1.103	1.729	2.545	0.535	−0.543
Switzerland	1.346	1.233	1.425	1.117	1.318	1.535	0.830	0.077
Thailand	1.146	0.619	1.432	0.883	0.991	2.451	0.955	0.042
Trinidad and Tobago	0.964	0.760	1.259	1.117	1.262	1.919	1.055	0.320
Turkey	1.181	1.216	1.643	1.056	1.685	1.795	1.400	0.518
Turkey*	0.808	1.002	1.295	0.811	1.565	2.289	1.043	−0.140
Ukraine	1.216	1.787	1.954	1.569	2.136	2.758	1.693	0.792
United Arab Emirates	0.727	0.887	1.391	1.068	1.555	2.069	0.894	0.000
United Kingdom	1.042	0.849	1.323	1.095	1.342	2.579	0.662	−0.447
United States of America	1.131	1.872	1.588	0.936	1.284	1.817	0.697	−0.438
Venezuela	0.701	0.793	0.924	1.049	1.600	2.578	0.811	−0.011

a. The higher the coefficient, the greater the weight attributed to any particular domain with respect to the base country domain (United Arab Emirates, support domain)

b. The survey covered three provinces in China, Shandong, Henan and Gansu, and one state in India (Andhra Pradesh).

*   Postal survey.

Figure 45.3 Domain weights under alternative anchor values

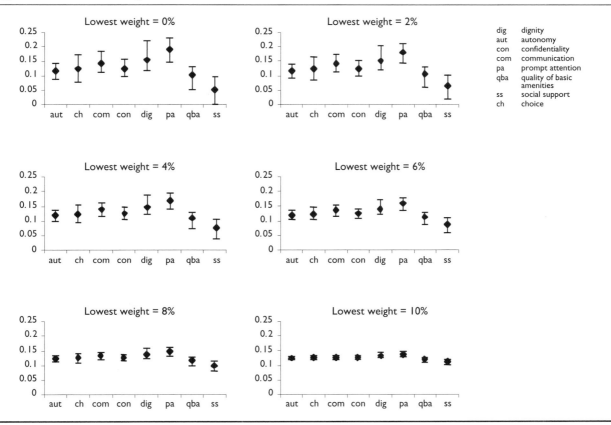

Each graph shows the range of weights (mean, minimum, and maximum) that are implied by choices for the lowest weight across all countries ranging from 0 to 10%, shown at 2% increments.

understanding variation in the weights that people from different countries and cultures place on different domains, this choice of a low value puts minimal constraint on the possibility of variation.

The average domain weights by country are shown in Table 45.3 for the base case anchor value of 2% (Denmark), along with summary statistics for the distribution of these weights across countries.

On average, the highest weight was attached to the domain of prompt attention (mean = 18%), with average weights for the other domains as follows: dignity (14.8 %), communication (14.0%), confidentiality

(12.4%), choice (12.3%), autonomy (11.7%), quality of basic amenities (10.6%), and access to support (6.3%).

Table 45.3 also shows the standard deviations of the domain weights across countries. There is some, albeit limited, variation in the weights across countries. This suggests, not surprisingly, that there is some variation in the way people in different countries view responsiveness, but that for the purposes of cross-country comparisons it would be reasonable to use a standard set of weights.

Figure 45.4 summarizes the country weights, with the survey results ordered from highest to lowest for prompt attention. The (Pearson's) correlations

Table 45.3 Domain weights for eight domains across 65 surveys[a]

Country	Autonomy	Choice	Communi-cation	Confidentiality	Dignity	Prompt attention	Quality of basic amenities	Support
Argentina	10.7	12.8	13.0	11.3	15.5	19.2	11.0	6.6
Austria	13.8	13.0	14.9	13.1	13.9	16.4	10.5	4.2
Bahrain	10.7	10.7	14.4	12.9	17.2	16.3	10.6	7.1
Belgium	12.6	12.8	13.7	14.1	14.8	17.4	7.3	7.4
Canada*	12.9	12.8	15.1	11.9	13.6	19.9	10.3	3.5
Canada	11.8	12.4	14.2	12.7	13.1	19.4	6.3	10.1
Chile	12.4	12.6	12.9	11.9	18.0	17.0	11.5	3.7
China (3 provinces)[b]	12.2	11.8	14.2	11.2	15.6	17.9	10.5	6.6
China (3 provinces)[b]*	13.4	12.6	13.4	11.3	17.4	14.8	12.6	4.4
Colombia	12.3	12.1	13.9	12.3	15.7	18.7	10.2	4.9
Costa Rica	11.4	11.0	14.8	12.3	14.7	17.6	10.8	7.4
Croatia	11.5	12.7	14.0	11.2	14.9	19.6	9.6	6.5
Cyprus	11.9	14.4	13.5	11.8	14.4	16.9	11.7	5.3
Czech Republic	11.2	12.9	12.2	12.8	13.8	19.9	11.0	6.1
Czech Republic*	12.0	14.0	15.7	12.0	13.7	17.4	11.5	3.7
Denmark	13.2	11.7	15.0	12.5	15.6	19.4	10.6	2.0
Egypt	11.1	12.2	12.8	13.2	19.6	14.5	10.1	6.5
Egypt*	9.3	12.0	12.5	14.0	18.6	14.3	12.1	7.2
Estonia	10.8	15.9	12.1	12.3	14.1	18.1	9.6	6.9
Finland	12.4	12.0	13.0	13.5	14.8	20.4	9.6	4.3
Finland*	12.5	11.6	15.5	13.7	13.6	19.0	9.6	4.6
France	12.1	13.0	14.2	14.2	14.3	18.3	6.8	7.0
France*	12.3	12.8	15.1	12.1	13.6	17.6	10.3	6.2
Georgia	9.9	13.6	15.3	10.3	16.0	15.4	11.8	7.6
Germany	12.5	13.8	12.5	14.7	13.5	17.1	9.7	6.1
Greece	11.1	13.6	13.5	11.4	14.5	18.8	12.2	4.8
Hungary	12.5	13.1	14.3	11.9	14.6	19.0	10.9	3.6
Iceland	12.5	11.9	13.9	15.1	16.1	15.8	8.6	6.2
India (1 province)[b]	11.0	9.3	15.9	11.5	13.4	20.1	11.7	7.0
Indonesia	11.0	10.6	14.2	10.5	14.9	21.3	11.4	6.2
Indonesia*	10.3	9.8	16.1	12.0	12.8	17.7	12.7	8.5
Ireland	11.7	13.5	12.9	13.1	14.9	18.4	9.3	6.1
Italy	11.4	12.9	12.7	12.0	13.4	21.1	9.8	6.7
Jordan	11.5	11.3	13.0	12.6	17.6	17.4	11.2	5.3

continued

between the country-specific weights and the global average weights are high, with an average correlation of 0.92.

For *The World Health Report 2000* (2), responsiveness was defined in terms of seven domains: dignity, autonomy, confidentiality, prompt attention, access to support, quality of basic amenities, and choice. The weights on these domains were derived from two sources: an internet survey (n = 1 007), and a survey of key health system actors in 35 countries (n = 1 791).

The combined weights derived from these two sources were 20% for prompt attention, 16.7% for dignity, autonomy, and confidentiality respectively, 15% for quality of basic amenities, 10% for access to support networks, and 5% for choice.

The mean values from *The World Health Report 2000* key informant surveys and the mean values and ranges from the WHO Multi-country Survey Study on Health and Responsiveness 2000–2001 of households are compared in Table 45.4. Communication was con-

Table 45.3 Domain weights for eight domains across 65 surveys *(continued)*

Country	Autonomy	Choice	Communi- cation	Confidentiality	Dignity	Prompt attention	Quality of basic amenities	Support
Kyrgyzstan	11.6	12.0	12.9	11.3	13.9	16.2	12.5	9.5
Latvia	10.0	14.8	13.6	11.4	15.2	17.7	8.6	8.7
Lebanon	11.4	11.7	14.6	11.8	18.8	14.7	11.0	6.0
Lithuania	11.4	13.3	13.8	10.1	15.1	18.4	10.6	7.2
Luxembourg	12.4	13.5	14.2	14.2	14.2	15.7	7.2	8.4
Malta	12.9	12.3	14.4	14.1	13.6	17.3	10.1	5.3
Mexico	11.4	10.7	14.1	12.8	15.7	18.6	9.8	6.9
Morocco	10.4	11.0	13.5	11.9	17.7	16.6	10.7	8.1
Netherlands	12.9	11.8	13.7	14.4	14.5	17.8	8.9	6.1
Netherlands*	13.8	11.7	14.9	12.5	14.1	18.5	10.6	3.8
New Zealand	13.1	11.9	14.9	12.3	14.2	19.7	10.2	3.8
Nigeria	10.5	8.5	15.3	12.0	11.8	20.5	12.6	8.8
Oman	10.4	10.7	15.1	13.2	16.1	17.0	11.7	5.9
Poland	12.2	13.9	12.7	12.0	13.7	19.5	11.3	4.7
Portugal	11.2	12.8	11.2	12.2	13.4	20.2	9.7	9.3
Republic of Korea	12.8	13.1	17.4	12.0	13.4	15.9	12.3	3.2
Romania	9.7	12.2	13.0	10.9	14.3	20.1	11.8	8.1
Russia	10.1	12.8	12.9	11.6	13.8	19.9	10.1	8.8
Slovakia	11.8	12.0	15.0	14.0	13.9	17.6	8.3	7.3
Spain	11.5	12.1	14.1	12.5	13.9	20.2	10.7	4.8
Sweden	13.4	10.8	14.2	12.5	15.7	20.0	9.5	3.9
Switzerland	13.7	13.1	14.1	12.5	13.6	14.7	11.0	7.1
Thailand	12.9	10.1	14.4	11.5	12.1	19.8	11.9	7.1
Trinidad and Tobago	11.9	10.8	13.4	12.7	13.4	16.9	12.4	8.5
Turkey	11.1	12.1	13.6	11.1	15.0	18.8	12.3	6.1
Turkey*	11.9	12.0	14.1	11.3	14.3	14.8	12.9	8.7
Ukraine	10.3	12.7	13.4	11.8	14.1	16.7	12.3	8.6
United Arab Emirates	10.7	11.5	14.2	12.5	15.0	17.7	11.6	6.8
United Kingdom	12.4	11.4	13.9	12.7	14.0	20.6	10.4	4.5
United States of America	12.6	16.4	15.0	11.6	13.4	16.2	10.4	4.5
Venezuela	10.6	11.1	11.8	12.5	15.4	20.6	11.2	6.8
Mean	11.7	12.3	14.0	12.4	14.8	18.0	10.6	6.3
Standard deviation	1.1	1.4	1.1	1.1	1.6	1.8	1.4	1.8

a. Weights were converted from the coefficients in Table 45.2 setting the lowest weight across domains and countries to 2%.

b. The survey covered three provinces in China, Shandong, Henan and Gansu, and one state in India, Andhra Pradesh.

* Postal survey.

sidered a sub-component of dignity and autonomy in *The World Health Report 2000*, but has since been added as a separate domain based on the recommendation of an expert consultation on responsiveness (4). For comparative purposes in Table 45.4, differences between the two sets of results have been computed by allocating a third of the weight for autonomy and a third of the weight for dignity in *The World Health Report 2000* to communication.

Four domains were allocated higher weights by key informants for *The World Health Report 2000* than by the respondents selected from the general population in the Multi-country Study: in descending order, quality of basic amenities (–4.4%), confidentiality (–4.3%), access to support (–3.7%), and prompt attention (–2%). Four domains were considered more important in the Multi-country Study. These were choice (7.3%), communication (2.9%), dignity (3.7%), and autonomy (0.6%). Finally, the relatively high weight (14%) attributed to communication supports the decision to include it as a domain in its own right.

The results of a simple (Pearson's) correlation of the domain weights with GDP per capita and health expenditure per capita are shown in Table 45.5. These variables were chosen to represent differences between countries with regards to socioeconomic levels and health system resources.

There is little association between the mean domain weights and the other variables, except in two cases. For quality of basic amenities, there is a strong negative correlation with GDP per capita (–0.56) and health expenditure per capita (–0.61). For autonomy, there is a moderate positive correlation with GDP

per capita (0.41) and health expenditure per capita (0.39). The negative relationships observed for quality of basic amenities are in line with the hypothesis that people in wealthier countries place less emphasis on the quality of basic amenities because good quality facilities already exist in these countries. Similarly with autonomy, it may be that individuals place more importance on autonomy where involvement in making decisions is more feasible, for example, in better-equipped health systems and in societies where higher levels of education prevail.

Discussion

This analysis of the relative importance of eight domains of responsiveness across 117 549 respondents from 56 different countries has yielded a number of surprising results. At the country level, there is some evidence of similarities between average domain weights, with the most important domain generally being prompt attention (for 54 out of 65 surveys) and the least important generally being access to support (for 60 surveys). The low standard deviation across countries of most of the domain weights provides some support for the use of a common set of global weights for comparative purposes, although further investigation of differences both within and across countries will be made possible by evaluation of variances at the individual level and by continuing data collection efforts in the World Health Survey (8).

Table 45.4 Comparison of responsiveness domain weights from 65 national sample surveys with the *World Health Report 2000* key informant survey results

	WHO Multi-country Study Results: mean*	World Health Report 2000 key informant survey results: mean	Difference
Prompt Attention	18.0	20.0	–2.0
Dignity	14.8	11.1	3.7
Communication	14.0	11.1	2.9
Confidentiality	12.4	16.7	–4.3
Choice	12.3	5.0	7.3
Autonomy	11.7	11.1	0.6
Quality of basic amenities	10.6	15.0	–4.4
Support	6.3	10.0	–3.7
Total	100.0	100.0	

* Weights are rounded to 1 decimal place. The summation based on the rounded values is 100.1.

Figure 45.4 Comparisons of eight domain weights across 65 surveys. Surveys in decending order based on prompt attention weights

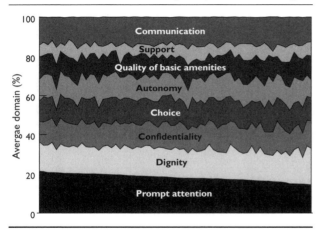

As more data become available on country-specific domain weights, sensitivity analyses for responsiveness assessments can be conducted to consider whether local variation in weights may affect policy conclusions in important ways.

Conceptually there has been some disagreement about whether communication was a domain in its own right, or a means to achieving better dignity, or better involvement in decision-making. The high weight assigned by individuals to communication (14%) seems to indicate that it should be a separate domain (4).

A comparison of the weights computed using the data and methods described in this chapter with those derived previously, from key informant surveys, revealed the largest discrepancy for the domain of choice. General population respondents in the WHO Multi-country Study gave this domain a much higher weight than respondents in the earlier key informant survey. This might be explained by the fact that key informants are less sensitive to constraints on choice of provider because they were themselves drawn largely from health services or provider groups, while respondents from a more general population sample value choice more highly. Comparison of the responses of people who work in the health system with those who do not is one way of exploring this question in more detail, an option pursued in the World Health Survey.

In interpreting the results, it is important to note several limitations. The study is based on artificially generated categorical ratings from questions on the most and the least important domains. A longer question for eliciting the relative importance of the domains has been included in the World Health Survey 2002, asking respondents to rate the importance of each domain on a five-point categorical response scale ranging from "extremely important" to "not at all important." It may also be useful to examine other possible models for deriving weights, including the analysis of direct rankings using variants of the discrete choice models introduced by McFadden (9). Another important limitation to be emphasized is that inferences regarding weights on different domains, given data only on the most important and the least important ones, require specification of at least one anchor weight in order to identify a unique scale. The basis for assigning this anchor weight deserves further consideration. Finally, additional enhancements to the statistical model should be explored, for example incorporation of other prior information about the weights in a Bayesian framework or combination of the two-step procedure of estimation and transformation into a single process.

Despite these limitations, the technique presented here allows a considerable amount of information to be extracted from a limited set of survey questions. This general approach may be useful in a number of other applications in which ordinal data are available, but these data are assumed to reflect an underlying set of weights.

ACKNOWLEDGEMENTS

The authors would like to acknowledge the special contribution of Charles Darby (Agency for Healthcare Research and Quality, USA) who was instrumental in developing the question on domain ranks in the responsiveness module of the Multi-country Survey Study. They would also like to thank Christopher J.L. Murray and David B. Evans of the World Health Organization, and Gouke J. Bonsel (Amsterdam Medical Centre, Holland) for their comments on earlier drafts.

NOTES

1 Responsiveness data from 65 out of 70 surveys containing the responsiveness module were available at the time of analysis.

REFERENCES

(1) Murray CJL, Frenk J. A framework for assessing the performance of health systems. *Bulletin of the World Health Organization*, 2000, 78(6):717–731.

Table 45.5 Correlation of responsiveness domain weights with GDP per capita and total health expenditure per capita for 65 surveys

	GDP per capita (US $)	Total health expenditure per capita (US $)
Autonomy	0.410	0.393
Choice	−0.092	−0.026
Communication	−0.011	0.055
Confidentiality	0.300	0.231
Dignity	−0.029	−0.054
Prompt attention	0.233	0.281
Quality of basic amenities	−0.562	−0.614
Support	−0.284	−0.318

(2) World Health Organization. *The World Health Report 2000. Health Systems: Improving Performance.* Geneva, World Health Organization, 2000.

(3) Häkkinen U, Ollila E, eds. *The World Health Report 2000: what does it tell us about health systems? Analyses by Finnish experts.* Helsinki, National Research and Development Center for Welfare and Health (STAKES), 2000.

(4) World Health Organization. Technical Consultation on Concepts and Methods for Measuring the Responsiveness of Health Systems. In: Murray CJL, Evans DB, eds. *Health systems performance assessment: debates, methods and empiricism.* Geneva, World Health Organization, 2003.

(5) Üstün TB et al. WHO Multi-country Survey Study on Health and Responsiveness 2000–2001. In: Murray CJL, Evans DB, eds. *Health systems performance assessment: debates, methods and empiricism.* Geneva, World Health Organization, 2003.

(6) Valentine NB et al. Classical psychometric assessment of the responsiveness instrument in the WHO Multi-country Survey Study on Health and Responsiveness 2000–2001. In: Murray CJL, Evans DB, eds. *Health systems performance assessment: debates, methods and empiricism.* Geneva, World Health Organization, 2003.

(7) Long JS. *Regression models for categorical and limited dependent variables.* Thousand Oaks, Sage Publications, 1997.

(8) World Health Organization. *World Health Survey.* Geneva, World Health Organization, 2003. URL: http://www3.who.int/whs/

(9) McFadden D. Conditional logit analysis of qualitative choice behavior. In: Zarembka P, ed. *Frontiers of econometrics.* New York, Academic Press, 1974: 105–142.

Chapter 46

Patient Experiences with Health Services: Population Surveys from 16 OECD Countries

Nicole B. Valentine, Juan Pablo Ortiz, Ajay Tandon, Kei Kawabata, David B. Evans, Christopher J.L. Murray

Introduction

One of the characteristics of the health sector is that health professionals have traditionally made decisions on what they think is in the best interest of the patient on the grounds that members of the general public lack the technical knowledge to make fully informed decisions themselves. Partly for this reason, attention has only recently focused on the perceptions of the public of their health systems, with patient satisfaction surveys and patient reports of their experiences with health care becoming more widely used for bench-marking purposes (1–6).

Estimates of patient satisfaction pose a number of problems for bench-marking. The most important is that satisfaction measures the discrepancy between expectations prior to an experience and the actual experience (7). This contains two pieces of information: expectations and the quality of the experience, making it difficult to determine if low satisfaction is due to high expectations or to interactions with the system that are of low quality. Additional problems are the lack of a comparable metric to measure satisfaction across settings and over time, and the difficulty of determining the reliability and validity of instruments due to the difficulty of establishing "truth." Patient satisfaction surveys have also been criticized for providing little direction on how to improve service quality (1;5).

For these reasons, increasing attention has focused on dimensions of people's experiences with the health system that can improve the well-being of the population independently of any resulting improvement in health. These dimensions characterize what is referred to here as health system responsiveness (8).

Two key principles guide the strategy for measuring responsiveness. First, it is measured from the perspective of the individual—how the individual describes the nature of his/her interaction with the health system. It is not measured from the perspective of an expert's evaluation of the technical quality of the interaction. Second, it is important to ensure comparability of measurement across populations and over time if responsiveness is to be used for bench-marking.

The results presented here focus on health system responsiveness in outpatient and inpatient service settings. Using a standardized questionnaire module fielded in a sample survey in 16 OECD countries in 2001, aspects of individuals' interactions with the system were measured on the following core domains: autonomy, choice of health care provider, communication, confidentiality of information, dignity, prompt attention, quality of basic amenities, and access to family and community support. This chapter reports the main results and compares the resulting estimates of health system responsiveness with earlier estimates of patient satisfaction in 15 of those countries.

Methods

Table 46.1 reports details of the survey study, including the countries involved, the survey modes, response rates, final sample sizes, and the percentage of respondents reporting an outpatient or inpatient experience in the previous 12 months.

All surveys used stratified, national sampling frames. Ten of the surveys involved face-to-face interviews, one was a random-digit telephone dialing survey (Luxembourg), and the remaining five were self-administered surveys posted to households. Surveys were conducted in the appropriate national

Table 46.1 Descriptive statistics of the responsiveness module for 16 OECD countries: survey mode, response rates, the number of respondents, and the percentage of respondents using health services

Country	Mode	Survey response rates (%)	Number of respondents (n)	Respondents with outpatient experience in the last 12 months (%)	Respondents with inpatient experience in the last 12 months (%)
Belgium	Face-to-face	48	1 100	56.2	12.2
Canada	Postal	55	407	61.4	10.6
Finland	Face-to-face	52	1 021	70.7	15.1
France	Face-to-face	77	1 003	65.0	13.1
Germany	Face-to-face	80	1 123	62.2	8.5
Greece	Postal	41	909	69.9	22.4
Ireland	Face-to-face	39	711	47.4	12.5
Italy	Face-to-face	61	1 002	45.0	6.9
Luxembourg	Telephone	72	719	71.2	13.4
Netherlands	Face-to-face	59	1 085	63.2	7.7
New Zealand	Postal	65	1 801	80.6	14.5
Portugal	Face-to-face	61	1 001	53.3	9.5
Spain	Face-to-face	75	1 000	61.9	8.5
Sweden	Face-to-face	53	1 000	56.4	10.7
United Kingdom	Postal	43	1 018	69.6	12.5
United States	Postal	36	588	75.9	13.8

language. Sampling frames excluded institutionalized populations.

The survey instrument built on the approach used to assess patient experience in the Consumer Assessment of Health Plans Survey (CAHPS) in the United States and in the surveys of the Picker Institute in the United States and Europe(*1;3;9*). Those surveys sought to ensure comparability by focusing on a specific, usually the most recent, visit and on clearly defined aspects of the process or outcome. The questions (items) included in the final instrument for our surveys were chosen after extensive field-testing and psychometric evaluation (*10–12*).

The responsiveness module consisted of items covering the domains of people's interactions with health systems in outpatient and inpatient settings. The same domains were covered in both settings, except quality of basic amenities in outpatient settings was replaced by access to family and community support in inpatient settings. Table 46.2 shows the specific items, with domains ordered as they appeared in the instrument.

The instrument also contained questions on the relative importance of the different responsiveness domains as perceived by each respondent (necessary for weighting the domains in the calculation of the overall inpatient and outpatient responsiveness results), health care utilization patterns, and socio-demographic variables. These questions were asked to all respondents (*12*).

Enhancing the cross-population comparability of the instrument built on the work on "anchoring vignettes," which required the inclusion in the questionnaire of a series of hypothetical stories or vignettes (*13*). Vignettes are short descriptions of people's experiences with health systems as they relate to the different domains of responsiveness. The respondent is asked to report the level of dignity, for example, with which the person in the vignette is being treated, answering on a scale of "very good," "good," "moderate," "bad," "very bad." This information provides a record of differences in the way people use verbal categories to evaluate a common stimulus.

For example, one person might categorize the scenario described in the vignette as "good," while another might consider the same scenario "very good." In the analysis of the results, the different response categories in the vignettes are used to adjust each respondent's description of his/her own experiences onto a common response scale.

Only the respondents who had used a health service in the previous 12 months were requested to complete the responsiveness questions. If they had visited both outpatient and inpatient services, they answered both sections. The number of responses obtained was, therefore, a function of the overall response rate as

Table 46.2 Wording of responsiveness module items and response options for inpatient and outpatient services in the Multi-country Survey Study for the domains of prompt attention, dignity, communication, autonomy, confidentiality, choice, quality of basic amenities, and support

	Section of questionnaire	Response categories
Prompt attention		
In the last 12 months, how long did you usually have to wait from the time that you wanted care to the time that you received care?	Outpatient	time
In the last 12 months, when you wanted care, how often did you get care as soon as you wanted?	Outpatient	never, sometimes, usually, always
Generally, how long did you have to wait before you could get the laboratory tests or examinations done?	Outpatient	same day, 1–2 days, 3–5 days, 6–10 days, more than 10 days (specify)
Did you get your hospital care as soon as you wanted?	Inpatient	yes, no
When you were in the hospital, how often did you get attention from doctors and nurses as quickly as you wanted?	Inpatient	never, sometimes, usually, always
Now, overall, how would you rate your experience of getting prompt attention at the health services (hospital) in the last 12 months?	Outpatient and Inpatient	very good, good, moderate, bad, very bad
Dignity		
In the last 12 months, when you sought care, how often did doctors, nurses or other health care providers treat you with respect?	Outpatient	never, sometimes, usually, always
In the last 12 months, when you sought care, how often did the office staff, such as receptionists or clerks there, treat you with respect?	Outpatient	never, sometimes, usually, always
In the last 12 months, how often were your physical examinations and treatments done in a way that your privacy was respected?	Outpatient	never, sometimes, usually, always
Now, overall, how would you rate your experience of getting treated with dignity at the health services in the last 12 months?	Outpatient and Inpatient	very good, good, moderate, bad, very bad
Communication		
In the last 12 months, how often did doctors, nurses or other health care providers listen carefully to you?	Outpatient	never, sometimes, usually, always
In the last 12 months, how often did doctors, nurses or other health care providers there, explain things in a way you could understand?	Outpatient	never, sometimes, usually, always
In the last 12 months, how often did doctors, nurses or other health care providers give you time to ask questions about your health problem or treatment?	Outpatient	never, sometimes, usually, always
Now, overall, how would you rate your experience of how well health care providers communicated with you in the last 12 months?	Outpatient and Inpatient	very good, good, moderate, bad, very bad
Autonomy		
In the last 12 months, how often did doctors, nurses or other health care providers there involve you as much as you wanted to be in deciding about the care, treatment or tests?	Outpatient	never, sometimes, usually, always
In the last 12 months, how often did doctors, nurses or other health care providers there ask your permission before starting tests or treatment?	Outpatient	never, sometimes, usually, always
Now, overall, how would you rate your experience of getting involved in making decisions about your care or treatment as much as you wanted in the last 12 months?	Outpatient and Inpatient	very good, good, moderate, bad, very bad
Confidentiality		
In the last 12 months, how often were talks with your doctor, nurse or other health care provider done privately so other people who you did not want to hear could not overhear what was said?	Outpatient	never, sometimes, usually, always
In the last 12 months, how often did your doctor, nurse or other health care provider keep your personal information confidential? This means that anyone whom you did not want informed could not find out about your medical conditions.	Outpatient	never, sometimes, usually, always
Now, overall, how would you rate your experience of the way the health services kept information about you confidential in the last 12 months?	Outpatient and Inpatient	very good, good, moderate, bad, very bad

continued

Table 46.2 Wording of responsiveness module items and response options for inpatient and outpatient services in the Multi-country Survey Study for the domains of prompt attention, dignity, communication, autonomy, confidentiality, choice, quality of basic amenities, and support *(continued)*

	Section of questionnaire	Response categories
Choice		
In the last 12 months, with the doctors, nurses and other health care providers available to you how big a problem, if any, was it to get to a health care provider you were happy with?	Outpatient	no problem, mild, moderate, severe, extreme
Over the last 12 months, how big a problem if any was it to get to use other health care services other than the one you usually went to?	Outpatient	no problem, mild, moderate, severe, extreme
Now, overall, how would you rate your experience of being able to use a health care provider or service of your choice over the last 12 months?	Outpatient and Inpatient	very good, good, moderate, bad, very bad
Quality of basic amenities		
Thinking about the places you visited for health care in the last 12 months, how would you rate the basic quality of the waiting room, for example, space, seating and fresh air?	Outpatient	very good, good, moderate, bad, very bad
Thinking about the places you visited for health care over the last 12 months, how would you rate the cleanliness of the place?	Outpatient	very good, good, moderate, bad, very bad
Now, overall, how would you rate the overall quality of the surroundings, for example, space, seating, fresh air and cleanliness of the health services you visited in the last 12 months?	Outpatient*	very good, good, moderate, bad, very bad
Support		
In the last 12 months, when you stayed in hospital, how big a problem, if any, was it to get the hospital to allow your family and friends to take care of your personal needs, such as bringing you your favourite food, soap etc.?	Inpatient	no problem, mild, moderate, severe, extreme
During your stay in hospital, how big a problem, if any, was it to have the hospital allow you to practice religious or traditional observances if you wanted to?	Inpatient	no problem, mild, moderate, severe, extreme
Now, overall, how would you rate your experience of how the hospital allowed you to interact with family, friends and to continue your social and or religious customs during your stay over the last 12 months?	Inpatient	very good, good, moderate, bad, very bad

*For all surveys run by INRA.

well as the rate of service utilization in the previous 12 months.

Data analysis was undertaken using Stata 7.0. The patient responsiveness domains were analysed using random-effects methods and a hierarchical ordered probit model (*13*). The steps from processing the raw data (responses) to the development of an average responsiveness score for the countries are described in Box 46.1.

Each domain mean score was age- and sex-standardized. All age-sex groups were assigned equal weights as each group's experience of responsiveness was considered of equal importance. Overall inpatient and outpatient responsiveness indices were calculated using weights obtained from the surveys for the different domains (in order of importance: prompt attention 0.180, dignity 0.148, communication 0.140, confidentiality 0.124, choice 0.123, autonomy 0.117, quality of basic amenities 0.106, support 0.063)(*14*).

RESULTS

A total of 27 521 (17 792 face-to-face and 9 729 postal) respondents were contacted in the 16 countries. Table 46.1 shows several survey statistics. The average response rate calculated on the basis of completed interviews as a percentage of effective contacts was 57%: 48% in the postal surveys and 60% in the interviewer administered surveys. The response rates are comparable to those observed for similar instruments in OECD countries (*5*). The average item missing rate was 4%, with a slightly higher average for the postal surveys (5%). Both rates were generally considered acceptable when compared with other studies (*4*). A total of 15 488 responses were eligible for analysis. The eligibility criterion was the completion of at least one of the questions on sex, age, health status, or one of the questions asking about utilization. Across all surveys, 10 088 respondents (65%) reported experi-

| **Box 46.1** | Steps for estimating the mean population level of responsiveness |

1 Run the compound hierarchical ordered probit model (CHOPIT) (*13*) to devise a common cross-country scale by domain.

    Model variables including age, sex, and education, interacted with country-reported health on the day (on 5-point "very good" to "very bad" scale).

2 Run a fixed random-effect CHOPIT model that generates 25 estimates per individual with

    2.1 Cut-points modelled using dependent variables: sex, years of education, and reported health.

    2.2 Responses on domain questions related to encounters modelled using dependent variables: age, sex, years of education and reported health.

3 Rescale domain results from 0 to 100 by setting the result corresponding to the coefficient of lowest vignette to 0, and the result corresponding to the highest vignette to 100.

4 Set any results over 100 to the maximum of 100 (truncation). Results above 100 imply that people had experiences that were better than the best vignette. This was considered an area of measurement akin to the measurement of "talent" in health (where a marathon runner is not considered "healthier" than someone who can run 5 kilometres) and therefore not of relevance for the study of the experiences of the general population (*11*).

5 Obtain survey means by taking an average of the mean 0 to 100 scores obtained for the following age and sex groups:

Male (yrs)	Female (yrs)
18–24	18–24
25–34	25–34
35–44	35–44
45–54	45–54
65+	65+

Equal weights were applied across all age and sex groups to reflect the notion that responsive treatment was given equal value regardless of sex or age.

6 Repeat steps 3 to 5 on the 25 estimates obtained for each survey respondent to obtain 25 survey means.

7 Obtain country means by taking an average of the 25 survey means.

8 Obtain confidence intervals by taking one standard deviation of the 25 survey means.

ences with health services in the previous 12 months: 1 856 as inpatients and 9 885 as outpatients, with an overlap of 1 653 answering both inpatient and outpatient sections of the questionnaire. The survey in Ireland coincided with the outbreak of foot-and-mouth disease when interviewers were not permitted to enter rural areas. The results for this country are applicable to urban areas only.

Tables 46.3 and 46.4 display the mean level of inpatient and outpatient service responsiveness and the associated confidence intervals by domain and by country. For inpatient services, responsiveness was relatively high in Ireland (urban), Luxembourg, Sweden, the United Kingdom, and the United States, while Greece, Portugal, and Italy reported relatively low levels. For outpatient services, the highest levels of overall responsiveness were reported in Ireland (urban), New Zealand, and the United States. Substantially lower levels were observed again in Greece, Portugal, and Italy.

Another way of looking at the responsiveness results is to compare the best and the worst performing domains overall. Across inpatient domains, the best performance was most often observed in support (seven countries out of 16 achieved the highest level on this domain) and choice (six countries). The worst performance was observed in the autonomy domain (10 countries). Across outpatient domains, the best performance was observed for choice (12 countries) and the worst for basic amenities (11 countries), followed by autonomy (five countries).

An interesting question to ask is whether countries are performing well on domains that are considered the most important. Table 46.5 shows the countries with the strongest and weakest performance in the two domains that were viewed as the most important: prompt attention (18%) and dignity (14.8%). If Germany is contrasted to the UK, outpatient confidentiality is lower in Germany, but prompt attention—the dimension that is most important to people—is rated at a much higher level. Partly as a result, Germany has a higher overall outpatient responsiveness score (89) than the UK (87).

The results within countries were also analysed to see whether it was possible to detect systematic relationship between responsiveness and common variables like sex, health status reported for the previous 30 days, and education. One systematic finding emerged. Reported health was positively associated with responsiveness in most countries across all outpatient domains (on average 10 countries per domain, with standard deviation of 1.4). The one exceptional domain was quality of basic amenities but this was not unexpected. Perceptions of facility cleanliness, for example, are unlikely to be affected by how a patient was feeling about their state of health, in contrast to perceptions of the promptness of attention.

The relationship between country responsiveness scores and total health expenditure per capita was also explored. Figure 46.1 shows the scatterplot of total health expenditure per capita with inpatient and outpatient responsiveness for the 16 countries in this study. Overall responsiveness increases with increases

Table 46.3   Responsiveness domain and overall results for inpatient services in 16 OECD countries: means an...

Survey	Autonomy			Choice			Communication			Confidentiality			Dignity		
	Mean	Lower bound	Higher bound	Mean	Lower bound	Higher bound	Mean	Lower bound	Higher bound	Mean	Lower bound	Higher bound	Mean	Lower bound	High bou...
Belgium	75	73	77	97	96	98	87	86	88	79	77	80	88	87	9
Canada	78	74	81	94	92	95	84	81	87	91	88	93	93	91	9
Finland	76	75	77	60	58	62	86	85	87	83	82	84	85	83	8
France	71	69	73	96	95	97	88	86	89	83	82	84	91	89	9
Germany	74	72	75	85	83	86	74	73	76	83	81	84	85	83	8
Greece	44	43	46	71	69	73	49	48	51	79	77	81	61	60	6
Ireland	75	73	77	88	85	90	91	90	93	92	90	93	91	90	9
Italy	53	51	56	90	88	92	74	72	76	68	66	69	74	72	7
Luxembourg	83	81	84	88	86	90	90	88	91	83	82	85	92	91	9
Netherlands	72	70	74	88	86	90	82	81	84	75	74	76	87	85	8
New Zealand	87	86	88	95	94	95	88	87	89	86	85	87	91	90	9
Portugal	66	63	68	78	76	81	71	69	73	70	68	71	66	65	6
Spain	61	59	63	82	80	84	84	83	86	83	81	84	85	83	8
Sweden	81	79	82	87	85	89	89	88	91	88	86	90	97	96	9
United Kingdom	81	79	82	93	92	94	85	83	87	90	89	91	94	93	9
United States	84	82	87	94	93	95	87	84	89	84	82	87	95	94	9
Average	72	70	75	87	85	88	82	80	83	82	81	84	86	84	87

Table 46.4   Responsiveness domain and overall results for outpatient services in 16 OECD countries: means an...

Survey	Autonomy			Choice			Communication			Confidentiality			Dignity		
	Mean	Lower bound	Higher bound	Mean	Lower bound	Higher bound	Mean	Lower bound	Higher bound	Mean	Lower bound	Higher bound	Mean	Lower bound	High bou...
Belgium	79	78	79	100	100	100	87	87	88	81	80	82	92	91	92
Canada	85	84	86	96	94	98	91	89	92	95	94	97	98	98	99
Finland	84	83	85	83	80	85	88	87	89	86	85	87	95	95	96
France	71	70	72	100	100	100	89	88	90	85	84	86	95	94	95
Germany	84	83	85	98	98	99	85	84	85	87	87	88	90	90	91
Greece	48	47	49	72	70	74	53	52	54	81	80	82	63	62	64
Ireland	87	86	88	98	98	99	94	93	95	94	93	95	98	97	98
Italy	58	57	59	98	96	99	73	72	74	69	69	70	73	72	74
Luxembourg	83	82	84	98	97	99	81	80	82	82	82	83	91	91	92
Netherlands	80	79	81	97	96	98	85	84	86	77	76	78	94	94	94
New Zealand	91	91	92	100	99	100	91	91	92	92	92	93	95	95	96
Portugal	67	66	68	85	82	87	76	75	77	71	71	72	71	71	72
Spain	64	63	64	85	83	87	79	78	80	83	82	83	83	82	83
Sweden	83	82	84	94	93	96	88	88	89	86	85	87	95	95	96
United Kingdom	81	80	82	98	97	98	85	84	86	96	95	96	95	95	95
United States	87	86	88	99	99	100	89	88	90	90	89	91	98	97	98
Average	77	76	78	94	93	95	83	83	84	85	84	86	89	89	90

in per capita health expenditure. This correlation was significant for inpatient services (Spearman's rho = 0.51, p = 0.04), but not significant for outpatient services (rho = 0.46, p = 0.07). At lower levels of expenditure, there appears to be a stronger relationship between health expenditure and responsiveness than at higher levels of expenditure.

RESPONSIVENESS VERSUS SATISFACTION

The responsiveness results reported to this point reflect people's experiences with the health system. To illustrate this, we compare the responsiveness results with results from recent representative surveys of patient satisfaction, available for 15 of the OECD countries in which the responsiveness surveys were undertaken standard errors, standardized by country, age and sex

	Prompt attention			Support			Overall inpatient	
Mean	Lower bound	Higher bound	Mean	Lower bound	Higher bound	Mean	Lower bound	Higher bound
73	72	74	91	90	93	83	83	84
71	69	72	96	93	99	85	84	86
81	80	81	87	85	88	79	79	80
72	71	73	90	89	92	83	83	84
85	84	86	89	88	91	82	81	82
61	61	62	78	77	79	62	62	63
82	81	83	90	89	92	87	86	87
78	77	80	79	77	81	74	73	74
83	81	84	94	93	96	87	86	88
85	85	86	96	95	97	83	82	84
78	77	79	83	82	84	87	86	87
71	70	73	74	72	76	71	70	71
78	77	79	80	79	82	79	79	80
74	73	75	95	94	96	86	86	87
82	81	83	95	93	96	88	87	88
79	77	80	91	88	93	87	86	88
77	76	78	88	86	90	81	81	82

standard errors, standardized by country, age and sex

	Prompt attention			Basic amenities			Overall outpatient	
Mean	Lower bound	Higher bound	Mean	Lower bound	Higher bound	Mean	Lower bound	Higher bound
84	83	85	75	74	76	86	85	86
81	80	82	77	75	79	89	88	90
86	86	87	72	71	73	86	85	86
81	81	82	77	76	78	86	85	86
94	93	94	83	82	84	89	89	90
71	70	71	59	59	60	64	64	65
95	94	95	88	86	90	94	93	94
75	74	75	61	60	62	73	72	73
82	81	83	74	73	75	85	84	85
89	89	90	73	72	74	86	85	86
89	88	89	77	76	78	91	91	91
76	75	77	65	64	66	73	73	74
83	82	84	71	70	72	79	78	79
82	81	83	74	73	75	86	86	87
81	80	81	77	76	78	87	87	88
90	90	91	81	80	83	91	90	92
84	83	84	74	73	75	84	84	85

(15). Simple Spearman's correlations were run between the satisfaction scores and each domain of responsiveness, as well as with overall responsiveness scores.

There was a significant correlation between the satisfaction measure and the inpatient domains of communication, prompt attention, and support, and with the outpatient domain of prompt attention (see

Table 46.5 Countries with high and low performance for two of the most important responsiveness domains: dignity and prompt attention

	Inpatient		Outpatient	
Performance	Dignity	Prompt attention	Dignity	Prompt attention
High	Sweden, UK, USA	Germany, Luxembourg, Netherlands	Canada, Ireland (urban), USA	Germany, Ireland (urban), USA
Low	Greece, Italy, Portugal	Greece, Canada, Portugal	Greece, Italy, Portugal	Greece, Italy, Portugal

Figure 46.1 National health expenditure compared with inpatient and outpatient responsiveness results for 16 OECD countries

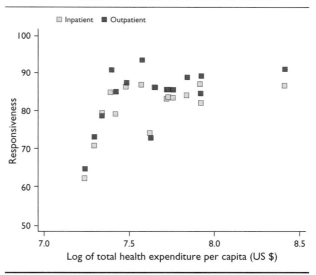

Table 46.6). No significant correlations were observed between satisfaction and the overall inpatient and outpatient responsiveness indices. This suggests that satisfaction might be determined more by the speed with which patients anticipate they can obtain care when they need it than by other facets of the interaction between the population and its health services.

The difference between responsiveness and satisfaction is further explored in Table 46.7 which groups the responsiveness and satisfaction results into three categories: where the poor have higher satisfaction or responsiveness than the rest of the population (or "wealthy"), where there is no statistically significant difference, and where the wealthy have higher satisfaction or responsiveness than the poor.

The poor were defined as respondents in the lowest two income quintiles for responsiveness (this was the

Table 46.6 Correlation of the percentage of the population "very satisfied or satisfied with the way health care runs in their country" and responsiveness domain-specific and overall inpatient and outpatient results

Domains and overall service levels	Spearman's correlation coefficient*	P-value
Autonomy	−0.23	0.41
Choice	0.14	0.62
Communication	0.58	0.02
Confidentiality	0.14	0.62
Dignity	0.31	0.27
Prompt attention	0.54	0.04
Social support	0.52	0.05
Overall inpatient services	0.36	0.18
Autonomy	0.35	0.21
Choice	0.29	0.30
Communication	0.44	0.10
Confidentiality	0.13	0.65
Dignity	0.40	0.14
Prompt attention	0.52	0.05
Quality of basic amenities	0.33	0.24
Overall outpatient services	0.26	0.35

* Excludes New Zealand because New Zealand was not included in the satisfaction data (*15*).

only breakdown available from the survey responses) and as those with incomes in the lowest quartile for the satisfaction work (again, the only possible breakdown from the available surveys). The responsiveness measure is based on an aggregation of the defined domains of people's interactions with the outpatient and inpatient health services (Box 46.1). The satisfaction measure is the percentage of respondents who were very or fairly satisfied "with the way health care runs in your country" (*15*).

In seven countries, the poor reported higher levels of satisfaction than the rest of the population (wealthy). It is unlikely that these systems treat the poor better than the rest of the population, and this result is probably related to the differential use of cut-points, lower expectations in the poor, or the fact that the construct includes many different, unspecified aspects of people's interactions with their health systems (*16*).

A different pattern is observed with responsiveness in Table 46.7, where the system is more responsive to the wealthy than to the poor only for outpatient responsiveness in Luxembourg. It must be remembered when interpreting these results that the responsiveness surveys had smaller sample sizes in general than the satisfaction surveys, so the power to identify significant differences was lower.

DISCUSSION

This is the first time that health system responsiveness has been measured and reported in a comparative way across countries from population surveys. It represents the actual experiences of the members of the population when they come in contact with the health system. Responsiveness differs from patient satisfaction, a construct that reflects people's expectations in addition to their experiences. The fact that poor people were shown in some countries to be more satisfied with their health systems than the rich is more likely to be due to differences in expectations—perhaps linked to what has been termed "happy slave" or "sour grapes" attitudes (*17*)—than to any preferential treatment of the poor.

Across 16 relatively rich OECD countries, there is substantial variation in the level of inpatient and outpatient responsiveness as reported by representative samples of the population and the scores on each component domain. These variations are likely to have been even greater if poorer countries were included in the analysis.

The countries with consistently lower results across all domains were Greece, Italy, and Portugal. The highest outpatient results were reported in Ireland, New Zealand, and the USA, although the results for Ireland should not be considered as representative of the country due to the urban bias described earlier. Inpatient responsiveness was highest in Luxembourg, New Zealand, Sweden, the UK, and the USA.

This analysis is only the first step towards policy dialogue and development, which can take three forms. First, the scores for the various domains and their relative weights can be evaluated for each country to determine priority areas for actions to improve responsiveness. For example, it was shown that Portugal and Greece consistently perform badly in several domains. If they wanted to improve their performance, however, they might consider focusing on improvements in the domains of prompt attention and dignity because these domains were valued more highly by people.

Some domain scores were relatively low in all countries. Autonomy is a case in point, for both inpatient and outpatient care. This suggests consistent failings by OECD health systems to involve patients in decision-making, a finding supported by previous research (*18;19*).

Second, personal characteristics associated with variations in responsiveness across individuals within a country can be explored. Few consistent patterns

Table 46.7 Responsiveness inpatient and outpatient results compared with satisfaction results for the poor and wealthy in 16 OECD countries[a]

	Poor have higher responsiveness/satisfaction than wealthy[b]	Poor and wealthy have equal responsiveness/satisfaction[b]	Wealthy have higher responsiveness/satisfaction than poor[b]
Responsiveness (2001)	Luxembourg (op)	Belgium (ip, op)	Germany (op)
		Canada (ip, op)	Greece (ip, op)
		Canada (ip, op)	Netherlands (op)
		Finland (ip, op)	
		Germany (ip)	
		Italy (ip, op)	
		Ireland (ip, op)	
		Luxembourg (ip)	
		Netherlands (ip)	
		New Zealand (ip, op)	
		Portugal (ip, op)	
		Spain (ip, op)	
		Sweden (ip, op)	
		UK (ip, op)	
		USA (ip, op)	
Satisfaction (1998, 2000[c])	France		Belgium
	Greece		Canada
	Ireland		Finland
	Italy		Germany
	New Zealand		Luxembourg
	Portugal		Netherlands
	Spain		Sweden
	UK		
	USA		

a. ip=inpatient services, op=outpatient services

b. Tested at the 5% significance level.

c. Data from 2000 for Canada and the USA, and 1998 for the remaining countries (15).

emerged from this analysis, the exception being the link between respondent's self-reported health status and some of the outpatient domain scores. This implies a need to identify people to whom the system responds less effectively on a country-by-country basis. This subject is discussed further elsewhere (20).

Third, it is important to understand the factors responsible for variations in responsiveness across countries and the extent to which they are amenable to change. While this is beyond the scope of the present chapter, a weak correlation between health expenditure and the responsiveness of inpatient services was observed. This provides the starting point for analysis of other system-wide variables that might determine differences in responsiveness, such as the extent of social health insurance, the availability and training of human resources, and the nature of incentives in public and private provision of health services in different settings.

ACKNOWLEDGEMENTS

The authors wish to extend special thanks to Charles Darby (Agency for Healthcare Research and Quality, USA) for assisting in the development of the questionnaire, and to Amala de Silva (University of Colombo, Sri Lanka) for conceptual guidance. The authors would also like to thank Lydia Bendib, Richard Poe, and René Lavallée for their technical assistance and comments.

REFERENCES

(1) Cleary P. The increasing importance of patient surveys. *British Medical Journal*, 1999, 319:721.

(2) Coulter A. After Bristol: putting patients at the centre. *British Medical Journal*, 2002, 324:648–651.

(3) Crofton C, Lubalin JS, Darby C. Consumer assessment of health plans study CAHPS. *Medical Care*, 1999, 37.

(4) McKinley RK et al. Reliability and validity of a new measure of patient satisfaction with out of hours primary medical care in the United Kingdom: development of a patient questionnaire. *British Medical Journal*, 1997, 314:193.

(5) Jenkinson C, Coulter A, Bruster S. The Picker patient experience questionnaire: development and validation using data from in-patient surveys in five countries. *International Journal for Quality in Health Care*, 2002, 14:353–358.

(6) Ware Jr JE et al. Defining and measuring patient satisfaction with medical care. *Evaluation and Program Planning*, 1983, 6:247–263.

(7) Sitzia J, Wood N. Patient satisfaction: a review of issues and concepts. *Social Science & Medicine*, 1997, 45: 1829–1843.

(8) Murray CJL, Frenk J. A framework for assessing the performance of health systems. *Bulletin of the World Health Organization*, 2000, 78(6):717–731.

(9) Sitzia J, Wood N. Response rate in patient satisfaction research: an analysis of 210 published studies. *International Journal for Quality in Health Care*, 1998, 10: 311–317.

(10) Üstün TB et al. WHO Multi-country Survey Study on Health and Responsiveness 2000-2001. In: Murray CJL, Evans DB, eds. *Health systems performance assessment: debates, methods and empiricism*. Geneva, World Health Organization, 2003.

(11) Valentine NB et al. Health system responsiveness: concepts, domains and operationalization. In: Murray CJL, Evans DB, eds. *Health systems performance assessment: debates, methods and empiricism*. Geneva, World Health Organization, 2003.

(12) Valentine NB et al. Classical psychometric assessment of the responsiveness instrument in the WHO Multi-country Survey Study on Health and Responsiveness 2000–2001. In: Murray CJL, Evans DB, eds. *Health systems performance assessment: debates, methods and empiricism*. Geneva, World Health Organization, 2003.

(13) Tandon A et al. Statistical models for enhancing cross-population comparability. In: Murray CJL, Evans DB, eds. *Health systems performance assessment: debates, methods and empiricism*. Geneva, World Health Organization, 2003.

(14) Valentine NB, Salomon JA. Weights for responsiveness domains: analysis of country variation in 65 national sample surveys. In: Murray CJL, Evans DB, eds. *Health systems performance assessment: debates, methods and empiricism*. Geneva, World Health Organization, 2003.

(15) Blendon RJ, Kim M, Benson JM. The public versus the World Health Organization on health system performance. Who is better qualified to judge health care systems: public health experts or the people who use the healthcare? *Health Affairs*, 2001, 20:10–20.

(16) Murray CJL, Kawabata K, Valentine NB. People's experience versus people's expectations. Satisfaction measures are profoundly influenced by people's expectations, say these WHO researchers. *Health Affairs*, 2001, 20:21–24.

(17) Johnson MD, Herrmann A, Gustafsson A. Comparing customer satisfaction across industries and countries. *Journal of Economic Psychology*, 2002, 23:749–769.

(18) Bruster S et al. National survey of hospital patients. *British Medical Journal*, 2002, 309:1542–1546.

(19) Coulter A, Entwistle V, Gilbert D. Sharing decisions with patients: is the information good enough? *British Medical Journal*, 1999, 318:318–322.

(20) Ortiz JP et al. Inequality in responsiveness: population surveys from 16 OECD countries. In: Murray CJL, Evans DB, eds. *Health systems performance assessment: debates, methods and empiricism*. Geneva, World Health Organization, 2003.

Chapter 47

Inequality in Responsiveness: Population Surveys from 16 OECD Countries

Juan Pablo Ortiz, Nicole B. Valentine, Emmanuela Gakidou, Ajay Tandon, Kei Kawabata, David B. Evans, Christopher J.L. Murray

Introduction

The World Health Organization has recently argued that responsiveness is one of the key goals to which health systems contribute in addition to improving population health (1). To facilitate its measurement in a systematic way across countries, a common set of domains was defined—autonomy, choice, communication, confidentiality, dignity, prompt attention, quality of basic amenities, and access to family and community support (2).

Estimates of the level of responsiveness of the health systems in 16 OECD countries have been reported by Valentine et al. (3). This chapter focuses on the distribution of responsiveness across individuals within countries, and develops indicators of inequality to describe this distribution. This is a critical step in improving the performance of health systems. After the inequality measure has been calculated, it is then possible to assess which of the various population subgroups are disadvantaged and how inequality can be reduced.

The first part of the present chapter explains the data and methods used to calculate responsiveness and its distribution for the 16 OECD countries. In the second part, different types of inequality measures are described and an inequality index for responsiveness is calculated for each country. The third section considers possible determinants of the observed levels of inequality and the implications of the results for policy and for further development of this work.

Data and Methods

Data Collection

The first attempt to measure the responsiveness of health systems in different settings in a comparable way was based on key informant interviews (4). It was criticized on a number of grounds, including the fact that the informants might not have been representative of the population as a whole (5–7). Accordingly, a responsiveness module was developed and included in 69 national sample surveys undertaken by 60 countries as part of the WHO Multi-country Survey Study on Health and Responsiveness 2000–2001 (8). During the preparation, several expert meetings and pilot studies were conducted to help refine the responsiveness methodology and concepts. One of the goals of this survey study was to develop a cross-culturally applicable instrument which could be used to measure the various domains of responsiveness, to investigate survey mode effects, and to test new strategies for enhancing the cross-population comparability of the results (9;10).

Selected Countries

Table 47.1 reports details of the representative surveys conducted in the 16 OECD countries, described in more detail in Valentine et al. (11). Self-administered postal surveys were used in Canada, the United States, the United Kingdom, Greece, and New Zealand, while face-to-face and telephone interviews were used in the remaining countries. Responsiveness was measured separately for inpatient and outpatient care.

Level of Responsiveness

Respondents reporting an experience with either outpatient or inpatient services in the previous 12 months were asked a series of questions on their experiences, the questions being divided into the different domains of responsiveness. Respondents were requested to rate their experiences in terms of one of five categorical responses—for example "very good," "good," "mod-

Table 47.1 Information on the countries analysed

Country	Completed responses	Experience in the last 12 months		% Male
		% Outpatients	% Inpatients	
Belgium	1 100	56	12	48
Canada*	407	61	11	46
Finland	1 021	71	15	44
France	1 003	65	13	48
Germany	1 123	62	9	48
Greece*	909	70	22	60
Ireland	711	47	13	50
Italy	1 002	45	7	48
Luxembourg	719	71	13	44
Netherlands	1 085	63	8	45
New Zealand*	1 801	81	14	43
Portugal	1 001	53	9	44
Spain	1 000	62	9	49
Sweden	1 000	56	11	46
United Kingdom*	1 018	70	12	45
United States of America*	588	76	14	55

* Postal

erate," "poor," "very poor." They were also asked to rate the experiences of hypothetical people in vignettes using the same categories. Different people rated any given vignette describing a particular experience into different categories. The differential use of categories can be conceptualized as the differential use of cutpoints between categories. This varied in a consistent manner across the population according to a set of personal characteristics (e.g. sex, education, and country of origin), and was used to adjust the responses to people's own reported experiences in order to obtain the final ratings of the system's responsiveness in each domain.

The compound hierarchical ordered probit (CHO-PIT) model (9) was used to do this. This model generates levels of the latent variable, responsiveness, on an unbounded scale, so the results were transformed to a scale of 0 to 100 for ease of interpretation. The value of the latent variable for the worst vignette was used to set the scale at zero, while the highest vignette set it at 100. The average levels of responsiveness on each domain were aggregated using weights also derived from questions in the surveys to obtain an aggregate responsiveness score, also from 0 to 100. This was done for inpatient and outpatient care separately, and the results were combined to obtain an overall responsiveness score (50% outpatient and 50% inpatient). Overall responsiveness scores and their associated uncertainty intervals for the 16 countries are reported in Table 47.2 (3). Responsiveness varied from a high of 90 for Ireland to a low of 63 for Greece.

MEASURES OF INEQUALITY

A variety of measures to summarize the inequality of any continuous distribution are available. They can be divided into two main groups: those measuring interindividual and those measuring individual-mean

Table 47.2 Overall outpatient and inpatient level of responsiveness for 16 OECD countries

Country	Mean level of responsiveness					
	Overall	Uncertainty	Outpatient	Uncertainty	Inpatient	Uncertainty
Belgium	85	84–85	86	85–86	83	83–84
Canada*	87	86–88	89	88–90	85	84–86
Finland	83	82–83	86	85–86	79	79–80
France	85	84–85	86	85–86	83	83–84
Germany	85	85–86	89	89–90	82	81–82
Greece*	63	63–64	64	64–65	62	62–63
Ireland	90	90–91	94	93–94	87	86–87
Italy	73	73–74	73	72–73	74	73–74
Luxembourg	86	85–86	85	84–85	87	86–88
Netherlands	85	84–85	86	85–86	83	82–84
New Zealand*	89	89–89	91	91–91	87	86–87
Portugal	72	71–73	73	73–74	71	70–71
Spain	79	79–80	79	78–79	79	79–80
Sweden	86	86–87	86	86–87	86	86–87
United Kingdom*	88	87–88	87	87–88	88	87–88
United States of America*	89	88–90	91	90–92	87	86–88

* Postal

differences (12;13). When applied to the distribution of responsiveness within a population, interindividual measures focus on differences in responsiveness between every pair of individuals in the population, while individual-mean difference measures are concerned about differences between individual levels and the mean level observed in that population.

The individual-mean difference measures take the following general form:

$$IMD(\alpha,\beta) = \frac{\sum_{i=1}^{n} |X_i - \overline{X}|^{\alpha}}{n\overline{X}^{\beta}}, \qquad [1]$$

while the inter-individual difference measures can be expressed as:

$$IID(\alpha,\beta) = \frac{\sum_{j=1}^{n}\sum_{i=1}^{n} |X_i - X_j|^{\alpha}}{2n^2 \overline{X}^{\beta}}, \qquad [2]$$

where X_i is the responsiveness level for individual i, n is the number of people in the population, and $\overline{X}$ is the average level of responsiveness in the population. The β coefficient determines the extent to which the inequality measures are relative to the mean or absolute. If $\alpha = \beta = 1$, the measure is strictly relative to the mean, concerned with percentage deviations from the mean (IMD) or percentage differences between individuals (IID). Such measures are invariant to proportionate changes in all observations. This property is called scalar invariance, or mean-independence, under which the inequality index remains unchanged if each individual's level of responsiveness is multiplied by the same positive scalar. In contrast, when $\beta = 0$, concern lies exclusively with absolute deviations from the mean (IMD) or absolute differences between individuals (IID). Such measures are invariant to the addition of a positive constant to each individual's observed responsiveness (12;13). A value of β between zero and one reflects a mix of concern between relative and absolute differences.

The choice of the parameter α is related to the significance attached to differences in responsiveness observed at the tails of the distribution, compared to those observed closer to the mean. The greater the concern with the tail, the higher is the resulting α. In the special case in which $\alpha = 2$, $IMD(2,\beta) = IID(2,\beta)$ for any. The choice of which measure to use to summarize inequality in responsiveness is determined, therefore, by three essentially normative considerations—the

choices of: interindividual versus individual-mean comparisons; the value of β; and the value of α.

A range of measures, including those used widely in quantifying income inequality, could be used to describe the distribution of observed inequality, each representing a different set of normative decisions.

The *relative mean deviation (M)* sums the absolute differences between individual observations and the mean, and divides the total by the total responsiveness in the population (equation [3]). A level of M = 0 implies perfect equality (14). This relative measure of inequality belongs to the IMD group where $\alpha = \beta = 1$.

$$M(\alpha,\beta) = \frac{\sum_{i=1}^{n} |X_i - \overline{X}|}{n\overline{X}} \qquad [3]$$

The variance (equation [4]), an absolute measure of inequality, is also from the IMD class with $\alpha = 2$ and $\beta = 0$. It can be expressed as:

$$V(\alpha,\beta) = \frac{\sum_{i=1}^{n} (X_i - \overline{X})^2}{n} \qquad [4]$$

The *standard deviation* (equation [5]) and the *coefficient of variation* (CV) (equation [6]) can be thought of as based on the variance with modifications. The standard deviation is equal to the square root of the variance, while the coefficient of variation is equivalent to the square root of the variance divided by the mean. The former, like the variance, is a strictly absolute measure and the latter is a strictly relative measure. In both cases, the smaller the estimate, the less is the inequality. Mathematically, the standard deviation can be expressed as:

$$\sigma(\alpha,\beta) = \sqrt{\frac{\sum_{i=1}^{n} (X_i - \overline{X})^2}{n}} \qquad [5]$$

while the coefficient of variation is:

$$CV(\alpha,\beta) = \frac{\sqrt{\dfrac{\sum_{i=1}^{n} (X_i - \overline{X})^2}{n}}}{\overline{X}} \qquad [6]$$

If the observations at the lower end of the distribution are important, then a logarithmic transformation is useful, and the corresponding measure of dispersion is the *standard deviation of logarithms* (SDL) (equation [7]). Another advantage of logarithms is that they eliminate the arbitrariness of the units, in contrast to the variance and the standard deviation (*14*). This measure is also from the IMD class (equation [7]).

$$SDL(\alpha, \beta) = \sqrt{\frac{\sum_{i=1}^{n}(\log X_i - \log \overline{X})^2}{n}} \quad [7]$$

Examples of interindividual measures are the *Gini coefficient* (G) (equation [8]) and *Theil's entropy index* (T) (equation [9]). Both belong to the group of relative inequality measures, most frequently used for measuring income inequalities so they are not sensitive to relative changes in the scale. The Gini coefficient is sensitive to inequality around the median, while Theil's index is more sensitive to inequality at the top part of the distribution (*15*).

$$G(\alpha, \beta) = \frac{\sum_{j=1}^{n}\sum_{i=1}^{n}\left|X_i - X_j\right|}{2n^2\overline{X}} \quad [8]$$

The Gini coefficient has $\alpha = \beta = 1$. It is bounded by zero and one, with zero representing perfect equality and one, perfect inequality.

Theil's entropy index can be expressed as:

$$T = (1/n)\sum_{i=1}^{n}\left(\frac{X_i}{\overline{X}}\right)\log\left(\frac{X_i}{\overline{X}}\right) \quad [9]$$

It can have any non-negative value. It equals zero when there is no inequality and it increases with more inequality.

AN INEQUALITY MEASURE FOR RESPONSIVENESS

To facilitate a decision about which measure of inequality would be most appropriate for responsiveness, a series of key informant surveys was undertaken in 2000–2001 (*8*). The results from the 37 countries from which a minimum of 100 responses were received, were used to decide the appropriate inequality measure.

To assist the respondents in choosing their preferences for each of these three normative choices, hypothetical populations were constructed (Annex 47.1). The choice for each respondent was between population A and population B, where one of the three normative issues was addressed in each of three scenarios. The first scenario (Figure 1 in Annex 47.1) dealt with the choice of the value of β. Populations A and B are at different average levels of responsiveness, but the distribution of individuals around these mean levels is the same for the two populations. The preference for one of them reflects the respondents' preference for

an absolute versus a relative measure of inequality. If the respondents express no preference for any of them, they are concerned with how the population is distributed around the mean but not where the mean is, which can be translated into a value of β equal to zero. If respondents have a preference for one of the two populations, when they think about "inequality" they think not only about how individuals are distributed around the mean, but also about where the mean is, implying a value of β greater than zero. Table 47.3 shows that only a third of respondents thought in terms of an absolute measure, so β should not be set at zero.

In the second scenario (Figure 2 in Annex 47.1), the choice involves how much weight should be assigned to the tails of the distribution, i.e. to outliers or subgroups of the population that are far from the average level. The change that happens in the two populations is the same in terms of absolute value, but it happens to individuals in different parts of the distribution. In population A, the transfers are given to individuals at the tails of the distribution, while in population B, the individuals receiving the transfers are closer to the mean. A preference for the transfer in A versus B indicates a preference for a value of α greater than one.

In the third scenario (Figure 3 in Annex 47.1), the choice is between individual-mean and interindividual measures. The populations are at exactly the same mean and the same transfer takes place in both of them. The only difference is how the rest of the individuals are distributed around the mean. Respondents who express no preference for the transfer in A versus B, are in reality preferring an individual-mean measure, since what they seem to consider important is the average value and the individuals affected by the transfer, but not the rest of the individuals in the population. Respondents with a preference for A over B, or B over A, are preferring interindividual measures as they are concerned not only with the individuals affected by

Table 47.3   Exercise based on key informants

| | Which population, A or B | | |
	Scenario 1	Scenario 2	Scenario 3
Answers	has more inequality	has a greater increase in inequality	experiences a greater increase in inequality
Population A	45%	35%	23%
Population B	17%	26%	38%
Both the same	38%	39%	39%

the transfer, but also with all other individuals in the population. Table 47.3 shows that a small majority of people preferred the individual-mean option.

On balance, the respondents did not support the option of $\beta = 0$, and they were evenly split on the choice of α and the choice of individual-mean versus interindividual measure. For this reason, the coefficient of variation has been chosen as the preferred summary measure. Because the preference between IMD and IID measures was not very strong from the survey responses, setting $\alpha = 2$ was an attractive option—it is the value of α at which IMD and IID measures are equal. Combining the preference for $\alpha = 2$ with the preference for a relative measure led to the choice of the coefficient of variation, shown in equation [6]. However, because the preferences for the different scenarios were relatively close, the results presented below based on the coefficient of variation are also compared with results based on other indicators of inequality.

RESULTS

INEQUALITY IN RESPONSIVENESS

The coefficient of variation for each of the 16 countries is reported in Table 47.4, for outpatient, inpatient, and overall responsiveness. Values for overall responsiveness range from a low (the most equal) of 0.061 in Germany to 0.137 (the least equal) for Greece. Greece has substantially higher levels of inequality than the

Table 47.4 Overall, outpatient, and inpatient inequality in responsiveness (coefficient of variation)

Country	Overall	Outpatient	Inpatient
Belgium	0.070	0.068	0.099
Canada*	0.072	0.068	0.117
Finland	0.079	0.070	0.138
France	0.068	0.067	0.106
Germany	0.061	0.055	0.124
Greece*	0.137	0.128	0.204
Ireland	0.084	0.074	0.155
Italy	0.095	0.086	0.174
Luxembourg	0.089	0.086	0.117
Netherlands	0.064	0.063	0.085
New Zealand*	0.065	0.061	0.108
Portugal	0.105	0.094	0.154
Spain	0.080	0.079	0.119
Sweden	0.090	0.092	0.089
United Kingdom*	0.080	0.080	0.092
United States of America*	0.068	0.064	0.120

* Postal

other countries for both inpatient and outpatient care. In all countries except Sweden, inequality is higher for inpatient than for outpatient services. Although this might reflect in part the smaller sample reporting on inpatient than outpatient experiences, countries like Sweden and the Netherlands show similar levels of inequality for both types of care, despite the differences in sample size. This suggests that the observed differences in inequality are not likely to be due solely to differences in sample sizes, but to reflect a greater degree of inequality in responsiveness in inpatient care.

Figure 47.1 helps to identify why one country ranks higher than others using the coefficient of variation as the summary measure of inequality. Because the coefficient of variation is of the IMD class, countries where observations are widely dispersed but with a lower mean will have more inequality than those with the same dispersion and a higher mean. Obviously, for any given mean, the greater the dispersion, the greater the inequality. The mean level of responsiveness in Sweden, for example, is relatively high, but there is more dispersion of the observations. This is why Sweden's coefficient of variation is higher than in other countries with similar mean levels of responsiveness. Spain, on the other hand, has a lower mean responsiveness but a more compact distribution than Sweden, with the result of less measured inequality in overall responsiveness using the coefficient of variation. In Greece, the mean is low and the distribution of observations is widely dispersed, accounting for the high measured inequality score.

INEQUALITY BY DOMAIN

Table 47.5 presents inequality results by domain. As with overall responsiveness, there is a general pattern of more inequality in inpatient than outpatient care on all domains. Again, this might be due partly to smaller sample sizes reporting on inpatient than outpatient experiences, but this cannot be the entire explanation. For example, there is less inequality in communication for inpatient than outpatient care in Portugal, Luxembourg, and France, despite the smaller sample size for inpatient care.

For outpatient care, the domains of choice and quality of basic amenities have less inequality than the other domains, while for inpatient care the domain with the greatest equality is confidentiality. Autonomy shows the most inequality for both inpatient and outpatient services. The relatively high levels of inequality for prompt attention were not expected, because the

Figure 47.1 Distribution of responsiveness for 16 countries

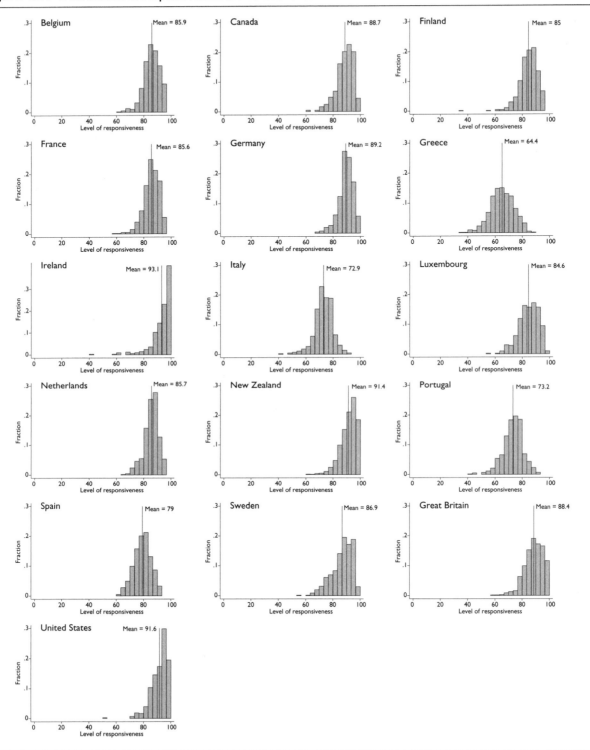

Table 47.5 Inequality in responsiveness by domain

Country	Autonomy Outpatient	Autonomy Inpatient	Choice Outpatient	Choice Inpatient	Communication Outpatient	Communication Inpatient	Confidentiality Outpatient	Confidentiality Inpatient	Dignity Outpatient	Dignity Inpatient	Quality of BA Outpatient	Quality of BA Inpatient**	Prompt attention Outpatient	Prompt attention Inpatient	Support Inpatient	Overall
Belgium	0.163	0.216	0.001	0.080	0.120	0.119	0.083	0.100	0.081	0.114	0.020	—	0.133	0.182	0.110	0.070
Canada*	0.145	0.205	0.073	0.119	0.109	0.168	0.066	0.116	0.035	0.087	0.041	—	0.174	0.220	0.068	0.072
Finland	0.162	0.226	0.113	0.428	0.113	0.142	0.073	0.085	0.069	0.148	0.036	—	0.140	0.189	0.155	0.079
France	0.161	0.260	0.003	0.096	0.118	0.145	0.092	0.090	0.076	0.093	0.029	—	0.135	0.171	0.113	0.068
Germany	0.125	0.241	0.036	0.207	0.108	0.162	0.074	0.120	0.076	0.125	0.030	—	0.073	0.125	0.129	0.061
Greece*	0.285	0.316	0.140	0.326	0.239	0.291	0.133	0.142	0.142	0.195	0.043	—	0.166	0.262	0.206	0.137
Ireland	0.182	0.301	0.055	0.235	0.121	0.199	0.078	0.112	0.061	0.134	0.054	—	0.116	0.231	0.142	0.084
Italy	0.211	0.328	0.020	0.189	0.149	0.258	0.125	0.135	0.121	0.205	0.025	—	0.173	0.228	0.213	0.095
Luxembourg	0.158	0.228	0.044	0.207	0.186	0.156	0.100	0.085	0.096	0.117	0.035	—	0.178	0.203	0.083	0.089
Netherlands	0.140	0.180	0.042	0.193	0.116	0.149	0.071	0.071	0.074	0.129	0.024	—	0.117	0.121	0.055	0.064
New Zealand*	0.111	0.149	0.010	0.111	0.104	0.135	0.085	0.108	0.065	0.099	0.036	—	0.120	0.189	0.153	0.065
Portugal	0.171	0.232	0.077	0.228	0.170	0.209	0.124	0.108	0.146	0.166	0.014	—	0.172	0.241	0.206	0.105
Spain	0.221	0.277	0.025	0.212	0.115	0.119	0.102	0.112	0.088	0.081	0.035	—	0.164	0.231	0.136	0.080
Sweden	0.175	0.186	0.068	0.201	0.137	0.124	0.090	0.104	0.088	0.058	0.056	—	0.184	0.187	0.068	0.090
United Kingdom*	0.176	0.174	0.045	0.123	0.142	0.147	0.063	0.069	0.066	0.089	0.061	—	0.161	0.145	0.062	0.080
United States of America*	0.145	0.198	0.028	0.118	0.117	0.171	0.095	0.150	0.038	0.085	0.053	—	0.110	0.182	0.123	0.068

* Postal; ** Quality of basic amenities inpatient is not available. Refer to chapter 46 of this volume (3).

sample of countries included in this analysis is limited to the high-income countries that spend relatively high levels on health per capita on a global basis. These countries were expected to be able to provide relatively rapid attention to most of their populations.

On a country basis, inequality is higher for most domains in Greece and Portugal than in the other countries, with some notable exceptions. For example, Finland reports very high levels of inpatient inequality on choice, while inequality in inpatient dignity is much higher in Italy than in the other countries. This provides a possible entry point for a more detailed analysis of the reasons behind unexpected patterns, and possible policy responses.

Different Inequality Measures

Table 47.6 compares the coefficient of variation with some other inequality measures commonly used to summarize inequality in other spheres. These include the Gini coefficient, the Theil index, the relative mean deviation, and the standard deviation of responsiveness (14;16). The different measures produce similar results—all show Greece to have the highest level of inequality in overall responsiveness and Germany to have the lowest. This is confirmed in Table 47.7 which shows that the rank order correlation between the different measures is very high. At least for this sample of countries, the assessment of inequality is not very sensitive to the choice of summary measure.

Determinants of Inequality

There are two possible approaches to analysing how best to reduce inequalities in responsiveness. The first is to examine whether there are any common characteristics of the people to which each system responds less well. This requires analysis of the characteristics of the people in the left-hand tail of the distributions of Figure 47.1—for example, although the mean level of responsiveness in the USA is high at 91.6, responsiveness is lower than 60 for some people. With sufficient information on the characteristics of the individual respondents, people in the left-hand tail of

Table 47.6 A comparison of different inequality measures (coefficient of variation, relative mean deviation, standard deviation of logs, Gini coefficient, Theil index, and mean)

Country	Coefficient of variation	Relative mean deviation	Standard deviation of logs	Gini coefficient	Theil index (GE(a), a = 1)	Mean
Belgium	0.070	0.028	0.072	0.039	0.003	85.9
Canada*	0.072	0.028	0.075	0.039	0.003	88.7
Finland	0.079	0.030	0.086	0.042	0.003	85.0
France	0.069	0.027	0.071	0.038	0.002	85.6
Germany	0.062	0.023	0.064	0.034	0.002	89.2
Greece*	0.137	0.055	0.142	0.077	0.010	64.4
Ireland	0.084	0.029	0.100	0.039	0.004	93.1
Italy	0.095	0.035	0.101	0.051	0.005	72.9
Luxembourg	0.089	0.036	0.092	0.050	0.004	84.6
Netherlands	0.064	0.024	0.066	0.035	0.002	85.7
New Zealand*	0.065	0.026	0.068	0.035	0.002	91.4
Portugal	0.105	0.041	0.111	0.058	0.006	73.2
Spain	0.081	0.032	0.082	0.046	0.003	79.0
Sweden	0.090	0.036	0.095	0.050	0.004	86.9
United Kingdom*	0.080	0.032	0.084	0.044	0.003	88.4
United States of America*	0.068	0.026	0.073	0.036	0.002	91.6

* Postal

Table 47.7 Rank correlation between different inequality measures

Measure	Coefficient of variation	Relative mean deviation	Standard deviation of logs	Gini coefficient	Theil index	Mean
Coefficient of variation	1					
Relative mean deviation	0.971	1				
Standard deviation of logs	0.971	0.916	1			
Gini coefficient	0.969	0.986	0.913	1		
Theil index	0.967	0.921	0.952	0.923	1	
Mean	−0.618	−0.670	−0.515	−0.737	−0.572	1

point for policy. The second approach is to determine if there are any system characteristics typically associated with high inequality in responsiveness, through the use of multivariate analysis across countries.

The first approach is illustrated here using sex differences in responsiveness as an example. Figure 47.2 shows the different distributions of responsiveness for males and females in Belgium, Portugal, and Finland. In Belgium, the distribution of responsiveness for males is generally to the left of that of females; in Portugal the distributions are very similar. In Finland the system seems more responsive on average to men than women, but the left-hand tail of the distribution is apparently longer for men than women. It is clear that in Belgium there are more men than women in the left-hand tail of the overall distribution.

The coefficient of variation is reported for all countries by sex in Table 47.8. For the three countries described above, the inequality in responsiveness for women is less than that for men. In Spain, Lux-

embourg, and Canada, on the other hand, inequality in responsiveness is greater for women than for men. A t-test on the pooled data found no consistent difference in inequality by sex across the 16 countries, suggesting the need for a country-by-country analysis for policy purposes.[1]

The second way of using the analysis for policy purposes is to examine whether there are characteristics of the health system that are consistently associated with higher levels of inequality. For example, Figure 47.3 shows a scatterplot with the coefficient of variation for responsiveness on the vertical axis and the proportion of GDP devoted to health (total health expenditure, denoted by THE, divided by GDP) (17) on the horizontal axis. There is an overall negative relationship, although Greece is a clear outlier. This relationship is confirmed in a multiple regression. Because there are only 16 countries in the sample used for this chapter, there is not a lot of power to identify system characteristics in a cross-country regression, but the coefficient

Figure 47.2 Distribution of responsiveness for Belgium, Portugal, and Finland for males and females

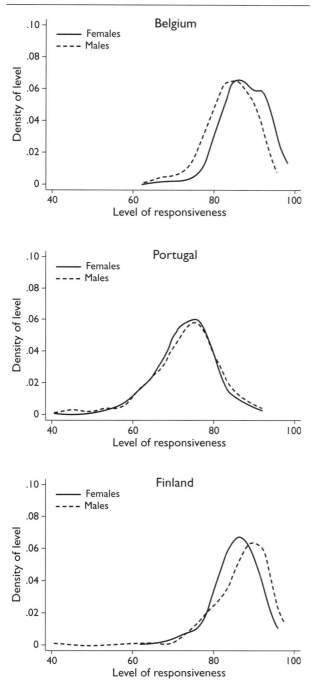

Table 47.8 Inequality of responsiveness by sex

	Overall level	
	Female	Male
Belgium	0.064	0.072
Canada*	0.072	0.071
Finland	0.071	0.087
France	0.069	0.067
Germany	0.059	0.064
Greece*	0.130	0.140
Ireland	0.092	0.074
Italy	0.095	0.095
Luxembourg	0.092	0.083
Netherlands	0.065	0.063
New Zealand*	0.064	0.064
Portugal	0.099	0.114
Spain	0.081	0.080
Sweden	0.092	0.087
United Kingdom*	0.079	0.080
United States of America*	0.068	0.067

* Postal

Figure 47.3 Inequality in responsiveness vs. total health expenditure as percentage of GDP

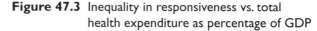
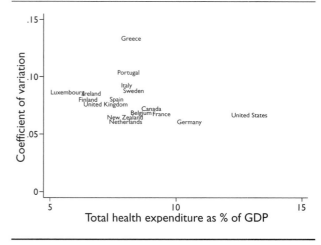

between inequalities in income (measured using the Gini coefficient) and inequality in responsiveness. As results become available from more countries, the possibility to identify additional system characteristics associated with higher inequality in responsiveness will increase.

of THE/GDP is negative and statistically significant (Figure 47.4). In addition, a World Bank indicator of government effectiveness (18;19) is inversely correlated with inequality in responsiveness, while there is a positive but statistically insignificant correlation

DISCUSSION AND CONCLUSIONS

Policy-makers are concerned not just with improving average levels of population health and health system responsiveness, but also with reducing inequalities in

Figure 47.4 Regression analysis using basic variables (inequality in responsiveness vs. Gini, total health expenditure as percentage of GDP and government effectiveness)

Dependent variable:	Coefficient of variation					
Independent variable:	Gini, THE/GDP 2000 and Government Effectiveness					
Coefficient of variation	**Coef.**	**Std. Err.**	**t**	**P>|t|**	**[95% Conf. Interval]**	
Gini	0.142	0.0868	1.64	0.128	–0.04716	0.33116
THE/GDP 2000	–0.007	0.0023	–2.88	0.014	–0.01141	–0.00159
Government Effectiveness	–0.033	0.0085	–3.89	0.002	–0.05169	–0.01457
_cons	0.137	0.0273	5.02	0.000	0.07756	0.19656

$$R\text{-squared} = 0.6119$$
$$\text{Adj } R\text{-squared} = 0.5149$$
$$\text{Number of obs} = 16$$

health and responsiveness. This requires the ability to measure inequality in responsiveness and to identify the people to which the system is least responsive. This chapter has reported inequalities in responsiveness for 16 OECD countries, based on representative household surveys undertaken as part of the WHO Multi-country Survey Study on Health and Responsiveness 2000–2001.

Even for countries with relatively high levels of health expenditure, there is considerable variation in the extent of inequality in responsiveness. In terms of health system characteristics, there is some evidence that higher levels of health expenditure as a proportion of GDP are associated with lower inequality, as are higher levels of government effectiveness. Other health system characteristics associated with lower or higher levels of inequality may well emerge as the results from surveys in additional countries become available.

Within individual countries, the measurement of responsiveness and its distribution across the population provides policy-makers with an entry point for developing strategies to reduce inequalities. This requires determining if there are common characteristics of people to whom the system is least responsive. These characteristics may well differ across various settings, as illustrated by the fact that the system was less responsive to men in Belgium and to women in Finland.

To increase the availability of key information on responsiveness to decision-makers, WHO has revised the responsiveness module of the 2000–2001 study for its incorporation in the World Health Survey. This survey is currently in the field in over 70 countries and will provide important information on the system characteristics associated with low inequality

in responsiveness, as well as information on which groups of people are faced with lower levels of responsiveness within a given system.

Notes

1   Note that the coefficient of variation may be identical for men and women, but one of the distributions could lie to the left of the other. This means that it is important to determine who is in the left-hand tail of the overall distribution as well as to consider the coefficient of variation by different characteristics.

References

(1)   Murray CJL, Frenk J. A framework for assessing the performance of health systems. *Bulletin of the World Health Organization*, 2000, 78(6):717–731.

(2)   Valentine NB et al. Health system responsiveness: concepts, domains and operationalization. In: Murray CJL, Evans DB, eds. *Health systems performance assessment: debates, methods and empiricism*. Geneva, World Health Organization, 2003.

(3)   Valentine NB et al. Patient experiences with health services: population surveys from 16 OECD countries. In: Murray CJL, Evans DB, eds. *Health systems performance assessment: debates, methods and empiricism*. Geneva, World Health Organization, 2003.

(4)   de Silva A, Valentine NB. *Measuring responsiveness: results of a key informants survey in 35 countries*. EIP Discussion Paper No. 21. Geneva, World Health Organization, 2000. URL: http://www3.who.int/whosis/discussion_papers/discussion_papers.cfm#

(5)   Almeida C et al. Methodological concerns and recommendations on policy consequences of the World

Health Report 2000. *The Lancet*, 2001, 357(9269): 1692–1697.

(6) Navarro V. Assessment of the World Health Report 2000. *The Lancet*, 2001, 356(9241):1598–1601.

(7) Blendon RJ, Kim M, Benson JM. The public versus the World Health Organization on health system performance. Who is better qualified to judge health care systems: public health experts or the people who use the healthcare? *Health Affairs*, 2001, 20(3):10–20.

(8) Üstün TB et al. WHO Multi-country Survey Study on Health and Responsiveness 2000–2001. In: Murray CJL, Evans DB, eds. *Health systems performance assessment: debates, methods and empiricism*. Geneva, World Health Organization, 2003.

(9) Tandon A et al. Statistical models for enhancing cross-population comparability. In: Murray CJL, Evans DB, eds. *Health systems performance assessment: debates, methods and empiricism*. Geneva, World Health Organization, 2003.

(10) King G et al. Enhancing the validity and cross-cultural comparability of measurement in survey research. *American Political Science Review*, 2003 (forthcoming).

(11) Valentine NB et al. Classical psychometric assessment of the responsiveness instrument in the WHO Multi-country Survey Study on Health and Responsiveness 2000–2001. In: Murray CJL, Evans DB, eds. *Health systems performance assessment: debates, methods and empiricism*. Geneva, World Health Organization, 2003.

(12) Gakidou E, Murray CJL, Frenk J. Defining and measuring health inequality: an approach based on the distribution of health expectancy. *Bulletin of the World Health Organization*, 2000, 78(1):42–54.

(13) Xu K et al. Summary measures of the distribution of household financial contributions to health. In: Murray CJL, Evans DB, eds. *Health systems performance assessment: debates, methods and empiricism*. Geneva, World Health Organization, 2003.

(14) Sen AK. *On economic inequality*. Oxford, Oxford University Press, 1973.

(15 Smeeding TM. Cross-national comparisons of inequality and poverty position. In: Osberg L, ed. *Economic inequality and poverty*. New York, M.E. Sharpe, Inc., 1991.

(16 Theil H. *Economics and information theory*. Amsterdam, North-Holland, 1967.

(17) World Health Organization. *The World Health Report 2002. Reducing Risks, Promoting Healthy Life*. Geneva, World Health Organization, 2002.

(18) Kaufmann D, Kraay A, Zoido-Lobatón P. *Aggregating governance indicators*. World Bank Policy Research Working Paper No. 2195. Washington, DC, World Bank, 1999.

(19) Kaufmann D, Kraay A, Zoido-Lobatón P. *Governance matters*. World Bank Policy Research Working Paper No. 2196. Washington, DC, World Bank, 1999.

Figure 1 Inequality scenario 1

Population A has an average level of responsiveness of 4 out of 10.
Population B has an average level of responsiveness of 7 out of 10.
In both populations A and B individuals are distributed similarly around the mean.

Which population, A or B, do you think has more inequality in responsiveness?

Population A has more inequality in responsiveness.
Population B has more inequality in responsiveness.
Both have the same inequality in responsiveness.

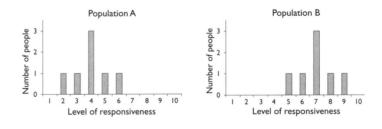

Figure 2 Inequality scenario 2

Populations A and B have exactly the same inequality of responsiveness.
Populations A and B have the same average level of responsiveness.
In both populations two individuals experience a transfer of 2 units of responsiveness.
In Population A, one person with 2 units loses 1 unit of responsiveness and another
    person with 8 units gains 1 unit of responsiveness.
In Population B, one person with 4 units loses 1 unit of responsiveness and another
    person with 6 units gains 1 unit of responsiveness.

Which population has a greater increase in inequality of responsiveness?

Population A has a greater increase in inequality of responsiveness.
Population B has a greater increase in inequality of responsiveness.
The increase is the same for both populations.

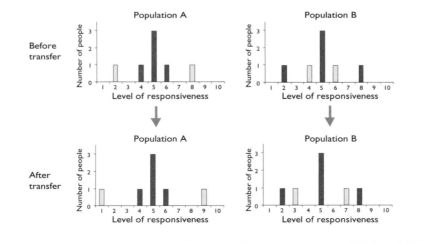

Figure 3 Inequality scenario 3

Populations A and B have the same average level of responsiveness.
Populations A and B have different inequality in responsiveness.
In both populations, there is a transfer of 8 units of responsiveness; one person with
5 units loses 4 units and another person with 5 units gains 4 units.

Which population experiences a greater increase in inequality of responsiveness?

Population A has a greater increase in inequality of responsiveness.
Population B has a greater increase in inequality of responsiveness.
The increase is the same for both populations.

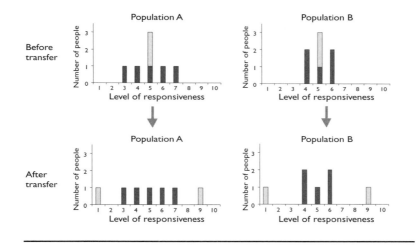

Chapter 48

QUALITY AND EQUITY: PREFERENCES FOR HEALTH SYSTEM OUTCOMES

EMMANUELA GAKIDOU, CHRISTOPHER J.L. MURRAY, DAVID B. EVANS

INTRODUCTION

Societies invest a large fraction of their available resources in health systems; nearly 8% of the global production of goods and services are spent on health (*1*). Not surprisingly, there is remarkable interest among policy-makers in having information on the performance of their health systems. Performance measurement can help them monitor the progress of their own systems over time, and allows them to compare their progress with that of other health systems. This information has the secondary benefit of contributing to the development of an evidence base on what works to improve health systems performance, and what does not. The lack of this type of information has been a major impediment to ensuring evidence-based policy development in the area of health system reform.

Measures of the outcomes of health systems are needed in order to allow comparisons across countries and populations in terms of overall goal attainment and the efficiency of achieving these goals. This means specifying the key social goals to which health systems contribute, country attainment on these goals, and their relative importance. The World Health Organization framework for assessing the performance of health systems(*1;2*) defines three main goals:

- Improving the health of populations. Population health should reflect the health of individuals throughout their life course and include both premature mortality and non-fatal health outcomes. Improving health entails raising its average level and reducing inequalities in it.

- Improving the responsiveness of the health system to the population it serves. When individuals interact with the health system it influences their well-being, partly through improvements in health and partly by other aspects of their personal interactions with the health system which is defined as responsiveness. Responsiveness has two components, respect for persons and client orientation. Respect for persons is meant to capture dimensions such as dignity, autonomy, and confidentiality. Client orientation includes promptness of attention, access to social support networks, basic amenities, and choice of provider. Both the level and inequalities in responsiveness are measured (*3*).

- Fairness in financial contribution is the extent to which the burden of paying for the health system is fairly distributed across households. This captures three related concerns: first, when some households are forced to pay a catastrophic share of their non-subsistence income (defined as being greater than 40%) to the health system; second, when households in similar circumstances contribute very different shares of their non-subsistence income to the health system; finally, the extent to which the poor contribute a larger share of their disposable income for health than the rich.

Figure 48.1 shows the five outcomes relevant to health systems in this framework. The level of health and responsiveness define the quality of the health system and the distributions of health, responsiveness, and financial burden relate to its equity.

The appropriate weights attached to the five outcomes in constructing a composite measure are fundamentally a normative choice. For global comparative purposes, a standard set of weights is needed, although country-specific weights can be used for local policy purposes. This standard set of weights should be the product of a deliberative debate informed as much as possible by empirical information on the preferences of the populations of countries around the world (*4*).

Figure 48.1 Health system goals as part of the performance assessment framework

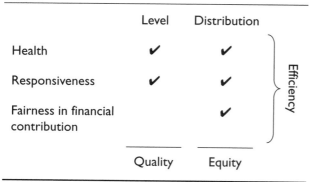

The choice of weights is important not only to set the balance between health, responsiveness, and fairness in financial contribution, but also to establish the balance between quality and equity. The World Health Organization has, for example, been criticized for being too egalitarian in its approach to health systems performance assessment on the one hand (5), while others have argued that the approach represents US market interests and does not adequately consider questions of equity (6). Empirical information on people's preferences for these outcomes in different societies can serve as a basis for a more informed and constructive global debate on the importance of these outcomes.

As a first step in the development of a long-term agenda to measure preferences for health system outcomes in various countries, preferences of informed individuals (rather than the general public) were used to derive the weights to measure composite attainment and efficiency by country, published in *The World Health Report 2000* (1). WHO's long-term goal is to measure the deliberative preferences of the general public for these outcomes. As an intermediate step, preferences of the general public were measured using nationally representative samples from 51 countries. This chapter presents the methods used and the major findings on preferences for health system goals.

METHODS

DATA

In 2000–2001, WHO conducted a Multi-country Survey Study in conjunction with relevant Member States of the Organization, research institutions, and survey organizations. The study was comprised of 71 surveys in 61 countries. It had a range of modules including health status description, health state valuations, responsiveness, adult mortality, health financing, and

preferences for health system goals. Information on the development of the content of the overall survey instrument, translation protocols, the various survey modes, selection of sites, sample frames, data collection and management, and quality of the data are detailed elsewhere[1] (7).

The module on health system goals preferences was included in 55 of the 71 population representative surveys, covering 51 countries and using 2 different modes—postal and brief face-to-face interviews. These included 36 brief household surveys (in-person interviews lasting approximately 35 minutes) and 19 postal surveys. On average, response rates were higher for the brief household surveys (64%) than for the postal surveys (46%). These response rates are similar to the ones observed for comparable instruments in OECD countries (8). Respondent missing data across all items were low, averaging 1.5% for the brief household surveys and 6.8% for the postal surveys. More details on the quality of the surveys are provided elsewhere (7).

Two different survey modes were used in four countries: the Czech Republic, Finland, France, and the Netherlands. Table 48.1 lists the country, survey mode, and sample size included in the subsequent analysis. In general, the data for each country are nationally representative of the non-institutionalized population over the age of 18 years.

SURVEY INSTRUMENT

To elicit relative weights on health systems performance, the questionnaire included word and graphics questions. In the textual question, respondents were asked to rank the health systems goals in order of importance. In the graphics question, respondents were shown seven pie charts with different values for the health systems goals and were asked to select the pie chart that best matched their preferences. Respondents also had the option to draw their own pie chart if they preferred. Because the cognitive load of asking participants to assign relative weights to five components was considered too large, three sets of pie charts were used to elicit relative weights between 1) health, responsiveness, and fairness in financial contribution, 2) average level of health and inequalities in health, and 3) average level of responsiveness and inequalities in responsiveness. The survey instruments are available on the internet at URL: http://www.who.int/evidence/hhsr-survey.

To arrive at the final weight for each component of health and responsiveness, the relative weight of average level versus inequalities was multiplied by the relative weight for the goal. The weight for fairness in financial contribution is taken from the pie chart of the three goals, without adjustment.

MODEL

A seemingly unrelated regression model was applied to check for systematic relationships between preferences for the five health system outcomes and respondent characteristics. The reported weight for each outcome was regressed on the respondent's personal characteristics, including age, sex, educational attainment, and self-rated health status, and a number of national characteristics, including average income per capita, average years of schooling, income inequality, and population density. The full set of variables included in the regression and the sources of data are found in Table 48.4.

Because the weights assigned to the five goals add up to one, the error terms of the equations are likely correlated with each other. Therefore, it is inappropriate to run five separate regressions on each of the goal weights. In contrast, a seemingly unrelated regression allows the error terms of each equation to be correlated, and estimates the full variance-covariance matrix of the coefficients (9). Seemingly unrelated regression can be applied using standard statistical packages such as Stata.

RESULTS

There were 53 024 respondents from the 51 countries. Their responses provide answers to two important questions. The first is the extent to which people assign greater weight to health, the defining goal of health systems, over the other two goals. The second is the extent to which respondents focus on quality versus equity. The average levels of health and responsiveness reflect system quality, while inequalities in health, responsiveness, and fairness in financial contribution are indicators of system inequity.

Table 48.2 shows the relative weights assigned to each of the three main health system goals—health, responsiveness, and fairness in financial contribution—by country and survey mode, ordered in terms of the weight attributed to health, from largest to smallest. The table also presents the sample standard deviations for each goal, which reflect the amount of variation in preferences within each country. All countries rated health as the most important of the three system goals, and all rated responsiveness as more

Table 48.1 Sample size and characteristics of surveys used

Country	Mode	Sample size
Argentina	Brief face-to-face	761
Australia	Postal	1 093
Austria	Postal	898
Bahrain	Brief face-to-face	577
Belgium	Brief face-to-face	1 042
Bulgaria	Brief face-to-face	999
Canada	Brief face-to-face	770
Chile	Brief face-to-face	962
China	Postal	1 358
Costa Rica	Brief face-to-face	712
Croatia	Brief face-to-face	1 465
Cyprus	Postal	578
Czech Republic	Brief face-to-face	1 072
Czech Republic	Postal	938
Denmark	Postal	1 493
Egypt	Postal	1 349
Estonia	Brief face-to-face	910
Finland	Brief face-to-face	966
Finland	Postal	1 132
France	Brief face-to-face	983
France	Postal	511
Germany	Brief face-to-face	1 031
Greece	Postal	782
Hungary	Postal	1 433
Iceland	Brief face-to-face	469
Indonesia	Brief face-to-face	2 373
Ireland	Brief face-to-face	624
Italy	Brief face-to-face	989
Jordan	Brief face-to-face	798
Korea, Republic of	Brief face-to-face	344
Kyrgyzstan	Postal	897
Latvia	Brief face-to-face	753
Lithuania	Postal	1 661
Luxembourg	Brief face-to-face	635
Malta	Brief face-to-face	500
Morocco	Brief face-to-face	721
Netherlands	Brief face-to-face	1 068
Netherlands	Postal	498
New Zealand	Brief face-to-face	1 479
Oman	Brief face-to-face	873
Poland	Brief face-to-face	777
Portugal	Brief face-to-face	972
Romania	Brief face-to-face	1 045
Russian Federation	Brief face-to-face	1 601
Spain	Postal	1 000
Sweden	Brief face-to-face	998
Switzerland	Postal	381
Thailand	Brief face-to-face	1 186
Trinidad and Tobago	Brief face-to-face	771
Turkey	Postal	1 610
Ukraine	Brief face-to-face	689
United Arab Emirates	Brief face-to-face	860
United Kingdom	Postal	852
USA	Postal	1 081
Venezuela	Brief face-to-face	704
Total		53 024

Table 48.2   Relative weights assigned to the three main health system goals

Country	Health		Responsiveness		Fairness in financial contribution	
	Average level	Sample standard deviation	Average level	Sample standard deviation	Average level	Sample standard deviation
Costa Rica	53.3	15.1	24.5	9.7	22.2	8.1
Venezuela	51.1	13.9	24.2	7.5	24.7	7.6
Czech Republic (postal)	50.9	12.5	25.3	7.1	23.9	6.9
Argentina	50.4	15.8	25.6	10.2	24.0	9.4
Spain	50.0	13.4	26.0	8.0	24.0	7.9
Czech Republic (face-to-face)	49.8	12.9	25.9	8.5	24.2	8.1
Korea, Republic of	49.0	12.8	25.4	7.5	25.5	7.5
Estonia	49.0	13.9	25.6	8.1	25.4	7.6
Portugal	48.9	14.3	25.7	8.8	25.4	7.7
Ireland	48.7	13.9	25.7	9.0	25.6	8.7
Luxembourg	48.5	15.5	26.1	10.1	25.4	10.0
France (face-to-face)	48.4	13.2	26.4	8.0	25.2	7.9
Croatia	48.3	12.8	26.2	7.0	25.5	6.8
Belgium	48.2	14.2	26.6	8.9	25.2	9.0
Ukraine	48.2	14.0	25.7	8.6	26.1	8.8
Malta	48.1	13.1	27.4	9.1	24.5	8.4
United Kingdom	48.1	12.0	25.9	6.7	26.0	7.2
China	47.9	12.1	27.1	7.8	25.0	7.3
Cyprus	47.8	13.0	27.3	7.4	24.9	7.7
Indonesia	47.7	10.5	28.2	6.8	24.1	6.6
Egypt	47.7	11.3	26.4	5.9	25.9	6.2
Italy	47.7	13.7	27.3	9.6	25.0	9.0
Bulgaria	47.5	12.9	26.0	7.2	26.5	7.9
Kyrgyzstan	47.4	13.8	26.3	8.2	26.3	8.0
Lithuania	47.1	13.2	28.2	7.8	24.7	8.7
Turkey	47.0	13.1	26.2	7.3	26.8	8.2
Romania	46.9	14.0	26.6	8.0	26.5	8.2
Denmark	46.9	11.0	27.9	5.9	25.3	6.6
Finland (face-to-face)	46.8	12.4	26.5	7.2	26.7	7.2
Poland	46.7	11.9	26.7	7.1	26.6	8.0
Bahrain	46.6	10.0	26.8	6.2	26.6	6.3
Iceland	46.5	13.0	27.8	8.3	25.8	8.3
Greece	46.4	14.0	27.6	8.9	26.0	8.2
Trinidad and Tobago	46.3	12.7	27.2	7.5	26.5	7.1
Finland (postal)	46.3	11.9	26.8	6.5	26.9	7.9
New Zealand	45.8	11.6	28.2	7.0	26.0	6.8
France (postal)	45.6	11.1	27.8	6.7	26.6	6.6
Germany	45.5	13.0	26.7	8.6	27.8	9.2
USA	44.7	18.3	30.9	15.1	24.4	13.9
Jordan	44.6	16.7	28.0	10.7	27.4	10.4
Australia	44.5	12.0	28.0	7.2	27.5	6.9
Hungary	44.4	11.8	28.9	6.6	26.7	7.9
Sweden	43.3	12.3	28.8	8.1	27.9	8.6
Latvia	43.3	14.1	26.4	8.7	30.4	11.4
Switzerland	43.2	11.2	29.9	7.8	26.9	6.9
Oman	43.2	15.9	32.2	14.8	24.6	10.9
Austria	43.1	10.7	28.9	5.8	28.0	6.1
Russian Federation	42.2	13.2	28.8	8.9	29.1	9.0
Canada	41.9	9.7	29.5	5.5	28.6	5.7
Netherlands (face-to-face)	41.5	12.1	30.9	9.2	27.7	7.9
Netherlands (postal)	41.5	10.8	30.6	7.2	27.9	6.7
Chile	41.3	11.5	29.7	6.6	29.0	7.2
United Arab Emirates	40.2	16.6	31.9	14.4	27.9	12.0
Thailand	39.9	14.5	32.1	11.4	28.0	11.8
Morocco	37.3	17.4	33.3	15.5	29.4	14.0

important than fairness in financial contribution, although the difference between these two goals was small. Health received an average weight of 46%, a proportion that varied across countries from a high of 53% in Costa Rica to a low of 37% in Morocco. The weights assigned to responsiveness varied less: from 24% in Costa Rica and Venezuela to 33% in Morocco, while the weights for fairness in financial contribution ranged from 22% in Costa Rica to 30% in Latvia.

Figure 48.2 presents a stacked bar chart containing the relative weights assigned to the five outcomes. Overall weights assigned to health and responsiveness are subdivided into the part attributed to level versus the part attributed to inequalities. The relative preferences for the five outcomes are shown by country and survey mode with countries ordered by the relative weight assigned to the level of health. The height of the bar equals 100% in all countries. While there are differences across countries in the relative weights assigned to the five outcomes, this variation is not very pronounced.

The results can be used to explore variations in the perceived importance of system quality compared to equity on a country basis. Table 48.3 contains the summed weights assigned to the average levels of health and responsiveness (system quality), and compares the result to system equity—the sum of the weights for the components dealing with system equity, namely health inequality, responsiveness

inequality, and fairness in financial contribution. Table 48.3 also shows the sample standard deviation for quality and equity within each country. All countries accord more importance to system equity than to system quality, with a great deal of consistency across settings. For example, the overall weight attached to system quality averages just under 40%, and varies between 36% and 44%.

The next step is to examine if there are characteristics of the countries that explain this variation. At the same time, it is important to identify if different groups of people in each country have different values. Table 48.4 reports the results of the seemingly unrelated regression analysis for each of the five outcomes.[2]

Some personal characteristics imply a preference for health over non-health goals, while others are correlated with a concern for system quality over system equity. For example, individual education is negatively correlated with a concern for health compared to non-health, while the higher the self-reported health status, the more responsiveness is valued compared to health. The concern with system equity compared to quality increases with age. In particular, older people are more concerned with health inequalities and less concerned with the level of responsiveness than younger people. Males also seem to be more concerned with the quality of the system than with equity, in this case rating the level of health more highly and inequalities in responsiveness less highly, than females.

Figure 48.2 Relative weights assigned to the five health system goals, by country and survey mode[a]

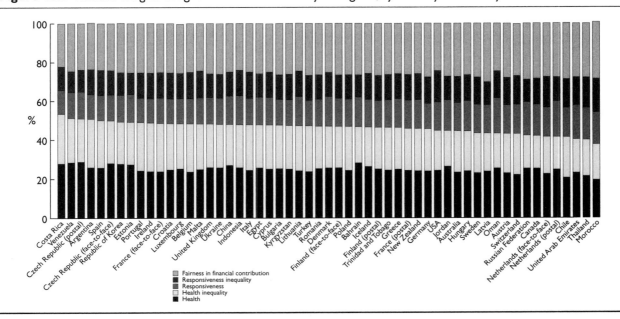

a. Countries are ranked by the highest score on health and health inequalities combined.

Table 48.3 Relative weights and sample standard deviations assigned to system quality vs. equity

Country	Quality		Equity	
	Average level	Sample standard deviation	Average level	Sample standard deviation
Oman	43.6	11.7	56.4	11.7
Bahrain	43.5	12.4	56.5	12.4
Netherlands (postal)	43.2	11.2	56.9	11.1
Czech Republic (postal)	42.7	11.8	57.3	11.8
Russian Federation	42.5	11.5	57.5	11.5
Jordan	42.2	11.5	57.8	11.5
Estonia	41.8	10.9	58.2	10.9
Venezuela	41.8	10.8	58.2	10.8
China	41.7	11.0	58.3	11.0
Korea, Republic of	41.5	10.0	58.5	10.0
Canada	41.5	7.6	58.5	7.6
Czech Republic (face-to-face)	41.4	10.1	58.6	10.1
Denmark	41.0	9.3	59.0	9.3
Indonesia	40.8	10.1	59.2	10.1
United Arab Emirates	40.7	12.3	59.3	12.3
Iceland	40.6	10.4	59.4	10.4
Finland (face-to-face)	40.2	9.8	59.8	9.8
Costa Rica	40.2	13.0	59.8	13.0
Egypt	40.0	10.5	60.0	10.5
Greece	39.8	10.4	60.3	10.5
Hungary	39.6	9.5	60.5	9.5
United Kingdom	39.5	9.4	60.5	9.4
Ukraine	39.4	10.0	60.6	10.0
Cyprus	39.3	10.1	60.7	10.1
Romania	39.3	11.7	60.7	11.7
Lithuania	39.2	9.8	60.9	9.9
Finland (postal)	39.0	10.2	61.0	10.2
New Zealand	39.0	9.5	61.0	9.5
France (postal)	38.9	8.8	61.2	9.0
USA	38.8	16.6	61.2	16.6
Spain	38.8	9.6	61.2	9.6
Bulgaria	38.6	10.2	61.4	10.2
Trinidad and Tobago	38.6	8.8	61.4	8.8
Latvia	38.5	12.3	61.5	12.3
Poland	38.5	9.4	61.5	9.4
Argentina	38.4	12.0	61.6	12.0
Malta	38.3	10.6	61.7	10.6
Luxembourg	38.2	12.8	61.8	12.8
Kyrgyzstan	38.2	9.9	61.8	10.0
Italy	38.2	10.0	61.8	10.0
Australia	37.9	9.0	62.1	9.0
Thailand	37.9	9.8	62.1	9.8
Sweden	37.8	9.9	62.2	9.9
Netherlands (face-to-face)	37.6	9.0	62.4	9.0
Austria	37.6	8.5	62.5	8.6
Croatia	37.5	9.7	62.5	9.7
Switzerland	37.2	8.7	62.8	8.7
France (face-to-face)	37.0	8.7	63.0	8.7
Turkey	36.9	10.2	63.0	10.3
Germany	36.9	10.0	63.1	10.0
Portugal	36.9	11.2	63.1	11.2
Belgium	36.6	10.7	63.4	10.7
Ireland	36.3	11.0	63.7	11.1
Morocco	35.9	14.2	65.0	14.0
Chile	35.6	7.5	64.5	7.6

Table 48.4 Results from the seemingly unrelated regression model

	Health	Health inequality	Responsiveness	Responsiveness inequality	Fairness in financial contribution
Age	0.0000	0.0001*	0.0001***	0.0000	0.0000
	(0.0000)	(0.0000)	(0.0000)	(0.0000)	(0.0000)
Sex	0.0019*	0.0009	0.0009	−0.0013*	0.0005
	(0.0009)	(0.0008)	(0.0005)	(0.0005)	(0.0008)
Self-reported health status	0.0005	0.0030**	0.0016*	0.0013*	0.0004
	(0.0010)	(0.0009)	(0.0006)	(0.0006)	(0.0008)
Education (individual)	0.0018	−0.0067***	0.0021***	0.0002	0.0027**
	(0.0010)	(0.0009)	(0.0006)	(0.0006)	(0.0008)
Average years of schooling (national)	0.0031***	0.0030***	0.0014***	0.0009***	0.0007*
	(0.0004)	(0.0004)	(0.0002)	(0.0002)	(0.0003)
Voice[1] [2]	−0.0089**	0.0046***	0.0017**	0.0045***	0.0016
	(0.0010)	(0.0009)	(0.0006)	(0.0006)	(0.0008)
% public health expenditure[4]	0.0241**	0.0403***	0.0283***	0.0308***	0.0052
	(0.0038)	(0.0035)	(0.0023)	(0.0022)	(0.0031)
Dependency ratio[4]	0.0472**	0.0085	0.0133**	−0.0031	0.0490***
	(0.0072)	(0.0065)	(0.0043)	(0.0041)	(0.0059)
Population density[3]	0.0021**	0.0040***	0.0024***	0.0002	0.0039***
	(0.0004)	(0.0004)	(0.0003)	(0.0003)	(0.0004)
Gini coefficient	−0.0291**	0.0362***	0.0174***	0.0184***	0.0293***
	(0.0082)	(0.0075)	(0.0049)	(0.0047)	(0.0067)
GDP per capita	0.0000	0.0000***	0.0000***	0.0000***	0.0000
	(0.0000)	(0.0000)	(0.0000)	(0.0000)	(0.0000)
Per capita out of pocket expenditure[4]	0.0000	0.0000***	0.0000***	0.0000	0.0000*
	(0.0000)	(0.0000)	(0.0000)	(0.0000)	(0.0000)
Constant term	0.1873***	0.2124***	0.1544***	0.1467***	0.2992***
	(0.0080)	(0.0073)	(0.0048)	(0.0046)	(0.0066)

* $P < 0.05$

** $P < 0.01$

*** $P < 0.001$

Sources of data:

[1] Kaufman D, Kraay A, Zoido-Lobatón P. *Aggregating governance indicators*. World Bank Policy Research Working Paper No. 2195. 1999.

[2] Kaufman D, Kraay A, Zoido-Lobatón P. *Governance matters*. World Bank Policy Research Working Paper No. 2196. 1999.

[3] *ESRI data and maps 1999*. Redlands, CA, Environmental Systems Research Institute, 1999. URL: http://www.esri.com/

[4] World Health Organization. *The World Health Report 2000. Health Systems: Improving Performance*. Geneva, World Health Organization, 2000.

Similar patterns can be found across all system characteristics that were tested. Interestingly, both the average educational level of the adult population and the dependency ratio are negatively correlated with a concern for system equity compared to quality. Countries in which each member of the working population supports a larger number of dependents are more concerned with improving the quality of the system, than with reducing inequalities. In contrast, countries where the population is seen to have an effective role in influencing government actions (the "voice" vari-able) feel that reducing inequities is more important than improving average levels.

Population density and the percent of health expenditure provided by the public sector are negatively correlated with a preference for non-health goals compared to health. On the other hand, countries with higher levels of GDP per capita and those with more income inequality are more likely to give higher weights to non-health goals than to health.

Even though the individual- and country-level characteristics of the respondents are associated with the weights assigned to the five outcomes of health systems, the resulting effect on the relative weights of the health system goals is not substantively significant in all cases. The coefficients on the variables in Table 48.4 are very small in magnitude so that, although the relationships are statistically significant, these variables rarely change the weight assigned to a goal by more than a few percentage points. This was reflected in Table 48.2 and Figure 48.2, where the range across countries in the weights is relatively small.

DISCUSSION

This chapter has presented results from the first attempt to measure preferences of the general public on the relative importance of the goals of health systems. Data from 51 countries and more than 53 000 respondents were analysed for this study.

This supplements the information on preferences obtained from informed respondents used in estimating the composite attainment of health systems in *The World Health Report 2000* (*10*). In that internet survey, the average weights from over 1 600 responses were 24% health, 25% health inequality, 13% responsiveness, 16% responsiveness inequality, and 22% fairness in financial contribution, very similar to the average of the respondents from the nationally representative surveys of the general public reported in this chapter (Table 48.2). Based on this evidence, informed respondents and the general public seem to differ very little in their preferences for health system goals.

Clearly, the preferences in the present analysis, derived from nationally representative samples, capture local preferences in a way that is impossible for a convenience sample of informed respondents. The overall similarity of the responses and the relatively small variation across countries is striking, and makes it more credible to use the average weights from an informed respondent study in places where it is not possible to conduct nationally representative surveys.

For global comparative purposes of health system attainment, a single set of weights might be desirable. It would be most appropriate to use the average or median weights from household surveys from around the world, although for the purposes of local policy-making, a locally derived set of weights has to be used. In either case, an analysis of how sensitive the substantive conclusions are to the choice of weights should be conducted. A preliminary analysis shows the encouraging result that substantive conclusions on health system attainment are not very sensitive to

the choice of set of weights for the five outcomes or to using the weights that are the most favourable to each individual country (*11*).

One limitation of the method used in the household surveys for this study is that time for deliberation was not built into the instrument. Modifications of the instrument might include the use of trade-off questions favoured by economists (*12–14*), in which respondents are explicitly asked to trade-off quantities of two types of benefits (e.g. health or health inequality reduction) under a particular resource constraint. On the other hand, this type of trade-off question tends to have poor psychometric properties in less educated respondents(*12–14*). Nonetheless, it would be very interesting to explore alternative methods of measuring preferences of health system goals and analyse whether responses differ depending on the survey instrument employed.

The results are striking for the substantial weight attached to health system equity. Health inequality (21%), responsiveness inequality (13%), and fairness in financial contribution (26%) combine to average 60% of the total weight. This heavy emphasis on equity was present in all groups of respondents. This orientation to equity is now being reflected in many countries by an increasing policy emphasis on reducing health inequalities (*15*).

Weights for the average level and distribution of health account for 46% of the total weight, but the goals of responsiveness and fairness in financial contribution together are considered more important. This may be surprising to many health practitioners who have traditionally focused only on health as the key goal of health systems. The importance given to non-health goals is consistent across different types of respondents and across all countries, and has significant implications not just for policy development, but also for data collection and measurement. It is only if attainment on these goals is routinely measured and monitored that the performance of health systems in the areas that people value will improve.

ACKNOWLEDGEMENTS

The authors wish to thank Margaret C. Hogan for research assistance, and Joshua A. Salomon and Ajay Tandon for helpful input.

NOTES

1   The survey instruments are available on the internet at URL: http://www.who.int/evidence/hhsr-survey/

2 The results are not substantively different using a wide variety of other functional forms of the model and five independent regression models.

REFERENCES

(1) World Health Organization. *The World Health Report 2000. Health Systems: Improving Performance*. Geneva, World Health Organization, 2000.

(2) Murray CJL, Frenk J. A framework for assessing the performance of health systems. *Bulletin of the World Health Organization*, 2000, 78:717–731.

(3) de Silva A. *A framework for measuring responsiveness*. EIP Discussion Paper No. 32. Geneva, World Health Organization, 2000. URL: http://www3.who.int/whosis/discussion_papers/discussion_papers.cfm#

(4) Hausman DM. The limits to empirical ethics. In: Murray CJL et al., eds. *Summary measures of population health: concepts, ethics, measurement and applications*. Geneva, World Health Organization, 2002:641–646.

(5) Helms RB. Health care à la Karl Marx. *The Wall Street Journal Europe*, 29 June 2000.

(6) Navarro V. Assessment of the World Health Report 2000. *The Lancet*, 2000, 356:1598–1601.

(7) Üstün TB et al. WHO Multi-country Survey Study on Health and Responsiveness 2000–2001. In: Murray CJL, Evans DB, eds. *Health systems performance assessment: debates, methods and empiricism*. Geneva, World Health Organization, 2003.

(8) Jenkinson C, Coulter A, Bruster S. The Picker Patient Experience Questionnaire: development and validation using data from in-patient surveys in five countries. *International Journal for Quality in Healthcare*, 2002, 14: 353–358.

(9) Greene WH. *Econometric analysis*, 4th ed. Upper Saddle River, NJ, Prentice-Hall, 2000.

(10) Gakidou E, Murray CJL, Frenk J. *Measuring preferences for health systems performance assessment*. EIP Discussion Paper No. 20. Geneva, World Health Organization, 2000. URL: http://www3.who.int/whosis/discussion_papers/discussion_papers.cfm#

(11) Murray CJL et al. *Overall health system achievement for 191 countries*. EIP Discussion Paper No. 28. Geneva, World Health Organization, 2000. URL: http://www3.who.int/whosis/discussion_papers/discussion_papers.cfm#

(12) Froberg DG, Kane RL. Methodology for measuring health state preference II: scaling methods. *Journal of Clinical Epidemiology*, 1989, 42:459–471.

(13) Nord E. Methods for quality adjustment of life years. *Social Science & Medicine*, 1992, 34:559–569.

(14) Richardson J. Cost utility analysis: what should be measured? *Social Science & Medicine*, 2000, 39:7–21.

(15) Lauer JA, Evans DB, Murray CJL. Measuring health system attainment: the impact of variability in the importance of social goals. In: Murray CJL, Evans DB, eds. *Health systems performance assessment: debates, methods and empiricism*. Geneva, World Health Organization, 2003.

Chapter 49

MEASURING HEALTH SYSTEM ATTAINMENT: THE IMPACT OF VARIABILITY IN THE IMPORTANCE OF SOCIAL GOALS

JEREMY A. LAUER, DAVID B. EVANS, CHRISTOPHER J.L. MURRAY

INTRODUCTION

Health decision-makers continue to seek timely and reliable information on the performance of their health systems and ways to improve performance. WHO recently defined a framework that can be used to measure performance in a comparable way across systems (1). The framework identified a parsimonious set of social goals to which health systems should contribute. They should contribute to improving population health, be responsive to the people they serve, and be financed fairly. Five outcome indicators were defined on this basis: the level of population health, inequalities in health, the level of responsiveness, inequalities in responsiveness, and fairness of financing. Estimates of attainment on these five indicators were made for the 191 countries which were Members of WHO at that time, and a composite (overall) attainment indicator was constructed for each country as a weighted average of attainment on the five indicators. Overall country attainment ranged from a minimum of 35.7 (Sierra Leone) to a maximum of 93.4 (Japan) on a scale from 1 to 100 (estimates for 1997).

The weights used in constructing the overall attainment indicator in *The World Health Report 2000* were based on the average results of a survey (2) in which participants were asked by means of an interactive pie chart to assign weights to the individual goals of the health system. A total of 1 007 people completed the survey, and small statistically significant differences were found between respondents from developed and developing countries in the weights assigned to health and inequality in responsiveness. These differences were on the order of two percentage points, and sensitivity analysis showed that the overall attainment scores were not sensitive to this magnitude of variation.

The publication of the report provoked considerable comments from governments, as well as debate in the academic press (3–9). One of the criticisms concerned the use of a uniform set of weights in the construction of the overall attainment index. It was argued that people from different cultural and social settings would value the individual goals of the health system in different ways (10). Our early results had showed that the overall attainment score was more sensitive to uncertainty in measurement of individual attainment indicators than to reasonable variations in the weights used to aggregate the individual scores, and this chapter accordingly does not address the question of how much it matters to be wrong about the (average) set of weights. Instead, it explores how much it matters if different countries are allowed to have different values for each of the components of health system attainment.

Whether values (as expressed in weights) do, in fact, differ substantively across countries is a testable hypothesis, which has recently been investigated by means of a series of household surveys conducted in 50 countries (see Chapter 48 for fuller discussion). Here, we explore whether the absolute and relative attainment of countries in terms of the overall indicator would differ substantively if country-specific weights had been used in constructing the composite measure.

The above-mentioned surveys suggest a natural strategy for estimating country-specific weights, i.e. to measure them in each individual country. However, here we adopt the device of using for each country the weights that would maximize its score on the overall attainment index. Such weights can be called "benefit of the doubt" weights (11), in that they implicitly allow for the possibility that a country may be maximizing its individual social preference function by its choices in the health system, or that health system decision-makers might be maximizing their own preference functions. The overall attainment scores resulting from the benefit of the doubt are country-specific global maxima conditional on the underlying levels of attainment on the individual country indicators, and subject to some necessary constraints explained below.

METHODS

WHO originally used fixed weights to aggregate the five outputs into a scalar health system attainment index. The weights were 0.25, 0.25, 0.125, 0.125, 0.25 for the level of population health, inequality in the distribution of health, the level of health system responsiveness, inequality in the distribution of responsiveness, and fairness in financial contribution, in turn. For the benefit of the doubt analysis, each country was assigned the set of weights giving it the highest possible attainment score. However, all countries were required to have all weights for individual indicators to be non-zero and to sum to one. Consequently, bounds on the maximum and minimum values for the individual weights are necessary, and the bounds we use are those that derive from the above-mentioned cross-population surveys. For each indicator, the lower bound is the minimum country-specific average weight across the sample, where the country-specific average weight is the average of the valuations provided by the respondents from that country. The upper bound was taken as the maximum of the average country-specific weights. The upper and lower bounds are found in Table 49.1.

Consequently, finding the maximum overall attainment score is a set of linear programming problems, one for each country. For the jth country, the goal is to determine the set of weights that maximizes overall attainment, subject to various constraints. Mathematically:

$$\max j \left(\Sigma w_i \times c_i \right), i = 1,\ldots,5; j = 1,\ldots,191$$

subject to:
$$0.19 \leq w_1 \leq 0.29$$
$$0.17 \leq w_2 \leq 0.25$$
$$0.12 \leq w_3 \leq 0.18$$
$$0.11 \leq w_4 \leq 0.17$$
$$0.22 \leq w_5 \leq 0.30$$
$$\Sigma w_i \leq 1, i = 1,\ldots,5$$

where c_i represents the attainment score on the five individual outcome indicators for country j and w_i is the weight for that component in the composite attainment index for that country (index "1" corresponds to health, "2" to health distribution, "3" to responsiveness, "4" to responsiveness distribution, "5" to fairness in financial contribution). Country attainment scores as measured according to this method of assigning weights will always be greater than or equal to country attainment scores using the original weights reported in *The World Health Report 2000 (1)*.

RESULTS

In Figure 49.1, country attainment scores obtained under the benefit of the doubt assumptions are plotted on the vertical axis against attainment scores reported in *The World Health Report 2000*, obtained using the original weights. If the two scores were the same, the plot would consist of points on the 45-degree line. However, attainment scores obtained using alternative weights always lie above the 45-degree line. The vertical difference of the alternative scores from the 45-degree line tends to be greatest for countries with relatively low attainment scores using the original weights—in other words, such countries have greater room for improvement than countries already scoring close to the maximum. The correlation between the alternative scores is 0.9978.

A histogram of the magnitude of the changes in the overall attainment score obtained under the benefit of the doubt is shown in Figure 49.2. The distribution of changes has a mean of 4.6 and a standard deviation of 1.39. No country's overall attainment score increases by more than 8.2 points. As can be seen in

Table 49.1   Original weights and benefit of the doubt weights with summary statistics

Variable	Original weight	Benefit of the doubt (Mean)	Benefit of the doubt (Standard deviation)	Benefit of the doubt (Minimum)	Benefit of the doubt (Maximum)
Responsiveness level	0.125	0.130	0.019	0.12	0.18
Responsiveness distribution	0.125	0.180	0.004	0.16	0.18
Fair financing (distribution)	0.250	0.291	0.025	0.22	0.30
Health distribution	0.250	0.200	0.036	0.17	0.25
Health level	0.250	0.200	0.028	0.19	0.29

the density plot (i.e. a smoothed histogram), showing a standard normal overlay (Figure 49.3), the distribution of changes in score is skewed slightly to the left and has a fat right-hand tail.

Countries are understandably concerned about their rank as compared with other, frequently closely ranked, countries. However, this can result in an undue emphasis on "local" comparisons, even though the main purpose of the attainment measurement exercise is to derive global policy implications about what types of health system strategies and policies work and what do not work. For example, when a country's rank under the benefit of the doubt is compared with

the original rank as reported in *The World Health Report 2000*, the great majority of countries show little or no change (Figure 49.4). Nearly 40 countries (20% of the sample) show no rank change at all under the benefit of the doubt, and 99 (52%) show changes of only one, two or three ranks (Figure 49.5).

However, in restricted rank-neighbourhoods, where there is clustering of the underlying overall attainment scores, rank changes naturally appear more substantial and the plot more dispersed. Overall, however, the

Figure 49.1 Alternative (maximum) attainment scores versus original (*World Health Report 2000*) scores, showing 45-degree line

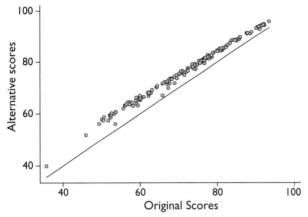

Figure 49.2 Histogram showing absolute differences in two sets of attainment scores: alternative (maximum) versus original (*World Health Report 2000*)

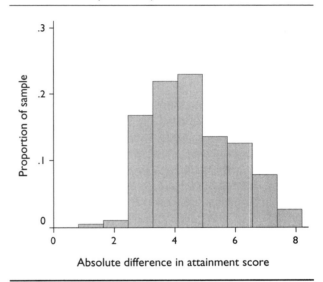

Figure 49.3 Density plot of the changes induced under benefit of the doubt, showing the standard normal distribution

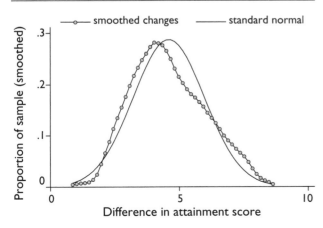

Figure 49.4 Alternative ranks (based on maximum scores) versus original (*World Health Report 2000*) ranks

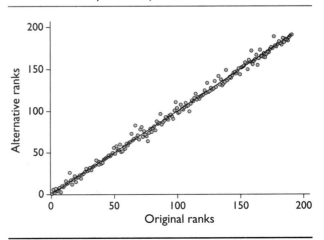

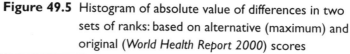

Figure 49.5 Histogram of absolute value of differences in two sets of ranks: based on alternative (maximum) and original (*World Health Report 2000*) scores

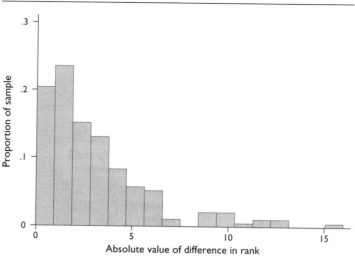

points in Figure 49.4 lie close to the 45-degree line (simple linear correlation, 0.9972). Since both positive and negative rank changes occur, points are scattered above and below the 45-degree line.

Like the histogram for changes in overall attainment score, the histogram in Figure 49.5 is skewed to the left and shows a fat right-hand tail, although both of these non-central tendencies are much more pronounced for rank than for score changes. Again, due to substantial clustering in scores, one country changes 16 ranks, and a number of countries make rank changes greater than 5. Nevertheless, all rank changes are within the rank uncertainty bounds reported in the original analysis (*1*).

Comparing the weights obtained under the benefit of the doubt to the original weights, interesting patterns emerge (Table 49.1). Most countries do better under the benefit of the doubt when the weights for responsiveness distribution and fair finance are at or near the upper bounds of their intervals, and when those for responsiveness level and health level are close to their lower bounds. This implies that most countries do relatively better on the first two indicators, and relatively worse on the second two. Interestingly, the lower bound for responsiveness is almost identical to the value used in *The World Health Report 2000*. On the other hand, the sample mean for health inequality under the benefit of the doubt is close to the middle of its range, but lower than the value assigned in the original calculations.

DISCUSSION

Overall attainment scores obtained under the benefit of the doubt put each country in the best possible light. All countries will benefit from this procedure unless the weights obtained under the benefit of the doubt happen to be the same as those used in the original analysis.

Weights obtained under the benefit of the doubt can be interpreted in two ways. First, they could be revealed social preference weights, at least for those social goals to which the health system contributes. Observed outcomes in terms of health level, health inequality, responsiveness level, responsiveness inequality, and fair financing could be interpreted as the result of a political and social maximization process, subject to a budget constraint which takes into account the relative weights that society places on those components. The linear program specified above simply identifies those implicit weights, assuming of course a linear social welfare function. Obviously, this interpretation ignores uncertainty, and it might be true that the actual observed outcomes do not fully reflect what social actors intended. The second possible interpretation is that they represent the values of the key decision-makers.

However, the most important point is that the use of variable weights across countries does not change substantively the pattern of either overall attainment scores or corresponding ranks. Moreover, the variation we find by allowing for intercountry differences in valuation of the individual attainment goals is well within the reported uncertainty intervals (1) calculated to reflect possible errors in the measurement of goal attainment. This conclusion is at odds with some of the assertions made in criticisms of *The World Health Report 2000* (3;4;9;12).

However, it also suggests that it may not be necessary to use fixed weights in future rounds of performance assessment. It might be effective to report overall attainment using average weights derived from the country surveys, as well as benefit of the doubt scores based on the upper and lower bounds for the weights that emerge from the country surveys.

Acknowledgements

We are indebted to William Greene, Philip Grossman, Kaliappa Kalirajan, C.A. Knox Lovell, Subal Kumbhakar, Christopher Tong, Marijn Verhoeven, and Paul Wilson for the discussions of the methods which led to the idea for this analysis and for the term "benefit of the doubt."

References

(1) World Health Organization. *The World Health Report 2000. Health Systems: Improving Performance.* Geneva, World Health Organization, 2000.

(2) Gakidou E, Frenk J, Murray CJL. *Measuring preferences on health system performance assessment.* EIP Discussion Paper No. 20. Geneva, World Health Organization, 2000. URL: http://www3.who.int/whosis/discussion_papers/discussion_papers.cfm#

(3) Navarro V. Assessment of The World Health Report 2000. *The Lancet*, 2000, 356:1598–1601.

(4) Williams A. Science or marketing at WHO? A commentary on 'World Health 2000'. *Health Economics*, 2001, 10(2):93–100.

(5) Van der SP, Unger JP. Improving the performance of health systems: The World Health Report as go-between for scientific evidence and ideological discourse. *Tropical Medicine and International Health*, 2000, 5:675–677.

(6) Ginter E. World Health Report 2000: the position of Slovak Republic. *Bratislavske Lekarske Listy (Bratislava Medical Journal)*, 2000, 101:477–483.

(7) Houweling TA, Kunst AE, Mackenbach JP. World Health Report 2000: inequality index and socioeconomic inequalities in mortality. *The Lancet*, 2001, 357: 1671–1672.

(8) Tangcharoensathien V, Lertiendumrong J. Health-system performance. *The Lancet*, 2000, 356 (Suppl.):s31.

(9) Almeida C, et al. Methodological concerns and recommendations on policy consequences of the World Health Report 2000. *The Lancet*, 2001, 357:1692–1697.

(10) Williams A. Science or marketing at WHO? Rejoinder from Alan Williams. *Health Economics*, 2001, 10:283–285.

(11) Melvyn W, Moesen W. *Towards a synthetic indicator of macroeconomic performance: unequal weighting when limited information is available.* Public Economics Research Paper No. 17. Centrum voor Economische Studien KUL, ed. Leuven, Belgium, Katholieke Universiteit Leuven, 1991.

(12) Navarro V. World Health Report 2000: responses to Murray and Frenk. *The Lancet*, 2001, 357:1701–1702.

Chapter 50

Health System Efficiency: Concepts

Ajay Tandon, Jeremy A. Lauer, David B. Evans,
Christopher J.L. Murray

Introduction

For much of the last two decades, health policy-makers have been concerned with the performance of their health systems and many countries have introduced reforms aimed at improving performance (1;2). However, it has been difficult to evaluate the impact of these reforms and to determine if performance has improved over time because of a lack of clarity about the goals of health systems against which outcomes should be judged, and a definition of health system performance which can be quantified (3).

The framework developed by WHO for measuring and assessing health system performance specifies three intrinsic goals of the health system: the defining goal is to improve population health, but health systems must also be responsive to the population and ensure that the financial burden of paying for health is fairly distributed. Both the level and distribution of health and responsiveness are important, resulting in five measurable indicators of health system outcomes: health level and distribution, responsiveness level and distribution, and fairness in financial contribution.

Health system efficiency is defined as attainment compared to the maximum that could have been achieved for the observed level of resource use. It relates the outputs of the health system to its inputs. This chapter describes how the definition of efficiency was operationalized in the first round of performance assessment using information about the inputs to the system and the system's achievements (4;5). Ways in which this framework could be modified to take into account some of the discussion and debate emerging from the initial work (6–10) are discussed in the next chapter (Chapter 51).

The Health System as a Production Unit

Measures of health system efficiency can be derived by conceptualizing the health system as a "production unit" the output of which is governed by certain functional relationships. A "production function" summarizes the relationship between the inputs and outputs of any production process. The *frontier* production function represents the maximum level of output that can be obtained from a given level of inputs. Different ways of estimating the frontier are discussed in a later section.

Health system attainment can be measured in terms of health or in terms of a composite index combining achievements on the five indicators described above. Figure 50.1 shows the relationship between the output of the system and the inputs used to achieve it. The vertical axis measures a country's goal attainment and the horizontal axis measures the amount of input(s).

Figure 50.1 The health system as a production unit

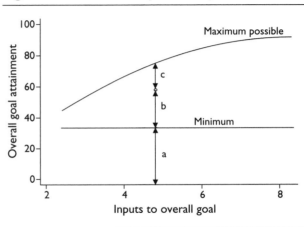

Inputs to overall goal

The line labelled "maximum possible" represents the frontier: the maximum level of goal attainment for given levels of inputs to the health system.

The distance between a country's actual level of goal attainment and the frontier is called its "efficiency" in the economics literature (*11*). Suppose a country is observed to achieve $(a + b)$ "units" in terms of goal attainment, efficiency is measured by the ratio $(a + b) / (a + b + c)$. If a country is on the frontier it is considered to be fully efficient, with an efficiency score of 1. Where the horizontal axis measures an individual input to the system, such as human resources, the ratio can be interpreted as measuring *technical efficiency*—that is, the output actually achieved compared to the maximum possible output for a given quantity of human resources. Where the horizontal axis represents the expenditures of the health system, the ratio $(a + b) / (a + b + c)$ reflects *economic efficiency*: in this case, measured inefficiency can be partly due to waste (technical inefficiency) and partly due to choosing the wrong mix of outputs (*allocative inefficiency*).

An important difference between traditional production situations (as for firms and farms) and the health system as a production unit is that in the latter case overall goal attainment will not be zero even in the absence of inputs. For example, the level of health in the population (one component of the overall attainment index) would not be zero even in the absence of a modern functioning health system—not all people would be dead. This fact implies the need for a definition of efficiency that takes into account the output that would be observed in the absence of inputs to the system. This output is defined here as the minimum possible, and is represented by the line labelled "minimum" in Figure 50.1. In terms of Figure 50.1, the efficiency of the health system is simply $b / (b + c)$, or:

$$Efficiency = \frac{(Attainment - Minimum)}{(Maximum\ Possible - Minimum)}$$

Measurement of efficiency is of considerable significance to policy-makers. First, it draws attention to the fact that a country may be able to achieve a higher level of overall goal attainment *without increasing its resource inputs*. Second, with the measurement of efficiency, it is then feasible to investigate exogenous *determinants of inefficiency*: it may be possible to identify, for instance, if low efficiencies are related to factors such as high AIDS prevalence, low levels of government effectiveness, high income inequality, or particular ways that the system is organized or financed. Third, the regular measurement of efficiency over time is important for monitoring the impact of policy reforms aimed at increasing technical and allocative efficiency.

Econometric Estimation of the Frontier

Before defining the inputs to the production of health system goals, methods of estimating the frontier—the maximum possible level of overall goal attainment for given resource levels—are considered. In principle, there are two possible strategies: a) a *micro-level* approach: determine the set of health system interventions that yields the maximum possible output for given inputs, and b) a *macro-level* approach: econometrically estimate the maximum possible output from a sample of observed data on inputs and outputs. The first (micro-level) approach is very data intensive. WHO is currently developing the framework and dataset for this approach under the WHO-CHOICE initiative described in Chapter 60, but this work is not yet complete. The second approach is described here.

Econometric measurement of efficiency can be undertaken by estimating either: a) a "deterministic" frontier, or b) a "stochastic" frontier (*12*). With the deterministic method, all observed data points are constrained to lie below the frontier, and all deviation from the frontier is attributed to inefficiency. With a stochastic frontier, some of the deviation from the frontier is attributed to "random factors." A further distinction can be made between parametric and non-parametric approaches: parametric approaches assume a functional form for the frontier, whereas non-parametric approaches allow the data to dictate the shape of the frontier.

Examples of non-parametric deterministic approaches include free disposal hull (FDH) analysis and data envelopment analysis (DEA). In FDH analysis, piece-wise linear segments are used to "wrap" the data. Figure 50.2 shows an example of FDH with healthy life expectancy (HALE) as the output of the health system, and health expenditure per capita as the input (*13*). By definition, all points on the frontier have an efficiency of 1, and the vertical distance of any given data point from the frontier gives a measure of inefficiency.

In DEA, the segments are estimated using linear programming methods. Figure 50.3 shows the frontier estimated using DEA; the dataset is the same as in Figure 50.2 so as to construct the convex hull of the data (14).

An example of a parametric deterministic approach is the corrected ordinary least squares (COLS) method where the average production function in the sample is estimated using ordinary linear regression methods. To find the frontier, the estimated function is "shifted up" by the value of the largest positive residual (Figure 50.4) (11).

Examples of parametric stochastic techniques are "error-decomposition models," where inefficiency is assumed to follow a one-sided distribution such as exponential or truncated-normal (Figure 50.5) (14). In stochastic models, some data points can be higher than the frontier if the "random error" portion of the residual is large enough (12).

Another parametric stochastic method uses panel data to estimate efficiencies using a standard fixed-effect model (Figure 50.6) (12;15). There are several advantages to using such models: a) multiple observations of inputs and outputs over time contain more information (i.e. it is easier to separate inefficiency from random noise), b) there is no need to make any kind of distributional assumption for inefficiency, and c) there is no need to assume that inefficiency is uncorrelated with inputs (11;12;15). In Figure 50.6, the frontier is estimated from the country having the maximum intercept and the distance of every other country's intercept from this maximum gives the technical efficiency.

Econometrically estimating a frontier using observed data probably results in the overestimation of efficiency. The true theoretical maximum level of output may be much greater than what is observed in

Figure 50.2 Efficiency: free disposal hull (FDH)

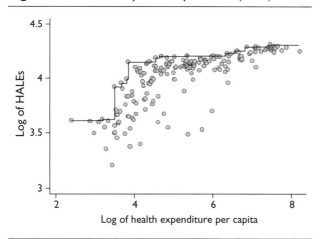

Figure 50.4 Efficiency: corrected ordinary least squares (COLS)

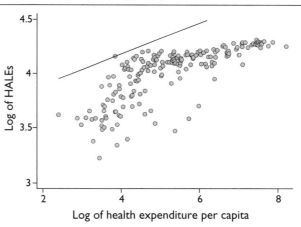

Figure 50.3 Efficiency: data envelopment analysis (DEA)

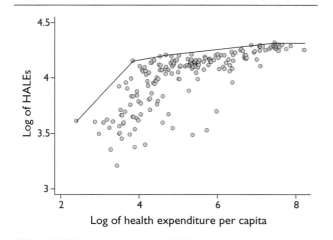

Figure 50.5 Efficiency: stochastic frontier truncated-normal model

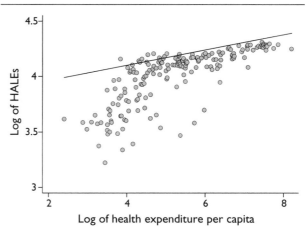

Figure 50.6 Efficiency: fixed-effect model

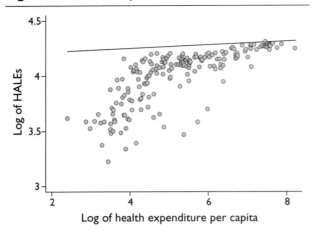

a given sample of data: this would certainly be the case where no country in the sample was able to attain its maximum level of output. An estimated efficiency of 1 does not necessarily mean that there is no room for improvement.

METHODOLOGY

In practical terms, the measurement of health system efficiency can be divided into five separate steps: a) specifying the inputs and outputs of production, b) estimating the production function, c) estimating the level of output that would have been achieved in the absence of a health system, d) uncertainty analysis, and e) analysis of the exogenous determinants of efficiency.

OUTPUTS

The level of composite health system goal attainment is the output of interest. Composite attainment is a weighted average of its five component goals: health, health distribution, responsiveness, responsiveness distribution, and fairness in financing. Details of the construction of this measure can be found in Gakidou et al. (16).

INPUTS

We distinguish two types of inputs to the production process: health system and non-health system inputs.

Health System Inputs

For the purposes of analysing the efficiency of the health system, we have represented all the factors

of production by means of the total dollar value of resources used in the system. It would be possible to undertake production function analysis separating the individual inputs such as human resources, drugs, physical infrastructure, etc., (17) or even distinguishing some factors of production as "intermediate inputs"—like tuberculosis treatment programmes. This is not feasible. Such detailed information is available for only a tiny handful of countries.

Non-health System Inputs

A long list of potential non-health system "inputs" could be incorporated, including educational attainment, food intake, quality of housing, tobacco consumption, the presence of various disease vectors, the seriousness of the HIV epidemic, income per capita, income inequality, and others. Some care must be taken, however, in selecting which ones to include.

Several questions are relevant to this choice:

Is the proposed variable truly a factor of production? In other words, does it directly enter the process of producing health, health inequalities, or responsiveness? We argue that only true factors of production should be included in the first phase of efficiency analysis, while other exogenous variables likely to influence efficiency should be introduced in the second phase of determinants of efficiency. On these grounds, the health system, food, housing, disease vectors, HIV prevalence, tobacco consumption, and education are probably direct "inputs" to the achievement of outcomes. By the same logic, income per capita is *not* a direct factor of production. In and of itself, income does not make people healthy. Although income is *correlated* with health outcomes, it is not itself an input to the production process. Figure 50.7 shows a very simple causal web. The diagram suggests that income makes it possible for people to afford better nutrition and housing. It enables society to develop better technologies. It allows for the purchase of inputs to the health system, but is not an input itself.

Levels of health have historically been highly correlated with income per capita (18–21). At the turn of the 19th century, increases in income primarily allowed people access to better housing and improved water and sanitation, which in turn contributed to better health. However, income simply allowed for the purchase of inputs that directly improved health and was not itself the direct input to those improvements. Moreover, efficiency analysis does not focus on factors historically correlated with health improvements. It is aimed at identifying direct inputs to the production of health system outcomes, and determining what is the maximum level of goal attainment which could have been achieved with those direct inputs. Thus, income as such should not be included in efficiency analysis.

Should the scope of accountability of the health system include or exclude the proposed variable? If the answer to this question is "yes" and the health system should be held accountable for that factor, then it should not be included as a separate input in efficiency analysis. To do so would have the effect of controlling for the proposed variable. For example, tobacco consumption affects health and health inequalities, but if it is included as a separate variable, the implication would be that the health system is not accountable for its reduction. However, WHO believes that one of the criteria for judging efficiency is whether the health system makes active efforts to discourage tobacco consumption. The same argument would apply to disease vectors and effects of the HIV epidemic.

Is measurement of the proposed variable feasible? If a factor such as food intake is potentially important but cannot be measured across a wide range of countries, then some proxy measure must be used. As explained subsequently, we used a proxy-variable approach to capture some important non-health system inputs.

Considering these three issues, in addition to health expenditure per capita, we included as inputs two non-health system factors: average educational attainment and a proxy variable designed to capture the impact of food, housing, and other income-related factors. With regard to educational attainment, an overwhelming body of evidence in developing and developed countries shows that education is correlated with better health outcomes and is also likely to be a causal factor in the production of health (*22–29*). However, the "stock" of education that has been achieved in a given setting can be measured in several ways. Literacy rates have a major disadvantage in that for many countries there is hardly any variation: for example, all rich countries report rates near 100% (Figure 50.8).

A more sensitive measure of educational stock is the average years of schooling in the population aged 15 years and over (Figure 50.9).

Since there are no widely available cross-population comparable data on other non-health system inputs such as food intake and housing, we constructed a proxy variable (called "Other") using the residual from a regression of income per capita on the other independent variables in the model, i.e. health expen-

Figure 50.8 Literacy rate versus GDP per capita, PPP

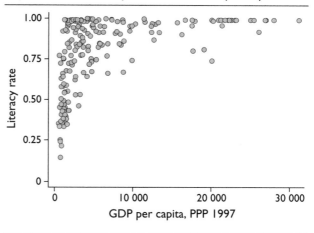

Figure 50.7 Causal web relating income to health

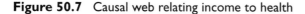

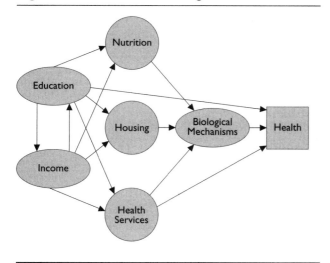

Figure 50.9 Educational attainment versus GDP per capita, PPP

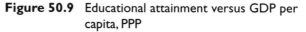

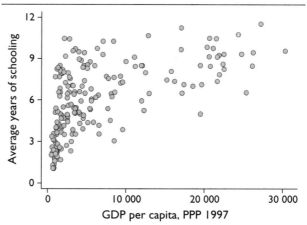

diture per capita and average years of schooling. The logic here is that, by construction, such a residual captures those aspects of income per capita that are not captured in health expenditure per capita and educational stock. In technical terms, the residual variable is orthogonal to health expenditure and average years of schooling. However, one limitation is that the residual variable is likely to capture some non-health system factors that should not reasonably be included in efficiency analysis by the three criteria mentioned above. In addition, there is a danger of "overdetermining" the efficiency of health systems by including too many factors as inputs to the production process.

ESTIMATING THE PRODUCTION FUNCTION

The general form of the production function can be written as:

Composite Goal = f (Health Expenditure,
Educational Attainment, Other)

The following figures (Figures 50.10–50.12) show a scatterplot of the composite goal and each of these three inputs. Figure 50.10 plots the composite attainment index versus health expenditure per capita in international dollars for 1997.

On average, attainment on the composite index is increasing with health expenditure per capita. However, there appear to be diminishing returns: the marginal increase in attainment is smaller at higher levels of health expenditure. But Figure 50.10 does not control for differences in the average years of schooling in populations. Overall attainment is also positively

correlated with the educational stock variable (Figure 50.11).

Finally, Figure 50.12 is a scatterplot of the overall attainment measure and our proxy variable "Other" (consisting of the residual from a regression of income on health expenditure and education). The plot shows a weak relationship and the correlation between the variables is close to 0.

The full "translog" (transcendental logarithmic) form of the above general production function is:

$$Y_{it} = \alpha_i + \beta_1 X_{1it} + \beta_2 X_{2it} + \beta_3 X_{3it} + \beta_4(X_{1it})^2 + \beta_5(X_{2it})^2 + \beta_6(X_{3it})^2 + \beta_7(X_{1it})(X_{2it}) + \beta_8(X_{1it})(X_{3it}) + \beta_9(X_{2it})(X_{3it}) + \upsilon_{it}$$

where Y_{it} is the composite index of attainment for country i at time t, X_1 is health expenditure per

Figure 50.11 Overall attainment versus educational attainment

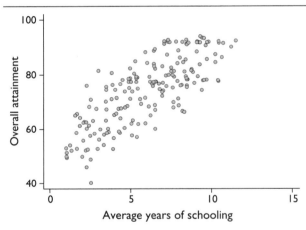

Figure 50.10 Overall attainment versus health expenditure per capita, 1997 international dollars

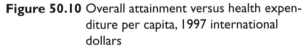
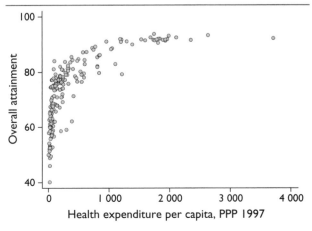

Figure 50.12 Overall attainment versus proxy "Other"

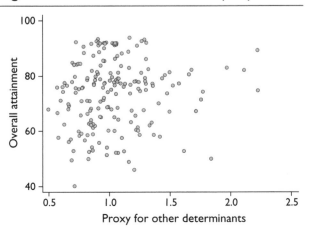

capita, X_2 is average years of schooling, and X_3 is a proxy variable for other determinants (all variables log-transformed). The translog production function is one of the most general formulations of a production function, and incorporates the Cobb-Douglas and the Constant Elasticity of Substitution forms as special cases (30;31).

After an extensive investigation of different specifications, the final model was chosen taking into account considerations of parsimony so as to match most closely the full translog specification. The rank correlation between the different translog specifications with and without the proxy variable "Other" was very high (around 0.99) (32;33). As a result of this finding, but also considering that the proxy variable captures more than the non-health system determinants of efficiency, we decided not to include the variable "Other" in the final formulation of the model.

OUTPUT IN THE ABSENCE OF A FUNCTIONING HEALTH SYSTEM

In the definition of efficiency, adjustment is made for the fact that output would not be zero in the absence of a modern health system. Two components of the composite index (i.e. "fairness in financial contribution" and "responsiveness distribution") are given full scores in determination of the minimum. This is because a non-existent system treats everyone totally equally—it is absolutely unresponsive to all people (so there is full equality), and if financial contributions are zero, it treats everyone exactly the same (completely fairly). Because of the way the composite index was measured, they contribute 37.5 units in the absence of a health system (i.e. $25 \times 1 + 12.5 \times 1 = 37.5$).

For converse reasons, the score for "health inequalities" and "responsiveness level" would be zero in the absence of a health system ($25 \times 0 + 12.5 \times 0 = 0$). That is, since a non-existent health system would clearly be completely unresponsive, "responsiveness level" receives a zero score, and although health inequalities would exist in the absence of a health system, with respect to the health system's goal of reducing inequalities, zero progress can be claimed. Thus, the only component variable that varies according to inputs at the minimum level of attainment is health level. The other goals contribute equally at all levels of input.

To measure the composite index, each of the five components is normalized on the [0,1] interval. Therefore, given that the weight on health level in the overall attainment measure is 25, the equation for the minimum level is:

$$\text{COMPOSITE}_{i\,\min} = 37.5 + 25 \times \left[\frac{(\text{HALE}_{i\,\min} - \text{HALE}_{\min})}{(\text{HALE}_{\max} - \text{HALE}_{\min})} \right]$$

The values of $\text{HALE}_{\min}$ and $\text{HALE}_{\max}$ were set at 20 and 80, respectively.

In order to obtain an expression for $\text{HALE}_{i\,\min}$—the hypothesized value that HALE would take in each country in the absence of a health system—a sample of countries for which data were available at around the turn of the century was investigated, and the minimum-frontier production function for health as a function of literacy was obtained. The estimated equation in the turn of the century sample was:

$$\text{HALE}_{1900} = 17.8 + 30.9 \times \text{Literacy}.$$

This relation was used to predict, for current observed levels of literacy, the health levels that would be achieved in the absence of a health system, $\text{HALE}_{i\,\min}$ (33).

UNCERTAINTY ANALYSIS

None of the five components of the composite index is known with certainty in a given country. Uncertainty intervals were generated for each component by taking 1 000 random draws from specified parameter distributions. This uncertainty was carried forward into calculation of the composite index by randomly drawing values for each component 1 000 times.

The efficiency measure was thus estimated 1 000 different times, where each regression used as its dependent variable a random draw from the composite index distribution. This resulted in a distribution for the efficiency measure for each country. Reported in the Statistical Annex of *The World Health Report 2000* was the mean value (and 80% confidence interval) of the efficiency distribution. The confidence interval was obtained by omitting the highest and lowest 10% of estimates of mean efficiency for each country. Country ranks on efficiency were based on the mean efficiency score, while uncertainty intervals on rank were similarly constructed by taking percentiles of the 1 000 individual estimates of rank for each country (4).

ANALYSIS OF THE DETERMINANTS OF EFFICIENCY

For *The World Health Report 2000*, two types of efficiency were estimated: efficiency in producing health, and efficiency in terms of composite goal attainment.

The former was reported in Evans et al. (5). Estimated levels of efficiency in producing the composite goal varied between close to 0% (Sierra Leone) to over 99% (France), with over 30 countries estimated to be producing less than 40% of their potential given their observed levels of inputs. To explain this variation, a second stage analysis was undertaken in which estimated levels of efficiency were regressed against a set of indirect (exogenous) determinants, i.e. factors not directly related to the production of health but nevertheless having influence on efficiency. This allowed hypotheses about the influence of institutional and organizational factors on efficiency to be explored. Other determinants might include intensity of the AIDS epidemic, inequality in income distribution, population density, etc. This analysis could be especially important for helping to design and implement policies for improving efficiency and is reported in Chapter 51.

DISCUSSION

Efficiency measurement of the type described in this chapter draws attention to the fact that, given their inputs, some countries are doing better than others at achieving their potential. Chapter 51 of this volume explores whether exogenous factors such as institutional quality, income distribution, or population density had an impact on the efficiency estimates emerging from *The World Health Report 2000*.

REFERENCES

(1) Maynard A, Bloor K. Health care reform: informing difficult choices. *International Journal of Health Planning and Management*, 1995, 10:247–264.

(2) Collins C, Green A, Hunter D. Health sector reform and the interpretation of policy context. *Health Policy*, 1999, 47:69–83.

(3) DeRosario JM. Healthcare system performance indicators: a new beginning for a reformed Canadian healthcare system. *Journal for Healthcare Quality*, 1999, 21:37–41.

(4) World Health Organization. *The World Health Report 2000. Health Systems: Improving Performance.* Geneva, World Health Organization, 2000.

(5) Evans DB, et al. Comparative efficiency of national health systems: cross national econometric analysis. *British Medical Journal*, 2001, 323:307–310.

(6) Hollingsworth B, Wildman J. The efficiency of health production: re-estimating the WHO panel data using parametric and non-parametric approaches to provide additional information. *Health Economics*, 2002, Published online: 23 Aug. 2002.

(7) McKee M. Measuring the efficiency of health systems. The world health report sets the agenda, but there's still a long way to go. *British Medical Journal*, 2001, 323: 295–296.

(8) Pedersen KM. The World Health Report 2000: dialogue of the deaf? *Health Economics*, 2002, 11:93–101.

(9) Jamison DT, Sandbu ME. Global health. WHO ranking of health system performance. *Science*, 2001, 293: 1595–1596.

(10) Appleby J, Street A. Health system goals: life, death and…football. *Journal of Health Services Research and Policy*, 2001, 6:220–225.

(11) Kalirajan KP, Shand RT. Frontier production functions and technical efficiency measures. *Journal of Economic Surveys*, 1999, 13:149–172.

(12) Kumbhakar SC, Lovell CAK. *Stochastic frontier analysis.* Cambridge, Cambridge University Press, 2000.

(13) Farrell MJ. The measurement of productive efficiency. *Journal of the Royal Statistical Society Series A*, 1957, 120:253–278.

(14) Coelli T, Prasada Rao DS, Battese G. *An introduction to efficiency and productivity analysis.* Boston, Kluwer Academic Publishers, 1997.

(15) Schmidt P, Sickles RC. Production frontiers and panel data. *Journal of Business and Economic Statistics*, 1984, 2:367–374.

(16) Gakidou E, Frenk J, Murray CJL. *Measuring preferences on health system performance assessment.* EIP Discussion Paper No. 20. Geneva, World Health Organization, 2000. URL: http://www3.who.int/whosis/discussion_papers/discussion_papers.cfm#

(17) Puig-Junoy J. Measuring health production performance in the OECD. *Applied Economics Letters*, 1998, 5: 255–259.

(18) Fogel RW. The contribution of improved nutrition to the decline in mortality rates in Europe and America. In: Simon JL, ed. *The economics of population: key modern writings.* Northampton, MA, Edward Elgar Pub., 1997.

(19) Preston SH. The changing relation between mortality and level of economic development. *Population Studies*, 1975, 29:231–248.

(20) Preston SH. *Mortality patterns in national populations.* New York, Academic Press, 1976.

(21) Preston SH. Mortality and development revisited. *Population Bulletin of the United Nations*, 1985, 18:34–40.

(22) Caldwell JC. Education as a factor in mortality decline:

an examination of Nigerian data. *Population Studies*, 1979, 33:395–413.

(23) Caldwell JC. Maternal education as a factor in child mortality. *World Health Forum*, 1981, 2:75–78.

(24) Caldwell JC, McDonald PF. Influence of maternal education on infant and child mortality: levels and causes. *Health Policy and Education*, 1982, 2:251–267.

(25) Caldwell JC, Caldwell P. Education and literacy as factors in health. In: Halstead SB , Walsh JA, Warren KS, eds. *Good health at low cost*. New York, The Rockefeller Foundation, 1985:181–185.

(26) Caldwell JC. Routes to low mortality in poor countries. *Population and Development Review*, 1986, 12: 171–220.

(27) Caldwell JC. Cultural and social factors influencing mortality levels in developing countries. *Annals of the American Academy of Political and Social Science*, 1990, 510:44–59.

(28) Caldwell JC. Health transition: the cultural, social and behavioural determinants of health in the Third World. *Social Science & Medicine*, 1993, 36:125–135.

(29) Caldwell JC. How is greater maternal education translated into lower child mortality? *Health Transition Review*, 1994, 4:224–229.

(30) Greene WH. *Econometric analysis*, 3rd ed. Upper Saddle River, NJ, Prentice Hall, 1997.

(31) Kmenta J. *Elements of econometrics*, 2nd ed. New York, Macmillan Publishing, 1986.

(32) Evans DB, et al. *The comparative efficiency of national health systems in producing health: an analysis of 191 countries*. EIP Discussion Paper No. 29. Geneva, World Health Organization, 2000. URL: http://www3.who.int/whosis/discussion_papers/discussion_papers.cfm#

(33) Tandon A et al. *Measuring overall health system performance for 191 countries*. EIP Discussion Paper No. 30. Geneva, World Health Organization, 2000. URL: http://www3.who.int/whosis/discussion_papers/discussion_papers.cfm#

Chapter 51

DETERMINANTS OF HEALTH SYSTEM PERFORMANCE: SECOND-STAGE EFFICIENCY ANALYSIS

DAVID B. EVANS, JEREMY A. LAUER, AJAY TANDON,
CHRISTOPHER J.L. MURRAY

INTRODUCTION

The analysis of economic efficiency is often considered a two-stage process. The first is estimation of the efficiency with which direct inputs to production are transformed into outputs. The second is explanation of the estimated levels of efficiency in terms of factors that are not direct inputs to production but nevertheless influence efficiency. Econometrically, the two steps can be performed either simultaneously or in two stages (1). Here we report the results from the second stage of a two-stage estimation process undertaken as part of the work published in *The World Health Report 2000* (2).

First-stage analysis includes direct inputs to the attainment of the health system goals. In the first round of health systems performance assessment undertaken by WHO (2), health expenditure per capita was used as an indicator of direct health system inputs, and the average level of education in the adult population was used to reflect non-health system determinants of health system attainment (3). However, nutrition, housing, disease vectors, the HIV/AIDS epidemic, and tobacco consumption might also be considered direct determinants of health system goals. Income per capita is not a direct factor because, in and of itself, income does not make people healthy. It allows people to obtain better food and housing, for example, which are direct determinants of the health system goals.

Variables such as housing and food consumption were not measured in enough Member States of WHO to allow incorporation into the first-round estimations. Accordingly, a variable to capture the effect of direct inputs that are mediated through income was developed. It was constructed as the residual from a regression of income per capita on health expenditure per capita and average years of education—in other words, that part of income variation that is not captured by the variation in the variables already included in the first-stage analysis.

For other health-related variables, such as tobacco consumption, a decision whether to include them in the first-stage analysis was made on the basis of whether the health system should reasonably be held accountable for their effects. If so, the variable should not be included as a separate input because this would have the effect of controlling for the variable in the assessment of efficiency. Tobacco consumption affects health and health inequalities, but if it is included in the first stage, efficiency measurements would not register the fact that failure to control tobacco consumption means that the system is not achieving as high a level of health as it could. Since a criterion for judging health system performance should be whether health policy-makers take active measures to encourage health promoting behaviours, tobacco consumption was omitted from the first-stage analysis. The same argument applies to the effects of the HIV epidemic where it can be argued that some decision-makers reacted quickly to the epidemic and others did not. Accordingly, the first-stage regressions were not controlled for the stage of the HIV epidemic.

Efficiency in first-stage analysis was measured as a function of health expenditures and the level of education of the adult population. The goal of second-stage analysis is to identify characteristics of the environment within which the health system operates that influence the resulting efficiency. The results of this analysis are presented in the subsequent sections.

DEPENDENT VARIABLES

For *The World Health Report 2000*, health system efficiency was measured in terms of two main outcomes. The first was health level and the second was a composite index of attainment on five outcome indicators (level and distribution of health, level and distribution of responsiveness, and fairness in financial contribution) (2;4;5). Efficiency was calculated for 191 WHO Member States by frontier production analysis (3;5). For efficiency on health, estimates ranged from a high of 0.992 for Oman to a low of 0.080 for Zimbabwe. For the composite outcome, estimates ranged from a high of 0.994 for France to a low of 0 for Sierra Leone. Accordingly, two sets of results on the determinants of efficiency are reported here: the first explaining estimated efficiencies in achieving health (where the output of the health system was specified as HALEs, i.e. healthy life expectancy), and the second explaining the estimated efficiencies in achieving the composite goal (called "overall efficiency").

As discussed elsewhere (4;5), efficiency scores are bounded between zero and one. Empirically, the distributions are skewed to the right (i.e. there are more high than low performers), resulting in significant non-normality. Figure 51.1 shows histograms of the distributions of efficiency scores on health and the composite measure.

Not surprisingly, the two efficiency scores are highly correlated, and the correlation is greater at higher levels of efficiency (Figure 51.2).

INDEPENDENT VARIABLES

Identification of the exogenous variables affecting health system efficiency can provide an important guide to policy-making. For example, if the health system operates in an environment of weak economic and political institutions, it may be difficult for policy-makers to influence the system to provide a more optimal mix of services, or to produce a given set at

the lowest possible cost. Low efficiency in the health sector might therefore be symptomatic of weak government stewardship in other sectors. Moreover, if high levels of inequality in income distribution are correlated with low health system efficiency, it is important to be aware that it may be difficult to improve efficiency without complementary action to improve the distribution of income, or to redress inequalities in levels of health, responsiveness or the financial burdens incurred in paying for health. The second-stage analysis should include as many explanatory variables with direct policy implications as possible.

Table 51.1 lists the dependent and independent variables for which data were obtained for the 191 countries. We hypothesize, for reasons explained below, that these variables will be correlated with the observed levels of efficiency. For independent variables, the hypothesized direction of the correlation

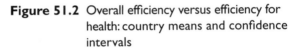

Figure 51.2 Overall efficiency versus efficiency for health: country means and confidence intervals

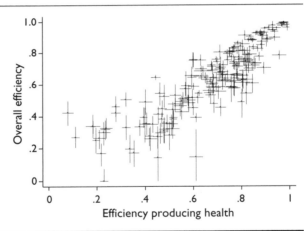

Figure 51.1 Distributions of estimated efficiency for health and overall attainment

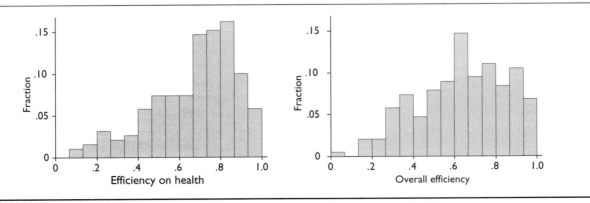

is indicated in the table. For all variables, the short name used in reporting results in a subsequent section is listed. Following the table, each variable and the sources from which it was obtained are described briefly.

We hypothesize that there is a minimum size below which a health sector cannot be efficient. Preliminary investigations suggest that below a spending level of $60 per capita in 1997 purchasing power parity (PPP) terms, it is very difficult for countries to be good performers (4). Indeed, a high proportion of low-performing countries have low levels of health expenditure per capita.

Accordingly, a dummy variable was defined for the hypothesized spending threshold below which it is difficult to be efficient. It was coded as "1" for countries with a health expenditure per capita below $60 (in 1997 PPP dollars), "0" otherwise. The sign of the binary variable is expected to be negative. Selected indicators of National Health Accounts were published in *The World Health Report 2000*, and this dataset formed the basis for construction of these binary spending variables (2).

The overall quality of government in a country determines its ability to play the important role of stewardship (2), influencing performance in all sectors. We consider here two published indexes of the quality of governance (6;7). Both are expected to be positively correlated with efficiency.

Inequalities in income distribution could affect health system performance adversely because high levels of income inequality could cause different levels of access to resources (including health system resources). In addition, stark inequalities might suggest a diminished general concern for fairness and human rights on the part of governments and policy-makers. An inverse correlation between income inequality and health system performance is expected and the Gini coefficient is used as a measure of income inequality.

The Gini coefficient represents the extent to which the distribution of income among individuals or households deviates from a perfectly equal distribution (8). A Gini coefficient of "0" indicates perfect equality and a Gini coefficient of "1", perfect inequality.

Part of the observed levels of efficiency could be due to lack of action in the past against particular diseases and risk factors such as HIV/AIDS and tobacco consumption. The variable used to investigate the effect of the former is the difference between the observed healthy life expectancy at birth in a country and the healthy life expectancy at birth estimated for that country netting out the impact of HIV/AIDS. Current smoking intensity is expected to have the same influence on efficiency as HIV/AIDS — countries with higher levels of smoking intensity would find it much harder to transform inputs into the outcome of population health.

A set of geographical and historical dummies was also defined to capture the impact of such diverse variables as climate, colonial history, and the way health and legal institutions developed. They comprised regional dummies for WHO Regions and World Bank databases indicating the presence of a French legal system and colonial history.

Several other variables were available for a considerable number of countries, including a World Bank index of voice and accountability, the public share of total health expenditure, the extent of urbanization, the demographic dependency ratio, and population density. None of these variables proved to be consistently significant in the different specifications of the equation, nor did they add explanatory power. They are not reported further.

Table 51.1 Variables used in the second-stage analysis

Independent variable	Short name	Hypothesized sign of coefficient	Dependent variable	Short name
Dummy for health spending below $60 per capita	d60	negative	Efficiency on health	ldmean
Index of government effectiveness	geff	positive	Overall efficiency	lcmean
Gini coefficient	gini	negative		
Impact of HIV/AIDS	diff	negative		
Income per capita in international dollars	gdpc	positive		
Latin American Region	latin	positive		
French legal system	leg_french	positive		
Former French colony	french	negative		

THE REGRESSION MODEL

The values of efficiency estimated in the first stage were regressed on the explanatory variables described above. The classical normal regression model was used (9), with a logistic transformation of the efficiency scores (10). The transformation entailed dropping an observation where overall efficiency had been measured as 0 (Sierra Leone). Figure 51.3 shows a smoothed histogram of the distribution of estimated efficiency scores after logistic transformation. Distributions are approximately normal.

EFFICIENCY ON HEALTH

Table 51.2 shows regression results for efficiency in terms of population health level. At the 5% significance level, efficiency in achievement of health is negatively correlated with health expenditures below $60 per capita, increasing income inequality, and high disease burden due to HIV/AIDS. It is positively cor-

related with income per capita and the presence of a French legal system. Smoking intensity showed the expected sign but was not significant. The overall model is significant ($F = 34.03$), and the independent variables explain most of the variation in the dependent variable ($R^2 = 0.6833$).

OVERALL EFFICIENCY

Similar patterns were found when regressing overall efficiency (Table 51.3). Government effectiveness and per capita income were positively correlated with efficiency, while significant negative correlations were observed for countries spending less than $60 per capita on health, with unequal income distribution, and with a high impact due to AIDS. Smoking intensity had an unexpected positive sign but was not significant.

The determinants model for overall efficiency is significant ($F = 42.42$) and the independent variables

Figure 51.3 Kernel density estimate of the distribution of logistic transformation of estimated efficiencies

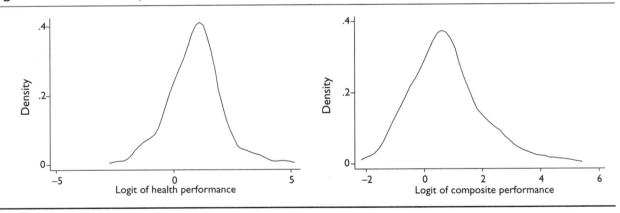

Table 51.2 Multivariate analysis for determinants of efficiency on health

Idmean	Coef.	Std. Err.	t	P >	t		95% Conf. Interval	
gini	−3.254193	.9519774	−3.42	0.001	−5.136072	−1.372313
geff	.2011822	.1067157	1.89	0.061	− .0097745	.4121388
gdpc	.0000333	.0000133	2.51	0.013	7.05e−06	.0000595
diff	− .1704684	.0241877	−7.05	0.000	−218283	−.1226538
d60	− .4619427	.1755737	−2.63	0.009	−.8090187	−.1148668
latin	.3378698	.2061774	1.64	0.103	−.0697039	.7454435
leg_french	.4391157	.1684353	2.61	0.010	.106151	.7720804
french	− .1965777	.2239268	−0.88	0.381	−.6392387	.2460834
smoktot	− .1280133	.7884938	−0.16	0.871	−1.686717	1.43069
cons	2.075001	.4032105	5.15	0.000	1.27793	2.872072

explain a high proportion of variation in the dependent variable ($R^2 = 0.7303$).

DETERMINANTS OF EFFICIENCY

Some of the results related to historical and geographical variables are not directly relevant to policy-making; they lead to a better understanding of the determinants of efficiency. Others have direct policy relevance. First, the positive correlation of "good governance" indicators with efficiency in a multivariate analysis lends support to the argument of *The World Health Report 2000* (2) that the stewardship function is important for improving health systems performance. Second, the HIV/AIDS epidemic has the predicted negative impact on efficiency independent of the other analysed variables. Countries clearly could have had much better levels of attainment given their resources if they had acted more effectively to reduce the spread of AIDS. However, since this did not happen in many cases, long-term assistance may be necessary to help such countries overcome the burden of HIV/AIDS. Third, the distribution of income is correlated with efficiency in the regression model. It will be important, however, to understand the causal pathways involved and to discover the extent to which reductions in income inequalities would be a cost-effective way of increasing health system performance. Finally, countries with very low levels of spending on health seem to have particular difficulty in performing efficiently — and the effect is more pronounced for overall goal attainment than simply for attainment of health outcomes. It is possible that recent attempts to scale up interventions for health in poor countries could have a complementary effect of improving health system efficiency.

This chapter presents a preliminary analysis of the determinants of the efficiency scores that were reported in *The World Health Report 2002* (2), an analysis based largely on explanatory variables that could be obtained from published sources. The analysis would undoubtedly be enriched by the inclusion of more policy relevant variables in it, as well as through simultaneous estimation of efficiency and its determinants in the one likelihood function. Future directions that this analysis may take are considered in Chapter 52 of this volume.

REFERENCES

(1) Kumbhakar SC, Lovell CAK. *Stochastic frontier analysis.* Cambridge, Cambridge University Press, 2000.

(2) World Health Organization. *The World Health Report 2000. Health Systems: Improving Performance.* Geneva, World Health Organization, 2000.

(3) Evans DB et al. Comparative efficiency of national health systems: cross national econometric analysis. *British Medical Journal*, 2001, 323:307–310.

(4) Evans DB et al. *The comparative efficiency of national health systems in producing health: an analysis of 191 countries.* EIP Discussion Paper No. 29. Geneva, World Health Organization, 2000. URL: http://www3.who.int/whosis/discussion_papers/discussion_papers.cfm#

(5) Tandon A et al. *Measuring overall health system performance for 191 countries.* EIP Discussion Paper No. 30. Geneva, World Health Organization, 2000. URL: http://www3.who.int/whosis/discussion_papers/discussion_papers.cfm#

(6) Kaufmann D, Kraay A, Zoido-Lobatón P. *Aggregating governance indicators.* Policy Research Working Paper No. 2195. Washington, DC, World Bank, 1999.

Table 51.3 Multivariate analysis for determinants of overall efficiency

ldmean	Coef.	Std. Err.	t	P > *t* OK?	95% Conf. Interval	
gini	−2.71348	.9894657	−2.74	0.007	−4.669585	−.7573738
geff	.3800862	.1059753	3.59	0.000	.1705803	.5895922
gdpc	.0000585	.0000131	4.47	0.000	.0000326	.0000844
diff	−.0780753	.0244095	−3.20	0.002	−.1263313	−.0298194
d60	−.5374407	.1752979	−3.07	0.003	−.8839926	−.1908887
latin	.1936916	.205724	0.94	0.348	−.2130827	.6003219
leg_french	.2953759	.1678074	1.76	0.081	−.0363679	.6271197
french	−.0729328	.2217784	−0.33	0.743	−.5113734	.3655078
smoktot	.5844514	.7781373	0.75	0.454	−.9538728	2.122776
cons	1.47173	.4078652	3.61	0.000	.6654084	2.278051

(7) Kaufmann D, Kraay A, Zoido-Lobatón P. *Governance matters*. Policy Research Working Paper No. 2196. Washington, DC, World Bank, 1999.

(8) World Bank. *World development indicators 1999*. Washington, DC, World Bank, 1999.

(9) Goldberger A. *A course in econometrics*. Cambridge, Harvard University Press, 1991.

(10) King G, Tomz M, Wittenberg J. Making the most of statistical analyses: improving interpretation and presentation. *American Journal of Political Science*, 2000, 44:341–355.

Chapter 52

HEALTH SYSTEM EFFICIENCY: TIME, ATTRIBUTION, AND MULTIPLE INDICATORS

DAVID B. EVANS, CHRISTOPHER J.L. MURRAY, AJAY TANDON

INTRODUCTION

For much of the last two decades, health policy-makers have been concerned with the performance of their health systems and many countries have introduced reforms aimed at improving performance (1). The desire to improve efficiency has been a central issue, but health system development has been hindered by the absence of an explicit, quantifiable definition of health system efficiency (2). It has not, therefore, been possible to demonstrate rigorously the association between any set of policies and changes in efficiency.

There is a long tradition of measuring efficiency in the fields of agricultural and industrial economics, which is useful for thinking about efficiency of health systems (3;4). The analytical framework traces its origins to Farrell (5) who defined technical efficiency as the ability to produce the maximum possible output from a given set of inputs. It is measured as the ratio of actual output to maximum possible output for a given use of resources. In Figure 52.1, M is the maximum level of goal attainment (output) possible for any input level. If observed output is A, technical efficiency would be $(a + b)/(a + b + c)$.

WHO has defined the components of health system performance in a similar manner (6–8). The vertical axis measures goal attainment or output[1], and inputs are measured on the horizontal axis. As in standard production theory, M represents the frontier, or the maximum possible level of goal attainment that can be achieved for given levels of inputs. However, health differs from other types of production in that some minimum level of population health would exist even in the absence of inputs to the system, e.g. the entire population will not be dead in the absence of a functioning health system. L in Figure 52.1 represents this minimum level of goal attainment. Observed

goal attainment at A is $(a + b)$, but only b has been produced in addition to the output that would have existed in the absence of the system (a). The contribution of the system, therefore, is b and the efficiency of the use of health system resources can be defined as $b/(b + c)$.

Country B achieves more than country A because it uses more resources. However, it is no more efficient than A attaining the same proportion of its potential contribution to health given the availability of resources—e.g. $b/(b + c) = d/(d + e)$. Attainment is a function of the level of resources available and the efficiency with which resources are used, and both attainment and efficiency are important concepts for health policy purposes.

EFFICIENCY AND THE HEALTH SYSTEM

Five characteristics of the health system influence the way that efficiency can be defined and measured. The

Figure 52.1 Defining health system efficiency

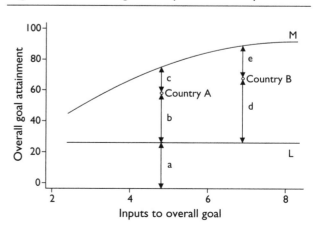

first has already been described, the fact that attainment would not be zero in the absence of health system inputs. The second relates to the question of whether it is possible to measure inputs and outputs of health production in physical units, the most obvious way to measure technical efficiency. For health, there are no datasets available across a large number of countries on the quantities of different types of inputs used to produce health outputs: for example, labour, capital, or the use of consumable such as pharmaceuticals. We are forced to use aggregate health expenditures as the single health system input for the moment, although WHO is attempting to develop a series on the physical inputs used by the health system.

This might suggest that we could estimate economic efficiency using a profit function approach where both inputs and outputs are measured in monetary units. While it would be technically possible to measure goal attainment (health, responsiveness, and fairness in financial contribution) in monetary units using some form of contingent valuation technique, there are several objections to using the resulting willingness to pay estimates in the analysis. The most important from our perspective is that this would value the preferences of rich people (and rich countries) more highly than the values of poorer people. We regard this as ethically unacceptable and choose to retain outcomes in physical units which represent the level of population health. This is the key variable of interest to health decision-makers.

Accordingly, the combination of health system inputs in monetary units with outcomes in physical units changes the interpretation of any efficiency estimate. Countries can be at a lower point that the theoretical maximum because they are technically inefficient. But they might also have chosen the wrong mix of physical inputs for the prices they face, or the wrong mix of health actions,[2] e.g. choosing high cost, low outcome interventions in preference to more cost-effective options. This type of misallocation of resources is often called allocative efficiency in the health economics literature on the grounds that interventions can be considered as inputs to the production of health outcomes.

The third difference between health and other systems relates to the lag between the application of inputs and the outputs. An intervention aimed at reducing the proportion of the population that smokes will not have an observable impact on health outcomes for several years (early effects being felt in relation to cardiovascular disease, for example), but its full impact (on lung cancer incidence) would take

30–40 years to be observed. Today's observed levels of goal attainment are, therefore, a function of inputs applied over a considerable period of time in the past. The corollary is that today's health system inputs will produce health benefits not just this year, but for many years into the future. This is similar to the case of perennial crops such as rubber where today's production is determined by past and present applications of fertilizer, and where today's application of fertilizer will influence production for many years into the future. This has implications for ways of estimating the relationship between inputs and outputs, and the data requirements.

Fourth, production of health is determined by factors outside the health system as well as by health system inputs. This is one of the reasons why health levels would not be zero in the absence of the health system. This is important to the definition of the minimum possible level of goal attainment—L in Figure 52.1—and, therefore, of efficiency. It is discussed in the fourth section of this chapter.

Fifth, the ability of a system to translate any given level of inputs (system and non-health system inputs) into goal attainment is mediated by factors other than efficiency. These might include climate, for example, which would moderate the ability of pathogens to multiply. Any measurement of health system efficiency must take into account non-health system inputs and the factors that make it more difficult for the system to translate inputs into outcomes. In the remainder of this chaper we refer to these variables as "difficulty" variables.

TIME AND THE MEASUREMENT OF EFFICIENCY

In view of the discussion above, two concepts of efficiency can be defined.

PREVALENCE EFFICIENCY

This approach asks the question: how efficiently have past and present health inputs been used to produce today's observed levels of population health? As suggested earlier, currently observed levels of health are a function of a stream of health actions taken now and in the past. Given that we must summarize this stream of actions by health expenditures, current levels of goal attainment are a function of the stream of present and past expenditures, with lags for the impact of some preventive interventions lasting decades. If the lags are long enough, this avoids the need for controlling for starting conditions at the beginning of the period, although it would be necessary to control for the difficulty of translating inputs into outcomes.

The maximum is defined as the maximum possible extent to which the health system could have contributed to goal attainment this period for a given stream of past and present health expenditures. It is the efficiency of the entire stream. The counterfactual used to define the minimum (L) would be the level of goal attainment that would be observed in the absence of the past stream of health expenditures, given current levels of non-health system inputs.

This concept of efficiency maps out the efficiency of an entire stream of health expenditures. It incorporates the fact that health actions influence outcomes over many time periods, and might encourage policy-makers to think of the impact of their actions on future health outcomes. On the other hand, only part of the measured inefficiency would be a result of actions undertaken by current policy-makers, so routine reporting using this definition might not give the desired signals to current decision-makers.

In many countries, historical expenditures are not available. To the extent that health expenditures are highly correlated over time, current year health expenditure can be interpreted as a summary indicator for historical expenditures and the results of the analysis interpreted as the efficiency of past and present health inputs. This is the approach taken in *The World Health Report 2000*.

INCIDENCE EFFICIENCY

This definition builds on the concept of incidence HALE (healthy life expectancy) under development in WHO. *It asks the question: conditional on the starting circumstances at the beginning of this time period, how efficiently are this time period's resources used to produce present and future health?*

At present HALE reflects the length of time a newborn child could expect to live in equivalent good health, faced with the same age and sex-specific death rates and rates of non-fatal health outcomes as people currently alive. This "period" measure is influenced by many health actions that occurred in the past. We propose to develop a standardized incidence-based HALE that extends the period measure to estimate the expected healthy years for a newborn child who experiences at each age the current incidence (rather than prevalence) of health problems and patterns of exposure to risk factors. This will allow the measure of health outcome to reflect current population risks and

health system activities, particularly those that are new or have long lag times to health outcomes, rather than population risks associated with past exposures.

Some of the present incidence is still determined by actions in the past. For example, risks of vector-borne diseases are related to the extent of vector control in the past, so some starting conditions would need to be controlled for in the estimation of incidence efficiency. It would also be necessary to control for the difficulty variables defined earlier. The minimum is the minimum level of incidence HALE that would exist if no health system inputs had been available this year, and the maximum is the maximum possible from this year's inputs. By taking into account the impact of today's health actions on people's health expectancies, it would incorporate the fact that preventive actions improve people's expectations of a healthy life.

The maximum would be defined as the highest possible level of present and future health associated with health actions this year. This is the preferred option for long-term development because it does not make current decision-makers responsible for activities undertaken in the past, but encourages them to think about the impact of their actions on present and future goal attainment. Ways in which incidence HALE might be calculated are currently being developed.

One practical problem is that incidence HALE must be estimated assuming something about the availability of curative interventions and living conditions in the future. The easiest is to assume a "business as usual" approach—that historical rates of income growth will continue and that currently available treatments will continue to be offered. Accordingly, the production function should be a mirror image of the prevalence production function—in this case incidence HALE is a function of present and future health expenditures. To the extent that current expenditures are correlated with future expenditures, current period expenditures could be taken as a summary indicator for the stream of future expenditures, and efficiency estimated using only current expenditures.

MULTIPLE INDICATOR MODELS

The approach used in *The World Health Report 2000* was based on the estimation of a frontier production function. HALE was modelled as a function of health expenditure and the stock of education. Difficulty variables were taken into account in a second-stage analysis but not incorporated into the overall efficiency index. Multiple indicator models (MIMs) offer an alternative approach.

They are based on the premise that health system output (Y) is a function of: a) direct "inputs" or positive determinants (X), b) the efficiency (E) of the health system in translating inputs into outcomes, and c) other factors (D) which may have a negative effect on outputs, signifying the difficulty of the environment within which the health system functions:

$$Y = f(X, E, D)$$

The efficiency of the health system is not directly observed (it is a latent variable). What is observed are multiple indicators of this latent variable ($E1, E2, E3, ...$), each being related to the underlying efficiency E:

$$E1 = f1(E)$$
$$E2 = f2(E)$$
$$E3 = f3(E)$$

Indicator 1 can be considered to be macro estimates of production using cross-country panel data similar to the way that was undertaken in *The World Health Report 2000*. Indicator 2 would be the effective coverage of critical interventions.[3] Information on the costs and effectiveness of interventions can help to determine the set of interventions that would maximize population health for the resources available to a country. The frontier M in Figure 52.2, which repeats Figure 52.1, now can be interpreted as the potential outcome if the most cost-effective mix of interventions had been used for the available resources, or ($a + b + c$) for country A. It also assumes that there is no technical inefficiency. The ratio of current coverage with

that set of interventions to optimal coverage must be directly related to observed efficiency as defined earlier $\{b/(b + c)\}$. This ratio provides information on the fraction of the potential health gain that has been achieved using the cost-effective set of interventions and can be used as another indicator of efficiency for the MIM estimation.[4]

We have experimented with runs of the model where efficiency itself is a latent variable but has, say, three measured indicators: incidence of TB, cervical cancer, and appendicitis. The determinants of the latent variable were chosen to be health expenditure per capita, population density, and an index of government effectiveness from the World Bank. There are still unresolved issues relating to the identification restrictions on the model that require further research. We believe that these models have the potential to make use of all possible sources of information relating to efficiency. However, many of the problems of timing discussed in the previous section still apply.

FURTHER DEVELOPMENTS

The efficiency of the health system can be defined in a similar way to the efficiency of any production process. However, the fact that outcomes would not be zero in the absence of the system requires an adjustment to the definition to incorporate both a minimum and a maximum possible level of goal attainment.

Moreover, the definition of efficiency changes because of the need to measure health system inputs in terms of aggregate health expenditure. The revised definition includes both technical inefficiency and inefficiency in the use of inputs and the choice of interventions.

The lags between inputs and outcomes in health are also found in other areas of production—perennial crops such as rubber or coconuts, forestry, and education, for example. The case of education is perhaps the closest to health. This year's examination results for a given cohort of children will not simply be a function of the quality and quantity of teaching inputs this year. They will also be determined in part by the quality and quantity of inputs in all previous years, as well as a set of variables which are not part of the education system. However, in these three areas we can find no published examples of frontier production function estimation using distributed lags of inputs. Most estimates of efficiency, even those using panel data, assume that output is a function of this year's inputs alone (e.g. Cooper and Cohn 1997

Figure 52.2 Efficiency and effective coverage of critical interventions

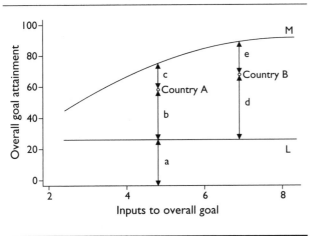

(9) and Chakraborty et al. 2001 (*10*) for education; Reddy & Yanagida 1999 (*4*) for sugar cane. This area requires further development of the models to allow lagged inputs to be included, as well as increasing the availability of data on health inputs and expenditures over time.

The MIM approach is promising and helps to address the debate about what variables should be included in the production function and what its specification should be (*11;12*). The MIM approach would allow true inputs, difficulty variables, and other indicators of efficiency such as coverage of key interventions to be considered at the same time. This also requires further development of both the methods and the available dataset.

NOTES

1 Goal attainment could be in terms of attainment on a single goal or a composite index of attainment on multiple goals.

2 A health action is any activity the prime intent of which is to improve health.

3 These models are related to multiple indicator multiple cause (MIMIC) models.

4 Point A in Figure 52.2 is no longer strictly equal to point A in Figure 52.1 where it was the observed level of goal attainment. This level could well have been achieved by using some interventions which are cost-ineffective. Here point A is the attainment from current coverage of interventions in the cost-effective set. The ratio of coverage of the cost-effective set to optimal coverage of this set must be directly related to efficiency.

REFERENCES

(1) Maynard A, Bloor K. Health care reform: informing difficult choices. *International Journal of Health Planning and Management*, 1995, 10:247–264.

(2) Collins C, Green A, Hunter D. Health sector reform and the interpretation of policy context. *Health Policy*, 1999, 47:69–83.

(3) Kao C. Measuring the performance improvement of Taiwan forests after reorganization. *Forest Science*, 2000, 46:1595–1596.

(4) Reddy M, Yanagida JF. Technical efficiency analysis of Fiji's sugar industry: an application of the stochastic frontier production function approach. *South African Journal of Economic and Management Sciences*, 1999, 2:77–92.

(5) Farrell MJ. The measurement of productive efficiency. *Journal of the Royal Statistical Society Series A*, 1957, 120:253–278.

(6) World Health Organization. *The World Health Report 2000. Health Systems: Improving Performance*. Geneva, World Health Organization, 2000.

(7) Evans DB, et al. Comparative efficiency of national health systems: cross national econometric analysis. *British Medical Journal*, 2001, 323:307–310.

(8) Murray CJL, Frenk J. A framework for assessing the performance of health systems. *Bulletin of the World Health Organization*, 2000, 78(6):717–731.

(9) Cooper ST, Cohn E. Estimation of a frontier production function for the South Carolina educational process. *Economics of Education Review*, 1997, 16:313–327.

(10) Chakraborty K, Biswas B, Lewis WC. Measurement of technical efficiency in public education: a stochastic and nonstochastic production function approach. *Southern Economic Journal*, 2002, 67:889–905.

(11) Jamison DT, Sandbu ME. Global health. WHO ranking of health system performance. *Science*, 2001, 293: 1595–1596.

(12) Holllingsworth B, Wildman J. The efficiency of health production: re-estimating the WHO panel data using parametric and non-parametric approaches to provide additional information. *Health Economics*, 2002, Published online: 23 Aug. 2002

Chapter 53

CROSS-POPULATION COMPARABILITY OF EVIDENCE FOR HEALTH POLICY[1]

CHRISTOPHER J.L. MURRAY, AJAY TANDON, JOSHUA A. SALOMON, COLIN D. MATHERS, RITU SADANA

INTRODUCTION

Across the various categories of evidence for health policy, including information on the levels of attainment on goals such as improving health and responsiveness, there is a fundamental need for cross-population comparable data. These data are essential for the purposes of measurement, monitoring, and evaluation of health systems performance. In the broadest sense, comparability is required not only across countries, but also within countries over time, or across different subpopulations delineated by age, sex, education, income or other characteristics.

Survey developers have emphasized the importance of establishing the validity of instruments and their reliability. Ensuring the cross-population comparability of results adds a third dimension to survey instrument development. The difference between comparability on the one hand and validity and reliability on the other can be illustrated using the example of two thermometers: one of which measures temperature in Celsius and the other in Fahrenheit. Both thermometers give valid and reliable measurements of temperature. However, 26 degrees on the Celsius thermometer is not comparable to 26 degrees on the Fahrenheit one. Comparability is fundamental to the use of survey results for the improvement of evidence for health policy, but has been under-emphasized in instrument development. Some have argued that estimates of quantities of interest do not need to be comparable. However, unless we compare estimates either across populations or across time, there is very little information content that can be used in health policy.

The fundamental challenge in seeking cross-population comparable measures is that the most accessible sources of data relating to many problems, such as health measurement or assessment of responsiveness, are categorical self-reported data. When categorical data are used as the basis for understanding quantities that are determined on a continuous, cardinal scale, the problem of cross-population comparability emerges from differences in the way individuals use categorical response scales. Efforts to ensure linguistic equivalence of questions across various settings may improve the psychometric properties of these questions in terms of traditional criteria such as reliability and within-population validity, but they will not resolve problems stemming from non-comparability in the interpretation and use of response categories. In the realm of health status measurement, for example, there has been great progress over the past three decades in developing instruments to measure the multiple domains of health that are reliable and demonstrate validity within a population (1–7). Even with these advances, however, results obtained using these instruments are usually not comparable across populations, as illustrated in Sadana et al. (8). Thus, cross-population comparability represents a more stringent criterion for evaluation of measurement instruments, beyond the traditional concepts of reliability and validity.

In this chapter, we begin by reviewing the general problem of cross-population comparability using a series of empirical examples. We introduce a conceptual framework for understanding the comparability problem in terms of differences in response category cut-points. We then examine the limitations of existing approaches to the problem. Finally, we outline a series of new strategies for enhancing the cross-population comparability of evidence for health policy using both new measurement instruments and new analytical tools.

THE PROBLEM OF CROSS-POPULATION COMPARABILITY

Empirical examples suggesting that self-reported categorical data lack cross-population comparability abound. In the area of health status measurement, for instance, a number of studies have pointed to likely differences in the use of response categories on self-reported assessments of general health, morbidity or levels on particular domains of health:

■ In Australian national health surveys comparing the self-reported health status of Aboriginals with that of the general population, only around 12% of the Aboriginal population characterized their own health status as fair or poor, while more than 20% of the general population rated their health in these low categories. By any other major indicator of mortality and morbidity, the Aboriginal population fares much worse than the general population, which suggests that there may be important differences in the interpretation of categorical responses in the various subpopulations due to shifts in response category cut-points (9).

■ Residents of the state of Kerala in India, which has the lowest rates of infant and child mortality and the highest rates of literacy in the country, consistently report the highest incidences of morbidity in India (10).

■ A series of studies from the Living Standards Measurement Surveys has examined the gradient of reported illness as a function of income and found that individuals in higher income quantiles consistently report more illness than those with lower income levels (11).

■ A recent article presenting self-reported data on the single question "How is your health in general?" and a five point Likert response scale "very "good," "good," "fair," "bad," "very bad" collected in 12 countries of the European Union, based on the same survey and methods in all countries, illustrates the problem of response category cut-point shift. Figure 53.1 shows the age-standardized proportion of the population reporting bad and very bad general health. It is unlikely that solely differences in the underlying true level of health status, language, or measurement error account for such large variations within the European Union, e.g. that the fraction of respondents reporting "very bad" or "bad" health varies from a high of 19% of the Portuguese to as little as 5% of the Irish

population (12). Such divergent levels of health are implausible, given other major health indicators.

■ A critical review and re-analysis of 64 datasets covering self-reported health status from population based surveys in 46 countries provide similar results. (8) Data concerning the level and distribution of health do not appear comparable across or even within populations, leading the authors to conclude that the information content of these surveys is suspect. Many surveys do not meet even the weakest form of criterion validity, i.e. that some decrements from "full health" are noted, and that self-reported health decreases with age, particularly in the oldest age groups. Figure 53.2 shows results by age groups and sex for China (from the Longitudinal Integrated Household Survey) and the United States of America (from NHANES III), with 100 equivalent to full health and 0 equivalent to the worst health state. Given that almost no decrements to health are reported in China, it is hypothesized that the Chinese "under-report" problems with their health status. Yet without external validation, to what degree cannot be gauged. Given findings on inconsistent reporting within the NHANES III (13),

Figure 53.1 Proportion of population ≥16 years of age, reporting bad and very bad general health, 12 European countries, 1994

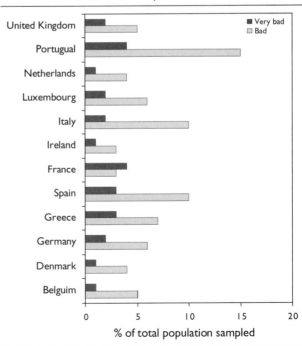

% of total population sampled

Source: (12)

we know that similar, even if potentially less pronounced reporting biases exist in the United States, i.e. with greater age, individuals assess their levels of non-fatal health more favourably in comparison to physical functioning tests (and therefore underreport conditions). It would be incorrect simply to take these data at face value and accept that individuals in older age groups in China have relatively few non-fatal health problems or conditions, or that their health status is significantly better than that of individuals living in the United States. Furthermore, the authors note that they have no reason to assume that reporting biases exist only in countries where it is clearly obvious, based on the lack of expected differences across age groups.

RESPONSE CATEGORY CUT-POINT SHIFTS

The problem of comparability can be conceptualized in terms of response category cut-point shifts across populations, across subgroups within a population, or within the same population over time. Figure 53.3 illustrates the primary challenge of using self-reported levels on a health status domain (even when reliability and within-population validity have been well established). For each domain, there is some true or latent scale that is, by definition, unobserved. For instance, imagine that there is a latent mobility scale depicted in the first column of Figure 53.3. Now imagine a self-reported survey question that asks respondents how much difficulty they have walking up stairs and offers five response categories: "no difficulty," "mild difficulty," "moderate difficulty," "severe difficulty," and

"extreme/cannot do." The second column in the figure shows the response category cut-points for population A. These are levels of mobility at which an individual will shift from one response category to another. The lowest cut-point in the figure shows the transition from answering "extreme/cannot do" to "severe difficulty." In population B, the response category cut-points are shifted relative to those in population A so that a higher level of mobility is associated with each of the response categories. Population C shows a third example with even more shift in the cut-points. The implication is dramatic. A response of "mild difficulty" walking up stairs, for instance, maps to a different level of mobility in populations A, B, and C. In this example, survey results may be reliable and valid within each population, but they cannot be compared across populations without adjustment.

We can hypothesize that cut-points may vary between populations because of different cultural expectations for domains of health. Cut-points are also likely to vary within a cultural group. The cut-points for older individuals may shift as their expectations for a domain diminish with age. Men may be more likely to deny declines in health so that their cut-points may be systematically shifted relative to those of women. Contact with health services may influence expectations for a domain and thus shift cut-points (11;14–18). Response category cut-point shift can make crude comparisons of results across populations nearly meaningless, even when exactly the same questions are used, as illustrated by some of the examples already provided.

An optimal strategy for equivalence of data (19;20) would require that all individuals with the same true

Figure 53.2 Comparison of average health levels by age and sex, China and the United States of America

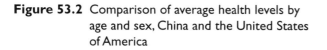

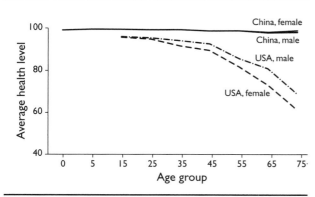

Source: (8)

Figure 53.3 Mapping from latent mobility variable to categories

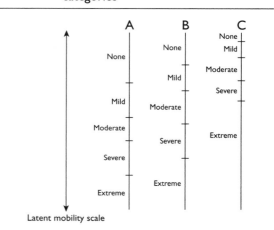

level of health, irrespective of their age, sex, cultural or geographical context, other socio-demographic characteristics, or time period, respond to an identical question addressing health as follows:

- Interpret the meaning of the question and response scale identically.

- Retrieve all relevant information with no loss of memory.

- Process all information, often contradictory, to form a single, integrated judgement or perception, in the same fashion, using cognitive processes that are unbiased.

- Convey this judgement as a final response in each survey context identically, i.e. using the same cut-points.

If so, individuals with exactly the same true level of health should then respond identically across and within populations, and no shift in response categories would occur. Obviously, this optimal strategy does not exist in practice.

STRATEGIES TO ENHANCE CROSS-POPULATION COMPARABILITY

Comparable measurement of health or responsiveness in different settings requires using the same questions or items in similar surveys. In addition, it requires explicit strategies to measure the response category cut-points of each item in different populations and socio-demographic groups. Methods to establish cut-points fall into two basic categories, each of which is discussed in detail below. The first strategy is to establish a scale that is strictly comparable across individuals and populations. Measurements on the comparable scale can then be used to establish the response category cut-points for each survey item. The second approach is to get categorical responses from different groups for a fixed level on the latent scale. If the level is fixed, variation in the responses provides information on the differences in cut-points across individuals and populations.

USING A COMPARABLE SCALE TO ESTABLISH RESPONSE CATEGORY CUT-POINTS

There are two main strategies for establishing a comparable scale of measurement: a) the use of multiple items (i.e. questions) for measuring a particular domain, and b) the incorporation of exogenous infor-

mation such as a measured performance test. In the following section, we begin by describing the general approach of using multiple domain items, consider the limitations of this approach, and introduce an alternative approach using measured tests to establish a comparable scale.

Item Response Theory

Psychometricians have over several decades developed powerful statistical models to establish response category cut-points for different items in a survey instrument by comparing each response category to the underlying factor in the data. This body of work is often associated with the term Item Response Theory (IRT). IRT has been widely used, for example, to establish the difficulty of different standardized scholastic test items (21). In a math test with 50 questions, what is the difficulty of each item? Is this difficulty the same for all types of respondents? There are many different statistical models used in the application of IRT, and the field is rapidly expanding (22;23). The basic building block for many of these models is the one-parameter Rasch model, which is a variant of the conditional logit model with a fixed effect. With more than two response categories, the Rasch model generalizes to the partial credit model (PCM).

Estimation of the Rasch-based PCM is based on specification of the probability of responding in a particular category rather than in the previous category, which is modelled as an increasing function of a person's "ability" (level on a particular domain) and a decreasing function of the item response "difficulty." The "difficulty" parameters specify the level on the latent variable at which an individual is more likely to respond in a specific category than in the previous one. It is worth noting that these difficulty parameters do not correspond exactly to the notion of response category cut-points described above, but they are conceptually related in that they refer to the probabilities of responding in each category.

The individual "ability" is captured through a fixed effect for each person, although in practice the use of the conditional logit means that these fixed effects are not directly estimated. The key insight in the model is that the response data can be used to estimate both the difficulties of various questions and the abilities of various individuals because the difficulties *for a particular question* are assumed to be the same for all individuals, and multiple responses per individual allows for estimation of their ability.

The key challenge in developing cross-population comparable measures from survey data is to detect systematic shifts in cut-points across different populations, or what is known as differential item functioning (DIF) in psychometric parlance. Various methods have been developed to identify DIF, but all of them assume that DIF applies only to a subset of items used to measure a domain, so that a comparable scale can be established using the underlying factor in the data from the remaining items. If all items suffer DIF in a systematic and correlated fashion, IRT is unable to identify this problem.

A simple thought experiment can prove that no statistical procedure can deal with this problem in its extreme form without the addition of exogenous information. Imagine a domain such as mobility. In population A the distribution of mobility on the latent scale is normal with mean 5 and standard deviation 2 (in units with interval scale properties on some arbitrary scale). In population B the distribution of mobility is normal with mean 8 and standard deviation of 2. In population B all the response category cut-points on all items about mobility are exactly 3 units higher than in population A. The net result is that the distribution of responses on all items in the survey in the two populations will be identical. In other words, population B has much higher mobility than A but the survey gives identical responses. No statistical method can identify this difference because the data are completely identical.

Because we have strong prior beliefs that cut-points on items are likely to shift systematically for a domain, we suspect that the potential to establish cross-population comparability using only the underlying factor in the response data without additional information is limited. For this reason, exogenous information is needed to aid in establishing cross-population comparability.

Measured Tests and the HOPIT Model

One type of exogenous information that could be used to establish a comparable scale is a measured calibration test for a particular domain. A calibration test can establish a comparable scale if: a) it adequately captures a domain, and b) it can be implemented in different settings without systematic bias in the results.[2] Such calibration tests are not feasible for a number of domains of health such as pain or affect. For some domains such as vision, hearing, cognition, mobility, and others, calibration tests are feasible. In the WHO Multi-country Survey Study on Health and Respon-

siveness 2000–2001 (24), low-cost calibration tests have been included for three domains of health:

- We use the Snellen's chart to measure visual acuity (distant vision). Since cross-national surveys include a range of literacy levels, we have selected the "tumbling E's" version of the Snellen's chart. Though more sensitive measures of visual acuity are available, such as LOGMAR charts, they require a set up that is not possible to replicate in large survey settings (25–28).

- In the domain of cognition, we have tested verbal fluency with a category naming task, vigilance with colour shape cancellation, and short-term memory with verbal recall. These tests were previously implemented by WHO in two large-scale international studies of cognitive impairments associated with HIV infections, and the development of a culture fair cognitive module to accompany assessments in neuropsychiatry. Tests of verbal fluency are consistently used to measure cognitive decline. We have used the task of naming animals within a one-minute period. For visual attention, the version of the test used in the WHO Multi-country Survey Study on Health and Responsiveness was adapted by de Viellers and Brandt for illiterate populations and has been field-tested by WHO. It consists of a series of three timed cancellation tasks involving symbols of four kinds, in four colours (blue, green, red, and orange) and two sizes distributed in a matrix on a single sheet of paper (29). Verbal learning tasks use a set of words to assess verbal learning and memory with immediate and delayed recall components. Several versions of these tasks such as the Rey Auditory Verbal Learning Task and the WHO-UCLA Auditory Verbal Learning Test, are available. We used a set of 10 words from the WHO-UCLA battery for our survey (30–32).

- Mobility involves a complex set of composite motor acts. Though many individual tests have been used in laboratory settings to assess individual mobility functions, we have implemented a modified version of the posturo-locomotion-manual (PLM) test, which has been used as a standard to measure movement patterns in neurological conditions. Though the original version of the test was designed for use in sophisticated laboratory conditions with computerized equipment, we have adapted this for use in survey settings to obtain gross measures of mobility. In the version of the test being used in the survey, subjects begin the test from a seated position, take one step, pick up an object of about two kilograms weight from the floor, walk six metres, place the object on a shelf at shoulder height, pick it up again, turn around and walk back, place the object back on the floor from where it was picked up, and sit down again. The test is repeated thrice and each trial is timed (33–35).

Test-retest reliability was found to be acceptable in pilot tests of these performance measurements. With more careful quality control on the calibration tests, we expect that test-retest will rise substantially. Further work on other calibration tests for other domains or alternatives for these domains will be needed. Additional calibration tests could be considered for hearing (audiometry), sleep (polysomnography), or exercise tolerance (treadmill).

Given a reliable and valid measured test for domains, variation in response category cut-points for the self-reported items on these domains may be estimated using the hierarchical ordered probit (HOPIT) model (36). The HOPIT model is a variant of the standard ordered probit model, which assumes that there is an unobserved latent variable that is normally distributed. Observed categorical responses depend on the categorical cut-points on this latent scale. The key difference between HOPIT and the standard ordered probit model is that these cut-points are allowed to vary as a function of covariates in the HOPIT model. In essence, this means that the mapping from the underlying latent variable to the categorical responses depends on individual characteristics.

Using Fixed Ability Comparisons to Assess Variation in Cut-Points

For some domains of health such as pain, reliable and valid measured tests may not exist, may not be affordable, or may be unethical, even for a subsample. An alternative strategy for establishing cross-population comparability is to fix the level of health on a domain and assess variation in the response categories across individuals, groups, and populations. In other words, if the level of mobility is fixed but one group says that this level maps to a response category of "no difficulty" and another says it maps to the category "some difficulty," this information can be used to assess the response category cut-points. Two strategies are available for fixed ability comparisons: vignettes and comparable homogeneous groups.

Establishing Cross-Population Comparability Using Vignettes

The primary strategy for using fixed ability comparisons to establish comparable scales is the use of vignettes, as described in detail in Salomon et al. (37). A vignette is a description of a concrete level of ability on a given domain that individuals are asked to evaluate using the same question and response scale as the self-reported question on that domain. For example, one self-report question on health in the WHO survey instrument is: *Overall in the last 30 days how much difficulty did you have with self-care?* (1 = Extreme/cannot do, 2 = Severe, 3 = Moderate, 4 = Mild, 5 = None). To assess the response category cut-points, each respondent is also asked to assess levels of self-care for hypothetical cases described with vignettes, for example:

> [John] cannot wash, groom or dress himself without personal help. He has no problems with feeding. How would you rate his difficulty with *self-care?*

Extreme/cannot do	1
Severe	2
Moderate	3
Mild	4
None	5

The vignette fixes a given level of self-care so that variation in the response categories is attributable to variation in the response category cut-points. When individuals are asked to evaluate a series of vignettes of varying severity, the cut-points can be evaluated using the HOPIT model (36). The vignette version of the HOPIT model is constructed such that the dependent variable is the categorical response for a given vignette, and the independent variables are simply indicator variables for each vignette. An underlying latent variable representing ability level on self-care is assumed to exist, with a fixed value associated with each vignette perceived with normal random error. The probability of responding in a particular category is then modelled in reference to individual cut-points expressed as a function of covariates such as country of residence, age, sex, education, and income.[3]

Using Comparable Homogeneous Groups to Establish Cross-Population Comparability

Another way to evaluate a fixed ability and thus variation in cut-points is to identify comparable homogeneous groups in different populations and compare their responses to an item. Recent acute changes in health status from injuries such as fractures might be used to identify reasonably comparable groups. Alternatively, some lifestyle or occupational characteristic might be used for example, elite athletes might constitute a relatively homogeneous group.

There are two main limitations to this strategy. First, identifying groups needs to be independent of any measurement of health status. Even when groups are identified through some factor such as an injury, doubts can always be raised about their true comparability. It may be difficult to persuade people that apparent differences in the responses are due to cut-point shift as opposed to differences in that domain between groups. Second, to be able to assess variation in response category cut-points for all response categories, a series of homogeneous groups must be used. Analytically, each homogeneous group is like one vignette. This means that the comparable group strategy can only work if several comparable groups are studied. Despite these limitations, it may be worthwhile assessing comparable groups as an adjunct to other methods.

DISCUSSION

One of the key conclusions of this chapter is that adjustments are needed to make survey results comparable across populations. In particular, when categorical variables are involved, differences in response category cut-points need to be accounted for. There is considerable evidence suggesting that response category cut-points are different across countries, and even across socioeconomic groups within a country. Therefore, until cut-points are assessed, one must start from a presumption that results are not comparable across populations.

Four strategies were identified to enhance cross-population comparability, of which the most promising, we believe, is to use calibration tests for some domains where possible (or for a representative subsample of the respondents), and to use vignettes for other domains. The use of vignettes is particularly attractive because vignettes are low-cost and involve no special work. This makes them potentially easy to implement across a variety of survey settings and domains.

The problem of cross-population comparability applies not only for comparison across countries, but also across different subpopulations defined by various socioeconomic or demographic variables. These differences can have important implications for the measurement of levels of inequality, which may be greater or smaller than measured before taking into account response category cut-point shifts. Cross-population comparability is also relevant for comparisons over time. Cut-points may systematically shift over time (e.g. due to rising income, education, and health norms), so long-term trends may be difficult to assess without correction.

There are several avenues to explore for future directions regarding this issue. One area that needs more analysis relates to measured calibration tests: different tests could be identified for calibration purposes, test-retest reliability has to be investigated further, and strategies for eliminating systematic bias in implementation of these tests need to be examined. Further research is also required for the strategy of using vignettes. Vignette results could be cross-validated with measured tests where both vignettes and measured tests are available.

NOTES

1 A version of this chapter was published previously as Murray CJL, Tandon A, Salomon JA, Mathers CD, Sadana R. New approaches to enhance cross-population comparability of survey results. In: Murray CJL et al., eds. *Summary measures of population health: concepts, ethics, measurement and applications*. Geneva, World Health Organization, 2002:421-431.

2 As long as the measurement error in the measured tests is white noise it should not create much bias in the results. However, the estimation will be more complicated if the measurement error is explicitly accounted for in the likelihood process (e.g. by using an error-in-variables type approach to estimation).

3 Vignettes can also be used with the PCM model. For details see Tandon et al. (*36*).

REFERENCES

(1) Bergner M et al. The sickness impact profile: conceptual formulation and methodology for the development of a health status measure. *International Journal of Health Services*, 1976, 6:393–415.

(2) Chambers LW, Sakett DL, Goldsmith CH. Development and application of an index of social function. *Health Services Research*, 1976, 11:430–441.

(3) Fanshel S, Bush JW. A health-status index and its application to health services-outcomes. *Operations Research*, 1970, 18:1021–1065.

(4) Feeney DH et al. Multi-attribute health status classification systems: health utilities index. *Pharmaco Economics*, 1995, 7:490–502.

(5) Hunt SM et al. The Nottingham Health Profile: subjective health status and medical consultations. *Social Science & Medicine*, 1981, 15:221–229.

(6) Krabbe PF et al. The effect of adding a cognitive dimension to the EuroQol multiattribute health-status classification system. *Journal of Clinical Epidemiology*, 1999, 52(4): 293–301.

(7) Ware JE. *SF-36 Health survey manual and interpretation guide*. Boston, Nimrod Press, 1993.

(8) Sadana R et al. Comparative analyses of more than 50 household surveys on health status. In: Murray CJL et al. *Summary measures of population health: concepts, ethics, measurement and applications*. Geneva, World health Organization, 2002:369–386.

(9) Mathers CD, Douglas RM. Measuring progress in population health and well-being. In: Eckersley R, ed. *Measuring progress: is life getting better?* Collingwood, CSIRO Publishing, 1998:125–155.

(10) Murray CJL. Epidemiology and morbidity transitions in India. In: Dasgupta M, Chen LC, Krishnan TN, eds. *Health, poverty and development in India*. Delhi, Oxford University Press, 1996:122–147.

(11) Murray CJL, Chen LC. Understanding morbidity change. *Population and Development Review*, 1992, 18(3):481–503.

(12) Eurostat. Self-reported health in the European Community. *Statistics in focus, population and social conditions*. ISSN 1024–4352. Eurostat, 1997.

(13) Iburg KM et al. Cross-population comparability of physician-assessed and self-reported measures of health. In: Murray CJL et al, eds. *Summary measures of population health: concepts, ethics, measurement and applications*. Geneva, World Health Organization, 2002:433–448.

(14) Caldwell J, Caldwell P. What have we learnt about the cultural, social and behavioral determinants of health? From selected readings to the first health transition workshop. *Health Transition Review*, 1991, 1:3–20.

(15) Findley SE. Social reflections of changing morbidity during health transitions. *Preceedings from the Health Transition Workshop*, vol. 1. Australia, 1990.

(16) Johansson SR. The health transition: the cultural inflation of morbidity during the decline of mortality. *Health Transition Review*, 1991, 1(1):39–68.

(17) Johansson SR. Measuring the cultural inflation of morbidity during the decline of mortality. *Health Transition Review*, 1992, 2(1):78–89.

(18) Riley JC. From a high mortality regime to a high mor-

bidity regime: is culture everything in sickness? *Health Transition Review*, 1992, 2(1):71–77.

(19) Tourangeau R. Cognitive sciences and survey methods. In: Jabine T et al, eds. *Cognitive aspects of survey methodology: building a bridge between disciplines*. Washington, DC, National Academy Press, 1984:73–100.

(20) Krosnick JA. Response strategies for coping with the cognitive demands of attitude measures in surveys. *Applied Cognitive Psychology*, 1991, 5:213–236.

(21) van der Linden WJ, Hambleton RK. Item response theory: brief history, common models, and extensions. In: van der Linden WJ, Hambleton RK, eds. *Handbook of modern item response theory*, New York, Springer-Verlag, 1997:1–28.

(22) Thissen D, Steinberg L. A taxonomy of item response models. *Psychometrika*, 1986, 51(4):567–577.

(23) van der Linden WJ, Hambleton RK. *Handbook of modern item response theory*. New York, Springer-Verlag, 1997.

(24) Üstün TB et al. WHO Multi-country Survey Study on Health and Responsiveness 2000–2001. In: Murray CJL, Evans DB, eds. *Health systems performance assessment: debates, methods and empiricism*. Geneva, World Health Organization, 2003.

(25) Ayed S et al. Prevalence and causes of blindness in the Tunisian Republic. *Santé*, 1998, 8(4):275–282.

(26) Coren S. Reporting the visual acuity of groups: the relation among alternate measures. *American Journal of Optometry and Physiological Optics*, 1987, 64(12): 897–900.

(27) Coren S, Hakstian AR. Validation of a self-report inventory for the measurement of visual acuity. *International Journal of Epidemiology*, 1989, 18(2):451–456.

(28) West SK et al. Function and visual impairment in a population-based study of older adults. *Investigative Ophthalmology and Visual Science*, 1997, 38(1):72–82.

(29) Wilson B, Cockburn J, Halligan PW. Development of a behavioural test of visuospatial neglect. *Archives of Physical Medicine and Rehabilitation*, 1987, 68:98–102.

(30) Laws KR. Gender affects naming latencies for living and nonliving things: implications for familiarity. *Cortex*, 1999, 35(5):729–733.

(31) Manly JJ et al. Effect of literacy on neuropsychological test performance in nondemented, education-matched elders. *Journal of the International Neuropsychological Society*, 1999, 5(3):191–202.

(32) Spreen O, Strauss E. *A compendium of neuropsychological tests*. Oxford, Oxford University Press, 1998.

(33) Guo X et al. A population-based study on motor performance and white matter lesions in older women.

Journal of the American Geriatrics Society, 2000, 48(8): 967–970.

(34) Kokko SM et al. The assessment of functional ability in patients with Parkinson's disease: the PLM-test and three clinical tests. *Physiotherapy Research International*, 1997, 2(2):29–45.

(35) Matousek M et al. Motor function in 90-year olds measured by optoelectronic kinesiology and activities of daily living. *Aging (Milano)*, 1994, 6(6):444–450.

(36) Tandon A et al. Statistical models for enhancing cross-population comparability. In: Murray CJL, Evans DB, eds. *Health systems performance assessment: debates, methods and empiricism*. Geneva, World Health Organization, 2003.

(37) Salomon JA, Tandon A, Murray CJL. *Using vignettes to improve cross-population comparability of health surveys: concepts, design, and evaluation techniques*. EIP Discussion Paper No. 41. Geneva, World Health Organization, 2001. URL: http://www3.who.int/whosis/discussion_papers/discussion_papers.cfm#

Chapter 54

Towards Evidence-Based Public Health

Christopher J.L. Murray, Colin D. Mathers, Joshua A. Salomon

Background

In the 1970s, the evidence-based medicine movement focused attention on the heterogeneous scientific underpinnings of common clinical practice (1–4). While there are still debates on the relative merits of different sources of evidence such as randomized clinical trials or observational studies (5–7), a common recognition of the importance of evidence has emerged. It is natural that the focus on evidence has spread from the world of clinical decision-making to public health decision-making (8–10). For example, in July 1998, Dr Gro Brundtland took over as Director-General of the World Health Organization (WHO) and began a systematic attempt to strengthen the evidence base and its use in decision-making for public health in the work of WHO. Journals (11) and conferences (12;13) devoted to the evidence-base for public health are also indications of the increase in interest in the scientific basis for decisions that can affect the health of populations.

Attempts to strengthen the evidence base for public health have, however, highlighted some important issues regarding the nature of evidence and how evidence should be strengthened. *The World Health Report 2000*, a first attempt to draw attention to the limited evidence base for decisions about the organization, financing and management of health systems, has generated an intense debate (14–20). Some of this debate has focused on the quality of evidence for monitoring versus strategic decision-making. Another issue is illustrated by calls for increased resource flows to fund health programmes in developing countries (21) that have led to a broad recognition of the need for independent authoritative monitoring of critical health outcomes. There has been less consensus on how to ensure independence for monitoring. Confusion also exists on the nature of evidence for different

tasks; the best available evidence to support strategic local, national or international decision-making may not be adequate to document significant changes for monitoring or evaluation purposes.

To stimulate a broader debate on the nature and role of evidence for public health action, in this chapter we outline four different uses of evidence and their interconnections. WHO promotes a consistent approach to generating and disseminating evidence for all four uses through five guiding principles: validity, reliability, comparability, consultation, and explicit audit trail. The potential of these principles to help clarify debates on the nature of evidence, differences between country data, and estimates and mechanisms to ensure independent monitoring are explored in the discussion section of the chapter.

Evidence for What?

Evidence can be used for at least four distinct purposes: strategic decision-making, programme implementation or management, monitoring of outcomes or achievements, and evaluation of what works and what does not. The time-frames for these different uses range from the immediate for strategic decision-making to the long-term for building a robust evidence base to evaluate alternative strategies to improve health or reduce health inequalities. Likewise, the requirements for strength of evidence vary for the distinct uses. In the following sections, we discuss in more detail the nature of evidence for each of these uses and the inter-relationships between them.

Strategic Decision-Making

A physician must often formulate a treatment plan with a patient based on all the evidence at hand. Sometimes that may include history and physical, blood tests and imaging studies; in other cases, decisions may be made only on the basis of a physical exam, e.g. a comatose patient in an airplane. Local, national and international decision-makers also must make key strategic choices about funding priorities for different programmes, targeting of actions to specific communities or groups, or the introduction or modification of regulations. Like the physician, a policy-maker must make these strategic decisions now and ideally should be equipped with the best available evidence.

Best available evidence is a key phrase meaning that all available sources should be used to provide relevant inputs for decision-making. Evidence on disease incidence or prevalence and its distribution in the population, on mortality by age, sex and cause, on current coverage of interventions, on the likely costs and benefits of pursuing different policies all may be relevant depending on the decision. Often data from vital registration systems, household surveys, censuses, and health service providers may give highly uncertain assessments of key parameters. Nevertheless, decisions must be taken and systematic assessments of the evidence—even if highly uncertain—are a better basis for decisions than no evidence at all. The need for the best available evidence means that assessments of any parameter should be based on the integration of all relevant information.

A good example of the ethos of using the best available evidence to inform strategic decision-making is provided by national and international assessments of population by age and sex. The centrality of population figures for a host of government and private sector decisions has led nearly every government to produce national population estimates and the United Nations to produce population figures for every country of the world from 1950 to 2050 (*22;23*). Figures for the next half-century, of course, are based on forecast models. Population estimates are developed using whatever sources are available. In some cases, the most recent census may be 30 or more years old so that there is considerable uncertainty about fertility, mortality and migration. Nevertheless, estimates are based on likely trends in the region, economic factors influencing fertility, mortality and migration, and geopolitical developments. This United Nations practice, which has been institutionalized for over 50 years, is no longer contentious (*23*). Yet in public health, providing figures for important quantities of interest based on the best available evidence is still debated (*24;25*).

PROGRAMME IMPLEMENTATION AND MANAGEMENT

Evidence is also needed to aid public health managers to implement programmes effectively. For example, the DOTS strategy for controlling tuberculosis has at its heart a real-time information system, which provides reports on the fraction of patients enrolled on short-course chemotherapy that have completed treatment each quarter at the district level (*26*). Regional and national supervisors react to poor treatment completion results through supervisory problem-solving visits. A number of examples from public health illustrate the use of information to guide programme management including: the seven-by-thirty cluster sample surveys for the implementation of childhood immunization programmes (*27*); surveillance systems for flaccid paralysis in the campaign against polio (*28*); and the complications of cardiovascular surgery monitoring system of the United States Veterans Administration (*29*).

While these examples illustrate the potential for timely evidence on key health system processes to improve programme implementation, they are perhaps the exception rather than the rule. The reality is that for a number of health system programmes, the information system may be too limited. Evidence for programme management often has to be available for districts or local areas. To be useful, the information systems need to be low-cost and able to provide timely input.

MONITORING CRITICAL OUTCOMES

Through a variety of international summits and agreements, the countries of the world have committed themselves to achieving a range of health targets. An important case is the Millennium Declaration, to which 189 countries have signed on to 8 goals for development and a set of 48 indicators for achievement of these goals. Seventeen of the indicators are health-related, which demonstrates the increasingly dominant role of health in the development agenda. New investment mechanisms like the Global Alliance for Vaccines and Immunizations and the Global Fund to Fight AIDS, Tuberculosis and Malaria are likely to be sustained if the initial investments can be proven to have had a real impact. The importance of monitoring is demonstrated by the proliferation of meetings and initiatives to strengthen national capacity to monitor critical heath outcomes.

Evidence for monitoring, however, must be of a different nature than the best available evidence for strategic decision-making. While population estimates based on a 30 year-old census and informed assumptions about fertility, mortality, and migration change in the last three decades may be essential for current investment decisions, using changes in these estimates to monitor the impact of national population policy would not be appropriate.

One way to understand the difference in the evidence required for strategic decision-making and the evidenced required for monitoring may be in terms of the width of uncertainty intervals.[1] Population figures based on a 30 year-old census have wide uncertainty intervals, and the uncertainty interval for the change in population over the last five years is likely to include no change at all. For monitoring progress towards national or international targets, narrower uncertainty intervals are often required in order to conclude whether progress is being made. Statements about time trends require much more evidence than informative statements about current levels. In reality, monitoring nearly always has to do with assessing the direction and magnitude of change.

The difference in the evidence necessary for monitoring versus strategic decision-making, however, is more a quantitative than a qualitative one. Even in the setting of uncertainty about trends, governments and other public health actors often need to make some judgement on the extent to which progress is being achieved. Such judgements may fuel reaffirmation of agreed-upon strategies or lead to widespread reappraisal. Monitoring feeds into an ongoing evidence-policy loop which is discussed more fully below.

EVALUATION AND BUILDING THE EVIDENCE BASE ON WHAT WORKS

The final purpose of evidence is to create the opportunity for shared learning so that local or national experience with policies and programmes in public health can be used to make critical judgements on what works and what does not. While the evidence-based medicine movement has stressed the importance of formal evaluation mechanisms like randomized clinical trials, similar rigor has not been widely applied to the assessment of public health interventions, health system financing and organization or regulation. The requirements for evidence for evaluation should be the most stringent. As with monitoring, evaluation of the effectiveness of various policies and programmes requires the assessment of change over time (i.e. before

and after implementing a policy or programme), but it also requires assessment of the counterfactual of not implementing. Randomization is rarely possible—although there have been a few examples of studies where communities have been randomized to different policies (30–32)—so more often than not, statistical models are required to estimate effectiveness in addition to robust monitoring of inputs, processes and outcomes.

EVIDENCE-POLICY CYCLE

The four uses of evidence are interconnected. Strategic decision-making is based on the cumulative knowledge built up from the evaluation of policies and programmes combined with the best available evidence on the current magnitude and distribution of health problems, health system inputs, processes, and outcomes. Implementation of strategic decisions requires good information and evidence that is used by managers at all levels of health systems. The impact of these programmes should be monitored. Monitoring information feeds back to managers and strategic decision-making directly, but it is also the basis for more systematic evaluation of programme and policy effectiveness.

Because there are many feedbacks in this process, different producers and users of evidence must at all times be aware of the strengths and limitations of the evidence at hand. Often because one group or discipline produces evidence and another uses this evidence in subsequent analyses, the pedigree or basis for evidence is lost. Economists may believe that demographic or health data are very robust with narrow uncertainty intervals relative to economic data, while public health analysts believe the opposite. Part of improving the production and use of evidence is to have some core principles that are widely accepted and understood.

The problems created when evidence is used across disciplines can be illustrated with two examples. First, economists have often used United Nations Population Division figures for child mortality and life expectancy in research studies that are meant to generate evidence on what works and what does not (33). The problem is that in some countries, assessments by the UN or others of the best available evidence take into account models explicitly relating income or education to expected levels of child mortality. This circularity in the generation of evidence by demographers and use by economists is clearly problematic. If analysts do not take this into account, the strength of relationships or at least the standard errors of some effect sizes may be seriously biased. Public health analysts often use income per capita in international dollars as an input to a variety of evaluation studies. Purchasing power parities, used in the calculation of international dollars, are based on price data collected five to ten years ago for some countries, but for the majority of countries they are based on regression models.

In both cases, evidence is produced to inform strategic decision-making and is subsequently used by others for evaluation purposes. The key challenge is to ensure a common language and approach to evidence for public health that clarifies the strengths and weaknesses of evidence and its appropriateness for different uses.

Towards Some Common Principles for Evidence

Broader discussion of the use of evidence in public health and some of the debates over *The World Health Report 2000* have helped clarify the different types and uses of evidence in the work of WHO. Based on the extensive series of regional and technical consultations on how to refine and improve health systems performance assessment and on the detailed report of the Scientific Peer Review Group, WHO has formulated five basic principles to inform the generation and dissemination of evidence. Not all these principles apply equally in all cases, but in general they lay the foundation for improved communication across disciplines, countries, and topics on the evidence for public health action.

The five principles are validity, quantified reliability, comparability, consultation, and explicit data audit trail. Each of these principles and their implications are explored in detail.

Proven Validity

While there are few champions of invalid measurements, there is a wide range of interpretations of what proven validity may mean. Blanket statements that something is invalid may actually mean that the results simply differ from the authors' opinions or may reflect judgements about reliability or comparability. A measurement is valid if it measures the construct that it was intended to measure (34;35). A corollary is that a valid measurement should in principle not be biased, although some amount of bias might be accepted for the sake of statistical efficiency. Producers and disseminators of evidence should establish the

validity of their measurement methods. Three of the many common limitations to the validity of evidence are worth noting here.

First, in public health and more generally in development, proxy measures are often used to assess an important quantity of interest. For example, some have argued that the infant mortality rate is a proxy indicator of general health status (36;37). For monitoring the spread of HIV/AIDS in Africa, data on HIV prevalence in pregnant women attending a small sample of antenatal care clinics have been used as a proxy for male and female adult HIV prevalence in many African populations (38). This latter example shows how what is available—prevalence data among a sentinel population that are relatively easier to collect—can become a proxy for what is of real interest—prevalence overall in the general population. To justify further interest in a proxy, the validity of this relationship should be established. Where the proxy is biased or likely to be biased, this should be quantified and attention paid to the fact that the relationship between the proxy and the true quantity of interest may change over time. Too often the fact that an indicator was justified as a proxy for another measure is forgotten and the proxy indicator assumes center stage. To remind users of the original purpose for measurements of an indicator and the evidence of the strength of the relationship between the proxy and the real quantity of interest, proxy measurements should be mapped back into estimates of the real quantity of interest. This mapping to the true quantity of interest should of course take into account known biases and uncertainty.

Second, validity of evidence on an important quantity of interest such as coverage with DTP3 immunization can also be profoundly affected by community level selection bias. For many diseases or risk factors, evidence may only be available from a limited number of local studies. For example, HIV sero-prevalence figures for Ethiopia are based on four antenatal clinics in Addis Ababa and another three to eight sites outside the capital (39). Community studies, however, are often conducted in settings where the investigators expect to find larger or smaller amounts of the disease or risk factor than expected. Overall, this creates a real prospect of selection bias when no national data are available. This problem is so common that efforts should be made to use more robust techniques to predict when selection bias is an issue.

Third, when analysis of data requires the use of statistical models, models that are consistent with known measurement errors should be used. Many statistical models assume that independent variables are measured without error. The discovery that measurement error for blood pressure and serum cholesterol leads to a systematic underestimation of these hazards due to regression dilution bias is one clear illustration of the problem (40;41). Unfortunately, much evidence is generated for which the potential bias introduced by measurement error in independent variables has not been adequately addressed.

Quantified Reliability

Reliability may be defined as the extent to which a quantity is free from random error (35). It thus may be related directly to the stochastic component of a measurement. For a given expected value, what is the distribution of the measure that would be observed with repeated measurement? In this sense, a measurement is never reliable or unreliable. Rather, reliability is an attribute of all measurements that should be explicitly quantified. For example, in routine epidemiological use, blood pressure is measured with a stochastic error that is normally distributed with mean zero and standard deviation 5 mmHg. Test-retest studies show that self-reported items on household surveys have relatively wide uncertainty intervals. This does not make the self-reported responses unreliable, but rather implies only that the magnitude of the stochastic measurement error should be recognized and reflected in subsequent analyses.

Quantifying reliability of evidence on a particular indicator must go beyond the reliability of the primary measurement instrument such as the sphygnometer. The reliability of evidence can be considered as inverse to the uncertainty of the evidence. Confidence intervals due to sampling error are familiar. Uncertainty, however, includes, in addition to sampling error, the measurement error associated with the instrument, parameter estimation error if statistical models are used in correcting the data, and uncertainty due to the possible choice of alternative plausible models.[2] These issues are explored in greater detail in the section below on quantifying reliability using uncertainty intervals.

Comparability

Evidence for monitoring or evaluation requires that it is comparable over time, across communities within a population, and across populations. To close the evidence-policy cycle, evidence for strategic decision-making should also be comparable. In clinical medicine, the importance of comparison (for example, via bench-marking across different patients) is deeply ingrained in practice. The accumulation of experience is, in part, tantamount to building up a personal set of bench-marks of how patients with particular measured characteristics may react in various settings. There are equally powerful arguments in favour of measurements and evidence that are comparable over time and across groups.

Comparability is an independent criterion from validity and reliability. Consider two thermometers that are both valid, with quantified measurement error, but one reports temperature in degrees Fahrenheit and the other in Celsius. Although each measurement instrument is reliable and valid, the results cannot be compared. Comparability requires a common scale. For many measurements, establishing comparability remains a major challenge. For example, problems of comparability in self-reported health status measures over time and across socioeconomic groups have been well-documented (42–48); however, recent methodological developments hold promise for enhancing comparability of these measures through novel survey instrumentation linked to new analytical models (49–51).

Consultation

With reference to evidence in which the unit of analysis is a country or a subnational unit within a country, WHO is committed to a process of explicit consultation with the relevant health authorities. This consultation provides an opportunity for national experts to identify new data sources, discuss limitations of the existing data sources, and recognize known biases that should be taken into account in the analysis. This dialogue also serves to reinforce a culture of evidence in international public health. WHO has used this explicit consultation process successfully in the production of the Annex Tables in *The World Health Report 2001* and *The World Health Report 2002*. This consultation has lead to a more informed debate and a broader ownership of the results for critical health outcomes. The nature of the dialogue focuses attention on the analysis of the available data and a common understanding of their strengths and weaknesses. Consultation with national health authorities is simply an application of a more general principle: those most centrally involved in the collection, collation and analysis of primary data should be consulted.

Explicit Data Audit Trail

In an era when there are calls on governments and international organizations for increased transparency, a very important principle for evidence is the concept of an explicit data audit trail. For every figure, whether evidence for strategic decision-making or evidence for evaluation or research, the trail from primary data collection, adjustments for known biases and statistical modelling should be replicable. For complete transparency, primary data should be in the public domain along with the analytical steps from primary data to the evidence on an indicator that is disseminated.

Implementation of a policy of an explicit data audit trail has an important implication for the practice of many public health organizations, and especially for WHO. The internet provides a practical mechanism through which the primary data and subsequent steps can be made available. But explicit data audit trails also imply a major change in the culture of medicine and public health. Frequently studies are reported in the medical and public health literature in which the primary data are not available. While this practice is uncommon in fields like physics or political science (52;53), it is still the norm in public health. Building the evidence base for public health implies that the principles of explicit data audit trail should not only apply to countries or international organizations, but should reasonably be adopted by the scientific community in general. Implementing a policy of explicit data audit trail for an organization like WHO will not be without considerable human and financial cost. Data systems, procedures for documentation, and the culture of analysis will need to be transformed. Nevertheless, in the long run these costs are a necessity.

A TYPOLOGY OF ESTIMATES

Given these principles, there are still questions that emerge on when it is appropriate to publish evidence. Is there a point at which uncertainty intervals are too large and uncertainty gives way to ignorance? To put it another way, is there a qualitative difference between different types of evidence or estimates for a quantity of interest that transcends the uncertainty interval[3]? We believe that while there are qualitatively different types of estimates, a quantified uncertainty interval provides the most useful unifying approach to communicating this information to the user. To help build this argument, however, we first present a typology of different types of estimates.

Table 54.1 identifies eight basic types of estimates defined in terms of data availability and its timeliness. It is useful to review each category and provide some examples from published data of this type of measurement. For any quantity of interest in a given place and time, direct measurement or measurements may be available. This situation is labelled as category 1A in the table. An example is the child mortality rate in a country with a complete vital registration system that provides information with a minimal time lag. For the WHO estimates of child mortality for 2000 (published in 2002), the United States had vital registration data available for the estimate. Uncertainty in the risk of child death in this case is simply a function of sample size. There are many cases, however, where more than one direct measurement from different national surveys may be available but give different results. In these cases, the uncertainty interval will need to reflect the range from all of the available high quality

Table 54.1   A taxonomy of evidence relating to population health and health systems

	Data time-frame	
	A. Data available for time period of interest	B. Data available for earlier time period
1. Direct unbiased measurement(s) available for population of interest	Evidence based on synthesis of available measurements	Evidence for earlier time period projected forward using model of time trends
2. Direct biased measurement(s) available for population of interest	Evidence based on synthesis of measurements adjusted for bias	Evidence for earlier time period (adjusted for bias) projected forward using model of time trends
3. Partial direct data available for population of interest	Partial data corrected for known biases and supplemented by evidence available for other similar populations, or use of prior knowledge and internal consistency requirements	Partial and other evidence used together with model to project forward to period of interest
4. Direct data not available for population of interest but information on covariates and evidence of their associations is available	Evidence based on observed relationship between measured covariates and quantity of interest	Evidence based on observed relationship between measured covariates and quantity of interest, and projected forward to period of interest

surveys. This is a common problem. For example, the population distribution of alcohol consumption has been measured in five separate national surveys for Australia in the mid-1990s and the resulting distributions are in some cases quite inconsistent (54).

In contrast to the US example, for a number of countries with complete vital registration data, these data may be collated with a considerable time lag. Figures for 2000 for the risk of child death may have to be based on a previous year and "updated" to a 2000 estimate. This updating or projecting forward a direct measurement is undertaken using a model based on observed empirical regularities in relationships between levels of child mortality and some set of covariates including time. This is an example of a Category 1B estimate, which uses a direct measurement of the quantity of interest in a previous time period and an updating model. The child mortality figure for Canada published for 2000 in *The World Health Report 2002* was based on data from 1950 to 1998 together with a projection model.

In some cases, direct measurement of the quantity of interest may be available but the measurement method may be subject to known biases. For example, household surveys asking about deaths in the last twelve months tend to report age-specific death rates that are systematically biased downwards due to under-reporting. In this case, demographers have developed techniques to measure the degree of under-reporting so that the direct data can be corrected to yield an unbiased estimate of mortality. There are many examples of this type of correction for known biases ranging from household health expenditures to self-rated health status. Examples of this type of situation include the correction of self-reported height and weight for known biases (55). Category 2B is where direct measurements requiring correction for known biases are available for a year prior to the reference year for the estimate, so that a model must be used to update the estimate.

Category 3 estimates are those for which only partial direct data are available with or without the need for corrections for known biases. Common examples are where survey data are available for one city or province in a country, or where one component of an aggregate is available but not the entire phenomenon. In measuring the burden of disease, survey data may be available for a range of disabling sequelae but not for all. In these cases, estimates are usually some hybrid of using the partial data corrected for known biases and using other sources from the region or models relating the missing information to certain covariates. An example of this situation is when only child mortality data are available for a country (such as Cameroon) and partial information on adult mortality is available (AIDS). A model life table system is used to predict the level of adult mortality (excluding HIV) associated with the observed level of child mortality, based on the associations observed for other countries. Separate estimates for HIV mortality are then added (56).

Estimates which are likely to have the largest uncertainty intervals are Category 4 estimates where no direct data are available for a country and the estimate is based exclusively on the observed relationship between measured covariates and the quantity of interest in other places. This type of estimate will probably have the largest degree of uncertainty, but the actual magnitude of the uncertainty interval depends critically on how adequately the model captures the observed variance in the quantity of interest in settings where direct measurements are available.

There is widespread use of evidence based on a mixture of estimates of the different types identified in Table 54.1. A good illustration is provided by national accounts information. This information is so critical for many types of economic planning that estimates are developed using various methods for nearly every country every year (57–59). For example, the World Bank develops its own estimates for countries of GDP in local currency units, which are often corrected for the size of the informal economy and other such adjustments based on specific staff country experiences. The resulting GDP estimates are converted to a common basis using purchasing power parity (PPP) exchange rate estimates, often based on regression extrapolations given that PPP data are not available for all countries. To compound these problems, PPP exchange rates come from two different sources using competing methods. Both base their observations on the same international price comparisons made intermittently for selected countries. These comparisons started in 1970 for only 10 countries and were repeated every 5 years until 1990 with an increasing number of countries. They are now being undertaken more regularly, but still not annually. For the 1993/1996 series of studies, 115 countries were included. For years between the actual observations, estimates are made assuming that GDP in PPP grew at the same rate as GDP in domestic currency units. So for years between the price surveys, GDP per capita figures for countries are based on no observations at all of purchasing price parities.

For those countries not included in the price comparison surveys, GDP in PPP is estimated using regression techniques to predict GDP based on a set of covariates observed to correlate with GDP for countries with price observations. Therefore, not only are there years for which no price observations were made for any country, there are countries for which GDP per capita in PPP are estimated, where no price comparisons have ever been made.

The qualitative typology of different types of estimates presented here can in large part be captured by appropriate quantification of the uncertainty interval. Uncertainty intervals are meant to capture much more than just sampling error. Uncertainty arises from the measurement error of an instrument (whether sphygmometer or self-reported symptom questions), sampling, a range of biases from study design, parameter uncertainty in the estimation of models, and model choice uncertainty. While methods to capture all these forms of uncertainty may be crude in some cases such as model choice, nevertheless the uncertainty interval can be a practical method to communicate the confidence a decision-maker should have in a measurement.

Table 54.2 classifies published life expectancy estimates for 191 countries from *The World Health Report 2002* for each of the eight qualitative categories of estimates. Table 54.3 shows the average uncertainty interval for countries in each of these categories. Not surprisingly, category 4 estimates have the larg-

est uncertainty intervals while 1A have the smallest. Although the complete ordering of the eight categories is likely to vary for different quantities of interest, the general principle that moving from column A to B will increase uncertainty and moving from row 1 to 4 will increase uncertainty as well, seems to hold. Tables 54.4 and 54.5 apply this taxonomy to estimates of maternal mortality ratios (MMR) per 100 000 women aged 15–44 years, prepared jointly by UNICEF and WHO for the year 2000 (60). As with the life expectancy estimates, there is a general increase in the relative uncertainty of these estimates for lower categories in the taxonomy. Since the countries where level 3 or 4 estimation processes have been used have much higher average MMRs than level 2 countries, the disparities in absolute uncertainty ranges for the MMR are even larger, ranging from 23 to 46 for group 2A to 100 to 970 for group 4A.

DISCUSSION

Debates over "what is evidence" are often caught up in three issues: claims in epidemiology that randomized

Table 54.2 Example of taxonomy for WHO estimates of life expectancy at birth for Member States for year 2000[a]

	Life tables—number of Member States		
	A	B	Total
1	34	13	47
2	42	44	86
3	12	41	53
4	5	—	5
Total	93	98	191

a. The World Health Report 2002, Annex Table 1.

Table 54.3 Average uncertainty range for life expectancy at birth (e_0) estimates (expressed as % of e_0)

	e_0 uncertainty range ±%	
	A	B
1	0.2	0.6
2	1.5	2.4
3	8.6	10.9
4	11.7	—

Table 54.4 Example of taxonomy for UNICEF/WHO joint estimates of maternal mortality ratios (MMRs) per 100 000 for Member States for year 2000[a]

	MMR—number of Member States		
	A	B	Total
1	—	—	—
2	71	23	94
3	20	29	49
4	49	—	49
Total	140	52	192

a. (60). Estimation process as follows:
  A2: Vital records for year 2000 adjusted for under-reporting
  B2: Vital records adjusted for under-reporting and RAMOS surveys in previous years
  A3: Adjusted incomplete vital records for year 2000
  B3: Sisterhood surveys in previous years (mostly in high mortality regions)
  A4: Model-based estimates

Table 54.5 Average uncertainty ranges for estimates of maternal mortality ratio (MMR) per 100 000 (expressed as % of MMR)

	MMR uncertainty range %	
	A	B
1	—	—
2	30	35
3	47	42
4	72	—

clinical trials are the only way to deal with unmeasured variables related both to the outcome of interest and to the factor being studied, namely confounders; claims that country data are fundamentally different than "estimates;" and concerns about how to ensure independence of evidence from those who may gain or lose by the results. The different uses of evidence and the implications of the five principles for each of these issues are worth exploring.

Randomized clinical trials (RCTs) can be a highly effective mechanism for dealing with unmeasured confounding, and if studies are large, then resulting effect sizes can be known with narrow uncertainty intervals. Strategic as well as clinical decision-making will always have to go beyond the RCT evidence. RCTs have exclusion criteria, and generalizing results to other patients or other populations necessarily introduces uncertainty about the effect size. Moreover, there are many population level interventions or combinations of strategies that cannot be tested in RCTs—for instance, taxes on tobacco or alcohol, or national legislation for speed limits or airbags. In reality, the challenge is to make sure that all possible efforts are undertaken to minimize the risk of biased results due to unmeasured confounding and to realistically capture the true range of uncertainty. Realistic assessments of uncertainty require the use of appropriate statistical models that allow the integration of different sources of data on the same effect.

In discussions of figures for a given health-related outcome such as the percentage of children who have been immunized with DTP3 before one year of age, some try to make a distinction between country data and what they call "estimates." This is a false dichotomy. Evidence is by its nature a public good. One can debate the nature of the primary data collection mechanism, adjustments for known biases, and statistical models used to make inference in terms of validity, reliability, and comparability. It is not meaningful to debate the quality of evidence in terms of who is the provider or disseminator. If the word "estimate" is used by some to imply there is uncertainty associated with the estimation process, then all figures are estimates. There is essentially no biological, physical or social quantity that can be known with absolute certainty. Adherence to the principle of an explicit data audit trail would help focus attention on the distinction between primary data and figures for a quantity of interest that are based on valid and comparable methods with quantified uncertainty. For example, vital registration data in Honduras are not complete, but these primary data have been analysed

by demographers using various techniques to generate a life table. Unadjusted death rates calculated from the vital registration data are clearly biased, while the life table is not, but the age-specific death rates have wide uncertainty intervals.

At a time when there is a considerable discussion of new resources from high-income countries flowing to help improve the health of the poor, there has been an upswing in the debate on the importance of authoritative, independent evidence to monitor critical health outcomes. What steps are required to ensure that evidence on changes in key outcomes is independent of groups who have a stake in the results? Groups that may have an interest range from technical specialists who have designed intervention programmes to industry or governments themselves. Three types of solutions are on offer to strengthen independence. One focuses on the need for independent governance of the institution or institutions that produce evidence. A second concentrates on the creation of processes such as peer review or scientific committees to safeguard evidence production. The third emphasizes transparency. It is likely that all three must be part of a solution.

This challenge is not new. Nearly every government monitors a range of critical outcomes of its own policies and programmes. Those applying the monitoring are sheltered from other considerations through a variety of mechanisms such as independent Central Statistical Bureaus or Audit Offices. Many examples demonstrate that such independence can be achieved through a diverse array of mechanisms. The systems in place to provide authoritative, independent evidence on intervention effectiveness are generally based on journals' peer review mechanisms or scientific review panels.

Regardless of the type of evidence or the institutional arrangements created to safeguard its generation, transparency will enhance the quality of evidence in the long run. The principle of an explicit data audit trail includes providing access to the primary micro-data used in generating evidence and all the intervening steps in the analysis. Given the potential benefits of transparency, why is it not a common practice? In public health, micro-data from epidemiological studies or intervention trials are rarely put in the public domain. While transparency is the norm in other fields of science, it is not yet the norm in public health. Likewise, international institutions rarely provide an explicit data audit trail. In the short run, transparency increases rather than decreases debate. *Ex-cathedra* statements are less often challenged when the details behind them are not revealed. This creates rather strong disincentives for institutions generating and disseminating evidence to provide complete transparency. Nevertheless, it is perhaps the only way to ensure that evidence which is valid, reliable, and comparable can be available to inform the range of key decisions that can make a difference to people's health.

The five principles put forward by WHO are implicitly part of a Bayesian framework for evidence. All relevant data and knowledge should be used to marshal the best available evidence. Users have to be fully informed of the nature of the evidence through quantification of uncertainty and an explicit data audit trail. Future efforts at strengthening the evidence base should be focused where assessments of what works and what does not are based on evidence with very wide uncertainty intervals.

Notes

1 There are a variety of types and sources of uncertainty. Uncertainty may arise from incomplete information (e.g. when we base estimates for a population on observations from a sample), from potential biases in information (e.g. how representative for a whole population are estimates from a study of a subgroup), from disagreements between information sources (e.g. when we have several studies giving different estimates for the same quantity), from model uncertainty (e.g. the type of function specified in a regression model), from uncertainty in preferences (e.g. in preferences for health states), or it may be inherent to the data generation process itself (e.g. we may only infer risks from event counts in a population, which means that we can never know the risks themselves with certainty).

2 Uncertainty is typically characterized using the language of probability (*61;62*). We may distinguish the classical or *frequentist* view of probability, which defines the probability of an event occurring in a particular trial or experiment as the frequency with which it occurs in a long sequence of similar experiments, from the Bayesian view, which interprets probability as the degree of belief a person has that an event will occur, given all the relevant information currently known to that person. The latter view is more easily reconciled with quantities of interest for which it is difficult to conceive of an infinite series of similar trials. Subjective probabilities in the Bayesian perspective must obey all the same axioms and rules as frequentist probabilities, and the practice of statistical inference is usually unaffected by these conceptual distinctions. Moreover, when an empirical series of data from trials become available, the Bayesian assessment of probability should converge to the frequentist assessment, assuming that the Bayesian analyst uses the data rationally to update the assessments.

3 Formally, ignorance is defined as having no knowledge of a phenomenon. This is equivalent to having no prior probability distribution (in Bayesian terms). For example, to say that we are ignorant of the prevalence of blindness in Bhutan implies that we have no beliefs that would support any particular prevalence between 0 and 100 per cent. This nonexistent prior seems quite implausible. The known range of blindness prevalence in countries with surveys is 0.2% to 3%. The biological processes that primarily account for blindness such as trachoma, congenital causes, diabetes, cataract and glaucoma are all likely to be present in Bhutan. More generally, it seems that, for biological phenomena, a state of complete ignorance is very unlikely. Even where there is ignorance (unknown prior), for all biological phenomena, the possible priors will be bounded, so that ignorance is not complete.

References

(1) Evidence-Based Medicine Working Group. Evidence-based medicine: a new approach to teaching the practice of medicine. *The Journal of the American Medical Association*, 1992, 268:2420–2425.

(2) Chalmers I, Dickersin K, Chalmers TC. Getting to grips with Archie Cochrane's agenda. *British Medical Journal*, 1992, 305:786–788.

(3) Davidoff F et al. Evidence based medicine: a new journal to help doctors identify the information they need. *British Medical Journal*, 1995, 310:1085–1086.

(4) Chalmers I, Sackett D, Silagy C. The Cochrane Collaboration. In: Maynard A, Chalmers I, eds. *Non-random reflections on health services research: on the 25 anniversary of Archie Cochrane's Effectiveness and Efficiency*. London, BMJ Books, 1997:231–249.

(5) McPherson K. The best and the enemy of the good; randomised trials, uncertainty, and assessing the role of patient preferences in medical decision making. *Journal of Epidemiology and Community Health*, 1994, 48:6–15.

(6) Marks HM. *The progress of experiment: science and therapeutic reform in the United States, 1900–1990*. Cambridge, Cambridge University Press, 1997.

(7) Vandenbroucke JP. Observational research and evidence-based medicine: what should we teach young physicians? *Journal of Clinical Epidemiology*, 1998, 51:467–477.

(8) Contributors to the Cochrane Collaboration and the Campbell Collaboration. *Evidence from systematic reviews of research relevant to implementing the 'wider public health' agenda*. York, NHS Centre for Reviews and Dissemination, 2001. URL: http://www.york.ac.uk/inst/crd/wph.htm (accessed 17 July 2001).

(9) Lancaster T et al. Effectiveness of interventions to help people stop smoking: findings from the Cochrane Library. *British Medical Journal*, 2000, 321:355–358.

(10) Beaglehole R, Bonita R. *Public health at the crossroads.* Cambridge, Cambridge University Press, 1997.

(11) *Evidence-based healthcare.* Elsevier Science, 2003.

(12) Kings Fund and NHS Health Development Agency. *Evidence into practice: challenges and opportunities for UK public health.* One Day Conference, London, 3 April 2001.

(13) International Union for Health Promotion and Education. *XVIIth World Conference on Health Promotion and Health Education Dissemination of Evidence for Effective Public Health.* Paris, July 2001.

(14) World Health Organization. *The World Health Report 2000. Health Systems: Improving Performance.* Geneva, World Health Organization, 2000.

(15) Blendon R, Kim M, Benson JM. The public versus the World Health Organization on health system performance. Who is better qualified to judge health care systems: public health experts or the people who use the healthcare? *Health Affairs,* 2001, 20(3).

(16) Almeida C et al. Methodological concerns and recommendations on policy consequences of the World Health Report 2000. *The Lancet,* 2001, 357(9269): 1692–1697.

(17) Navarro V. Assessment of the World Health Report 2000. *The Lancet,* 2000, 356(9241):1598–1601.

(18) Murray CJL, Frenk J. World Health Report 2000: a step towards evidence-based health policy. *The Lancet,* 2001, 357(9269):1698–1700.

(19) Williams A. Science or marketing at WHO? A commentary on "World Health 2000." *Health Economics,* 2001, 10(2):93–100.

(20) Murray CJL et al. Science or marketing at WHO? A response to Williams. *Health Economics,* 2001, 10(4): 277–282.

(21) Commission on Macroeconomics and Health. *Macroeconomics and health: investing in health for economic development.* Geneva, World Health Organization, 2001.

(22) U.S. Census Bureau. *International Data Base (IDB).* Washington, DC, U.S. Census Bureau Population Division, International Programs Center (IPC), 2002. URL: http://www.census.gov/ipc/www/idbnew.html

(23) United Nations. *World Population Prospects—the 1998 revision Volume III: Analytical Report.* New York, United Nations, 2000.

(24) Cooper RS et al. Disease burden in sub-Saharan Africa: what should we conclude in the absence of data? *The Lancet,* 1998, 351:208–210.

(25) McKee M. Measuring the efficiency of health systems. The World Health Report sets the agenda, but there's still a long way to go. *British Medical Journal,* 2001, 323(7308):295–296.

(26) World Health Organization. *An expanded DOTS framework for effective tuberculosis control* (WHO/CDS/TB/2002.297). Geneva, World Health Organization, 2002.

(27) Hoshaw-Woodard S. *Description and comparison of the methods of cluster sampling and lot quality assurance sampling to assess immunization coverage.* The Ohio State University for Department of Vaccines and Biologicals, Geneva, World Health Organization, 2001.

(28) World Health Organization. *Polio Eradication.* URL: http://www.polioeradication.org/

(29) Demakis JG et al. Quality Enhancement Research Initiative (QUERI): a collaboration between research and clinical practice. *Medical Care,* 2000, 38(6 Suppl.1): 117–25.

(30) Farquhar J et al. Effects of community-wide education on cardiovascular disease risk factors. The Stanford five city project. *The Journal of the American Medical Association,* 1990, 264:359–365.

(31) Luepker R et al. Community education for cardiovascular disease prevention: risk factor changes in the Minnesota heart health program. *American Journal of Public Health,* 1994, 84:1383–1393.

(32) Newhouse JP et al. Some interim results from a controlled trial of cost sharing in health insurance. *New England Journal of Medicine,* 1981, 305:1501.

(33) Murray CJL. A critical review of international mortality data. *Social Science & Medicine,* 1987, 25(7): 773–781.

(34) Kirshner B, Guyatt G. A methodological framework for assessing health indices. *Journal of Chronic Diseases,* 1985, 38(1):27–36.

(35) Nunnally JC, Bernstein IR. *Psychometric theory,* 3rd ed. New York, McGraw Hill, 1994.

(36) Reidpath DD, Allotey P. Infant mortality rate as an indicator of population health. *Journal of Epidemiology and Community Health,* 2003, 57(5):344–346.

(37) Mathers CD, Salomon JA, Murray CJL. Infant mortality is not an adequate summary measure of population health. *Journal of Epidemiology and Community Health,* 2003, 57(5):319.

(38) Zaba B, Boerma T, White R. Monitoring the AIDS epidemic using HIV prevalence data among young women attending antenatal clinics: prospects and problems. *AIDS,* 2000, 14(11):1633–1645.

(39) UNAIDS. *Epidemiological fact sheets on HIV and sexually transmitted infections—Ethiopia, 2002 update.* Geneva, UNAIDS, 2002.

(40) MacMahon S et al. Epidemiology: blood pressure,

stroke, and coronary heart disease. Part I: prolonged differences in blood pressure: prospective observational studies corrected for the regression dilution bias. *The Lancet*, 1990, 335:765–774.

(41) Clarke R et al. Underestimation of risk associations due to regression dilution in long-term follow-up of prospective studies. *American Journal of Epidemiology*, 1999, 150:341–353.

(42) Moriyama IM. Problems in the measurement of health status. In: Sheldon EB, Moore WE, eds. *Indicators of social change: concepts and measurement.* New York, Russell Sage Foundation, 1968.

(43) Murray CJL, Chen LC. Understanding morbidity change. *Population and Development Review*, 1992, 18(3):481–503.

(44) Johansson SR. Measuring the cultural inflation of morbidity during the decline of mortality. *Health Transition Review*, 1992, 2(1):78–89.

(45) Murray CJL. Epidemiology and morbidity transitions in India. In: DasGupta M, Chen LC, Krishnan TN, eds. *Health, poverty and development in India.* Delhi, Oxford University Press, 1996:122–147.

(46) Mathers CD, Douglas RM. Measuring progress in population health and wellbeing. In: Eckersley R, ed. *Measuring progress: is life getting better?* Collingwood, CSIRO Publishing, 1998:125–155.

(47) Sen A. Health: perception versus observation. *British Medical Journal*, 2002, 324:860–861.

(48) Sadana R et al. Comparative analyses of more than 50 household surveys of health status. In: Murray CJL et al, eds. *Summary measures of population health: concepts, ethics, measurement and applications.* Geneva, World Health Organization, 2002:369–386.

(49) Murray CJL et al. Cross-population comparability of evidence for health policy. In: Murray CJL, Evans DB, eds. *Health systems performance assessment: debates, methods and empiricism.* Geneva, World Health Organization, 2003.

(50) Tandon A et al. Statistical models for enhancing cross-population comparability. In: Murray CJL, Evans DB, eds. *Health systems performance assessment: debates, methods and empiricism.* Geneva, World Health Organization, 2003.

(51) Salomon JA et al. Unpacking health perceptions using anchoring vignettes. In: Murray CJL, Evans DB, eds. *Health systems performance assessment: debates, methods and empiricism.* Geneva, World Health Organization, 2003.

(52) King G. The future of replication. *International Studies Perspectives* (forthcoming). Cambridge, Harvard University, 2003. URL: http://gking.harvard.edu/files/replvdc.pdf

(53) King G. Replication, replication. *PS: Political Science and Politics*, with comments from nineteen authors and a response. A revised proposal, proposal, 1995, 28(3):443–499. URL: http://gking.harvard.edu/data.shtml#repl

(54) Mathers CD, Vos T, Stevenson C. *The burden of disease and injury in Australia.* Canberra, Australian Institute of Health and Welfare, AIHW, 1999.

(55) Villanueva EV. Validity of self-reported weight in US adults: a population based cross-sectional study. *BMC Public Health*, 2001, 1:11.

(56) Lopez AD et al. *World mortality in 2000: life tables for 191 countries.* Geneva, World Health Organization, 2002.

(57) World Bank. *World development indicators.* Washington, DC, World Bank, 2001.

(58) International Monetary Fund. *World economic outlook.* Washington, DC, International Monetary Fund, 2001.

(59) Ahmad S. *Regression estimates of per capita GDP based on purchasing power parities.* World Bank International Economics Department Policy, Research Working Paper 956. Washington, DC, World Bank, 1992.

(60) WHO/UNICEF/UNFPA. *Maternal mortality in 2000: estimates developed by WHO, UNICEF and UNFPA.* Geneva, 2003 (forthcoming).

(61) King G. *Unifying political methodology: the likelihood theory of statistical inference.* Michigan, University of Michigan Press, 1998.

(62) Morgan MG, Henrion M. *Uncertainty: a guide to dealing with uncertainty in quantitative risk and policy analysis.* Cambridge, Cambridge University Press, 1990.

Chapter 55

STATISTICAL MODELS FOR ENHANCING CROSS-POPULATION COMPARABILITY

AJAY TANDON, CHRISTOPHER J.L. MURRAY, JOSHUA A. SALOMON, GARY KING

INTRODUCTION

Measuring the health state of individuals is important for the evaluation of health interventions, monitoring individual health progress, and as a critical step in measuring the health of populations. Self-report responses in household survey data are widely used for assessing the non-fatal health status of populations. These data typically take the form of ordered categorical (ordinal) responses. Over the past three decades, there has been great progress in developing instruments to measure the multiple domains of health that are reliable and demonstrate within population validity (1;2).

One key analytical issue is that these self-report ordinal responses are not comparable across populations primarily because of response category cut-point shifts. Conceptualizing the observed responses as resulting from a mapping between an underlying unobserved latent variable (e.g. ability on the domain of mobility) and categorical response categories, cut-points are threshold levels on the latent variable that characterize the transition from one observed categorical response to the next. If cut-points differ systematically across populations, or even across socio-demographic groups within a population, then the observed ordinal responses are not cross-population comparable since they will not imply the same level on the underlying latent variable that we are trying to measure (Figure 55.1). Another way of characterizing this problem is that, for the same level of the latent variable on any given domain, the probability of an individual responding in any given response category is different across populations. This issue of cross-population comparability is not limited to health surveys: it is of equal relevance to self-report surveys on responsiveness of health systems, as well

as to numerous other questions that rely on ordinal responses.

One example of self-report health data comes from the WHO Multi-country Survey Study on Health and Responsiveness 2000–2001 (3). The main self-report question on the domain of mobility is: "Overall in the past 30 days, how much difficulty did you have with moving around?" Respondents are asked to classify themselves using one of five response categories: "1=Extreme/Cannot do; 2=Severe difficulty; 3=Moderate difficulty; 4=Mild difficulty; 5=No difficulty." We can hypothesize that cut-points may vary between populations because of different cultural or other expectations for domains of health. Cut-points are also likely to vary within a cultural or socio-demographic group. The cut-points for older individuals may shift as their expectations for a domain diminish with age. Men may be more likely to deny declines in health so that their cut-points may be systematically shifted rela-

Figure 55.1 Mapping from unobserved latent variable to observed response categories

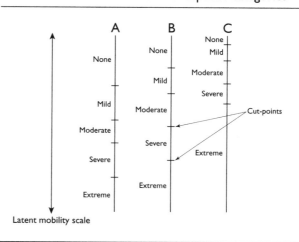

tive to those of women. Contact with health services may influence expectations for a domain and thus shift cut-points (4).

Empirical examples suggesting cross-population cut-point shifts in health surveys abound. For instance, in Australian national health surveys comparing the self-reported health status of Aboriginals with that of the general population, only around 12% of the Aboriginal population characterized their own health status as fair or poor, while more than 20% of the general population rated their health in these low categories (5). By any other major indicator of mortality and morbidity, the Aboriginal population fares much worse than the general population, which suggests that there may be important differences in the interpretation of categorical responses in the various subpopulations due to shifts in response category cut-points. Residents of the state of Kerala in India—which has the lowest rates of infant and child mortality and the highest rates of literacy in India—consistently report highest incidences of morbidity in the country (6).

The object of this chapter is to elaborate on several statistical models used in the analysis of survey data. First, we focus on off-the-shelf models that are widely available as part of any standard statistical software. In particular, we demonstrate the problems of inference that arise from these standard methods when the underlying data are not cross-population comparable. In later sections, we introduce methods that modify these standard routines to enhance the cross-population comparability of survey analyses.

MODELS FOR ANALYSING ORDINAL SURVEY RESPONSES

We begin by describing the application of existing statistical models for the analysis of ordinal survey data. These models serve as the building blocks for the methodological innovations introduced in subsequent sections. In particular, the focus is on two off-the-shelf methods: a) the *ordered probit model* (widely used by econometricians and other social scientists), and b) the *partial credit model* (from psychometrics). Both these models are used in the analysis of ordered categorical response data. The partial credit model is a multiple-category generalization of the Rasch model and is part of a large body of literature—often referred to as Item Response Theory (IRT)—which has its roots in educational testing using standardized exams (7;8).

One needs to be careful, though, in using these standard models in the analysis of data that may not be cross-population comparable. In other words, if there are good reasons to believe that respondents saying they are in "good" health in Ethiopia and in Denmark mean very different things in terms of an underlying latent variable measure, then the use of these methods without correction may lead to very misleading conclusions regarding the actual levels of health in these two populations. In order to better demonstrate this point, and to subsequently introduce some methodological innovations dealing with cross-population comparability, a simulated dataset is utilized. This dataset consists of 1 000 respondents each from two hypothetical populations (countries A and B) for which the level of health on a domain, say mobility, is to be estimated based on self-report categorical responses to three questions (one core question, and two auxiliary questions). These questions are: [1]

Main Question: "Overall in the past 30 days, how much difficulty did you have moving around?"

Auxiliary Question 1: "Overall in the past 30 days, how much difficulty did you have standing for long periods such as 30 minutes?"

Auxiliary Question 2: "Overall in the past 30 days, how much difficulty did you have climbing several flights of stairs or walking up a steep hill?"

Each of the questions asks the respondents to pick one of five responses:

1 = Extreme/cannot do
2 = Severe
3 = Moderate
4 = Mild
5 = None

Since these are simulated data, the true mobility levels are known for each respondent. This enables a comparison of the estimated mobility levels versus truth for the different models. The simulated data are generated based on the assumption that true mobility is a function of age, sex, education, and country of residence for each respondent. An individual-level random effect term is also added to represent other individual-specific unobserved factors that might affect mobility. Table 55.1 reports the mean age, education level, and sex distribution in the simulated sample.

In addition, the simulation allows cut-points for each question to differ by socio-demographic group. The response category cut-points are generated as functions of age, sex, education, and country of residence. Figure 55.2 plots the distribution of the simulated "observed" categorical responses for the three

Table 55.1   Descriptive statistics (simulated data)

Country	Mean age	Mean education	Female	N
A	38.72	4.72	500	1 000
B	38.63	7.33	492	1 000

questions for countries A and B.[2] At first glance, the distribution of self-report responses in the two countries does not look very different.

In the next two subsections, these data are analysed using both the ordered probit model and the Rasch-based partial credit model. It is assumed that the data analyst has access to the self-report categorical responses as well as standard demographic variables such as age, sex, education, and country of residence for each of the respondents. The goal is to estimate mobility levels in the two simulated populations using these data. In later sections, we introduce models that allow response category cut-points also to be functions of covariates (9). In such models, the direction of shift for the response category cut-points is also of substantive interest (e.g. to test the hypotheses that more educated respondents have higher cut-points indicative of higher norms, or that older individuals respond based on norms for their age category, and so on). Of course, such models can also be used for testing hypotheses relating to causal inferences and other tests of statistical significance.

THE ORDERED PROBIT MODEL

The ordered probit model assumes there is an unobserved latent variable Y_i^* (mobility) distributed with mean μ_i and variance 1, where i refers to the respondent.[3] The mean level of the latent variable is a function of individual-level socio-demographic characteristics such as age, sex, education, and country of residence,

$$Y_i^* \sim N(\mu_i, 1), \qquad i = 1, \dots, N$$
$$\mu_i = Z_i\beta.$$

Let y_i be the observed categorical response of individual i to the main self-report question. The ordered probit model stipulates an observation mechanism such that:

$$y_i = k \text{ if } \tau^{k-1} \leq Y_i^* < \tau^k;$$
$$\text{for } \tau^0 = -\infty, \ \tau^5 = \infty, \ \forall \ i \ \& \ k = 1, \dots, 5.$$

Also, it follows from the set-up of the model that $\tau^1 < \tau^2 < \tau^3 < \tau^4$. Given this structure, the probabilities of responding in any given category $k = 1, \dots, 5$, conditional on a vector of covariates Z_i, can be derived as:

$$\Pr(y_i = k) = \begin{cases} F(\tau^1 - Z_i'\beta), & k=1 \\ F(\tau^2 - Z_i'\beta) - F(\tau^1 - Z_i'\beta), & k=2 \\ F(\tau^3 - Z_i'\beta) - F(\tau^2 - Z_i'\beta), & k=3 \\ F(\tau^4 - Z_i'\beta) - F(\tau^3 - Z_i'\beta), & k=4 \\ 1 - F(\tau^4 - Z_i'\beta), & k=5, \end{cases} \quad [1]$$

where $F(\cdot)$ is the standard normal cumulative distribution function.

Figure 55.2   Distribution of responses for three self-report questions in countries A and B

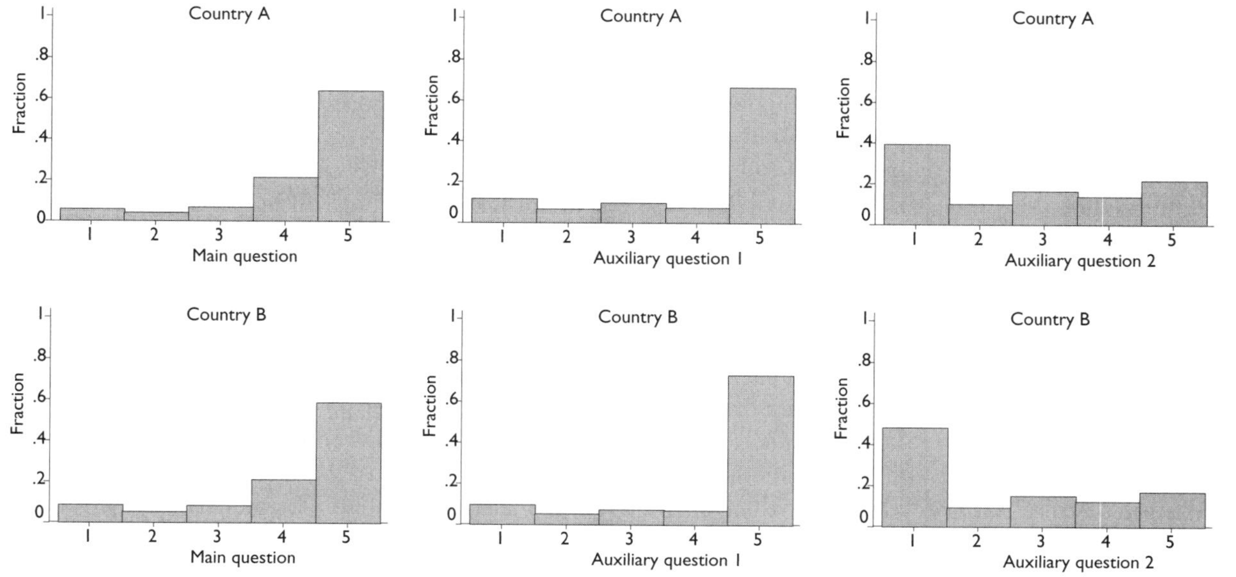

If the observations are assumed independent across individuals, then the likelihood function is simply the product of the probabilities of observing each value of y_i in the dataset. Estimates of the β vector as well as the cut-points τ^k may then be obtained using maximum likelihood methods. It is important to note that the standard ordered probit model assumes the same set of cut-points for the entire sample. Table 55.2 reports the results from a run of the ordered probit model for our simulated data for the main question in both countries.

Figure 55.3 plots the cut-points estimated from the ordered probit model versus true cut-points for the main question. Because the true cut-points may vary across individuals but the model assumes that they are fixed, each predicted cut-point is associated with a range of different true values. Figure 55.4 is a plot of true mobility versus estimated average mobility using the standard ordered probit model. As reported in the graph, the R-squared value is only about 0.011. Not only does the ordered probit model predict the mean mobility poorly, it also predicts that the average mobility is lower in country B (see coefficient on country B in Table 55.2) even though the true level of mobility is higher in country B in the simulated data. The basic point of this simulation experiment is simple: if there are significant cut-point shifts in the underlying data-generating mechanism, then using standard procedures such as the ordered probit model to analyse the data can be very misleading.

Since the ordered probit model is a probability model, we can also obtain the predicted probabilities of responding in each of the five categories for the main question, given any particular level on the underlying latent variable scale (Figure 55.5). We have used only the main question for analysing the data using the ordered probit model. One way to analyse multiple

questions using this model would be to pool the data and allow for a dummy variable per question (since the cut-points will be assumed to be the same for all questions). However, doing this will yield a different mean value of the latent variable per question for each individual. Running the model in this way is potentially confusing, since we assume that an individual has a single value on the latent variable of interest that informs answers to all three questions, but this procedure would allow estimates of this latent variable to differ by question.

THE PARTIAL CREDIT MODEL

A second model that is often used in the analysis of ordinal data is the partial credit model from Item

Figure 55.3 Predicted versus true cut-points: ordered probit for main question

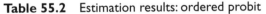

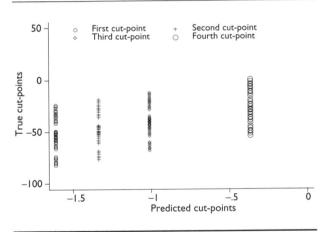

Figure 55.4 Predicted versus true mobility: ordered probit for main question

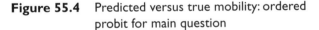

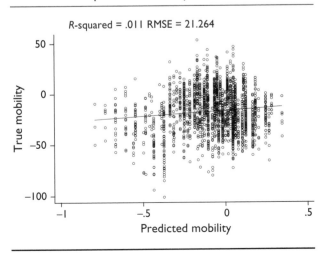

Table 55.2 Estimation results: ordered probit

Variable	Coefficient	(Std. Err.)
Age 30–44	–0.079	(0.065)
Age 45–59	–0.166	(0.077)
Age 60+	–0.498	(0.088)
Male	–0.062	(0.053)
$1 < \text{Educ} \leq 6$	0.124	(0.091)
$6 < \text{Educ} \leq 11$	0.245	(0.096)
$\text{Educ} > 11$	0.344	(0.113)
Country B	–0.232	(0.056)
τ^1	–1.612	(0.102)
τ^2	–1.335	(0.100)
τ^3	–1.010	(0.098)
τ^4	–0.365	(0.096)

Response Theory. This is basically a polytomous extension of the binary-response Rasch model $(10–12).$[4] Suppose there are N respondents, each answering J questions on a given domain. Individual $i=1,...,N$ chooses response category $k=1,...,5$ for question $j=1,...,J$. The partial credit model conceptualizes the ordinal nature of the categorical data as a series of dichotomies or "steps."[5] These dichotomies are modelled such that the probability that a respondent chooses response category k, given the choice between response category k or $k-1$, is:

$$\phi_{ij}^k = \frac{\Pr(y_{ij}=k)}{\Pr(y_{ij}=k-1)+\Pr(y_{ij}=k)} = \frac{\exp(\beta_i-\delta_j^k)}{1+\exp(\beta_i-\delta_j^k)}$$

Here, $\Pr(y_{ij}=k)$ is the probability that individual i responds in category k for question j, and ϕ_{ijk} is the corresponding probability of responding in category k conditional on responding either in category $k-1$ or k. β_i is the "ability" of individual i, and δ_j^k is the "difficulty" associated with the k-th step in question j. In other words, the probability of responding in category k, conditional on responding either in category $k-1$ or k, is modelled as a positive function of a person's ability and a negative function of the difficulty for the question category. Making use of the condition that the probabilities of responding in a category must sum to 1 across all five categories for each individual i and question j, i.e.

$$\Pr(y_{ij}=1)+\Pr(y_{ij}=2)+\Pr(y_{ij}=3)+\Pr(y_{ij}=4)+\Pr(y_{ij}=5)=1,$$

a general expression for the probability of respond-ing in the k-th category (where $k=1,...,5$) can be derived:

$$\Pr(y_{ij}=k) = \frac{\exp[(k-1)\beta_i-\sum_{m=0}^{k-1}\delta_j^m]}{\sum_{s=1}^{5}\exp[(k-1)\beta_i-\sum_{m=0}^{s-1}\delta_j^m]}$$

where, for notational convenience, $\sum_{m=0}^{0}\delta_j^0 \equiv 0$. For the case of five categories, the probabilities of responding in each category can be written as:

$$\Pr(y_{ij}=k) = \begin{cases} 1/A, & k=1 \\ \exp(\beta_i-\delta_j^1)/A, & k=2 \\ \exp(2\beta_i-\delta_j^1-\delta_j^2)/A, & k=3 \\ \exp(3\beta_i-\delta_j^1-\delta_j^2-\delta_j^3)/A, & k=4 \\ \exp(4\beta_i-\delta_j^1-\delta_j^2-\delta_j^3-\delta_j^4)/A, & k=5, \end{cases} \quad [2]$$

where A is the expression:

$$A \equiv 1+\exp(\beta_i-\delta_j^1)+\exp(2\beta_i-\delta_j^1-\delta_j^2) \\ +\exp(3\beta_i-\delta_j^1-\delta_j^2-\delta_j^3)+\exp(4\beta_i-\delta_j^1-\delta_j^2-\delta_j^3-\delta_j^4)$$

For a fixed number of questions, the unconditional estimation of the likelihood function yields difficulty parameters that are inconsistent $(10;15)$. Consistent estimates of the difficulty parameters can be obtained by conditioning on the raw score (i.e. on the sum of responses across questions for each individual). So, for example, the conditional probability that a person responds in category 2 for all 3 questions is calculated as the joint probability divided by the probability of getting a raw score r of 6 across the questions:

$$\frac{\Pr(y_{i1}=2)\Pr(y_{i2}=2)\Pr(y_{i3}=2)}{\Pr(r=6)}$$

The likelihood written in this manner is free of the ability parameter β. Once the difficulty parameters have been estimated using the conditional approach, estimates of β_r can be obtained using the unconditional likelihood derived from:

$$\Pr(y_{ij}=k) = \begin{cases} 1/A, & k=1 \\ \exp(\beta_r-\hat{\delta}_j^1)/A, & k=2 \\ \exp(2\beta_r-\hat{\delta}_j^1-\hat{\delta}_j^2)/A, & k=3 \\ \exp(3\beta_r-\hat{\delta}_j^1-\hat{\delta}_j^2-\hat{\delta}_j^3)/A, & k=4 \\ \exp(4\beta_r-\hat{\delta}_j^1-\hat{\delta}_j^2-\hat{\delta}_j^3-\hat{\delta}_j^4)/A, & k=5, \end{cases}$$

The notation changes to β_r because this method requires only one estimate of ability for every possible raw score of responses across all questions.

In the partial credit model, the difficulty param-eters are points on the latent variable scale where the

Figure 55.5 Predicted probabilities: ordered probit for main question

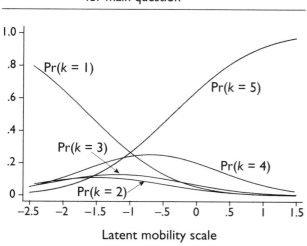

Latent mobility scale

probabilities of responding in one category or the next are equal. Alternatively, the difficulty parameters are points where the probability of responding in category k, conditional on responding in categories $k-1$ or k, is 0.5. The ability parameters can be thought of as estimates of the individual's underlying latent variable. The estimates of ability levels can be compared to true mobility for the simulated data to assess the performance of this model. This simple version of the partial credit model assumes that the difficulty parameters do not vary by socio-demographic characteristics which—in the language of psychometrics—is akin to saying that it assumes there is no "differential item functioning."

Table 55.3 reports the difficulty parameters for the simulated data obtained by running the conditional likelihood procedure in Stata (for identification, δ^1 is set to zero for the main question).[6] Figure 55.6 plots the estimated ability parameters versus the true mobility. As with the ordered probit model, Figure 55.7 reports the predicted probabilities from the model for given values of ability. The predicted probabilities are quite similar to those that are predicted by the ordered probit model (Figure 55.1). As the value of the latent variable increases, the probability of responding in the lowest category becomes small and the probability of responding in higher categories increases.

The partial credit model does better than the ordered probit model in predicting the true level of mobility. The R-squared value is much higher than that of the ordered probit model. However, the comparison between the two models is not entirely fair

since we only use one question for the ordered probit model and all three questions in the partial credit model.

In the formulation introduced here, the partial credit model uses no extraneous information (i.e. covariates such as sex, age, and education) in the estimation of the abilities. In the next subsection, we present an alternative specification of the model that includes covariates.

The Partial Credit Model with Covariates

The partial credit model can be reformulated so that instead of having a dummy variable per individual β_i, variables such as age, sex, education, and country of residence can be introduced. Such a modification

Figure 55.6   Predicted versus true mobility: two-stage partial credit

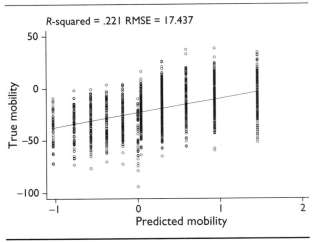

Table 55.3   Estimation results: two-stage partial credit

Variable	Coefficient	(Std. Err.)
δ^1		
Dummy Aux 1	0.207	(0.183)
Dummy Aux 2	1.615	(0.178)
δ^2		
Dummy Aux 1	0.225	(0.186)
Dummy Aux 2	0.723	(0.183)
Main question	−0.795	(0.267)
δ^3		
Dummy Aux 1	1.277	(0.154)
Dummy Aux 2	1.797	(0.151)
Main question	−0.933	(0.187)
δ^4		
Dummy Aux 1	−1.267	(0.110)
Dummy Aux 2	1.291	(0.131)
Main question	−0.544	(0.175)

Figure 55.7   Predicted probabilities: two-stage partial credit for main question

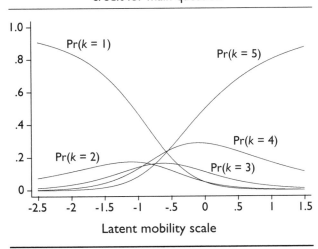

to the partial credit model is especially useful in the analysis of health survey data given that socio-demographic variables are usually collected in such surveys. Equation [2] with covariates can be written as the probability that individual i responds in category k for each of the questions j, conditional on a vector of covariates Z_i:

$$\Pr(y_{ij}=k) = \begin{cases} 1/A, & k=1 \\ \exp(Z_i'-\delta_j^1)/A, & k=2 \\ \exp(2Z_i'-\delta_j^1-\delta_j^2)/A, & k=3 \\ \exp(3Z_i'-\delta_j^1-\delta_j^2-\delta_j^3)/A, & k=4 \\ \exp(4Z_i'-\delta_j^1-\delta_j^2-\delta_j^3-\delta_j^4)/A, & k=5, \end{cases} \quad [3]$$

where A is the expression:

$$A \equiv 1 + \exp(Z_i'\beta-\delta_j^1) + \exp(2Z_i'\beta-\delta_j^1-\delta_j^2) \\ + \exp(3Z_i'\beta-\delta_j^1-\delta_j^2-\delta_j^3) \\ + \exp(4Z_i'\beta-\delta_j^1-\delta_j^2-\delta_j^3-\delta_j^4)$$

Assuming independence across observations and questions, estimates can be computed using maximum likelihood. The mean predicted level of mobility versus truth is plotted in Figure 55.8 and the estimates are in Table 55.4.

The mean level of the estimated latent variable that is plotted in Figure 55.8 does not account for the fact that the deterministic variation in the latent variable will be imperfectly captured by the limited set of included covariates. In the absence of a random effect, the model will overestimate the amount of stochastic variability in the data. The next subsection introduces a method for accounting for this by using Bayes' Theorem to estimate the predicted mobility.

RANDOM EFFECTS AND LATENT VARIABLE ESTIMATION USING BAYES' THEOREM

If there is an individual-level random effect in the data—i.e. when covariates in our model do not capture all the systematic variation in the latent variable—then there remains information content in the set of responses across questions for each individual that has not been fully exploited. The partial credit model with covariates *and* a random effect v_i with mean zero and variance σ_v^2 can be written out as follows:

$$\Pr(y_{ij}=k) = \begin{cases} 1/A, & k=1 \\ \exp[(Z_i'\beta+v_i)-\delta_j^1]/A, & k=2 \\ \exp[2(Z_i'\beta+v_i)-\delta_j^1-\delta_j^2]/A, & k=3 \\ \exp[3(Z_i'\beta+v_i)-\delta_j^1-\delta_j^2-\delta_j^3]/A, & k=4 \\ \exp[4(Z_i'\beta+v_i)-\delta_j^1-\delta_j^2-\delta_j^3-\delta_j^4]/A, & k=5, \end{cases} \quad [4]$$

where A is the expression:

$$A \equiv 1 + \exp[(Z_i'\beta+v_i)-\delta_j^1] + \exp[2(Z_i'\beta+v_i)-\delta_j^1-\delta_j^2] \\ + \exp[3(Z_i'\beta+v_i)-\delta_j^1-\delta_j^2-\delta_j^3] \\ + \exp[4(Z_i'\beta+v_i)-\delta_j^1-\delta_j^2-\delta_j^3-\delta_j^4]$$

Table 55.4 Estimation results: partial credit with covariates

Variable	Coefficient	(Std. Err.)
Mean		
Age 30–44	−0.134	(0.024)
Age 45–59	−0.203	(0.028)
Age 60+	−0.336	(0.032)
Male	−0.077	(0.019)
1 < Educ ≤ 6	0.049	(0.033)
6 < Educ ≤ 11	0.109	(0.034)
Educ > 11	0.160	(0.041)
Country B	−0.075	(0.020)
δ^1		
Dummy Aux 1	0.274	(0.185)
Dummy Aux 2	1.261	(0.163)
Main question	0.272	(0.144)
δ^2		
Dummy Aux 1	0.092	(0.185)
Dummy Aux 2	−0.076	(0.166)
Main question	−0.747	(0.140)
δ^3		
Dummy Aux 1	1.261	(0.151)
Dummy Aux 2	1.247	(0.126)
Main question	−1.124	(0.100)
δ^4		
Dummy Aux 1	−1.319	(0.109)
Dummy Aux 2	0.746	(0.099)
Main question	−1.202	(0.066)

Figure 55.8 Predicted versus true mobility: partial credit with covariates

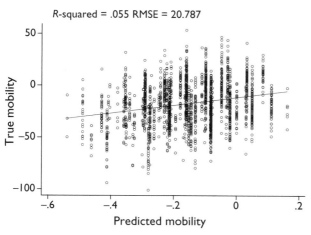

R-squared = .055 RMSE = 20.787

In order to exploit the information content in the set of responses, we can make use of Bayes' Theorem to obtain estimates of the mean level of mobility conditional of the observed set of responses. That is, we can estimate $\Pr(\mu_i \mid y_i)$ using Bayes' formula:

$$\Pr(\mu_i \mid y_i) = \frac{\Pr(\mu_i \mid y_i)\Pr(\mu_i)}{\int \Pr(\mu_i \mid y_i)\Pr(\mu_i)d\mu_i} \qquad [5]$$

where y_i represents the vector of categorical responses on all questions for individual i. The way this can be implemented is as follows. First, we use the model with a random effect and estimate all the parameters including the variance of the random effect. This estimate of the variance can be used to simulate 100 different values of μ_i around the predicted $Z_i'\beta$ of the latent variable for each individual in the sample. Hence, for each simulated value of μ_i, $\Pr(\mu_i)$ can be calculated. $\Pr(y_i \mid \mu_i)$ can be calculated using the probability specifications given in equation [4]. Integrating over all simulated values of μ_i for each individual gives us the denominator of equation [5].

In the absence of a model that estimates the variance of this individual-specific random effect, one can assume that the random effect captures about 50% of the variation in estimated variance of the error term. Under this assumption, the Bayesian predication of mobility conditional on the observed pattern of responses is plotted in Figure 55.9 for the partial credit model with covariates.[7]

It is quite remarkable that the Bayesian correction significantly improves the estimation of mobility (Figure 55.9) when compared with the estimation of abilities using the two-step conditional procedure for the partial credit model (Figure 55.6), as judged by the R-squared values. In other words, if the goal of the analyst is to estimate the underlying latent variable, then a modification of the partial credit model that allows for covariates and a random effect outperforms the simple version of the partial credit model.

Ordered Probit versus Partial Credit

We have introduced two basic types of models that are widely used in the analysis of categorical data, namely the ordered probit model and the partial credit model (with ability dummies and with covariates). Fundamentally, both models assume some sort of latent variable that gives rise to an observation mechanism governed by probabilities given in equations [1] and [2]. Viewed this way, the two models are quite similar, differing only with respect to the functional form for the data generating mechanism and in their approach to modelling the probabilities: these being derived from differences in the cumulative probability function for the ordered probit model versus the focus on adjacent categories in the partial credit model.

Apart from poor predictions of the underlying latent variable, both the ordered probit and the partial credit models suffer from the problem that one cannot allow the response category cut-points (τ's), or the so-called difficulty parameters (δ's), to be functions of the same covariates as the mean value of the latent variable. This is because there will be a clear identification problem if one does so: in the absence of additional exogenous information, neither model will be able to detect whether the effects of the covariates are on the mean value of the latent variable or on the cut-points or difficulties. This is easy to see from the equations for the predicted probabilities, equations [1] and [2]. This is likely to be a serious shortcoming of both models in estimating cross-population comparable differences in the latent variable of interest. In simple terms, these models do not allow for a world in which the Danish not only have a higher health status, but also have different expectations for their health status relative to Ethiopians.

In the next section, we introduce an innovation to both the ordered probit and partial credit models that allows for the introduction of exogenous information in the form of vignettes. Analysing the self-report questions in conjunction with responses to vignettes allows us to identify the model such that the same set of covariates can be used to assess differences in the

Figure 55.9   Predicted versus true mobility: partial credit with covariates (Bayesian)

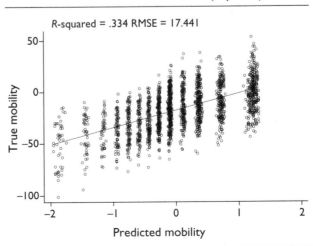

R-squared = .334 RMSE = 17.441

mean level of the underlying latent variable as well as in cut-points or difficulties.

VIGNETTES

We now introduce the use of vignettes as a means of correction of self-report responses in order to make them cross-population comparable. A vignette is a description of a concrete level of ability on a given domain that respondents are asked to evaluate with relation to the same main question and on the same categorical response scale as the main self-report question (16). The vignette fixes the level of ability such that variations in categorical responses are attributable to variations in response category cut-points. This introduction of exogenous information in the form of responses to vignettes allows us to identify the effects of a set of socio-demographic covariates (such as age, sex, education, country of residence, etc.) on both the level of the underlying latent variable that is being estimated as well as on the cut-points (in the ordered probit version of the model) and difficulties (in the partial credit version of the model).[8]

In the WHO Multi-country Survey Study, there are six vignettes for the domain of mobility, each designed to capture a different level of ability on this domain. The vignettes are:

Vignette 1: [Paul] is an active athlete who runs long distance races of 20 kilometres twice a week and engages in soccer with no problems.

Vignette 2: [Mary] has no problems with moving around or using her hands, arms and legs. She jogs 4 kilometres twice a week without any problems.

Vignette 3: [Rob] is able to walk distances of up to 200 metres without any problems but feels breathless after walking one kilometre or climbing up more than one flight of stairs. He has no problems with day-to-day physical activities, such as carrying food from the market.

Vignette 4: [Margaret] feels chest pain and gets breathless after walking distances of up to 200 metres, but is able to do so without assistance. Bending and lifting objects such as groceries produces pain.

Vignette 5: [Louis] is able to move his arms and legs, but requires assistance in standing up from a chair or walking around the house. Any bending is painful and lifting is impossible.

Vignette 6: [David] is paralysed from the neck down. He is confined to bed and must be fed and bathed by somebody else.

Respondents are asked to classify each of these vignettes on the same five-point response category scale as the main question. So, for each individual, we not only have categorical responses to their self-report main question and several auxiliary questions, but we also have their categorical responses to a set of vignettes (ranging in number from six to eight across the different domains for health and responsiveness in the WHO Multi-country Survey Study).

In order to introduce statistical models designed around the use of vignettes, we have extended the simulated dataset to include hypothetical ratings of seven mobility vignettes in countries A and B by assigning "true" mobility scores to the different vignettes and assuming that individuals will use the categorical response scale the same way in assessing vignettes as they do in assessing their own levels of mobility on the main question. This assumption is critical for the estimation of the models, as discussed below.

The simulated vignette ratings for the two countries are summarized in Figures 55.10 and 55.11. Each figure shows the distribution of categorical responses for the set of vignettes (lighter colours signifying worse responses). The vignettes are ranked from 1 to 7 in decreasing order of ability: i.e. vignette 1 refers to a higher level of mobility than vignette 2, vignette 3 is higher than vignette 2, and so on. From these figures, it is clear that there are important differences in the cut-points between country A and country B. At lower levels of mobility, respondents in country B are more likely to characterize a vignette unfavourably

Figure 55.10 Distribution of vignette responses for country A

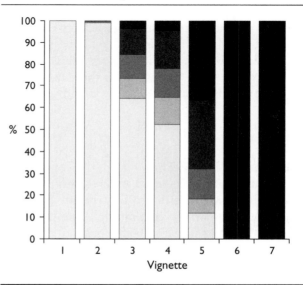

Figure 55.11 Distribution of vignette responses for country B

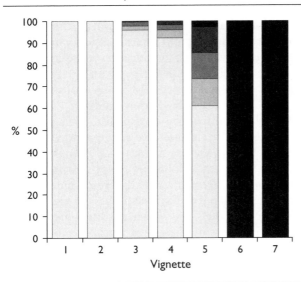

than respondents in country A. In addition, the compression of the middle categories in country B suggest cut-points that are more narrowly spaced than those in country A.

The types of variation in vignette ratings that we have generated in the simulated dataset closely parallel the variation observed in actual data from the WHO Multi-country Survey Study. In a later section, we show the response distributions for China versus those for India for mobility vignettes. In the following sections we describe how variants of the ordered probit model and partial credit model may be used in conjunction with vignette ratings in order to characterize these systematic cut-point differences more precisely. Both models are modified such that: a) information from responses to vignettes is introduced in the likelihood function, and b) cut-points and difficulties are allowed to be functions of the same covariates as those used in the estimation of the mean value of the latent variable.

HIERARCHICAL ORDERED PROBIT MODEL (HOPIT)

The hierarchical ordered probit (HOPIT) model is a modification of the standard ordered probit model described earlier. In order to incorporate information on vignette ratings and multiple questions, the expanded model has several components to the likelihood function: the first component refers to estimation of cut-points using responses to vignettes, and the second component utilizes responses on the self-

report main question. The remaining components are for auxiliary questions. In formal terms, the first component of the likelihood function assumes there is an unobserved latent variable $Y_{ij}^{v^*}$ distributed with mean μ_{ij}^v and variance 1. Here, i refers to the respondent, j refers to the vignette number, and the v superscript indicates that this refers to the vignette component of the model. In mathematical terms,

$$Y_{ij}^{v^*} \sim N(\mu_{ij}^v, 1), \; i = 1, \ldots, N; j = 1, \ldots, V$$

$$\mu_{ij}^v = J_i \alpha,$$

where J_i is a vector of indicator variables for each of $V-1$ vignettes. Letting y_{ij}^v denote the observed categorical response by individual i to vignette j, the observation mechanism is defined as follows:

$$y_{ij}^v = k \; \text{if} \; \tau_i^{k-1} \le Y_{ij}^{v^*} < \tau_i^k;$$
$$\text{for} \; \tau_i^0 = -\infty, \; \tau_i^5 = \infty, \; \forall \; i, j \; \& \; k = 1, \ldots, 5.$$

In addition, the cut-points are allowed to be functions of covariates (9):

$$\tau_i^k = X_i \gamma^k.$$

As before, $\tau_i^1 < \tau_i^2 < \tau_i^3 < \tau_i^4$.

The second component of the likelihood function utilizes information from the respondent's main self-report question (the one that is tied to the vignettes) and assumes there is an unobserved latent variable $Y_i^{s^*}$ distributed with mean μ_i^s and variance σ^2. Here, the s superscript indicates that this component refers to self-report questions. This formulation is slightly different from the standard ordered probit model: since we are allowing the vignettes to drive the cut-point estimation, this second component of the likelihood function has more in common with an interval regression model (i.e. an ordered probit model with known cut-points). Since the cut-point estimation is being driven by vignettes and the scale is set by the first estimation component, we are now able to obtain estimates of the variance of the latent variable (i.e. there is no need to set the variance equal to 1 as before). In mathematical terms, the model is:

$$Y_i^{s^*} \sim N(\mu_i^s, \sigma^2), \quad i = 1, \ldots, N$$

$$\mu_i^s = Z_i \beta.$$

Let y_i^s be the observed categorical responses on the self-report such that:

$$y_i^s = k \; \text{if} \; \tau_i^{k-1} \le Y_i^{s^*} < \tau_i^k;$$
$$\text{for} \; \tau_i^0 = -\infty, \; \tau_i^5 = \infty, \; \forall \; i \; \& \; k = 1, \ldots, 5$$

Similarly for the auxiliary questions, let a_i^j be the observed categorical responses on the j-th auxiliary question such that:

$$a_i^j = k, \text{ if } \tau_i^{j,k-1} \le Y_i^{s*} < \tau_i^{j,k};$$
$$\text{for } \tau_i^{j,0} = -\infty, \ \tau_i^{j,5} = \infty, \ \forall \ i \ \& \ k = 1,\dots,5$$

and

$$\tau_i^{j,k} = X_i \gamma^{j,k}$$

It is assumed that Y_i^{s*} & Y_i^{s*} are independent $\forall \ i = i$, conditional on X_i. Y_{ij}^{v*} & Y_i^{s*} are independent $\forall \ i,j$ conditional on X_i, J_i and Z_i. The probabilities associated with the observed responses to vignettes, the main question, and the auxiliary questions can be computed as in equation [1] with the adjustment for cut-point shifts being functions of covariates. The likelihood function can be written using these probabilities as three separate components. The three components of the likelihood function are additive in logs and can be jointly maximized to yield the parameter estimates. There is explicit parametric dependence between the different components of the likelihood function. The cut-points to be estimated from the vignettes component are the same as those in the main question component. In addition, μ_i^s is the same for both the main question and all the auxiliary questions. This ensures that the estimated cut-points for both the main question and the auxiliary questions are on the same scale to enable meaningful comparisons.

Tables 55.5 to 55.9 report the results of the estimation in Annex 55.1. Figure 55.12 plots the estimates of the mean level versus truth. The R-squared for the prediction has improved when compared with the simple ordered probit model as well as with the partial credit models with and without covariates. Figure 55.13 reports the true versus estimated cut-points for the main question. These differ by socio-demographic group in that they are also functions of the same covariates (age, sex, education, and country of residence) as the mean level of the mobility. As can be seen, the model is able to recover the cut-point differences quite well. Figures 55.14 and 55.15 report the comparison of estimated cut-points to truth for the two auxiliary questions. The recovery here is not quite as good as that for the main question. This is to be expected since the information in the vignettes is directly driving the main question cut-points, whereas the estimation of the cut-points for the auxiliary questions is more indirect and is not anchored to the cut-

Figure 55.13 Predicted versus true cut-points: HOPIT main question

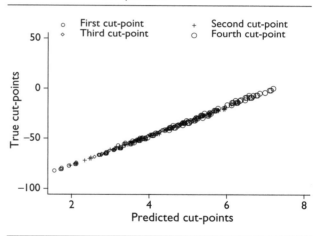

Figure 55.12 Predicted versus true mobility: HOPIT

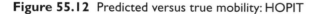
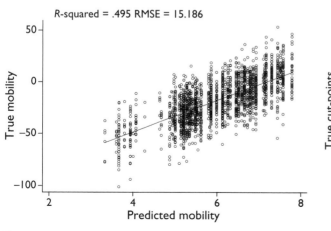

Figure 55.14 Predicted versus true cut-points: HOPIT auxiliary question 1

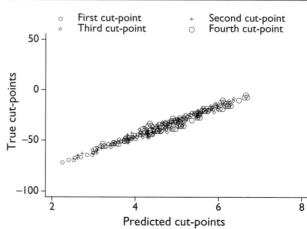

Figure 55.15 Predicted versus true cut-points: HOPIT auxiliary question 2

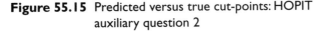
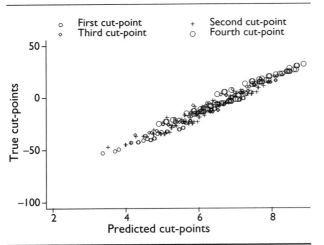

Figure 55.16 Predicted versus true mobility: HOPIT (Bayesian)

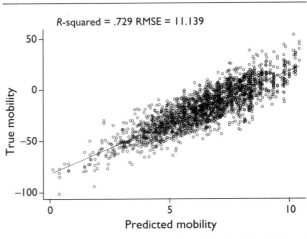

points derived from vignette responses. The estimation of the latent variable using Bayes' Theorem (Figure 55.16) improves the R-squared quite significantly, yielding estimates of mobility that are very close to the true mobility levels in the underlying simulated data.

HIERARCHICAL PARTIAL CREDIT MODEL

In analogy to the HOPIT model, we implement the use of vignettes in exactly the same way for the Rasch-based partial credit model. We allow for responses to vignettes to set the difficulty levels and estimate differences across socio-demographic groups in the first component of the likelihood function. In the other components of the likelihood, we utilize information from the main and auxiliary questions. The logic is the same as before: we are using information on difficulty parameters from responses on vignettes to allow us to have covariates that affect both the mean level of the estimated latent variable and the difficulty parameters. For all vignette questions, i.e. for $j=1,\dots,V$:

$$\Pr(y_i^v = k) = \begin{cases} 1/A, & k=1 \\ \exp(J_i'\alpha - \delta_i^1)/A, & k=2 \\ \exp(2J_i'\alpha - \delta_i^1 - \delta_i^2)/A, & k=3 \\ \exp(3J_i'\alpha - \delta_i^1 - \delta_i^2 - \delta_i^3)/A, & k=4 \\ \exp(4J_i'\alpha - \delta_i^1 - \delta_i^2 - \delta_i^3 - \delta_i^4)/A, & k=5, \end{cases} \quad [6]$$

where J_i is a vector of indicator variables for each of $V{-}1$ vignettes, and A is the expression:

$$A \equiv 1 + \exp(J_i'\alpha - \delta_i^1) + \exp(2J_i'\alpha - \delta_i^1 - \delta_i^2) \\ + \exp(3J_i'\alpha - \delta_i^1 - \delta_i^2 - \delta_i^3) \\ + \exp(4J_i'\alpha - \delta_i^1 - \delta_i^2 - \delta_i^3 - \delta_i^4)$$

and,

$$\delta_i^k = X_i'\beta^k$$

Similarly, the probabilities for the main question (the one which is tied to the vignettes):

$$\Pr(y_i^s = k) = \begin{cases} 1/A, & k=1 \\ \exp(Z_i'\beta - \delta_i^1)/A, & k=2 \\ \exp(2Z_i'\beta - \delta_i^1 - \delta_i^2)/A, & k=3 \\ \exp(3Z_i'\beta - \delta_i^1 - \delta_i^2 - \delta_i^3)/A, & k=4 \\ \exp(4Z_i'\beta - \delta_i^1 - \delta_i^2 - \delta_i^3 - \delta_i^4)/A, & k=5, \end{cases} \quad [7]$$

where Z_i is a vector of individual-level covariates, and A is the expression:

$$A \equiv 1 + \exp(Z_i'\beta - \delta_i^1) + \exp(2Z_i'\beta - \delta_i^1 - \delta_i^2) \\ + \exp(3Z_i'\beta - \delta_i^1 - \delta_i^2 - \delta_i^3) \\ + \exp(4Z_i'\beta - \delta_i^1 - \delta_i^2 - \delta_i^3 - \delta_i^4)$$

And for the j-th auxiliary question:

$$\Pr(y_{ij}^s = k) = \begin{cases} 1/A, & k=1 \\ \exp(Z_i'\beta - \delta_{ij}^1)/A, & k=2 \\ \exp(2Z_i'\beta - \delta_{ij}^1 - \delta_{ij}^2)/A, & k=3 \\ \exp(3Z_i'\beta - \delta_{ij}^1 - \delta_{ij}^2 - \delta_{ij}^3)/A, & k=4 \\ \exp(4Z_i'\beta - \delta_{ij}^1 - \delta_{ij}^2 - \delta_{ij}^3 - \delta_{ij}^4)/A, & k=5, \end{cases} \quad [8]$$

where Z_i is a vector of individual-level covariates, and A is the expression:

$$A \equiv 1 + \exp(Z_i'\beta - \delta_{ij}^1) + \exp(2Z_i'\beta - \delta_{ij}^1 - \delta_{ij}^2) \\ + \exp(3Z_i'\beta - \delta_{ij1}^1 - \delta_{ij2}^2 - \delta_{ij}^3) \\ + \exp(4Z_i'\beta - \delta_{ij}^1 - \delta_{ij}^2 - \delta_{ij}^3 - \delta_{ij}^4)$$

Tables 55.10 to 55.14 in Annex 55.1 report the results of this estimation. Figures 55.17 and 55.18 show the predicted mobility versus the true mobility before and after the Bayesian correction. The R-squared values obtained from the hierarchical ordered probit model for predicted mobility are similar in magnitude for the pre-Bayesian estimates obtained using the HOPIT model. The post-Bayesian estimation appears to be slightly higher for HOPIT than for the hierarchical partial credit model. This may result from the fact that the hierarchical partial credit model, in the way we have formulated it, does not estimate the variance of the stochastic term. This constraint will inhibit the model from fitting the data as well as it could if the variance were included as a parameter.

GOODNESS-OF-FIT

Assessing goodness-of-fit for categorical data is not straightforward. One can compute a simple count-R^2 which is a measure of the proportion of correct responses obtained for a given sample. For ordinal data, the predicted categorical response would be the one associated with the maximum predicted probability. Other options include a pseudo-R^2 measure, which in software such as Stata, is a likelihood-based comparison of the model with all the parameters to one with only the intercept (17). Rasch-based models use measures of fit such as "outfit" and "infit": "outfit" is a chi-square test based on the sum of the standardized deviation of observed versus expected values of a response. "Infit" is also a chi-square test which utilizes an information-weighted sum by adjusting for extreme responses using weights (18).

In order to assess model fit, a standard likelihood ratio test can be used. These tests compare the log-likelihood value of the full model with a constrained version of the same model (i.e. a model that is nested within the full model) to assess the contribution of the dropped covariates to the likelihood function. Assume L_0 is the log-likelihood value associated with the full model and L_1 is the log-likelihood value of the constrained model. Then $-2(L_1-L_0)$ is distributed χ^2 with d_0-d_1 degrees of freedom, where d_0 and d_1 are the model degrees of freedom associated with the full and the constrained models, respectively (17).

UNIDIMENSIONALITY

Both the HOPIT model and the Rasch-based models in IRT assume some form of unidimensionality. In formal terms, unidimensionality can be defined as the assumption that any dependence between different questions tapping into a given domain is solely due to the existence of a single underlying latent trait. Tests of unidimensionality are often based on uncovering this assumed factor that underlies observed responses to multiple questions. Mathematically, the assumption of unidimensionality can be worked out by assuming responses to all questions on a given domain are tapping this latent trait.

In the WHO Multi-country Survey Study, test-retest data are available from a subsample of respondents who were revisited and administered the survey questionnaire for a second time. This availability of test-retest data can be used to design a test of unidimensionality. Suppose we get latent variable estimates from two separate questions on any given domain, Y_1^* and Y_2^*. Each of these estimates of the latent variable

Figure 55.17 Predicted versus true mobility: partial credit model

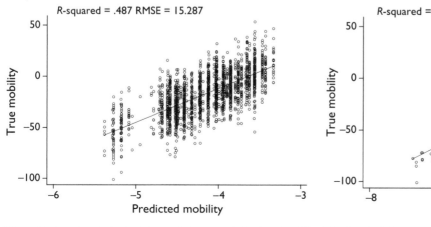

Figure 55.18 Predicted versus true mobility: partial credit model (Bayesian)

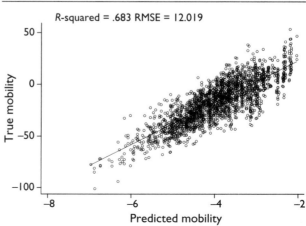

represents some measure of "truth" with error. That is, if truth were denoted by Y^*_{true}, then:

$$Y^*_{1test} = Y^*_{true} + \varepsilon_{1test}$$
$$Y^*_{1retest} = Y^*_{true} + \varepsilon_{1retest}$$

and

$$Y^*_{2test} = Y^*_{true} + \varepsilon_{2test}$$
$$Y^*_{2retest} = Y^*_{true} + \varepsilon_{2retest}$$

Here, ε_1 and ε_2 are the question-specific error terms for both test and retest questions, $\varepsilon_1 \sim N(0, \sigma^2_{\varepsilon 1})$, $\varepsilon_2 \sim N(0, \sigma^2_{\varepsilon 2})$. The correlation coefficient ρ between the measured Y^*'s is:

$$\rho = \frac{\mathrm{cov}(Y^*_1, Y^*_2)}{\sigma_{Y^*_1} \sigma_{Y^*_2}} \quad [9]$$

Rewriting [9],

$$\rho = \frac{\mathrm{cov}(Y^*_1, Y^*_2)}{\sigma_{Y^*_1} \sigma_{Y^*_2}} = \frac{\mathrm{cov}(Y^*_1, Y^*_2)}{\sqrt{\sigma^2_{Y^*_{true}} + \sigma^2_{\varepsilon_1}} \sqrt{\sigma^2_{Y^*_{true}} + \sigma^2_{\varepsilon_2}}} \quad [10]$$

Similarly,

$$\rho^* = \frac{\mathrm{cov}(Y^*_{true}, Y^*_{true})}{\sigma_{Y^*_{true}} \sigma_{Y^*_{true}}} \quad [11]$$

Dividing [11] by [10],

$$\frac{\rho^*}{\rho} = \frac{\sqrt{\sigma^2_{Y^*_{true}} + \sigma^2_{\varepsilon_1}} \sqrt{\sigma^2_{Y^*_{true}} + \sigma^2_{\varepsilon_2}}}{\sigma_{Y^*_{true}} \sigma_{Y^*_{true}}}$$

since $\mathrm{cov}(Y^*_1, Y^*_2) = \mathrm{cov}(Y^*_{true}, Y^*_{true})$ if the error terms are assumed to be uncorrelated. Therefore,

$$\rho^* = \sqrt{\frac{\sigma^2_{Y^*_{true}} + \sigma^2_{\varepsilon_1}}{\sigma^2_{Y^*_{true}}}} \cdot \sqrt{\frac{\sigma^2_{Y^*_{true}} + \sigma^2_{\varepsilon_2}}{\sigma^2_{Y^*_{true}}}} \cdot \rho = 1$$

where $\sigma^2_{\varepsilon_i} = \frac{\mathrm{var}(Y_{itest} - Y_{iretest})}{2}$ for $i = 1, 2$. Given that both $\sigma^2_{Y^*_{true}} = \mathrm{cov}(Y^*_1, Y^*_2)$ and ρ are observed, the above expression should equal 1. This can form the basis of a test of unidimensionality using information from test-retest data.

DISCUSSION

One of the key conclusions of this chapter is that adjustments are needed to make survey results comparable across populations. In particular, when cat-egorical variables are involved, analyses must account for differences in response category cut-points. There is considerable evidence suggesting that response category cut-points are different across countries. Therefore, until variation in cut-points is addressed, one must start from a presumption that results are not comparable across populations.

The problem of cross-population comparability also appears to apply within populations across different socioeconomic and demographic groups. This has important implications for the measurement of inequality, which may be greater or smaller than measured before taking into account response category cut-point shifts. It also has critical implications for comparisons over time. Cut-points may systematically shift over time (e.g. due to rising income, education, and health norms) so long-term trends may be difficult to assess without correction.

NOTES

1 The questions mirror those in the WHO Multi-country Survey Study on Health and Responsiveness 2000–2001.

2 In generating the categorical responses, a stochastic error term with variance ranging from 15 to 25 units was used (assumed different across questions, with auxiliary question 2 being the "noisiest" question).

3 Since the latent variable is unobserved, the variance of the latent variable, conditional on determinants, is arbitrarily set to 1 in the ordered probit model. In addition, in order to identify the model, the constant term is set to 0. These conventions produce a scale that is unique up to any positive affine transformation, i.e. the latent scale has so-called interval properties.

4 The Rasch model is a fixed-effect logit model and can also be reformulated as a quasi-symmetry loglinear model (13;14).

5 In this sense, the partial credit model can be viewed as an adjacent category logit model.

6 Estimates of the difficulty and ability parameters using Stata were of the same magnitude as those obtained using IRT software such as WINMIRA and RUMM.

7 We have developed working versions of the models with random effects. However, they are very slow to run and we are currently trying to improve the speed of estimation.

8 An alternative method to set a comparable scale such that response category cut-point differences can be recovered is to use measured tests.

REFERENCES

(1) Ware JE, Gandek B. Overview of the SF-36 health survey and the International Quality of Life Assessment (IQOLA) project. *Journal of Clinical Epidemiology*, 1998, 51(11): 903–912.

(2) Rabin R, deCharro F. EQ-5D: a measure of health status from the EuroQol Group. *Annals of Medicine*, 2001, 33: 337–343.

(3) Üstün TB et al. WHO Multi-country Survey Study on Health and Responsiveness 2000–2001. In: Murray CJL, Evans DB, eds. *Health systems performance assessment: debates, methods and empiricism*. Geneva, World Health Organization, 2003.

(4) Murray CJL et al. Cross-population comparability of evidence for health policy. In: Murray CJL, Evans DB, eds. *Health systems performance assessment: debates, methods and empiricism*. Geneva, World Health Organization, 2003.

(5) Mathers CD, Douglas RM. Measuring progress in population health and well-being. In: Eckersley R, ed. *Measuring progress: is life getting better?* Collingwood, CSIRO Publishing, 1998:125–155.

(6) Murray CJL. Epidemiology and morbidity transitions in India. In: DasGupta M, Chen LC, Krishnan TN, eds. *Health, poverty and development in India*. Delhi, Oxford University Press, 1996.

(7) van der Linden W, Hambleton RK, eds. *Handbook of modern item response theory*. New York, Springer-Verlag, 1997.

(8) Andrich D. *Rasch models for measurement*. Newbury Park, Sage Publications, 1988.

(9) Groot W. Adaptation and scale of reference bias in self-assessments of quality of life. *Journal of Health Economics*, 2000, 19:403–420.

(10) Masters GN. A Rasch model for partial credit scoring. *Psychometrika*, 1982, 47(2):149–174.

(11) Masters GN. A comparison of latent trait and latent class analyses of Likert-type data. *Psychometrika*, 1985, 50(1):69–82.

(12) Masters GN, Wright BD. The partial credit model. In: van der Linden W, Hambleton RK, eds. *Handbook of modern item response theory*. New York, Springer-Verlag, 1997.

(13) Tjur T. A connection between Rasch's item analysis model and a multiplicative Poisson model. *Scandinavian Journal of Statistics*, 1982, 9:23–30.

(14) Kelderman H. Loglinear Rasch model tests. *Psychometrika*, 1984, 49:223–245.

(15) Chamberlain G. Analysis of covariance with qualitative data. *Review of Economic Studies*, 1980, 47: 225–238.

(16) Salomon JA, Tandon A, Murray CJL. *Using vignettes to improve cross-population comparability of health surveys: concepts, design, and evaluation techniques*. EIP Discussion Paper No. 41. Geneva, World Health Organization, 2001. URL: http://www3.who.int/whosis/discussion_papers/discussion_papers.cfm#

(17) Long JS, Freese J. *Regression models for categorical dependent variables using Stata*. College Station, Stata Press, 2001.

(18) Wright BD, Mok M. Rasch models overview. *Journal of Applied Measurement*, 2000, 1(1):83–106.

Table 55.5 Estimation results: HOPIT

Variable	Coefficient	(Std. Err.)
Vignettes		
_Ivignette_2	−0.035	(0.146)
_Ivignette_3	−4.033	(0.117)
_Ivignette_4	−5.116	(0.122)
_Ivignette_5	−5.341	(0.123)
_Ivignette_6	−7.458	(0.175)
_Ivignette_7	−7.643	(0.195)
Mean		
Age 30-44	−0.488	(0.085)
Age 45-59	−0.715	(0.1)
Age 60+	−1.656	(0.113)
Male	0.174	(0.068)
1<Educ≤6	0.185	(0.115)
6<Educ≤11	0.332	(0.122)
Educ>11	0.521	(0.147)
Country B	0.996	(0.074)
Intercept	−2.985	(0.166)
log(s)	0.061	(0.043)

Table 55.6 Estimation results: HOPIT τ^1

Variable	Coefficient	(Std. Err.)
Main question		
Age 30–44	−0.504	(0.046)
Age 45–59	−0.569	(0.054)
Age 60+	−1.282	(0.062)
Male	0.25	(0.037)
1<Educ≤6	0.079	(0.061)
6<Educ≤11	0.072	(0.065)
Educ>11	0.129	(0.079)
Country B	1.296	(0.041)
Intercept	−4.662	(0.134)
Auxiliary question 1		
Age 30–44	−0.384	(0.132)
Age 45–59	−0.544	(0.156)
Age 60+	−1.172	(0.170)
Male	0.227	(0.106)
1<Educ≤6	0.056	(0.175)
6<Educ≤11	0.161	(0.185)
Educ>11	0.196	(0.227)
Country B	0.928	(0.113)
Intercept	−4.312	(0.223)
Auxiliary question 2		
Age 30–44	−0.099	(0.113)
Age 45–59	−0.159	(0.134)
Age 60+	−0.768	(0.155)
Male	0.464	(0.092)
1<Educ≤6	0.249	(0.157)
6<Educ≤11	0.242	(0.166)
Educ>11	0.395	(0.197)
Country B	1.260	(0.099)
Intercept	−3.777	(0.202)

Table 55.7 Estimation results: HOPIT τ^2

Variable	Coefficient	(Std. Err.)
Main question		
Age 30–44	−0.441	(0.048)
Age 45–59	−0.551	(0.056)
Age 60+	−1.283	(0.063)
Male	0.25	(0.038)
1<Educ≤6	0.053	(0.062)
6<Educ≤11	0.059	(0.066)
Educ>11	0.072	(0.081)
Country B	1.259	(0.043)
Intercept	−4.399	(0.134)
Auxiliary question 1		
Age 30–44	−0.356	(0.125)
Age 45–59	−0.402	(0.145)
Age 60+	−1.232	(0.164)
Male	0.271	(0.100)
1<Educ≤6	−0.117	(0.165)
6<Educ≤11	−0.005	(0.175)
Educ>11	0.104	(0.212)
Country B	0.839	(0.107)
Intercept	−3.922	(0.210)
Auxiliary question 2		
Age 30–44	−0.152	(0.112)
Age 45–59	−0.224	(0.133)
Age 60+	−0.845	(0.155)
Male	0.460	(0.092)
1<Educ≤6	0.324	(0.157)
6<Educ≤11	0.346	(0.165)
Educ>11	0.458	(0.196)
Country B	1.258	(0.098)
Intercept	−3.579	(0.201)

Table 55.8 Estimation results: HOPIT τ^3

Variable	Coefficient	(Std. Err.)
Main question		
Age 30–44	−0.395	(0.051)
Age 45–59	−0.537	(0.059)
Age 60+	−1.160	(0.065)
Male	0.227	(0.040)
1<Educ≤6	0.089	(0.065)
6<Educ≤11	0.079	(0.070)
Educ>11	0.136	(0.087)
Country B	1.252	(0.046)
Intercept	−4.074	(0.135)
Auxiliary question 1		
Age 30–44	−0.271	(0.118)
Age 45–59	−0.388	(0.138)
Age 60+	−1.262	(0.158)
Male	0.217	(0.095)
1<Educ≤6	−0.093	(0.159)
6<Educ≤11	0.031	(0.168)
Educ>11	0.073	(0.204)
Country B	0.836	(0.101)
Intercept	−3.611	(0.203)
Auxiliary question 2		
Age 30–44	−0.120	(0.113)
Age 45–59	−0.250	(0.136)
Age 60+	−0.883	(0.162)
Male	0.345	(0.093)
1<Educ≤6	0.206	(0.160)
6<Educ≤11	0.259	(0.168)
Educ>11	0.367	(0.200)
Country B	1.235	(0.100)
Intercept	−2.945	(0.203)

Table 55.9 Estimation results: HOPIT τ^4

Variable	Coefficient	(Std. Err.)
Main question		
Age 30–44	−0.371	(0.059)
Age 45–59	−0.526	(0.069)
Age 60+	−1.095	(0.074)
Male	0.188	(0.046)
1<Educ≤6	0.054	(0.076)
6<Educ≤11	0.090	(0.081)
Educ>11	0.199	(0.101)
Country B	1.223	(0.057)
Intercept	−3.364	(0.139)
Auxiliary question 1		
Age 30–44	−0.285	(0.115)
Age 45–59	−0.371	(0.135)
Age 60+	−1.263	(0.155)
Male	0.290	(0.093)
1<Educ≤6	0.004	(0.157)
6<Educ≤11	0.081	(0.166)
Educ>11	0.127	(0.200)
Country B	0.822	(0.100)
Intercept	−3.498	(0.201)
Auxiliary question 2		
Age 30–44	−0.097	(0.118)
Age 45–59	−0.221	(0.143)
Age 60+	−0.842	(0.178)
Male	0.371	(0.098)
1<Educ≤6	0.161	(0.170)
6<Educ≤11	0.118	(0.178)
Educ>11	0.339	(0.212)
Country B	1.263	(0.106)
Intercept	−2.461	(0.212)

Table 55.10 Estimation results: hierarchical partial credit

Variable	Coefficient	(Std. Err.)
Vignettes		
_Ivignette_2	−0.181	(0.349)
_Ivignette_3	−4.975	(0.264)
_Ivignette_4	−5.665	(0.265)
_Ivignette_5	−5.809	(0.265)
_Ivignette_6	−8.535	(0.362)
_Ivignette_7	−8.814	(0.394)
Mean		
Age 30–44	−0.29	(0.066)
Age 45–59	−0.461	(0.074)
Age 60+	−1.052	(0.079)
Male	0.096	(0.051)
1<Educ≤6	0.108	(0.082)
6<Educ≤11	0.198	(0.088)
Educ>11	0.333	(0.111)
Country B	0.563	(0.056)
Intercept	−4.327	(0.277)

Table 55.11 Estimation results: hierarchical partial credit δ^1

Variable	Coefficient	(Std. Err.)
Main question		
Age 30–44	−0.708	(0.126)
Age 45–59	−0.614	(0.151)
Age 60+	−1.196	(0.176)
Male	0.233	(0.100)
1<Educ≤6	0.177	(0.161)
6<Educ≤11	0.150	(0.171)
Educ>11	0.394	(0.223)
Country B	1.383	(0.110)
Intercept	−3.664	(0.316)
Auxiliary question 1		
Age 30–44	−0.306	(0.326)
Age 45–59	−0.910	(0.352)
Age 60+	−0.515	(0.427)
Male	−0.034	(0.251)
1<Educ≤6	0.558	(0.363)
6<Educ≤11	0.669	(0.395)
Educ>11	0.429	(0.502)
Country B	0.827	(0.266)
Intercept	−3.961	(0.481)
Auxiliary question 2		
Age 30–44	0.225	(0.215)
Age 45–59	0.222	(0.258)
Age 60+	0.022	(0.320)
Male	0.339	(0.179)
1<Educ≤6	−0.161	(0.346)
6<Educ≤11	−0.322	(0.357)
Educ>11	−0.017	(0.419)
Country B	0.799	(0.188)
Intercept	−3.038	(0.446)

Table 55.12 Estimation results: hierarchical partial credit δ^2

Variable	Coefficient	(Std. Err.)
Main question		
Age 30–44	−0.042	(0.158)
Age 45–59	−0.188	(0.187)
Age 60+	−0.841	(0.204)
Male	0.175	(0.123)
1<Educ≤6	−0.153	(0.199)
6<Educ≤11	−0.082	(0.213)
Educ>11	−0.330	(0.273)
Country B	0.396	(0.135)
Intercept	−5.569	(0.341)
Auxiliary question 1		
Age 30–44	−0.477	(0.333)
Age 45–59	−0.037	(0.365)
Age 60+	−0.998	(0.466)
Male	0.455	(0.260)
1<Educ≤6	−0.451	(0.383)
6<Educ≤11	−0.402	(0.416)
Educ>11	0.258	(0.532)
Country B	0.300	(0.275)
Intercept	−4.512	(0.497)
Auxiliary question 2		
Age 30–44	−0.486	(0.235)
Age 45–59	−0.558	(0.287)
Age 60+	−1.111	(0.366)
Male	0.408	(0.198)
1<Educ≤6	0.649	(0.370)
6<Educ≤11	0.754	(0.383)
Educ>11	0.693	(0.452)
Country B	0.688	(0.209)
Intercept	−5.606	(0.464)

Table 55.13 Estimation results: hierarchical partial credit δ^3

Variable	Coefficient	(Std. Err.)
Main question		
Age 30–44	−0.195	(0.134)
Age 45–59	−0.331	(0.156)
Age 60+	−0.529	(0.159)
Male	0.143	(0.102)
1<Educ≤6	0.195	(0.168)
6<Educ≤11	0.076	(0.180)
Educ>11	0.161	(0.224)
Country B	0.775	(0.114)
Intercept	−5.62	(0.322)
Auxiliary question 1		
Age 30–44	−0.014	(0.304)
Age 45–59	−0.449	(0.350)
Age 60+	−1.168	(0.417)
Male	−0.414	(0.244)
1<Educ≤6	−0.504	(0.444)
6<Educ≤11	−0.289	(0.468)
Educ>11	−0.423	(0.572)
Country B	0.556	(0.235)
Intercept	−3.342	(0.545)
Auxiliary question 2		
Age 30–44	−0.089	(0.205)
Age 45–59	−0.354	(0.253)
Age 60+	−0.855	(0.329)
Male	−0.150	(0.175)
1<Educ≤6	−0.044	(0.288)
6<Educ≤11	0.289	(0.306)
Educ>11	0.156	(0.359)
Country B	0.512	(0.184)
Intercept	−4.00	(0.398)

Table 55.14 Estimation results: hierarchical partial credit δ^4

Variable	Coefficient	(Std. Err.)
Main question		
Age 30–44	−0.167	(0.110)
Age 45–59	−0.286	(0.127)
Age 60+	−0.526	(0.133)
Male	0.044	(0.085)
1<Educ≤6	−0.069	(0.139)
6<Educ≤11	−0.002	(0.148)
Educ>11	0.101	(0.186)
Country B	0.665	(0.096)
Intercept	−5.130	(0.298)
Auxiliary question 1		
Age 30–44	−0.086	(0.243)
Age 45–59	−0.005	(0.274)
Age 60+	−0.588	(0.321)
Male	0.536	(0.196)
1<Educ≤6	0.497	(0.379)
6<Educ≤11	0.396	(0.397)
Educ>11	0.365	(0.466)
Country B	0.343	(0.203)
Intercept	−7.336	(0.482)
Auxiliary question 2		
Age 30–44	0.060	(0.198)
Age 45–59	0.023	(0.249)
Age 60+	−0.386	(0.347)
Male	0.308	(0.171)
1<Educ≤6	0.028	(0.291)
6<Educ≤11	−0.293	(0.307)
Educ>11	0.133	(0.359)
Country B	0.856	(0.181)
Intercept	−4.947	(0.397)

Chapter 56

Estimating Permanent Income Using Indicator Variables

Brodie D. Ferguson, Ajay Tandon, Emmanuela Gakidou, Christopher J.L. Murray

Introduction

The empirical examination of the impact of economic and social policy on the objective of poverty alleviation—especially at the micro level—requires appropriate instruments and other mechanisms to measure poverty. This has become especially relevant in recent years given the increasing use of household survey data in research. Although economists have traditionally relied on reported income and expenditure as the preferred indicators of poverty and living standards, the use of such indicators is problematic. Not only does their measurement require lengthy modules and detailed questions which are not practical for household surveys with other priorities such as health, but the data resulting from such modules are fraught with substantial measurement error and are subject to systematic reporting biases (1). For these reasons, a number of analysts have developed methods to estimate household wealth or permanent income using information on the ownership of selected assets or on the use of certain services that correlate with permanent income. In addition to being consistent with a broader definition of poverty which has become increasingly prominent, such indices have enabled the analysis of poverty and inequality using otherwise rich household surveys that do not include income or expenditure modules. Such methods have been applied using the Demographic and Health Surveys (DHS) which provide consistent instruments and sampling frames, as well as information on durable goods and dwelling characteristics (2–4).

Often developed by means of principal components or factor analysis, these asset and permanent income indices have a number of limitations. First, if the principal components or factor analysis is performed on a country by country basis using data from different survey instruments, it is not possible to compare the results across countries. An index of household wealth estimated in such a manner can neither be compared across populations nor over a period of time in the same population. Even when the same survey instrument is used, the tendency to acquire an asset such as a boat or air conditioning unit is certain to differ among households of different cultural backgrounds living in different environments. Similarly, supply and demand for assets such as electronic devices can change rapidly in the same setting over even a few years time, rendering inter-temporal comparisons invalid. Second, principal components and factor analysis do not provide information on the level of income at which different assets or goods and services will be purchased. Finally, these two approaches do not provide prospective guidance on the best assets or goods and services to include in future surveys in order to obtain more refined estimates of household permanent income.

In this chapter, we use a dichotomous variant of the hierarchical ordered probit (DIHOPIT) model to develop an indicator of permanent income using household survey data from Greece, Peru, and Pakistan. The HOPIT model was originally developed to enhance the cross-population comparability of self-report survey data (5). We apply the model in order to estimate the cut-points for different indicator variables for each of the three surveys, which are combined with the household's responses to each question to calculate an estimate of permanent income for that household. We then validate these estimates against reported household income and expenditure. Further analysis will demonstrate that the permanent income for each household can be estimated using different subsets of indicators and that systematic analysis of the indicator variable cut-points will enable more parsimonious design of future questionnaires. Only those indicators that are relevant for mapping the range of permanent income for a given country need then be included in the survey questionnaire.

BACKGROUND

Modelling unobservables, such as permanent income and permanent consumption, is a long-standing issue in economics and econometrics. Friedman's permanent income hypothesis states that consumption is a function of permanent income. The central argument is that consumption decisions are made in a forward-looking manner and that current (measured) income is a poor determinant of consumption patterns (6). This, combined with the fact that observed income shows considerable measurement error and is a poor proxy of permanent income since it does not incorporate expectations, has spawned a large literature on the measurement of permanent income. Though permanent income is not directly observable, there is general agreement that it is determined by physical and human resources, such as property, education or experience which enable income generation. Standard economic theory would argue for specifications in which permanent income (Y) is a function of household characteristics, education, the stock of physical assets, and community and environmental characteristics (7). For a variety of reasons, such definitions cannot be used to derive estimates of permanent income in cross-country settings. Arguably, one problem is that the stock of physical assets is not simply a causal determinant of permanent income, but rather also an observed indicator of permanent income. This is especially true in less-developed economies characterized by poorly developed financial sectors, which makes household physical asset ownership more of a correlate of permanent income than a determinant. A second problem is that the same bundle of physical assets may map to different levels of permanent income in different countries. Due to norms, expectations, price distortion, and other environmental factors, the same level of permanent income in two countries may imply a different probability of ownership of any given physical asset. Hence, the use of physical asset ownership as a determinant of permanent income may lead to estimates that are simply not comparable across populations.

Due to the abundance of household survey data on asset ownership and the considerable biases and measurement error associated with reported income, a substantial literature has developed on asset-based measures of income. Several approaches, ranging from very simple to fairly complex, have been employed to approximate permanent income using asset, housing quality and other indicators from household surveys that do not include information on income or expenditure. One of the more simple approaches is that utilized by Townsend (8) who proposes a set of five simple indicators to distinguish among households: the ratio of household rooms to persons; car ownership; number of economically active persons seeking work; children aged 5 to 15 who receive school meals free, and number of times the household experienced disconnection of electricity in the previous 12 months. Townsend finds a high consistency of ranking across these five indicators. Another approach by Montgomery et al. (9) aims to control for the effect of permanent income by including a series of separate indicator variables for durable goods and housing quality measures in a multivariate regression. While this method allows the researcher to test whether consumption's effect on the dependent variable is statistically different from zero, it is not possible to isolate the direct effect of each indicator variable on the dependent variable from its indirect effect through household income.

Adams et al. (10) and Takasaki et al. (11) adopt and validate a qualitative approach for stratifying households into wealth groups. Their method, consistent with the general approach known as Rapid Rural Appraisal (RRA), involves training interviewers in wealth ranking who then assign households to a wealth group according to pre-identified criteria. The key informant interviewers must reach consensus on the wealth group assigned to each household. The studies conclude that key informants can accurately differentiate households according to an array of culturally appropriate criteria of wealth. However, it is difficult to establish the content validity of the wealth ranking technique, as the extent to which one criterion might have predominated over others in the process of decision-making (i.e. implicit weighting of criteria) and the extent to which these wealth groups might be comparable across populations are unknown. A more common approach in the literature is to construct an index using the indicator variables available in a particular survey. The indices that have been proposed range from the seemingly simple to the computationally more complex. Muhuri (12) uses an indicator of whether the household owns at least one of five durable goods or receives remittances. Jensen (13) and Havanon et al. (14) construct indices by equally weighting items such as durable goods and housing quality variables. Several researchers have constructed an index based on the sum of the number of consumer durable goods and other indicator variables for land ownership, quality of drinking water, and sanitation facilities (15–18).

Additional approaches involve weighting the indicator variables used in the estimation of the index. Some researchers have tried to approximate household consumption using indices where each item owned by the household is weighted by its value (19); however, a significant limitation of this approach is that information on the value of indicator variables is not widely available from surveys or other sources of information. Layte et al. (20) have constructed a relative deprivation index in which each individual item is weighted by the proportion of households possessing that item in each country. As a consequence, not possessing an item is considered a more substantial deprivation in a country where a higher proportion of the population owns one. As pointed out by the authors, this relative deprivation index is not suitable for comparisons of absolute levels of deprivation across countries.

Similarly, Morris et al. (21) propose an index where they assign to each item in the list of assets (g) a weight equal to the reciprocal of the proportion of the households which own one or more of that item (w_g), then multiplying that weight by the number of units of asset g owned by the household (f_g), and summing the product over all possible assets. The resulting index proposed by Morris et al. for a household j would then be:

$$\text{score} = \sum_{g=1}^{G} f_{gj} w_g$$

In addition to the asset score, the total value of household assets owned can be calculated by summing—over all assets owned—the reported current values of those assets (V_g). This approach is based on the assumption that households with greater resources will purchase and own a greater number of durable goods. This weighting of the household assets assumes that households are progressively less likely to own a particular item the higher its monetary value, as pointed out by Morris et al. The authors also found that the household asset score is correlated highly with household asset values, indicating that the two measures classify households in a similar manner.

Principal components analysis and principal factors analysis are two methods which have been used to derive individual weights for items in the construction of a wealth index. The principal components analysis approach to deriving weights employed by Filmer and Pritchett has been widely used by the World Bank in their analyses of socioeconomic inequalities in health

based on the DHS surveys (22). Gakidou and King apply a similar approach based on principal factors analysis to the DHS in order to analyse the components of inequality in child survival (23). Sahn and Stifel also use factor analysis in their multi-country study of poverty in Africa, and note that there is a high rank correlation between the index created from this method and that resulting from principal components analysis (4). It is interesting to note that Bollen et al. (24) find that simple proxies, such as the sum of durable goods and housing quality indicators, perform almost as well as these more complex data reduction methods, and that indices incorporating information on asset values seem to perform worse. They also find that adding more consumer durable questions to the core set available in most surveys does not substantially improve the estimates of permanent income. Unfortunately these methods provide little guidance with respect to the number of questions which should be used, as well as how questions appropriate for a specific country might be selected.

In a subsequent section, we elaborate a model which combines information from indicator variables such as assets with other determinants to derive estimates of permanent income. The model assumes permanent income to be a function of household composition (such as household size and number of dependents), household characteristics (such as age and education of the household head), environmental factors (such as urban or rural residence), plus an unobserved component (or random effect) the magnitude of which is derived from the multiplicity of indicator variables available per household. Hence, the model uses information on asset ownership or access to services in order to estimate the magnitude of other unobserved factors that may help determine permanent income. Subsequently, using Bayes' Theorem, this information on the magnitude of unobserved determinants is incorporated to yield posterior estimates of permanent income. This approach builds on several of the existing measures mentioned earlier, such as the asset index proposed by Filmer and Pritchett. Analysis will show that the approach performs comparably with existing approaches, while offering the potential for substantially enhanced comparability across populations. A further advantage is the capability of achieving more parsimonious survey instruments and more refined estimates of permanent income through item reduction methods.

METHODS

The statistical model utilized in this analysis is developed in terms of a latent variable, y_i^*, which denotes the permanent income of household i. This variable is, by definition, unobserved. What is observed is a series of asset and other indicator variables for each household i. These dichotomous variables take the value of 0 if the household does not possess or have access to the good or service, and 1 if it does. Examples of these indicators include whether the household has a separate kitchen, hot running water, a television, an automobile, and so on. In addition, we utilize a series of socio-demographic covariates that are expected to be correlated with permanent income such as education, age, sex, household size, or the number of adults in the household. The model can be formulated in terms of the latent variable, along with an observation mechanism for each of the assets and indicator variables. In mathematical terms, we assume that the latent variable y_i^* is a function of a vector of covariates X_i', a household-level random effect v_i with mean 0 and variance σ_v^2 which captures other systematic unobserved factors that affect permanent income for a given household, plus an error term with mean 0 and variance set to 1. Since this is a latent variable model, the variance is unobserved, and the assumption of variance set to 1 is one of mathematical convenience. The coefficients on the covariates adjust in response to differences in variance of the error term in the underlying data generating mechanism.

$$y_i^* = X_i'\beta + v_i + \varepsilon_i \qquad i = 1,...,N$$
$$v_i \sim N(0,\sigma_v^2)$$
$$\varepsilon_i \sim N(0,1)$$

The observation mechanism is specified for each indicator variable $a = 1,..., A$ such that the indicator variable y_i^a:

$$y_i^a = 0 \quad \text{if} \quad -\infty < y_i^* \le \tau^a$$
$$y_i^a = 1 \quad \text{if} \quad \tau^a < y_i^* \le +\infty$$

where τ^a is an indicator-specific cut-point. The model specifies that there is some indicator-specific threshold τ^a such that a household is more likely to respond affirmatively than not when its permanent income exceeds this threshold. Figure 56.1 visualizes the model. The solid line on the left of the graph represents the latent variable, while the line to the right shows the estimated cut-points for certain indicators such as ownership of a car, television or bicycle, or having electricity in the

household. These indicator cut-points represent "ownership thresholds" on the underlying latent variable of permanent income.

Given this set-up, we can derive the probability of an affirmative response conditional on covariates as follows:

$$\Pr(y_i^1,...,y_i^A \mid X_i, v_i) = \prod_{a=1}^{A} [d_i^a \cdot \Pr(\tau^a < X_i'\beta + v_i + \varepsilon_i \le +\infty)$$
$$+ (1 - d_i^a) \cdot \Pr(-\infty < X_i'\beta + v_i + \varepsilon_i \le \tau^a)]$$

where $d_i^a = 0$ if $y_i^a = 0$ and $d_i^a = 1$ if $y_i^a = 1$ for all $a = 1,...,$ A. Given the normal distribution assumption for error term ε, this implies,

$$\Pr(y_i^1,...,y_i^A \mid X_i, v_i) = \prod_{a=1}^{A} [d_i^a \cdot \Phi(-\tau^a + X_i'\beta + v_i) + (1 - d_i^a)$$
$$\cdot \Phi(\tau^a - X_i'\beta - v_i)]$$

where $\Phi(\cdot)$ is the cumulative normal distribution. Conditioning out the random effect v_i, the probabilities can be written as:

$$\Pr(y_i^1,...,y_i^A \mid X_i) = \int_{-\infty}^{+\infty} \varphi(v_i) \left\{ \prod_{a=1}^{A} [d_i^a \cdot \Phi(-\tau^a + X_i'\beta + v_i) \right.$$
$$\left. + (1 - d_i^a) \cdot \Phi(\tau^a - X_i'\beta - v_i)] \right\} dv_i$$

where $\varphi(\cdot)$ is the normal probability density function. Rewriting, we have

$$\Pr(y_i^1,...,y_i^A \mid X_i) = \int_{-\infty}^{+\infty} \frac{e^{-v_i^2/2\sigma_v^2}}{\sqrt{2\pi\sigma_v^2}} \left\{ \prod_{a=1}^{A} [d_i^a \cdot \Phi(-\tau^a + X_i'\beta + v_i) \right.$$
$$\left. + (1 - d_i^a) \cdot \Phi(\tau^a - X_i'\beta - v_i)] \right\} dv_i$$

Figure 56.1 Hypothetical indicator cut-points on the permanent income latent variable

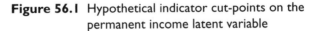

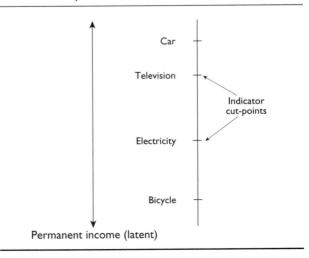

The integral can be approximated using M-point Gauss-Hermite quadrature,

$$\int_{-\infty}^{+\infty} e^{-x^2} f(x)dx \approx \sum_{m=1}^{M} \varpi_m^* f(a_m^*)$$

where the ϖ_m^* denote the quadrature weights and the a_m^* denote the quadrature abscissas. Estimation of parameters can be done using standard maximum likelihood methods. The likelihood is simply the product of all the individual probabilities since these are independent after conditioning on the covariates and the random effect.

If there is a household-level random effect in the data—i.e. when covariates in the model do not capture all the systematic variation in the latent variable permanent income—then there remains information content in the set of responses across indicators for each household that has not been fully exploited. In order to exploit the information content in the set of responses we can make use of Bayes' Theorem to obtain estimates of the mean level of permanent income conditional on the observed set of responses for a given household. Let $\mu_i \equiv X_i'\beta + v_i$ be the mean level of permanent income predicted by the model. Then $\Pr(\mu_i \mid y_i)$ can be estimated using Bayes' formula:

$$\Pr(\mu_i \mid y_i) = \frac{\Pr(y_i \mid \mu_i)\Pr(\mu_i)}{\int \Pr(y_i \mid \mu_i)\Pr(\mu_i)d\mu_i} \qquad [1]$$

where y_i represents the vector of categorical responses on all indicator questions for household i. The way this is implemented is as follows. First, using the model with the random effect, all parameters are estimated including the variance of the random effect σ_v^2. This estimate of the variance of the random effect is then used to simulate one hundred different values of μ_i around the predicted $X_i'\beta$ of the latent variable for each individual in the sample. Hence, for each simulated value of μ_i, $\Pr(\mu_i)$ can be calculated. $\Pr(y_i \mid \mu_i)$ can be derived using the probability specifications as elaborated earlier. Integrating over all simulated values of μ_i for each individual yields the denominator of equation [1].

We contrast the results obtained using the above model with those obtained by calculating a weighted index using principal components analysis (PCA). PCA is an exploratory multivariate statistical technique for simplifying complex datasets (25;26). The defining characteristic that distinguishes PCA from principal factors analysis is that in PCA it is assumed that all of the variability in an item should be used in the analysis, while in principal factors analysis the con-

cern is only the variability in an item which is shared with other items. The two methods generally yield similar results, but PCA is often preferred as a method for data reduction, while principal factors analysis is preferred where there is a need to detect structure. Given m observations on n variables, the goal of PCA is to reduce the dimensionality of the data matrix by finding r new variables, where r is less than n. Termed principal components, these new r variables together account for as much of the variance in the original n variables as possible while remaining mutually uncorrelated and orthogonal. Each principal component is a linear combination of the original variables, such that researchers often ascribe meaning to what the variables represent. PCA has been applied to asset questions in household surveys under the assumption that it is long-run wealth or permanent income that is the phenomenon attributable to the linear index of variables with the largest amount of information common to all of the variables. The result of such application of PCA is an asset index for each household according to the formula:

$$A_i = f_1(a_{i1} - a_1)/(s_1) + \ldots + f_N(a_{iA} - a_A)/(s_A)$$

where f_1 is the scoring factor for the first asset as determined by the procedure, a_{i1} is the i-th household's value for the first asset and a_i and s_i are the mean and standard deviation of the first asset variable over all households. In a subsequent section, we provide the results of our assessment of the degree of correlation of the PCA and latent variable approaches with reported household income and expenditure.

DATA

Data for this analysis come from nationally representative surveys carried out in three countries with considerably different socioeconomic characteristics: Greece, Peru, and Pakistan. The surveys were selected based on their inclusion of questions or modules on either income or expenditure, or both, as well as a number of indicator variables covering items such as household ownership of durable goods, characteristics of the neighbourhood and dwelling, and access to services such as water, sanitation, and electricity.

The data for Greece form part of the European Community Household Panel Survey (ECHP). In 1991, Eurostat, the Statistical Office of the European Communities, completed a comprehensive review of existing data on income at the household and individual levels among EU Member States. One of the outcomes of this review was the decision to launch the ECHP survey, which was intended to allow flexibility for adaptation to national specificities despite being designed centrally at Eurostat (27;28). The ECHP contains a wide range of comparable social statistics on income including social transfers, labour, poverty and social exclusion, housing and health, as well as several other indicators of living conditions. The longitudinal design of the ECHP (a total of three waves were carried out in 1994, 1995, and 1996) makes it possible to study relationships and transitions in these indicators over time at the micro level. A total of 16 countries participated in the ECHP, from which we have selected Greece for analysis. In addition to information on living conditions and durable goods, the ECHP data for Greece contain reported household income, which can be analysed for a particular household over the three-year period for approximately 4 400 households.

The data for Peru come from the National Living Standards Measurement Survey (LSMS) carried out in 2000, based on the methodology developed by the World Bank to measure the well-being and quality of life of households in developing countries. Six such surveys have been carried out in Peru: in 1985–86, 1991, 1994, 1996, 1997, as well as 2000. The most recent national LSMS collected data on the levels of education, health, labour activity, and migration for approximately 4 000 households, from which estimates of total household income and expenditure can be derived (29).

Data for Pakistan were collected through the 1991 Pakistan Integrated Household Survey (PIHS) which was conducted jointly by the Federal Bureau of Statistics (FBS), Government of Pakistan, and the World Bank (30). This nationwide survey gathered individual- and household-level data on topics including housing conditions, education, employment characteristics, health, consumption, and household energy consumption for approximately 4 800 households. Community-level and price data were also collected during the course of the survey, and estimates of total monthly income and expenditure have been calculated for each household.

EMPIRICAL ASSESSMENT

In this section, we validate the use of the DIHOPIT model to calculate an estimate of household permanent income in three different economic contexts: a high-income country, Greece, a low-income country,

Pakistan, and a middle-income country, Peru. Household surveys from these countries were selected because they included items on a range of consumer durables and household services or physical attributes, plus full-scale modules on income as well as modules on expenditure in the case of Pakistan and Peru (see Table 56.1 for a complete list of variables used). For each country, we have analysed the validity of the estimates of household permanent income through comparisons to reported income or expenditure of the household. For comparison, we have also examined the results of principal components analysis. As part of the analysis of the Peru household survey data, we demonstrate that reasonably comparable results for household permanent income can be obtained using two completely different sets of consumer durables or household services.

GREECE (ECHP, 1994–1996)

Household permanent income has been estimated for the ECHP sample for 1995 in Greece using responses for 23 different consumer durables, household services or household attributes. The ECHP dataset includes three waves for 1994, 1995, and 1996. Income between waves is highly correlated reflecting the combination of small measurement error and relatively stable income for most households. Reported income for 1995 has a correlation coefficient with the average for households over the three waves of 0.90. In the analysis below, we make use of the average reported income for the three waves of the panel as an indicator that is likely to be more highly correlated with permanent income than income reported in any one year.

Table 56.2 shows the output of the DIHOPIT model applied to the data for 4 413 households in Greece. For this initial assessment, we have omitted the covariates on the latent variable and used only the random effect outlined above. More specifically, the model we estimate is:

$$y_i^* = v_i + \varepsilon_i \qquad i = 1, \ldots, N$$
$$v_i \sim N(0, \sigma_v^2)$$
$$\varepsilon_i \sim N(0, 1)$$

The observation mechanism remains as described earlier. The cut-point on the latent variable of permanent income for each indicator variable was statistically significant for all except indicators 3 (indoor flushing toilet) and 12 (telephone). $\ln(\sigma_v)$ is the log of the estimated standard deviation of the household-level random effect. Figure 56.2 shows for Greece the

Table 56.1 Variables used in the estimation and validation of permanent income using DIHOPIT

Greece ECHP, 1994–1996	Pakistan IHS, 1991	Peru LSMS, 2000
Predictors		
Age of household head	Number of household adults	Age of household head
Employment of household head	Number of household children	Religion of household head
Medium education attainment	Literacy of household head	Ethnicity of household head
Higher education attainment	Numeracy of household head	Civil status of household head
Household size		Language of household head
Number of household adults		
Indicators		
Separate kitchen	Walls made of concrete material	Radio
Bath or shower	Finished floors	Colour television
Indoor flushing toilet	Covered windows	Blender or food processor
Hot running water	Private tap water	Refrigerator
Heating or storage heaters	Soak pit or better sanitation	Sewing machine
Place to sit outside	Open drains or better sanitation	Gas stove
Automobile	Underground drains	Record player
Colour television	Truck-collected garbage	Bicycle
Video recorder	Communal latrine or better toilet	Electric fan
Microwave oven	Private latrine or better toilet	Telephone (fixed-line)
Dishwasher	Private flush toilet	Telephone (mobile)
Telephone	Telephone	Washing machine
Second home	Household member worked abroad	Clothing dryer
Can afford keeping home warm	Electricity	Vacuum cleaner
Can afford annual holiday	Refrigerator	Videocassette recorder
Can afford replacing furniture	Freezer	Automobile
Can afford new clothes	Air conditioner	Therma
Can afford to eat meat often	Room heater	Personal computer
Number of rooms (dichotomized)	Water heater	Microwave oven
	Television	Knitting machine
	Sewing machine	Iron
	Gas stove	Cable television
	Cylinder gas stove	Company or business
	Does not own a kerosene lamp	Urban property
	Number of rooms (dichotomized)	
Validation		
Total household income, 1994	Total household income	Total household income
Total household income, 1995	Total household expenditure	Total household expenditure
Total household income, 1996		
Avg. total household income (1994–1996)		

name of each indicator variable on the latent variable at its estimated cut-point. The vertical line represents the permanent income latent variable, while the horizontal dashes are the estimated cut-points. These cut-points represent points on the underlying scale above which the household is more likely than not to respond affirmatively to the question regarding ownership of a good or access to a service. In other terms, if the predicted permanent income is greater than the cut-point for a given asset, then the probability that this household responds affirmatively is greater than 0.5. In Figure 56.2, we see that the cut-points for the number of rooms in the house increase with permanent income. Ownership of a dishwasher or microwave occurs at a higher level of household permanent income than a television or telephone. Living in a home with two rooms or less, having an indoor flush-

Table 56.2   Results of application of random-effect DIHOPIT to Greece ECHP, 1995

Variable	Coefficient	Std.Error
Cut-points		
Separate kitchen	−1.800	0.034
Bath or shower	−0.263	0.049
Indoor flushing toilet	−0.078	0.046
Hot running water	2.489	0.039
Heating or storage heaters	1.752	0.038
Place to sit outside	−0.188	0.047
Automobile	1.541	0.038
Colour television	0.113	0.044
Video recorder	2.182	0.039
Microwave oven	3.949	0.051
Dishwasher	3.036	0.042
Telephone	0.071	0.044
Second home	3.112	0.042
Afford keeping home warm	1.675	0.038
Afford annual holiday	2.018	0.039
Afford replacing furniture	2.823	0.041
Afford new clothes	1.277	0.039
Afford meat often	1.371	0.038
Home has 2+ rooms	−0.394	0.051
Home has 3+ rooms	1.010	0.039
Home has 4+ rooms	2.482	0.039
Home has 5+ rooms	3.601	0.046
Home has 6+ rooms	4.522	0.065
$\ln(\sigma_v)$	−0.450	0.027
rho	0.389	0.007

Figure 56.2   Indicator variable ladder for 23 indicators, Greece ECHP, 1995

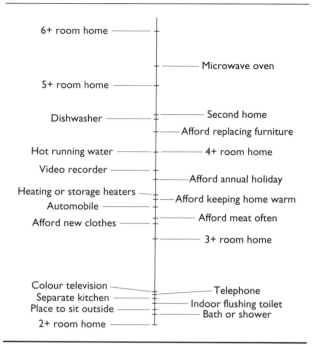

Table 56.3   Correlation of estimated permanent income with reported income measures, Greece ECHP, 1995

Variable	Pearson's r	Spearman's rho
Household income (1994)	0.50	0.61
Household income (1995)	0.57	0.65
Household income (1996)	0.55	0.62
Average household income (1994–1996)	0.60	0.67
Average household income per capita (1994–1996)	0.41	0.47
Average household income per adult equivalent (1994–1996)	0.56	0.63

ing toilet, having a bath or shower, and having a separate kitchen are relatively low on the indicator ladder.

The next step in this analysis is to validate the estimation of permanent income from the model. Using the ECHP data for Greece, this can be done by comparing the correlations of the estimated permanent income (using indicator responses from 1995) with household income for the individual years 1994–1996, as well as with the average household income over this period. Table 56.3 shows these correlations as well as the correlation of estimated permanent income with total household income per adult consumption equivalent and total household income per capita.

As can be seen from the table, the highest correlation of estimated permanent income with household income for any of the three individual years of data is 0.57 in 1995. If we instead compare the permanent income estimate with the average reported household income over the three-year period, the correlation improves to 0.60. In all cases, the rank (Spearman) correlation is considerably higher than the Pearson's correlation suggesting that the relationship between

estimated permanent income and reported household income is somewhat non-linear. The rather high degree of correlation between the permanent income estimate and reported household income, together with the observation that this correlation increases as income is averaged over a period of time, would support the assumption that it is permanent income or long-term wealth that is being measured. The higher correlation of estimated permanent income on the latent variable with household income rather than total household income per capita or per adult consumption equivalent confirms the theoretical premise of the model that consumer durables and household services are a function of household permanent income rather than attributes of particular individuals in the household.

It is also worth noting that the estimated cut-points are highly stable over the three years of data. The correlation of the indicator cut-points using data from 1994 with those using data from 1995 is 1.00, as is the correlation for estimates using data from the years 1995 and 1996. The correlation between estimates from 1994 and 1996 is 0.99. Another comparison of interest would be how well the DIHOPIT model performs relative to a similar and commonly used approach based on principal components analysis. The correlation coefficient and Spearman's rho values of the rank correlation between average reported income and the principal component analysis give nearly identical results, 0.61 and 0.68 respectively.

The results above were obtained from application of DIHOPIT without including any covariates on the latent variable, thereby allowing the random effect to capture as much of the systematic variance as possible. When additional variables such as age, employment status, educational attainment, and household size (see Table 56.1) are included as predictors, the resulting correlations of the estimated permanent income with reported income in 1995 or average income for 1994–1996 are only slightly improved. While the addition of such information presumably increases validity, the increase is so slight that the results can be interpreted as being basically robust to the specification of covariates on the latent variable.

Pakistan Integrated Household Survey, 1991

For the second validation study, we examine how estimates of permanent income based on the application of the DIHOPIT model function in a low-income setting. Household surveys in populations with lower levels of education, less formal sector employment and in some cases, less interaction with the monetized market often have much higher levels of measurement error, especially for reported income (31). The challenges of income and expenditure surveys are illustrated by the 1991 Pakistan Integrated Household Survey in which the correlation of reported income and expenditure was only 0.15. The Spearman's rho was 0.46 reflecting the non-linear relationship in the data between reported income and expenditure. Not surprisingly, average income was 94% of average reported expenditure. Given the presumed high level of measurement error in both reported income and expenditure, we would expect estimates of permanent income to have

lower correlations with these two variables than in Greece or Peru.

Table 56.4 provides the results from the application of random effect DIHOPIT without covariates on the latent variable for 4 752 households. We see that the cut-points are statistically significant for all 30 indicator variables on the latent variable permanent income. Figure 56.3 represents each consumer durable, household service or household attribute shown on the latent variable. In addition to the statistical significance of the cut-points, their ordering has face validity—households with low levels of permanent income are more likely to have a home with a soak pit or communal latrine than a private flush toilet. At the other end of the spectrum, only those households with the highest levels of permanent income in this

Table 56.4 Results of application of random-effect DIHOPIT to Pakistan IHS, 1991

Variable	Coefficient	Std.Error
Cut-points		
Walls made of concrete material	0.133	0.025
Finished floors	−0.072	0.030
Covered windows	−0.220	0.030
Home has 2+ rooms	−0.994	0.031
Home has 3+ rooms	0.289	0.030
Home has 4+ rooms	1.104	0.033
Home has 5+ rooms	1.773	0.038
Home has 6+ rooms	2.270	0.045
Home has 7+ rooms	2.701	0.055
Private tap water	0.388	0.030
Soak pit or better sanitation	−0.808	0.031
Open drains or better sanitation	−0.543	0.031
Underground drains	1.114	0.033
Garbage collected by truck	1.562	0.036
Private flush toilet	0.354	0.031
Private latrine	−0.585	0.031
Communal latrine	−0.708	0.031
Telephone	2.036	0.042
Household member has worked abroad	2.200	0.043
Electricity	−1.179	0.039
Refrigerator	1.201	0.034
Freezer	2.812	0.059
Air conditioner	2.630	0.054
Room heater	2.670	0.054
Water heater	3.346	0.084
Television	0.430	0.031
Sewing machine	2.451	0.049
Gas stove	1.210	0.034
Cylinder gas stove	1.866	0.038
Kerosene lamp (inverted)	0.400	0.030
$\ln(\sigma_v)$	−0.027	0.021
rho	0.493	0.005

Figure 56.3 Indicator variable ladder for 30 indicators, Pakistan IHS, 1991

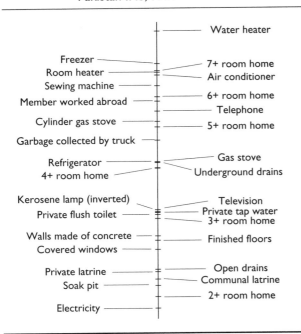

Table 56.5 Correlation of permanent income estimates with reported household income and expenditure, Pakistan IHS, 1991

Variable	Pearson's r	Spearman's rho
Household income	0.17	0.53
Household expenditure	0.33	0.53
Household income per capita	0.18	0.47
Household income per adult equivalent	0.18	0.52
Household expenditure per capita	0.30	0.43
Household expenditure per adult equivalent (1994–1996)	0.34	0.52

of household permanent income as covariates on the latent variable (see Table 56.1). As expected, the addition of covariates leads to a negligible increase in the Pearson's correlation of estimated permanent income and reported income and expenditure, equal to 0.17 and 0.34, respectively. In general, we believe that adding covariates related to permanent income to the model ought to improve estimation of household permanent income, but the improvement is relatively small in the cases we have investigated. Estimates of household permanent income or wealth using principal components analysis yield very similar correlation coefficients (0.16 for reported household income and 0.34 for total household expenditure). Both the DIHOPIT model and the PCA model in this case are capturing similar information about household permanent income or wealth.

survey are likely to have an air conditioner, freezer or telephone.

Table 56.5 provides a summary of the validation of the estimates of permanent income for Pakistan based on the application of the DIHOPIT model. The correlation with reported household income is 0.17 which is much lower than in Greece but consistent with the low correlation between reported income and expenditure. The relationship is quite non-linear so that the Spearman's rho for reported income and estimated permanent income is 0.53. Notably, estimated permanent income has a closer relationship to reported income than reported total household expenditure. Simultaneously, estimated permanent income has a correlation coefficient with total household expenditure of 0.33 and a Spearman's rho of 0.53. In other words, the estimated household permanent income is more closely related both to reported income and expenditure than they are to each other. This is consistent with a hypothesis that both are in truth related to permanent income but measured in the survey with substantial error. As for Greece, the results in Table 56.5 illustrate that the latent variable appears to be measuring household permanent income rather than permanent income per capita or per adult consumption equivalent.

As before, we have rerun the DIHOPIT model to determine the effect of including certain predictors

PERU LIVING STANDARDS MEASUREMENT SURVEY, 2000

Our final validation study included in this chapter is Peru. Income and expenditure in this LSMS survey are strongly related (correlation coefficient of 0.79), suggesting that there is a combination of more stable income for many households and lower levels of measurement error. Reported household income is 121% of total household expenditure on average. Table 56.6 shows the output of the model when applied without covariates to the Peru LSMS data using 24 indicator variables. The full list of indicator variables can also be found in Table 56.1 as well as in Figure 56.4, which shows the indicator variable ladder resulting from the cut-points predicted by the model.

Estimated permanent income using the DIHOPIT model (Table 56.7) demonstrates a strong relationship to reported income (correlation coefficient of 0.59) and to reported expenditure (correlation coefficient of 0.61). The corresponding Spearman's rho are 0.72 and 0.73 for income and expenditure respectively. Results

Table 56.6 Results of application of random-effect DIHOPIT to Peru LSMS, 2000

Variable	Coefficient	Std. Error
Cut-points		
Radio	−1.500	0.033
Colour television	1.660	0.037
Blender or food processor	1.601	0.037
Refrigerator	1.877	0.038
Sewing machine	2.197	0.038
Gas stove	1.603	0.037
Record player	2.590	0.040
Bicycle	2.315	0.038
Electric fan	2.939	0.042
Telephone (fixed line)	2.614	0.040
Telephone (mobile)	3.883	0.055
Washing machine	3.501	0.049
Clothing dryer	4.596	0.078
Vacuum cleaner	3.687	0.051
Video cassette recorder	3.274	0.046
Automobile	3.545	0.049
Therma	3.931	0.056
Personal computer	3.916	0.056
Microwave oven	4.076	0.060
Knitting machine	4.539	0.075
Iron	1.164	0.037
Cable television	4.128	0.060
Company or business	2.073	0.037
Urban property	0.847	0.037
$\ln(\sigma_v)$	−0.133	0.0028
rho	0.467	0.007

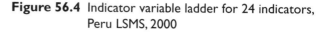

Figure 56.4 Indicator variable ladder for 24 indicators, Peru LSMS, 2000

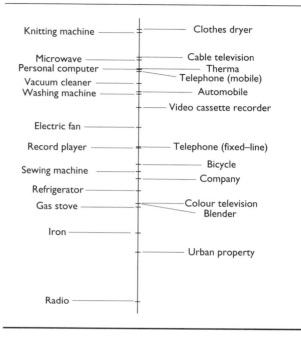

Table 56.7 Correlation of permanent income estimates with reported household income and expenditure, Peru LSMS, 2000

Variable	Pearson's r	Spearman's rho
Household income	0.59	0.72
Household expenditure	0.61	0.73
Household income per capita	0.52	0.69
Household income per adult equivalent	0.58	0.73
Household expenditure per capita	0.48	0.66
Household expenditure per adult equivalent (1994–1996)	0.59	0.73

from application of principal components analysis to the Peru dataset are again similar to the results using the DIHOPIT approach, with Spearman correlation coefficients of 0.72 for household income and 0.73 for household expenditure. The analysis for Peru has been rerun with covariates on the latent variable in addition to the household random effect. Results from this application of the model made no difference to the correlation of estimated permanent income with reported income or total household expenditure.

Using the Peru survey, we can illustrate one of the main advantages of this approach to the estimation of permanent income using indicator variables on ownership of consumer durables, household services and household attributes. From the 24 original indicator variables used, we have created two non-overlapping sets of 12. The two sets, shown in Table 56.8, have been created by assigning each indicator in an alternating fashion as one moves of the indicator ladder in Figure 56.4 to one group or the other. The DIHOPIT model has been rerun for each set of indicator variables separately as if only that set of variables was

available. The resulting estimates of household permanent income can be compared both to the original estimation using 24 indicator variables and to reported income and total household expenditure. Remarkably, both estimates based on only 12 indicator variables are highly correlated with the estimation based on 24 variables, with an average correlation coefficient of 0.94 for the two subsets. This underlines the potential to undertake item reduction in surveys and obtain similar estimates of household permanent income or wealth using many fewer variables. Table 56.9 shows that both sets of 12 indicator variables yield estimates of permanent income that are equally highly correlated with reported income and expenditure. In other words, estimates of household permanent income do not seem to be biased by the particular set of indicator variables used in the analysis. The combination of the potential for item reduction illustrated in moving from 24 indicators to 12 with minimal loss of information and the robustness of the estimation of permanent income to changing the set of indicator variables used provides substantial flexibility in both survey design and analysis.

DISCUSSION

This chapter has demonstrated the use of the DIHOPIT model to estimate permanent income from household surveys where information on dwelling characteristics, durable goods, and other indicator variables is routinely collected. The implications of this analysis are that with appropriate data, the indicator variables for a particular country can be mapped onto a latent variable which is a measure of permanent income. The model is able to identify indicator-specific points on the latent variable scale which mark the transition such that at values of the latent variable higher than the cut-point, the household is more likely to have access to the good or service than not. Given that we let the data tell us the extent to which any given indicator variable maps to the latent variable, one major advantage of this approach is that the set of indicator variables need not be the same across countries. Designers of future surveys can choose the most appropriate set of indicator variables based on this analysis to better understand the role of the indicator and its relation to permanent income in any given country. In this sense, the approach is analogous to adaptive testing in edu-

cational surveys where items are allowed to vary by specific criteria such as respondent ability.

In addition, our analysis shows that there is significant potential for item reduction in that similar results are obtained using fewer questions. This also has implications for questionnaire design: if preliminary analysis suggests that certain items are redundant—in that they do not have a significant marginal contribution in the (posterior) estimation of permanent income—then these items may be removed from future rounds of the survey. In the case of Peru, reduction of the number of indicator variables by half yields unbiased estimates of permanent income which show a high degree of correlation with those of the full set. It is likely that discrimination between the permanent income of different households depends on the location on the latent variable of the various indicator variables used. The high correlation achieved with two distinct sets of indicator variables may in part be due to the fact that each set of 12 was spaced from low levels of permanent income to high levels. This type of consideration will be important in the prospective design of surveys that want to include a short list of these indicator variables.

Furthermore, the comparison with estimates produced using principal components analysis shows that our approach is at least as good as this method in terms of estimating permanent income. Due to norms, price distortion and other factors, however, the same level of permanent income in two countries is likely to imply a different probability of ownership of any given physical asset. Hence, one of the key limitations of the principal components analysis approach is that use of physical asset ownership as a determinant of permanent income may lead to estimates which are not comparable across populations. This analysis has not explicitly addressed the problem of cross-population comparability; however, the DIHOPIT model used to estimate permanent income has the potential

Table 56.8   Item reduction subsets, Peru LSMS, 2000

Item subset #1	Item subset #2
Radio	Urban property
Iron	Blender or food processor
Gas stove	Colour television
Refrigerator	Company or business
Sewing machine	Bicycle
Record player	Telephone (fixed line)
Electric fan	Video cassette recorder
Washing machine	Automobile
Vacuum cleaner	Telephone (mobile)
Personal computer	Therma
Microwave oven	Cable television
Knitting machine	Clothing dryer

Table 56.9   Spearman rank correlation of permanent income estimated from indicator subsets with full-set permanent income, household income and household expenditure, Peru LSMS, 2000

Variable	Subset #1	Subset #2
Household income	0.67	0.66
Household expenditure	0.68	0.67
Estimated household permanent income (full set)	0.93	0.93

to be modified so that estimates of permanent income can be directly compared across countries. There are three possible paths that could be pursued to enhance the comparability of permanent income estimates: 1) an exogenous estimate of the average level (mean) and variance of the permanent income distribution by country can be used to adjust the latent scale of permanent income to a comparable scale across countries, in the units of income; 2) the level on the permanent income scale for two or more of the indicator variables can be fixed across countries; or 3) the cut-points on the permanent income scale for the indicator variables can be allowed to vary across socioeconomic variables but not across countries. Any of these three methods would place the permanent income estimates on the same scale across countries, thus enhancing the cross-population comparability of the estimates.

The approach proposed in this chapter is similar to previously proposed asset indices in that it has the potential to provide a more accurate measurement of permanent income than values of reported current income from survey questionnaires, as it is likely that the measurement error in these indicator variables is much less than the error associated with reported income. More research is required to further validate this approach in a larger number of countries, enhance the item-reduction analysis to define the optimal set of indicator questions to ask in each country, and finally to make estimates of permanent income directly comparable across countries.

REFERENCES

(1) Moore J, Stinson L, Welniak E. Income measurement error in surveys: a review. *Journal of Official Statistics*, 2000, 16(4):331–361.

(2) Filmer D, Pritchett L. Estimating wealth effects without expenditure data—or tears: an application to educational enrolments in states of India. *Demography*, 2001, 38:115–132.

(3) Hammer J. *Health outcomes across wealth groups in Brazil and India.* DECRG, Washington, DC, World Bank, 1998.

(4) Sahn D, Stifel D. Poverty comparisons over time and across countries in Africa. *World Development*, 2000, 28(1):2123–2155.

(5) Tandon A et al. Statistical models for enhancing cross-population comparability. In: Murray CJL, Evans DB, eds. *Health systems performance assessment: debates,*

methods and empiricism. Geneva, World Health Organization, 2003.

(6) Friedman M. *A theory of the consumption function.* Princeton, Princeton University Press, 1957.

(7) Singh I, Squire L, Strauss J. *Agricultural household models: extensions, applications and policy.* Baltimore, Johns Hopkins University Press, 1986.

(8) Townsend P, Simpson D, Tibbs N. Inequalities in health in the city of Bristol: a preliminary review of statistical evidence. *International Journal of Health Services*, 1985, 15(4):637–663.

(9) Montgomery M et al. Measuring living standards with proxy variables. *Demography*, 2000, 37(2):155–174.

(10) Adams A et al. Socioeconomic stratification by wealth ranking: is it valid? *World Development*, 1997, 25(7):1165–1172.

(11) Takasaki Y, Barham B, Goomes O. Rapid-rural appraisal in humid tropical forests: an asset possession-based approach and validation methods for wealth assessment among forest peasant households. *World Development*, 2000, 28(11):1961–1977.

(12) Muhuri P. Estimating seasonality effects on child mortality in Bangladesh. *Demography*, 1996, 33(1):98–110.

(13) Jensen E. The fertility impact of alternative family planning distribution channels in Indonesia. *Demography*, 1996, 33(2):153–165.

(14) Havanon N, Knodel J, Werasit S. The impact of family size on wealth accumulation in rural Thailand. *Population Studies*, 1992, 46:37–51.

(15) Guilkey D, Jayne S. Fertility transition in Zimbabwe: determinants of contraceptive use and method choice. *Population Studies*, 1997, 51(2):173–190.

(16) Bollen K, Guilkey D, Mroz T. Binary outcomes and endogenous explanatory variables—tests and solutions with an application to the demand for contraceptive use in Tunisia. *Demography*, 1995, 32(1):111–131.

(17) Gorabach P et al. Contraception and abortion in two Vietnamese communes. *American Journal of Public Health*, 1998, 88(4):660–663.

(18) Razzaque A et al. Sustained effects of the 1974–75 famine on infant and child mortality in rural area of Bangladesh. *Population Studies*, 1990, 44(1):145–54.

(19) Dargent-Molina P, et al. Association between maternal education and infant diarrhœa in different household and community environments. *Social Science & Medicine*, 1994, 38(2):343–350.

(20) Layte R et al. Persistent and consistent poverty in the 1994 and 1995 waves of the European Community Household Panel. *International Association for Research*

in Income and Wealth, New York. *Review of Income and Wealth*, 2001, 47(4).

(21) Morris S et al. Validity of rapid estimates of household wealth and income for health surveys in rural Africa. *Journal of Epidemiology and Community Health*, 2000, 54(5):381–387.

(22) World Bank. *Country reports on health, nutrition, population and poverty.* Washington, DC, World Bank, 2000. URL: http://www.worldbank.org/poverty/health/data/intro.htm

(23) Gakidou E, King G. Measuring total health inequality: adding individual variation to group-level differences. *International Journal for Equity in Health*, 2002, 1:3.

(24) Bollen K, Glanville J, Stecklov G. *Economic status proxies in studies of fertility in developing countries: does the measure matter?* MEASURE Evaluation Working Paper, WP-01-38. Chapel Hill, Carolina Population Center, 2001.

(25) Lawley D, Maxwell A. *Factor analysis as a statistical method.* London, Butterworth, 1971.

(26) Basilevsky A. *Statistical factor analysis and related methods: theory and applications.* New York, John Wiley & Sons, 1994.

(27) Eurostat. *European Community Household Panel (ECHP).* Volume 1—*Survey methodology and implementation.* Theme 3, Series E. Luxembourg, Eurostat, OPOCE, 1996.

(28) Eurostat. *European Community Household Panel (ECHP).* Volume 1—*Survey questionnaires: Waves 1–3.* Theme 3, Series E. Luxembourg, Eurostat, OPOCE, 1996.

(29) *Peru National Living Standards Measurement Survey (LSMS).* LSMS Data Manager, DECRG, Washington, DC, The World Bank, 2000.

(30) *Pakistan Integrated Household Survey (PIHS).* PIHS Section, Islamabad, Federal Bureau of Statistics, G-8 Markaz, 1991.

(31) Deaton A. *The analysis of household surveys: a microeconometric approach to development policy.* Baltimore, Johns Hopkins University Press, 1997.

Chapter 57

WHO Multi-country Survey Study on Health and Responsiveness 2000–2001

T. Bedirhan Üstün, Somnath Chatterji, Maria Villanueva, Lydia Bendib, Can Çelik, Ritu Sadana, Nicole B. Valentine, Juan Pablo Ortiz, Ajay Tandon, Joshua A. Salomon, Yang Cao, Wan Jun Xie, Emre Özaltin, Colin D. Mathers, Christopher J.L. Murray

Summary

In order to develop various methods of comparable data collection on health and health system responsiveness, WHO started a scientific survey study in 2000–2001. This study has used a common survey instrument in nationally representative populations with modular structure for assessing health of individuals in various domains, health system responsiveness, household health care expenditures, and additional modules in other areas such as adult mortality and health state valuations.

The health module of the survey instrument was based on selected domains of the International Classification of Functioning, Disability and Health (ICF) and was developed after a rigorous scientific review of various existing assessment instruments. The responsiveness module is the result of ongoing work over the past two years that has involved international consultations with experts and key informants and has been informed by the scientific literature and pilot studies. Questions on household expenditure and proportionate expenditure on health have been borrowed from existing surveys. The survey instrument has been developed in multiple languages using cognitive interviews and cultural applicability tests, stringent psychometric tests for reliability (i.e. test-retest reliability to demonstrate the stability of application), and most importantly, utilizing novel psychometric techniques for cross-population comparability.

The study was carried out in 61 countries completing 71 surveys. Two different modes were intentionally used for comparison purposes in 10 countries. Surveys were conducted in different modes: in-person household 90-minute interviews in 14 countries; brief face-to-face interviews in 27 countries; computerized telephone interviews in 2 countries; and postal surveys in 28 countries. All samples were selected from nationally representative sampling frames with a known probability so as to make estimates based on general population parameters.

The survey study tested novel techniques to control the reporting bias between different groups of people in various cultures or demographic groups (i.e. differential item functioning) so as to produce comparable estimates across populations. To achieve comparability, the self-reports of individuals of their own health were calibrated against well-known performance tests (i.e. self-report vision was measured against standard Snellen's visual acuity test), or against short descriptions in vignettes that marked known anchor points of difficulty (e.g. people with different levels of mobility such as a paraplegic person or an athlete who runs 4 km each day) so as to adjust the responses for comparability. The same method was also used for self-reports of responsiveness of their health systems, where vignettes on different responsiveness domains describing different levels of responsiveness were used to calibrate the individual responses.

These data are useful in their own right to standardize indicators for various domains of health (such as cognition, mobility, self-care, affect, usual activities, pain, social participation, etc.), but also provide a better measurement basis for assessing health of populations in a comparable manner. The data from the surveys can be fed into composite measures such as healthy life expectancy and improve the empirical data input for health information systems around the world. Data from the surveys are also useful to improve the measurement of the responsiveness of health systems to the legitimate expectations of the population.

INTRODUCTION

Countries need timely information on critical outcomes to evaluate their health policies, manage their health systems, and monitor progress. Routine health information systems are meant to provide affordable and timely information. In most developing countries, these have long focused on civil registration systems for vital events and registries of services delivered through publicly owned facilities. Developed and developing countries, however, have increasingly recognized the role of periodic household surveys to fill critical information gaps in the data provided by the health information system. The large number of general and specialized household surveys fielded in countries at all levels of development, used to measure child mortality, utilization, health financing, mental health, disease-specific outcomes etc., are an indication of the potential role of surveys in filling critical information gaps. In addition, information on aspects such as responsiveness of a health system is unavailable from health information systems and needs to be collected through surveys designed for this purpose.

Data from surveys in different countries, however, often have a serious problem of comparability. For example, responses of individuals vary by country or by population subgroups due not only to real differences in the quantity of interest, but also to differences in norms and expectations, or cognitive processing of survey questions. The general health reporting in EUROSTAT[1] surveys in 12 European countries has revealed a six-fold difference between the proportion of people reporting good or very good health in Denmark and Portugal. Similarly there is a four-fold difference between the proportion reporting bad or very bad health. This fact is not congruent with other health correlates like mortality or health service use and may create serious problems if such data are utilized as a basis for comparison across countries or population groups *(1–5)*. Such examples are manifold, indicating the need to improve the comparability of self-reported health data.

To obtain comparable data, it is essential to pay great attention to questionnaire development. This requires clarity in what is meant by the concept under measurement (e.g. what domains should be included) and its operationalization in a survey instrument (e.g. question wording, response categories, the meaning of responses, use of a comparator against which individuals report their experiences, translation protocols, and classical techniques for psychometric equivalence are all important). In addition, there is the need to control for possible "differential item functioning" which involves a shift in the response category cut-points between populations or subgroups. This occurs when people at similar levels of health give different answers to describe their health *(6)*.

In order to develop methods to gather comparable data across populations, WHO launched the WHO Multi-country Survey Study in 2000–2001 through a series of carefully designed steps. The study attempts to deal with the shortcomings in existing methods and to arrive at common instrument modules and techniques suited to multiple user needs to measure health system performance outcomes. The first step in the process was to review existing survey instruments and cultural comparison techniques. More than 300 international tools used in more than 50 countries were systematically reviewed to identify their items, their utility in survey conditions, and psychometric properties *(7)*. These included whether the questions were clear and unambiguous, if they were translated in a meaningful way, and whether they have an identically interpreted response scale, good test-retest reliability, and validity (e.g. concurrent validity with known reference tests or construct validity to predict other impacts). Where possible, we examined the calibration properties of different instruments using methods derived from Item Response Theory, which indicated whether different populations use similar cut-points in their rating of responses *(8)*. We then took into account well known sources of bias in questionnaires including "social desirability," "central tendency" (i.e. aversion to endpoints), and other framing effects such as the "halo effect," "carry-over effect," and "positive bias" (e.g. answers to questions are affected by other questions or by interview style) *(9)*.

It is clear that measurements of health and health-related parameters need to be applicable cross-culturally, reliable, calibrated for relevant response categories, and valid[2] *(10)*. However, these characteristics are not sufficient to ensure cross-population comparability. In addition to the classical psychometric criteria, to make meaningful international and cross-population comparisons, an instrument should have a common metric in different populations, i.e. the same response level should correspond to the same level of health (or responsiveness) in a given domain. Evidence of equivalent metric properties should be shown by external calibration tests and other possible mechanisms. Comparability of results adds a new dimension to international survey instrument development. The difference between comparability on the one hand, and validity and reliability on the other, can be illustrated with two thermometers, one of which measures temperature in Celsius, the other in Fahrenheit. Both thermometer measures give valid and reliable measurements of temperature. However, 26 degrees on one thermometer is not comparable to 26 degrees on the other.

Comparability is fundamental to the use of survey results for bench-marking and evaluation but has been under-emphasized in instrument development. WHO is trying to focus attention on the importance of comparability in instrument development. An example of a monitoring task that puts a premium on comparability and the gaps in existing health information systems is the comparative reporting by WHO of healthy life expectancy and responsiveness in *The World Health Report 2000 (11)*. Such comparative reporting highlights the need for valid, reliable, and comparable survey instruments to measure these outcomes. The list of outcomes for which valid, reliable, and comparable survey instruments are needed is not restricted to health state and responsiveness, but also includes coverage of critical health interventions, utilization of services, risk factors such as tobacco or alcohol use, and disease specific outcomes. Notably, instruments with established validity, reliability, and comparability (i.e. the generalizability of findings across diverse populations) are not widely available.

Though WHO has been, as part of its mandate, collecting systematic information with regard to causes of death and morbidity in its Member States around the world, more recently there has been a clear recognition that the impact of health conditions is perhaps better understood when non-fatal health outcomes are taken into account, over and above mortality. Health is an abstract and complex concept, yet there is an expectation that we all have an intuitive universal understanding of health. Moreover, our notion of well-being encompasses areas beyond health, and health is a fundamental human capacity that interacts with other areas of well-being. The challenge is to separate the constituents of a health experience that are intrinsically health from those that are non-health or health-related, in clear recognition of the fact that health experiences are not context-free *(12)*.

It is now recognized that building a scientific base to inform policies, strategies, and programmes is essential. In this context, WHO is operationalizing a framework for the measurement of health and the impact of all actions whose primary intent is to improve, restore or maintain health. To catalyze the development of valid, reliable, and comparable survey instruments to measure key outcomes, WHO launched the multi-country national household survey study in 2000–2001. The purpose of this paper is to report on the objectives, design, instrument development, and execution of this multi-country study.

OVERALL GOALS OF THE SURVEY STUDY

The WHO Multi-country Survey Study was a research exercise to develop instruments that would allow the measurement of health, responsiveness, and other health-related parameters in a comparable manner, and would provide useful information to refine this methodology. The Study focused on the way populations report their health and value different health states, the reported responsiveness of health systems, and the modes and extent of payment for health encounters through a nationally representative general population-based survey.

The WHO Multi-country Survey Study had as its first objective the *assessment of health* in different domains using self-reports by people in the general population. The International Classification of Diseases (ICD) was used as the framework to gather information on mortality in the households and self-reported morbidity (such as the diagnosis of depression, alcohol-related problems, and other chronic health conditions) *(13)*, and the revised International Classification of Functioning, Disability and Health (ICF) was used to describe the essential elements of non-fatal health outcomes *(14)*. The survey also included vignettes and some measured tests on selected domains, intended to calibrate the way respondents categorized their own health. This part of the survey allowed for direct comparisons of the health of different populations across countries.

A related objective of the WHO survey was to measure the value that individuals assign to descriptions of health states and to test if these varied across settings. These health states were described as decrements in major domains of body functions and activities. This allows the construction of summary measures of population health taking into account both fatal and non-fatal health outcomes.

The second overall objective of the WHO Multi-country Survey Study was to test instruments to measure the *responsiveness of health systems*. The concept of responsiveness is different from people's satisfaction with the care they receive, in that it examines what actually happens when the system comes in contact with an individual. It includes two major categories:

respect for persons, which comprises the respect for the dignity of the individual, confidentiality, communication, and autonomy; and client orientation, which consists of prompt attention, amenities of adequate quality, access to social support networks, and the choice of institution and care provider.

Additionally, the WHO Study aimed to test instruments in areas such as health expenditures, adult mortality, birth history, various risk factors, and assessment of main chronic health conditions with additional modules.

Specific Aims of the WHO Multi-country Survey Study

More specifically, the aims of the WHO Multi-country Survey Study were to:

- Develop valid, reliable, and comparable instruments to describe individual health states and health system responsiveness on a core set of domains, and to test these in household surveys.

- Test the validity of different modes of survey implementation including long-form household, short-form household, self-administered postal, and computer-assisted telephone interview.

- Contribute to the development of WHO's and Member States' capacity to field surveys with quality control, appropriate sampling, and data management strategies, as well as to build capacity to analyse data from complex surveys.

- Address critical methodological issues related to: identifying the most parsimonious set of questions that would suffice to adequately measure the health of a population in an efficient and cost-effective manner; and maintaining cross-population comparability.

- Test other candidate modules including adult mortality and health expenditure.

The focus of the current survey study has been to collect data in different modes across the world on a core set of health domains as well as on domains related to responsiveness. This is superior to analysing existing data sets that have been collected in different parts of the world using a range of methods (4). The survey study achieves a better representation of multiple dimensions of health and health systems, and obtains comparable data across countries. One basic objective is to systematically address issues related to the most parsimonious set of questions that could

adequately measure the health of a population and the responsiveness of a health system in an efficient and cost-effective manner, and maintain cross-population comparability.

The Specific Aim of Cross-Population Comparability

There is sufficient evidence indicating that self-reports on health (or responsiveness or other quantities of interest) may not be comparable across countries or even across different socioeconomic subgroups within a population (6). The problem of comparability can be conceptualized in terms of response category cut-point shifts. Even when reliability and within population validity have been well-established, the meaning that different groups attach to the labels used for each of the response categories in self-reported questions can vary greatly (Figure 57.1).

For each domain, there is some "latent scale" for that domain that represents the true level, which by definition is unobserved. For example, let us assume that there is an underlying health domain for "mobility" and we attempt to assess mobility by asking respondents how much difficulty they have climbing stairs. For this self-reported survey question, the response categories are labelled by order of difficulty as "no difficulty," "mild difficulty," "moderate difficulty," "severe difficulty," and "extreme/cannot do," and A, B, and C represent three different populations. When different individuals respond as "mild difficulty" in climbing stairs, the response could indeed map to different levels of mobility in different populations (e.g. from climbing a few steps to a few flights of stairs depending on their norms). The survey results

Figure 57.1   Response category shift — different rulers

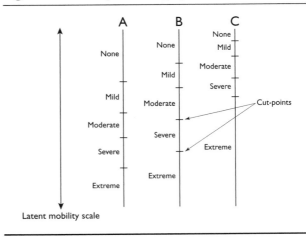

would be reliable and valid within each population but the results cannot be compared across populations without adjustment.

We hypothesize that cut-points vary between populations because of different cultural or other expectations. Cut-points are also likely to vary within cultural, socio-demographic or other groups within populations: the cut-points for older individuals may shift as their expectations for a health domain diminish with age; men may be more likely to deny declines in health so that their cut-points may be systematically shifted as compared to women; contact with health services may influence expectations for a domain and thus shift cut-points.

Comparable measurement of individual and population health, or any other such quantity that is assessed through self-reports (e.g. responsiveness), therefore, requires explicit strategies to measure the response category cut-points of each item in different populations and socio-demographic groups. Methods to establish cut-points fall into two basic categories:

■ a scale that is strictly comparable across individuals and populations is established and measurements on this comparable scale are used to establish the response category cut-points for each survey item; or

■ categorical responses are obtained from different groups for a fixed level on the latent scale. If the level is fixed, variation in the responses provides information on the differences in cut-points across individuals and populations.

A comparable scale of measurement can be achieved in two different ways:

■ when a domain is measured using multiple items, the underlying factor in the data may be, under certain assumptions, comparable; or

■ when a measured test—such as a Snellen's eye chart for vision or the posturo-locomotion-manual (PLM) test for mobility—can be used to establish a comparable scale. However, for some domains of health such as pain, reliable and valid measured tests may not exist or be affordable, or may even be unethical.

An alternative strategy for establishing cross-population comparability is to fix the level on a given domain and assess variation in the response categories across individuals, groups, and populations. In other words, if the level of mobility is fixed but one group gives the response category of "no difficulty"

while another gives the response category of "some difficulty," that information can be used to assess the response category cut-points. The same strategy can be used to assess notions such as dignity or promptness of attention where the responses may range from "very good" to "very bad." Two ways of evaluating a fixed level comparisons and thus variation in cut-points, are available: *vignettes* and assessment of *comparable homogeneous groups*.

A *vignette* is a description of a concrete level of ability on a given domain that individuals are asked to evaluate. To assess the response category cut-points, each respondent is asked to assess the level for a hypothetical case described in a vignette. The vignette fixes a given level in the domain of interest such that variation in the response categories is attributable to variation in the response category cut-points. Vignettes fix the level on a domain and only cut-points need to be estimated.

Comparable homogeneous groups in different populations are used for comparing responses to an item. For example, for health states, recent acute changes in health from injuries such as fractures might be used to identify reasonably comparable groups. Alternatively, some lifestyle or occupational characteristic might be used to identify these groups, such as a group of elite athletes. Similarly for responsiveness, all attendees at a given facility can be asked about their experience, for example, of prompt attention or dignity with an assumption that the facility treats all users belonging to a homogenous population (as defined by ethnicity, income, etc.) in more or less the same way.

The comparable homogenous group approach has limitations for two reasons. First, identification of the groups needs to be independent of any measurement of health status. Even when groups are identified through some factor such as an injury, doubts can always be raised as to the true comparability of groups. In the same way, one can well imagine that a given facility indeed treats people belonging to different categories such as income or ethnic groups differently. It may be difficult to persuade people that apparent differences in the responses are due to cut-point shifts as opposed to true differences in that domain between groups. Second, to be able to assess variation in response category cut-points for all response categories, a series of homogeneous groups must be used. Analytically, each homogeneous group is like one vignette. This means that the comparable group strategy can only work if several comparable groups are studied. Despite these limitations, it may be worthwhile assessing comparable groups as an adjunct to other methods.

The current set of surveys uses the vignette and measured test approach to calibrate self-report on health domains and the vignette approach alone for the responsiveness domains in order to make cross-population comparable analyses (6).

DEVELOPMENT AND CONTENT OF THE SURVEY INSTRUMENT

HEALTH MODULE SELECTION OF HEALTH DOMAINS

In preparation for the module on health in the WHO Multi-country Survey Study, an extensive review of existing instruments was carried out. This review was closely synchronized with the revision of the International Classification of Functioning, Disability and Health (ICF), which is a classificatory framework for components of health. ICF describes health and health-related domains (14). An item pool was constructed and the published psychometric properties of each question documented. Qualitative research identified the core constructs in different countries (7). In addition, the health section of the interview was presented to a WHO Committee of Experts that met in Geneva in August and September 2000. This list of domains was then presented to a group of experts in the measurement of health from all WHO regions at a UN/OECD meeting in Ottawa in October 2000. From the above item pool and based on the qualitative research, the health domain questions were selected according to the following criteria:

- they should be linked to a conceptual framework of the ICF;

- they should have face and construct validity, i.e. they must be linked to the intuitive, clinical, and epidemiological concepts of health; and together the questions should be comprehensive enough to reflect major health conditions;

- they should be amenable to self report;

- they should build on the existing knowledge base of common questionnaires;

- they should be cross-population comparable; and

- it should be possible for some domains to be linked to a calibration test.

The domains included in the WHO Survey Instrument are listed in Table 57.1.

FORMULATION OF QUESTIONS

Based on the selected health domains, the questions were chosen with reference to existing survey research instruments mainly from the work based on the WHO Disability Assessment Schedule (WHO-DAS II). The following guidelines were used in the construction of the health module for achieving reliable and valid assessment of health in different populations:

- Clear and unambiguous questions to allow for similar cognitive processing by the respondents, translation across different languages, and application in different cultures.

  The language of the questions in the survey was intentionally chosen to reflect the "extent of difficulty" actually experienced by the individual in carrying out the tasks or actions. Further, the questions were framed so that the response categories were uniform and the referents used were as concrete as possible (e.g. how much difficulty do you have in seeing and recognizing a person across the road, i.e. from a distance of about 20 meters?).

- Reliable recall period used as a timeframe.

  For the purposes of this survey, a period of one month was chosen, as recall is known to rapidly deteriorate beyond this period.

- Basic test-retest reliability as proof of consistent application.

  Questions that have earlier been demonstrated to have good reliability were preferred.

Table 57.1   Assessment instrument domains

Health domains	Health-related domains
Vision	Self-care: daily activities including eating
Hearing	Usual activities: household activities;
Speech	work or school activities
Digestion	Social functioning: interpersonal relations
Bodily excretion	Participation: societal participation
Fertility	including discrimination and stigma
Sexual activity	
Skin and disfigurement	
Breathing	
Pain	
Affect	
Sleep	
Energy/vitality	
Cognition	
Communication	
Mobility and dexterity	

- Basic concurrent validity with known reference tests (or in-depth expert evaluations).

    There are limited data with regard to this area. However, wherever possible, questions that have been demonstrated to have good correlation with measured performance on tests for that domain were chosen.

- Construct validity to predict other impacts, consequences or determinants (e.g. such as outcomes, service use, costs or other known variables).

- Invariance in the measurement properties across different populations.

    Modern psychometric techniques such as Item Response Theory (IRT) provide tools to detect relative shifts in cut-points (8). Each item in a questionnaire can be examined by its difficulty and the respondents' ability. Such analysis may display the items that work similarly across groups and those that demonstrate differential item functioning (DIF). However, if all items suffer DIF in a systematic and correlated manner, usual IRT methods fail to identify this problem, because these models assume that cut-points on a scale are independent of each other and not a systematic function of the characteristics of individual respondents. Therefore, newer techniques using item response modelling approaches need to be developed to deal with response category cut-point shifts to make meaningful comparisons of data.[3]

OPERATIONALIZATION OF CROSS-POPULATION CRITERIA

The criteria above are necessary yet not sufficient for cross-population comparability. When systematic reporting biases occur (e.g. when poor people report their health to be better than the "truth" since they may have lower expectations, or in certain cultures where people report their health to be worse than the "truth" since reporting good health is thought to bring bad luck) some external mechanism must be found to get additional information that allows for making adjustments for these reporting biases. Specific approaches were used in the WHO Multi-country Survey Study to achieve cross-population calibration properties in different populations:

- *Calibration tests* for some of the key domains that summarize overall health, such as the domains of vision, cognition, and mobility, were selected. Tests for these domains were chosen as they are relatively easy to carry out in a large-scale survey setting, do not require very specialized interviewer training, are not dependent on equipment infrastructure, and have been used in other surveys comparing self-report with performance. For near and distant vision, standard vision charts that use symbols were chosen instead of letters in order to ensure applicability in illiterate populations. For cognition, standard tests of verbal fluency, immediate and delayed recall of a word list, and a cancellation task for attention were chosen. Finally, the posturo-loco-motion-manual task was chosen for mobility as a composite task involving different aspects of moving. These tests were discussed with international experts such as WHO's prevention of blindness programme, neuropsychologists, and movement experts from the NINDS, USA (15–19).

    Calibration tests are an objective measurement of what the survey questions basically intend to measure in different cultures, and can be used as a closer approximation of "truth." Performance on these allows one to adjust for biases in self-report. For example, the responses to the question on how well a person can see an object at arm's length can be calibrated against standard near vision tests.

- *Standard case vignettes* are well-described case stories with precise concrete levels of health status. They can be applied in different cultures and calibrations can be obtained. Each vignette is a description of a specific level of ability on a given domain that individuals are asked to evaluate. By using vignettes, the level on a domain is fixed and only the cut-points need to be estimated. Vignettes were developed for the seven major domains of health: mobility, self care, pain, affect, cognition, usual activities, and vision. The vignettes spanned the breadth of the scale ("no difficulty or problem" to "extreme difficulty or problem") and were discussed with international experts to ensure cross-cultural applicability and understandability.

HEALTH STATE DESCRIPTIONS

The health domains and questions were developed based on experience in the revision of the International Classification of Functioning, Disability and Health (ICF) (14) and the development of assessment instruments linked to ICF such as the WHO Disability Assessment Schedule (WHODAS II). The WHODAS II was conceived as a general health state assessment measure capable of being used for multiple purposes including epidemiological surveys. It covers the major domains of cognition, self care, mobility, interpersonal relationships, daily activities at work and in the household, and social participation and impact. Prior to the WHO Multi-country Survey Study, during 1997–2000 the WHODAS II was *separately* piloted in 21 centres across 19 countries in 1 431 subjects that spanned the adult age group (≥ 18 years of age). The analysis examined reliability, convergent validity with other assessment instruments as well as other performance measures, sensitivity to change following intervention, and relationships to valuation of health states. Findings from the field trials show a stable factor structure that is replicable across countries and population groups, unidimensionality of domains, and good test-retest reliability with a Kappa 0.65 to 0.91. Twenty-three items from the final version of the WHODAS II, as well as items that were used for the WHODAS II development item pool during early phases of testing, were used in the survey study questionnaire in the domains of pain, vision, hearing, cognition, self-care, mobility, usual activities, interpersonal relations, and social participation.

HEALTH STATE VALUATIONS

Health state valuations, (also known as preferences or disability weights) represent overall assessments of the levels of health associated with different states. They provide the critical link between the non-fatal health experience and mortality in summary measures of population health (such as healthy life expectancy or Disability-Adjusted Life Years, among others).

Measurement of health state valuations depends not only on assessments of the health levels in different states, but also on other values such as attitudes toward risk and uncertainty, distributional concerns, or preferences for immediate rather than future outcomes (referred to as time preference). A related issue is that measurement methods are highly abstract and cognitively demanding, and have demonstrated poor reliability and validity in the general community.

In order to address these problems, the WHO Multi-country Survey Study, besides obtaining actual self-reports on different domains of health, asked respondents to value their own, as well as a set of other, health conditions. A brief description of each health condition was provided and respondents were asked to rate each of these on the seven core domains. Respondents were afterwards asked to rank the different health conditions and then rate them on a visual

analogue scale where 0 is death and 100 is perfect health.

In addition, more detailed surveys using multiple methods for valuation, such as Time Trade Off (TTO), Person Trade Off (PTO), and Standard Gamble (SG), were carried out among respondents with high levels of educational attainment in the same sites. The primary objective of the population-based surveys was to collect information on health state valuations in the general population in order to better understand differences across countries and within countries by age, sex, education, income, and other variables. The multi-method study was designed to allow empirical adjustment of the valuations obtained in the general population surveys to account for the scaling properties of the simple measurement instrument used in these surveys. Because the multi-method exercise involves valuation methods that are abstract and cognitively demanding, it was implemented among individuals who were educated and willing to undertake such a task, and included students, journalists, policy-makers, care providers and health care professionals. Some individuals with physical (such as diabetes or fractures) and mental (such as depression or substance use disorders) health conditions were also able to undertake these exercises with adequate explanations and visual props.

The simple visual analogue scale used in the general population surveys provides a relatively simple measurement tool for assessing the valuation of health levels associated with the hypothetical states. The scaling properties of the visual analogue scale have been challenged: mild states may be overvalued due to scale distortions. Nevertheless, once the nature of the distortion has been defined as a function, it allows for empirical adjustment of valuations. The study provided information on how the visual analogue scale relates to other valuation techniques in order to estimate the underlying health state valuations that inform responses to all different measurement methods. By formalizing the relationships between the different valuation techniques and the underlying quantity of interest based on previous theoretical and empirical findings, statistical methods were used to recover these underlying valuations and to simultaneously characterize the nature of the scale distortion in visual analogue scale responses (as well as to quantify other values such as risk aversion, distributional concerns, and time preference). The product of this analysis is a function that may be used to adjust visual analogue responses to the appropriate scale for valuations (21).

RESPONSIVENESS

DEVELOPMENT OF THE RESPONSIVENESS MODULE

Responsiveness of health systems to the legitimate expectations of populations is recognized as an important element of health systems performance. To operationalize this concept and measure it meaningfully in different settings, a survey instrument was developed for the long household, postal, and brief household surveys. The content of the household and postal instruments did not differ greatly, but there were fewer items in the postal and brief household questionnaires.[4]

The questions in the responsiveness module were field-tested and comments on the questionnaire were taken from a number of experts. As part of the development of the existing questionnaire, a key informant survey was run initially in 35 countries across 1 791 individuals. In addition, three pilot household surveys were conducted in Tanzania, Colombia, and the Philippines (about 150 individuals per country). Based on this experience, and in consultation with several international experts, a new questionnaire was developed.

The questions in the current household and postal survey were field tested prior to their finalization as part of the pre-testing of the entire survey study instrument (22).

CONTENT OF THE RESPONSIVENESS MODULE

Within the responsiveness section of the survey, subjects were asked if they had had an outpatient, home care or inpatient contact with the health system. They had to name the last place of care they went to and to identify whether this was their usual place of care. They were then asked to rate their experiences over the past 12 months and about their utilization of health services over the last 30 days. The questions on responsiveness covered eight domains, all relevant to inpatient visits, but only seven used for outpatient visits. Social support was the domain asked only to inpatients. The eight domains and the corresponding number of questions per outpatient and inpatient domain were: prompt attention (four outpatient, one inpatient), dignity (four outpatient, one inpatient), communication (four outpatient, one inpatient), autonomy (four outpatient, one inpatient), confidentiality (two outpatient, one inpatient), choice of institution and care provider (three outpatient, one inpatient), and basic amenities of acceptable quality (three outpatient, one inpatient).

All domains included a summary rating question (scaled one to five, "very good" to "very bad"). In addition, several domains included report questions on how often a particular experience had occurred during encounters with the health system (scaled one to four, "always" to "never").

All questionnaires on responsiveness included vignettes, i.e. descriptions of hypothetical scenarios which respondents are asked to rate using the same rating scale as in the responsiveness questions ("very good" to "very bad"). These vignettes were pre-tested on a small group of people.

OTHER MODULES

MENTAL HEALTH (DEPRESSION AND ALCOHOL USE)

The survey questionnaire, based on WHO Composite International Diagnostic Interview (CIDI)'s Depression and Alcohol Sections, specifically screened for depression and alcohol use disorders using questions that have formed part of many international studies (24). Since depression and alcohol related disorders are a major cause of health burden worldwide, it was felt necessary to measure these in a comparable manner across countries. Further, since these conditions are associated with stigma in all societies and produce substantial restrictions in participation, it was necessary to also measure health state valuations associated with them.

CHRONIC HEALTH CONDITIONS

Though there is conflicting evidence on the reliability of self-reported morbidity in different surveys, information was gathered on this area in the current survey using a checklist of chronic health conditions (25). In addition, to improve the validity of the information, respondents were asked whether the diagnosis was made by a doctor, what investigations were carried out, whether any specific treatment was received, and what impact the health condition had on the person's life. This allowed for the relationship between self-reported health status and morbidity to be estimated across different populations.

ADULT MORTALITY

The Multi-country Survey Study included a module that asked questions related to adult mortality in the past two years in each household. This was to supplement information on overall rates of adult mortality in countries where these data were not available from vital registration systems, and to explore if it was possible to obtain reliable information on some of the causes. Information from the head of the household was collated with information from other sources such as medical records wherever available (26). Attempts were made to compare the information thus obtained with the life tables available for each country to determine the validity of this mode of data collection on mortality.

HEALTH RELATED AREAS: ENVIRONMENTAL FACTORS

The survey questionnaire also collected some basic information related to environmental risk factors in the form of mode and place of cooking, and the kinds of fuel used for cooking. In addition to providing minimal information about the risks to health depending on the cooking environment, it was expected that this information would also be correlated with socioeconomic status (27).

HEALTH FINANCING

The WHO Multi-country Survey Study included questions on health expenditure and financing within the context of the interview. Respondents were also asked to provide information on the relative proportion of household income that is spent on health as compared to accommodation and food (28). Since respondents answer the questions within a health survey, and therefore in the context of health, it is estimated that the information obtained is more relevant to the health experience than other expenditure and income surveys.

MODES USED IN THE WHO MULTI-COUNTRY SURVEY STUDY

The WHO Multi-country Survey Study provided survey content in different modes with different possible sampling strategies. The modes were in-person individual interviews, telephone surveys, and mail surveys, with a view to test the mode effect on the parameters in question as well as the comparison of efficiency and cost of various applications. The basic modes that were used are described below and shown in the summary in Figure 57.3.

HOUSEHOLD INDIVIDUAL INTERVIEWS

Interviews for the household survey were conducted face-to-face using paper and pencil questionnaires. In each household a single adult individual (> 18 years) was selected by a random process (i.e. Kish Table, which identifies a predefined individual in the household with a known probability) after completing a full household roster. The survey protocol specified that all interviews should be conducted in privacy. Where members of the household, neighbours or friends were present, the interviewers requested privacy and, where necessary, steps were taken to ensure that interviewers were the same sex as the respondent.

HOUSEHOLD BRIEF FACE-TO-FACE INTERVIEWS

In view of the costs of carrying out a full face-to-face interview (lasting around 90 minutes) and the need to carry out the survey in as many countries as possible, a briefer version of the questionnaire (around 30 minutes) was carried out in a face-to-face interview in several countries. This version focuses on selected key domains of health and responsiveness.

COMPUTER ASSISTED TELEPHONE INTERVIEW (CATI)

In two countries where telephone coverage is extensive, the brief survey (30 min) described above was administered using this format. The telephone interviews use computer technology to automatically sequence and branch questions, which eliminates interviewer error in failing to ask questions. They can achieve a better sampling coverage because of the known sampling frame and random digit dialing.

POSTAL SELF-ADMINISTERED SURVEYS

Since it is relatively inexpensive to carry out a postal survey in countries where literacy levels are high and the reach of the postal system is good, the brief survey questionnaire was used in a mail format in many countries. In some countries (i.e. Turkey and Egypt), the survey was hand-couriered to the respondents and collected back from them.

The survey was carried out in some countries using more than one mode. This has allowed the data from the different modes to be compared in order to estimate the effect of the mode of the survey.

INITIAL TESTING OF THE QUESTIONNAIRE

TRANSLATION AND COGNITIVE INTERVIEWING

The survey questionnaire was translated using a translation and linguistic analysis protocol developed by WHO. Forward translation was carried out by health experts, and a bilingual group examined the accuracy and appropriateness of the translation. A report on linguistic analysis and translation of all key terms used in the questionnaire was requested from all sites. Back-translations were made by an independent group of linguistic experts. A team at WHO reviewed the reports and finalized the questionnaires.

Following translation, the instrument was pilot tested on 100 subjects at each site. During this test, the respondents were asked specific debriefing questions in order to determine if the survey questions were understood and if the intent of the question was accurately conveyed. Respondents were also asked to elaborate on the reasons why a particular response category was chosen for a question. This information was analysed to see if the instrument was being used in the same manner across sites and if it was feasible to obtain information in a consistent manner.

TRANSLATION AND BACK-TRANSLATION

Sites were asked to translate and back-translate a list of 145 items from the questionnaire. The aim of this process was to achieve different language versions of the English questionnaire that are conceptually equivalent in each of the countries. The focus was on cross-cultural and conceptual, rather than on literal/linguistic, equivalence.

Some words or phrases were somehow problematic and did not convey the concept addressed by the original item. In some countries (e.g. Indonesia), scales of time (some of the time, a good bit of the time, most of the time) were back-translated as scales of frequency (occasionally, often, every time). Other terms gave a similar, yet different, meaning. For example "distress" was back-translated as "pain, anguish, stress or difficult/dangerous situation." Some items had no equivalent in the local language and were difficult to translate. For example, in Nigeria, the term "bipolar disorder," when back-translated gave the equivalent of "mental problem."

PILOT TESTS

The instrument was piloted in 100 respondents at each household survey site (10 countries) and 50 respondents were also retested to determine reliability. Feedback was given to sites based on the qualitative experiences as well as the quantitative results. In countries that applied other modes (brief face-to-face, telephone, and postal surveys) a limited number of pilot tests were completed (between 10–50 interviews) to test the adequacy of translations and feasibility of applications.

The pilot study was very informative and provided valuable information for modification of substantial portions of the interview. The results of the pilots indicated that the test-retest reliability of self-report, vignettes, and the calibration tests were high, though the test-retest for calibration tests varied by country. In view of the findings of the pilot work, the vignettes were modified and the manner of implementation of the performance tests was discussed with each site. Further quality assurance steps were introduced, including a detailed video for training, supervising tests during site visits, and standardizing these tests in each country with self-report and vignettes in controlled conditions.

The pilot data also served to reduce the questionnaire length by about 30%. Items that had very poor reliability and were not providing additional information on a domain were either deleted or combined. Questions that were unclear were rephrased. The pilot highlighted problems related to the length of the overall questionnaire and hence, in the main study respondents were allocated to different rotations in the modules of the questionnaire (e.g. half the respondents were asked the valuation module and the other half were administered the calibration tests.) The pilot clearly demonstrated the value of vignettes and calibration tests: vignettes were added for multiple domains of health and responsiveness, and modified to reflect more clearly a level of function in the specific domain.

SITES

SELECTION OF PARTICIPATING COUNTRIES

Identifying potential survey partners was based on interest in the study, previous survey experience, capability for conducting high-quality surveys at the national level, available resources, and acceptable budget proposals and timeframe. An extensive search was done among universities, research institutions, and other international agencies. Potential collaborators were asked to provide details on the surveys they had carried out, submit a sampling frame, a detailed budget breakdown, and a plan of action for conducting the survey. Geographic distribution and country development were also taken into account. Overall, more than 400 contacts were made in over 100 countries and this process took around four months. On average, three proposals per country were received. Criteria for site selection included:

- Former experience in health surveys in various modes.

- Quality of the proposal in terms of its response to technical specifications.

- Ability of the institution to carry out the survey in a timely manner.

- Survey costs.

- Access to representative general population samples.

Based on evaluation of the proposals, consultations with technical experts, and feedback from WHO Regional Offices, country representatives, and consultants, decisions were made with regard to which sites to select. Seventy-one surveys were conducted in 61 countries.

SAMPLING PLANS

To develop sampling plans, an up-to-date registry of all persons residing in the country was preferred as the sampling frame. When such listings were not available, registries providing postal coverage or post office listings were considered.

The sampling plans were implemented in different survey modes as follows. Post stratification corrections were made based on the population data available from the UN Population Databases.

Household Survey

Generally, sample sizes of between 5 000 to 10 000 male and female adults aged above 18 years, non-institutionalized and living in private households, were obtained (with the exception of Slovakia where 1 183 respondents were sampled) as a multistage stratified probability sample that was reasonably representative of the country's population. In each sampling stage of the design, probability methods were implemented to ensure that a representative sample of the target popu-

lation was obtained. Each site was asked to develop a sampling plan together with WHO and submit the final sample description and calculation of weights according to the technical specifications. Some countries already had a sampling frame in place used at the government level, e.g. Central Agency for Public Mobilization and Statistics (CAPMAS) in Egypt. One respondent per household was randomly selected using the Kish tables (29), which allocates equal probability of selection to each eligible individual within the household. Quota sampling methods or other respondent selection procedures that are not probabilistic were considered unacceptable.

In three countries (China, India, and Nigeria) survey samples were not representative of the whole country because of the size of the countries and language barriers. In China, the study was carried out in the provinces of Gansu, Henan, and Shandong; in India—in the state of Andhra Pradesh; and in Nigeria—in the Yoruba speaking regions of Ibadan, Iseyin, Ido, and Ogo of Oyo state.

Brief Face-to-Face Survey

Male and female adults older than 18 years, non-institutionalized and living in private households were selected as a multistage random cluster sampling. The number of respondents ranged from 489 in Iceland to 3 000 in Croatia. The sampling points represented the whole territory of the country surveyed and were selected proportionally to the distribution of the population. Metropolitan, urban, and rural areas were covered with the exception of a few countries, where only urban areas were selected as they represented most of the country, or where rural areas were remote and difficult to access. Sample weights based on probability of sampling for each individual were estimated.

Postal Survey

Male and female adults older than 18 years, non-institutionalized and living in private households, were taken into the sampling frame from existing address lists and mailed the questionnaire. In those cases where an acceptable sampling frame of individuals was unavailable, households were selected. In that case, the recipient of the mailed survey was then asked to select household members older than 18 years and ask the person with the closest birthday to complete the questionnaire. The questionnaire included a question on the number of people aged 18+ residing in the household, to help develop weights for the data. Around 5 000 questionnaires were mailed in each country (except Canada where around 1 500 questionnaires were sent). The sample sizes ranged from 705 (out of 3 000 mailed questionnaires) in the Republic of Korea to 4 524 (out of 5 000 mailed questionnaires) in Turkey. In some countries (i.e. Turkey and Egypt), the survey was hand-couriered to the respondents and personally collected from them (30).

Computer Assisted Telephone Interview (CATI)

One thousand male and female adults aged over 18 years, non-institutionalized and living in private households were taken into the sampling frame. Two variations of the random digit dialling (RDD) were used in both countries in which CATI was implemented.

Random digit dialling was used in Luxembourg to include new and unlisted numbers. This procedure is designed to overcome problems of sampling from telephone directories, which is the usual sampling frame for telephone surveys. Directories are often inaccurate and out-of-date. They are also incomplete because of unlisted numbers (31).

In Canada, telephone numbers were selected from the most recently published telephone directories, with a fixed number of telephone numbers per sampling unit, to provide a probability sample.

In both countries, from within each household contacted, respondents were selected using the "most recent birthday" method.

TRAINING OF INTERVIEWERS AND TRAINERS

A training workshop for the Household Survey countries was held at WHO in Geneva from 3–6 July 2000, and two participants per country were invited to act as trainers for the country survey teams. The ten participating countries were China, Colombia, Egypt, Georgia, India, Indonesia, Lebanon, Nigeria, Slovakia, and Turkey. The purpose of the workshop was to train the trainers in conducting the household survey, and share ideas and concerns in a multicultural setting. The training covered sampling, interviewing techniques, questionnaire review and practice, and general issues related to the survey.

Additionally, training manuals and videos were distributed to each site for ongoing training. The training manuals clearly described the question-by-question specifications for the survey instrument and gave instructions to interviewers in terms of the "dos and don'ts" for the interview. It also provided guidance as to what clarifications the interviewers could provide if asked by the respondents. The videos illustrated basic interviewing techniques and some difficult interview situations, and clarified issues related to specific questions. They also demonstrated how the calibration tests and valuation exercises were to be carried out. All this material was made available on different media as well.

In countries where brief face-to-face surveys were undertaken, interviewers were trained to follow standard instructions in a rigorous manner under the responsibility of the Project Manager and the Fieldwork Supervisors. Site visits for training and supervision of interviews were carried out in all countries for quality assurance purposes.

IMPLEMENTATION OF SURVEY IN THE FIELD

Surveys were conducted in various countries in three different modes. Sampling plans approved by WHO were implemented with specifications of the sampling units and stratification procedures at each sampling stage (primary, secondary, and tertiary sampling levels). Several contact calls (at least four in the BFTF and ten in the household mode) were attempted and interviewers tried to contact each selected household at different times of the day and days of the week. Each contact call was recorded together with reasons for non-response.

Interviewers were supervised on a regular basis during fieldwork to ensure that expectations and production requirements were met, interviewers were performing well, information was kept confidential and professional ethics were followed, questionnaires and other materials were completed accurately and submitted on time, and lastly, that any problems were reported as soon as they arose. WHO asked supervisors to sit in on at least 10 interviews during the pilot phase to check that interviews were conducted in a standardized way. The data were entered in the following days of paper-pencil instrument finalization after editing and approval by the supervisors. Each country reported on the following aspects of the survey implementation:

- Details on each stage of sampling;

- Quality control procedures implemented in the fieldwork;

- Response rates and efforts undertaken to increase this, and the effects of these incentives;

- Qualitative reports on the implementation process from the fieldworkers.

QUALITY ASSURANCE

In order to monitor the quality of the data and ensure that countries complied with WHO guidelines in all household surveys, the conditions under which the interviews were conducted and the problems that survey teams encountered were observed by supervisors first hand. Supervisors reviewed 10% of the questionnaires to check if options had been recorded appropriately and if questions were skipped correctly. About 10% of respondents were called or visited by the supervisor to ensure that the interview had been done, and 10% of all interviews were repeated by another interviewer within a period of one week to check for the reliability of the interview.

In addition, a site visit was scheduled to all full-length household survey sites during data collection. During these site visits several activities were undertaken:

- Overall survey management: sampling procedures, training/supervision, selection of respondent, and timing of survey were discussed.

- Interview assessment: the WHO staff sat in at least four interviews to see how the interview was conducted, the interaction between the interviewer and the respondent, and the timing of the interview.

- A meeting with the survey team was held to discuss contacting procedures, interviews, data, and logistics.

- The data in questionnaires were checked by examining the survey records and data entry program.

Site visits made in the early phases of data collection detected any problems, ensured that the questionnaire was administered and completed correctly, and confirmed that calibration tests were performed according to the instructions provided by WHO.

FEEDBACK DURING DATA COLLECTION

The data were sent to WHO in a weekly or fortnightly basis, such that a quick assessment could be made of the survey for each country in terms of missing information, reliability, use of appropriate skips, etc. Following data submission, certain computerized algorithms were run to identify possible errors while the survey teams were in the field. Feedback regarding the data quality was routinely given to the site coordinator who took relevant action to ensure good quality data.

ETHICAL ASPECTS

To ensure that the set of survey studies was carried out with the highest standards, a working group was established with varied expertise in carrying out large-scale multinational surveys. This group met on a weekly basis to review the state-of-the-art in survey design and implementation so that benefits of the surveys to the participants and public were maximized and potential hazards minimized. In addition, consultations were held with a committee of experts who agreed to the overall design of the questionnaire. Periodically, on an as-and-when-needed basis, discussions were also held with international experts to get further guidance with regard to this survey. The survey study core protocol and processes were cleared by the Sub-Committee for Research Involving Human Subjects (SCRIHS) at the World Health Organization.

Informed consent was obtained from every respondent in the survey. The consent form was carefully drafted in keeping with internationally accepted standards and in discussion with WHO's SCRIHS. Further, confidentiality agreements with each collaborating site were executed whereby the principal investigator at each site assured confidentiality of the data. A draft confidentiality declaration from collaborators was discussed with SCRIHS and agreed upon. Ethical bodies at each site also reviewed the confidentiality issues of particular local relevance as part of the process of obtaining local ethical clearance.

Some personal identifying information was required for purposes of re-contact for testing the validity of the questions. However, once data were collected from the respondent they were stored in an anonymous manner with all identifying information stripped from the dataset. Data transmitted to the World Health Organization contained no personal identifying information. Locally stored data were under the personal control of the principal investigator at each site and kept secure in agreement with local ethical committees.

DATA COLLECTION AND MANAGEMENT

DATA CODING

At each site, the data were coded by investigators to indicate the respondent status and the selection of the modules for each respondent within the survey design. After the interview was edited by the supervisor and considered adequate, it was entered locally.

DATA ENTRY PROGRAM

A data entry program was developed in the World Health Organization specifically for the survey study and provided to the sites. It was developed using a database program called the *I-Shell* (short for Interview Shell), a tool designed for easy development of computerized questionnaires and data entry (*32*). This program allows for easy data cleaning and processing.

The data entry program checked for inconsistencies and validated the entries in each field by checking for valid response categories and range checks. For example, the program did not accept an age greater than 120. For almost all of the variables there existed a range or a list of possible values that the program checked for.

In addition, the data were entered twice to capture other data entry errors. The data entry program was able to warn the user whenever a value that did not match the first entry was entered at the second data entry. In this case the program asked the user to resolve the conflict by choosing either the 1st or the 2nd data entry value to be able to continue. After the second data entry was completed successfully, the data entry program placed a mark in the database in order to enable the checking of whether this process had been completed for each and every case.

DATA TRANSFER

The data entry program was able to export the data that were entered into one compressed database file which could be easily sent to the World Health Organization using email attachments or a file transfer program onto a secure server, no matter how many cases were in the file.

The sites were allowed the use of as many computers and as many data entry personnel as they wanted. Each computer used for this purpose produced one file and the files were merged once they were delivered to the World Health Organization with the help of other programs built for automating the process.

The sites sent the data periodically as they collected them, thus enabling checking procedures and preliminary analyses in the early stages of the data collection.

DATA QUALITY CHECKS

Once the data were received, they were analysed for missing information, invalid responses, and representativeness. Inconsistencies were also noted and reported back to sites.

DATA CLEANING AND FEEDBACK

After receipt of cleaned data from sites, another program was run to check for missing information, incorrect information (e.g. wrong use of center codes), duplicated data, etc. The output of this program was fed back to sites regularly. Mainly, this consisted of cases with duplicate IDs, duplicate cases (where the data for two respondents with different IDs were identical), wrong country codes, and missing age, sex, education, and some other important variables.

QUALITY ASSURANCE STEPS FOR DATA COLLECTION

As noted above, each record was entered twice, using the data entry program that checked for inconsistencies between the two entries in order to minimize errors. The steps outlined above ensured periodic corrections and checking as well.

Figure 57.2 summarizes the steps in the quality assurance process.

DATA ANALYSIS STRATEGIES

BASIC DESCRIPTIVE ANALYSIS

Univariate, Bivariate, and Multivariate Statistics

Once the data had been cleaned using standard procedures, univariate (i.e. frequencies, descriptives, etc.), bivariate (i.e. Pearson's and Spearman's correlation coefficients, cross-tabulations, etc.), and multivariate (i.e. analysis of variance, regression analysis) analyses were carried out overall, for each country, and between countries using a pooled sample.

Item Analysis: Classical Approach

All the items of the survey were subject to traditional item analysis using standard statistical procedures.

Endorsement rates were determined for each survey item by calculating the proportion (p) of people choosing a particular answer (i.e. "*Yes*").

Cronbach's alpha coefficient was calculated on the scales (factors) resulting from the exploratory factor analysis (EFA) and confirmatory factor analysis (CFA), to estimate the internal consistency of each new composite score. The classical index of discrimination was obtained by calculating the corrected item-total correlation coefficients (r) for each item with its scale.

Figure 57.2   Quality assurance steps for data

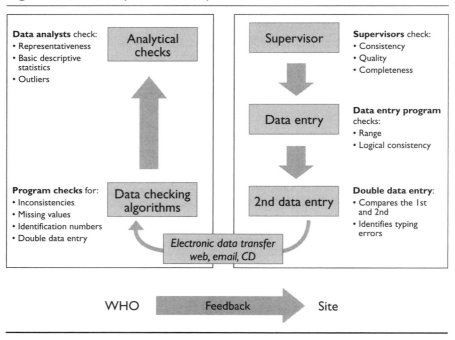

Test-retest reliability indices were computed within and across populations using *Kappa statistics* for categorical and *intraclass correlation coefficient* for continuous variables to give estimates of chance corrected agreement rates for concordance between test and retest applications to indicate the stability of the application. These were estimated only for the full-length household surveys.

Item Analysis: Item Response Theory Approach and HOPIT

In addition to the methods described above, the items from the health status description section were also calibrated using the responses from the subjects on the vignettes and the performance tests. Since self-reports are dependent on the semantic value ascribed to words in a rating scale, in order to make valid comparisons between subjects within and across populations, it is imperative to correct for systematic biases in self-report such that comparisons indeed reflect true similarities and differences in the underlying trait of interest, in this case "health." Strategies such as the IRT approach and a hierarchical ordered probit model (HOPIT), developed by the World Health Organization for this purpose, were used. These strategies are designed to correct for biases in cut-points in rating scales and are fully described elsewhere (20).

SPECIFIC ANALYSES FOR HEALTH STATE VALUATIONS

The results of the valuation component of the survey were descriptions and valuations of 11 health states by each respondent. The 11 health states include the individual's own health state plus 10 other hypothetical states drawn from four different sets. Health state descriptions consist of levels on each of the seven domains of health included in the survey. The first level of analysis was an examination of the different descriptions provided by respondents for the health state labels. Frequency distributions and summary statistics were compared across sites, and analysis of determinants of variation both across and within sites were undertaken using ordered probit and other models. This analysis was combined with the analytical efforts to estimate cut-points on underlying domain scales using calibration vignettes and tests as mentioned above.

Health state valuations for each state, obtained from the visual analogue thermometer scale, were examined for differences across and within sites. The primary analytical objective in the valuation section was to estimate the valuation function through which health state profiles are mapped to valuations, i.e. the relative weights and interactions of different domains. Hierarchical models were developed in order to estimate these valuation functions in a way that accounts for variation in these functions according to different locations and individual characteristics such as age, sex, etc.[5]

SPECIFIC ANALYSES FOR HEALTH SYSTEM RESPONSIVENESS

As in the case of health state measurements, an important part of the measurement and analysis strategy for

responsiveness was the inclusion of vignettes which described different responsiveness experiences. Analyses of responsiveness scores (inpatient and outpatient) for all elements with the variables of sex, age, health state, health service utilization, income, rural/urban, and education were conducted to see how responsiveness results differ across these subgroups. Inpatient and outpatient element scores were compared across all elements. Classical test theory approaches were used to examine the factor structure of the construct of responsiveness. If a unidimensional structure is demonstrated, and a set of common items is identified that have similar properties across populations, the scale cut-off points for the responsiveness vignettes across countries are calculated using HOPIT and compound HOPIT (or CHOPIT) techniques. This exercise enabled calibration of the results if necessary, improving the interpretation of cross-country comparisons.

PRELIMINARY RESULTS

The WHO Multi-country Survey Study in 2000–2001 was carried out in 61 different countries using 71 surveys. There were a total of 188 307 respondents in different modes including 14 full-length household surveys, 27 brief face-to-face surveys, 28 postal surveys, and two telephone (CATI) surveys. Figure 57.3 shows the different modes and Figure 57.4 shows the regional distributions with Table 57.2 summarizing the geographical distribution by WHO regional offices.

Figure 57.3 Different survey modes in the WHO Multi-country Survey Study, 2000–2001

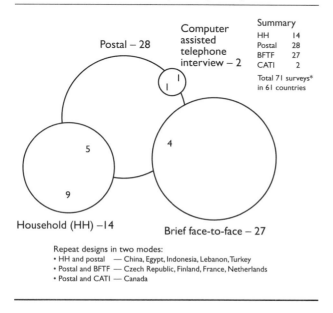

Postal – 28

Computer assisted telephone interview – 2

Summary
HH	14
Postal	28
BFTF	27
CATI	2
Total 71 surveys*	
in 61 countries	

1

5

4

9

Household (HH) –14

Brief face-to-face – 27

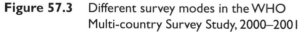

Repeat designs in two modes:
• HH and postal — China, Egypt, Indonesia, Lebanon, Turkey
• Postal and BFTF — Czech Republic, Finland, France, Netherlands
• Postal and CATI — Canada

Figure 57.4 WHO Multi-country Survey Study, 2000–2001

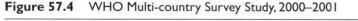

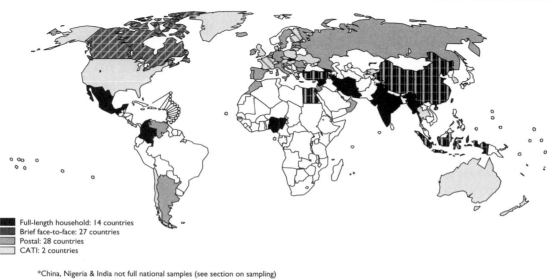

Full-length household: 14 countries
Brief face-to-face: 27 countries
Postal: 28 countries
CATI: 2 countries

*China, Nigeria & India not full national samples (see section on sampling)

Table 57.2 Distribution of survey countries by WHO regions

Region	Total countries	Number of survey countries	% Region coverage (by country)
AFRO	46	1	2.2
AMRO /PAHO	35	11	31.4
EMRO	22	8	36.4
EURO	51	33	64.7
SEARO	10	3	30.0
WPRO	27	5	18.5
Total	191	61	31.9

Full household surveys are currently in progress in Iran, Lebanon, Singapore, and Syria.

PARTICIPATING COUNTRIES

Table 57.3 lists the countries that have participated in the survey study.

RESULTS BY SURVEY MODES

Household Mode

In the household mode, trained interviewers carried out a face-to-face detailed interview with one randomly selected respondent from each household in the sample. Calibration tests were also carried out at the respondents' houses.

For brief descriptions of survey samples in each country, see EIP Discussion Paper No. 37 at URL: http://www3.who.int/whosis/discussion_papers/discussion_papers.cfm#. The sampling was done as a general multistage cluster sampling. The quality of the sample to represent the general population was monitored through the Sample Population Deviation Index, which shows the proportion of age and sex strata in the sample in comparison to the general population as taken from UN population statistics (refer to Figure 57.5 for further explanation). In general, the duration of the household surveys ranged between 65 and 119 minutes with an average of 87 minutes (see also the section on survey length for detailed information on duration).

The average household response rate across all countries was 84%. The missing data rate overall was less than 5%, where missing data is defined as proportion of respondents missing greater than 10% of items in household, 2% of items in BFTF, and 5% of items in postal modes. Test-retest reliability calculated by chance corrected agreement rates was in general higher than 0.6 which indicated overall good

Table 57.3 Countries participating in the survey study

Household	Brief Face-to-Face	CATI	Postal
China*	Argentina	Canada	Australia
Colombia	Bahrain	Luxembourg	Austria
Egypt	Belgium		Canada
Georgia	Bulgaria		Chile
India*	Costa Rica		China
Indonesia	Croatia		Cyprus
Iran	Czech Republic		Czech Republic
Lebanon	Estonia		Denmark
Mexico	Finland		Egypt
Nigeria*	France		Finland
Singapore	Germany		France
Slovakia	Iceland		Greece
Syria	Ireland		Hungary
Turkey	Italy		Indonesia
	Jordan		Kyrgyzstan
	Latvia		Lebanon
	Malta		Lithuania
	Morocco		Netherlands
	Netherlands		New Zealand
	Oman		Poland
	Portugal		Rep. of Korea
	Romania		Switzerland
	Russian Federation		Thailand
	Spain		Trinidad and Tobago
	Sweden		Turkey
	United Arab Emirates		Ukraine
	Venezuela		United Kingdom
			USA
14	27	2	28

* Not full national sample

reliability. Design effects (i.e. the ratio of sampling variance in comparison to simple random sample) ranged between three and eight in selected key variables. While most surveys make sample size estimates based on design effect estimates of around two, the results of this study suggest that design effect for many items may indeed be much higher; the WHO Multi-country Survey Study had calculated required sample sizes based on a conservative design effect estimate of 2.5. All these summary diagnostic variables for different modes of surveys are shown in Table 57.4. Detailed findings for each country are given in the Tables 57.10A through 57.10C.

Brief Face-to-Face Mode

In the brief face-to-face mode, trained interviewers carried out a face-to-face short interview (on average 35

Table 57.4 Summary survey diagnostics for different modes

Survey mode	Duration (min.)	Sample deviation index	Response rate (%)	Respondent missing data* (%)	Reliability	Design effects
Household	87 [65–119]	2.06 [0.67–3.84]	84 [82–99]	12.1 [0.8–31.9]	0.67 [0.43–0.87]	5.85 [2.0–10.7]
BFTF	35 [15–40]	2.28 [0.89–6.57]	64 [35–80]	1.5 [0–17.6]	Not done	Not applicable
Postal	45 (estimated)	2.91 [0.86–7.95]	46 [24–92]	6.8 [0–26]	Not done	Not applicable
CATI	30 [18–42]	2.18 [1.50–2.87]	40 [25–55]	2.1 [1.6–2.6]	Not done	Not done

* Respondents with missing data 10% in household, 2% in BFTF and CATI, 5 % in postal surveys.

minutes) with one randomly selected respondent from each household in the sample, using either the birthday method (an adult member of the household whose birthday was closest to the date of the interview was requested to complete the questionnaire) or the Kish Method (28). The response rates for the brief face-to-face interviews ranged between 35–80% with a mean value of 64%. In comparison to longer household surveys, this response rate is lower mainly because of the fact that fewer calls were made to households in the case of non-response (three calls versus ten) and possibly because of the selection of countries for this mode (western countries tend to have higher refusal rates). The BFTF mode had a missing data rate of 1.5%, the lowest of all modes, and a SDI of 2.28, lower than the postal mode and not significantly different from the household mode ($p = 0.61$).

Postal Mode

Using a well described sampling frame of addresses, questionnaires were mailed or couriered to respondents. Either the respondent to whom the questionnaire was addressed or the person with the closest birthday answered the questionnaire. The questionnaires were mailed back in most countries, and collected in person in China, Egypt, and Turkey. Personal collection yielded a very high response rate (over 90%). According to the reports from sites, it took on average 45 minutes for the respondents to fill in the questionnaires. Postal mode application had higher levels of missing data since there was no interviewer assistance to explain questions and individuals on their own took more liberty not to respond. The postal mode had a missing data rate of 6.8% and a SDI of 2.91, both higher than the household and brief face-to-face modes.

Representativeness of Samples

The sampling procedure used aimed to create a representative subgroup of the whole population from which population-based estimates can be generated. A simple indicator of representativeness is the sex ratio in the sample and the general population. Table 57.5 provides a comparison of the sex ratio between the population in the respective countries as reflected in the UN Population Database and that in the samples from the household surveys.

Table 57.5 reveals that at some sites post-stratification strategies may have to be employed to correct for less than perfect representativeness. For example, in Turkey, Mexico, and China, the male population was over-represented, while in Colombia the female population was over-represented. In most countries women in the age groups between 35–54 were over-represented.

In addition to sex, the age distribution is an important indicator of the representativeness of the sample. We computed a "Sample Population Deviation Index" by age categories which shows how closely the distribution of the study sample in the different age groups by sex matches that of the general population distribution as available in the UN Population Database. A perfect match between the study population and the UN database is indicated by 1, whereas values greater than 1 indicate that the population in that age group

Table 57.5 Sex ratio (male/female) in the UN Population Database and in the household survey country samples

Country	Population	Survey (unweighted)	Survey (weighted)
China	1.04	1.14	1.29
Colombia	0.94	0.53	0.48
Egypt	1.01	0.78	0.80
Georgia	0.87	0.73	0.96
Indonesia	0.97	0.83	1.13
India	1.06	0.86	0.83
Mexico	0.94	1.47	1.39
Nigeria	0.96	0.64	0.82
Slovakia	0.92	0.82	0.80
Turkey	1.00	1.72	1.92
Overall	0.97	0.95	1.04

has been over-sampled in the survey. Similarly, values less than 1 indicate that the population in that group is under-represented in the study sample.

An example of a country-specific sample population deviation index is shown in Figure 57.5. The sample population deviation indexes for all countries participating in the household, BFTF, and postal surveys are provided in EIP Discussion Paper No. 37 at URL: http://www3.who.int/whosis/discussion_papers/discussion_papers.cfm#.

Figure 57.5 provides a comparison of the sex-age ratio between the WHO sample for the postal survey in a country and the UN Population Database for 2000. It is evident that between the ages of 20 to 74, the sample surveyed for the WHO postal survey for this particular country closely approximates UN population data. Further, the sex distribution (i.e. ratio of males to females) for the WHO postal survey is comparable to the UN Population Database.

SURVEY LENGTH

For the full-length household surveys, the interview length varied by country, taking between an hour to nearly two hours to complete with an average of 87 minutes. Table 57.6 provides a more detailed view of the length of different sections of the interview duration for each section during the pilot phase of the study. Table 57.7 shows the average interview dura-

tion for the main phase of the study by country for the full-length household countries.

Given that the pilot phase of the study was intended to develop the survey instrument, it is understandable that the interviews lasted this long. Since individual modules will be used singly or in combination, the duration of the interview can be tailored according to the needs of countries and existing resources.

RELIABILITY OF THE SURVEY INSTRUMENT

Reliability of the items in the survey instruments is measured using chance-corrected agreement rates. Kappa (κ) statistics were used for categorical variables, and intraclass correlation coefficients (ICC) for

Table 57.6 Timing of individual sections of full-length household interviews, pilot phase (data from 10 countries)

Section	Timing (minutes)	
	Average	Range
Demographics	8	5–12
Health state description	15	12–23
Health conditions	4	3–7
Screening	4	3–6
Health state valuations	24	15–40
Health system responsiveness	20	15–30
Adult mortality	4	3–7
Calibration tests	15	10–19
Total (minutes)	94	66–144

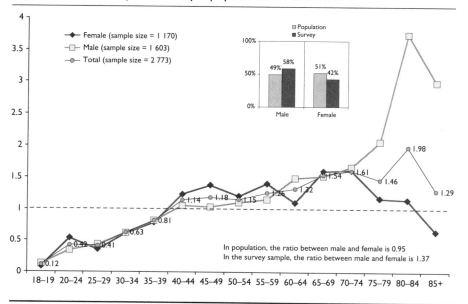

Figure 57.5 Example of a sample population deviation index

continuous variables. These measures assess reliability as a relative measure of agreement between observers compared to the agreement that can occur by mere chance. A weighted Cohen's Kappa analysis (33) was employed to determine the test-retest reliability of the items. The differences between the multiple categorical responses at time 1 and time 2 were weighted such that a greater discrepancy on the categories across the two applications (e.g. between 2 and 4 compared to between 3 and 2) would receive a greater weight.

Reliability coefficients can range from +1 to –1. A Kappa coefficient of +1 means that there is complete agreement, while a coefficient close to 0 is consistent with the hypothesis that agreement occurs by chance. Any Kappa coefficient less than 0 suggests that any agreement that occurs is less than that due to chance alone. Kappa values less than 0.0 indicate poor reliability; 0.0 to 0.2 slight reliability; 0.21 to 0.4 fair reliability; 0.41 to 0.6 moderate reliability; 0.61 to 0.80 substantial agreement; and 0.81 to 1.00 almost perfect agreement (34). Table 57.8A summarizes the reliability statistics for major sections of the health component of the survey study. Table 57.8B summarizes the reliability statistics for major sections of the responsiveness component of the survey study. The retest sample size was 5 684 (range 98–1 040) individuals in 10 countries for the health domains and 4 625 (range 96–940) for the responsiveness domains. All retest subjects were readministered the original interview in its entirety.

Most values reported in Tables 57.8A and 57.8B are within acceptable ranges. Some countries such as Colombia and Nigeria have lower reliabilities across a large number of variables. Tables 57.10A to 57.10C present the reliability coefficients for each country.

Implementation of Measured Calibration Tests

The calibration tests were tested in pilot studies. In order to ensure their uniform application, all principal investigators from household study sites were trained in their implementation at a workshop in July 2000 in Geneva. A training video demonstrating the implementation of the tests was also prepared and distributed to all sites. Further, during each of the site visits made by HQ staff, the actual implementation of the calibration tests was observed and suggestions were provided for a standardized application. In spite of these methods, it was noted that the calibration tests were not being consistently applied at some sites because the lay-trained interviewers were not accustomed to carrying out such tests in the field.

The measurement properties of the calibration tests are reported in Table 57.9. They are within acceptable ranges and are comparable to Kappas for self-report

Table 57.7 Mean interview duration (minutes) of full-length household interviews, main phase (data from 10 countries)

Country	Mean duration (minutes)
China	97
Colombia	68
Egypt	71
Georgia	97
Indonesia	119
India	87
Mexico	90
Nigeria	79
Slovakia	102
Turkey	65
Average	87

Table 57.8A Reliability statistics for major sections of the health component of the survey (data from 10 countries in full-length household interview mode)

	Overall average Kappa value across all countries	Range
Health items		
Mobility	.71	.37–.92
Self-care	.60	.32–.95
Work and household activities	.69	.24–.93
Pain or discomfort	.67	.36–.94
Distress, sadness, worry	.65	.31–.93
Concentrating and remembering	.62	.16–.95
Personal relationship; community participation	.58	.20–.93
Vignettes		
Self-care	.53	.38–.54
Pain	.56	.47–.56
Mobility	.49	.45–.56
Affect	.51	.41–.52
Usual activities	.55	.52–.63
Cognition	.55	.49–.63
Vision	.58	.46–.62
Performance tests		
Verbal fluency	.83	.35–.95
Immediate recall	.57	.30–.86
Delayed recall	.63	.26–.86
Cancellation	.66	.30–1.00
PLM	.39	.30–.98
Vision	.80	.34–.92

described above. Completion rates were over 95% for all calibration tests.

Some practical problems will have to be dealt with during the refinement of their implementation in the future. Almost all the calibration tests (except for vision) are timed tasks. The timing of these tests

Table 57.8B Reliability statistics for major sections of the responsiveness component of the survey

	Average Kappa	Range	
		min	max
Utilization	0.80	0.78	0.84
Discrimination	0.50	0.00	0.80
Responsiveness items—Outpatient			
Dignity	0.65	0.63	0.69
Confidentiality	0.75	0.74	0.76
Quality of basic amenities	0.73	0.73	0.74
Choice	0.75	0.71	0.77
Autonomy	0.74	0.70	0.78
Prompt attention	0.77	0.63	0.88
Responsiveness items (Total)—Inpatient	0.73	0.63	0.81
Vignettes			
Communication	0.57	0.48	0.58
Dignity	0.53	0.43	0.60
Confidentiality	0.55	0.54	0.66
Quality of basic amenities	0.48	0.45	0.61
Choice	0.54	0.50	0.57
Social support	0.56	0.48	0.57
Autonomy	0.60	0.48	0.62
Prompt attention	0.59	0.53	0.65
Importance	0.54	0.49	0.60

need to be recorded accurately using stop watches, and a failure to use them in all settings may have led to some inaccuracies. The implementation of the Posturo-locomotion (PLM) test requires a distance of 6 metres as well as a standard weight of 2 kgs. In most households interviewers were able to find an object of that weight but variation may have occurred in the non-standard shape and size of the objects. This is also true for the seating from which the test is begun. For vision tests, in some households it was difficult to find a space six metres long, and this instruction may have therefore not been followed accurately. More rigorous training will probably be required to standardize the methods in future studies.

Vignette Implementation

Though care was taken to ensure that the vignettes were written in a culturally sensitive manner and were reviewed by all study sites, the very nature of the task is unfamiliar in some study settings. Some respondents in some settings might not have wanted to think of such situations, lest they became ill themselves. Others responded by saying that they could not say how much difficulty the person described in the vignette would have because this depends on many other factors such as the person's life circumstances. However, overall the vignettes show good repeatability (demonstrated in Tables 57.8A and 57.8B), suggesting that respondents understand the task and are able to provide meaningful responses.

Overall Survey Metrics

To assess the quality of the survey process, the survey metrics of the WHO Multi-country Survey Study

Table 57.9   Summary results of calibration tests

Calibration test	Description	Measurement results	Reliability (Kappa/ICC)
Vision	Near vision	20% of sample better than 6/6 10% of sample worse than 6/60	0.80 [0.34–0.92]
	Distant vision	70% of sample better than 6/6	
PLM	Mean time to stand-up	2.4 seconds	0.39 [0.30–0.98]
	Mean time to complete test	13.4 seconds	
Verbal fluency	Mean # of animals correctly named	16.7	0.83 [0.35–0.95]
	Errors	0.7	
Verbal recall	Immediate recall—mean # of words	6.4	0.57 [0.30–0.86]
	Delayed recall—mean # of words	5.5	0.63 [0.26–0.86]
Cancellation test	Mean time to complete test	33 seconds	0.66 [0.30–1.00]
	Mean # of errors in cancellation	2.3	

were examined in a systematic fashion using four components: 1) an aggregate or summary sample population deviation index[6] and the deviation from the UN Population Database as expressed in terms of chi-square values 2) response rate (i.e. those who completed the interviews among eligibles), 3) item missing values (i.e. percentage of items with > 5% missing data), as well as the percentage of respondents with missing data (> 10% for household surveys, > 2% for the BFTF surveys and > 5% for the postal surveys), and 4) reliability coefficients (i.e. percentage of items which have higher than 0.4 Kappa values or equivalent chance-corrected concordance coefficients). Tables 57.10A–57.10C provide a detailed description of these survey metrics.

The tables reveal that the survey samples were fairly representative of the national population structure as estimated by the summary sample population deviation indices. The household samples were closer to the UN Population Database figures than the postal survey samples. In Slovakia, the population was the closest to that in the UN Database. Whether this was a function of the smaller sample size in Slovakia is unclear.

The response rates for the full-length household survey were much higher than for the other two modes (with the exception of the Egypt and Turkey couriered postal surveys as mentioned earlier). This was perhaps a function of the more rigorous interviewer training and call back attempts described earlier.

The missing rates at the respondent- and item-levels are higher for the full-length survey than for the brief survey. Interestingly, the item-level missing data rate is the highest for the postal survey, although the respondent-level missing data is highest for the full-length survey. A possible interpretation is that the length of the full version may have been more than optimal. However, the presence of an interviewer (unlike the way a postal survey is conducted) leads to more complete data collection on all items.

Figure 57.6 illustrates the country- and mode-specific chi-square values for the deviation of the WHO sample (observed) from the UN Population Database for the year 2000 (expected), collapsed across all age groups between 20 and 74 years. Within each survey mode, the countries are rank ordered according to their aggregate chi-square. For every survey mode, the average chi-square across all countries is also indicated. It is evident that there is variation in the aggregate chi-square among countries within each survey mode, the greatest variation being among countries in the postal survey mode. In the countries with the greatest deviation from the expected sample age and sex

Table 57.10A Survey metrics for the household survey, health and responsiveness components

Country	Summary SPDI (un-weighted)	Summary SPDI (weighted)	Deviation from UN Population Chi-square critical value = 49.58 (29 df, p = 0.01)	Response rate (%)	Health module Individuals with > 10% of missing data	Health module Items with > 5% missing data	Responsiveness module Individuals with > 10% of missing data	Responsiveness module Items with > 5% missing data	Health module Overall items	Health module % of items > 0.40	Outpatient Overall items	Outpatient % of items > 0.40	Inpatient Overall items	Inpatient % of items > 0.40
China	1.95	3.62	425.2	99.0	10.0	4.6	21.1	7.3	0.75	99.0	0.8	100.0	0.8	100.0
Colombia	1.70	1.38	201.8	82.0	31.9	1.7	52.0	5.2	0.43	49.0	0.4	12.0	0.5	75.0
Egypt	1.77	1.39	283.9	99.0	12.1	6.1	59.2	1.0	0.75	97.0	0.8	100.0	0.9	100.0
Georgia	1.00	0.91	214.3	87.0	5.4	6.0	24.7	4.2	0.53	69.0	0.4	52.0	0.6	92.0
India	2.29	2.84	309.9	98.0	0.8	4.7	31.3	4.2	0.66	91.0	1.0	100.0	1.0	100.0
Indonesia	1.69	1.69	512.7	99.0	6.4	7.3	23.7	3.1	0.81	98.0	0.7	100.0	0.7	100.0
Mexico	3.30	3.47	408.6	96.0	3.9	10.5	—	4.2	0.83	98.0	N/A	N/A	N/A	N/A
Nigeria	2.36	2.80	411.6	98.0	11.5	5.6	21.2	14.6	0.37	45.0	0.3	36.0	0.1	8.0
Slovakia	0.67	1.08	28.8	84.0	16.5	6.0	43.9	7.3	0.87	97.0	0.9	100.0	0.9	83.0
Turkey	3.84	3.96	171.5	90.0	22.6	8.0	65.5	8.3	0.66	93.0	0.8	100.0	0.5	8.0
Overall	2.06	2.31	296.83	93.2	12.12	6.1	34.2	5.9	0.67	83.6	0.6	70.0	0.6	66.6

Table 57.10B   Survey metrics for the brief face-to-face survey, health and responsiveness components

Country	Deviation from UN Population			Response rate %	Health module		Responsiveness module	
	Summary SPDI	Chi-square critical value = 49.56 (26 df, p = 0.01)	Chi-square p-values		Individuals with > 5% of missing data	Items with > 5% missing data	Individuals with > 6% of missing data	Items with > 5% of missing data
Argentina	1.31	62.0	3.5 E-4	36	3.9	2.4	0.0	9.1
Bahrain	4.23	408.8	0.0 E-6	35	0.2	3.5	0.2	3.0
Belgium	1.36	83.6	0.0 E-6	48	5.5	1.7	8.3	15.9
Bulgaria	0.91	46.7	7.6 E-3	88	1.7	3.5	14.2	27.0
Costa Rica	1.33	36.4	8.5 E-2	37	2.1	0.8	0.0	1.5
Croatia	0.83	94.3	0.0 E-6	68	0.5	4.1	5.6	13.6
Czech Republic	1.39	54.2	9.6 E-4	60	0.4	1.0	16.5	36.0
Estonia	2.42	120.2	0.0 E-6	71	0.0	2.0	17.2	33.3
Finland	1.86	70.1	0.0 E-6	52	0.2	2.1	9.7	14.4
France	1.59	104.2	0.0 E-6	77	1.0	1.4	5.1	10.6
Germany	1.28	63.5	5.6 E-5	80	3.7	2.0	6.1	16.3
Iceland	1.44	77.1	0.0 E-6	53	0.8	2.0	20.0	33.0
Ireland	1.99	69.8	0.0 E-6	39	0.0	1.8	6.5	21.2
Italy	1.22	118.0	0.0 E-6	61	0.2	1.6	7.4	19.3
Jordan	3.19	149.4	0.0 E-6	74	0.0	2.7	0.2	4.5
Latvia	2.18	190.9	0.0 E-6	53	0.0	2.2	87.6	4.5
Malta	2.19	64.1	4.6 E-5	63	0.2	1.3	5.0	12.1
Morocco	1.57	72.2	3.0 E-6	69	0.0	1.4	0.1	3.0
Netherlands	0.86	115.0	0.0 E-6	59	0.4	2.1	12.1	17.4
Oman	6.00	437.9	0.0 E-6	71	0.0	3.2	0.2	3.0
Portugal	1.53	62.5	4.6 E-5	61	0.0	1.6	9.2	20.1
Romania	2.58	99.5	0.0 E-6	52	1.0	2.9	10.8	40.5
Russian Federation	0.89	166.8	0.0 E-6	25	0.1	1.6	14.5	22.4
Spain	6.57	59.4	2.0 E-4	75	1.6	1.4	6.8	15.5
Sweden	1.45	59.6	1.9 E-4	53	0.1	1.3	13.5	21.2
United Arab Emirates	4.90	469.5	0.0 E-6	72	17.6	3.4	0.9	3.0
Venezuela	4.49	232.3	0.0 E-6	66	0.4	6.8	0.1	1.5
Overall	2.28	132.9	0.0 E-6	59	1.5	2.3	10.3	15.66

Table 57.10C Survey metrics for the postal survey, health and responsiveness components

Country	Summary SPDI	Deviation from UN Population — Chi-square critical value = 49.56 (26 df, p = 0.01)	Chi-square p-values	Response rate (%)	Health module — Individuals with > 5% missing data	Health module — Items with > 5% missing data	Responsiveness module — Individuals with > 10% missing data	Responsiveness module — Items with > 5% missing data
Australia	3.00	746.0	0.0E-6	35	0	13.0	N/A	N/A
Austria	3.93	310.0	0.0E-6	56	7.3	15.1	0.0	31.3
Canada	3.68	158.4	0.0E-6	55	2.4	4.8	0.0	20.2
Chile	4.80	410.7	0.0E-6	42	4.2	8.4	0.0	29.8
China	7.86	1 969.3	0.0E-6	50	0.4	4.1	0.3	12.6
Cyprus	2.95	331.8	0.0E-6	27	3.2	2.2	0.0	17.7
Czech Republic	3.24	359.8	0.0E-6	40	4.0	1.7	0.1	42.2
Denmark	0.98	91.9	0.0E-6	54	5.3	9.7	0.1	42.7
Egypt	1.00	85.1	0.0E-6	92	1.9	1.2	0.1	19.7
Finland	1.49	300.8	0.0E-6	54	10.1	8.1	0.3	23.2
France	2.13	239.3	0.0E-6	31	6.3	6.5	0.2	25.3
Greece	3.19	359.6	0.0E-6	35	3.3	2.6	1.2	38.4
Hungary	0.86	171.6	0.0E-6	72	4.1	15.6	0.0	29.3
Indonesia	3.40	986.5	0.0E-6	60	6.1	5.8	0.2	13.6
Kyrgyzstan	2.94	273.1	0.0E-6	44	13.2	9.0	0.6	32.8
Lebanon	3.19	66.4	2.2E-5	44	1.4	5.1	N/A	N/A
Lithuania	1.13	120.9	0.0E-6	70	4.6	6.5	1.4	10.6
Netherlands	0.96	275.2	0.0E-6	40	5.0	6.1	0.5	17.7
New Zealand	2.81	474.2	0.0E-6	68	5.5	1.7	0.2	22.5
Poland	1.52	370.9	0.0E-6	34	4.7	6.2	0.1	26.8
Rep. of Korea	7.95	506.4	0.0E-6	24	0	1.2	0.4	18.7
Switzerland	1.85	63.4	5.8E-5	38	9.7	16.9	0.3	41.0
Thailand	1.89	179.4	0.0E-6	46	0	1.0	0.5	26.5
Trinidad & Tobago	2.48	231.7	0.0E-6	52	22.3	7.9	0.3	53.3
Turkey	3.57	511.4	0.0E-6	90	23.9	10.1	0.1	70.5
Ukraine	1.02	129.9	0.0E-6	31	4.5	15.0	0.4	54.3
United Kingdom	2.26	182.7	0.0E-6	40	26.7	16.5	0.0	30.3
USA	5.28	857.5	0.0E-6	35	10.9	2.5	0.0	48.5
Overall	2.91	384.43	0.0E-6	48.54	6.82	7.31	0.3	30.8

Figure 57.6   Sample population representativeness by survey mode

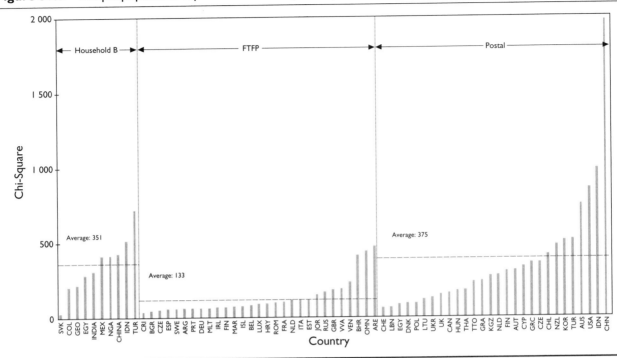

distribution, attempts are being made to understand what happened and how this can be overcome.

COMPARISON OF SURVEY MODE EFFECTS

One of the objectives of the WHO Multi-country Survey Study was to compare the feasibility and efficiency of different survey modes, therefore it is of scientific interest to consider the survey metrics in countries where multiple modes were used.

Figure 57.7A provides a comparison of the chi-square values of the deviation of the samples from the UN Population Database for 2000 for countries that participated in both the postal and household surveys. This figure illustrates that for Egypt and Turkey the WHO sample deviation from the UN Population Database for the postal surveys was considerably less than that for the household surveys, perhaps because the postal surveys were hand delivered in these countries using a sample frame of postal addresses. In contrast, for Indonesia and China, the postal surveys had a much higher deviation from the UN Population Database than the household surveys. This is possibly due to the fact that the postal surveys were actually mailed and the sampling frame may not have been adequate. Also, the response rates for the mailed surveys in China and Indonesia were much lower than

the ones for the household surveys (50–60% compared to 99%).

Figure 57.7B compares the chi-square for countries that participated in both the postal and brief face-to-face (BFTF) surveys. In all countries, but particularly in the Czech Republic and Finland, the sample deviation from the UN Population Database was considerably higher for the postal surveys than for the brief face-to-face (BFTF) surveys. This is perhaps due to the lack of an adequate sampling frame for the postal surveys.

Figures 57.8A–57.8F provide an overview of the performance of survey metrics in countries participating in the household surveys, in terms of their population deviation (chi-square), their test-retest reliability as measured by the Kappa coefficient, the missing values, and the response rates. The five figures show the relationship between these four quality metrics of the surveys.

From these figures it appears that the different survey modes performed differently depending on the metric examined. For example, though the surveys in India and Mexico had very little missing data and high reliabilities, the survey samples in these countries were not as representative of the overall country population, as, for example, the ones in Slovakia. Though the survey in Turkey had acceptable reliability, the missing

Figure 57.7A Comparison of household vs. postal surveys for representativeness

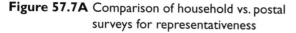

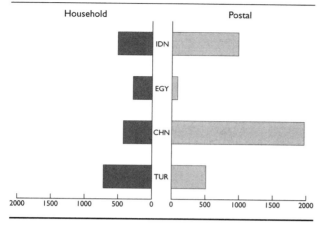

Figure 57.7B Comparison of brief face-to-face vs. postal surveys for representativeness

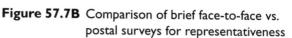

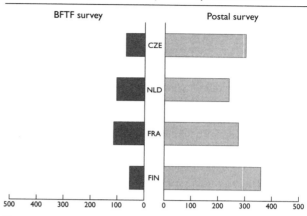

Figure 57.8A Summary quality assessment of household surveys by reliability and missing value

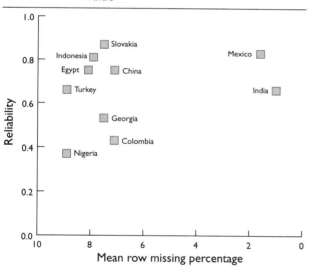

Figure 57.8B Summary quality assessment of household surveys by reliability and representativeness

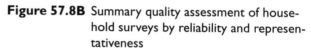

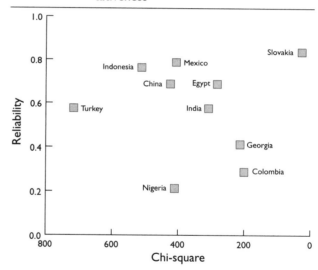

data and deviation from the country population were relatively high. The survey in Nigeria had higher missing values and lower reliabilities, while the chi-square values were close to the overall average.

Overall, the results suggest that there is no consistent relationship between the different survey metrics for any mode, e.g. reliability is not correlated with missingness or with representativeness. Brief face-to-face interviews have higher response rates and less missing data relative to the other modes, but the trade-off is that they collect less data. We are in the process of developing a single index of quality that can combine all these different parameters using multiple-indi-cator models, and examining how costs, sample size, country of implementation, etc. relate to that index.

COMPARISON TO OTHER MULTI-COUNTRY SURVEYS

The results of the survey study in terms of the quality metrics can be better understood when they are compared with surveys such as the LSMS (35) and the DHS (36). For example, in the DHS surveys the proportion of missing items that have more than 5% missing data ranges from 0.82% for Colombia in DHS III to 25.24% for Thailand in DHS I. There is

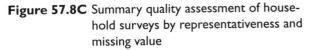

Figure 57.8C Summary quality assessment of household surveys by representativeness and missing value

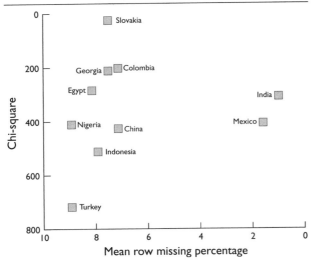

Figure 57.8D Summary quality assessment of WHO surveys by representativeness and missing value

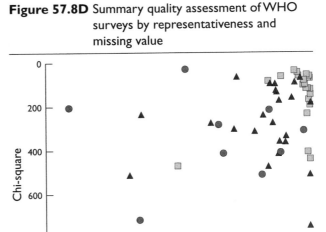

Household (missing > 10%)
BFTF (missing > 2%)
Postal (missing > 5%)

Figure 57.8E Summary quality assessment of WHO surveys by response rate and missing value

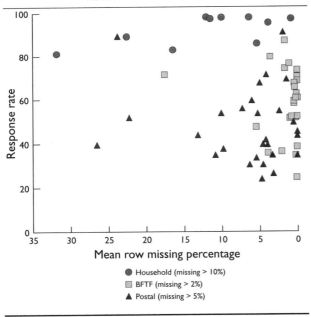

Household (missing > 10%)
BFTF (missing > 2%)
Postal (missing > 5%)

Figure 57.8F Summary quality assessment of WHO surveys by representativeness and response rate

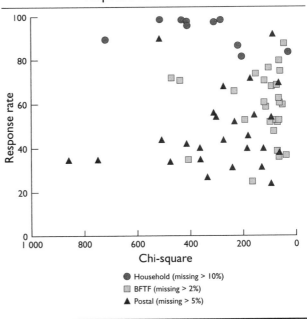

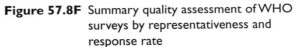

Household (missing > 10%)
BFTF (missing > 2%)
Postal (missing > 5%)

a substantial decrease in the percentage of items with more than 5% missing data over the three waves of the DHS. The chi-square values comparing the observed survey sample with the expected values obtained from the UN Population Database for 2000 for the DHS surveys (when considering all women in the age group 15–49 years, critical value = 26.22, 6df, p = .01) range between 6.21 for El Salvador in DHS I to 351.03 for Mali in DHS III. This is shown below in Figures 57.9A and 57.9B.

Figure 57.9A Representativeness of DHS surveys by country

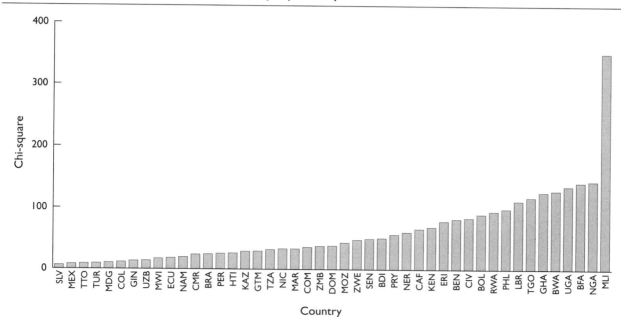

Figure 57.9B Relationship between missing data and representativeness for DHS surveys

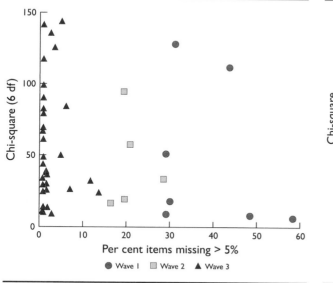

Figure 57.10 Comparison of representativeness across different surveys

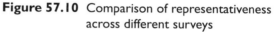

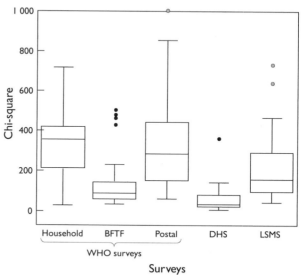

Similarly for the LSMS and related surveys, the chi-squares for the representativeness of the sample ranged between 46.28 for Guyana to 1 609.28 for the Lebanon Family Expenditure Survey (critical value = 44.31, 25df, p = .01).

Figure 57.10 shows the comparisons in the chi-square values as measures of representativeness of the samples across the WHO and other surveys. The DHS surveys have a very narrow range of chi-square values as compared to the LSMS or WHO surveys, and are the least deviant from the UN Population Database. Though the BFTF surveys also have a narrow range and smaller chi-square values, all the WHO and LSMS surveys are within overlapping ranges, suggesting that all the surveys were comparable in terms of their deviation from the UN population data.

Costs

It is difficult to compare the costs of surveys in different contexts because many factors vary across sites (for example, the equivalence of modes, variation in purchasing power, and individual arrangements with the sites). Nonetheless, it is still important to give an idea for the WHO Multi-country Survey Study, since there is a general erroneous belief that surveys are costly. The average in-country interview is shown in Table 57.11.

The findings confirm that face-to-face surveys are generally more expensive than postal surveys. The costs of the BFTF surveys, on average, were higher, perhaps because they were carried out mainly in European countries. Nonetheless, the overlapping ranges suggest that costs are comparable across survey modes (see Figure 57.11).

It is useful to compare these costs with other various survey programmes, although detailed costs are not always available. The average cost in the European Social Survey was about $222 for a completed interview. The Multiple Indicator Cluster Survey (MICS) of UNICEF cost about $112 000 on average per country, excluding costs for UNICEF staff, etc., for between 4 000 and 8 000 interviews per country (37). Comparatively, surveys in the WHO study ranged between $16

000 to $180 000 for sample sizes between 1 200 and 10 000 respondents. This information is not easily available for the other major surveys. If a conclusion could be drawn from these comparisons, WHO surveys are probably less costly than other survey programmes partly because they were conducted directly through governmental agencies or universities rather than intermediary agencies, and partly because they do not rely on expensive international consultants to maintain them. More importantly, these survey costs are quite reasonable and affordable in view of the information gains and they therefore offer a good means of supporting routine HIS.

Selected Results on the Health Module

One of the main aims of the results of the WHO Multi-country Survey Study has been developing appropriate analytical methods to ensure cross-population comparability of the survey data. The analytical methods reported in sections *The Specific Aim of Cross-population Comparability* and *Item Analysis: Item Response Theory Approach and HOPIT* served to ensure that the same level of "true" health can be estimated in different populations from self-reported data in order to make valid comparisons. Figure 57.12 illustrates the results for difficulties in moving around in a given country. The circles show the mean response by age and the triangles show the adjusted responses. There is only a slight decrease in average mobility with age without any adjustment. Once the way in which respondents use the categorical scale is determined by way of HOPIT, the drop-off in mobility with age is more pronounced. This indicates that the methods developed to adjust self-reports for ensuring cross-population comparability seem to adjust self-

Table 57.11 Average cost per completed interview

Survey mode	Average cost per final case [range]
Household	$16 [8–35]
Brief face-to-face	$34 [6–59]
CATI (avg. 30 minutes)	$30 [27–33]
Postal	$15 [5–43]

Figure 57.11 Comparison of cost by mode

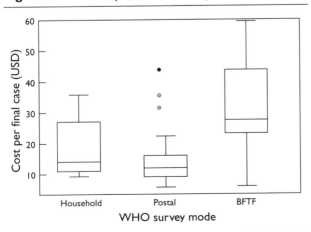

Figure 57.12 Adjusted and unadjusted mobility by age

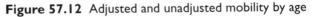
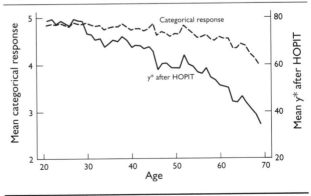

reports in the expected directions, allowing for more appropriate comparisons.

Figure 57.13 illustrates similar findings with self-care. The adjustment shows that mean responses decline much more rapidly with age than unadjusted self-reports.

SELECTED RESULTS ON THE RESPONSIVENESS MODULE

Figure 57.14 illustrates an example of using vignettes to enhance cross-population comparability. The model employed in this analysis (HOPIT) was developed to adjust self-reported data using vignettes. In the data shown in the figure, before adjustment (circles) there are no significant changes with age in the way that respondents describe their experience of being treated with dignity when they come into contact with the health services. However, once the results are adjusted (triangles) it is clear that older people in this sample actually experience that they are treated with less dignity by the health care services than younger people. Once again, the methods identify differences that were not evident before the results were adjusted for the cut-point shifts.

SELECTED RESULTS ON THE ADULT MORTALITY MODULE

Results from the full version of the household surveys were analysed for the information regarding adult mortality. Information gathered from the household surveys was compared to the estimates made by the World Health Organization from all other data sources such as vital registration, census, UN Population Database, etc. Figure 57.15 illustrates that data

gathered from the surveys on mortality for females in Nigeria compare favourably with other WHO estimates for the adult female age groups in Nigeria. This is one piece of evidence that suggests surveys may be an accurate and efficient way to supplement information on mortality in countries where vital registration data are limited or unavailable in order to construct life tables for the population.

DISCUSSION AND CONCLUSIONS

FEASIBILITY AND UTILITY

The WHO Multi-country Survey Study has demonstrated the feasibility of carrying out large surveys on selected outcomes to which the health system contributes, in a way that supplements the information provided by routine national health information systems. This was necessary because some data, such as those

Figure 57.14 Adjusted and unadjusted dignity by age

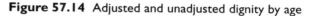
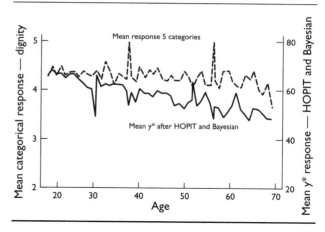
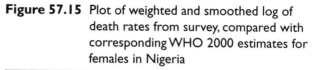

Figure 57.13 Adjusted and unadjusted self-care by age

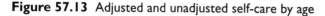

Figure 57.15 Plot of weighted and smoothed log of death rates from survey, compared with corresponding WHO 2000 estimates for females in Nigeria

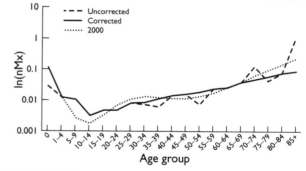

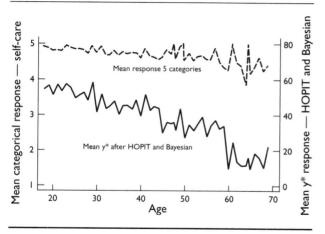

on responsiveness, are not routinely collected. It was also necessary because the data on health that are collected are not standardized, do not include multiple domains, and are not cross-population comparable.

The collaborating sites in countries have shown great interest in being a part of this endeavour. They participated actively in all phases of the survey and completed the data collection in a timely manner. The survey study used a rather complex design with many different modules and randomization of respondents across various components of the survey. Despite these complexities, completion rates have been high and the rate of missing data has been within acceptable limits.

The implementation of a complex survey study involving 61 countries and 71 surveys within 18 months requires substantial organizational skills on the part of the collaborating partners and continuous monitoring and support from the World Health Organization. This has been ensured through periodic phone conversations, email contacts, and actual visits to sites for on-site observation. The logistics of the WHO Multi-country Survey Study have been examined and several lessons learnt for future applications.

USE OF DATA

The WHO Multi-country Survey Study has proven useful in providing reliable and relevant data on health of populations, responsiveness of health systems, adult mortality, and health care expenditure modules for international comparisons. The annex tables included in *The World Health Report 2000* were based largely on secondary analyses of existing data sources. The World Health Organization has now developed an instrument which can be used to collect primary data on key aspects of health system performance.

APPROACHES FOR CROSS-POPULATION COMPARABILITY

In the analysis, use of novel techniques such as the vignettes and the calibration techniques have proven effective to achieve cross-population comparability. Using these data and novel statistical methods (i.e. HOPIT), we were able to overcome the known biases in the self-report data such as those between people from different cultural and educational backgrounds.

The study has demonstrated the feasibility and utility of using vignettes and performance tests to subsequently adjust self-reports. However, further work

is necessary in this area. The current set of vignettes needs to be expanded to capture the breadth of each domain better. In addition, some of the domains of health are inherently multidimensional (e.g. "vision," which may be a combination of near and distant vision, colour vision and adaptation to light). This leads to difficulties in rating vignettes according to severity since the different aspects of a domain may be viewed as independent from each other. Further, the questions asked to each respondent also need to span all levels of difficulty such that segments of the population that are in good health can be discriminated from those that are in average health and in turn from those in poor health.

Performance tests have also been implemented effectively in this study. The feasibility of lay interviewers using them in the general population in survey settings has been demonstrated. However, tests have also shown variation across sites in the manner in which they were conducted, and steps need to be taken to ensure they are more uniformly executed. More rigorous training of interviewers with periodic supervision to maintain quality might be the appropriate response.

SURVEY COSTS

The overall cost of carrying out the study has been considerably lower than the prices of comparable surveys such as the Living Standards Measurement Survey (LSMS). The latter costs between 500 000–1 000 000 USD per country (36). However, survey costs cannot be compared directly given the differences in the nature of various surveys. Nonetheless, the surveys in this study have maintained similar standards of quality. This suggests that surveys of this kind may be an efficient way of gathering data. The implementation of such surveys may often be the best method to collect in a reliable manner specific data not available from routine health information systems.

PLANS FOR THE WORLD HEALTH SURVEY (2002–2003)

The demand for internationally comparable information on health and health systems requires a search for low cost ways of supplementing the information routinely gathered by national health information systems (HIS). Based on the experience gained in the WHO Multi-country Survey Study 2000–2001, the World Health Survey (WHS) has been designed specifically to fill these critical information gaps in routine HIS. The Director–General of the World Health Organization has decided to launch the WHS. This will systematically gather data from representative populations to facilitate the task of monitoring health and the components of the health system. In addition, it will be an ideal platform from which to obtain information on health system performance.

The WHO Multi-country Survey Study has provided valuable scientific opportunities for testing different survey modes, developing appropriate questions and techniques for ensuring cross-population comparability. It has also proved to be a low-cost way of obtaining data. Some important lessons have been learned that have helped develop the WHS.

Questionnaires

The WHO Multi-country Survey Study provided extensive empirical data on the applicability and psychometric properties of individual survey questions. It identified certain questions that have low reliabilities and response rates across several sites (e.g. question on overall health, or overall interpersonal relationships and participation in the community; questions related to alcohol and substance use; vignettes describing risky sexual behaviour, etc.). Such questions have been rephrased to ensure better measurement qualities and uniform applicability across cultures. Questions that are long or complicated were shortened and made more precise.

Measuring Health in the Relatively Well Populations

It is also important to capture the health level of the relatively well members of the population—in technical terms, avoid ceiling effects in the questionnaire. Given that the respondents were selected randomly from the general population, most were in a relatively well functioning level in any given health domain. Traditional health survey questions are designed to pick up problems, and they worked well with people who have moderate and severe problems but do not discriminate between relatively mild problems. Thus, more specific questions have been developed that attempt to capture this range of the health spectrum. Given the existing database, it will now be possible to develop adaptive questioning strategies allowing us to tailor the questionnaires to the respondents' experience and facilitate the discrimination of the health states of persons who are at the relatively healthy end of the continuum.

Modes

Given the survey quality metrics in the postal surveys, we plan to focus mainly on in-person household or telephone interviews. Although this will slightly increase the costs of the surveys, the increase would be offset by the corresponding gains in quality.

Sampling

- We used vigorous sampling techniques to ensure that the sample is representative of the general population. However, further work is necessary to ensure that the elderly and the more sick members of the population are not excluded from the surveys. Because these populations may not be in households, we need to sample from institutions or over-sample the elderly so as to provide information on the health of this segment of the population.

- The current phase of the study has focused exclusively on the adult population. Inclusion of youth and children in the World Health Survey would be valuable since data on this age group are particularly scarce. More importantly, in developing countries, a large proportion of the population (30–50%) is in this age group.

- We also plan to geo-code the data and to use a Geographical Information System (GIS) in order to improve the sampling designs. This would reduce possible clustering effects as well.

Vignettes

The WHO Multi-country Survey Study has demonstrated the feasibility and utility of using vignettes for cross-population comparability. To be useful, vignettes need to span the whole continuum of a given domain. Some of the sets of vignettes that were piloted did not do this adequately. In addition, some domains of health are inherently multidimensional (e.g. the domain of "vision" which may be a combination of near and distant vision, colour vision and adaptation to light). Vignettes need to yield a unidimensional stimulus to respondents for comparability purposes.

Performance Tests

To calibrate the range of responses, known tests were used in the survey study (e.g. Snellen eye chart for vision, and some mobility and cognition tests). We have demonstrated that they can be applied to the general population by lay interviewers in survey settings, suggesting that they can be introduced in a larger survey programme. However, these tests have also shown variation across sites in the manner in which they are implemented (e.g. measured mobility tests showed variability because respondents were asked to walk on different types of surfaces). Therefore, these tests need to be more uniformly executed in different sites. More rigorous training of interviewers specifically on performance tests, with periodic supervision to maintain quality, is required as well.

New Survey Modules

Given the modular design, there has been a demand from countries to develop new modules.

Coverage—Access—Utilization

The ways of ensuring the effective coverage of health interventions have long been a concern of health policy-makers. Despite separate studies on particular aspects of coverage such as immunization and antenatal care, no overall framework allowing regular measurement of what proportion of the population is effectively covered by the needed critical interventions is available. Conceptual development work is under way, and following pilot studies, such a module will be incorporated in the survey instrument.

Risk Factors

Given the importance of risk factors in explaining the current and future health status of individuals and populations, it is useful to describe the risk factors influencing health in a survey module. Such a module would include risk factors in detail, such as water and sanitation, air pollution, malnutrition, lack of breast-feeding, smoking, alcohol and drugs, physical activity, obesity, unsafe sex, behavioural factors, cholesterol, and blood pressure, etc. The current survey questionnaire contains several questions on these topics, but a more systematic approach to the measurement of risk factors is under development.

Health Financing

The Multi-country Study questionnaire included several questions on household income and health expenditures. With the demonstration of the feasibility of this approach, it will be useful to gather more information on health expenditures from all sources in countries that do not collect this information routinely.

Capacity Building and Sustainability

In the future waves, it is important to establish the common goals of the survey programme with outside partners, taking into account their information needs. Given the need for comprehensive health systems performance assessment at the national and subnational levels, it is important to build capacity to carry out periodic surveys in countries and sustain this platform with appropriate resources and skills. Clear strategies for moving from diagnosis to intervention with regard to health systems need to be identified as well, such that the survey results are used as the evidence to inform policy, and to monitor and evaluate performance.

The WHS platform will thus provide a modular approach that will allow Member States to prioritize the areas of immediate concern for the purpose of data collection in order to inform and monitor decisions. It will be an ongoing programme such that Member States can decide the frequency with which the survey needs to be carried out in their respective countries. Attempts will be made to incorporate these surveys into national HIS and to harmonize data elements already being gathered as part of national HIS with those included in the WHS.

The World Health Survey offers an ideal platform to seek information on the prevalence of health states, health state valuations, responsiveness levels and distributions, household health expenditures, risk factors, coverage, basic demography, and permanent income, all of which can be useful for health systems performance assessment.

Special efforts to build consensus on collaborative approaches with other agencies sponsoring or conducting surveys will be made, e.g. with Demographic and Health Surveys, Living Standards Measurement Surveys, EURO Barometer, and national surveys.

NOTES

1 Statistical Office of the European Communities, European Commission.

2 *Validity* is the extent to which a survey instrument measures what is intended to measure. It describes how actually the instrument is able to capture the real nature of what is measured. This can be measured for an item, a series of items or overall instrument level. *Reliability* is the extent to which repeated use of the instrument gives the same result. Reliability is the consistency of the measurement, or the degree to which an instrument measures the same way each time it is used under the same condition with the same subjects. In short, it is the repeatability

of the measurement. A measure is considered reliable if a person's score on the same test given twice is similar. One can think of reliability as measurement invariance or conversely the extent to which a measurement is subject to random measurement error. Validity is the extent to which a measurement correcting for random measurement error is correlated to the true level. In other words, validity can be understood as lack of bias. Validity is the strength of our conclusions, inferences or propositions. It is the best available approximation to the truth or falsity of a given inference, proposition, or conclusion. Construct validity is the degree to which inferences we have made from our study can be generalized to the underlying concepts in the first place. For example, if we are measuring mobility as an outcome, can our definition (operationalization) of that term in our study be generalized to the rest of the world's concept of mobility?

2 The methods developed by WHO such as HOPIT and CHOPIT can be conceptualized as modified IRT models (20).

4 In addition, a "Key Informant Survey" with similar questions, given to selected key informants (e.g. providers, consumers, policy-makers, media workers etc.), was also developed to test possible concurrence of its results with the personal report of responsiveness construct in the same set of countries. Key informants gave their opinions of their health system responsiveness of the public and private sectors, the extent of unequal treatment and experiences for different population groups within their country, how they measure and value different states of inequality in responsiveness, and how they value the importance of the different responsiveness domains within the overall construct (URL: http://snow.who.int/whosis_stage/menu.cfm?path=hsr (23)).

3 In WHO Multi-country Survey Study Household sites, an additional multi-method valuation study among educated respondents was undertaken in order to estimate the relationship between health state valuations elicited using the visual analogue scale and the underlying strength of preference function that is required in the construction of summary measures of population health.

4 Aggregate Deviation Index or summary index is calculated using the following formula:

$$\text{Summary Index} = \Sigma \mid 1 - \text{Age Group Index} \mid$$

The summary index was calculated for all age groups between 20 and 74, as they represent the most stable age groups across survey countries and modes.

REFERENCES

(1) Eurostat. *Self-reported health in the European community: statistics in focus, population and social conditions.* ISSN 1024-4352. Eurostat, 1997.

(2) Mathers CD et al. *Estimates of DALE for 191 countries: methods and results.* EIP Discussion Paper No. 16. Geneva, World Health Organization, 2000. URL: http://www3.who.int/whosis/discussion_papers/discussion_papers.cfm#

(3) Mathers CD et al. *Estimates of healthy life expectancy for 191 countries in the year 2000: methods and results.* EIP Discussion Paper No. 38. Geneva, World Health Organization, 2001. URL: http://www3.who.int/whosis/discussion_papers/discussion_papers.cfm#

(4) Sadana R et al. Comparative analyses of more than 50 household surveys on health status. In: Murray CJL et al., eds. *Summary measures of population health: concepts, ethics, measurement and applications.* Geneva, World Health Organization, 2002:369–386.

(5) Mathers CD et al. Healthy life expectancy in 191 countries, 1999. *The Lancet*, 2001, 357:1685–1691.

(6) Murray CJL et al. *Enhancing cross-population comparability of survey results.* EIP Discussion Paper No. 35. Geneva, World Health Organization, 2000. URL: http://www3.who.int/whosis/discussion_papers/discussion_papers.cfm#

(7) Üstün TB et al. *Disability and culture: universalism and diversity.* Gottingen, Hogrefe and Huber, 2001.

(8) Hambleton RK, Swaminathan H, Rogers HJ. *Fundamentals of item response theory.* Newbury, Sage Publications, 1991.

(9) Streiner DL, Norman GR. *Health measurement scales: a practical guide to their development and use,* 2nd ed. Oxford, Oxford University Press, 1995.

(10) Graziano AM, Raulin ML. *Research methods: a process of inquiry.* New York, Longman, 1997.

(11) World Health Organization. *The World Health Report 2000. Health Systems: Improving Performance.* Geneva, World Health Organization, 2000.

(12) Chatterji S et al. *The conceptual basis for measuring and reporting on health.* EIP Discussion Paper No. 45. Geneva, World Health Organization, 2002. URL: http://www3.who.int/whosis/discussion_papers/discussion_papers.cfm#

(13) World Health Organization. *International Classification of Diseases and Related Health Problems—Tenth Revision (ICD-10).* Geneva, World Health Organization, 1992.

(14) World Health Organization. *International Classification of Functioning, Disability and Health (ICF).* Geneva, World Health Organization, 2001.

(15) Coren S. Reporting the visual acuity of groups: the relation among alternate measures. *American Journal of Optometry & Psychological Optics*, 1987, Dec. 64(12): 897–900.

(16) Kokko SM et al. The assessment of functional ability in patients with Parkinson's disease: the PLM-test and three clinical tests. *Physiotherapy Research International*, 1997, 2(2):29–45.

(17) Spreen O, Strauss E. *A compendium of neuropsychological tests.* Oxford, Oxford University Press, 1998.

(18) Trennery MR et al. *Visual search and attention test.* Odessa: Psychological Assessment Resources, 1990.

(19) Wilson B, Cockburn J, Halligan PW. Development of a behavioural test of visuospatial neglect. *Archives of Physical Medicine and Rehabilitation*, 1987, 68:98–102.

(20) Tandon A et al. Statistical models for enhancing cross-population comparability. In: Murray CJL, Evans DB, eds. *Health systems performance assessment: debates, methods and empiricism.* Geneva, World Health Organization, 2003.

(21) Salomon JA et al. Health state valuations in summary measures of population health. In: Murray CJL, Evans DB, eds. *Health systems performance assessment: debates, methods and empiricism.* Geneva, World Health Organization, 2003.

(22) Valentine NB, de Silva A, Murray CJL. *Estimating responsiveness level and distribution for 191 countries: methods and results.* EIP Discussion Paper No. 22. Geneva, World Health Organization, 2000. URL: http://www3.who.int/whosis/discussion_papers/discussion_papers.cfm#

(23) World Health Organization. *Health systems responsiveness.* URL: http://snow.who.int/whosis_stage/menu.cfm?path=hsr

(24) World Health Organization. *Composite International Diagnostic Interview (CIDI).* Geneva, World Health Organization, 1992 (Updated 2000). URL: http://www.who.int/msa/cidi/

(25) Murray CJL et al. Adult morbidity: limited data and methodological uncertainty. In: Feachem RG et al., eds. *The health of adults in the developing world.* New York, Oxford University Press, 1992:113–160.

(26) Lopez AD et al. Life tables for 191 countries for 2000: data, methods, results. In: Murray CJL, Evans DB, eds. *Health systems performance assessment: debates, methods and empiricism.* Geneva, World Health Organization, 2003.

(27) World Health Organization. *Environmental health indicators: framework and methodologies.* Protection of the Human Environment Occupational and Environmental Health Series. Geneva, World Health Organization, 1999.

(28) Xu K et al. Household health system contributions and capacity to pay: definitional, empirical, and technical challenges. In: Murray CJL, Evans DB, eds. *Health systems performance assessment: debates, methods and empiricism.* Geneva, World Health Organization, 2003.

(29) Kish L. *Survey sampling.* New York, John Wiley & Sons, 1965.

(30) Dillman DA. *Mail and internet surveys: the tailored design method*, 2nd ed. New York, John Wiley & Sons, 2000.

(31) Dillman DA. *Mail and telephone surveys: the total design method.* New York, Wiley-Interscience, 1978.

(32) World Health Organization. *I-Shell.* URL: http://www.who.int/evidence/hhsr-survey/

(33) Cohen J. A coefficient of agreement for nominal scales. *Educational and Psychological Measurement*, 1960, 20:37–46.

(34) Fleiss JL. *Statistical methods for rates and proportions*, 2nd ed. New York, John Wiley & Sons, 1981.

(35) Grosh M, Glewwe P. *Designing household survey questionnaires for developing countries: lessons from 15 years of the Living Standards Measurement Study.* Washington, DC, World Bank, 2000.

(36) Macro International Inc. *Demographic and Health Surveys.* URL: http://www.measuredhs.com/

(37) United Nations Children's Fund. *Evaluation of multiple indicator cluster surveys.* New York, UNICEF, 1997.

Chapter 58

The World Health Surveys

T. Bedirhan Üstün, Somnath Chatterji, Abdelhay Mechbal, Christopher J.L. Murray, WHS Collaborating Groups[1]

The World Health Surveys (WHS) are an initiative launched by the World Health Organization to strengthen national capacity to monitor critical health outputs and outcomes through the fielding of a valid, reliable, and comparable household survey instrument. To provide the context for the WHS, we first discuss the role of household surveys in national health information systems. The remainder of the chapter gives an overview of the objectives of the WHS, the development and rationale for the WHS modules, the current status of implementation of the WHS, and the WHS methods. Some reflections on the relevance of the WHS to policy formulation are provided at the end.

Role of Household Surveys in Health Information Systems

Health information systems (HIS) are the set of data collection instruments, actors, resources, and institutions whose primary purpose is to inform strategic decision-making, support programme management, monitor progress towards agreed targets, and provide the basis for the evaluation of what works and what does not in health systems. National health information systems need to give information on a wide range of topics including levels, causes and patterns of health, use and effectiveness of health interventions, client experience of health services, financial, physical and human resource inputs, and a range of other health system activities.

A key aspect of health information systems is the mode through which needed information is collected for a range of purposes, topics, and levels of aggregation. Figure 58.1 illustrates the seven main modes of information gathering that should be part of any national health information system.

Vital registration systems, which capture events such as birth and death, and attribute deaths based on the International Classification of Diseases, are the backbone of most national health information systems. Irrespective of whether a Ministry of Health manages vital registration, it is an integral component of a functioning health information system.

The second main mode is information collected from purchasers of health interventions, including Ministries of Health, which allocate budgets to their own hospitals and clinics. Purchaser information comprises budgets, expenditure accounts, staff lists, and the more richly detailed information purchasers in some high- and middle-income countries on specific health system transactions through, for example, insurance records.

In many countries, HIS investments are focused on the third mode of data collection: provider registries and case reporting. This information, collected at the point of service by health providers, includes case notifications meeting specified criteria as well as registries of specific interventions such as DTP3. Providers can be categorized into Ministry of Health, other public sector, and private sector. In the vast majority of countries, provider registry information is often received only from Ministry of Health providers, giving an incomplete picture of morbidity and intervention delivery.

Fourthly, health information systems also collect information from a number of actors and institutions whose primary role is stewardship. Examples of information collected from stewards of the health system include nurse or physician licensing, hospital accreditation, or occupational safety inspections.

The fifth mode is collecting information directly from households through national censuses, or more commonly through household surveys. Household sur-

Figure 58.1   Different information collection modes
for health information systems

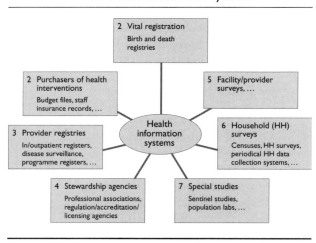

vey data may be collected as part of a broader national survey or may be focused only on health topics. A well-designed household survey can address many of the selection bias problems that plague both vital registration and provider registries in many countries. Similarly, information on quality, resourcing, and efficiency can be collected through facility surveys, which can be considered a separate mode of data collection.

Household surveys have an important role to play in national health information systems. They represent a low-cost method of addressing the selection bias inherent in provider registries in nearly all countries; effective coverage of health interventions delivered by private providers is a good example of this. Collecting information directly from households also provides a practical strategy for dealing with the poor coverage of vital registration data in many low-income countries. Household surveys are the only method of obtaining some important types of information, such as household out-of-pocket payments to providers or patient experience of the full spectrum of health system providers. With increasing policy concern in health and health system outcomes in the poor and other disadvantaged groups, household surveys are the most practical and low-cost approach to measuring key outcomes for different socio-demographic subgroups including the poor.

Household surveys are currently used in nearly all health information systems, but their full potential is often unrealized. Well-established health information systems in high-income countries use household surveys routinely to provide essential information. For example, the National Health Interview Survey in the United States has been implemented annually since

1957 (*1*). In low- and middle-income countries, a large number of household surveys focusing on health topics are undertaken every year. This major investment by nearly all countries includes a wide range of narrow surveys on particular topics such as nutritional status, oral health, chronic disease risk factors, adolescent health, or integrated management of childhood illness. The opportunity presented through each contact with a household in existing surveys could be better used if valid and reliable standardized instruments were available for a wide range of topics.

The Demographic and Health Surveys (DHS) have been an important effort to create and implement standardized modules for measuring child and maternal health, and household characteristics including assets, environmental risk factors, nutritional status, reproductive behaviour, children's health, status of women, AIDS, and other sexually transmitted infections (*2*). The implementation of the DHS in over 50 countries over the last 20 years has added substantially to global knowledge on child mortality and fertility. Standardized modules built on multi-country implementation, however, are not available for a range of important topics such as multidimensional health status, patient experience, household health expenditures, coverage of interventions for non-communicable conditions or some risk factors that can be captured through household surveys in a cost-effective manner. In some cases, existing standardized modules in use in various survey programmes have not undergone extensive psychometric evaluation.

When household survey instruments are designed to enhance comparability of responses across individuals within a population and across different cultural groups, the utility of the information can be greatly increased. Valid, reliable and comparable information can be used to bench-mark important health or health system outcomes, inputs and processes. When information is valid, reliable and comparable, data collected for monitoring and evaluation purposes can also contribute to the global evidence base on what works and what does not. Comparability can often be obtained in household surveys at relatively low cost through the appropriate design of the instrument and the inclusion of specific testing in development of the comparability of results. The World Health Survey is the first major survey programme to explicitly recognize the importance of comparability in the development of the instrument, in addition to the important concerns about validity and reliability.

OBJECTIVES OF THE WHS

Recognizing both the central role of regular household surveys in an effective national health information system and the under-utilized potential of existing household surveys in most countries, the World Health Organization launched the World Health Survey (WHS) in August of 2001. The programme of work in support of the WHS has the following specific objectives:

■ To develop valid, reliable, and comparable household survey modules for a wide range of priority topics that can be used by countries as an integral part of their health information systems in a cost-effective manner.

■ To define a set of quality assurance protocols and reporting strategies, including visits by technical advisers, in order to ensure satisfactory survey design and implementation.

■ To formulate a strategy for building national capacity and expertise to conduct surveys and develop long-term sustainable platforms to share this information in public.

■ To encourage the formation of links with international and regional networks to build national and regional research capacity.

■ To provide a dynamic data collection platform that can be continuously developed with a transparent audit trail and availability of data in the public domain as an international public good.

■ To facilitate the use of information collected through the WHS in appropriate strategic planning, programme management, monitoring, and evaluation. Particular emphasis is placed on policy use of the monitoring of the Millennium Development Goal indicators and on the critical outcomes concerning the poor.

MODULAR DESIGN

In order to enhance the utility of the World Health Survey, its development, testing and implementation have been formulated on a modular basis. The intention is that each module may be used as a stand-alone product in a variety of household survey contexts. New modules will be added to the initial set of modules incorporated into the first round of the WHS. Participating countries can choose from these modules in any combination according to their policy needs. They can add their own modules if they wish, or add WHS modules to existing survey platforms in their countries.

The existing set of modules included in the WHS is listed in Table 58.1. The current WHS modules address different aspects of health and health systems, and are organized in two sections, the household questionnaire and the individual questionnaire.

INSTRUMENT DEVELOPMENT

In this section, we briefly review the origin, testing, and revision of the WHS modules. Special emphasis is given in this discussion to the health state description and the health system responsiveness modules, since these are relatively innovative and underwent a longer process of development and testing. An important aspect of the development of the WHS has been the use of the anchoring vignette strategy to enhance the comparability of self-responses for health state descriptions, responsiveness, and social capital. Instrument development should be seen as a continuous process. Each wave of empiricism has to be used to revise and improve the instrument for subsequent waves. The focus of this section, therefore, is on the development of the WHS instrument used in the first wave of surveys fielded in 2002 and 2003.

INSTRUMENT DEVELOPMENT PROCESS

The health state description and responsiveness modules began with an extensive review of the available items in common use in health and patient experience

Table 58.1   Modules of the WHS instrument in 2002–2003

The Household Questionnaire	Roster of all the individuals in the household
	Household health intervention coverage
	Health insurance
	Health expenditure
	Indicators of permanent income
	Health occupations
The Individual Questionnaire	Socio-demographics
	Health state description
	Health state valuation
	Risk factors
	Mortality
	Coverage of health interventions
	Health system responsiveness
	Health system goals and social capital
	Interviewer observations

instruments. The review of existing health instruments was facilitated by the ongoing work on developing the *International Classification of Functioning, Disability and Health* (ICF) (3). The ICF provides a coherent framework and terminology for the multiple domains of health. Based on this systematic review and consultations with experts in the field, a pilot instrument was tested in household surveys in Tanzania, the Philippines, and Colombia in 1999. Following analysis of the preliminary data and consultations in expert meetings, the instrument was thoroughly revised. The major development was the inclusion in the instrument of panels of anchoring vignettes (see Chapters 30 and 31 in this book for details (4;5)). Anchoring vignettes are meant to help understand how respondents in diverse socioeconomic, demographic, and cultural settings may use response categories in different ways. The information collected through anchoring vignettes can be used non-parametrically or with appropriate statistical models such as CHOPIT, to enhance response comparability (6).

The health state description and responsiveness modules including panels of anchoring vignettes, along with modules on mortality, socio-demographics, health system goals, and mental health, were included in the WHO Multi-country Survey Study on Health and Responsiveness 2000–2001 (MCSS). Seventy-one surveys were completed in 61 countries using face-to-face, postal, and telephone interviewing modes (see Chapter 57 (7)). A 90-minute long version of the interview and a shorter 30-minute version were used. The purpose of this study was to develop a valid, reliable, and comparable instrument to describe individual health and responsiveness, and to test the effects that the interviewing mode may have on data quality and self-report. The study was also intended to develop a comprehensive methodology for WHO to gather data on important indicators of interest and to assist countries with the fielding of household surveys. The survey was designed to be implemented with careful quality control, appropriate sampling, and data management strategies. Another major goal was to build capacity in countries to analyse data from complex surveys. The MCSS provides the first comprehensive data set that allows the adjustment of self-reports based on shifts in cut-points using the anchoring vignettes methodology. The MCSS collected 188 307 cases and 10 309 retest cases who were given the same questionnaire twice within a week. Such retest data provides a much richer basis for formal psychometric evaluation of instrument properties.

Analysis of the MCSS provided an extensive empirical basis for modifying items and reducing the number of domains and/or items per domain for the health state description, health state valuation, health system goals, and responsiveness modules. Kappas and intra-class correlation coefficients allowed identification of items with particularly low test-retest reliability. Data on item missingness also provided insights into the psychometric properties of items or groups of items. Formal item and domain reduction methods were used on the MCSS data to suggest ways to decrease substantially the overall length of these modules.

With the public announcement of the WHS and reporting of the results of the WHO Multi-country Survey Study, the discussion platform was widened to include multiple inputs to improve the content and style of the WHS. Demands for information that could be used in national health policy debates and monitoring exercises from national decision-makers led to the development of new draft modules to more systematically collect information from households. These new modules included expanded information on health insurance, household members working in the health sector (health occupations), indicators of permanent income, risk factors, and coverage of health interventions. Items in these modules were taken from existing surveys such as the DHS, or developed by working groups of WHO technical staff from a range of departments.

Between February and April 2002, revised modules for health state description, health state valuation, responsiveness, and health system goals, along with new draft items for modules on health expenditures, health insurance, health occupations, indicators of permanent income, risk factors, and health intervention coverage, were fielded in a 12-country WHS pilot study. Because of the length of some of the draft modules, not all modules were fielded in all sites. Health state description, risk factors, and mortality, along with all the modules at the household level, were fielded in China (467 respondents), Myanmar (599 respondents), Pakistan (549 respondents), Sri Lanka (594 respondents), Turkey (600 respondents), and the United Arab Emirates (595 respondents). Responsiveness, coverage, and all other modules excluding health state description, risk factors, and mortality, were fielded in Cote d'Ivoire (598 respondents), India (649 respondents), Malaysia (602 respondents), Mexico (604 respondents), South Africa (585 respondents), and Spain (592 respondents). As these were pilot studies to allow formal psychometric evaluation of the modules, they were not random sample surveys. In all, 7 043 respondents were surveyed and 1 200 were retested within two weeks.

Based on careful analysis of the WHS pilot data, working groups for each module proposed a draft final instrument. These proposals were timed and an overall steering group for the WHS made further reductions in the instrument length, so that all modules could be fielded in an average of 90 minutes. In addition, a 30-minute version was developed for use in countries where costs of a 90-minute interview would be prohibitive. The final WHS wave I instrument was available in August 2002. This instrument has been translated into multiple languages following a standardized protocol including back translation (8).

CURRENT WHS MODULES AND RATIONALE FOR THEIR CONTENT

In this part of the chapter, we review each module of the WHS and give a brief explanation of its content.

The first section, the *Household Questionnaire,* takes a roster of all individuals in the household and examines common features of the household. This section of the WHS provides important information on household composition and characteristics. In detail, it includes the following modules:

- Household roster. The informant gives information on members of the household, their relationship to the informant, age, education, marital status, and whether they have worked in a health occupation. The adult member of the household who will be interviewed as the primary respondent for the individual questionnaire, is selected using a Kish table.

- Household health intervention coverage. In this module, selected health interventions that are household interventions by nature are explored. These include, for example, use of insecticide-impregnated bednets for children and pregnant women in the household. Household members who are institutionalized for health reasons are also recorded.

- Health insurance. For each household member, the informant is asked whether he or she is covered by a health insurance plan and what are the various characteristics of this health insurance, including premiums. In selected countries, this module is extended to collect detailed information on participation in community health insurance schemes.

- Health expenditure. Information on total expenditure broken down into food, housing, education, health care, and all other expenditures is collected in this module. Health expenditure is further divided into a range of categories.

- Indicators of permanent income. Robust estimates of household permanent income can be obtained with information on the ownership of selected assets such as radios, televisions, cars, or chairs, as well as access to household services such as electricity, running water, and sewerage (9;10). This module uses a standard set of dichotomous questions about household assets and services. The exact set of items is adjusted to national levels of income per capita. Permanent income estimates provide important information for the measurement of health of the poor and the analysis of inequalities in health, coverage, and responsiveness.

- Health occupations. For any household member identified in the household roster as having worked in a health related occupation, a series of items on the type of employment and employer, educational experience, and compensation mechanism is collected. This module is meant to provide information on a cross-section of health workers in a country including public and private sectors.

The second section, the *Individual Questionnaire,* covers the following aspects:

- Socio-demographics. This module collects information on age, sex, education, employment status, and ethnicity.

- Health state description. Self-assessed health levels are elicited for each of the eight domains of health—mobility, self-care, pain and discomfort, cognition, interpersonal activities, vision, sleep, and energy and affect. For each domain, two items are included to reduce measurement error and improve the efficiency of statistical models used to analyse these data. In addition, respondents provide answers to five vignettes relating to two of the eight domains. Respondents are randomized to answer vignettes for one of four combinations of two domains.

- Health state valuation. Respondents rank a series of hypothetical health states and provide associated detailed descriptions of those hypothetical states. This can be used to understand how individuals combine information on levels of different domains of health into an overall assessment of health.

- Risk factors. Items in this module cover tobacco use, alcohol consumption, fruit and vegetable intake, physical activity, water and sanitation, and indoor air pollution. These risks have been selected taking into account the risk factors that are the largest worldwide and for which self-report is a reasonable method of data collection. Responses can be used as inputs to comparative risk assessment exercises.

- Mortality. Primarily intended for use in countries with incomplete vital registration systems, this module includes a complete birth history, sibling survivorship history, and a brief verbal autopsy designed to identify selected leading causes of death. Measurements of adult mortality are particularly weak in many low-income countries; the sibling survival items may provide an important input to demographic assessments of adult mortality in these settings.

- Coverage of health interventions. This module is intended to collect information that can be used to assess the coverage or effective coverage of certain key health interventions. Coverage is the probability that an individual who needs an intervention will receive it. For interventions that an entire target population is meant to receive, such as immunization, assessment of coverage requires information on who received the immunization. For interventions directed at particular diseases, the coverage module collects information on the prevalence or incidence of a condition and whether the respondent received treatment. The module includes items on immunization, treatment of childhood illnesses, safe motherhood interventions, DOTS for tuberculosis, STD and HIV/AIDS prevention, and treatment of angina, asthma, arthritis, depression, road traffic injuries, and others.

- Health system responsiveness. The responsiveness module gathers basic information on health care utilization for inpatient and outpatient services. For health system contacts, two items are collected on the eight domains of responsiveness—autonomy, dignity, communication, confidentiality, basic amenities, prompt attention, choice, and social support. For two of the eight domains, each respondent also answers these items for five vignettes (*11*).

- Health system goals and social capital. Because many health systems performance assessment schemes have a composite measure combining different aspects of health systems such as health of the population, responsiveness, and financing of the system (*12;13*), it is useful to obtain the preferences of the respondents on these components. WHS modules ask about the relative importance of the key goals of a health system: level and distribution of health, level and distribution of responsiveness and fairness in financial contribution. In addition, given the importance of interdependencies between social capital and health, this module includes a range of questions on social capital, e.g. relating to stress, security, and participation in community, plus corresponding anchoring vignettes to enhance the cross-population comparability of these data.

- The WHS interview schedule ends with a section to record interviewer observations regarding the interview context and quality of responses.

The short version of the interview is nested within (i.e. includes a subset of questions from) the long version, which enables a direct comparison of data collected using the different versions. The short version takes about 30 minutes to complete and is administered to a single respondent in its entirety. It excludes questions on insurance, valuation of health, risk factors, mortality, and social capital, and has abbreviated coverage and responsiveness sections.

Ongoing Instrument Development and Modification

The WHS instrument is envisaged as an evolving product. As country needs arise, new WHS modules will be developed following the same principles of rigorous psychometric testing and piloting on a large scale. As lessons are learned, items and vignettes will be modified. Individual items will be changed, added, or dropped depending on the way they have performed psychometrically and based on the information they provide. Systematic testing (see Chapter 30 in this book (*4*)) will detect items that perform particularly poorly across populations or in selected situations, and these items will be modified or replaced. Vignettes will continue to be improved in order to achieve the goal of comparability. Every new module that is developed will have to pass the same stringent tests before being implemented on a wide scale. It will be carefully developed on the same principles as the core of the WHS instrument, and will be extensively pre-tested in several languages and regions.

NATIONAL PARTICIPATION IN THE WHS

WHO recognizes that the WHS must lead to the building of collaborations and partnerships that will strengthen survey capacity and improve data quality in Member States. With this goal in mind, participation in the WHS is based on the desire of Ministries of Health to use the survey for national needs. Ministries of Health that expressed an interest in participating in the WHS have worked with WHO to identify partners to implement the WHS in their countries. Given the needs of the complex survey infrastructure, it is essential to involve multiple parties such as the National Statistical Offices, Census Bureaus and Survey Institutions, to collaborate and implement the various steps of the survey.

The World Health Survey Programme will continue to be developed in individual countries through consultation with policy-makers, particularly those involved in planning the scaling-up of health activities in response to the prospective increase in available resources. It will also be undertaken in collaboration with the people involved in routine health information systems. It will be complementary to their efforts to ensure periodic data input in a cost-effective way so that important gaps in health information are covered.

It will also establish a baseline for efforts to scale-up health activities.

The WHS will be implemented within a comprehensive programme with a long-term view on the development of national health information systems. Appropriate use of household surveys as a key form of data collection in an overall national health information system requires national capacity building and sustaining continued survey programmes.

Currently, World Health Surveys are being conducted in different modes of in-household 90-minute interviews in 55 countries (including a computerized personal interview in one country); 30-minute long brief face-to-face interviews (BFTF) in 13 countries; and computer assisted telephone interviews (CATI) in four countries. Table 58.2 lists the countries that are participating in the WHS in different WHO regions, and Figure 58.2 shows their geographical distribution.

WORLD HEALTH SURVEY METHODS

MODE

Given the importance of health issues, complex information requirements, and the length of the WHS interview, the basic survey mode is in-person interview. There is a choice of survey modes available for the

Table 58.2   Countries participating in the WHS 2002–2003

		EURO				
AFRO	AMRO	Common survey platform for short form	Other EURO countries	EMRO	SEARO	WPRO
Burkina Faso	Brazil	Austria	Bosnia	Morocco	Bangladesh	Australia*
Chad	Chile	Belgium	Croatia	Pakistan	India	China
Comoros	Dominican Rep.	Denmark	Czech Rep.	Tunisia	Myanmar	Lao (PDR)
Congo	Ecuador	Finland	Estonia	United Arab	Nepal	Malaysia
Côte d'Ivoire	Guatemala	France	Georgia	Emirates	Sri Lanka	Philippines
Ethiopia	Mexico	Germany	Hungary			Viet Nam
Ghana	Paraguay	Greece	Israel*			
Kenya	Uruguay	Ireland	Kazakhstan			
Malawi		Italy	Latvia			
Mali		Luxembourg*	Norway*			
Mauritania		Netherlands	Russian Fed.			
Mauritius		Portugal	Slovakia			
Namibia		Sweden	Slovenia			
Senegal		United Kingdom	Spain			
South Africa			Turkey			
Swaziland			Ukraine			
Zambia			Yugoslavia			
Zimbabwe						
18	8	14	17	4	5	6

Total number of countries: 72

* Australia, Israel, Luxembourg, and Norway are implementing the WHS short form through CATI (Computerized Telephone Interviews).

Figure 58.2 The WHS 2002–2003 geographical distribution of participating countries

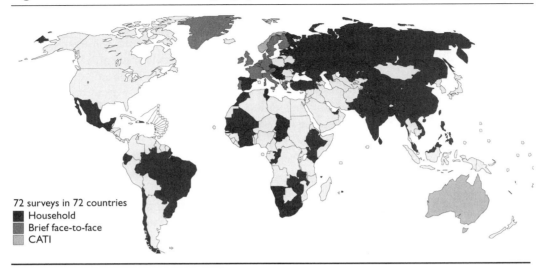

72 surveys in 72 countries
■ Household
▨ Brief face-to-face
□ CATI

The boundaries and names shown on this map do not imply the expression of any opinion whatsoever on the part of the World Health Organization concerning the legal status of any country, territory, city or area or of its authorities; or concerning the delimitation of its frontiers or boundaries.

Dotted lines on maps represent approximate border lines for which there may not yet be full agreement.

© WHO 2002. All rights reserved.

WHS implementation in a country. All modes have been pre-tested in the WHO Multi-country Survey Study as well as other pilot work for the WHS. All modes involve random selection of respondents on a nationally representative sampling frame. The choice will depend on the most practical and cost-effective mode in different settings.

■ Household face-to-face surveys. In most countries, randomly selected households are contacted and a single person from each household is interviewed. This mode can be either 90 minutes or a 30-minute, brief version.

■ Telephone surveys. When there is good coverage of a telephone network, surveys can be conducted via phone, using computerized systems. Telephone surveys use the same instrument as the 30-minute face-to-face surveys.

SAMPLE SIZE

To be useful for policy, responses should be representative of the population under consideration. It is recommended that samples be drawn by scientific principles of random selection to avoid any bias, and that quality assurance procedures be conducted during survey implementation to ensure that accurate and reliable data are obtained. Depending on the information needs and the amount of detail required, sample size

may vary between 1 000 and 10 000 for each country survey. This first wave of the WHS covers adult populations (i.e. older than 18 years). All samples were selected from nationally representative frames with a known probability in order to obtain estimates based on general population parameters. The sample sizes drawn for the longer household questionnaires ranged between 5 000 and 10 000, based on feasibility and survey costs. Brief face-to-face and CATI interviews generally had between 1 000 and 1 500 respondents (except in Luxembourg, which included a sample of 600). Details of country samples are documented on the WHS web site (8).

QUALITY ASSURANCE

To implement the WHS with high quality, intensive consultations with survey countries were undertaken to understand and improve survey implementation. A large-scale exercise was built with participation of countries, international survey experts, and regional advisors on *WHS Quality Assurance Standards & Guidelines*. This exercise has led to the examination of country needs and survey procedures to ensure appropriate sampling, efficient survey implementation, high quality data management, and analysis strategies.

The *WHS Quality Assurance Standards & Guidelines* identify explicitly the operational criteria as quality standards (14). The best practices to achieve these standards are also defined, together with assessment strategies for monitoring and evaluation procedures. These guidelines will be implemented locally by national institutions and monitored by external peer review. Figure 58.3 depicts the different stages of quality assurance procedures.

Each step of the survey production process involves a certification of quality. The instrument design requires careful consideration to ensure that the questions are easily understood, the concepts are transferable across languages, and the measurement properties are stable across populations and over time. Attention needs to be paid to the design and implementation of the survey with adequate supervision and training of interviewers. Troubleshooting on-site with actual observations of the implementation is a prerequisite. In large multi-country surveys, uniform procedures for data entry, cleaning, and archiving are necessary. Ongoing monitoring of this process during the data collection phase, with a regular feedback loop from the site to the central monitoring centre and back, ensures that all analytical strategies can be executed with minimal error. All methodologies to analyse the data should be clearly documented and reviewed for appropriateness. Audit trails must be established to ensure transparency in the final analysis since these data will often have important policy implications and potentially far-reaching impacts in public health.

As an example of monitoring the end result of survey data, the following standard indicators are currently being used to monitor the survey data quality:

■ Sample Population Deviation Index (SDI) shows the proportion of age and sex strata in the sample in comparison to the general population, here taken from the UN population database. It indicates the quality of the sample in terms of its representativeness. A ratio of one shows that the survey sample matches the characteristics of the general population, whereas deviations from one indicate over- or under-sampling from that age or sex group. The expected value of one (i.e. ideal representativeness) is rarely observed in surveys because of sampling errors. Figure 58.4 shows the SDI for one of the postal surveys indicating under-representation at younger ages and over-representation at older ages, particularly for older men.

■ Response rate shows the completion rate of interviews in the selected sample—the number of completed interviews among eligibles. This indicator illustrates how well the survey has covered its defined sampling frame.

■ Rate of missing data is defined as the proportion of missing items in a respondent's interview. We measured the number of people failing to complete a selected acceptable range of items to indicate the

Figure 58.3 WHS quality assurance procedures

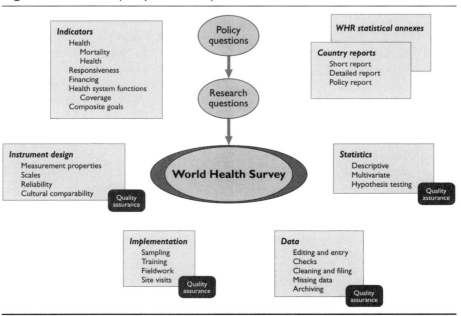

Figure 58.4 Example of a sample population deviation index

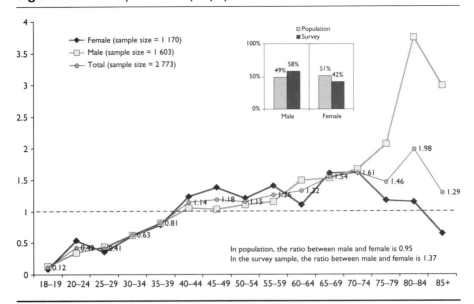

quality of the interviews (e.g. 10% in the household face-to-face interviews).

■ Reliability coefficients for test-retest interviews demonstrate the standardization and stability of interview administration. These are calculated as chance-corrected concordance rates (i.e. *kappa statistics* for categorical, and *intra-class correlation coefficients* for continuous variables). This indicator refers to the standard application of the interview, i.e. how well a given interview could be repeated yielding the same results. Generally a score greater than 0.4 is acceptable, greater than 0.6 is fair, and higher than 0.8 is excellent (*3;12*).

In addition, design effect coefficients (DEFF) for the multi-stage cluster samples will be calculated where appropriate. This measure compares the actual sample to an assumed true simple random sample. Since a true simple random sample is not practicable in large-scale surveys due to costs and transportation, it is customary to calculate the variance estimation in comparison to a random sample (*15*). A DEFF of between 1 and 6 is generally considered acceptable for this sample size.

CAPACITY BUILDING

In order to build capacity in WHO Member States to implement the WHS with high quality and sustainability, intensive consultations with survey countries were undertaken. Training courses for participating country teams were organized by WHO regions. These courses used standardized training materials. Survey-monitoring tools were also developed and implemented. Collaborating sites worked hard to obtain a representative sample and to ensure participation of selected respondents in the survey. This required substantial organizational skills on the part of the collaborating partners. Ongoing support from WHO was provided through periodic phone conversations, email contacts, and site visits for on-site monitoring, problem solving, and constant quality improvement. The quality of survey implementation at sites has been continuously monitored through electronic data delivery.

To make a meaningful impact and reach country-relevant conclusions from the World Health Surveys, WHO has established a mechanism to publish national reports based on data analysis in collaboration with countries themselves and international advisors. These reports will translate the findings of the WHS into practical suggestions for policy formulation. There will be different types of WHS reports:

■ Country-specific reports. Brief National Reports will summarize the main findings for policy-makers, media, and other stakeholders. A detailed National Report will give richer findings on health system properties, poverty and health, and other country-relevant issues.

■ Reports on specific issues. These reports will make comparisons within and across countries either globally or regionally, to facilitate learning from each other by focusing on similarities and differences in findings.

WHO will assist countries in producing their own national reports and will support local country teams to conduct in-depth analysis of WHS data. In this way, the WHS will be useful for locally relevant policy questions. To support such activities, many tools for training, as well as courses and workshops are planned, focusing on data analysis, production of country reports, and discussion forums for better dissemination and assimilation of results.

ENSURING POLICY RELEVANCE

The WHS provides important information on inputs, coverage of interventions, and critical outputs of health systems. The results can be of immediate policy relevance to countries and could in some cases allow appropriate policy implementation. For this to happen, however, WHO needs to also focus energy on strengthening national capacity to analyse household survey data and to draw policy conclusions. This general need for national capacity to use data for policy purposes is particularly important for two priority areas.

With growing interest in health and poverty, the WHS has the potential to provide cross-country comparable information on health status and access to effective health interventions for the poor versus the non-poor within each country. The inclusion of indicators of permanent income in the WHS strengthens considerably the ability of governments to diagnose the health challenges of the poor and to monitor the efforts of the health system to deliver services to the poor. Detailed information on insurance and geographical, financial, and cultural access, included in the WHS, can be extremely useful in developing pro-poor health policies.

With increasing recognition of the central role of the government as the steward of the health system, information on subnational performance is essential. Such subnational performance assessment frameworks can be particularly important as a policy tool in countries that have undergone considerable decentralization. The WHS, with adjustments for sample size or the adoption of Bayesian methods, can be used as an effective tool for collecting information on subnational performance assessment (16). As a result, a country can make comparisons of key variables such as the levels and distributions of health of the population, responsiveness, coverage, financing, mortality, risk factors and others accordingly (see Chapter 59 in this book (16)).

A third area of particular policy relevance is the focus of the world's nations on achieving the Millennium Development Goals (MDG) (17). These goals show that health is at the centre of development; three of eight goals for development are health goals. Eighteen of 48 MDG indicators are health indicators. Nearly two-thirds of the health-related MDG indicators can be monitored using the WHS instrument. Robust monitoring of the health-related MDGs is an essential requirement to be able to advocate for continued increases in resources for improving the health of the poor in the poorest countries.

FUTURE OF THE WHS

In developing the WHS, WHO has a vision of a series of valid, reliable, and comparable survey modules covering the full range of relevant health information that can be collected from households. A country considering implementing a household survey, irrespective of funding sources, could draw on this international resource. The instrument is designed to be valid and reliable, and to generate data that allow meaningful comparisons over time, across subgroups within a country and across countries. The library of standardized modules is far from being complete. The WHS instrument currently in use in wave I of the survey represents a first step to fulfil this vision.

Further empirical work will lead to improvements in the instrument. Demands from users of health information will lead to the development of new modules. Implementation of the WHS will, we hope, lead to enhanced country capacity to field high quality household surveys and, ultimately, to effective policy formulation. WHO is committed over the long term to ensuring that the WHS is an effective tool for national health information systems.

NOTES

1   Including WHS Collaborators in WHO: Can Çelik, Ajay Tandon, Joshua A. Salomon, Wan Jun Xie, and the following working group members:

Sampling: Somnath Chatterji, Emre Özaltin, Lydia Bendib, Marguerite Schneider, T. Bedirhan Üstün

Socio-Demographics: William D. Savedoff, Somnath Chatterji, Brodie D. Ferguson, Emmanuela Gakidou, Jan Klavus, Mario Dal Poz, Ke Xu, Kei Kawabata, T. Bedirhan Üstün

Health: Somnath Chatterji, Lydia Bendib, Maria Villanueva, Colin D. Mathers, Joshua A. Salomon, Marguerite Schneider, T. Bedirhan Üstün, Emre Özaltin, Ajay Tandon, Christopher J.L. Murray

Valuation: Joshua A. Salomon, Somnath Chatterji, Emmanuela Gakidou, Christopher J.L. Murray

Mortality: Alan D. Lopez, Colin D. Mathers, Andre L'Hours, Mie Inoue, Emmanuela Gakidou, Margaret C. Hogan, Emre Özaltin, Chalapati Rao, Christopher J.L. Murray

Responsiveness: Nicole B. Valentine, Kei Kawabata, Juan Pablo Ortiz, René Lavallée, Lydia Bendib, Somnath Chatterji, T. Bedirhan Üstün, Ajay Tandon, Christopher J.L. Murray

Risk Factors: Alena Petrakova, Majid Ezzati, Alan D. Lopez, Maria Villanueva, Kathleen L. Strong, Annette Pruess, T. Bedirhan Üstün

Coverage: Bakhuti Shengelia, Somnath Chatterji, Neeru Gupta, Saba Moussavi, Alena Petrakova, Elena A. Varavikova, Orvill B. Adams, T. Bedirhan Üstün, Ajay Tandon, Christopher J.L. Murray

A full list of the WHS Collaborators in WHS Member States (see Table 58.1) can be found on the WHS web site at URL: http://www.who.int/whs.

REFERENCES

(1) National Center for Health Statistics. *National Health Interview Survey* (NHIS). National Center for Health Statistics, Division of Data Services, Hyattsville, MD. URL: http://www.cdc.gov/nchs/nhis.htm

(2) Macro International Inc. *Demographic and Health Surveys.* 2001. URL: http://www.measuredhs.com/

(3) World Health Organization. *International Classification of Functioning, Disability and Health (ICF).* Geneva, World Health Organization, 2001.

(4) Murray CJL et al. Empirical evaluation of the anchoring vignette approach in health surveys. In: Murray CJL, Evans DB, eds. *Health systems performance assessment: debates, methods and empiricism.* Geneva, World Health Organization, 2003.

(5) Salomon JA et al. Unpacking health perceptions using anchoring vignettes. In: Murray CJL, Evans DB, eds. *Health systems performance assessment: debates, methods and empiricism.* Geneva, World Health Organization, 2003.

(6) Tandon A et al. Statistical models for enhancing cross-population comparability. In: Murray CJL, Evans DB, eds. *Health systems performance assessment: debates, methods and empiricism.* Geneva, World Health Organization, 2003.

(7) Üstün TB et al. WHO Multi-country Survey Study on Health and Responsiveness 2000–2001. In: Murray CJL, Evans DB, eds. *Health systems performance assessment: debates, methods and empiricism.* Geneva, World Health Organization, 2003.

(8) World Health Organization. *World Health Survey.* Geneva, World Health Organization, 2003. URL: http://www3.who.int/whs/

(9) Ferguson BD et al. Estimating permanent income using indicator variables. In: Murray CJL, Evans DB, eds. *Health systems performance assessment: debates, methods and empiricism.* Geneva, World Health Organization, 2003.

(10) Filmer D, Pritchett L. Estimating wealth effects without expenditure data—or tears: an application to educational enrolments in states of India. *Demography*, 2001, 38: 115–132.

(11) Valentine NB, de Silva A, Murray CJL. Estimating responsiveness level and distribution for 191 countries: methods and results. EIP Discussion Paper No. 22. Geneva, World Health Organization, 2000. URL: http://www3.who.int/whosis/discussion_papers/discussion_papers.cfm#

(12) World Health Organization. *The World Health Report 2000. Health Systems: Improving Performance.* Geneva, World Health Organization, 2000.

(13) Schieber GP, Poullier JP, Greenward LM. Health system performance in OECD countries, 1980–1992. Organisation for Economic Co-operation and Development. *Health Affairs,* 1994, 13(4):100–112.

(14) World Health Organization. *World Health Survey. Quality assurance standards & guidelines: procedures for quality assurance implementation by country survey teams and quality assurance advisors.* Geneva, World Health Organization, 2002.

(15) Kish L. Design effect. In: Kotz S, Johnson NL, eds. *Encyclopedia of statistical sciences,* vol. 2. New York, Wiley, 1982:347–348.

(16) Travis P et al. Subnational health systems performance assessment: objectives, challenges and strategies. In: Murray CJL, Evans DB, eds. *Health systems performance assessment: debates, methods and empiricism.* Geneva, World Health Organization, 2003.

(17) United Nations. *UN Millenium Development Goals.* URL: http://www.un.org/millenniumgoals/

Chapter 59

Subnational Health Systems Performance Assessment: Objectives, Challenges and Strategies

Phyllida Travis, Abdelhay Mechbal, Ajay Tandon,
Brodie D. Ferguson, Michel Thieren, Christopher J.L. Murray

Introduction

The WHO health systems framework (1) provides a systematic approach to analysing different aspects of health systems performance: from *inputs*, through health system *functions* and achievements in intermediate goals such as *coverage* and *provider performance*, to overall health system *goals* and *efficiency*. Commentators have suggested that the national level framework should be adapted so that policy-makers and managers can use it to monitor subnational performance regularly—for a variety of strategic and operational purposes (2).[1]

For analytic purposes, any health system can be subdivided in many different ways: by geographical area, sub-system, programme, facility or population subgroup. The discussion here focuses on the performance of health systems within any of the geographically defined political and administrative entities that may exist—states, regions, provinces, districts, municipalities, communes, etc. These may of course be of very different population sizes, and services may be arranged in many different ways. This diversity has some practical implications for the methods and indicators used, but at any level the basic conceptual approach can, and indeed we argue should, remain the same.

Currently WHO's work is focusing more on what one needs to know about the performance of local health systems so as to make better informed *strategic* decisions, rather than for day to day management, though there is certainly some overlap. In addition to the work described here, facility assessment tools are being developed, so that ultimately there will be a portfolio of practical instruments and indicators based on the concepts elaborated in the WHO health systems framework, from which countries can select those best suited to their needs.

WHO's work on subnational assessment is guided by three main considerations. The first is that if the aim is to monitor performance regularly, the burden of effort should be as small as possible. Therefore, WHO is exploring what information decision-makers consider "essential," and efforts are being made to ensure that methods and tools are as simple and low-cost as possible, subject to being "fit-for-purpose" (3). The second consideration is that in order to interpret results and compare between areas, the approach used should be consistent with the national performance assessment approach. Third, any assessment should be comprehensive, or system-wide, in its scope. Many useful tools already exist for monitoring specific programmes and sub-systems (4). However, by design, these give a partial view of a health system's performance. This may result in a "tunnel vision," with problems elsewhere in the system going undetected. The work reported here contributes to the less well charted territory of system-wide performance monitoring.

The present chapter is organized in six sections. The first one addresses the purposes and uses of subnational performance assessment. Section two explores the types of information that may be needed at the subnational level. Mapping the national WHO health systems assessment framework to the local level is addressed in the following section. Section four discusses a range of options to use existing data and to collect new data in a cost-effective manner in order to address data gaps. Other issues and challenges for regular subnational performance assessment are presented in section five, and the last section focuses on future developments.

PURPOSE AND USES OF SUBNATIONAL PERFORMANCE ASSESSMENT

Before embarking on any discussion about indicators or methods, it is important to consider in more detail the objectives and possible uses of subnational health systems performance assessment. The applications that have been suggested by national policy-makers fall into two broad categories: as a tool for more effective stewardship and as a management tool.

Such information may help decision-makers in a variety of tasks, especially if generated regularly enough to have a picture of trends. First, in national policy formulation, by providing information on variations in health system inputs, functions, achievements, and efficiency across a country and over time. It can assist oversight of policy implementation by monitoring the adherence to and effects of health sector policies and reforms. It may also be used to create incentives for change, and to promote transparency and accountability—both to the legislature and to the population. Information can be used to mobilize resources and assist resource allocation decisions. Lastly, it may help provincial/district level managers to identify operational problems.

These are all challenges faced regularly by decision-makers. For example, in some countries that are going through a process of decentralization, direct central control over the use of inputs is reduced. As a result, there is a wish by the central Ministry of Health to monitor the performance of lower levels of the health system in order to ensure that some measure of accountability is retained. Some countries with more centralized health systems are also interested in monitoring variations in performance across the country, because they remain heterogeneous geographically or by level of development. Some countries have new policies and strategies to improve the health of the poor and their access to services, and want to know how effective these are. From a more international perspective, systematic subnational assessment has the potential to enhance understanding of a country's progress towards internationally agreed pro-poor health and development targets, such as the Millennium Development Goals (5). And if comparable approaches are used in different countries, subnational monitoring efforts will contribute to building a more robust international evidence base, still rather limited, on the relationships between similar health system reforms in various settings and their effects on performance.

In all cases, monitoring the performance of the heath system at the subnational level is seen as a way to track progress and detect whether the desired results are being achieved. The spectrum of potential users and uses is wide, from local health managers to national health policy-makers; from civil society to national politicians; from operational to more strategic decisions; from advocacy to accountability for results.

WHAT TO ASSESS: WHAT DOES ONE NEED TO KNOW?

Users need different sorts of information, depending on what they are responsible for. For example, what the central level needs to know about a district's performance differs from what the district health manager needs to know, at least in the level of detail required. What the district manager needs to know will in part be influenced by whether he can actually do something about it directly: i.e. by the degree of control held over key resources, especially money and staff. Differences in information needs, however, should not be exaggerated, e.g. comparisons of cost and quality are of interest to both district managers and national policy-makers. And part of the responsibility of both central and district level decision-makers is to negotiate and influence other key actors in the allocation and use of resources to improve health, even where they do not have direct control over them. Information on needs, inputs, and results can considerably strengthen their ability to be more effective stewards.

For more effective stewardship, it is important to know about the performance of the *whole* health system within any given area. This includes private and non-profit actors, who can constitute a major but often rather neglected part of a country's health system. Such breadth in scope does not automatically mean that a large number of measures are needed. However, in the quest for a parsimonious set of indicators, balance is required. Too much information can be unmanageable and key findings might be ignored. Too little can bias behaviour in unwanted ways: people may be encouraged to over-focus on certain policy priorities at the expense of other desirable actions, or to manipulate results in order to get promised rewards. A first challenge is to obtain an overview across the health system which signals where important problems may be arising; the latter can then be investigated in more detail if needed. As with any assessment, time series of data will be more informative than one-off exercises.

To come back to the initial question of this section, what does one need to know to obtain a reliable overview of how different health regions or districts are operating? We use the four components in the WHO health systems framework to approach this. They are:

- Health system inputs
- Health system functions
- Health system outcomes/goals
- Health system efficiency

This section first considers what sort of information for each of these components might be considered essential by decision-makers. Contextual information (for example, on economic trends, political opportunities) is also needed, but is not discussed further here. The section then summarizes some of the debates around different types of indicators and their uses. Thinking on indicators for some components is more advanced than for others. As experience with use accumulates, indicators may need to be revised.

HEALTH SYSTEM INPUTS

There are many different inputs to a local health system: money, staff, equipment, drugs and other consumables, infrastructure. We focus here on money and staff.

Information on health expenditures has several possible uses. One is to simply know variations in the level of funding. Another is to track whether resource allocation policies are being observed. For example, in some countries going through a process of decentralization, the delegation of budgets to local authorities was accompanied—contrary to national policy—by decreases in budgets for some types of health services. This was detected by monitoring the patterns of local health expenditures. Another use is to advocate for maintaining or increasing annual health budgets in negotiations with the Ministry of Finance. A third is to gain insights into factors, such as resource availability, that might explain performance. Lastly, information on expenditures is used in the WHO framework to obtain a measure of overall health system "efficiency," because health system achievements are related to available resources.

While highly detailed subnational health accounts may not be feasible, certain critical information is required, such as the levels of public sector expenditure on health, out-of-pocket payments, and donor assistance (if present). In many countries even such basic information is limited. A more detailed analysis of resource flows to different providers and for dif-

ferent interventions may also be useful. Whether the investment required is justified will depend on the context.

The second key input is human resources. Nothing happens without health workers and they also affect the use of other resources. Monitoring the total numbers of key categories of personnel in the public and private sectors in an area is likely to be considered a minimal requirement. There are of course many other concerns related to human resources: skill-mix in relation to needs, their quality, productivity, the effects of rewards and sanctions, etc. In the WHO framework issues concerning the *management* of human resources are addressed under Provision.

HEALTH SYSTEM FUNCTIONS

In order to improve health systems performance, four key elements, or "functions" need attention: provision, resource generation, financing, and stewardship. For monitoring purposes, what is it that decision-makers might need to know about these different functions in order to detect problems in good time? In many ways, the minimum information sought is again likely to be similar at the national and subnational levels, even if it is broken down or presented in different ways. In the first instance, indicators that reveal critical aspects of the operation of health system functions are required. The Report of the Scientific Peer Review Group on Health Systems Performance Assessment provides a useful checklist of basic principles[2] for choosing indicators of functions (3). Current thinking is as follows.

Provision

Any subnational assessment is likely to want to include information on coverage. A key concern for many decision-makers is the level of *effective coverage*: the extent to which people are able to receive care when they need it. A second is to know of any significant inequalities in coverage, for example, by area or income group. The set of interventions for which coverage is monitored will vary to some extent, because it should be related to local priorities. But in all cases it should include interventions that, if delivered, make a major difference to population health. Monitoring coverage may require information beyond public sector service registries to adequately reflect the effects of the entire local health system. This is often limited. One module of the World Health Survey (6) will provide new coverage information that is population rather than provider based. The survey assesses coverage with effective interventions for a range of major communicable and non-communicable conditions, and some major risk factors, e.g. physical activity, water, sanitation, that can be adapted to local circumstances.

A second common concern is the *performance of providers* themselves. Some measure of the quality of care delivered and of provider efficiency, is frequently wanted. Any assessment of provider performance should include both public and private providers in the area concerned. Adams et al. summarize WHO's current work on monitoring personal and non-personal service provision (7).

When "drilling down" in an assessment to understand *why* rather than just *how* a system is operating, information on different aspects of staff management is often sought. Many existing district, facility, and programme management tools have extensive lists of possible indicators (4). Rigorous consideration of the added value of trying to routinely collect data for these types of indicators is needed. Such detail may be more appropriate to "second level" assessment, brought into play only when problems are flagged from a smaller set of overview indicators.

Resource Generation

What local information might be wanted? Some basic information on capital stock and drug availability is frequently cited as desirable at the subnational level, in order to detect variations in available resources and the balance between resources, which may account for differences in the observed achievements. These would also reflect resource generation and distribution capacity. Adams et al. discuss this further (8).

Financing

As mentioned above, knowing the proportion of funding from various sources of financing is critical. A more detailed analysis of resource flows to different providers and for different interventions and financial management can also be useful, but whether the effort required is justified for routine monitoring will depend on the context. Indicators considered at the national level that might be relevant and useful subnationally include the share of total health expenditures that are pre-paid, and the share of total funds allocated by inputs, outputs, and outcomes. Savedoff et al. discuss these in more detail (9).

Stewardship

Stewardship is about oversight of the health system and its guidance in the public interest. For example, public policy objectives not uncommonly include reducing the existing inequities between rich and poor, and promoting quality and efficiency in the use of limited resources. WHO has identified six core domains that together appear to constitute "good" stewardship: generation of intelligence; formulation of strategic policy direction; ensuring tools for implementation: powers, incentives, and sanctions; coalition building and conflict resolution; ensuring a fit between strategy and structure, and accountability (10). While the ultimate responsibility for stewardship lies with the government, its execution is not a purely national level function. It is possible to envisage important differences in health system stewardship between provinces or districts, especially in a country that is very decentralized. WHO's work in developing stewardship assessment tools is less advanced than in other areas. WHO is now investigating which might be the critical aspects of these domains in order to help governments detect where there are problems in stewardship. Qualitative approaches may be the most appropriate.

HEALTH SYSTEM OUTCOMES

What health system outcomes can or should be assessed at the subnational level? And how sophisticated do the measures need to be for policy purposes? The WHO framework identifies three goals of health systems: health, responsiveness, and fairness in financial contribution. These concepts and their measurement approaches are described in detail elsewhere (11–13). To summarize, responsiveness is considered a health system goal because the way people are treated when they come into contact with the health system can improve or reduce their well-being independently of whether or not their health improves. It captures concerns people have about whether they are treated with dignity, that confidentiality is observed, etc.— eight "domains" of responsiveness have been defined. The concept of fairness in financial contribution is considered a goal on the grounds that the way funds are raised for the health system also affects people's well-being. People are concerned that this is done in a fair way and that they are not pushed into poverty as a result of health spending. This particular measure does not take account of the utilization of services; the latter is captured under provision and provider performance.

In terms of *summary* measures of health system outcomes, current thinking about what could usefully be monitored at the subnational level and how it might be reported, is as follows.

It is essential to measure the *levels of health and responsiveness of the health system* in an area. This information can also be used to detect differences or inequalities *between* subnational entities. Measuring the *complete distribution of health or responsiveness within an area* may not be as essential. The effort and resources required to characterize the complete distribution of these outcomes may not be justified, if the population sizes are small, or relatively homogeneous. Less sophisticated measures could be used for the monitoring of local level inequalities in health or responsiveness, that broadly capture the information in the complete distribution.

For example, it may be more appropriate and relevant to policy objectives to measure the fraction of the population falling above or below a critical threshold set by policy-makers, instead of using the local equivalent of the national "equality index." To illustrate, for health one could report the percentage of the population whose risk of death or ill-health is greater than some critical level, rather than measuring the inequality in the distribution of health. For example, the fraction of children facing risks of death greater than 100 per 1 000. The actual threshold would be specific to the country and would presumably be the same for all districts in it. Whatever way the information is reported, it is thought important that non-fatal as well as fatal outcomes are included in any measure. This is because inequalities in life expectancy can be falling, while differences in healthy life expectancy remain large. For responsiveness, one can use the same logic as for health, and ask what fraction of the population has health system responsiveness levels below some critical level. This "national norm" could be taken from the national average.

With fairness in financial contribution, policy concerns that are addressed include: the extent to which people are contributing to the financing of the health system according to their ability to pay, and the various determinants of this. In terms of possible measures, the fraction of a local population incurring catastrophic spending (spending more than 40% of their "disposable" or non-subsistence income on health) is easier to measure than the fairness in financial contribution index, and closely resembles it except in very high-income countries. Ways to measure determinants of catastrophic expenditures are also being developed (*14*). Other information that may be useful includes the types of health expenditures leading to catastrophic payments, such as payments for drugs, outpatient service or hospitalization.

It may also be useful to report a simple disaggregation of the summary measure for a specific goal, for example of the individual domains of health or responsiveness, in order to identify or track changes in key problem domains, or with regard to vulnerable groups such as the poor, or specific services. As always, the trade-off will be the extra cost and effort required to provide that extra detail. Any decision will be influenced by the size of the population under consideration and the current policy importance of the issue. Table 59.1 summarizes current thinking of minimum information needs for "first-level," regular assessment purposes irrespective of any additional specific concerns.

Subnational information on risk factors is also useful in order to develop relevant health promoting policies. What health risk factors should be routinely monitored at the subnational level? It would seem sensible to choose risk factors that are considered priority problems—nationally or subnationally. *The World Health Report 2002* suggests that priority should in general be given to controlling those risks that are common, substantial, widespread, and for which effective and acceptable risk reduction strategies are available (*15*). While there is no standard list of risk factors to monitor, current evidence suggests the following are important candidates to consider in both developing and industrialized countries: underweight, unsafe sex, unsafe water and sanitation, alcohol, blood pressure, tobacco, cholesterol, indoor air pollution, iron deficiency, and overweight.

SUBNATIONAL EFFICIENCY

In the WHO framework, a single measure of health system efficiency is calculated. This provides a snapshot of how well the system is doing compared to its best possible performance, given the resources it has. The approach used at the national level could

Table 59.1 Assessment of health system outcomes

	Level	Distribution
Health	X	Per cent with health worse than threshold
Responsiveness	X	Per cent with responsiveness worse than threshold
Fairness in financial contribution		Per cent incurring catastrophic spending

be adapted for the subnational one, and would allow comparisons of performance across provinces or districts. Provided that a sufficient number of local areas are included in the subnational performance assessment, a *national* frontier production function can be estimated (*16*). This will give useful information on the levels of efficiency of different districts relative to the most efficient local area in the country. It will still be important to compare local areas to the more global frontier production function, using a similar approach.

If subnational performance assessment is evaluated on a regular basis, the focus will shift from cross-area comparison to improvements in achievements and efficiency over time by the individual districts/provinces.

TYPES OF INDICATORS TO USE

There is a long standing debate about the relative merits of disaggregated and more aggregated or summary measures. Disaggregated indicators are widely used in health. Summary measures are becoming increasingly available as well—currently more for health system outcomes than health system functions. Table 59.2 provides a few examples of both types.

In practice, both types are useful and necessary, for different purposes. Both also have their limitations. Summary measures are exactly that: they summarize a large amount of information into a few manageable indicators and provide a strategic overview of the situation. They do not necessarily change slowly—the changes in life expectancy in the Newly Independent States are one example of rapid change. They can be used to flag policy issues, but are not enough on their own for policy development purposes. However, neither are disaggregated indicators which are, by design, more partial. WHO proposes that whatever the indicator used, it should meet five basic quality criteria: validity, comparability, reliability, audit trail, validation at country level (*17*). Given that countries have different systems and needs, the aim is to put together a coherent family of validated indicators ranging from summary to the more disaggregated, from which countries can select.

WAYS TO USE AVAILABLE DATA AND TO ADDRESS DATA GAPS

USING AVAILABLE DATA

In many countries a lot of data are collected, sometimes with considerable duplication of effort, but little are actually used. Any strategy for monitoring performance should obviously make as much use of the existing data as possible.

Some of the relevant data for assessing subnational health systems performance exist in all countries, though they are of variable completeness. Sources include: routine activity reporting from health facilities, disease registers, surveillance systems including sentinel surveillance, vital registration systems, one-off or regular household and facility surveys, and periodic programme assessments. Serious biases can arise where only facility reported data are used. Murray et

Table 59.2   Illustration of types of indicators[3]

Health System	Indicator	
	Disaggregated	*Aggregated / Summary*
Inputs	% expenditure on drugs, salaries, etc.	Total health expenditure per capita
	Specific cadres of workers/1 000	Total number of health workers/1 000
Functions		
Financing	Membership of prepayment pools	% prepayment
Resource generation	Ratio of new doctors/total number	% total health expenditure in basic health worker training and education
Provision	Immunization coverage	
	% Caesarian sections	Effective coverage
	% returns to operating theatre	Some summary measure of hospital quality
Outcomes	Infant mortality, maternal mortality	HALE incidence and prevalence
	Waiting time	Inequality in life expectancy
	Out of pocket expenditure by specific income groups	Responsiveness index
		FFC index
		Health systems performance index

al have demonstrated differences between DTP3 coverage reported from facility routine reporting systems and coverage estimated from data in Demographic and Health Surveys in 45 countries. Figure 23.2 in Chapter 23 suggests that estimates derived mainly from routine reporting systems tend to over-report coverage, if the DHS is taken as a gold standard (18).

It is not always easy to make better use of the existing data. Challenges include fragmented data collection systems; a tendency to aggregate subnational data as they move up through the system in such a way that they cannot be readily disaggregated by geographical area; and lack of information about or easy access to data collected outside one's own institution.

Even so, much more use can be made. In particular, national health and income and expenditure surveys are often carried out routinely at one to five year intervals, and these provide a rich source of critical population based information. We find it conceptually useful to consider both data collected routinely by facilities and data collected through regular surveys—by programmes, projects or other institutions, simply as different sources of routine data. This is because a more comprehensive view of what constitutes routine health information could—indirectly—help rationalize data collection and facilitate better use of the existing data.

Finally, as the next section will show, where subnationally representative surveys do not exist, available national data can still be used to develop rough subnational estimates (otherwise known as priors) that can then be made more precise in a variety of low-cost ways.

ADDRESSING DATA GAPS: TECHNIQUES USED TO REDUCE COSTS

Application of the WHO health systems performance framework at any level below province/region is likely to entail some new data collection because several key variables are not well captured by the existing data systems. Many factors influence how one does this. They include: population size of the areas (for cost and effort rather than for statistical reasons); the health system's organization; the policy issues on which information is sought; the level of detail required for data credibility; available human and financial resources; and the existing information gathering systems. Different strategies may be needed for the immediate versus longer term.

Whatever the local context, it will rarely be cost-effective to undertake representative sample surveys in every local area. Fortunately, there are several possible strategies which could be combined to minimize time and cost. Although some are conceptually quite sophisticated, relatively simple applications are possible. Broadly, they fall into two groups: techniques to reduce the cost of data collection per person in a sample, and techniques to reduce the number of individuals that need to be sampled.

Three different strategies have been identified that could lower the cost and effort required per person in a sample survey collecting information on local health system inputs, coverage, and outcomes. The first is to reduce the cost per person through alternative approaches to sampling such as modified cluster sampling or longitudinal panels. The other possible strategy to reduce the cost per person sampled is the application of careful *item reduction strategies,* to shorten the questionnaires used without compromising beyond the "acceptable" limits on validity and reliability.

Two examples of existing applications to reduce the cost per person sampled are the use of panel data in Thailand and the use of cluster surveys by the Expanded Programme of Immunization (EPI). Panel data are collected from the same subset or "panel" of households from a larger survey sample, over several time periods. They can help to obtain more immediate trend information in a less expensive way. In countries where there is relatively less mobility, the costs of identifying households are lower. Thailand conducts socioeconomic surveys with a sample size of 46 000 every two years. Following the introduction of the Government's poverty reduction policy in 1994/1995, a smaller panel of 1 000 households across 76 provinces was selected from the original sample frame to be resurveyed every six months in order to promptly detect provincial trends in household income, expenditure and debt, especially in rural areas. This approach is now being adapted by the Ministry of Public Health for monitoring provincial health systems performance following a recent resource allocation reform. Changes in household income, health expenditure, health risk behaviour, and access to care will be monitored. There are some known trade-offs in the use of panel data: sample attrition, complicated sampling design, costs of data storage. Still, panel data are a promising avenue to explore.

The 30 cluster 7 child survey was developed for the Expanded Programme of Immunization in the 1970's (*19*). It was designed to estimate vaccination coverage to within ±10 percentage points of the true proportion, with 95% confidence. The survey is a two-stage cluster sample. The population is subdivided into a set of non-overlapping clusters, for example districts. In the first stage, 30 of these clusters are sampled with probability proportionate to the size of the population in the cluster. Sampling this way allows the larger clusters to have a greater chance of being selected. In the second stage of sampling, 7 subjects are selected within each cluster. Only the first subject is randomly selected. The following six are taken from the nearest households, until 7 eligible subjects are found. This approach meant that implementation costs were rather low due to the sampling strategy. For a population, a reasonable estimate of immunization coverage needs only 210 children to be sampled.

Item reduction techniques have been used to decrease costs by reducing the number of questions needed. Item reduction should not be a random process; it should be based on eliminating redundant items to the extent possible, e.g. a) eliminating items that have little or no marginal impact on estimates of the underlying variable of interest, and b) eliminating items that do not help discriminate among respondents. In addition, "noisy" items, i.e. those that exhibit no systematic relation with other items that measure the same latent trait. There are different methods available, all of which examine the relation between individual items and the larger instrument (*20–23*). They examine different properties and therefore, have different limitations and are often used together. One example of their application is in the Short Form Health Survey, which has long been used in the US and in European countries. This survey, known as the SF-36, consists of 36 questions that assess physical and mental health states in the general population. Ware et al. (*24*) describe how regression methods were used on the original SF-36 to create a highly correlated 12 item questionnaire (SF-12). Correlations were also high when cross-validated against other existing datasets in the Medical Outcomes study (0.905 for the physical component and 0.938 for the mental health component) (*25*). Country specific scores were highly correlated as well. Average scores for the two summary measures of physical and mental health closely mirrored the SF-36 results, and showed comparable sensitivity to change. Because of the high degree of correspondence, Ware et al. concluded that the SF-12

is a practical alternative to SF-36 for the purposes of large group comparisons where the focus is on overall physical and mental health outcomes.

The second approach to lower overall costs is to reduce the number of individuals that need to be sampled. To achieve this, two main options are available. First, the quantity of interest can be modified to contain less information. For example, a continuous variable can be changed to a dichotomous one. As an example of this information reduction approach, EPI also uses another small sample approach called Lot Quality Assurance Sampling (LQAS). The basic concept is to define a desired threshold for the item one wishes to measure, and then simply count the proportion falling below that threshold. Because the response required is "binary," i.e. above or below the threshold, smaller sample sizes can be used. However, for LQAS the sample selection must be strictly randomized, which may actually increase costs.

The second option is to reduce the number of individuals that need to be sampled by using existing information to inform estimates of the quantity of interest. How can this be done systematically? WHO is exploring the use of a statistical approach known as Bayesian analysis (*26–28*). To date, this has been less used in health systems analysis, but is regularly used in other fields such as economics. In general terms, Bayesian analysis is a statistical approach in which an approximate or "prior" estimate of the item of interest is combined with some additional empirical information to obtain a more precise estimate, known in technical terms as the "posterior." The simple intuitive notion is that prior knowledge about a quantity, such as the poverty rate in a community, can reduce the required sample size for measurement. Box 59.1 illustrates the concept. Examples are given in the next section.

POTENTIAL APPLICATIONS TO SUBNATIONAL ASSESSMENT: ILLUSTRATIONS FROM RECENT WHO WORK

WHO has been investigating the potential uses of some or all of these different techniques in the monitoring of subnational performance: developing priors, developing small sample surveys, combining data from different sources using Bayes' Theorem, and item reduction techniques. The results of using these techniques are being compared with "the truth"—data from representative surveys. This section provides illustrations of the work to date which suggests that these approaches

---

Box 59.1   Application of Bayesian analysis: an illustration

Peter is asked by Paul to bet on whether the coin he is about to flip will come up heads or tails. Peter starts to work out his chances of winning. He uses Bayes' Theorem. He first develops his *prior*. Peter knows that for a fair coin there is an even or 50:50 chance that the coin will fall heads. But given what he knows of Paul, Peter thinks that there is a small chance that Paul has fixed the coin so that it is more likely (though not guaranteed) to fall one way than the other. Peter's prior probability distribution is that the coin has a 90% chance of being fair, a 5% chance of being biased to tails, and a 5% chance of being biased to heads. Peter also assumes that the coin has one of three probabilities of falling heads. 50% if it is a fair coin, 45% if it is biased to fall tails, and 55% if it is biased to fall heads. Peter then watches Paul tossing the coin: this is his "small sample survey." Eighteen out of 20 times he sees that the coin comes up heads. Peter decides he must take this additional information into account. He calculates the *likelihood* that the coin would come up 18 times heads out of 20 for all three probabilities of the coin coming heads, namely 45%, 50% ,and 55%. Clearly, 18 heads is a lot. It suggests that the coin has been tampered with to fall heads (probability of falling heads of 55%).

	If biased to fall tails	If a fair coin	If biased to fall heads	
True probability of coin falling heads	0.45	0.5	0.55	
	Of coin being biased to tails	Of coin being fair	Of coin being biased to heads	
Prior probability	0.05	0.9	0.05	
Likelihood	Number of coin tosses		20	
	Number of heads		18	
Likelihood	0.000033	0.000181	0.000816	
	0.000002	0.000163	0.000041	0.000206
	Of coin being biased to tails	Of coin being fair	Of coin being biased to heads	
Posterior probability	0.008006	0.793471	0.198523	1

Peter therefore changes his original *prior* on the nature of the coin, using this new information from his small survey to calculate his *posterior* on the coin's probability of coming up heads. In fact, this information leads him to a posterior that there is a 1% chance the coin is biased to tails, a 20% chance the coin is biased to heads, but there is still a 79% chance the coin is fair. He can therefore bet more confidently, though not certainly, that the coin will fall heads.

---

offer a real promise for developing feasible subnational monitoring strategies.

As was described in the preceding section, a "prior" is an estimate of an indicator constructed from other existing related data sources. For example, to construct a district level prior for health, sources could include the national or provincial health indicator, adjusted by relevant district level variables such as income, education, etc. In a related approach, priors can be formed based on expert opinion or common sense. Such prior estimates can then be made more precise by combining them with a small amount of additional district level data specifically collected for the indicator concerned. The two distributions are combined to obtain the "posterior" distribution by using Bayes' Theorem. The challenge is to find the smallest sample size which will still provide a reasonable estimate when combined with a prior. To summarize, the Bayesian approach can be visualized as an updating mechanism in which prior data are revised in light of new evidence from sample data to produce better estimates. The purpose of constructing priors is to allow a smaller sample size to be used for any required additional data collection.

The types of data that can be used to construct priors are well illustrated by the development of priors for poverty and health, at the subnational level.

For both quantities of interest, national estimates normally exist: for poverty, it may be based on the proportion of the population living below $1 a day; for health, life expectancy or child mortality is often used.

To calculate provincial or district priors for poverty, the following variables could be used as indicators in the model: household asset information, such as whether households have electricity, a television, a car, or other consumer durable or living standards indicators; and community based information, such as quality of roads, proportion of households having electricity, presence of street lighting, etc.

To calculate provincial or district priors for health, the following variables could be used as indicators in the model: health service delivery data, average household size, health infrastructure availability and coverage information, any available provincial or district level mortality data.

Using Priors Combined with Small Samples: Results from a Simulation Model

Figure 59.1 shows the results of a simulation study to investigate the effects of different sample sizes on the robustness of the posterior estimates produced using Bayesian analysis. In the simulation, a population of 1 million is divided into ten regions. In each region, the population is 100 000. There is a national survey of 5 000 available. From the national survey, a prior can be derived for each region based on the relationships in the national survey between the outcome one is interested in and covariates. One can also estimate confidence intervals for the estimates in order to see how precise they are.

In Figure 59.1 the effect of increasing the sample size on the precision of the sample and posterior estimate for a given prior for one of those regions is illustrated. The x axis represents different sample sizes from 5 to 50. The y axis shows the extent to which the prior, sample and posterior estimates differ from "the truth"—which lies at 0 on the y axis.

When prior estimates are combined with a small amount of additional data collected from the region concerned, the final or posterior estimates are nearer truth in all cases, and progressively nearer truth as

the sample size increases. Improvement in the prior estimates of the variance of the outcome of interest can be achieved using the same approach.

Using Priors Combined with Small Samples: Illustration Using Real Data

The first example was based on a simulated population. What happens when real data are used? The next example illustrates how the techniques were used to estimate provincial poverty rates. In Figure 59.2 three curves are shown that have been plotted from actual survey data. The left-hand curve is a plot of the prior distribution for the poverty rate for a province in Indonesia, calculated based on analysis of asset data from the 1997 Demographic and Health Survey. Note that the wider these uncertainty intervals in prior subnational poverty estimates (that is, the wider the curve), the less informative are the priors in a Bayesian framework.

These priors were then combined with additional province-level estimates of poverty derived from separate micro-samples (e.g. from a small representative sample of households in each province). The right-hand curve in Figure 59.2 represents the estimated poverty rate from the micro-sample.

The taller, thinner central curve in the figure represents the result of combining prior and micro-sample estimates to obtain a poverty rate estimate for which there is less uncertainty (i.e. there is more precision) than there was for both of the single sets of data.

Effects of Item Reduction: Illustration Using Estimates of Economic Status

As already stated, the basic principle behind item reduction is to estimate the quantity of interest with the fewest possible items, without compromising on criteria such as validity and reliability of the measurement. Figure 59.3 reports the results of applying item reduction techniques to estimate the economic status of respondents using a series of asset and other indicator variables (such as ownership of a bicycle, car, TV, electricity, etc.) from the Indonesian Demographic and Health Survey. The x-axis reports the number of asset indicator variables that were used in the estimation of the economic status of respondents and the y-axis is the Spearman's correlation. As the graph demonstrates, there is a decline in the correlation of the estimates of economic status as measured using 20 asset indicator variables rather than 10, 9, and so on down to 5. However, that decline is very small: there remains a remarkably high correlation (almost 0.9),

Figure 59.1 Effect of increasing sample size on accuracy of sample and posterior estimates for a given prior estimate

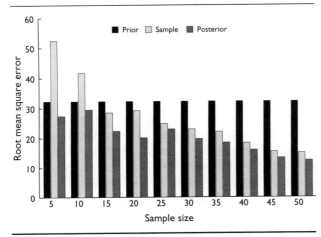
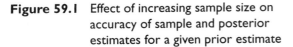

Figure 59.2 Proportion of a provincial population estimated to be poor

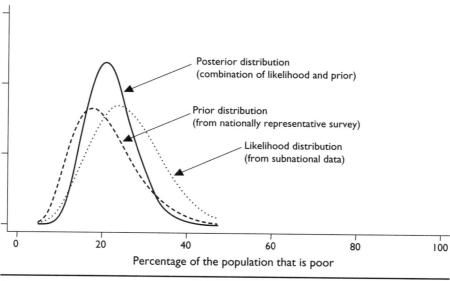

Source: Indonesia DHS 1997

even if the number of assets used in the estimation drops down to 5 versus the estimation using 20 assets. This example underscores the importance of considering item reduction techniques in micro-samples for subnational assessment, since there may be considerable cost and time efficiency gains—with a relatively minimal loss of information content—in implementing such techniques. A more detailed discussion is provided by Ferguson et al (29).

ROUTINE MONITORING OF HEALTH SYSTEMS PERFORMANCE: OTHER ISSUES AND CHALLENGES

PERIODICITY OF DATA COLLECTION

In terms of the periodicity of monitoring, there is a number of issues to consider. First, the country specific circumstances. For example, whether the health system is in a period of relative stability or rapid change, its capacity to collect and analyse data. Second, the nature of the indicators and the type of data required. A case can be made for monitoring inputs and selected aspects of the four functions on an annual basis, on the grounds that these give "early warning" signals to managers and policy-makers, and because the channels through which the data are obtained may already exist, or should be developed anyway for other purposes. For outcomes assessment, especially where survey data will always be needed, one could argue that a

two-year interval is a reasonable compromise between the effort involved and monitoring, with sufficient frequency to detect trends in a timely fashion.

IMPROVING THE COMMUNICATION AND USE OF FINDINGS

As was mentioned earlier, even when information is available, it is often not used, either by decision-makers or the general public. Why is this so? Many different reasons have been suggested, a few of which

Figure 59.3 Effects of item reduction: deriving estimates of economic status from asset questions

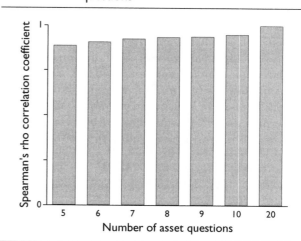

Source: Indonesia DHS 1997

are listed here. Decision-makers may be unaware of the fact that the information exists, or it may be hard to find. The information is not what decision-makers or the general public want. The system may not be producing the information when it is wanted. It could be presented in a way that is hard to understand. Finally, decision-makers may not want the information because they do not know what to do with it; they have no possibility to use it; they have no incentives to use it, or may even have incentives not to use it.

There is much rhetoric about the need to find ways to communicate results more effectively to decision-makers. This is certainly an important and complex issue, of which only a few aspects are touched on here.

The preceding sections have explored ways to synthesize a large amount of information from different sources, and summarize it in a few manageable indicators so that main messages come across clearly in the first instance. Another challenge is to present results in ways that make intuitive sense to the target audience. In terms of data presentation, experience teaches that the simpler the better. And it also suggests that this is possible even for somewhat complex concepts such as inequalities in health and responsiveness. For example, the notion of "threshold" measures was mentioned earlier as being reasonably easy to communicate: one can report on the number of people who fall below a certain agreed threshold level for that measure. Language is also critical, e.g. when trying to explain current problems with financial risk protection, the notion of "catastrophic expenditures" is more easily understood at the start of a discussion than is the index of fairness in financial contribution. The last aspect discussed here is that bringing decision-makers and data collectors together early on in any debate about information needs and system development, pays dividends later on in terms of the usefulness and use of the information subsequently produced.

CHALLENGES AND FUTURE DEVELOPMENTS

This chapter has explored the sort of information thought useful to monitor overall health systems performance at the subnational level for stewardship purposes. It has outlined what can be done from data that exists, and illustrated the potential of techniques already used in other fields to help develop practical, low-cost tools for regular subnational performance monitoring. Many challenges remain. They are being

tackled through a programme of work that is intended to have direct national and also cross-national benefits.

The first challenge is to further elaborate the critical aspects of performance to monitor regularly at different subnational levels, and devise indicators that reflect these concerns. The continuing wider work in the WHO to develop and refine measures of individual health system inputs, outcomes, and especially functions, at the national level is an essential input to this debate.

The second is to address the problem of critical data gaps. One route is through the World Health Survey (WHS). The latter has been designed to complement the existing survey and routine reporting systems, which have a number of important limitations in scope. The World Health Survey covers health, risk factors, responsiveness, coverage, access and utilization of key services, health care expenditures and assets. Its approach is modular and individual modules can be used with other existing survey platforms. There is a choice of survey delivery methods. If all modules are taken together, the World Health Survey captures many elements of health systems performance. It also captures 13 of the 17 health related Millennium Development Goals. Its predecessor, the WHO Multi-country Survey Study on Health and Responsiveness was tested in 2000–2001 by 71 surveys in 61 countries (*30*). In 2003 the World Health Survey is being implemented in over 70 countries. It will help build a stronger baseline for monitoring at the subnational as well as at the national level.

The third challenge is to move further ahead with the development of simple, reliable, and low-cost methods and tools that can be used regularly at the subnational level. Some techniques have been illustrated here. Further practical application is beginning. One activity is that in 2003, three countries will implement the World Health Survey using subnationally representative sampling strategies, and it will be possible to test different item reduction and small sampling techniques for subnational monitoring using data from these surveys.

The last two challenges are even bigger: to improve the communication and use of findings, and to strengthen country capacity to monitor subnational performance. WHO is working with several countries to support the analysis of subnational data by national teams using WHO methods, and then present findings to decision-makers. All countries have identified some specific policy uses they want from the exercise, in addition to building skilled teams who can do their own analyses. The exercise is also expected to help strengthen—and in some instances the framework is expected to help "rationalize"—the existing information systems. The initial focus is on generating information that is useful for primarily strategic or stewardship purposes: getting the "big picture," strengthening advocacy on health issues to other key actors, tracking whether their health system is moving in line with stated policy objectives, and promoting accountability. Feedback from these teams will help ensure the policy relevance and usability of the methods and tools.

In each country, a series of questions are being considered. What do decision-makers really need to know in order to make health policy decisions that lead to better health and health systems performance? Can a small set of indicators be devised, that, if reported for all areas, would give a more reliable and complete picture of performance than is currently available? What data already exist; how useful are they; what are the gaps? Are the trade-offs between cost, repeatability, quality, and level of detail acceptable? How can findings be more effectively communicated to decision-makers and to the public. What factors enhance the chances of their use? How can the exercise be institutionalized, so that monitoring becomes a regular rather than a research activity? A monograph on subnational health systems performance will be brought out in 2003, which will include case studies of the experience with application in countries.

NOTES

1 This chapter is largely based on presentations and discussions at the International Technical Meeting on Subnational Health Systems Performance Assessment, organized by the World Health Organization/Secretaria de Salud, México. Oaxaca, Mexico, 24–26 April 2002.

2 The policy principles are: policy relevance, easy to use and understand, sensitive to change in both directions, provide clues about the factors influencing level and change, sustainable, compatible with local culture and systems.

3 Adaptation of a slide presented by Julio Frenk at the International Technical Meeting on Subnational Health Systems Performance Assessment, organized by the World Health Organization/Secretaria de Salud, México. Oaxaca, Mexico, 24–26 April 2002.

REFERENCES

(1) Murray CJL, Frenk J. A framework for assessing the performance of health systems. *Bulletin of the World Health Organization*, 2000, 78(6):717–731.

(2) Wibulpolprasert S, Tangcharoensathien V. Health systems performance—What's next? *Bulletin of the World Health Organization*, 2001, 79(6):489.

(3) Anand S et al. Report of the Scientific Peer Review Group on health systems performance assessment. In: Murray CJL, Evans DB, eds. *Health systems performance assessment: debates, methods and empiricism*. Geneva, World Health Organization, 2003.

(4) Travis P, Weakliam D. *Tools and methods for health system assessment: inventory and review.* Geneva, World Health Organization, 1998.

(5) United Nations. *Road map towards the implementation of the United Nations Millennium Declaration. Report of the Secretary-General. General Assembly. Fifty-sixth session.* New York, United Nations, 2001.

(6) Üstün TB et al. The world health surveys. In: Murray CJL, Evans DB, eds. *Health systems performance assessment: debates, methods and empiricism*. Geneva, World Health Organization, 2003.

(7) Adams OB et al. Provision of personal and non-personal health services: proposal for monitoring. In: Murray CJL, Evans DB, eds. *Health systems performance assessment: debates, methods and empiricism*. Geneva, World Health Organization, 2003.

(8) Adams OB et al. Human, physical, and intellectual resource generation: proposals for monitoring. In: Murray CJL, Evans DB, eds. *Health systems performance assessment: debates, methods and empiricism*. Geneva, World Health Organization, 2003.

(9) Savedoff WD et al. Monitoring the health financing function. In: Murray CJL, Evans DB, eds. *Health systems performance assessment: debates, methods and empiricism*. Geneva, World Health Organization, 2003.

(10) Travis P et al. Towards better stewardship: concepts and critical issues. In: Murray CJL, Evans DB, eds. *Health systems performance assessment: debates, methods and empiricism*. Geneva, World Health Organization, 2003.

(11) Salomon JA et al. Quantifying individual levels of health: definitions, concepts, and measurement issues. In: Murray CJL, Evans DB, eds. *Health systems performance assessment: debates, methods and empiricism*. Geneva, World Health Organization, 2003.

(12) Valentine NB et al. Health system responsiveness: concepts, domains and operationalization. In: Murray CJL, Evans DB, eds. *Health systems performance assessment: debates, methods and empiricism*. Geneva, World Health Organization, 2003.

(13) Murray CJL et al. Assessing the distribution of household financial contributions to the health system: concepts

and empirical application. In: Murray CJL, Evans DB, eds. *Health systems performance assessment: debates, methods and empiricism*. Geneva, World Health Organization, 2003.

(14) Xu K et al. Understanding household catastrophic health expenditures: a multi-country analysis. In: Murray CJL, Evans DB, eds. *Health systems performance assessment: debates, methods and empiricism*. Geneva, World Health Organization, 2003.

(15) World Health Organization. *The World Health Report 2002. Reducing Risks, Promoting Healthy Life*. Geneva, World Health Organization, 2002.

(16) Evans DB et al. Comparative efficiency of national health systems: cross national econometric analysis. *British Medical Journal*, 2001, 323:307–310.

(17) World Health Organization. *WHO's contribution to the achievement of the development goals of the United Nations Millenium Declaration. Report by the Secretariat.* Executive Board, 111th Session. Geneva, World Health Organization, 2002.

(18) Murray CJL et al. Validity of reported vaccination coverage in 45 countries. In: Murray CJL, Evans DB, eds. *Health systems performance assessment: debates, methods and empiricism*. Geneva, World Health Organization, 2003.

(19) Hoshaw-Woodard S. *Description and comparison of the methods of cluster sampling and lot quality assurance sampling to assess immunization coverage*. The Ohio State University for Department of Vaccines and Biologicals, Geneva, World Health Organization, 2001.

(20) DeVellis RF. *Scale development: theory and applications*. Newbury Park, Sage Publications, 1991:7–12, 58, 74–78, 86–89,106.

(21) Marx RG et al. Clinimetric and psychometric strategies for development of a health measurement scale. *Journal of Clinical Epidemiology*, 1999, 52(2):105–111.

(22) Feldt LS. The relationship between the distribution of item difficulties and test reliability. *Applied Psychological Measurement*, 1993, 6:37–49.

(23) Fischer GH, Molenaar IW, eds. *Rasch models: foundations, recent developments, and applications*. New York, Springer-Verlag, 1995.

(24) Ware J Jr, Kosinski M, Keller SD. A 12-item short-form health survey: construction of scales and preliminary tests of reliability and validity. *Medical Care*, 1996, 34(3):220–233.

(25) Gandek B et al. Cross-validation of item selection and scoring for the SF-12 health survey in nine countries: results from the IQOLA Project. International Quality of Life Assessment. *Journal of Clinical Epidemiology*, 1998, 51(11):1171–1178.

(26) Black J. *A dictionary of economics*. Oxford, Oxford University Press, 1997.

(27) Pearce DW. *The MIT dictionary of modern economics*. Cambridge, The MIT Press, 1992.

(28) Kennedy P. *A guide to econometrics*. Cambridge, The MIT Press, 1998.

(29) Ferguson BD et al. Estimating permanent income using indicator variables. In: Murray CJL, Evans DB, eds. *Health systems performance assessment: debates, methods and empiricism*. Geneva, World Health Organization, 2003.

(30) Üstün TB et al. WHO Multi-country Survey Study on Health and Responsiveness 2000–2001. In: Murray CJL, Evans DB, eds. *Health systems performance assessment: debates, methods and empiricism*. Geneva, World Health Organization, 2003.

Chapter 60

WHO-CHOICE: CHOosing Interventions That Are Cost-Effective

Raymond C.W. Hutubessy, Rob M.P.M. Baltussen, Tessa Tan Torres–Edejer, David B. Evans, WHO-CHOICE Working Group[1]

Introduction

Cost-effectiveness analysis (CEA) provides one means by which decision-makers can assess and potentially improve the performance of their health systems. The process can help to ensure that health system resources are achieving the maximum possible benefit in terms of outcomes that people value. In Figure 60.1, the level of goal attainment is measured on the vertical axis and input use on the horizontal one. M shows the maximum possible level of goal attainment for the available resources, and L the minimum. L is not zero in health because health outcomes would not be zero in the absence of health system inputs.

Efficiency can be defined as the ratio of attainment (above the minimum) to the maximum possible attainment (also above the minimum), i.e. what proportion of the potential health system contribution to goal attainment is actually achieved for the observed level of resources. For a country at A it is b/(b + c).

If the horizontal axis measures total health expenditures to summarize all inputs to the health system, inefficiency could be due to two causes. The first is waste, e.g. over-staffing of hospitals, or *technical inefficiency*. The second is that the wrong mix of interventions is undertaken for the health problems of the country and the available resources. This is sometimes called *allocative efficiency*.[2]

If attention is restricted to health on the vertical axis, the frontier M is the potential attainment if the most cost-effective mix of interventions had been used for the available resources, or (a + b + c). The maximum possible contribution of the system is (b + c), the contribution above the minimum. Current outcome A is determined by the mix of interventions that is actually used, so observed health system efficiency is related to actual coverage of the optimal mix of interventions. Information on the costs and effectiveness on a range of interventions is, therefore, valuable to policy-makers seeking ways of improving goal attainment and efficiency.

In response to this need, over the past three decades there has been considerable growth in the number of economic appraisals performed in health care. Following standard textbooks on economic evaluations, most of these CEA studies pursue an incremental approach which requires comparison of the additional costs of an intervention (compared to current practice) with the additional health benefits (*1;2*). Such an incremental approach, however, is unable to provide policy-makers with information on whether the resources currently devoted to health achieve as much as they could. In addition, the results of an incremental analysis undertaken in one setting are not generalizable to other settings because results are sensitive to variables such as the level of infrastructure and the history of disease control activities (*3*).

Figure 60.1 Health system efficiency

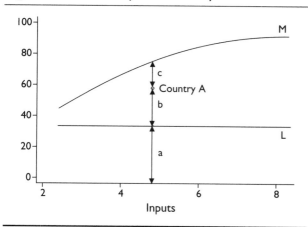

This chapter describes a broader sectoral approach via the application of a generalized CEA framework which allows existing inefficiencies in the health system to be identified, as well as decisions to be made about how best to use any additional resources that become available. It does this by comparing current and possible future interventions to a common counterfactual, which is the situation of not doing the intervention or interventions under discussion.

The chapter presents some evidence of existing inefficiencies in health care at both the macro and micro levels, indicating the need for a reallocation of health resources. It then discusses sectoral cost-effectiveness attempts made in the past to focus on allocative efficiency questions, and their shortcomings. In a subsequent section, the WHO generalized cost-effectiveness framework is described. The implementation and operationalization of this framework are illustrated by presenting ongoing activities and future plans of the programme of work relating to WHO-CHOICE (CHOosing Interventions that are Cost-Effective). Its application is demonstrated using cardiovascular (CV) diseases as an example showing how WHO-CHOICE can be used to define the most cost-effective mix of interventions at different resource levels, and the frontier M in Figure 60.1.

EXISTING INEFFICIENCIES IN HEALTH SYSTEMS

Both at the macro and the micro levels there is ample evidence on existing inefficiencies in the health system. At the macro level, health systems have multiple goals, yet their defining objective is to improve health. Despite this common aim, health systems with very similar levels of health expenditure per capita can show wide variations in population health outcomes. *The World Health Report 2000* published a first attempt to measure the attainment of the proposed health system goals in 191 countries, and considered how well countries were performing, given the resources available (4). Evans et al. (4;5) showed that countries like Sri Lanka and China, which were previously believed to have been efficient in producing health, performed less well than other countries at similar levels of development.

The authors concluded that efficiency is positively correlated with health expenditure per capita, especially at low expenditure levels, and that performance increases sharply with expenditure up to about I$80 per capita a year.[3] These findings can in part be explained by variation in non-health system factors such as the level of education of the population. However, a further part can be explained by the fact that some systems devote resources to expensive interventions with small effects on population health, while at the same time low-cost interventions which would result in relatively large health improvements are not fully implemented or ignored.

At the micro level, Tengs (6) and Murray et al. (7) argued that health both in the United States and sub-Saharan Africa could be greatly improved by reallocating available resources from interventions that are not cost-effective to those that are more cost-effective but not fully implemented. In the case of the United States, it was estimated that about US$214.4 billion was spent each year to fund a set of 185 interventions. Between them, they saved 592 000 years of life, but reallocating those funds to the most cost-effective set of interventions could save additional 638 000 life years (6).

SECTORAL COST-EFFECTIVENESS ANALYSIS INITIATIVES

One approach to help policy-makers in decisions about resource reallocation is the construction of a league table that rank-orders interventions by their cost-effectiveness ratios (cost per unit of health outcome). Many published league tables have been criticized for including only a few interventions (8–10), or for including interventions within only one disease area. For example, Pinkerton et al. (11) recently constructed league tables to compare interventions to prevent sexual transmission of HIV. Only rarely has the league table approach been applied in a broader sectoral perspective, in which cost-effectiveness results are compared on a wide range of health interventions. Notable exceptions are the work of Oregon Health Services (12), the Harvard Life Saving Project (13), and World Bank Health Sector Priorities Review (HSPR) (14). What these studies have in common is their aim to provide information which will help decision-makers allocate health care resources across many interventions and population groups to generate the highest possible overall level of population health. Each study will be described in more detail in turn.

WORLD BANK HSPR PROJECT

The first attempt to undertake a comprehensive sectoral CEA on a global level was the World Bank HSPR. It began in 1987, and in 1993 reported on the cost-effectiveness of more than twenty conditions or clusters of conditions. The resulting global league table was used as the basis for proposing a minimum package of basic public health and curative interventions in the *World Development Report 1993* (*15*).

The study results suggested that categorical assessments such as "prevention is more cost-effective than cure" are too simplistic. Some preventive interventions proved to be cost-effective and some not; some curative interventions were cost-effective and some were not. Another key finding was that many of the interventions undertaken then were very expensive ways of improving health, while many of the low-cost ways of improving health were not fully funded, implying that there was considerable room to improve allocative efficiency.

Oregon Health Plan

The objective of the "Oregon Experiment" was to try to extend the coverage of Medicaid, the US government programme that funds health for the poor, to more people without increasing the budget. It did this by restricting the services that people eligible for coverage could have funded under the plan. It proposed rationing services based on an elaborate technical analysis, one that merged cost-effectiveness analysis and medical outcomes research with public participation in policy-making decisions. A Health Services Commission was organized to compile clinical information from physicians, treatment costs and benefit data, and community values from the public. Initially, the list of conditions was based on CEA ranking, and then the list was revised through a process of community consultations. The final list was very different from the initial ranking. On one hand, the evidence from Oregon suggests that CEA had a limited impact on priority-setting. However, from a broader perspective, the process of using CEA brought the concepts of scarcity and choice to the forefront of the debate (*16;17*).

The Harvard Life Saving Project

A project at the Harvard Center for Risk Analysis was undertaken to review the published literature on the cost-effectiveness of interventions that reduce mortality (*13;18*). It was based on published papers, with minor amendments for differences in methods, and did not include non-fatal health outcomes. It reported its results in 1996, and like the HSPR, showed a substantial range of cost-effectiveness ratios across interventions that were then undertaken in the USA. The

investigators estimated that reallocating resources from cost-ineffective to cost-effective interventions in the US, just focusing on primary prevention, would save additional 600 000 years of life annually for the same level of investment (*18*).

A Critique of Previous Sectoral CEA Initiatives

The sectoral CEA studies presented in the previous section showed major inefficiencies in the allocation of resources in the health system at that time, implying that countries could make significant gains in population health by shifting resources from high-cost, low-effect interventions currently in use, to low-cost, high-effect interventions that are not used, or underutilized. However, each study has methodological flaws which make the results of it difficult to recommend for use by policy-makers in setting priorities.

Firstly, the studies included in the analyses are typically based on the incremental CEA approach that is appropriate in settings where policy-makers are constrained not only by the availability of resources, but also by the current level of and mix of interventions. However, this type of analysis ignores the question of whether current interventions themselves are cost-effective. As shown above, there is considerable evidence that some interventions currently undertaken are not cost-effective.

Secondly, incremental analysis has only limited use to decision-makers in settings other than the one in which a study is undertaken. The starting points for an incremental analysis vary across settings (for example, the current state of infrastructure and the current mix of interventions), while the additional health effect achieved from a given increase in resource use is dependent on what is currently done and the local epidemiology. This makes it very difficult for policy-makers in one setting to be sure that the ranking of interventions in another setting also applies to them.

Thirdly, in all the sectoral studies, the comparison of a wide range of interventions was based on studies using varying methods to estimate costs and health effects, undertaken at different points in time. The HSPR also compared cost-effectiveness ratios of studies undertaken in totally different settings in its league table. While comparisons over time will be inevitable in any sectoral analysis, standardized methods must be used consistently across CEA studies to ensure comparability (*19;20*).

Fourthly, previous sectoral CEAs did not consider synergistic effects between interventions. In reality, interventions can interact in terms of both costs and effectiveness. For example, passive case detection and treatment with directly observed therapy, short course (DOTS) interacts with BCG vaccination in terms of costs and outcomes. If BCG is delivered, the number of cases of tuberculosis that will occur will decline so that the variable cost component of the treatment programme will decline. Likewise, health benefits of BCG in the presence of a treatment programme will be less because many of the deaths from tuberculosis expected in the absence of treatment will be avoided (3).

Finally, uncertainty around cost-effectiveness ratios (CER) did not receive much attention in the above studies. For example, the *World Development Report 1993* reported only point estimates of the CERs with no indication of how large the uncertainty interval was likely to be. This information is particularly important for risk-averse decision-makers.

Generalized CEA and WHO-CHOICE

The shortcomings of previous sectoral CEA initiatives in health are closely related to the use of league tables in general. Many commentators have cautioned against the unthinking use of league tables because of non-comparability of methods, inappropriate comparators, and non-generalizability of results (8;10;21). WHO-CHOICE applying the framework of generalized cost-effectiveness analysis, has been designed to address some of these shortcomings (3;22). It allows existing and new interventions to be analysed at the same time. Using WHO-CHOICE, the analyst is no longer constrained by what is already being done, and policy-makers can revisit and revise past choices if necessary and feasible. Further, the use of a common methodology, that of generalized CEA, enhances comparability among interventions targeting a wide range of health problems and transferability of findings across countries within regions. Bearing in mind that obtaining evidence on context-specific cost-effectiveness information is time consuming and costly, the issue of generalizability of information is important, in particular for low- and middle-income countries.

WHO-CHOICE also introduces stochastic league tables to inform decision-makers about the probability that a specific intervention would be included in the optimal mix of interventions for various levels of resource availability, taking into account the uncer-

tainty around estimates of the costs and effectiveness of different interventions (23;24).

WHO-CHOICE has been developing tools and methods for generalized CEA since 1999. Its objectives are to:

- develop a standardized method for cost-effectiveness analysis that can be applied to all interventions in different settings (22);

- develop and disseminate tools required to assess intervention costs and impacts at the population level;

- determine the costs and effectiveness of a wide range of health interventions, undertaken by themselves or in combination;

- for transparency summarize the results in subregional databases that will be available on the World Wide Web;[4]

- assist policy-makers and other stakeholders in interpreting and using the evidence.

WHO-CHOICE has developed the following computer-based tools that will be available for use by analysts:

- PopMod® is a standard multi-state modelling tool in which health effects are estimated by tracing what would happen to each age/sex cohort of a given population over 100 years, with and without each intervention. It allows the health effects of interventions to be calculated in terms of DALYs averted or healthy years of life gained, thereby measuring intervention effectiveness in terms of comparable units across different types of interventions and diseases (25).

- COST-IT® is a costing spreadsheet based on a standardized ingredient approach that facilitates the analysis and reporting of intervention costs (26;27).

- The MCLeague® program presents the cost-effectiveness results in a stochastic league table, i.e. explicitly taking into account uncertainty surrounding cost and effectiveness estimates of many interventions at the same time (23;24).

WHO-CHOICE develops league tables of the cost-effectiveness of interventions (expressed in terms of cost per DALY averted) for 14 epidemiological subregions of the world (Annex 60.1) defined by the Global Burden of Disease Study (28). Subregions have been chosen to ensure the maximum amount of comparability between countries in terms of health systems and epidemiological profiles. Groups of interventions that interact are analysed together to account for synergies: for example, interventions to improve the health of children under five years of age (e.g. treatment of diarrhœal diseases and pneumonia, food supplementation, and micronutrient supplementation and fortification); and those to reduce the risks of cardiovascular disease (blood pressure and cholesterol lowering activities including medication, interventions to reduce smoking). The interventions range from prevention to curative to rehabilitative to palliative, from individual to packaged (e.g. oral rehydration therapy to integrated management of childhood illness), from those addressing infectious to non-communicable diseases, including injuries.

Subregional databases represent a compromise between a single global database that is not applicable locally in any setting, and the ideal of a separate database for each country, which is not feasible in the short run. To help analysts in countries use the results, WHO-CHOICE provides information in a way that enables them to modify the results of the subregional databases to their country. The databases include the raw cost and effect data, as well as the method and calculations that were used to obtain the summary cost-effectiveness ratios. The costing template accompanying all interventions uses an ingredients approach: quantities of resources used and prices are recorded separately. Effectiveness data are presented in a similarly transparent format.

The WHO-CHOICE databases should not be used in a formulaic way. They reveal a menu of interventions that are cost-effective in each subregion, a menu of interventions that are not, and another set of interventions in-between. Policy-makers would then assess the appropriate mix for their settings, taking into account other goals of the health system in addition to the improvement of population health. WHO works closely with policy-makers on ways of using the evidence WHO-CHOICE provides to achieve social goals.

GENERALIZED CEA: STRATEGIES TO REDUCE THE RISKS OF CARDIOVASCULAR DISEASE

The initial focus of the CHOICE project is to evaluate the costs and effectiveness of interventions targeting major causes of health burden across the world. The tools and methods described in the previous section have to date been used to analyse a range of interventions that address some of the leading risks to health. WHO's *World Health Report 2002 (29)* was devoted to quantifying major risks to health in the 14 subregions, and the effectiveness and costs of selected interventions to reduce the health impact of these risks. The report covers 28 major risks to health grouped under the following headings: environmental, occupational, addictive substances, childhood and maternal undernutrition, other nutrition-related risk factors and exercise, sexual and reproductive health, health practices (such as unsafe injections), and abuse and violence. It shows, for example, that in high mortality developing countries, undernutrition, unsafe sex and unsafe water, sanitation and hygiene are the three most important risks to health, while in developed regions, tobacco, blood pressure, and overuse of alcohol are the most important (Table 60.1). The report contains the best available evidence on the cost and effectiveness of selected interventions to reduce some

Table 60.1 Leading 10 selected risk factors as per cent of disease burden measured in DALYs*

Developing countries				Developed countries	
High mortality		Low mortality		Developed countries	
Underweight	14.9%	Alcohol	6.2%	Tobacco	12.2%
Unsafe sex	10.2%	Blood pressure	5.0%	Blood pressure	10.9%
Unsafe water, sanitation & hygiene	5.5%	Tobacco	4.0%	Alcohol	9.2%
Indoor smoke from solid fuels	3.6%	Underweight	3.1%	Cholesterol	7.6%
Zinc deficiency	3.2%	Body mass index	2.7%	Body mass index	7.4%
Iron deficiency	3.1%	Cholesterol	2.1%	Low fruit and vegetable intake	3.9%
Vitamin A deficiency	3.0%	Low fruit and vegetable intake	1.9%	Physical inactivity	3.3%
Blood pressure	2.5%	Indoor smoke from solid fuels	1.9%	Illicit drugs	1.8%
Tobacco	2.0%	Iron deficiency	1.8%	Unsafe sex	0.8%
Cholesterol	1.9%	Unsafe water, sanitation & hygiene	1.8%	Iron deficiency	0.7%

* Source: WHO 2002 (29)

of the major risk factors. The list of interventions is not exhaustive and it does not include all the risk factors. The ones for which interventions are considered in *The World Health Report 2002* (29) are highlighted in bold type in Table 60.1.

In this chapter, blood pressure and cholesterol are used to illustrate the approach to developing a frontier (M in Figure 60.1) using CEA. They are among the top 10 risks to health identified in the report in all parts of the world. The costs, effects, and cost-effectiveness of 17 interventions have been evaluated. The results from one representative subregion—AmrA (in the Americas with very low adult and child mortality)—are discussed in detail here, although the costs and effectiveness estimates for all 14 subregions have been published elsewhere (30).

INTERVENTIONS

Evaluation of the costs and effects of the major intervention strategies for reducing the burden attributable to blood pressure and cholesterol must address two

key debates. First, what is the relative role of non-personal health services such as mass media messages to change diet or legislation to reduce the salt content of processed foods, and personal health services such as the pharmacological management of cholesterol and hypertension?(31–33) Second, should management of blood pressure and cholesterol be based on thresholds for each risk factor seen in isolation, such as treating for a systolic blood pressure over 160mmHg, or should management be based on the absolute risk of cardiovascular disease for a given individual taking into account all his/her known determinants of risk?(34) Here we analyse the population health effects and costs of non-personal health measures, treatment of individual risk factors, and treatment based on different levels of absolute risk (35).

A variety of non-personal and personal interventions were evaluated individually, and a mix of strategies was also assessed (Table 60.2). Non-personal strategies included health education through the mass media focusing on blood pressure, cholesterol and body mass, and either legislation or voluntary

Table 60.2 Interventions evaluated

Intervention	Description
Non-personal interventions (N)	
Salt reduction through voluntary agreements with industry (N1).	Cooperation between government and the food industry for stepwise reduction of salt in processed foods and labelling.
Population-wide salt reduction—legislation (N2).	Legislation to reduce salt content in processed foods and appropriate labelling.
Health education through mass media (N3).	Health education through broadcast and print media focusing on body mass index, cholesterol.
Combined intervention of N2 and N3 (N4).	Combination of N2 and N3.
Personal interventions (P)	
Individual-based hypertension treatment and education (P1 and P2).	Treatment of people with systolic blood pressure (BP) above 160mmHg (P1) or above 140mmHg (P2) on a standard regimen of beta-blocker and diuretic.
Individual treatment for high cholesterol and education (P3 and P4).	Treatment with statins for people with total cholesterol levels above 240 mg/dl (6.2 mmol/L) (P3) and above 220 mg/dl (5.7 mmol/L) (P4).
Individual treatment and health education for systolic blood pressure and cholesterol (P5).	The combination of P2 and P3, with treatment thresholds of 140mmHg systolic BP and 240 mg/dl (6.2 mmol/L) for total cholesterol.
Absolute risk approach (P6 to P9).	People with an estimated combined risk of a cardiovascular event* (acute myocardial infarction; angina pectoris; congestive heart failure; first-ever fatal stroke; long-term stroke survivors) over the next decade above a given threshold are treated for multiple risk factors—with statin, diuretic, beta blocker and aspirin—regardless of their observed levels on individual risk factors. Four different thresholds were evaluated—35% (P6), 25% (P7), 15% (P8) and 5% (P9).
Combined personal and non-personal interventions (C)	
Building the absolute risk approach at the four thresholds on to the combined non-personal health intervention (C1 to C4).	The combination of N4 with P6 to P9.

* The definition of a cardiovascular event differs across studies, so the results reported here might not be strictly comparable with those of similar studies (37).

agreements on salt content to ensure appropriate labelling and stepwise reductions of the salt content of processed foods. Personal interventions included treating people with elevated levels of cholesterol and systolic blood pressure in turn, and treatment based on an assessment of an individual's absolute risk of a cardiovascular event in the next 10 years (called the "absolute risk" approach (36)) using different absolute risk thresholds.

EFFECTIVENESS

For estimating population health effects, generalized CEA involves two fundamental processes: 1) construction of the counterfactual—or what would have happened in the absence of the intervention; and 2) consideration of the consequences of an intervention, relative to the counterfactual. These two processes must be carried out for both costs and health outcomes.

PopMod was used to translate age and sex specific changes in the risk of cardiovascular disease events into changes in population health quantified in terms of DALYs (25). The parameters reflecting the natural history of the disease were estimated by back-adjusting current rates using coverage and known effectiveness of interventions. The most important side effect, relating to the consequences of bleeding associated with the use of aspirin, was included in the model. The entire population is subjected to background mortality and morbidity, which is assumed to be independent of the cardiovascular disease states explicitly modelled. For example, high blood pressure increases the risk of dying from cardiovascular diseases (CVD). The impacts of beta-blockers and diuretics are then mediated in the model by a decrease in incidence rate of CVD. Effectiveness data came from systematic reviews where available. The difference in the healthy life years gained by the population with and without the intervention is the impact of the intervention and is entered as the denominator of the cost-effectiveness ratio.

COSTS

Costs include programme-level costs associated with running the intervention, such as administration, training and media, and patient-level costs, such as primary care visits and hospitalizations. These costs have been based on a standardized ingredients by using Cost-It® (26). The units of physical inputs required were assessed and multiplied by the unit price for each input. For programme costs, the quantities of the required inputs (such as labour, vehicles, office space) were identified from the literature with additional details provided by programme staff in various parts of the world. The quantity of patient-level resource inputs required for a given health intervention, e.g. hospital inpatient days, outpatient visits, medications, laboratory tests etc., was identified in a similar manner.

Unit costs of programme-level and patient-level resource inputs, such as the salaries of central administrators, the capital costs of vehicles, offices and furniture, or the cost per outpatient visit, were obtained from a review of the literature and supplemented by primary data from programme staff in several countries. Costs of drugs were based on the price of off-patent drugs from the lowest cost vendor of high-quality drugs. Information on the costs and effectiveness of interventions that are undertaken inefficiently is of little value to decision-makers. For that reason we assume capacity utilization of 80% in most settings, e.g. that health personnel are fully occupied for 80% of their time. The results identify, therefore, the set of interventions that, if done relatively efficiently, would be cost-effective in the different settings.

COST-EFFECTIVENESS

Information on the total costs of each intervention with information on the total health effects in terms of DALYs averted from these interventions is combined into average cost-effectiveness ratios. In addition, using a standard approach, we have evaluated what set of interventions a subregion should purchase to maximize health gain for different budget levels. The order in which interventions would be purchased is called an "expansion path" and is based on the incremental costs and benefits of each intervention compared to the last intervention purchased. Based on the Commission on Macroeconomics and Health, we label interventions that have a cost-effectiveness ratio of less than three times Gross Domestic Product (GDP) per capita as "cost-effective" (38). Further, we use the label "very cost-effective" to refer to interventions that cost less than one times GDP per capita.

UNCERTAINTY ANALYSIS

Multivariate uncertainty analysis was undertaken to assess the impact of uncertainty in the assumptions on the baseline levels of risks and intervention effect sizes on the cost-effectiveness ratios. Effect size of changes in risk factors and population risk factor distributions are modelled as random variables so as to obtain mean estimates of incidence after intervention. Draws were made from limits developed from the literature review producing upper and lower confidence bounds on the mean incidence. This also includes the effects on costs because different numbers of people will be covered by an intervention under the different scenarios. At the same time, the price of medicines—the key cost driver—was allowed to vary from half to double the base estimate.

In order to report the impact of these confidence intervals around the mean costs and health benefits on the optimal mix of cardiovascular risk interventions at increasing levels of resources availability, we used MCLeague® to develop stochastic league tables (24). Here random sampling (up to 10 000 iterations) draws were taken from generated truncated distributions based on the upper and lower confidence limits of intervention effect sizes and prices of medicines. We assumed that costs and health benefits have a normal distribution.

RESULTS

Average Cost-Effectiveness Ratios

Table 60.3 provides the total annualized costs, total annual health effect in terms of DALYs averted, and the average cost-effectiveness ratio for each of the 17 interventions in subregion AmrA. All 17 interven-

Table 60.3 Annual costs, effects, and cost-effectiveness of interventions for AmrA

Intervention*	Costs ($ in millions)	DALYs (100 000s)	Cost/DALY ($)
Non-personal (N)			
N1: voluntary salt red.	92	4	229
N2: legislated salt red.	92	8	119
N3: mass media	114	11	106
N4: N2 and N3	207	18	115
Personal (P)			
P1: BP at 160	6 136	50	1 224
P2: BP at 140 mmHg	19 669	60	3 294
P3: cholesterol at 240	7 716	52	1 475
P4: cholesterol at 220	13 776	60	2 280
P5: P2 with P3	27 384	90	3 059
P6: Absolute risk 35%	9 614	81	1 181
P7: Absolute risk 25%	13 278	88	1 512
P8: Absolute risk 15%	18 498	95	1 953
P9: Absolute risk at 5%	29 728	103	2 882
Combined Interv. (C)			
C1: N4 then P6	9 117	85	1 077
C2: N4 then P7	12 783	91	1 409
C3: N4 then P8	17 931	97	1 845
C4: N4 then P9	29 142	105	2 767

tions are cost-effective according to the Commission on Macroeconomics and Health criterion.

When considered individually, non-personal health interventions to reduce blood pressure and cholesterol are very cost-effective. Measures to reduce salt intake are potentially very cost-effective, with legislation being more cost-effective than voluntary agreements under the assumption that it would lead to the larger reduction in dietary salt intake. Mass media interventions to reduce cholesterol alone, then mass media in combination with legislation to reduce salt content in processed foods would be the first two strategies chosen in the subregion.

On the other hand, adding personal health service strategies involving medication will reduce the burden of disease substantially more than the initial non-personal interventions, even though they are slightly less cost-effective. The most efficient option is to add treatment based on the absolute risk approach to the non-personal interventions. People identified (using information on their age, sex, body mass index, serum total cholesterol, systolic blood pressure levels, and smoking status) to have an elevated risk of vascular disease over the next 10 years are provided with low dose combination treatment using diuretics and beta-blockers (to lower blood pressure), statins (to lower cholesterol) and aspirin (to reduce blood thickness). This reflects recent evidence that such therapy benefits all groups at elevated risk, even those with average or below average blood pressure or cholesterol.

In AmrA it is cost-effective to provide such therapy to all people with a risk in excess of 5%.

Treatment using the absolute risk approach is always more efficient than treatment of systolic blood pressure alone or treatment of people with total cholesterol levels above standard thresholds.

Incremental Cost-Effectiveness Ratios

Figure 60.2 plots the annual cost and DALYs averted for each of the 17 interventions in AmrA. The slope of the line connecting the origin to each point is the cost-effectiveness ratio. The steeper the slope, the more expensive the intervention per DALY averted. These figures can also help visualize the incremental cost and incremental health gain of moving from one intervention strategy to another.

From the perspective of how best to maximize population health for the available resources, the appropriate overall strategy is a combination of the non-personal and personal based interventions. The solid lines joining the most cost-effective points in

Figure 60.2 Annual costs and effectiveness for CVD risk factor interventions, AmrA

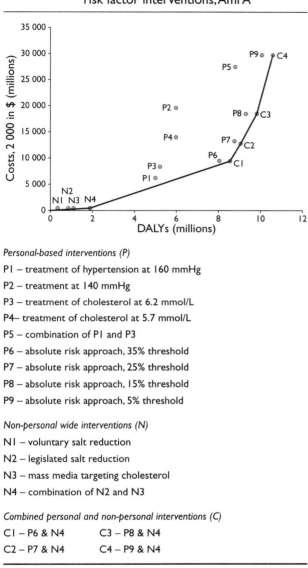

Personal-based interventions (P)

P1 – treatment of hypertension at 160 mmHg

P2 – treatment at 140 mmHg

P3 – treatment of cholesterol at 6.2 mmol/L

P4– treatment of cholesterol at 5.7 mmol/L

P5 – combination of P1 and P3

P6 – absolute risk approach, 35% threshold

P7 – absolute risk approach, 25% threshold

P8 – absolute risk approach, 15% threshold

P9 – absolute risk approach, 5% threshold

Non-personal wide interventions (N)

N1 – voluntary salt reduction

N2 – legislated salt reduction

N3 – mass media targeting cholesterol

N4 – combination of N2 and N3

Combined personal and non-personal interventions (C)

C1 – P6 & N4   C3 – P8 & N4

C2 – P7 & N4   C4 – P9 & N4

Figure 60.2, the "expansion path," show the interventions that would be selected for increasing levels of resource availability. The slopes between each point represent the "incremental cost-effectiveness ratio"—or the additional costs required to avert each additional DALY by moving from the lower to the higher cost intervention. If resources are extremely scarce, the non-personal interventions would be chosen first and then the absolute risk approach added with the threshold determined by the available resources.

Although the patterns of CVD risk vary across subregions as do cost-effectiveness ratios, the findings for AmrA are typical for most of the other subregions. In settings of extreme resource constraints, one of the

non-personal interventions to reduce salt or cholesterol would be purchased first. Decision-makers who want to maximize health gain for available resources would next move to a combined strategy of legislated salt reductions in processed foods with mass media campaigns, and then add the absolute risk approach to managing blood pressure and cholesterol. Depending on the resources available, the absolute risk threshold for a cardiovascular event that would trigger intervention with beta-blockers, diuretics, statins, and aspirin would be lowered. While the total costs, total effects, and cost-effectiveness ratios vary considerably across subregions, the sequence of intervention strategies that would be purchased is similar.

Uncertainty Analysis

The multivariate uncertainty analysis illustrates that the cost-effectiveness ratios vary—for AmrA they can be up to 85% higher or 55% lower. Figure 60.3 depicts the stochastic league diagram for the cluster of interventions focusing on blood pressure and cholesterol for the same subregion when low (Figure 60.3A) and high (Figure 60.3B) levels of resources are available. The vertical axis shows the probability that an intervention will be included in the optimal package for the level of the resource constraint on the horizontal axis, taking into account uncertainty around the input parameters. The results are remarkably robust to changes in assumptions at most levels of resource availability—for example, between $1.3 and $1.8 billion, mass media campaign targeting cholesterol would be chosen over 90% of the time (Figure 60.3A). At any level of resource availability over $750 billion, the combination of both non-personal interventions with treatment using the absolute risk approach at a 5% threshold would be chosen more than 90% of the time. It is only at intermediate levels of resource availability, for example between $75 and $250 billion, that uncertainty arises (Figure 60.3B).

USING CEA TO ESTIMATE A FRONTIER

For sector-wide priority setting, cost-effectiveness information should be collected in a way that will allow policy-makers to address two critical questions: "Do the resources currently devoted to health achieve as much as they could?" and "How best to use additional resources if they become available?" WHO-CHOICE provides information which is an important input to policy-makers in all settings considering these two questions and interested in devising ways of making their health systems more efficient.

This chapter has shown that WHO-CHOICE can be used to identify the most cost-effective mix of interventions at different resource levels. This is the micro approach to defining a production frontier (line M in Figure 60.1)—the maximum possible health output achievable for a specific level of input. Once the frontier for a health system, or a discrete part of a health system (e.g. decentralized administrative unit or hospital) has been defined, it can be used as a basis for evaluating overall health system efficiency.

To illustrate this with the CVD example, Figure 60.4 illustrates the production frontier for the interventions evaluated for AmrA above. The vertical axis depicts healthy years of life (HALE) gained (obtained by transforming DALYs averted for each intervention to HALEs gained) and resource use or costs are shown on the X axis. Available data on current coverage of the interventions in AmrA and their costs and effectiveness allow current attainment and costs to be estimated, represented as point •. The higher line shows the frontier estimated from information about the costs and effects of the most efficient mix of interven-

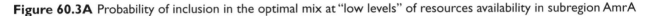

Figure 60.3A Probability of inclusion in the optimal mix at "low levels" of resources availability in subregion AmrA

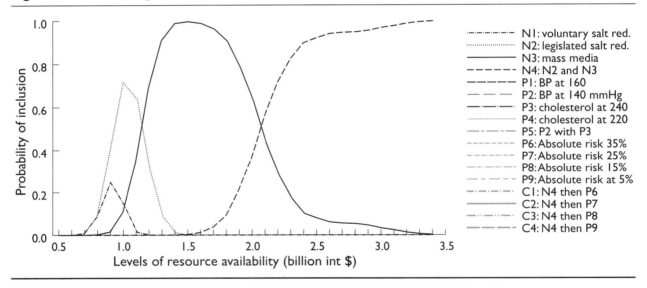

Figure 60.3B Probability of inclusion in the optimal mix at "high levels" of resources availability in subregion AmrA

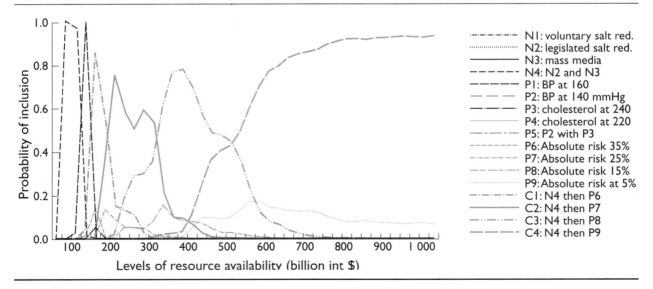

tions at any given level or resource availability. The point • is below the frontier, suggesting that they are not achieving their full potential in terms of reducing the risks associated with high blood pressure and cholesterol.

Clearly, information in addition to cost-effectiveness estimates is crucial to any final decision about how to allocate scarce resources. Health systems seek not only to improve population health, but also to be responsive to people's non-health expectations, reduce inequalities in health outcomes and in responsiveness, and ensure that household financial contributions are fairly distributed (39). Other political, ethical, and social issues also influence practical policy-making (40;41). Cost-effectiveness information should not be used mechanistically to allocate resources, but it can provide vital information on the efficiency of current resource use and on how to improve population health.

ACKNOWLEDGEMENTS

The worked example relating to strategies to reduce cardiovascular risks is based on the work by the WHO-CHOICE working group in collaboration with Niels Tomijima (WHO/GPE), Louis Niessen (University Medical Centre Rotterdam, Netherlands), Anthony Rodgers and Carlene Lawes (University of Auckland, New Zealand).

NOTES

1 The WHO-CHOICE Working Group consists of the following people in addition to the named authors: Taghreed Adam, Moses Aikens, Dan Chisholm, Chika Hayashi, Benjamin Johns, Jeremy A. Lauer, Kenji Shibuya, and Christopher J.L. Murray.

2 Allocative efficiency is achieved when the mix of inputs minimizes the cost for a given level of output. If interventions are viewed as inputs, allocative efficiency can be considered as the mix of interventions that are the most cost-effective. This is how the term is often used in the health economics literature.

3 International dollars are derived by dividing local currency units by an estimate of their purchasing power parity (PPP) compared to a US$. PPPs are the rates of currency conversion that equalize the purchasing power of different currencies by eliminating the differences in price levels between countries.

4 URL: http://www.who.int/evidence/cea

Figure 60.4 Maximum possible health gains from selected CVD risk factor interventions, subregion AmrA

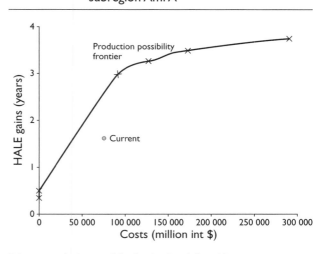

Points on production possibility frontier, from left to right:

N3 – mass media targeting cholesterol

N4 – combination of legislative salt reduction (N2) and mass media targeting cholesterol (N3)

C1 – combination of N4 and absolute risk approach, 35% threshold

C2– combination of N4 and absolute risk approach, 25% threshold

C3 – combination of N4 and absolute risk approach, 15% threshold

C4 – combination of N4 and absolute risk approach, 5% threshold

REFERENCES

(1) Drummond M et al. *Methods for the economic evaluation of health care programmes*, 2nd ed. Oxford, New York, Torronto, Oxford Univeristy Press, 1997.

(2) Gold MR et al. *Cost-effectiveness in health and medicine*. New York, Oxford University Press, 1996.

(3) Murray CJL et al. Development of WHO guidelines on generalized cost-effectiveness analysis. *Health Economics*, 2000, 9:235–251.

(4) World Health Organization. *The World Health Report 2000: Health Systems: Improving Performance*. Geneva, World Health Organization, 2000.

(5) Evans DB et al. Comparative efficiency of national health systems: cross national econometric analysis. *British Medical Journal*, 2001, 323:307–310.

(6) Tengs TO. *Dying too soon: how cost-effectiveness analysis can save lives*. NCPA Policy Report No. 204. Dallas, USA, National Center for Policy Analysis, 1997.

(7) Murray CJL, et al. Cost effectiveness of chemotherapy for pulmonary tuberculosis in three sub-Saharan African countries. *The Lancet*, 1991, 338:1305–1308.

(8) Drummond M, Torrance G, Mason J. Cost-effectiveness league tables: more harm than good? *Social Science & Medicine*, 1993, 37:33–40.

(9) Birch S, Gafni A. Cost-effectiveness ratios: in a league of their own. *Health Policy*, 1994, 28:133–141.

(10) Mason J, Drummond M, Torrance G. Some guidelines on the use of cost effectiveness league tables. *British Medical Journal*, 1993, 306:570–572.

(11) Pinkerton SD et al. Using cost-effectiveness league tables to compare interventions to prevent sexual transmission of HIV. *AIDS*, 2001, 15:917–928.

(12) Blumstein JF. The Oregon experiment: the role of cost-benefit analysis in the allocation of Medicaid funds. *Social Science & Medicine*, 1997, 45:545–554.

(13) Tengs TO et al. Five-hundred life-saving interventions and their cost-effectiveness. *Risk Analysis*, 1995, 15:369–390.

(14) Jamison DT et al. *Disease control priorities in developing countries*. New York, Oxford University Press, 1993.

(15) World Bank. *World development report 1993: investing in health*. New York, Oxford University Press, 1993.

(16) Blumstein JF. The Oregon experiment: the role of cost-benefit analysis in the allocation of Medicaid funds. *Social Science & Medicine*, 1997, 45:545–554.

(17) Dixon J, Welch HG. Priority setting: lessons from Oregon. *The Lancet*, 1991, 337:891–894.

(18) Tengs TO. Enormous variation in the cost-effectiveness of prevention: implications for public policy. *Current Issues in Public Health*, 1996, 2:13–17.

(19) Walker D, Fox-Rushby J. Economic evaluation of parasitic diseases: a critique of the internal and external validity of published studies. *Tropical Medicine & International Health*, 2000, 5:237–249.

(20) Walker D. Cost and cost-effectiveness guidelines: which ones to use? *Health Policy and Planning*, 2001, 16:113–121.

(21) Gerard K, Mooney G. QALY league tables: handle with care. *Health Economics*, 1993, 2:59–64.

(22) Baltussen RMPM et al. *Generalized cost-effectiveness analysis: a guide*. Geneva, World Health Organization, 2003. URL: http://www.who.int/evidence/cea

(23) Baltussen RMPM et al. Uncertainty in cost-effectiveness analyses: probabilistic uncertainty analysis and stochastic league tables. *International Journal of Technology Assessment in Health Care*, 2002, 18(1):112-119.

(24) Hutubessy RCW et al. Stochastic league tables: communicating cost-effectiveness results to decision-makers. *Health Economics*, 2001, 10:473–477.

(25) Lauer JA et al. PopMod: a longitudinal population model with two interacting disease states. *Cost-Effectiveness and Resource Allocation*, 2003, 1(6). URL: http://www.resource-allocation.com/content/1/1/6

(26) Adam T, Evans DB, Murray CJL. Econometric estimation of country-specific hospital costs. *Cost-Effectiveness and Resource Allocation*, 2003, 1(3). URL: http://www.resource-allocation.com/content/1/1/3

(27) Johns B, Baltussen R, Hutubessy RCW. Programme costs in the economic evaluation of health interventions. *Cost-Effectiveness and Resource Allocation*, 2003, 1(1). URL: http://www.resource-allocation.com/content/1/1/1

(28) Murray CJL, Lopez AD. Global mortality, disability, and the contribution of risk factors: Global Burden of Disease Study. *The Lancet*, 1997, 349:1436–1442.

(29) World Health Organization. *The World Health Report 2002: Reducing Risks, Promoting Healthy Life*. Geneva, World Health Organization, 2002.

(30) Murray CJL et al. Reducing the risk of cardiovascular disease: effectiveness and costs of interventions to reduce systolic blood pressure and cholesterol–a global and regional analysis. *The Lancet*, 2003, 361:717-725.

(31) Puska P. Development of public policy on the prevention and control of elevated blood cholesterol. *Cardiovascular Risk Factors*, 1996, 6:203–210.

(32) World Health Organization. *Innovative care for chronic conditions: building blocks for action*. Document No. WHO/MNC/CCH/02.01. Geneva, World Health Organization, 2002.

(33) Martin I. Implementation of WHO/ISH Guidelines: role and activities of WHO. *Clinical and Experimental Hypertension*, 1999, 21:659–669.

(34) Law MR, Wald NJ. Risk factor thresholds: their existence under scrutiny. *British Medical Journal*, 2002, 324:1570–1576.

(35) Cooper RS et al. Hypertension treatment and control in sub-Saharan Africa: the epidemiological basis for policy. *British Medical Journal*, 1998, 316:614–617.

(36) Jackson R et al. Management of raised blood pressure in New Zealand: a discussion document. *British Medical Journal*, 1993, 307:107–110.

(37) Anderson KM et al. Cardiovascular disease risk profiles. *American Heart Journal*, 1991, 121:293–298.

(38) WHO Commission on Macroeconomics and Health. *Macroeconomics and health: investing in health for economic development. Report of the Commission on Macroeconomics and Health*. Geneva, World Health Organization, 2001.

(39) Murray CJL, Frenk J. A framework for assessing the

performance of health systems. *Bulletin of the World Health Organization*, 2000, 78:717–731.

(40) Callahan D. Ethics and priority setting in Oregon. *Health Affairs (Millwood)*, 1991, 10:78–87.

(41) Daniels N. Is the Oregon rationing plan fair? *The Journal of the American Medical Association*, 1991, 265: 2232–2235.

Annex 60.1
Epidemiological Subregions

Region*	Mortality stratum**	Countries
AFR	D	Algeria, Angola, Benin, Burkina Faso, Cameroon, Cape Verde, Chad, Comoros, Equatorial Guinea, Gabon, Gambia, Ghana, Guinea, Guinea-Bissau, Liberia, Madagascar, Mali, Mauritania, Mauritius, Niger, Nigeria, Sao Tome and Principe, Senegal, Seychelles, Sierra Leone, Togo
AFR	E	Botswana, Burundi, Central African Republic, Congo, Côte d'Ivoire, Democratic Republic of the Congo, Eritrea, Ethiopia, Kenya, Lesotho, Malawi, Mozambique, Namibia, Rwanda, South Africa, Swaziland, Uganda, United Republic of Tanzania, Zambia, Zimbabwe
AMR	A	Canada, United States of America, Cuba
AMR	B	Antigua and Barbuda, Argentina, Bahamas, Barbados, Belize, Brazil, Chile, Colombia, Costa Rica, Dominica, Dominican Republic, El Salvador, Grenada, Guyana, Honduras, Jamaica, Mexico, Panama, Paraguay, Saint Kitts and Nevis, Saint Lucia, Saint Vincent and the Grenadines, Suriname, Trinidad and Tobago, Uruguay, Venezuela
AMR	D	Bolivia, Ecuador, Guatemala, Haiti, Nicaragua, Peru
EMR	B	Bahrain, Cyprus, Iran (Islamic Republic of), Jordan, Kuwait, Lebanon, Libyan Arab Jamahiriya, Oman, Qatar, Saudi Arabia, Syrian Arab Republic, Tunisia, United Arab Emirates
EMR	D	Afghanistan, Djibouti, Egypt, Iraq, Morocco, Pakistan, Somalia, Sudan, Yemen
EUR	A	Andorra, Austria, Belgium, Croatia, Czech Republic, Denmark, Finland, France, Germany, Greece, Iceland, Ireland, Israel, Italy, Luxembourg, Malta, Monaco, Netherlands, Norway, Portugal, San Marino, Slovenia, Spain, Sweden, Switzerland, United Kingdom
EUR	B	Albania, Armenia, Azerbaijan, Bosnia and Herzegovina, Bulgaria, Georgia, Kyrgyzstan, Poland, Romania, Slovakia, Tajikistan, The Former Yugoslav Republic of Macedonia, Turkey, Turkmenistan, Uzbekistan, Serbia and Montenegro
EUR	C	Belarus, Estonia, Hungary, Kazakhstan, Latvia, Lithuania, Republic of Moldova, Russian Federation, Ukraine
SEAR	B	Indonesia, Sri Lanka, Thailand
SEAR	D	Bangladesh, Bhutan, Democratic People's Republic of Korea, India, Maldives, Myanmar, Nepal
WPR	A	Australia, Japan, Brunei Darussalam, New Zealand, Singapore
WPR	B	Cambodia, China, Lao People's Democratic Republic, Malaysia, Mongolia, Philippines, Republic of Korea, Viet Nam Cook Islands, Fiji, Kiribati, Marshall Islands, Micronesia (Federated States of), Nauru, Niue, Palau, Papua New Guinea, Samoa, Solomon Islands, Tonga, Tuvalu, Vanuatu

* AFR = Africa Region; AMR = Region of the Americas; EMR = Eastern Mediterranean Region; EUR = European Region; SEAR = South-East Asia Region; WPR = Western Pacific Region

** A = subregions have very low rates of adult and child mortality; B = low adult, low child; C = high adult, low child; D = high adult, high child; E = very high adult, high child mortality.

Part V

Report
of the
Scientific
Peer
Review
Group
on
Health
Systems
Performance
Assessment

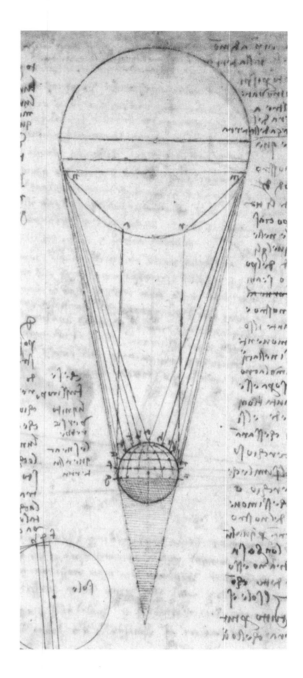

Chapter 61

Report of the Scientific Peer Review Group on Health Systems Performance Assessment[1]

Sudhir Anand, Walid Ammar, Timothy Evans, Toshihiko Hasegawa, Katarzyna Kissimova-Skarbek, Ana Langer, Adetokunbo O. Lucas, Lindiwe Makubalo, Alireza Marandi, Gregg Meyer, Andrew Podger, Peter Smith, Suwit Wibulpolprasert

Acknowledgements

Dr John Eisenberg, who was appointed to SPRG at its inception, regretfully passed away on 10 March 2002. SPRG wishes to place on record its appreciation for his participation, and expresses its condolences to his family.

A very large number of people provided input, both written and oral, to SPRG on different aspects of HSPA. This contributed substantially to SPRG's understanding of the scope and depth of the scientific debate. There are too many contributors to name individually, but SPRG is enormously grateful for their inputs. A special note of thanks is due to the Ministry of Health, Brazil for inviting the chair of SPRG to a special two day workshop, hosted by the Oswaldo Cruz Foundation (FIOCRUZ) in March 2002, to discuss technical issues related to HSPA.

Executive Summary

The Scientific Peer Review Group (SPRG) on Health Systems Performance Assessment (HSPA) was set up by the Director-General at the end of October 2001. The list of 13 members of SPRG is attached as Annex 1. Its terms of reference were:

- To review the scientific merit of methods proposed by the WHO Secretariat for the next round of HSPA, building on the suggestions made in the technical, regional and country consultations, in ongoing research and the general academic debate;

- To propose revisions, as necessary, to the methods that improve their scientific merit, and work with the WHO Secretariat to assess the feasibility and impact of any revision;

- To advise the Director-General of the scientific merit of the final methods emerging from this process.

SPRG met for the first time in December 2001, and prepared an interim report that was presented to the WHO Executive Board in January 2002. The Group had two subsequent meetings in February and April 2002. Each of the three SPRG meetings was attended in person by at least nine members, with most of the others participating via a video-conference or tele-conference link.

This is the final report of SPRG, presented to the Director-General in May 2002. The report has been prepared with input from every member, and the conclusions and recommendations in it are unanimous.

SPRG considers that the objectives of the HSPA initiative are valid, and that the provision of comparative data on health-system characteristics is a vital component of securing health-system improvements. In its deliberations SPRG has therefore sought to apply the following overarching criterion to inform its recommendations: that all future HSPA activity should be judged by the extent to which it effects an improvement in health systems performance worldwide, particularly in countries with low levels of attainment.

SPRG welcomes the opportunity it has been given to contribute to the HSPA process. WHR 2000 made an important breakthrough in seeking to provide an integrated quantitative assessment of health systems performance, and bringing the topic of health-system performance to the attention of policy makers worldwide.

SPRG considers that many of the important issues that have been raised in the public debate about HSPA are strategic policy concerns rather than scientific concerns. The strategic concerns may be matters on which WHO will need to determine a policy, but are in general beyond the remit of SPRG. The Group has therefore sought wherever possible to focus only on the scientific aspects of HSPA.

Within the limited time and resources at its disposal, SPRG has sought to review the scientific evidence from five main sources:

1. Published and unpublished documents and presentations by WHO staff.

2. The reports of the WHO regional consultations and technical workshops.

3. The reports of the WHO meetings of experts.

4. Commentaries by national governments and agencies.

5. Published literature in peer-reviewed journals and unpublished working papers by external commentators.

In addition, during the review process, the Group has been open to considering comments and criticisms received in the form of personal communications from various quarters—researchers, academics, and professionals in the public policy area.

SPRG wishes to congratulate and thank the WHO Evidence and Information for Policy (EIP) Cluster for the breadth and quality of the materials presented. An enormous volume of material has been made available to SPRG, and members of all Departments in the Cluster were unfailingly helpful in making themselves available and responding to requests for clarification and additional material. Without this responsiveness, our job would have been impossible.

The responsiveness of the EIP staff was an immensely encouraging aspect of the SPRG process. Paradoxically, however, it did generate problems for SPRG, in the sense that the Group frequently found itself commenting on what one member referred to as a 'moving target'. WHO proposals were refined over the course of the review process, leading to the production of numerous new working papers as the review process progressed.

The general approach adopted by SPRG has been to follow the template set out by the WHO Secretariat in its Summary Document "Proposed Strategies for Health Systems Performance Assessment" (in Background Documentation for Scientific Peer Review Group Meeting, Geneva, 7–8 December 2001). This included 15 topic areas, which correspond to the sections set out in the main body of this report. For each topic we have sought to describe the approach taken

in WHR 2000, summarize the criticisms that WHR 2000 attracted, outline the subsequent response by WHO, and put forward our comments and recommendations.

In reviewing the material made available, SPRG also developed some overarching recommendations that apply across a wide range of HSPA activity. They can be summarized as follows.

1. The development of local capacity to provide and interpret comparative data is essential to the effectiveness and sustainability of HSPA. It is also likely to be a highly cost-effective use of HSPA resources. Attention should be given to mechanisms of developing capacity at regional and country level, through processes such as "Enhancing Health Systems Performance Initiative" (EHSPI), promoting regional networks, nurturing academic networks, implementing training courses, and encouraging active user engagement.

2. HSPA should be a dynamic, interactive process in which users and other stakeholders are actively involved at both conceptual and implementation stage. HSPA may induce beneficial responses within nations, but unless carefully designed it has the risk of being ineffective, or of inducing undesirable outcomes, such as lack of attention to long-term health system goals. Therefore, in order to achieve its goals, it is imperative that HSPA has a positive influence on Ministries of Health and other key stakeholders. WHO should consider whether it is possible systematically to evaluate the impact of HSPA on Member States.

3. WHO should use rigorous scientific methods in developing and implementing new measurement tools. WHR 2000 was criticized for inadequate engagement with, and recognition of the contributions of, experts in the field. SPRG recognizes that, like all scientific endeavours, the methods will evolve over time. The Group considers it imperative that future methodology is developed in collaboration with relevant outside experts, and welcomes the recent consultative processes initiated by WHO. Mechanisms to secure expert engagement include expert panels, independent peer review, and secondments to and from relevant institutions. SPRG also encourages WHO to work closely with other international bodies with expertise in this area, such as OECD.

4. Numerous technical judgements have to be made at every stage of the HSPA methodology. There is

a need for WHO to prepare a careful audit trail of such judgements, and to make this available for public scrutiny.

5. Notwithstanding the need for scientific rigour, the methods used should be as simple as possible, subject to being fit-for-purpose. HSPA introduces many new concepts and methodologies that are challenging for governments and other stakeholders, and any unnecessary complexity is a serious impediment to communication. The final product should be a set of scientifically sound, practical, user-friendly tools that achieve the objectives of HSPA in enhancing health-system performance.

6. The research function implicit in HSPA should be distinguished carefully from operational implementation. Methods and data sources should be robust, credible, sustainable, and cost-effective before full implementation. In the meantime, they should be presented as work-in-progress, and should be developed using the collaborative and open research process advocated above. It may be helpful for WHO to develop explicit criteria against which it can evaluate initiatives being considered for implementation within HSPA.

7. Great care should be taken with the dynamic aspects of health-system performance. Many actions, particularly in the domain of public health, may have effects on outcomes only after a considerable time lag, and the methodologies used should reflect this complication. Furthermore, policy makers are naturally concerned with national trends over time. Therefore, as methodologies and datasets change, there will arise an important need to ensure that consistent time-series of data are made available to countries.

8. There is an urgent need to improve the quality and continuity of the data on which HSPA is based. Detailed recommendations are given in relevant sections of this report. Particularly important means to this end will include nurturing the development of sustainable health-information systems within countries, development of user skills and capacity, implementation of new data collection tools, and use of cost-effective quality assurance instruments.

9. The World Health Survey (WHS) is a particularly important new development within HSPA. SPRG welcomes the introduction of WHS, acknowledging its potential to inform diverse constituencies concerned with the performance of health systems. SPRG recommends that developmental work to ensure its effectiveness and reliability must continue over time, and its detailed recommendations are given in Section XII. The Group noted that WHS should wherever possible build on existing survey platforms, be useful for local purposes, and not put an unsustainable burden on local capacity for data collection. SPRG also notes that WHS is likely to be of greatest benefit in countries with poor information systems and low levels of health-system attainment. It therefore recommends that WHO gives priority in WHS and its implementation to the needs of such countries.

10. SPRG welcomes the WHO proposal to develop a parsimonious set of indicators related to the financing, service provision and resource generation functions (in the form of a 'dashboard' approach). The Group offers detailed recommendations in the relevant sections of this report, but considers that the development of a set of reliable, valid, cost-effective, and comparable indicators of health-system functions is an urgent requirement to enhance the usefulness of HSPA.

11. WHO should consider publishing an HSPA report card for every country, which offers a diagnostic tool in the form of a commentary on issues such as measured performance and prospects for improvement. The exact content of these should be determined in consultation with Member States, and should reflect the criterion of cost-effective use of WHO resources. SPRG suggests that the report cards could include a commentary on data quality and assumptions, on progress made since the last HSPA, and on aspects of performance that appear to merit further investigation.

12. SPRG has examined carefully the role of "league tables" of health-system performance within the HSPA process. It considers that the decision as to whether or not to publish such league tables is ultimately a policy and strategic decision for WHO rather than a technical issue. However, there were serious technical questions raised about the WHR 2000 methodology relating to the weights used in the composite index, the scaling of the component indicators, and the treatment of missing data. These criticisms have been documented in the subsequent sections of this report, which also give our detailed response to the WHO proposals for addressing these criticisms.

The following sections report the results of our detailed scrutiny of each of the 15 topic areas. They bear testimony to the extraordinary breadth and richness of the agenda unleashed by WHR 2000. Within the limited time and resources available, SPRG has found it extremely challenging to cover all the issues raised. We nevertheless hope that the treatment of the topics can serve as an adequate basis for informing progress on HSPA in the near future. We have sought to reflect the major issues raised in WHR 2000, and have made numerous detailed recommendations. The main messages from our review are now briefly noted under the 15 headings.

I. SPRG broadly endorsed the framework for HSPA, but in Section I makes some detailed comments designed to clarify and refine the concept.

II. SPRG noted the extensive work that has already gone into the development of measures of health system inputs, in the form of the national health accounts. Section II offers a large number of detailed observations and suggestions for improvement.

III. SPRG welcomes the attention now placed on the resource generation function, but considers current WHO thinking to be at an early stage of development. Section III offers some preliminary observations, but we recommend that this topic should be developed in full consultation with relevant users and experts.

IV. SPRG considers that the service provision and coverage function is particularly important for nations seeking to understand the reasons for their measured level of health-system performance. In particular, WHO has started to develop an ambitious methodology that contains promising implications for operational measurement. However, the methodology will need continued elaboration, refinement, and clarification.

V. We agree that WHO should continue to develop operational measures relating to the financing function. There is a need for research that provides evidence on how the financing function affects health-system performance.

VI. SPRG welcomes the emphasis on the stewardship function in WHR 2000. Although it considers that the measurement of stewardship poses serious challenges and could be a sensitive area, SPRG suggests that WHO should develop and test the proposed new tools.

VII. Methodology for the measurement of average level of population health is relatively advanced. A number of technical issues have been raised concerning the estimation of Health-Adjusted Life Expectancy (HALE), and these are treated in detail in Sections VII and XIII.

VIII. The concept and measurement of health inequality have generated some of the most contentious debates arising from WHR 2000. This HSPA goal poses epistemological as well as policy challenges, and introduces serious practical measurement difficulties. SPRG is not aware of any current data sources that allow international measurement of inequality in the chosen measure for 'average level of population health', HALE (rather than inequality in child survival to age 2 as used in WHR 2000). Hence, SPRG recommends that the 'pure health inequality' approach to examining 'health inequalities' should be developed further at both a methodological and statistical level, and acknowledges that measuring 'socioeconomic inequalities in health' is a valuable additional approach.

IX. The treatment of level and distribution of responsiveness in WHR 2000 was weak, relying on Key Informant surveys administered in only a fraction of Member States. The introduction of the World Health Survey will for the first time provide population-based information on responsiveness. However, further work is required to define the concept of responsiveness and identify its importance in different cultural settings and at different stages of development.

X. The concept and measurement of the fairness of financial contributions have attracted a great deal of debate since WHR 2000 was published. Although there are some as yet unsettled technical questions, many of the concerns expressed in the debate relate to policy choices that WHO will have to make and defend.

XI. SPRG considers that the decision on whether or not to continue to publish a composite index of health-system performance is ultimately a policy decision for WHO rather than a technical issue. However, there were serious technical questions raised about the WHR 2000 methodology, which are addressed in Section XI.

XII. Data inadequacies were a chief source of concern in commentaries on WHR 2000. In response,

WHO has launched a major initiative on data quality and data collection strategies, including the World Health Survey. As noted above, SPRG welcomes this development, but has raised serious concerns that are detailed in Section XII. SPRG recommends that WHO makes intensive efforts to obtain household survey data in as many countries as possible, and reduces the need to estimate missing data to a minimum.

XIII. SPRG considers that the methods proposed to achieve cross-population comparability are necessary and innovative. The methodology represents a major advance in comparing self-reported survey responses of different population groups (countries). The methods are still at a developmental stage, and require extensive further testing for robustness.

XIV. SPRG acknowledges the usefulness of seeking to measure health-system efficiency. However, the measurement of efficiency gives rise to a large number of technical problems that have yet to be resolved, as explained in Section XIV. This work requires further development and consultation, and WHO should recognize that it is work-in-progress in any tables it produces.

XV. SPRG considers that enhancing policy relevance is an essential aspect of the HSPA exercise, without which the finest technical endeavours will be irrelevant. WHO has made a number of recommendations for country support and capacity building, all of which appear to offer promise. Their implementation will require careful design and evaluation.

We feel that the independent peer review process has been illuminating and valuable to both WHO and SPRG members, and that the WHO consultation process has already enhanced the effectiveness of the HSPA initiative. We believe that adoption of our recommendations will further enhance the longer-term effectiveness of HSPA, and are pleased to note that many of our comments and suggestions during the review process have already been incorporated into the WHO methodology. More generally, we hope that the usefulness of the peer review process will encourage WHO to embrace the principle of engaging with independent outside expertise on specific HSPA topics, whenever appropriate.

NOTES

1   This is the original version of the SPRG report that was presented to the Director-General in May 2002. Only very minor editorial changes have been made for publication in this volume.

I. The Framework for HSPA

1. WHR 2000

WHR 2000 defined the health system to include personal medical care, public health interventions and intersectoral actions designed primarily to improve health. It was recognized that the health system contributes towards many outcomes that are socially desirable, including improving health, educational attainment, and individual incomes. WHR 2000 specified a parsimonious set of these goals where the contribution of health actions is sufficiently large to warrant measuring the goals regularly.

A goal was defined as intrinsically valued if raising the level of attainment on that goal is desirable in and of itself. To ensure that each goal measures a different outcome, it was further specified that each intrinsic goal must be at least partially independent of all others, i.e. it is possible to raise the level of attainment of the goal while holding the level of all other intrinsic goals constant. Instrumental goals were defined as outcomes that are desirable because they contribute to attainment of an intrinsic goal.

To warrant measuring attainment of an intrinsic goal regularly, two additional criteria were proposed. The health system must be able to make a large enough contribution to the goal to warrant the expense of measuring it regularly, and it must be feasible to measure the health-system impact on a regular basis.

Using these criteria, three intrinsic goals were identified. The defining goal was to improve health, both the average level of population health and its distribution (i.e. to reduce health inequality). The second intrinsic goal was to enhance the responsiveness of the health system to the legitimate expectations of the population for the non-health improving dimensions of their interaction with the health system. Responsiveness also had two components—the average level of and inequality in responsiveness.

The third intrinsic goal was the fairness in household financial contributions to the health system. Although it was recognized that other goals, such as educational attainment and income-earning potential, might meet the criteria of an intrinsic goal, it was judged that it was impractical to measure the impact of the health system on them on a regular basis.

A number of instrumental goals, such as the coverage of health services, were discussed in the text of WHR 2000. But the level of attainment on these goals was not measured in the annex tables. WHR 2000 also defined four basic functions which contribute to intrinsic goal attainment—financing, service provision, resource generation, and stewardship. The text of the report summarized the available evidence relating these functions to goal attainment and efficiency, but did not define or measure indicators of performance for the functions.

The final concept proposed in the framework was called performance—equivalent to the economic concept of efficiency. It was defined as the system's contributions to the intrinsic goals taking into account the inputs used to achieve them. The efficiency of systems in producing health and the composite attainment index (made up of the three intrinsic goals) was estimated.

2. Main Commentaries and Criticisms

There are eight commentaries and four responses that relate to the issue of framework (Almeida et al. 2000; World Health Organization 2001a; DfID 2000; McKee 2001; Murray and Frenk 2001; Navarro 2000; Navarro 2001; Oswaldo Cruz Foundation 2000; Travassos and Buss 2000; World Health Organization 2001b; Williams 2000, 2001; Murray et al. 2001). Only general issues relating to the framework are discussed here. Debates and suggestions on specific indicators, overall attainment, and efficiency are discussed later in this report.

Definition of the health system

Two opposing definitions were expressed. One was that the boundaries of the health system should be drawn tightly around the activities under the direct control of the Ministry of Health—largely personal medical services (WHO Regional Office for the Americas, 2001a). The other extreme was that the boundaries used in WHR 2000 were too narrow, focusing largely on medical interventions and ignoring the broader social and perhaps spiritual components (Navarro 2000; WHO Regional Office for the

Americas, 2001b; Ugá et al. 2001; Oswaldo Cruz Foundation 2000).

Goals

Some debate focused on the appropriate intrinsic goals to include for routine monitoring. Again, two opposing views were expressed. The first was that health systems should be concerned with, and judged on, their contributions to population health alone so that population health should be the only intrinsic goal. The opposing view was that not only should health, responsiveness and fairness of financial contributions be included as intrinsic goals, but others should be added as well (WHO Regional Office for the Americas 2001b). The OECD (Hurst 2002), for example, has adopted the concept of responsiveness in its proposed health-system performance framework, but called it "responsiveness and access". (Access was defined by WHO as an intermediate goal rather than an intrinsic goal—more access is only valued if it contributes to furthering one of the intrinsic goals). In addition, the OECD has included the level of health financing as an intrinsic goal, although it has not attempted to identify the optimal level for each country.

Other approaches to identifying indicators that could be potentially useful for HSPA include the Essential Public Health Functions (EHPF) of the WHO Regional Office for the Americas. That approach defines 11 key functions involving a mix of inputs, functions and outcomes without a composite index or an explicit statement of which ones contribute more or less to health-system performance. The "benchmarks of fairness" approach of Daniels et al. (2000) is similar. In it, nine benchmarks are used to evaluate the impact of health-system reforms on "fairness"—including assessing the impact on: coverage of key interventions both within and outside the health sector (e.g. literacy, education); barriers and inequalities in access; equitable financing; efficacy, efficiency and quality of care; democratic accountability and empowerment; and autonomy. Each benchmark contains many components and sub-indicators which raters must evaluate subjectively and incorporate into a composite rating for each benchmark on a scale from −5 to +5. No weighting is suggested for possible aggregation across indicators. The benchmarks and their components include indicators that would be labelled intermediate goals in the WHO framework as well as components of WHO's intrinsic goals (e.g. autonomy is a component of responsiveness in the WHO framework). These approaches focus on very important

questions related to the functioning of the health system and, in the case of the benchmarks project, the impact of reforms on fairness. They do not purport to be a comprehensive framework for assessing health-system performance.

Attribution and measurement

All regional consultations pointed out that goal attainment is influenced not only by health actions but by non-health system actions as well. WHO used multivariate statistical analysis to separate the influence of the health system from other possible determinants. Some commentators suggested that it would be useful for decision-making to define and measure indicators of that part of overall goal attainment believed to be determined largely by the activities of the Ministry of Health, either instead of, or in addition to, the outcome indicators defined by WHO. One possible example is the number of deaths due to medical errors which is more directly under the control of the Ministry of Health than all-cause mortality.

Inputs

There was little published criticism of the use of health expenditure per capita as an aggregate indicator of the inputs available to the system, although questions of timing between inputs and outcomes have been raised (Williams 2000; Ministry of Health, Vietnam 2001), which are considered in Section XIV on Efficiency. Regional consultations also suggested the need to measure inputs to the production of health such as human resources (WHO Regional Office for the Americas 2001b).

Health system functions

Many commentators argued that while information on intrinsic goal attainment was important, it was only a starting point. It was necessary to develop indicators that allowed policy makers to "drill down" so as to discover possible causes of poor performance and ways in which that might be improved (WHO Regional Office for the Americas 2001b; WHO Regional Office for the Eastern Mediterranean 2001). These indicators should be linked to the key function of the health system, which would make the measurement exercise more policy-relevant (Ollila and Koivusalo 2000).

Performance and efficiency—terminology

In WHR 2000 the term "performance" was used as a synonym for "efficiency" (Williams 2000). At a number of the regional consultations it was suggested that "health system performance assessment" should be defined to include the measurement of goal attainment, as well as the efficiency of input use and the way the system is functioning (WHO Regional Office for the Americas 2001b; WHO Regional Office for Europe 2001), whereas the term "efficiency" should be used in the narrower sense of how well resources are used to produce the desired outcomes.

Focus

Participants in the South-East Asian Regional Consultation suggested that it would be useful to extend the performance assessment exercise to the sub-national level (WHO Regional Office for South-East Asia 2001), while Wibulpolprasent and Tangcharoensathien (2001) argued it could also be used to assess the performance of particular programmes or interventions.

3. WHO RESPONSES AND PROPOSALS

WHO proposes to retain the definition of the health system used in WHR 2000 and to retain the three intrinsic goals. Although WHO recognizes the desire for policy makers to define an appropriate level of health spending, appropriate ways of operationalizing the concept need to be developed. Since publication of WHR 2000, WHO has attempted to make the framework more policy-relevant by defining a set of intermediate indicators that can be of immediate use to policy makers, allowing them to drill down to possible causes of poor performance. They are linked to the four key functions of health systems and are discussed later in this report. It has also begun to develop ways of assessing the inputs of human resources to the system (see Section III).

4. SPRG COMMENTS AND RECOMMENDATIONS

Definitions

The definition of health systems as proposed by the Secretariat in WHR 2000 is clear and acceptable. The three levels of health attributes, i.e. personal medical, non-personal health services, and intersectoral actions, are acceptable and should be used as the 'operational framework'. Given the definition of 'health' in the WHO constitution, which encompasses physical, mental and social well-being, it is suggested that WHO

could work with other international agencies to ensure that the impact of health on education and income could be assessed at regular intervals. Some members of SPRG felt that WHO might consider interacting with UNDP to explore if it were possible to modify the Human Development Index (HDI) into something like a Health-Adjusted Human Development Index (HAHDI) by substituting HALE for Life Expectancy in the HDI.

In interacting with other international agencies, it was also suggested that they might do a 'health impact assessment' of their activities on a routine basis.

Goals

The three intrinsic goals—i.e. health, responsiveness and fairness of financial contributions—are operational and acceptable. Countries do care about the level of financing as well, but there is no easy way to operationalize the ideal level of health financing for every country, and inclusion of this might have to be postponed.

SPRG members nonetheless agreed on the importance of retaining measures of the level of financing in future reports (as WHO proposes), and on the benefits of WHO collaborating with any future OECD work on optimal levels of health spending.

Attribution and measurement

SPRG agrees with the Secretariat's proposal to measure the system's contribution to the desired final outcomes. Although this may be a difficult task in developing countries with limited capacity, efforts should be commenced. SPRG also commends the attempt at regular measurement of intermediate goals as proposed by the Secretariat. Data availability and accuracy, scientific soundness of method, including transparency of the processes, are major concerns. Responses by the WHO Secretariat to these questions have been encouraging in that weaknesses in WHR 2000 have been acknowledged and steps have been taken for improvement.

Inputs

It is reasonable to use health expenditures as the main input. However, data availability in this area is critical and in many countries either there are no reasonable estimates or there are competing estimates. WHO should work with international agencies to standardize methods and estimates on variables such as GDP, expenditures and purchasing-power-parity exchange rates. It should also build capacity in countries in this area. SPRG also commends the Secretariat's attempts to explore the possibility of estimating the quantities of labour and capital stock for all Member States.

Functions

The four main functions are acceptable. SPRG commends the Secretariat's proposal to measure routinely a set of instrumental goals linked to each of the four functions as well as to selected attributes of these functions. It suggests that the work of the benchmarks-for-fairness exercise (Daniels et al. 2000) could provide useful insights. Some members of SPRG suggested that WHO might consider adding one more function, the organization of health resources as suggested by Kleczkowski, Roemer, and Van der Werff (1984). This function may be inserted between resource generation and service provision. It is quite logical to think that after we generate resources, we organize them, and then they provide services. However, other members felt that this is really part of each of the other functions.

Performance

SPRG recommends that the term 'performance' should be redefined to include the measurement of goal attainment, as well as the efficiency of input use and the way the system is functioning. 'Efficiency' should then be used more narrowly to represent the concept of value for money.

A strategic plan

SPRG recognizes that the HSPA exercise of WHR 2000 stimulated fresh thinking about health-system performance, and awareness and concerns for better health information (particularly vital registration, health-care financing, morbidity and mortality data, and responsiveness.) It recommends that WHO develop a strategic plan to improve data availability and accuracy of all variables at the global, regional and country levels. Specific plans, including the World Health Survey, should be developed and implemented with clear targets of achievement. Additional resources from funding agencies could also be mobilized for this purpose.

REFERENCES

Almeida, CM, P Braveman, MR Gold, CL Szwarcwald, J M Ribeiro, A Miglionico, JS Millar, S Porto, NR Costa, VO Rubio, M Segall, B Starfield, C Travassos, A Ugá, J Valente, and F Viacava (2001): Methodological concerns and recommendations on policy consequences of the World Health Report 2000. *Lancet* 357(9269): 1692–1697.

Daniels, N, J Bryant, RA Castano, OG Dantes, JS Khas, and S Pannarunnothai (2000): Benchmarks of fairness for health care reform: A policy tool for developing countries. *Bulletin of the World Health Organization* 78(6): 740–750.

Other suggestions

Issues	Improvements
Measurements	■ Request for further dissaggregation should be handled with great care. Only very important variables should be measured routinely.
	■ Improvement of indicators through more interactive peer review and user feedback.
Data non-availability and accuracy	■ Provide more support to sustain national information systems in increasing coverage and accuracy of available data.
	■ Improve estimation through more peer review process on scientifically sound techniques.
	■ Transparency through detailed explanation of data sources and estimation techniques.
Methodologies	■ Demystification through capacity-strengthening, creation of global, regional, sub-regional and country networks/institutes for HSPA. More training, publications, surveys and research are needed.
	■ Involve more researchers in future rounds.
	■ Use more extensive peer review on methodologies.
	■ Description of methods used and commentaries, as well as current improvement strategies, should be presented and open to the public.
League tables	■ The decision to continue with the league table is a strategic one, which it is up to WHO to make. If WHO decides to continue publishing league tables, it should include more explanations and precautions. More detail on this issue is discussed in Section XI on 'Composite Indicators'.
	■ Incentives may be offered to those at the bottom of the list, e.g. more WHO support, more financial support from donors, reward for improvement in the next round of assessment.

DfID (Department for International Development, UK Health Systems Resource Center) (2000): World Health Report 2000: Summary and comments. Draft 10 July 2000.

Hurst, J (2002): Performance measurement and improvement in OECD health systems: Overview of issues and challenges. Measuring Up: Improving Health System Performance in OECD Countries. Organization for Economic Co-operation and Development.

Kleczkowski, BM, MI Roemer, and A Van der Werff (1984): National Health Systems and their reorientation towards health for all guidelines for policy-making. Public Health Papers, No. 77. Geneva, Switzerland: World Health Organization. *http://whqlibdoc.who.int/php/WHO_PHP_77.pdf*

McKee, M (2001): Measuring the efficiency of health systems. *British Medical Journal*, 323(7308): 295–296.

Ministry of Health, Vietnam (2001): Comments and suggestions of Vietnam Ministry of Health/Health Policy Unit as regards the World Health Report 2000.

Murray, CJL and J Frenk (2001): World Health Report 2000: A step towards evidence-based health policy. *Lancet* 357(9269): 1698–1700.

Murray, CJL, J Frenk, D Evans, K Kawabata, A Lopez, and O Adams (2001): Science or marketing at WHO? A response to Williams. *Health Economics* 10(4): 277–282.

Navarro, V (2000): Assessment of the World Health Report 2000. *Lancet* 356(9241): 1598–1601.

Navarro, V (2001): World Health Report 2000: Responses to Murray and Frenk. *Lancet* 357(9269): 1701–1702.

Ollila, E and M Koivusalo (2000): Values, ideologies and evidence-based recommendations—The World Health Report 2000: WHO's health policy drifting off course. In eds. U Häkkinen and E Ollila. The World Health Report 2000: What does it tell us about health systems? Analyses by Finnish Experts. Helsinki: National Research and Development Center for Welfare and Health (STAKES). *http://www.stakes.fi/english/publicati/Publications.htm*

Oswaldo Cruz Foundation, Brazilian Ministry of Health (2000): Report of the workshop "Health Systems Performance: The World Health Report 2000". 14-12-2000, Rio de Janeiro.

Travassos, C and M Buss (2000): The controversial World Health Organization report. Editorial. *Cadernos de Saude Publica* 16(4): 890–891.

Ugá, AD, CM Almeida, CL Szwarcwald, C Travassos, F Viacava, JM Ribeiro, NR Costa, PM Buss, and S Porto (2001): Considerations on methodology used in the World Health Organization 2000 Report. *Cadernos de Saude Publica* 17(3): 705–712.

Wibulpolprasert, S and V Tangcharoensathien (2001): Health systems performance: what's next? *Bulletin of the World Health Organization* 79(6): 489.

Williams, A (2000): Science or marketing at WHO? A Commentary on 'World Health 2000'. Health Economics 10(2): 93–100.

Williams, A (2001): Science or marketing at WHO? Rejoinder from Alan Williams. Health Economics 10(4): 283–285.

World Health Organization (2001a): The methods and data used in the World Health Report 2000: A response to Almeida et al. Geneva, Switzerland: World Health Organization.

World Health Organization (2001b): The methods and data used in the World Health Report 2000: A response to the commentary made by the Brazilian delegation to the Executive Board, 17 and 19 January 2001.

WHO Regional Office for the Americas (2001a): Regional consultation of the Americas on Health Systems Performance Assessment, Background Document: Critical issues in health systems performance assessment. Washington, D.C.

WHO Regional Office for the Americas (2001b): Regional consultation of the Americas on Health Systems Performance Assessment: Final Report. 8-5-2001, Washington, D.C.

WHO Regional Office for the Eastern Mediterranean (2001): Report on the Regional Consultation on the Conceptual Framework for Health System Performance Assessment. 9-7-2001, Ain Saadeh, Lebanon.

WHO Regional Office for Europe (2001): Report of the Regional Consultation on Health Systems Performance Assessment. 3-9-2001, Copenhagen.

WHO Regional Office for South-East Asia (2001): Report of the regional consultation and technical workshop on health systems performance assessment. 18-6-2001, New Delhi, India.

II. Health System Inputs

Health system inputs include both physical and financial resources. The concepts and measurements related to these inputs play two distinct roles in WHR 2000. First, they are important to estimating the efficiency of the health system. WHR 2000 explicitly utilized total health spending as the aggregate input in its efficiency estimates, but spending was implicitly being used to reflect the application of physical resources toward improving health. Secondly, health system inputs were discussed in terms of health system functions. In the case of physical inputs, the conceptual framework discussed both their supply (resource generation) and utilization (under service provision). This section focuses specifically on the WHR 2000 report of financial inputs through the use of National Health Accounts.

1. WHR 2000

Concepts

National Health Accounts (NHA) are a method for quantifying the financial flows of the health system in a comprehensive, consistent, and integrated manner. In WHR 2000 and WHR 2001, the estimates of health expenditure for 191 countries are reported and disaggregated by source. The principal categories are public and private spending, which are further disaggregated into tax-funded, social insurance, out-of-pocket, and private insurance expenditures. WHR 2000 presented the first global NHA estimates using data for 1997. These data have been revised using additional statistical sources. The revised data for 1997 and new estimates for 1998 are presented in WHR 2001. WHR 2001 also included a new sub-category: externally-financed health spending.

Methods

The health system is quite complex, but the nominal value (and, where unavailable, the imputed value) of resources funded and spent in a health system have to be equal to the sum of the value of all goods and services delivered. Using this identity to enforce consistency, NHAs organize health financing information by selecting a group of dimensions that are useful for analysing this complexity. These dimensions are then summarized in a series of matrices that provide information on expenditures by source, financing agents, providers, and uses. By using common classifications, it becomes possible to learn through comparisons across countries and over time. Efforts are made to report expenditures on an accrual basis (i.e. when the resources are consumed not when payments are made) wherever possible (Poullier and Hernandez 2000).

Data/Evidence/Sources

Complete data were not available for all countries. For WHR 2000, the information was based on 67 country NHA reports for various years. Of these, 30 traced expenditures through the main components of health-care financing: resource mobilization, resource allocation, and service and goods provision. Estimates had to rely on partial information for 124 countries, for which various sources of information on health expenditure were consulted. Figures presented in the WHR are in US dollars at official exchange rates, and also in international dollars converted at purchasing power parities (PPP).

2. Main Commentaries and Criticisms

Concepts

No one questioned the usefulness of NHA for estimating health expenditure per capita as an aggregate indicator of the inputs available to the system. Nevertheless, some comments were made on the basic concepts, methods and data.

Some reviewers were concerned that WHR 2000 assigned too much importance to the data reported in the National Health Accounts, particularly as the single most important input in calculating the efficiency of health systems. One article stated that "NHAs seem to be treated as a sort of panacea...for the purpose of restoring productivity in the Member States' health systems" (DfID 2000).

Another criticism was that NHA are not fully consistent with the WHO definition of the health system (McKee 2001). The reported NHA data concentrate mainly on personal medical and non-personal health-services expenditure. Intersectoral actions and the production of resources, which are emphasized in WHR 2000 as integral parts of the health system, are not always included. The figure for health expenditure on all the activities of intersectoral actions in promoting health "is nowhere to be found in any national health accounts" (McKee 2001). Therefore, using NHA data to measure health-system resources is misleading since it forces a comparison of outcomes with health services inputs rather than with health system inputs.

Methods

A range of criticism focused on the non-comparability of expenditure categories and definitions. Different agencies classify expenditures differently, and do not have the same definition for functions and services (Ministry of Health, Lebanon 2000). Comparability is difficult because of diverse national standards, in addition to differing concepts of boundaries, dimensions, and classification systems. Furthermore, standardized regional reporting systems are lacking, and it is very difficult to achieve consensus by policy makers regarding the framework and content of NHA (WHO Regional Office for South-East Asia 2001).

Due to the important role played by these figures, and the questions regarding methodology and data sources, it was argued that future reporting needs to discuss explicitly levels of uncertainty for expenditure estimates. This is highlighted by the debates around WHR 2000 on the assessment of outcomes, inputs and efficiency with widely varying uncertainty intervals.

Data/Evidence/Sources

There is lack of comparability between the different data sets. Collecting information on the distribution of expenditures by function, and linking expenditures with utilization is difficult given the state of most countries' health financing data. The NHA estimates were questioned on the basis that the quality, validity and reliability of the data available in the countries is variable and frequently poor. They noted that discrepancies exist between expenditure data from different sources and questioned the process of reconciling these varying estimates.

Sources used to estimate health expenditures are not always complete. Sometimes they provide data only on the public sector while others concentrate on private expenditures. There is double-counting as well as gaps in coverage. Estimations of private spending were a particular subject of such criticism. The quality and reliability of such estimates remains uncertain because of incomplete coverage, unrepresentative surveys, and the likelihood of double counting expenditures (WHO Regional Office for South-East Asia 2001). For example, some commentators argued that reliable estimates of out-of-pocket expenditure were unavailable in up to 75% of countries (WHO Regional Office for South-East Asia 2001). Development of better methods to estimate private spending were recommended.

Some countries disagreed with the estimates of health expenditure reported in WHR 2000, on account of the data being outdated, the source of data being insufficient, and methods applied.

Some countries also disagreed with estimates of exchange rates (official and/or PPP), and the sources of PPP exchange rates used to convert local currency units into international dollars were questioned.

Countries argued that WHO had a responsibility to provide necessary technical assistance to prepare or improve NHA data. They argued that WHO's data collection efforts should more closely integrate with capacity-building in the countries. Regional activities may be needed to ground NHA in countries and to build better evidence for policy.

Specific problems were cited in WHO's estimation of external resources applied to health in WHR 2001. It was noted that there are large discrepancies between NHA surveys and data on public expenditure on health reported in national and international publications ("The Health Dime"). The problem cannot be ignored because in some cases external resources account for a third or more of total resources spent on health. Some of the limitations include:

- Disadvantages of the existing registration system: data reported under the IMF classification of expenditure by function appear in many countries to be institutional rather than functional, and omit expenditure on health-enhancing interventions by ministries other than the Ministry of Health. They frequently report planned rather than actual outlays.

- The multiple channels through which external resources flow into a country are not always reported.

- There are problems in tracing and valuing in-kind flows. For instance, donations of equipment, stocks of vaccines, and medicines are not always reported or given a value.

- Private grants and loans are not registered.

Overall, the importance of explaining the findings and checking their validity was emphasized.

3. WHO Responses and Proposals

Concepts

WHO maintained that the concept used in NHA is close to the definition of the health system and argued that much of what gets reported depends on the availability of data. WHO recognizes that statistical imperfections exist and in order to address the criticism of inconsistencies in the definition of the health system, the new framework for NHA incorporates further breakdowns of expenditure.[1]

WHR 2001 introduced two additional categories of expenditures, viz. external resources for health as a percentage of public expenditure on health, and private insurance and other pooled expenditure. A further enlarged dataset is anticipated for WHR 2002 which will include a broader time-frame (1995–1999). Also, trends for 1970–2000 are in the process of estimation (with completion planned after 2002). WHO also proposes the introduction of further breakdowns of expenditure to the extent possible:

(i)   by type of function or provider (inpatient, outpatient, long-term care);

(ii) by type of resource (capital, labour, consumables);

(iii) by type of provider.

In order to improve cross-country consistency and provide technical assistance, WHO is in the process of preparing a Producer's Guide to offer a common framework for NHA. WHO has also initiated a capacity-building programme at regional and national levels (Africa and Eastern Europe) with other activities also to respond to demands from the Americas, the East Mediterranean, and Asia. WHO is collaborating with other international organizations on developing the methodology for NHAs and on technical training.

Methods

A prototype NHA has been initiated because of large gaps in data (particularly for the private sector), non-availability of required disaggregations, cash- and not accrual-data. Boundaries reflect different degrees of the private-public mix ("in search of commonality").

Data/Evidence/Sources

WHO has redoubled its efforts to interact with national authorities and other international agencies in a continuing process of updating estimates. WHO has specifically initiated a consultation process with countries in order to validate the information compiled. For example, estimates for 1998 and the revisions for 1997 were sent to countries for comment, and the changes agreed with them were reported in WHR 2001.

Since WHR 2000, WHO is working on a method to improve the calculation of purchasing power parities, and is collaborating with the World Bank for the next round of the International Comparisons Project.

To deal with the problems identified in estimating external resources, WHO suggests that:

- Data should be collected from both the external agencies and the recipient countries (through the questionnaire listing input categories using the major functional classifications);

- The value of in-kind transfers should be calculated at replacement cost;

- The resources allocated only by the external agency directly to the population and health institutions—as cash or in-kind—should be counted.

4. SPRG Comments and Recommendations

In the new framework of the NHA, WHO intends to incorporate the main indicators concerned with inputs examination for the purposes of HSPA. This is evident from an examination of the modified template for NHA, which is closer to the classifications in the Producer's Guide. The purpose is to document (through the NHA) the problem of existing imbalances between different types of resources. However, NHA provide only one-year expenditures, whereas for the purposes of investment planning the stock of available capital is needed—which incorporates past investment decisions too. Preparing a time-series of NHA will indicate the changing demands and supplies of the health system over time.

NHA are based on accountancy principles which do not readily offer estimates of data uncertainty. This may conflict with the statistical methods used in other aspects of HSPA. There is a problem with the availability and accuracy of the data being presented. No explanation is available on the methods used to estimate missing data (when the nominal values are not available). There is little or no information on the approach that is applied to choose among different values reported by different sources, and to decide on the level of expenditure when no information exists (e.g. expert opinion, imputed from international patterns, some sort of average, etc). WHO should consider developing methodologies for indicating uncertainty in the financial data.

WHO is attempting to enter into a dialogue with countries for continuous improvement of NHA. However, more transparency is needed. WHO is consulting countries to establish whether the series are plausible and to fill gaps. Basic macro-variables—such as general government total expenditure—should be reviewed, and information to fill missing data should be obtained at the national level. WHO has to specify the procedures for examining the accuracy in the NHA data.

It is extremely important that WHO work towards the standardization of classifications. The classifications applied are usually country-specific, adopting the OECD International Classification of Health Expenditures' system to the country's own situation. Also, the number and scope of breakdowns presented are different, depending on the data available.

Apart from standardizing classifications, the definitions of categories have to be uniform. Different items that are similarly labelled may be included in health-care costs. SPRG recommends that in order to achieve uniformity among expenditures labelled identically and to ensure comparability across countries, WHO should clarify the content of each category incorporated into the NHA template. Explicit definitions are needed. Clarification is also needed to ensure the consistency of NHA with the definition of the health system, so as to be able to identify the inputs to the health system from which the outcomes are evaluated.

The weak basis of PPP estimates can be highly influential on a country's measured performance. However, it remains a preferable alternative to conversion using official exchange rates. We would encourage WHO to continue actively exploring improved PPP estimates.

Additional household surveys are often undertaken to elicit private out-of-pocket expenditures. Unfortunately, attention is not always paid to capital investment in private facilities, and to the health expenditure incurred by a country's citizens when they are abroad. Another problem is health spending by citizens of neighboring countries (especially living in border areas) who work and pay health insurance premiums in one country but live and use health services in another. WHO should determine whether such spending should be included.

In terms of basic accounting principles, income and expenditure must be balanced in the NHA. The value of resources funded and spent in a health system should be equal to the sum of the value of all goods and services delivered (Poullier, Hernandez, and Kawa-

bata 2001). However, expenditures (consumption and investment) are not necessarily equal to the sum of the value of goods and services provided. The amount of investment in resource generation (for training and construction) is usually different from the cost of factors employed, for the following reasons:

- migration and unemployment of human resources in the health system;

- unfinished construction;

- buildings are not depreciated (no consumption of fixed capital is taken into account) until they are finished.

WHO should examine further the most appropriate treatments of these complications.

There is an extremely important role for WHO to play in capacity-building of countries.

- We propose that WHO publish the Producer's Guide as soon as possible, in order to increase capacity-strengthening in countries;

- WHO should work for greater harmonization across international agencies;

- WHO should strengthen support to the NHA regional networks and find ways of improving interaction among users of NHA. This will also help in capacity-building.

- For countries with limited capacity, the measurement process for health expenditure flows should be incorporated into the regular UN System of National Accounts.

NOTES

1   These will appear in the NHA Producer's Guide currently under preparation. It is co-funded by the World Bank, WHO and USAID, and is being jointly prepared by those agencies and a team from the Harvard School of Public Health.

REFERENCES

Anonymous (2000): The Health Dime, No. 1. Geneva, Switzerland.

DfID (Department for International Development, UK Health Systems Resource Center) (2000): World Health Report 2000: Summary and comments. Draft 10 July 2000.

Dorabawila, T, S De Silva, J Mendis, and E Rasell (2001): WHO Fairness in Financing Study: Estimates for Sri Lanka 1995/96 using WHO methodology. Colombo, Sri Lanka: Institute of Policy Studies of Sri Lanka.

McKee, M (2001): Measuring the efficiency of health systems. *British Medical Journal*, 323(7308): 295–296.

Meerding, WJ, L Bonneux, JJ Polder, MA Koopmanschap, and PJ Van der Maas (1998): Demographic and epidemiological determinants of health care costs in Nederlands: Cost of illness study. *British Medical Journal*, 317: 111–115.

Ministry of Health and Institute of Policy Studies (2001): Sri Lanka National Health Accounts: Sri Lanka National Health Expenditures 1990–1999. Colombo, Sri Lanka: Institute of Policy Studies of Sri Lanka.

Ministry of Health, Lebanon (2000): Lebanon National Health Accounts: Executive Summary (Working Draft).

Poullier, JP and P Hernandez (2000): Estimates of National Health Accounts for 1997. Global Programme on Evidence for Health Policy Discusion Papers, No. 27. Geneva, Switzerland: World Health Organization.

Poullier, JP, P Hernandez, and K Kawabata (2001): National Health Accounts: Concepts, data sources and methodology. Global Programme on Evidence for Health Policy Discussion Papers, No. 47. Geneva, Switzerland: World Health Organization.

Poullier, JP, P Hernandez, K Kawabata, W Savedoff, C Indikadahena, and R Zeramdini (2001): Global and national spending patterns: Results from National Health Accounts.

WHO Regional Office for South-East Asia (2001): Report of the regional consultation and technical workshop on health systems performance assessment. 18-6-2001, New Delhi, India.

III. Resource Generation Function

1. WHR 2000

In WHR 2000 the available evidence on the links between the resource generation function and health-system performance was summarized. WHO argued that whatever the level of inputs, there was an efficient way to combine them. Significant imbalances between different types of productive resources existed in many settings, and countries must address a number of complex questions such as:

■ What is the most cost-effective balance between different types of productive resources and how can this be achieved?

■ How much effort should be devoted to developing new resources (e.g. investment) compared with developing strategies and incentives to improve the use of existing resources?

No attempt was made to define or measure indicators of how the resource generation function was being performed. Health expenditure per capita was the only source of information on health-system inputs used for performance assessment.

2. Main Commentaries and Criticisms

There were few comments and criticisms of the WHO approach to this function apart from the general comment that WHO needed to develop the links between each of the four key functions and the performance of the system as a whole (WHO Regional Office for the Americas 2001).

Human resources were seen as particularly important because health systems are labour-intensive and expenditure on personnel is usually the largest single item of recurrent health expenditure. Health systems require not only a sufficient number of qualified and experienced staff to function well, but an appropriate mix between the different types of human resources. Changing the mix will not, however, solve all problems and some commentators (e.g. DfID 2000) suggested that special attention should also be paid to the following issues:

■ the difficulty of reorienting staff from one activity to another;

■ the problem of low productivity of human resources which was seen to be linked closely to the issue of remuneration;

■ development of ways to measure and improve the quality of human resources, perhaps linked to realistic estimates of the level of outputs that the various inputs might be expected to deliver (DfID 2000).

Similar comments were made in relation to physical capital where deficits in the stock of assets (e.g. buildings and equipment) can be a real constraint to the delivery of effective interventions. Conversely, it is not uncommon to find health systems where there has been significant investment in physical infrastructure but where recurrent budgets do not allow for staff costs or the maintenance of the physical capital stock, which results in efficiency losses. Goal attainment is a function of the number and type of health facilities and equipment available. Various types of incentives and legislation influence how capital is purchased, used and maintained. Hence it is not just a matter of counting the availability of resources, but of ensuring that the mix is appropriate and the resources are used efficiently (Anell and Willis 2000).

3. WHO Responses and Proposals

WHO has proposed a set of indicators for each of the four key functions, which will help decision makers identify practical areas where performance can be improved. For the resource-generation function, WHO proposes to focus on investment in the production of resources and maintenance of their quality and productivity. The management and deployment of resources will be assessed under the service-provision function.

Generation of human resources for health

The following indicators are proposed:

■ Total annual investment in human resources (HR) as a percentage of total health expenditure;

- The number of new entrants to educational institutions that train health-care professionals divided by the total stock of health-care personnel;

- The total stock, composition and distribution of human resources for health;

- Migration of human resources. As an input to this exercise, it will be necessary to explore the feasibility of estimating the quantity of different types of labour inputs currently available to the health systems of Member States. To do this, WHO will develop a global database on human resources. Data will be collected on the quantity and characteristics of different provider groups, partly through the World Health Survey (for which a draft survey module has been developed).

WHO also proposes to develop a human resources policy. The purpose will be to synthesize the evidence on the effects of different human resources policies on the performance of health systems. This will allow different parts of WHO to work together to develop a coherent set of strategies that can help Member States to improve the performance of this function. The Organization acknowledges that there is a strong need for capacity building in countries to achieve effective policy-making in this area.

Physical resource generation

The following activities are proposed by WHO:

(i) To explore the feasibility of estimating the quantity of different types of capital stock (e.g. health facilities, equipment).

(ii) To develop and apply methods for measuring the physical capital stock available to the health system (e.g. the value of buildings and equipment).

(iii) To monitor:
   - Annual new investments in health facilities as a percentage of total health expenditure;
   - Annual expenditure on maintenance as a percentage of annual investment in health facilities;
   - The total stock of facilities (current value) as a proportion of GDP. Pharmaceuticals and medical devices

WHO proposes to measure investment in medical devices as a component of its work on health facilities. Measuring the availability and utilization of essential drugs and other consumables is included in WHO proposals to define indicators of the health services provision function (Section IV).

Knowledge

WHO proposes to measure total annual investment in health research and development. WHO has also started a process to develop the performance assessment of health research systems, and plans to publish its findings in WHR 2004.

4. SPRG COMMENTS AND RECOMMENDATIONS

Human resource generation

SPRG supports the need to develop indicators for each of the four functions of the health system, including resource generation. Inter alia, this will help to generate evidence about the influence of the composition of human resources on the attainment of health-system goals.

Among the problems related to human resources, the lack of standardization in definitions of human resource categories needs to be addressed. More attention also needs to be paid to non-medical professionals and the migration of human resources.

The methodology proposed by WHO for estimating National Health Accounts (NHA) incorporates an additional category of expenditure—investment for human resource generation (production and continuing development). SPRG believes that 'annual investment in human resource generation as a percentage of total health expenditure', one of the indicators proposed by the Secretariat, is too general as an indicator of efficiency for the human resource generation function. The inclusion of maintenance costs for human resources is also desirable in an assessment of efficiency, even though it may be difficult to collect these data. WHO should explore whether maintenance costs could be included as part of NHA.

Concerning the breakdown of human resources categories, SPRG questions whether the six provider categories proposed by WHO are sufficient. Other categories such as public-health physicians, preventive-care professionals and traditional health-care providers might also be important. On the other hand, SPRG recognizes that too many categories may overburden health-information systems and make data collection difficult.

Owing to the functional substitution between different categories of human resources, which often occurs in resource-poor areas, data on the quantity and characteristics of selected categories may not represent the functional profile of human resources in certain areas.

There is concern about the apparent tendency of WHO to follow the trend of focusing on curative care that is observable in many countries. It is recommended that WHO should pay more attention to traditional public-health occupations in its work on human resources.

SPRG recommends that WHO reviews its work on the migration of human resources with a view to developing an indicator that takes into account the dynamic character of the process.

Indicators to assess performance of human-resource generation should follow the general framework of HSPA, i.e. they should include the quantities of resources available, their distribution, and their efficiency.

Members of SPRG expressed the need for a parsimonious set of indicators related to shortage (demand minus supply), equity (distribution), and efficiency of human resource generation. One possible approach may be summarized in tables 61.1 and 61.2.

These suggestions are made for consideration and further development by WHO.

Physical resources

Investment decisions have an impact on the type of services provided and the geographical distribution of the services. The health system needs to take account of the current condition of the health-care facilities infrastructure, i.e. the physical capital stock.

For operational efficiency, no standards exist either on the proportion of total health expenditure that should be devoted to investment in physical infrastructure, or on the ratio of maintenance and operating costs to investment.

SPRG welcomes the approach proposed by WHO to establish a core set of equipment to be measured, which can be used to assess resource availability, and to test the feasibility of collecting such information in demonstration countries.

Table 61.1   Matrix for the assessment of human resource generation

	Level			Equity		
Selected categories	Adequacy (number, density)	Skill mix	Quality	Fairness of finance of HR production	Distribution of new entrants	Efficiency of production
Doctors					Composition (social, demographic, income)	Per capita investment (Investment per trained person)
Nurses						
Midwives						
Public-health workers						
Dentists						
Pharmacists						
Managers						
Traditional health workers						
Etc.						

Table 61.2   Matrix for the assessment of human resource maintenance and utilization

	Level		Equity	
Selected categories	Remuneration	Incentives	Distribution	Productivity
Doctors	Possible indicators:	Non-pecuniary	Distribution among socio-demographic groups	Possible indicators:
Nurses	■ Range			■ No. of Full-Time Equivalents (FTE) per bed occupancy in hospital
Midwives	■ Timelines (are the salaries paid on time, regularity of payments)			
Public-health workers				■ No. of FTE per visit
Dentists	■ Adequacy (e.g. in comparison with other countries in the region or countries with similar national income)			
Pharmacists				
Managers				
Traditional health workers				
Etc.				

Specific comments on data for indicators:

(i)   What to collect. For estimation of the current value of physical inputs, a standard procedure needs to be applied so as to assure comparability across countries. In the first instance, WHO should collect data only on the number and type of selected facilities, equipment, etc., their anticipated physical depreciation, and their distribution in each country. Subsequently, appropriate modelling needs to be undertaken for the imputation of values.

(ii) Sources of data. In general, no agency collects data on the number and types of all fixed assets. Central and local governments often have statistics on specific equipment, e.g. MRI and CT scans. WHO should collect the necessary data but avoid duplication with other data-collection bodies. Financial reports to statistical authorities are a cheaper source of data than direct measurement strategies, although they may be partial. Given different arrangements in countries concerning ownership and management of buildings, information on public facilities may be available only in separate reports (provider reports show only maintenance and operating costs; local government reports include the value of buildings and their depreciation). In consequence, additional surveys may have to be undertaken.

Pharmaceuticals and medical devices

SPRG supports WHO proposals for including pharmaceuticals and medical devices as important resources to be measured.

Knowledge

SPRG commends the WHO initiative to measure the performance of national health-research systems and publish its findings in WHR 2004. The lessons learned from HSPA will be useful in this respect.

REFERENCES

Anell, A and M Willis (2000): International comparison of health care systems using resource profiles. *Bulletin of the World Health Organization*, 78(6): 770–778.

DfID (Department for International Development, UK Health Systems Resource Center) (2000): World Health Report 2000: Summary and comments. Draft 10 July 2000.

WHO Regional Office for the Americas (2001): Regional consultation of the Americas on Health Systems Performance Assessment: Final Report. 8-5-2001, Washington, D.C.

IV. Service Provision Function

1. WHR 2000

WHR 2000 described four functions of the health system—financing, resource generation, service provision, and stewardship—and summarized the available evidence about their links to outcomes and health-system performance. In the text of the Report, service provision was defined as the way inputs are combined to allow the delivery of a series of interventions or health actions.

Three main aspects of health-service provision were identified:

- Priority setting—choosing the appropriate mix of interventions;

- Organization of service delivery—choosing the appropriate level for delivering interventions and the degree of integration;

- Aligning provider incentives to ensure that performance is optimized.

Coverage was seen as an intermediate goal, something that was valuable because it contributed to the intrinsic goals. No attempt was made to define and measure indicators of how this function was being performed, or to assess the coverage of key interventions.

2. Main Commentaries and Criticisms

Assessing service provision attracts attention because it is directly related to the daily management of the health system, and impacts are immediate and visible. WHR 2000 focused mainly on the measurement of intrinsic goals. As with the other functions, Member States and policy makers expressed a desire for practical applications of the assessment exercise. During the regional and technical consultations on HSPA, the development of instrumental goals has been consistently emphasized as a way of allowing policy makers to 'drill down' to find practical ways of improving system performance. At all regional consultations coverage was recognized as one of the key intermediate goals that should be routinely monitored.

3. WHO Responses and Proposals

WHO proposed three focus areas for health-service provision: (i) health-system inputs, (ii) organizational structure and processes, and (iii) the quantity and quality of personal and non-personal health services in relation to the health-care needs of the population (Adams et al. 2000).

Nine domains are proposed for these areas in order to assess and monitor the management and development of the health system. Health-system inputs are measured through: (i) recurrent costs of service provision; (ii) physical availability of inputs; (iii) skill mix of health-care personnel; and (iv) utilization of medical equipment and structures. The organizational structure of the system and the process of health-service delivery are assessed through: (i) the level and type of autonomy and integration; and (ii) incentive structures. The outcomes of the service-provision function will be reflected in the intrinsic goals of health and responsiveness, both in terms of overall level and distribution. Two concepts—effective coverage and provider performance—are proposed as instrumental goals.

The concept of effective coverage was developed at a technical consultation in Brazil in August 2001. WHO subsequently proposed that it should incorporate the traditional concepts of access, utilization, and effectiveness (Shengelia et al. 2001). Coverage is an integrated concept using these three traditional elements, and is defined as the probability of receiving a necessary health intervention conditional on the presence of a certain health problem or health-care need. WHO further proposes five domains of coverage—availability, accessibility, affordability, acceptability and effective coverage.

Effective coverage can be estimated at the population level or at the individual level. WHO recommends estimation at the individual level, allowing the estimation of inter-individual inequality in (the probability of) coverage. Effective coverage at individual level can be measured by five steps using data on: prevalence and incidence of diseases; occurrence of interventions in the population; individual observable and unobservable characteristics; health-system characteristics; and effectiveness of intervention (Murray et al. 2001). The Secretariat further proposes that reducing inequality of effective coverage should be an instrumental goal, measured using methods developed previously

Eight areas and 19 indicators are proposed for regular measurement using the criteria suggested by experts at the technical consultation.

4. SPRG COMMENTS AND RECOMMENDATIONS

The conceptual frame that WHO proposes for considering the service-provision function, consisting of three focus areas and nine measurement domains, seems to be useful. But the relationship between personal and non-personal health services needs further development, particularly in respect of the instrumental goals proposed by WHO for this function, i.e. effective coverage and provider performance. In the domain for management of service provision, management-oriented concepts such as autonomy, integration and incentives should be more clearly delineated.

Because targets for intermediate goals of the health system are more manageable in the short term than targets for intrinsic goals, outcome-related process indicators such as effective coverage will be very useful for policy makers and field workers. The assembly of a parsimonious set of indicators of the intermediate goals is an essential step towards enhancing the policy relevance of HSPA.

SPRG agrees that it is highly desirable for WHO to develop indicators of service provision. The categories of inputs, organizational structure, and health services appear to be conceptually sound. However, considerable further work is needed to develop operational indicators. WHO should develop a set of criteria for evaluating such indicators. The indicators should be clear, appropriate, understandable, measurable, and where necessary country-specific.

The process of indicator selection is important, and must involve relevant specialists and field workers. In presenting these indicators, their relationship to other functions such as resource generation—and to the intrinsic goals of health and responsiveness—has to be spelt out. To enhance policy relevance, it would be useful in some settings to measure these indicators at the sub-national level or even at the level of health institutions.

There has recently been a worldwide concern for improvement in the quality of health care, and in several countries quality of care has been redefined to include patient safety (IOM/NAS 2001). SPRG endorses the proposal to develop the notion of pro-vider performance as an instrumental goal, including the concepts of quality and safety.

The analytical framework being developed by WHO for the other instrumental goal of effective coverage holds great promise, but needs to be exposed to detailed peer scrutiny and to incorporate feedback from external experts.

The concept of effective coverage can be important in quantifying the gap between efficacy and effectiveness of many interventions. However, the way that the proposed components of coverage—availability, accessibility, affordability, acceptability and effective coverage—relate to the more traditional concepts of access, utilization and effectiveness, needs to be explained clearly to policy makers.

SPRG endorses the development of carefully chosen measures of coverage that can be shown from research evidence to be linked to the achievement of the intrinsic goals. The use of such indicators is an important step in addressing the difficulty that some outcome indicators relate not only to the current period but reflect the results of health-system activity in the past. The choice of the type of interventions that are routinely monitored for coverage should be guided by the criterion that these interventions are expected to be significant determinants of population health (HALE).

The development of indicators of coverage not yet linked through research to the achievement of the intrinsic goals should be approached with caution. Use of such indicators may encourage some nations to introduce interventions that are subsequently shown to be ineffective. We suggest instead that appropriate research be commissioned to identify effective interventions.

Some care is needed in the presentation of coverage data. Interventions that are cost-effective in some countries may not be so in others, and crude rankings will be inappropriate.

Measuring inequality in effective coverage is useful because it is directly amenable to policy and is a determinant of inequality in health outcomes. But the method of measurement should be carefully developed and different alternatives explored.

Finally, in keeping with the general approach of WHO to examine both inequality and deprivation in the intrinsic goals (e.g. fairness in household financial contributions), SPRG recommends that deprivation in coverage should be measured alongside inequality. This will require specifying a minimum threshold level of coverage and estimating the percentage of individuals who fall below it. Identifying individuals with a low probability of coverage of key interventions would be very useful for policy purposes.

REFERENCES

Adams, O, B Shengelia, B Stilwell, I Larizgoitia, A Issakov, S Kwankam, and F Jam (2000): Provision of personal and non-personal health services: Proposal for monitoring. Global Programme on Evidence for Health Policy Discussion Papers, No. 25. Geneva, Switzerland: World Health Organization.

IOM/NAS (2001): Crossing the Quality Chasm: A New Health System for the 21st Century.

Murray, CJL, B Shengelia, N Gupta, and O Adams (2001): Inequality in coverage: concepts and measurement strategies. Global Programme on Evidence for Health Policy, mimeo. Geneva, Switzerland: World Health Organization.

Shengelia, B, O Adams, M Thieren, Y Berchmans, Y Kwankam, and CJL Murray (2001): Measuring the coverage of critical interventions through household surveys. Global Programme on Evidence for Health Policy, mimeo. Geneva, Switzerland: World Health Organization.

V. Financing Function

1. WHR 2000

WHR 2000 (Chapter 5) analysed health financing as one of the four principal functions of health systems. It categorized financing into the collection of funds, pooling of resources, and purchasing of services. It highlighted the advantages of health financing mechanisms that collect resources from a wide base, pool risk between the sick and the healthy and between rich and poor, and that allocate resources and purchase services strategically.

2. Main Commentaries and Criticisms

Overall, there was almost no direct criticism of the financing function part of WHR 2000. Nevertheless, references in some of the broader critiques of the report drew on several aspects of the financing function chapter.

The main criticisms relating to the chapter on the financing function were that the analysis was ideologically driven and not based on evidence. Some commentators viewed the framework as inherently biased towards increasing private sector involvement in insurance and health financing (Almeida et al. 2001; Oswaldo Cruz Foundation 2000; Navarro 2000; Navarro 2001a; Navarro 2001b; Häkkinen and Ollila 2000; Van der Stuyft and Unger 2000). Such critiques noted the attention given to the analytical separation of financing and purchasing, the high fairness-in-financing ranking of certain countries (such as Colombia) that have engaged in market-oriented reforms, as well as discussions of a role for private provision. These papers argued that the Report ignored evidence regarding problems with managed competition, private insurance, and other kinds of market-oriented reforms.

An opposing view was expressed by Helms (2000) who perceived the health financing approach taken in WHR 2000 to be inherently biased against private sector involvement. The author argued that if countries followed this approach to health financing they would dull incentives for progress in medical technology and health-service provision.

The response to these arguments of ideological bias towards either "market orientation" or "central planning" was summed up by Murray and Frenk (2001). They argue that the WHR was not advocating any particular policy stance, but rather calling for more systematic evidence in how health systems affect the final goals. According to them, WHR 2000 states "... there is no evidence that systems relying a great deal on public funding will necessarily be more efficient than systems with a greater degree of private sector involvement, or vice versa. Whether this is seen as a Marxist or capitalist conclusion depends entirely on the ideology of the commentator and the motivations for their commentaries. We see it simply as a summary of the best available evidence at present."

Another criticism was that the Report did not link the analysis of the financing function with health-system goals—and, in particular, with the fairness-in-financial-contribution goal (Walt and Mills 2001). This criticism was reiterated in the regional consultations and later discussions in which critiques of ideological bias gave way to discussions of how best to improve analysis and measurement of the function in order to generate an objective evidence base for policy advice.

In particular, WHO was requested to develop ways of measuring the effectiveness of different financing mechanisms towards achieving system goals (WHO Regional Office for the Americas 2001; WHO Regional Office for Europe 2001). Through such measurement, it would be possible to 'drill down' and understand why a particular country was performing well or poorly with regard to its health-system goals.

3. WHO Responses and Proposals

In order to deepen work in this area, WHO has initiated a series of technical papers to review the evidence on well performing financing functions as part of the development of a health financing policy. The technical papers are aimed at a policy audience and seek to synthesize existing evidence on high-priority topics for Member States such as the right amount of funding for health, minimum spending on health, user fees, community financing, and private insurance.

In parallel, WHO has developed a strategy for measuring and characterizing the health financing function with the aim of relating its effectiveness to the health system's intrinsic goals. WHO proposes to undertake pilot activities in a small set of countries in which both "core" variables and country-specific information would be collected and analysed. This work will be undertaken jointly with national governments, policy makers, and local research institutions. The measures will also be submitted for expert review. As a result of this work, refined "core" variables will gradually be generalized for measurement in other countries.

4. SPRG COMMENTS AND RECOMMENDATIONS

These dimensions and a proposed set of potential variables were discussed with SPRG and are presented in Table 61.3. They were also discussed at an internal WHO consultation (in March 2002) that included staff from regional and country offices. There was general agreement that the chosen variables should be useful for measuring the function's performance in a variety of dimensions, and should control for important contextual factors. In broad terms, the measurements should help assess how well the system collects, pools, and allocates funds to service provision. This

Table 61.3 Indicators discussed with the Scientific Peer Review Group, Dec. 2001

Indicators proposed by WHO	Purpose	SPRG Comments
(a) Revenue Collection		The proposed indicators do not measure:
■ The formal sector share of GDP ■ Natural resource revenues as a share of total public sector income	Potential resources available to finance public health spending	1. The minimum threshold for health-sector funding (minimum expenditure) 2. The degree of revenue collection progressivity or regressivity *(The FFC index does not distinguish between progressivity and regressivity; it is affected even if the better-off pay a larger proportion of their ability to pay than the poor)*
■ Public sector expenditures as a share of GDP ■ External health sector aid as a share of total public health expenditures	To measure resources specifically available to the public sector	
■ The share of public health expenditures in total public expenditure ■ Total health expenditure (per capita level and share of GDP)	To measure public sector allocation decisions, additional resources, and potential constraints	3. The cost of revenue collection
The share of total health expenditures that are prepaid (as against those which are paid out-of-pocket at time of service)	A broad measure of financial protection against out-of-pocket expenses	
(b) Pooling		The proposed indicators do not reflect:
Means and concentration indices of: ■ Share of copayments to total health expenditure in each pool ■ Membership in each pool ■ Per capita spending in each pool	Measures of the scale, depth of financial coverage, and existence of compensatory mechanisms across pools	1. Those who do not belong to any pool, are eligible to public services without paying contributions or fee-for-service (waivering system) 2. Risk distribution among pools (prohibitive measures and exclusions) 3. Pools overlapping 4. Differences in benefit packages between pools 5. Pools administrative costs
(c) Purchasing		The following issues need to be treated:
■ Number of purchasers ■ Means and distribution of total expenditure across purchasers ■ Mean and distribution of the number of providers who are contracted or hired by each purchaser	To characterize the structure of interactions between purchasers and providers	1. Incentives through payment mechanisms *(To what extent do they: contain costs, encourage over- or under-utilization, hinder access, or affect quality of care?)* 2. Transparency and accountability
■ Share of total funds allocated by inputs (e.g. salaries and traditional budgets), outputs (e.g. fee-for-service) and outcomes (e.g. capitation)	To measure the financial incentives embedded in payments to providers	

should enable better targeting of appropriate policy actions needed to improve the financing function. SPRG also recommended that WHO draw on the work of other agencies working in this area such as the OECD Health Project (Hurst and Jee-Hughes 2001; Hurst 2002).

In the course of these discussions, the following issues were raised.

■ Minimum threshold of funding for the health sector. Can WHO provide guidance on what countries should minimally spend on health?

■ Cost of revenue collection. Any measures of the financing function should include the costs of administering revenue collection because they are a measure of the effectiveness of the collection subfunction.

■ Uncovered population. The proposed indicators do not appear to measure the number of people who do not belong to any pool, or who are eligible for free public services. This will depend on the definition adopted for "pool", and the kind of data from which the indicators will be derived. It was also noted that people covered by a public "safety net" are implicitly in a "pool". In any case, the indicators should include some measure to reflect this potential failure of a health-financing system.

■ Progressivity of financing. The financing function is closely tied to the goal of fairness-in-financing. There is concern that the Fairness in Financing Index (FFI) is misleading because the formula can rank an extremely progressive system as being just as 'unfair' as a very regressive one.

■ Differences in benefit packages between pools. The indicators need to address not only how many people are in the pools, but also what services are covered. When benefit packages differ, the implications for the effectiveness of the financing function will also differ.

■ Risk distribution among pools. It was noted that the financing function will behave very differently depending on whether there are constraints to adverse selection or exclusion. How will these institutional features be incorporated in the indicators?

■ Overlapping pools. The indicators will have to take into account the fact that in many countries pools overlap.

■ Payment mechanisms. The final indicator was unclear. The purpose here will be to analyse how the incentives generated by payment mechanisms affect costs, as well as the amount, kinds and quality of health services provided.

■ Transparency and accountability. It is important to find ways to measure the transparency and accountability of the financing function since these factors probably have a large impact on its effectiveness.

■ Sources of funds. Measurements need to capture the wide range of sources for funds flowing into the health sector, including external aid which is significant in many low-income countries.

■ Indicators for research vs. policy guidance. Questions were raised regarding whether these indicators are sufficiently "universal" to measure cross-country differences. The extent to which they are aimed at supporting research or monitoring policy also requires clarification.

■ Links with other work. The financing indicators work needs to be well-coordinated with other work on FFC, provision, coverage, and responsiveness.

Recommendations

■ WHO should continue to develop measurements of the health-financing function and address the concerns listed above.

■ WHO should produce technical papers aimed at consolidating the evidence on the health-financing function and how it affects health-system performance.

References

Almeida, C, P Braveman, MR Gold, CL Szwarcwald, JM Ribeiro, A Miglionico, JS Millar, S Porto, NR Costa, VO Rubio, M Segall, B Starfield, C Travassos, A Ugá, J Valente, and F Viacava (2001): Methodological concerns and recommendations on policy consequences of the World Health Report 2000. *Lancet*, 357(9269): 1692–1697.

Häkkinen, U and E Ollila, eds. (2000): The World Health Report 2000: What does it tell us about health systems? Analyses by Finnish experts. Helsinki: National Research and Development Center for Welfare and Health (STAKES). *http://www.stakes.fi/english/publicati/ Publications.htm*

Helms, R (2000 August): Sick list: health care à la Karl Marx. *Wall Street Journal.*

Hurst, J (2002): Performance measurement and improvement in OECD health systems: Overview of issues and challenges. In Measuring Up: Improving Health System Performance in OECD Countries. Paris, France: Organization for Economic Co-operation and Development (OECD).

Hurst, J and M Jee-Hughes (2001): Performance measurement and performance management in OECD health systems. Labour Market and Social Policy—Occasional Papers, No. 47. Paris, France: Organization for Economic Co-operation and Development (OECD).

Murray, CJL and J Frenk (2001): World Health Report 2000: A step towards evidence-based health policy. *Lancet*, 357(9269): 1698–1700.

Navarro, V (2000): Assessment of the World Health Report 2000. *Lancet*, 356(9241): 1598–1601.

Navarro, V (2001a): The new conventional wisdom: an evaluation of the WHO report, Health Systems: Improving Performance. *International Journal of Health Services*, 31(1): 23–33.

Navarro, V (2001b): World Health Report 2000: Response to Murray and Frenk. *Lancet*, 357(9269): 1701–1702.

Oswaldo Cruz Foundation, Brazilian Ministry of Health (2000): Report of the workshop "Health Systems Performance: The World Health Report 2000". 14-12-2000, Rio de Janeiro.

Van der Stuyft, P and JP Unger (2000): Improving the performance of health systems: The World Health Report as go-between for scientific evidence and ideological discourse. *Tropical Medicine and International Health*, 5(10): 675–677.

Walt, G and A Mills (2001): World Health Report 2000: Comments. *Lancet*, 357(9269): 1702–1703.

WHO Regional Office for the Americas (2001): Regional consultation of the Americas on Health Systems Performance Assessment: Final Report. 8-5-2001, Washington, D.C.

WHO Regional Office for Europe (2001): Report of the Regional Consultation on Health Systems Performance Assessment. 3-9-2001, Copenhagen.

VI. Stewardship Function

1. WHR 2000

WHR 2000 introduced the concept of stewardship as one of the four essential functions of the health system: service provision, resource generation, financing and stewardship. In the Introductory chapter, the Director-General highlighted this new concept noting that the function involves "setting and enforcing the rules of the game and providing strategic direction for all the different actors involved". The concept was developed further in chapter six. Here stewardship was defined as "the careful and responsible management of the well-being of the population, the very essence of good government". The text continued "This does not, of course, mean that the government needs to fund and provide all health interventions. It needs, however, to set the direction for both public and private sectors and ensure that the health system contributes to the socially desired intrinsic goals. How well or poorly a government executes its stewardship role can influence all aspects of health system performance". It also stated that ultimate responsibility for the overall performance of a country's health system lies with government, which in turn should involve all sectors of society in its stewardship. Within government, Ministries of Health must take on a large part of the stewardship of health systems and should direct/coordinate intersectoral action for health.

2. Main Commentaries and Criticisms

Although various individuals and groups had commented extensively on aspects of the WHR 2000, there was little published comment on stewardship. Only two articles have been identified. Saltman and Ferroussier-Davis (2000) discuss the concept of stewardship in health policy as proposed in WHR 2000, and conclude that the concept "holds substantial promise if adequately developed and effectively implemented". An editorial in the European Journal of Public Health (McKee 2001a) also discusses the potentially major implications of the concept of 'stewardship' of health systems, both for countries and for WHO as it seeks to strengthen its role as a credible advocate for global health.

The Regional Consultations on health-system performance assessment did discuss stewardship. In addition to statements about the importance of the notion of stewardship, it featured in general discussions on the need to better map all the health system functions, their linkages with each other, and their relation to outcomes. Participants in the EMRO consultation observed the need for better definition of each of the components of stewardship (WHO Regional Office for the Eastern Mediterranean 2001). In AFRO and SEARO, participants recommended that in future work on performance assessment, WHO and Member States should pay special attention to developing methods for assessing the stewardship function of health systems (WHO Regional Office for Africa 2001; WHO Regional Office for South-East Asia 2001). In the EURO consultation, it was stressed that assessment should not be seen as an isolated exercise, but explicitly linked to efforts to strengthen stewardship (WHO Regional Office for Europe 2001). More general comments were also made on the need to develop complementary and qualitative measures of functions, not just pursue quantitative dimensions of analysis. PAHO/AMRO proposed the use of a 'dashboard' approach to assessing functions (WHO Regional Office for the Americas 2001). In the WPRO consultation, the participants commented on WHO's own stewardship role in the international health arena (WHO Regional Office for the Western Pacific 2001).

The most extensive debate on stewardship has been the international technical consultation on stewardship in September 2001 at which the participants reviewed the definition of the term and discussed its relation to governance (World Health Organization 2001). They also noted the difficulty in preserving the idea when translating the term into other languages. Participants referred to it metaphorically as combining three elements ("the 'glue' that holds the health system together; the 'oil' that keeps it running smoothly, and the 'energy' that gives it ethical direction and momentum"). They generated a list of possible stewardship tasks that fitted within the three-part classification that WHR 2000 set out:

■ formulating health policy;

- exerting influence; and

- collecting and using intelligence.

Participants agreed that some form of descriptive characterization of approaches to stewardship would be useful, and counselled against measurement of stewardship as an isolated exercise. They emphasized that a clearer understanding is needed of relationships between approaches to stewardship, the resultant effectiveness of the stewardship function, and the performance of health systems.

The few comments on assessment of stewardship have noted that this will be an important yet challenging task. Some have commented on the importance of ensuring that any assessment is useful in the first instance to nationals in their own efforts to improve stewardship.

3. WHO Responses and Proposals

Stewardship: conceptual issues

Building on the work of other organizations as well as the recommendations of the meeting on the stewardship function held in September 2001, WHO staff prepared a paper in November 2001 that further developed the concept (Travis et al. 2002). The paper tentatively identifies a number of essential ingredients or "core domains" that appear to constitute good stewardship. Domains are conceived as relatively well defined, distinct areas of responsibility that collectively constitute effective stewardship. The six domains or sub-functions that constitute effective health system stewardship, i.e. that lead to better outcomes to achieve the goals of health systems are referred to as:

- Generation of intelligence

- Formulating strategic policy direction

- Ensuring tools for implementation: powers, incentives and sanctions

- Coalition building / Building partnerships

- Ensuring a fit between policy objectives and organizational structure and culture

- Ensuring accountability

The paper states that it is desirable to increase capacity within the health systems of Member States with regard to each of these domains. The assumption is that, collectively, the better these sub-functions are carried out, the more effective health system stewardship will be and the higher attainment of intrinsic goals. These domains, attributes and relationships are based on prevailing notions of effective stewardship, and the paper emphasizes that all should be considered "testable hypotheses". The concept of stewardship has evolved in the course of the consultations and analyses (see table 61.4).

The scope and core attributes of each domain are outlined briefly here and described in more detail in the background paper.

Generation of intelligence

This domain responds to the concern "to what extent do health system actors have useful intelligence at their disposal?"; and do key actors have reliable, up-to-date information on current and future trends in health and different aspects of health system performance, important contextual factors and actors, possible policy options based on national and international experience?

Formulating strategic policy direction

This domain responds to the concern "to what extent is there a clear sense of vision and strategic direction for the health system?":

Table 61.4   Three classifications of tasks for stewardship

WHR 2000	Consultation	Travis et al. (2002)
Collecting and using information	Collecting and using intelligence	Generation of intelligence
Defining the vision and direction of health policy	Formulating health policy	Formulating strategic policy direction
Exerting influence through regulation and advocacy	Exerting influence	Ensuring tools for implementation: powers, incentives and sanctions
		Coalition building / Building partnerships
		Ensuring a fit between policy objectives and organizational structure and culture
		Ensuring accountability

■ Is there clear articulation of health system objectives?

■ Is there a clear definition of roles and responsibilities of public and private actors in all four functions?

■ Has there been a clear identification of policy instruments and institutional arrangements required to achieve improvements?

■ Have the authorities developed strategies for making the required changes? and

■ Have they provided guidance for prioritizing health expenditures based on realistic resource and needs assessment, and for monitoring effects of changes on performance?

Ensuring tools for implementation: powers, incentives and sanctions

This domain addresses the concern "to what extent is there a regulatory framework that facilitates implementation of health policy, i.e. steers different actors in the desired direction?". "Regulatory framework" refers to the spectrum of rules, procedures, laws, codes of conduct, standards, etc., that exist. This will involve looking at the scope of existing regulation, conflicts or contradictions between stated policy and the regulatory framework (whether powers and responsibilities are matched); and the extent to which they are enforced.

Coalition building/Building partnerships

This domain addresses the concern "to what extent does capacity exist to create alliances of individuals, groups or organizations for joint action around strategic health and health system priorities?"

Ensuring a fit between policy objectives and organizational structure and culture

This domain addresses two questions: "To what extent do organizational structures and management systems fit with policy objectives so that they help rather than hinder policy implementation?"; and "to what extent have conditions been created by government that allow stewards themselves to be effective?".

Ensuring accountability

This is considered a separate domain at present on the grounds that it is a stewardship responsibility to ensure that all health system actors are held accountable for their actions. This will also contribute to consumer protection.

Assessing stewardship

WHO states that the objective of its work is to support health systems' performance improvement at country level by providing evidence-based advice on the relationships between stewardship and health system outcomes. Travis et al. (2002) rightly point out that whilst the importance of many of the activities thought to contribute to effective stewardship have long been written about, as a whole it is a new construct in health systems and there are no tools for looking at all its different aspects. They referred to studies in other areas which have attempted to measure some of the elements of stewardship. In particular, they noted the work done on governance, and work to define an instrument for measuring 'Essential Public Health Functions' (Pan American Health Organization et al. 2001) that may assess selected aspects of stewardship. WHO proposes to explore this and other approaches in the development of credible stewardship assessment tools. Based on WHO's recent experience with measuring responsiveness, one approach that is being considered is to develop a survey instrument that would include questions on all domains of stewardship, accompanied by vignettes, that could be administered to all main groups of health system actors, including households if appropriate.

Development of an instrument to assess stewardship

Descriptive and analytical approaches will require qualitative and quantitative assessments. The analyses required, audience and intended use will guide the selection of approaches. Therefore, rather than one single instrument, a set of assessment approaches will be developed and tested.

WHO has developed a provisional programme of work to further develop the concept of stewardship and its assessment based on the comments thus far received.

Proposed outputs by December 2003

■ Revised conceptual paper and broad-based consensus on domains and assessment indicators.

■ Tools for assessing stewardship developed and used in around 15 interested countries.

■ Series of country reports on key findings of the stewardship assessment for in-country discussions and policy dialogue.

- Valid and meaningful approach to analyses, for in-country, regional and cross-national use.

- Set of training modules for capacity building on stewardship related to health systems' performance.

- Dissemination and public access to information and linking various research results across functions and goals.

4. SPRG Comments and Recommendations

Conceptual issues

- *What is the value of this new concept?*
  Several commentators (McKee 2001b) see it as an important development. "WHO has clearly stated that governments have a responsibility for their health systems. Stewardship implies a much more active involvement in promoting health than most governments have previously assumed" (McKee 2001a). Not all commentators have seen it as such a departure. In the discussions of SPRG, it was observed that WHO as a technical and political organization has long had an obligation to produce reliable evidence on health or health system issues, and to 'speak up' and publicize that evidence. One WHO Regional Office commentator pointed out that it builds on previous efforts by WHO to strengthen ministries of health and their 'leadership' role. Another noted that there are many examples of current market or political failures arising from the lack of stewardship within ministries of health. Some commentators have requested that WHO provides examples of effective stewardship when different actors in public and private settings have conflicting goals or interests, as a means to illustrate good stewardship more concretely (Saltman and Ferroussier-Davis 2000).

- *The definition of stewardship*
  SPRG consider that the concept is well defined. They considered whilst it is not that distinct from governance, the word stewardship may better reflect the element of directing a health system. In the Technical Consultation, the ethical foundation of the concept was stressed (World Health Organization 2001). One commentator observed that it is the 'moral' aspect of stewardship that distinguishes it most from governance, which is seen as a more procedural notion. Another distinction has been drawn between stewardship as an 'intelligent' func-tion and governance as a more structural one—a set of activities that have to happen.

- *Who is responsible for stewardship?*
  Governments have the primary responsibility for discharging the stewardship function of the health system. The expectation is that each government will ensure that it meets the legitimate health needs and expectations of the population in the context of available resources. This does not imply that the government will be solely responsible for performing all the essential tasks. In discharging its stewardship role, the government develops partnerships, works with civil society and with the private sector, but such linkages cannot dilute the fact that governments are primarily responsible for discharging the function of stewardship. Active participation by civil society can be of great value in developing national goals and in ensuring good stewardship by government. The active involvement of civil society and the contributions of the private sector are vital components of the health system but the people have the right to hold their governments account-able for the operation of the health system as a whole. Responsibility refers to who must ensure that justifiable expectations are met and it identifies who must take the blame when things go wrong.

The proposed domains/sub-functions of stewardship

SPRG supports the six elements of stewardship and proposes an interconnected framework for these six elements (see figure 61.1).

More work is required to characterize each domain more clearly. Aspects of stewardship that are currently insufficiently addressed or unclear include:

- The need for a clearer link between the generation and use of intelligence.

- The need to be clear that stewardship is not only about central control.

- The early warning / detection function of steward-ship—for example of harmful practices.

- The refereeing function—detection and dealing with conflicts of interest.

Assessment issues

In the SPRG discussion, WHO emphasized that the work being proposed was mainly aimed at improving understanding of the different components of stew-

Figure 61.1 A framework for stewardship

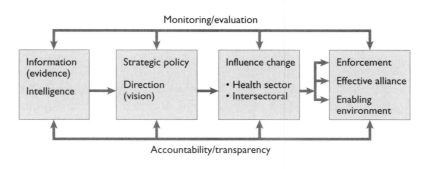

ardship, so that action could be taken by countries. Qualitative as well as quantitative approaches are likely to be needed.

On the question about the use of surveys to measure stewardship, SPRG raised several issues:

■ Who should be surveyed—key informants, households, or a mix?

■ Who should carry out such surveys?

■ Would assessment from household surveys be useful to governments who may have to make unpopular decisions?

The reliability, validity and comparability of any survey approach were viewed as key issues in ensuring acceptability and use of results. A note of caution was provided by SPRG that whatever aspects of stewardship are selected for assessment, these will automatically be assumed to be important or desirable, when there is still little evidence.

SPRG commends the Secretariat's initiative to measure the level of stewardship. The Group suggests that in addition to subjective measurements, some objective indicators should also be developed. The key stakeholders who will be the respondents should be clearly defined and identified and conflict of interests avoided. A composite index on stewardship may be developed. However, as this is quite a sensitive area involving the function and responsibility of national health leaders, great care should be accorded to the methodology, the measurements, and the publication.

REFERENCES

McKee, M (2001a): The challenge of stewardship. *European Journal of Public Health*, 11: 122–123.

McKee, M (2001b): Measuring the efficiency of health systems. *British Medical Journal*, 323(7308): 295–296.

Pan American Health Organization, World Health Organization, Centers for Disease Control and Prevention, and Centro Latinoamericano de Investigaciones en Sistemas de Salud (2001): "Public Health in the Americas" Initiative: Instrument for Performance Measurement of Essential Public Health Functions.

Saltman, RB and O Ferroussier-Davis (2000): The concept of stewardship in health policy. *Bulletin of the World Health Organization*, 78(6): 732–739.

Travis, P, D Egger, P Davies, and A Mechbal (2002): Towards better stewardship: concepts and critical issues. Global Programme on Evidence for Health Policy Discussion Papers, No. 48. Geneva, Switzerland: World Health Organization.

World Health Organization (2001): Report on WHO meeting of experts on the stewardship function in health systems. 10-9-2001, Geneva, Switzerland. (unpublished document HFS/FAR/STW/00.1).

WHO Regional Office for the Eastern Mediterranean (2001): Report on the Regional Consultation on the Conceptual Framework for Health System Performance Assessment. 9-7-2001, Ain Saadeh, Lebanon.

WHO Regional Office for Africa (2001): General Report on the Regional Consultative Meeting on Health Systems Performance Assessment: Final Report. 18-5-2001 Harare, Zimbabwe.

WHO Regional Office for the Americas (2001): Regional consultation of the Americas on Health Systems Performance Assessment: Final Report. 8-5-2001, Washington, D.C.

WHO Regional Office for Europe (2001): Report of the Regional Consultation on Health Systems Performance Assessment. 3-9-2001, Copenhagen.

WHO Regional Office for the Western Pacific (2001): Report of the regional consultation on health system performance. 3-7-2001, Manila, Philippines.

WHO Regional Office for South-East Asia (2001): Report of the regional consultation and technical workshop on health systems performance assessment. 18-6-2001, New Delhi, India.

VII. Average Level of Population Health

1. WHR 2000

WHO has reported indicators of population health for each Member State for many years, including child and adult mortality risks and life expectancy at birth. In addition, for over a decade WHO has been involved in the development of summary measures of population health (SMPH), which combine information on mortality and non-fatal health outcomes to represent population health as a single number. WHR 2000 reported disability-adjusted life expectancy (DALE) at birth and at age 60, for males and females, with uncertainty intervals around the most likely estimates.

As part of this process, new life tables and life expectancies were estimated for all 191 Member States. Data were taken from different sources. For example, vital registration data were available for 80 countries. In other countries, indirect information on mortality—infant, child and/or adult—was available. At times, UN Population Division estimates of adult mortality were used where no direct sources of data were available. For countries without adequate vital registration data or surveys, estimates were based on regional logit models.

To estimate DALE for each country, the life table data were supplemented with information on age- and sex-specific prevalences of non-fatal health outcomes and appropriate health-state valuations. Health-state valuations were estimated for each major non-fatal health outcome for five standard age groups, by sex, in eight regions. Where the data were available, detailed information on the epidemiology of the major conditions in countries was used to construct prevalence of non-fatal health outcomes, along with the earlier Global Burden of Disease (GBD) estimates. Existing health surveys were also used, but the additional information they provided was limited by problems of cross-population comparability.

2. Main Commentaries and Criticisms

Summary Measures of Population Health

Much of the discussion about the indicator of the level of health used in WHR 2000 was a continuation of the long-standing debate about the value of summary measures of population health (SMPH). For example, it was argued that SMPH do not describe health in sufficient detail to be useful for policy makers. Reporting the components separately is of more value, e.g. mortality, and prevalence, incidence duration and severity of various non-fatal health outcomes (Navarro 2001a; Rosén 2001; WHO Regional Office for Africa 2001). Some commentaries criticized disability-adjusted life years (DALYs), stating that by themselves they should not be used for resource allocation decisions (Almeida et al. 2001; Häkkinen 2000; Rissanen and Sintonen 2000). SMPH were seen to be too complex for policy makers to understand (Almeida et al. 2001; Oswaldo Cruz Foundation 2000) and the fact that Life Expectancy at birth (LE) and Disability-Adjusted Life Expectancy (DALE) were highly correlated led some critics to argue that DALE added little that was not already captured by LE (Oswaldo Cruz Foundation 2000; Häkkinen 2000, McKee 2001a; Ugá et al. 2001).

Another concern with SMPH surrounded the valuation of non-fatal health outcomes on the same scale as death and full functioning. Critics of summary measures argued that this type of assessment undervalued the lives of disabled people (Almeida et al. 2001; Oswaldo Cruz Foundation 2000) and also raised other ethical problems (Oswaldo Cruz Foundation 2000; Rissanen and Sintonen 2000; Nord 2002). Others claimed that the valuations used in WHR 2000 did not capture all aspects of quality-of-life or heterogeneity across countries in the way people understood and valued health (DfID 2000; Oswaldo Cruz Foundation 2000; Rissanen and Sintonen 2000; WHO Regional Office for the Americas 2001; Nord 2002). Still others argued that weights should ideally be obtained from representative population groups rather than from a limited group of experts (Almeida et al. 2001; Oswaldo Cruz Foundation 2000; Rissanen and Sintonen 2000; WHO Regional Office for the Eastern Mediterranean 2001).

The word "disability" in DALE also raised concerns: "disability" could be seen as a pejorative term and was not an appropriate word to use to describe a state that is less than full health. Moreover, it does not well capture the idea that health is a multidimensional and complex concept (Oswaldo Cruz Foundation 2000; Häkkinen and Ollila 2000; Van der Stuyft and Unger 2000).

As a key goal in assessing the performance of health systems, a number of authors pointed out that measures such as DALE reflected past as well as current performance, and hence cannot be interpreted as being a function only of current performance (Almeida et al. 2001; DfID 2000; McKee 2001b; Oswaldo Cruz Foundation 2000; Rosén 2001; Häkkinen 2000; WHO Regional Office for Europe 2001; Ministry of Health, Vietnam 2001; McKee 2001a).

A series of specific technical points were also raised about the construction of DALE. For example, life tables estimated for countries where vital registration data did not exist do not fit the oldest age groups well in some countries (WHO Regional Office for Africa 2001; WHO Regional Office for the Americas 2001; WHO Regional Office for the Eastern Mediterranean 2001; WHO Regional Office for Europe 2001; WHO Regional Office for South-East Asia 2001; WHO Regional Office for the Western Pacific 2001). The way in which the estimates of the prevalence of non-fatal health outcomes were obtained, and co-morbidity was handled in developing the overall severity-adjusted prevalence of non-fatal health outcomes, was seen as simplistic (Navarro 2001a; Rosén 2001; Rissanen and Sintonen 2000; World Health Organization 2001). For example, the prevalence of different types of disability was assumed to be the same in all countries with similar life expectancies (Oswaldo Cruz Foundation 2000; Ugá et al. 2001). In addition, McKee (2001a) argued that in estimating uncertainty intervals around the estimates, all possible sources of uncertainty had not been considered.

The final set of commentaries concerned data sources. It was generally agreed that epidemiological data were sparse and of variable quality in many countries, and that the use of more vital registration data would greatly improve the estimates (McKee 2001b; Oswaldo Cruz Foundation 2000; Williams 2001; Häkkinen 2000; Rissanen and Sintonen 2000; WHO Regional Office for Africa 2001; WHO Regional Office for the Eastern Mediterranean 2001; WHO Regional Office for Europe 2001; Ugá et al. 2001). The available data on child and adult mortality, as opposed to infant mortality, were particularly poor (WHO Regional Office for Africa 2001). WHO had used UN Population Division estimates at times, and the sources and methods underlying them were seen to be unclear (WHO Regional Office for Europe 2001; McKee 2001a).

3. WHO Responses and Proposals

Noting that there are large variations in DALE for any given level of LE, the WHO Secretariat argued that DALE does indeed provide additional information to that contained in LE. It proposed to SPRG that it should continue to use SMPH to measure and monitor population health. In doing this, it was important to be clear that the question of measuring and monitoring population health was not the same as the question of resource allocation. The criticism that DALYs should not be used for resource allocation was not relevant to this debate—as this was not being proposed. To help policy makers identify the possible causes of changes in health outcomes, WHO proposes to continue publishing the components of DALE separately—i.e. mortality and non-fatal health outcomes. SMPH is a complement to, but not a substitute for, information on the separate components.

In recognition of the problems associated with the term "disability", and the fact that health is a multidimensional concept, WHO proposes to accept the advice that the name of the indicator should be changed from DALE to health-adjusted life expectancy (HALE).

To respond to criticisms related to health valuation a more precise definition of its conceptual basis was provided. Part of the WHO Multi-Country Survey Study 2000–2001 involved detailed questionnaires in 12 countries designed to explore if people from different cultures rated the domains of health differently. WHO used these results to develop a method for estimating new health-state valuations (Salomon et al. 2002). The Secretariat proposes to apply it to the data from the World Health Survey (WHS): a global average valuation function will be applied to the individual domain levels estimated using the HOPIT model (Section XIII) in order to derive severity-adjusted prevalences of health states by age and sex for each survey country. At present, the prior estimates of severity-weighted prevalences derived from the GBD study use the disability weights from GBD 1990, together with weights from the Dutch disability weights study (Stouthard et al. 1997). WHO plans to revise all disability weights used in the GBD study from the population-based valuations that are obtained from WHS.

The question of timing is taken up again in Section XIV on 'Efficiency' in the SPRG report. To complement the prevalence-HALE that is already reported routinely, WHO proposes to explore the feasibility of developing an incidence-HALE based on current incidence and transition rates and information on cur-rent exposures to major risk factors. It would then be determined largely by actions undertaken in the cur-rent time period.

WHO has undertaken intense efforts to obtain more and better data. This started with consultations between WHO and Member States to verify the best sources of recent data on vital registration and causes of death. The number of countries with relatively complete vital registration or cause-of-death data has increased from 80 in 2000 to 110 in 2002. New life tables for the year 2000 have been constructed for all 191 Member States using these data. A modified logit life table model was developed for countries with incomplete registration or survey data. It employed a much larger empirical database of observed life tables than any previous model life table system, and has resulted in much better estimates of mortality at older ages. Separate estimates of HIV mortality were made for countries with high HIV mortality.

In addition to methods development for life tables, WHO has introduced ways of taking co-morbidity into account in estimating HALE. This was facili-tated partly by the Multi-Country Survey Study, which included instruments and analytical tools for improving cross-population comparability of survey data. Comparable data on the prevalence of non-fatal conditions from 63 surveys in 55 countries were used to estimate HALE for WHR 2001. (The new statistical methods to establish cross-population comparability are discussed in Section XIII.) The other components of the calculations were:

(a) Direct estimates of prevalence for major disease and injury sequelae.

(b) Country-level prevalence data for selected condi-tions.

(c) Regional information, specific epidemiological studies, and available country information on cause-specific mortality to estimate morbidity in countries with poor information about causes.

(d) Adjustment by known under-registration for highly stigmatized causes of morbidity and mor-tality such as abortion, HIV/AIDS, and suicide.

(e) For estimating health-state prevalences, data from the Multi-Country Survey Study were used (cross-population comparable prevalences, and valua-tions based on population preferences) together with severity-weighted prevalences derived from epidemiological analyses in GBD 2000. In addi-tion, improved Bayesian methods were used to compute posterior health-state prevalences that combine GBD 2000-based 'prior' estimates with prevalence estimates from the Multi-Country Survey Study. For those countries with no survey results, a relationship between posterior and prior estimates of prevalences for the survey countries was used to update the priors.

Finally, improved methods for uncertainty analysis were used, including more explicit and comprehen-sive treatment of uncertainty in various inputs. The uncertainty interval of 80% used in WHR 2000 was increased to 95% in WHR 2001. WHO proposes to continue calculating and reporting uncertainty inter-vals in a systematic manner so that different users can make their own assessment of the estimates.

4. SPRG Comments and Recommendations

(i) WHO is playing a leading role in the development of new concepts and health measures that incor-porate non-fatal outcomes into SMPH. Consider-ing the complexity of the issues, it is natural that there will be debate about these innovations—and some policy makers will prefer to use indicators of individual components of health rather than sum-mary measures. Moreover, SMPH are sometimes seen as having less validity than the single com-ponent measures, especially for Member States where both morbidity and mortality estimates have wide uncertainty intervals. WHO should continue to emphasize that SMPH complement rather than compete with the disaggregations of the component parts, and it should continue to take steps to make more detailed disaggregations of SMPH available.

(ii) SMPH require valuation of health outcomes to allow non-fatal conditions to be combined with mortality. WHO should take additional steps to explain and clarify the concept of health-adjusted life expectancy. This should be distinguished from the complexity of the methods needed for esti-mation where appropriate data are not available, and from the issue of cross-population compar-ability.

(iii) Despite these difficulties, WHO should continue to improve the conceptual and technical aspects of health measurement, engage in external debate and consultation, and obtain better data.

(iv) SPRG recommends that WHO take steps to strengthen local capacity to build and use these measures, particularly in developing countries. Related to this, SPRG believes that it would be valuable for WHO to establish a permanent forum for discussion of conceptual and methodological aspects of health measurement, and promote the participation of academics, policy makers and civil society—especially from developing countries. As part of this process, there should be a continuing dialogue with social scientists from subject areas such as ethics, anthropology and sociology, so as to take into account insights from these disciplines on the 'value' of health.

(v) The modified logit life tables provide a reasonable methodology for countries where vital registration data are not available, but the assumptions behind their construction and use should be made more comprehensible for non-expert audiences.

(vi) Vital statistics registration (VSR) systems are complex and expensive, and do not exist in many developing countries. WHO should encourage the establishment of these registries and provide the necessary technical assistance. Considering the inevitable time lags to establish a functioning VSR system, the use of indirect methods is acceptable as an intermediate solution.

(vii) In relation to WHS, SPRG believes it is important to increase the number of participating countries, especially those with inadequate health-information systems. The face validity of the WHS data is still an issue. Although the inclusion of vignettes in the questionnaire facilitates the comparability of self-report data between countries, further development and testing of the methods is recommended.

(viii) Data on adult mortality are still scarce. The WHO Multi-Country Survey Study 2000-2001 found that questions on deaths in households provided some useful information, but that there was underreporting of deaths. An expanded module on adult mortality should be included in WHS and validated in countries with good vital registration data. Improved methods should be developed to maximize the usefulness of this information for estimation of adult mortality.

(ix) It is important that WHO clarifies the methods and procedures used to estimate causes of death by age and sex for countries without vital regis-

tration data or with only partial data, and that it intensifies data collection efforts in such countries.

(x) HALE incorporates prevalences and valuations of health states from population surveys and from GBD 2000. Currently, the weights used in the GBD 2000 study are predominantly based on the GBD 1990 weights with some additional weights from a Dutch study (Stouthard et al. 1997). Examination of GBD 1990 and Dutch weights (Mathers et al. 1999) suggest that these weights are comparable. SPRG welcomes the effort made by WHO to improve the health-state valuation methods and endorses the proposal to revise the GBD disability weights using valuations derived from the forthcoming WHS.

(xi) The difference between the uncertainty analysis proposed by WHO and statistical confidence intervals should be made clear in WHO publications.

(xii) National simulations based on regional or global estimates can be a good starting point to encourage National Burden of Disease studies.

References

Almeida, C, P Braveman, MR Gold, CL Szwarcwald, JM Ribeiro, A Miglionico, JS Millar, S Porto, NR Costa, VO Rubio, M Segall, B Starfield, C Travassos, A Uga, J Valente, and F Viacava (2001): Methodological concerns and recommendations on policy consequences of the World Health Report 2000. *Lancet*, 357(9269): 1692–1697.

DfID (Department for International Development, UK Health Systems Resource Center) (2000): World Health Report 2000: Summary and Comments.

Häkkinen, U (2000): Assessment of the goal attainment and efficiency of health systems in the World Health Report 2000. In eds. U Häkkinen and E Ollila. The World Health Report 2000: What does it tell us about health systems? Analyses by Finnish Experts. Helsinki: National Research and Development Center for Welfare and Health (STAKES). [http://www.stakes.fi/english/publicati/Publications.htm]

Häkkinen U and E Ollila, eds. (2000): The World Health Report 2000: What does it tell us about health systems? Analyses by Finnish experts. Helsinki: National Research and Development Center for Welfare and Health (STAKES). [http://www.stakes.fi/english/publicati/Publications.htm]

Mathers, C, T Vos, and C Stevenson (1999): The burden of

disease and injury in Australia. Canberra, Australia: Australian Institute of Health and Welfare.

McKee, M (2001a): The World Health Report 2000: Advancing the debate. Prepared for the European Regional Consultation on Health Systems Performance Assessment. 3-9-2001, Copenhagen.

McKee, M (2001b): Measuring the efficiency of health systems. *British Medical Journal*, 323(7308): 295–296.

Ministry of Health, Vietnam (2001): Comments and suggestions of Vietnam Ministry of Health/Health Policy Unit as regards the World Health Report 2000.

Navarro, V (2000): Assessment of the World Health Report 2000. *Lancet*, 356(9241): 1598–1601.

Navarro, V (2001a): The new conventional wisdom: an evaluation of the WHO report, Health Systems: Improving Performance. *International Journal of Health Services*, 31(1): 23–33.

Navarro, V (2001b): World Health Report 2000: responses to Murray and Frenk. *Lancet*, 357(9269): 1701–1702.

Nord, E (2002): Measures of goal attainment and performance: A brief, critical consumer guide. *Health Policy*, 59(3): 183–191.

Oswaldo Cruz Foundation, Brazilian Ministry of Health (2000): Report of the workshop "Health Systems Performance: The World Health Report 2000". 14-12-2000, Rio de Janeiro.

Rissanen, P and H Sintonen (2000): Measurement of the state of health in the World Health Report 2000. In eds. U Häkkinen and E Ollila. The World Health Report 2000: What does it tell us about health systems? Analyses by Finnish Experts. Helsinki: National Research and Development Center for Welfare and Health (STAKES). [*http://www.stakes.fi/english/publicati/Publications.htm*]

Rosén, M (2001): Can the WHO Health Report improve the performance of health systems?. *Scandinavian Journal of Public Health*, 29(1): 76–80.

Salomon, J, CJL Murray, B Üstün, and S Chatterji (2002): Health state valuations in summary measures of population health. Global Programme on Evidence for Health Policy, mimeo. Geneva, Switzerland: World Health Organization.

Stouthard, MEA, ML Essink-Bot, GJ Bonsel, JJ Barendregt, PGN Kramer, HPA van de Water, LJ Gunning-Scheppers, and PJ Van der Maas (1997): Disability Weights for Diseases in the Netherlands. Rotterdam, The Netherlands: Department of Public Health, Erasmus University.

Ugá AD, CM Almeida, CL Szwarcwald, C Travassos, F Viacava, JM Ribeiro, NR Costa, PM Buss, and S Porto (2001): Considerations on methodology used in the World Health Organization 2000 Report. *Cadernos de Saude Publica*, 17(3): 705–712.

Van der Stuyft, P and JP Unger (2000): Improving the performance of health systems: the World Health Report as go-between for scientific evidence and ideological discourse. *Tropical Medicine and International Health*, 5(10): 675–677.

Williams, A (2000): Science or marketing at WHO? A Commentary on 'World Health 2000'. Health Economics, 10(2): 93–100.

Williams, A (2001): Science or marketing at WHO? Rejoinder from Alan Williams. Health Economics, 10(4): 283–285.

World Health Organization (2001): Report on WHO meeting of experts on statistical methods for enhancing the cross-population comparability of survey results. 1-10-2001, Cambridge, MA, USA.

WHO Regional Office for Africa (2001): General Report on the Regional Consultative Meeting on Health Systems Performance Assessment: Final Report. 18-5-2001, Harare, Zimbabwe.

WHO Regional Office for the Americas (2001): Regional consultation of the Americas on Health Systems Performance Assessment: Final Report. 8-5-2001, Washington, D.C.

WHO Regional Office for the Eastern Mediterranean (2001): Report on the Regional Consultation on the Conceptual Framework for Health System Performance Assessment. 9-7-2001, Ain Saadeh, Lebanon.

WHO Regional Office for Europe (2001): Report of the Regional Consultation on Health Systems Performance Assessment. 3-9-2001, Copenhagen.

WHO Regional Office for South-East Asia (2001): Report of the regional consultation and technical workshop on health systems performance assessment. 18-6-2001, New Delhi, India.

WHO Regional Office for the Western Pacific (2001): Report of the regional consultation on health system performance. 3-7-2001, Manila, Philippines.

VIII. HEALTH INEQUALITY

1. WHR 2000

WHR 2000 defined 'total health inequality' as 'inter-individual variation in healthy life expectancy', thus basing inequality assessment on between-individual and not between-group variation in health expectancy. An important conceptual characteristic of this approach arises from the fact that an individual's health expectancy cannot be observed, but must be estimated. The Report argues that the ideal approach is to combine individual risks of ill-health and death across ages in a measure of healthy life expectancy, and summarize the distribution of these risks into a measure of inter-individual inequality. However, owing to lack of international data on individual risks across the age groups, WHR 2000 was only able to estimate inequality in the probability (duration) of child survival to age 2.

The index of inequality used in WHR 2000 is as follows:

$$II[\alpha, \beta] = \frac{\sum_{i=1}^{n} \sum_{j=1}^{n} |h_i - h_j|^\alpha}{2n^2 \bar{h}^\beta}$$

where h_i is the expected survival time for child i, n is the number of children in the population, and $\bar{h}$ is the average expected survival time for all children. The alpha parameter is derived from interviews aimed at assessing aversion to inequality, and the beta parameter is similarly derived from individual preferences for a relative versus absolute measure of inequality. The alpha and beta parameters were estimated from information obtained through internet interviews of approximately 1,600 persons.

The above index of inequality was applied to child survival to age 2, and is called the Index of Child Survival Inequality. The individual survival rates and risk profiles for children were estimated from maternal birth histories and other covariates, using the Demographic and Health Surveys (DHS) database for 50 countries. As mentioned earlier, no measures of adult health inequality were developed for WHR 2000.

2. MAIN COMMENTARIES AND CRITICISMS

Total or partial health variation

A concern with the concept of total health inequality is that it includes all variation in health in a population, without making any judgements as to which part of the variation is unfair. For example, during the technical consultation on health inequalities it was debated whether voluntary or genetic risks should be excluded from the assessment of total variation, indicating a discomfort with the notion that all inter-individual variation is unfair.

Inter-individual and/or social group approaches to inequality

The inter-individual approach to inequality in WHR 2000 has generated impassioned debate about the appropriateness and relevance of inter-individual versus social-group inequality measurement. A number of analyses (Braveman et al. 2001; Houweling et al. 2001; Ugá et al. 2001; Szwarcwald 2002) have shown the relative independence of the social-group measures of inequality from the index reported in WHR 2000, and have argued for both social group and inter-individual assessments of inequality.

Inequality in risks of healthy life expectancy

It is not clear whether the methods employed by WHO to estimate the underlying distributions of risk are applicable to settings where there are no data at the individual level. Wolfson and Rowe (2001) raise concerns about using small geographic area data in these models, as the models are based on the assumption that the population within the areas is homogeneous; in cases where this assumption does not hold, these methods should not be used.

Index of child survival inequality

Szwarcwald (2002) emphasizes the fact that for a majority of countries the index of child survival inequality was not based on child survival data, but estimated using a regression model. This is viewed as a major weakness of WHR 2000.

The choice of the age group (survival up to age 2) has been justified on the basis that mother's recall of child survival beyond age 2 may be defective, and that the survival risks and their distribution are not significantly different for older children (up to age 5). However, there are significant differences in the causes and risks of child death at different ages (neo-natal, infant, and child) and at different levels of overall mortality (high and low), thus calling into question the appropriateness of this age-grouping to capture inequality in child survival.

As the index of child survival inequality (a generalized Gini coefficient) is homogeneous of degree 2.5, it matters whether survival time is measured in months or years (Szwarcwald 2002). Moreover, defining the index of child survival equality as the complement of the index of child survival inequality (1 minus the index of inequality) would be strictly correct only if the latter is a relative measure (Szwarcwald 2002). Both these considerations affect the scale used to measure inequality.

As the index is a generalized Gini coefficient, it will not be decomposable into additively separable components (with the between- and within-components adding up to total inequality). This makes the measured contributions of the different 'components' of inequality dependent on the order in which they are introduced into the decomposition exercise (e.g. holding income constant first and then education, or vice-versa). Hence the magnitude of the components will be difficult to assess unambiguously.

The empirical values of the inequality measure demonstrate a very tight range across countries with low child mortality. However, it has been remarked in the literature that significant residual social-group inequalities in child survival do exist in these low mortality countries but are not captured by the WHO inequality index (Houweling et al. 2001; Leon et al. 2001; Szwarcwald 2002).

The specification of the risks of child survival that are related to maternal characteristics may not include important residential and environmental covariates. As noted by Wolfson and Rowe (2002), the cross-sectional DHS data may not be of sufficiently high quality to estimate inequality in risks.

DHS data are used to derive the measure of child survival inequality in the year 2000. However, DHS data are collected infrequently in most countries, and the year 2000 estimates of inequality cover a wide range of years (e.g. 1975–1985, 1985–1995). Szwarcwald (2002) raises questions about what these estimates actually represent in terms of the data

under consideration, and about what the realistic time interval should be for the calculation of inter-temporal change.

As pointed out by Braveman et al. (2001), Houweling et al. (2001), Leon et al. (2001), Ugá et al. (2001) and Szwarcwald (2002), the policy value of the WHO measure of 'total health inequality' relies on an analysis of its determinants, which was not included in WHR 2000.

Key technical issues

Equality standard. The current WHO approach to health inequality measurement is based on the total inter-individual variation in health for a population. The unresolved question is whether there is an appropriate common fairness standard for all countries against which to assess this variation.

Alpha parameter—aversion to inequality. The values of this parameter are likely to be dependent on the age group and type of health outcome under consideration. For example, populations may have more aversion to a certain level of inequality in children's health compared with a similar level of inequality in adults' health. Similarly, the alpha parameter may be more sensitive to inequality in survival than in states of (ill-) health.

Beta parameter—absolute versus relative measures. It is important to note that the WHO measure of total health inequality falls between a purely absolute and a purely relative measure. As such it is different from most measures used in the literature and WHO should be clear as to its interpretation.

Estimation of alpha and beta. On the empirical side, a more transparent estimation procedure for the alpha and beta parameters is desirable. At present, it is not clear that the information obtained through the internet surveys uniquely identifies a person's alpha and beta parameters in the inequality formula.

3. WHO RESPONSES AND PROPOSALS

Total or partial health variation

WHO suggests that social-group inequalities in health outcomes ignore the within-group inequalities that exist in social groups, and argues that the poor health expectancy of individuals should be of concern independently of their membership of a social group. Therefore, WHO proposes to continue to measure overall or total health inequality in a population, ideally in terms of inequality in health-adjusted life expectancy (HALE). In addition, it proposes to introduce a special focus on the health of the poor, using data on assets ('permanent income') from the World Health Survey to identify the poor.

WHO has intensified efforts to increase the availability of data through multiple sources including DHS, the Pan-Arab Project on Children, the UNICEF Multiple Indicator Cluster Surveys (MICS), and an abridged birth history module in WHS (for countries that do not have a recent DHS). Relevant birth history data from up to 120 countries should be available for the next round of estimation of inequality in child survival.

The covariates of risk of child mortality have been used in a 'decomposition' analysis to identify the effect of changing one covariate on the inequality index, e.g. removing inequality in income or improving education levels. This work represents an explicit response by WHO to the critique concerning the policy relevance of measuring pure inter-individual inequality. The analysis attempts to identify the main sources of inequality in a population with a view to suggesting policies and interventions to reduce these inequalities. For example, improving access to health care appears to lower the inequality index of child survival.

Inequality in adult health

In response to the criticisms about the lack of relevance of the indicator for high-income countries, WHO is proceeding with the development of methods to estimate inequality in healthy life expectancy. A survival analysis model has been developed to estimate the distribution of adult mortality risk. This model is similar to the one used for children, and can be used on individual level data from health surveys and censuses that have been linked to vital registration information in some Member States. The survival analysis model includes a shared frailty component that is able to capture unmeasured community effects on adult mortality.

This approach, while appropriate for high-income countries with sophisticated vital registration systems and computerized census and health survey databases, is difficult to apply in the majority of Member States. For Member States where individual-level data are not available, statistical techniques are being developed by WHO to estimate the distribution of mortality risk from small-area data. Wolfson and Rowe (2002) and Szwarcwald (2002) note that the approach of

using small-area data depends on the construction of the geographical areas and the homogeneity of the population in them. Inevitably, small-area data will underestimate the true level of inequality. In order to quantify the extent of under-estimation, WHO proposes to compare results from small-area data analysis with results from individual-level data analysis for about 10 Member States where both types of data are available.

Statistical models and micro-simulation techniques developed and already in use at Statistics Canada will help in the implementation of this strategy. If a systematic relationship is found between the estimates from the two types of data, small-area data can be used with more confidence to estimate the distribution of mortality risk for adults where individual-level data are not available. In this case, WHO would proceed with small-area analysis of health inequality in a number of Member States (approximately 50 to 60) where vital registration and health data exist for relatively homogeneous small areas, such as municipalities or counties.

Inequality in health states

In WHR 2000 there were no measures of health inequality related to non-fatal health outcomes. This not only reflects the absence of data for such an assessment but also the challenge of identifying an appropriate indicator of non-fatal health that is amenable to inequality measurement.

In its Multi-Country Survey Study 2000–2001, WHO has collected data on health states for nationally representative samples of males and females of all ages in a manner that allows for cross-country comparisons. WHO proposes to incorporate the distribution of health states by age and sex into the estimation of HALE for Member States. Preliminary results from the analysis of these data suggest that the observed trends in survival, where there is more variation for males than for females, are different from trends in non-fatal health outcomes, where there is more variation for (adult) females than for (adult) males. This highlights the importance for WHO to complete this analysis and continue with the implementation of WHS for reporting on health inequality in the future.

4. SPRG COMMENTS AND RECOMMENDATIONS

Total or partial health variation

The concept of total health inequality defined as 'inter-individual variation' raises the question of the purpose of measuring inequality in health. Are health systems interested in assessing distributional performance by describing total variation (which is perhaps an over-inclusive notion of inequality)? Or are health systems interested in assessing distributional performance by describing inequalities that are thought to be unfair (which are a sub-set of the total variation)? SPRG recommends that WHO should continue to foster open debate on these two approaches.

Single *or multiple measures of inequality*

We acknowledge that WHO needs to use a single measure of inequality in its final estimation of health-system attainment. But as the average level of population health is reported separately by WHO, this measure can be a purely relative one. In addition to the single measure used in HSPA, WHO should also report on health inequality using alternative summary measures such as the inter-quartile range, the Gini coefficient, and the coefficient of variation. A combination of measures may need to be calculated to encompass concerns about distinct aspects of inequality.

Social group measures of inequality

SPRG endorses WHO plans to estimate separately the health of the poor and the non-poor in Member States. SPRG also recommends that a broader range of social inequalities in health be assessed, including gender and racial (or ethnic) inequalities. These social groupings raise fundamental issues related to the norms against which the inequalities are assessed, e.g. genetic differentials in survival between the sexes. WHO should take account of the current policy environment to assess which of these group stratifiers is most useful in identifying inequalities. For example, the pervasive move towards decentralized health systems raises the importance of being able to identify both within- and between-district inequalities in health. SPRG noted that there was no conceptual or empirical attempt to assess gender inequalities in health in WHR 2000.

Inequality in individual risks

Further validation of the approach proposed by WHO to measure inequality in the distribution of health expectancy is recommended. It should be sensitive to the extreme ranges in levels of mortality across countries, and not overly dependent on the level of healthy life expectancy.

Index of child survival inequality

A number of technical recommendations on the index of child survival inequality follow:

- More explicit deliberation is needed about the equality standard against which inequality in health performance is assessed.

- Further estimates of the alpha parameter used to incorporate aversion to inequality are required for different age groups and for different health outcomes.

- Instead of relying exclusively on a hybrid absolute-relative measure, separate indices of relative and absolute inequality would help to clarify the different impact they have on assessing both the level of, and trends in, inequality.

- The robustness of the current index should be evaluated further by comparing it to more tightly defined age-group measures of inequality, e.g. neonatal, infant, and child.

- The sensitivity of the index to inequality in high-, medium- or low-mortality settings should be explored, and if necessary an index developed that is appropriately sensitive.

- The current risk model (based on cross-sectional DHS data) should be validated by using longitudinal data on child survival from demographic surveillance sites such as Matlab, Bangladesh or Navrongo, Ghana.

- Approaches to reporting the inequality index for estimates based on data collected in different years and in different countries, but reported for a single year (e.g. 2000), should be standardized.

- Given the rate at which new child survival data are generated, guidelines for the frequency of reporting on the 'Index of Inequality in Child Survival' should be developed.

Decomposition of the inequality index

Further work should specify whether the models of the determinants of inequality in child survival perform differently from the models of the determinants of average child survival. WHO should take advantage of longitudinal data to develop more robust models of the determinants of inequality to understand better the extent to which modifying risk factors alters inequality.

Adult health inequality

SPRG recommends that WHO proceeds with the evaluation of small area variation as a basis for deriving reliable estimates of adult inequality.

Data requirements

Given the number of countries in WHR 2000 for which data were missing for the estimates of child survival inequality, it is likely that an absence of data will limit more ambitious inequality measurement efforts, e.g. for a broader range of age-sex groups and health states. The data intensity of these methods raises significant concerns about whether countries, especially those with limited health-information systems, will be able to invest in such data. WHO should propose strategies for the sustainability of the assessment of health inequality at regular time intervals.

General recommendations for future development

Although fairness in the distribution of health is a key performance criterion of health systems, it is not clear that the current 'Index of Inequality in Child Survival' actually informs the fairness in health outcomes component of HSPA. The literature, experts and members of SPRG have raised a considerable number of conceptual and technical challenges, some of which have been addressed, while others are only beginning to be explored. For these reasons SPRG believes that the health inequality aspect of HSPA would benefit from further conceptual, technical and practical discussion and development in collaboration with international experts.

Given the extent to which other inequality measures—e.g. effective access and coverage inequality—draw on the conceptual framework of the approach to health inequality (inter-individual inequality in the probability of an event), these measures too should be included in a robust indicator development process that engages appropriate technical and country-based constituencies.

REFERENCES

Braveman, P, B Starfield, and HJ Geiger (2001): World Health Report 2000: How it removes equity from the agenda for public health monitoring and policy. *British Medical Journal*, 323(7314): 678–681.

Houweling, TA, AE Kunst, and JP Mackenbach (2001): World Health Report 2000: inequality index and socioeconomic inequalities in mortality. *Lancet*, 357(9269): 1671–1672.

Leon, DA, G Walt, and L Gilson (2001): International perspectives on health inequalities and policy. *British Medical Journal*, 322: 591–594.

Szwarcwald, CL (2002): On the World Health Organisation's measurement of health inequalities. *Journal of Epidemiology and Community Health*, 56: 177–182.

Ugá AD, CM Almeida, CL Szwarcwald, C Travassos, F Viacava, JM Ribeiro, NR Costa, PM Buss, and S Porto (2001): Considerations on methodology used in the World Health Organization 2000 Report. *Cadernos de Saude Publica*, 17(3): 705–712.

Wolfson, M and G Rowe (2001): On measuring inequalities in health. *Bulletin of the World Health Organization*, 79(6): 553–560.

IX. Responsiveness: Level and Distribution

1. WHR 2000

Responsiveness was included as an intrinsic goal in the health systems performance framework because the way people are treated when they come into contact with the system can improve or reduce their well-being independently of health outcomes. There were seven domains of responsiveness: dignity, autonomy, confidentiality of information, prompt attention, access to social-support networks, quality of basic amenities, and choice of health-care provider. For WHR 2000, WHO obtained data on responsiveness through key informant surveys for 35 out of 191 countries. Within each of the 35 countries, a single focal person was canvassed. Each focal person selected an average of 50 key informants from a broad range of health-system stakeholders, including consumer groups, to answer a short questionnaire. Focal persons oversaw data capture and submission of data to WHO. Data from two such surveys was not of sufficient quality to be used in WHR 2000.

For the overall measure of responsiveness, key informants were asked to provide a general rating of the health system in their country with respect to the seven domains after they had answered specific questions on each domain. The specific questions were used to ensure that key informants correctly identified the various components of the domains. Correlation and exploratory factor analysis were undertaken to check for consistency. There was a high degree of consistency between the responses to the specific domain questions and the general rating questions.

In the final analysis, the overall domain scores were regressed on a set of covariates for the 33 surveyed countries, and from these regressions the missing data for the remaining 158 countries were imputed. For the distribution of responsiveness, key informants were asked to identify marginalized groups. This information was used together with the information on the size of those groups in the country to develop a responsiveness inequality score (distribution). Once again, the information was imputed for the 158 non-surveyed countries.

2. Main Commentaries and Criticisms

Data sources

Many criticisms were raised on this method of obtaining information (Almeida et al. 2001; Navarro 2001; Blendon et al. 2001a) and estimating the missing data (Williams 2000; Almeida et al. 2001; Aalto 2000). Criticisms included the fact that the method was biased because most of the key informants were WHO people; that the method was inherently flawed as it was not a representative sample of the population; that only seven questions out of 42 were used for the index; and that too many imputations were made from too little data. In particular, it was noted that the data and methods used to estimate responsiveness inequality for the unsurveyed countries resulted in multiple tied ranks (Williams 2000).

Relative weight of responsiveness

Commentators from regional consultations questioned the relative importance of having responsiveness in the framework (WHO Regional Office for the Eastern Mediterranean 2001).

Domain weights

Several commentators questioned the relative weights of the seven domains in the aggregation for an index of overall responsiveness (WHO Regional Office for Europe 2001; WHO Regional Office for South-East Asia 2001; WHO Regional Office for the Western Pacific 2001; WHO Regional Office for Africa 2001).

Responsiveness of the broader health system

Comments were made in regional consultations (WHO Regional Office for Europe 2001; WHO Regional Office for South-East Asia 2001) that responsiveness needed to reflect the broader boundaries of the health system, including public access to information and other services of health protection and promotion (see also Ugá et al. 2001; Travassos 2001; Oswaldo Cruz Foundation 2000).

Sources of information

The Blendon et al. (2001a) critique addresses the issue of who is better qualified to judge health-care systems—key informants or users of the system. Blendon et al. (2001b) state that both satisfaction and responsiveness measures are important when information is canvassed from the population.

Translation, validity and reliability

The critique of Aalto (2000) covers questions related to translating the concept of responsiveness and cross-cultural validity. The issue of cross-cultural validation was also raised in several regional consultations (WHO Regional Office for Europe 2001; WHO Regional Office for South-East Asia 2001; WHO Regional Office for the Western Pacific 2001). Participants in the regional consultations (WHO Regional Office for Africa 2001; WHO Regional Office for the Western Pacific 2001) felt that translation might be a slightly more difficult problem for responsiveness than for other modules owing to the abstractness of the concepts involved (see also Almeida et al. 2001). Aalto (2000) and participants in regional consultations (WHO Regional Office for South-East Asia 2001; WHO Regional Office for the Western Pacific 2001) criticized the availability of standard instrument psychometric data on the responsiveness key informant instrument. Aalto (2000) and the SEARO and WPRO regional consultations (WHO Regional Office for South-East Asia 2001; WHO Regional Office for the Western Pacific 2001) indicated that this type of data should be available for any subsequent responsiveness questionnaire instruments (e.g. in household surveys).

Universality of domains

Aalto (2000) commented extensively on the need to provide a convincing rationale for the choice of domains. The change to household surveys was commended but WHO was cautioned that cross-cultural validation of survey questions on domains should be ensured in any future household survey work. (To some extent this is linked to the issue of translation.) At some of the regional consultations, participants raised the issue of relevance of the domains in different cultural settings (WHO Regional Office for Africa 2001; WHO Regional Office for the Western Pacific 2001; WHO Regional Office for South-East Asia 2001). The critique of Williams (2000) also touched on this issue.

Non-users

A commentary of the Brazilian Ministry of Health (Oswaldo Cruz Foundation 2000) criticized the responsiveness work on the grounds that the WHO indicator was limited to measuring the experiences of people who actually use health services.

3. WHO RESPONSES AND PROPOSALS

Data sources

In order to improve data sources, WHO has focused on developing survey instruments to obtain information from households. The number of countries covered by household surveys will be increased substantially. Some 60 countries have already been surveyed through the Multi-Country Survey Study, and the World Health Survey will cover a further 70 countries. Using the Multi-Country Survey Study data, distributional measures of responsiveness are being developed and tested.

Relative weight of responsiveness

The relative importance of responsiveness within the overall framework is being tackled with new survey questions in the World Health Survey, which are currently being tested.

Domain weights

Since WHR 2000, WHO has launched the Multi-Country Survey Study in which households were asked directly about their relative weights for each domain. In analysing the data from this study, WHO has found that they indicate a common set of rankings of domains across countries, and possibly a tendency towards a common set of weights. However, conclusions on the weight structure across countries are limited by the structure of the original question. New questions to elicit weights from respondents for the domains are being tested in the World Health Survey pilots.

Responsiveness of the broader health system

New questions on heath promotion and support structures for families looking after ill family members at home are being tested in the World Health Survey pilots.

Satisfaction versus responsiveness

The WHO responsiveness survey module is designed using the latest thinking in the field of patient assessment measurement, based on patients' interactions with the health-care system. Satisfaction remains an interesting measure for other reasons because it solicits people's opinions about the system, rather than their reports of personal interactions with it. More work is being done to test the use of techniques to improve cross-population comparability of results from surveys of people's experiences.

Translation, validity and reliability

Since WHR 2000, WHO has developed an extensive translation protocol for the Multi-Country Survey Study, which has been improved further in the piloting of the World Health Survey instrument. In addition, facility surveys are being developed to collect evidence on the validity of the questionnaire instrument. These surveys will enable the comparison of observations on certain domains of responsiveness in facilities with reports from individuals using those facilities. Other standard validity strategies recommended by Aalto (2000) and mentioned by participants in regional consultations (WHO Regional Office for South-East Asia 2001; WHO Regional Office for the Western Pacific 2001), such as comparisons with similar data series, are being pursued. WHO is also continuing to document the results of standard psychometric tests of the household survey instruments.

Universality of domains

WHO has produced a paper documenting the criteria for selection of the domains (De Silva 2000). Since WHR 2000, an eighth domain of responsiveness—clarity of communication—has been included. Questions relating to this new domain were developed in response to consultations and included in the Multi-Country Survey Study. A group of ethicists was asked to review the cross-cultural dimensions of the responsiveness domains. Their findings were submitted to the technical consultation on responsiveness (World Health Organization 2001). In addition, further work is currently underway to map the responsiveness domains to UN and other international conventions and treaties on human rights. More cognitive testing is planned for the responsiveness module items in the World Health Survey.

Non-users

With respect to this critique, efforts have concentrated on finding ways to include non-user and low-user groups. As a first attempt at addressing the non-user

and low-user problem, models to predict responsiveness for non-users and low-users were developed. This proposal was discussed at the technical consultation on responsiveness (World Health Organization 2001), and goes some way to addressing the problem of non-users and low-users. Both the Multi-Country Survey Study and the piloted World Health Survey instruments have included questions regarding utilization.

4. SPRG COMMENTS AND RECOMMENDATIONS

Data sources

SPRG members agree with the criticisms made by external commentators about the data sources. In particular, SPRG members concur that people using health systems should be asked their opinion about it, rather than relying on information from key informants. They recommend that if the indicator of responsiveness is to be utilized in future, it will be necessary for WHO to obtain representative household-level data for all countries.

Relative weight of responsiveness

Some SPRG members were concerned with the inclusion of 'responsiveness' for the evaluation of health-systems performance. Responsiveness as defined by WHO is meant to deal with the interactions of users with the health system, and includes features such as respectful treatment, confidentiality of information, prompt attention, and involvement in decision-making. Such features apply to many service activities, e.g. educational services, transportation services, etc. Some SPRG members therefore felt that it might be better to deal with issues of responsiveness generically, i.e. at the national (or even international) level rather than at the health-system level. Other members rejected this notion and pointed out that if responsiveness was measured at the national level, accountability could only be attributable at that level—and not at the health-system level.

SPRG members were also surprised that the weight on responsiveness in the composite indicator was as high as 25%, the same weight as for average health level. This implies that a one-point increase in responsiveness is valued as highly as a one-point increase in the scale used for health (equivalent to almost one year of health-adjusted life expectancy). In view of the implied trade-off, SPRG members wondered whether appropriate questions had been asked to elicit the relative weights for responsiveness and the intrinsic goal of average health level. SPRG members also wondered whether it might have been appropriate to incorporate a changing set of weights for responsiveness at different stages of health-system development. (The present set of weights is constant for all levels of development.) It could be argued that a greater weight attaches to pure health goals relative to responsiveness at low levels of life expectancy (e.g. 50 years) than at high levels of life expectancy. Once life expectancy reaches 70 or more years, as in the OECD countries, it may be more appropriate to use a relatively larger weight on responsiveness. At high levels of life expectancy the room for further improvement in health is limited, and other goals—such as responsiveness of the health system—may assume greater importance.

Domain weights

Several commentators (WHO Regional Office for Europe 2001; WHO Regional Office for South-East Asia 2001) suggested that the responsiveness domains should be given country-specific weightings in the aggregation of the domains into an index of overall responsiveness (while maintaining the relative weight of overall responsiveness vis-à-vis other goals of the health system). SPRG members also recommend that WHO experiments with a non-linear system of weights to reflect changing priorities that might attach to responsiveness relative to pure health goals at different stages of development. It was recognized that some of the responsiveness measures deal with human rights issues, such as dignity and confidentiality, which need to be addressed at all stages of development. An appropriately specified non-linear system of weights can accommodate constant linear weights on certain domains of responsiveness.

Some SPRG members suggested that WHO assess the relationship between the level of responsiveness (by domain) in a country and the level of financial resources available to its health system. This approach will help assess whether there is a differential capacity in countries for producing responsiveness.

Responsiveness of the broader health system

Some SPRG members also questioned the use of the term 'responsiveness'. Responsiveness of the health system could be construed to include several other features apart from interactions with the population—such as the delivery of health services, health promotion and protection, and health education. The term has often been confused with the notion of how well the health system 'responds'. In consequence, some SPRG members suggested that WHO should consider

changing the term 'responsiveness' to something like 'interactions with users'. Other SPRG members suggested that possibly a term like 'patient-/people-centredness' or 'patient rights' might work.

Some SPRG members suggested that WHO should conduct a thorough survey to identify potential questions that address responsiveness as it relates to health promotion and disease prevention.

Based on the critiques and their own assessment, SPRG felt that the present WHO questionnaire on responsiveness was geared to eliciting information mainly on personal health services, and that health promotion and protection activities were relatively neglected. Some SPRG members also wished to see the responsiveness of financing activities assessed.

Taken together, SPRG felt that there was a case for extending the responsiveness domains to aspects of health-system activities beyond personal health-care services—e.g. early warning systems in the case of epidemics or other biological or environmental health threats, health promotion and protection, health education in schools, research, etc.

Satisfaction versus responsiveness

SPRG agrees with Blendon et al. (2001a) that users rather than key informants should be the judges of the health-care system. SPRG acknowledges the usefulness of satisfaction measures in general, but feels they are not necessarily a substitute for responsiveness in the framework of HSPA. For example, a person might feel satisfied because he was cured, but he may not have received prompt attention or have been treated with respect. Alternatively, a person might feel satisfied if he were prescribed drugs, even if these drugs were unnecessary, or harmful, for his condition.

In this regard it should be noted that, unlike responsiveness, measures of satisfaction do not adjust for people's differing expectations of the health system. This adjustment is made through the HOPIT approach (see Section XIII on Cross-Population Comparability).

SPRG recommends that WHO should continue work on developing experience measures and the use of vignettes and other techniques for dealing with cultural differences in expectations and response tendencies.

Translation, validity and reliability

Ensuring the accuracy of translation is a difficulty faced by all surveys administered in multiple languages. In particular, in a country with many dialects, the infeasibility of issuing a questionnaire in all its languages and dialects presents obvious problems in administering interviews. (For example: Was the interviewer able to communicate in the respondent's dialect? How well was the interviewer able to translate concepts and questions on the spot? Did he use exactly the same wording for different households?) SPRG members as well as participants in the regional consultations (WHO Regional Office for Africa 2001; WHO Regional Office for the Western Pacific 2001) felt that translation might be a slightly more difficult problem for responsiveness than for other modules owing to the abstractness of the concepts involved.

SPRG recommends that WHO conducts more extensive cognitive testing to evaluate how respondents interpret the survey items. In addition, rigorous interviewer training protocols need to be developed, tested and applied. Training and management of interviews must meet high standards to try to ensure the consistent application of the survey protocols.

Universality of domains

SPRG recommends that WHO should document the mapping of cultural influences on responsiveness domains as well as the mapping of domains onto UN and other international conventions and treaties on human rights.

Non-users

In noting the Brazilian comments (Oswaldo Cruz Foundation 2000, Travassos 2001), SPRG felt that there were indeed serious problems in using an indicator that was limited to measuring the experiences only of people who use health services, especially when making cross-country comparisons. For example, it could turn out that only 20% of the population of country A used its health-care system, and this system was judged to be perfectly responsive by its users (according to the scoring criteria). In contrast, in country B, 80% of the population used its health-care system, which was judged to be only 50% responsive by its users. Which system is more responsive?

According to the WHR 2000 definition of responsiveness (experience of users), the health-care system of country A is more responsive. Several SPRG members expressed unease with this logical conclusion. However, the conclusion is inevitable if coverage is not a part of the definition of responsiveness. Indeed, according to some SPRG members, the term 'responsiveness' evokes the idea of a health-care system responding to people's needs. Hence, if people in country A have been put off from using the system

(because of out-of-pocket costs, lack of knowledge, high transport costs, previous bad experience, etc.), this should be reflected in any measure of the responsiveness of the system.

SPRG noted the development of an approach by WHO to predict responsiveness among non-users. However, if the WHO maintains its current approach to measuring responsiveness among the actual users of the system, SPRG recommends that measures of responsiveness should be accompanied by measures of utilization.

REFERENCES

Aalto, AM (2000): Measuring the responsiveness of health care system in the World Health Report 2000. In eds. Häkkinen, U and Ollila, E. The World Health Report 2000: What does it tell us about health systems? Analyses by Finnish Experts. Helsinki, Finland: National Research and Development Center for Welfare and Health (STAKES). *http://www.stakes.fi/english/publicati/Publications.htm*

Almeida, C, P Braveman, MR Gold, CL Szwarcwald, JM Ribeiro, A Miglionico, JS Millar, S Porto, NR Costa, VO Rubio, M Segall, B Starfield, C Travassos, A Ugá, J Valente, and F Viacava (2001): Methodological concerns and recommendations on policy consequences of the World Health Report 2000. *Lancet*, 357(9269): 1692–1697.

Bernard, RH (1994): Research Methods in Anthropology. Qualitative and Quantitative Approaches. AltaMira Press.

Blendon, RJ, M Kim, and JM Benson (2001a): The public versus the World Health Organization on health system performance. *Health Affairs*, 20(3): 10–20.

Blendon, RJ, M Kim, and JM Benson (2001b): Authors respond to WHO critics. *Health Affairs*, 20(4): 253.

Darby, C, N Valentine, and CJL Murray (2000): WHO strategy on measuring responsiveness. Global Programme on Evidence for Health Policy Discussion Papers, No. 23. Geneva, Switzerland: World Health Organization.

De Silva, A (2000): A framework for measuring responsiveness. Global Programme on Evidence for Health Policy Discussion Papers, No. 32. Geneva, Switzerland: World Health Organization.

De Silva, A and N Valentine (2000b): Measuring responsiveness: results of a key informant survey in 35 countries. Global Programme on Evidence for Health Policy Discussion Papers, No. 21. Geneva, Switzerland: World Health Organization.

Häkkinen, U and E Ollila, eds. (2000): The World Health Report 2000: What does it tell us about health systems? Analyses by Finnish experts. Helsinki: National Research and Development Center for Welfare and Health (STAKES). *http://www.stakes.fi/english/publicati/Publications.htm*

Murray, CJL, J Frenk, D Evans, K Kawabata, A Lopez, and O Adams (2001): Science or marketing at WHO? A response to Williams. *Health Economics*, 10(4): 277–282.

Murray, CJL, K Kawabata, and N Valentine (2001): People's experience versus people's expectations. *Health Affairs*, 20(3): 21–24.

Navarro, V (2002): The World Health Report 2000: Can health care systems be compared using a single measure of performance? *American Journal of Public Health*, 92(1): 31–34.

Navarro, V (2001): World Health Report 2000: Response to Murray and Frenk. *Lancet*, 357(9269): 1701–1702.

Navarro, V (2000): Assessment of the World Health Report 2000. *Lancet*, 356(9241): 1598–1601.

Oswaldo Cruz Foundation, Brazilian Ministry of Health (2000): Report of the workshop "Health Systems Performance: The World Health Report 2000". 14-12-2000, Rio de Janeiro.

Travassos, C (2001): Assessing health systems performance—a critical appraisal about the WHO World Health Report 2000 and future developments. Paper presented at Conference on Restructuring of Health Services and Corporate Public Health in the Era of Reforms. 5-7-2001, Maastricht, The Netherlands.

Ugá, AD, CM Almeida, CL Szwarcwald, C Travassos, F Viacava, JM Ribeiro, NR Costa, PM Buss, and S Porto (2001): Considerations on methodology used in the World Health Organization 2000 Report. *Cadernos de Saude Publica*, 17(3): 705–712.

Ustün B, S Chatterji, M Villanueva, L Bendib, C Celik, R Sadana, N Valentine, C Mathers, JP Ortiz, A Tandon, J Salomon, Y Cao, XW Jun, and CJL Murray (2000): WHO multicountry household survey study on health and responsiveness 2000–2001. Global Programme on Evidence for Health Policy Discussion Papers, No. 37. Geneva, Switzerland: World Health Organization.

Ustün, B and CJL Murray on behalf of the World Health Organization Survey Programme (2001): World Health Survey: objectives, design, modules. Global Programme on Evidence for Health Policy, mimeo. Geneva, Switzerland: World Health Organization.

Valentine, N, JP Ortiz, A Tandon, K Kawabata, and CJL Murray (2001): Health System Responsiveness: Evidence from Population Surveys in 15 Countries. Global Programme on Evidence for Health Policy, mimeo. Geneva, Switzerland: World Health Organization.

Valentine, N, J Salomon, and CJL Murray (2001): Weights for responsiveness domains: analysis of country variation in 57 national sample surveys. Global Programme on Evidence for Health Policy, mimeo. Geneva, Switzerland: World Health Organization.

Williams, A (2000): Science or marketing at WHO? A Commentary on 'World Health 2000'. *Health Economics*, 10(2): 93–100.

World Health Organization (2001): Report on WHO meeting of experts: Responsiveness. 13-9-2001, Geneva, Switzerland.

WHO Regional Office for Africa (2001): General Report on the Regional Consultative Meeting on Health Systems Performance Assessment: Final Report. 18-5-2001, Harare, Zimbabwe.

WHO Regional Office for the Americas (2001): Regional consultation of the Americas on Health Systems Performance Assessment, Background Document: Critical issues in health systems performance assessment. Washington, D.C.

WHO Regional Office for the Eastern Mediterranean (2001): Report on the Regional Consultation on the Conceptual Framework for Health System Performance Assessment. 9-7-2001, Ain Saadeh, Lebanon.

WHO Regional Office for Europe (2001): Report of the Regional Consultation on Health Systems Performance Assessment. 3-9-2001, Copenhagen.

WHO Regional Office for South-East Asia (2001): Report of the regional consultation and technical workshop on health systems performance assessment. 18-6-2001, New Delhi, India.

WHO Regional Office for the Western Pacific (2001): Report of the regional consultation on health system performance. 3-7-2001, Manila, Philippines.

X. Fairness in Financial Contribution

1. WHR 2000

WHO began its analysis of the fairness of household financial contributions to a health system by asking the question: Taking society's efforts to redistribute income as a given, what are fair contributions by households to the health system? As a normative claim, WHO proposed that the sacrifice created by contributing to the health system should be equalized across households independent of their health status or their utilization of health services. This 'equal sacrifice' was interpreted as an equal share of each household's capacity to pay. The goal of the health system was not seen to involve the redistribution of income, but was based on the notion that a health system should be financed in a fair manner.

Household payments to the health system included all financial contributions attributable to the household through taxes, social-security contributions, private insurance, and direct out-of-pocket payments. Household capacity-to-pay was defined as household effective income net of subsistence expenditure, where effective income was taken to be the level of consumption of the household (or 'permanent income' in a life-cycle perspective). Subsistence expenditure typically includes spending on food, basic shelter and minimal clothing, but not on health. However, in WHR 2000, it was not possible to obtain estimates of spending for basic shelter and minimal clothing, so capacity-to-pay was measured simply as total consumption expenditure minus food consumption, and a household's financial contribution (HFC_i) was measured as its total payments to the health system divided by its capacity-to-pay (CTP_i).

A fairness of financial contribution index was constructed to measure inequality in the distribution of household financial contributions. As catastrophic spending was considered to be the first concern of the health-financing system, WHO argued that households with catastrophic health expenditure should be given more weight in the index of inequality. The index should take into account catastrophic expenditure (extreme horizontal inequality) as well as moderate horizontal inequality, and incorporate people's expectations that the rich should pay more in absolute terms than the poor.

The formula used to calculate the Fairness of Financial Contribution Index was

$$FFC = 1 - 4\left(\frac{\sum_{i=1}^{n}\left|HFC_i - \overline{HFC}\right|^3}{0.125n}\right)$$

where

$$\overline{HFC} = \frac{\sum HFC_i}{n}$$

This is an index of individual-mean differences rather than an index of inter-individual differences, and was built on the assumption that people care about their place in relation to the average contribution and judge inequality accordingly. The alternative would be that people care about their place relative to other individuals, and not to the average. The choice of the former index was made after conducting an internet survey of over 1,600 people in which a majority of people appeared to care more about the difference between their contribution and the average for the population than the difference between their contribution and that of every other individual in the population.

The index was estimated for 21 countries which had recently conducted household income and expenditure surveys. The results for these countries were used in a regression analysis to identify critical covariates of the FFC index, and this regression was used to estimate FFC for the remaining 170 countries.

2. Main Commentaries and Criticisms

The commentaries and criticisms covered three general areas: technical questions about the index used in WHR 2000; problems with data availability; and the policy relevance of the FFC index.

The FFC index

The first technical question raised about the FFC index used in WHR 2000 was that it could penalize countries with very progressive payment systems because perfect fairness was defined as the situation in which all households contribute an equal share of their capacity-to-pay. Countries with very progressive payments where the rich pay a higher proportion of their capacity-to-pay than the poor would then be shown as having an unfair health system (Shaw 2001; Wagstaff 2001; Ministry of Health, Vietnam 2001; Wagstaff and Van Doorslaer 2001; Travassos 2001; Ugá et al. 2001; WHO Regional Office for the Americas 2001; World Health Organization 2001).

Secondly, the FFC index is found to be relatively insensitive to vertical inequality (Ammar and Kasperian 2001), an aspect that policy makers can target—as opposed to horizontal inequality, which they cannot so easily target.

Thirdly, measuring capacity-to-pay as total expenditure minus food consumption was criticized because much of the food consumption of the rich is not subsistence spending (Klavus 2000; Navarro 2000). Subtracting food consumption from total expenditure may underestimate the capacity-to-pay of rich households (Ammar and Kasperian 2001).

Fourthly, the technical consultation and some of the regional consultations suggested that the interval-scaling properties of the FFC index had not been established and that the units of the index were not interpretable (Szwarcwald 2002).

Data availability

Household income and expenditure surveys that had appropriate information for the construction of the index were available for only 21 countries. This was not seen as sufficient for estimating an FFC index for all 191 Member States—there was simply too much missing data (Williams 2000; Nord 2002).

Policy relevance of the FFC index

Some commentators at the regional consultations suggested that policy makers needed to have the ability to drill down to the components of the index and to identify the impact on vertical inequality, horizontal inequality and catastrophic payments separately. A second issue was whether policy makers might be interested in the income redistributive effects of health payments in addition to inequality in the financial burden of payments (Wagstaff 2001).

Thirdly, the FFC index does not take account of the utilization of health services (Travassos 2001). A system in which all people pay the same low proportion of their capacity-to-pay would be fair according to the index, but would give no indication about whether people were unable to obtain the care they needed because of its cost.

3. WHO RESPONSES AND PROPOSALS

Since publication of WHR 2000, WHO has undertaken a considerable body of analytical work to explore the implications of the commentaries, criticisms and suggestions made at the consultations, in the literature, and by SPRG members. This has led to a number of background documents being prepared for SPRG and the following proposals have been put to SPRG for the next round of performance assessment.

WHO proposes to report routinely on four indicators of the fairness of financial contributions. The FFC index focuses on the impact of payments on a household's financial burden—in what is referred to as the 'burden space'. In addition to the FFC index, which summarizes inequality in the distribution of financial burdens, a threshold measure—the proportion of households facing catastrophic expenditures due to health payments—will also be reported. Because of interest expressed by policy makers and researchers since WHR 2000, WHO also proposes to estimate and report the impact of health payments in the 'income space'. Two indicators would be used—the impact of health payments on the overall income distribution, and the percentage of households who fall below the poverty line due to health payments. WHO background documents prepared for SPRG showed that it is feasible to use both indicators with the available data, although the different indicators do attempt to capture different concepts.

For the FFC index, WHO proposes to change the mathematical formula by using a cube root function to transform the index back into natural units, thereby improving its interpretability.

$$FFC = 1 - \sqrt[3]{\frac{\sum_{i=1}^{n} \left| HFC_i - HFC_0 \right|^3}{n}}$$

where

$$HFC_0 = \frac{\sum HE_i}{\sum CTP_i}$$

This index still belongs to the individual-mean family and it is an absolute measure of inequality. It retains the property of the earlier FFC index in that it places a larger weight on households with catastrophic expenditure.

WHO also proposes to change the measure of household capacity-to-pay (CTP) in response to the criticism that food expenditure is not a good indicator of subsistence expenditure. CTP will be redefined as total household expenditure minus the level of expenditure corresponding to the international poverty line (in local currency), as long as total expenditure exceeds this poverty line. In households where total expenditure is less than the estimated poverty line, CTP will be taken to be total expenditure minus the actual food expenditure of the household. The poverty line estimate of 'subsistence' is lower for rich households than the total food expenditure that was used in WHR 2000 to define 'subsistence', which increases the apparent capacity-to-pay of the rich.

Perfect fairness is still defined as each household contributing an equal share of its (redefined) CTP. Although it is theoretically possible that countries with very progressive tax systems may depart from total fairness according to this definition, preliminary empirical results from 55 countries suggest that this does not happen in practice.

WHO also reported to SPRG the results of decomposition of the FFC index into different components—those due to extreme horizontal inequality related to catastrophic health expenditure, to mild horizontal inequality, and to vertical inequality. Vertical inequality has a small measured component relative to horizontal inequality. For countries with a low value of the FFC index, inequality is primarily attributable to household catastrophic spending.

Since the publication of WHR 2000, intensive efforts have been made in collaboration with countries to identify new data sources. Currently 104 surveys from 80 countries are available and WHO proposes to continue to seek new sources of data. This will be in addition to questions included in the World Health Survey on assets.

Finally, it is possible that two health systems have the same FFC score—for example, in one system everyone can afford health services, but in the other system a part of the population cannot. WHO proposes, however, that in the second case the population will show poorer levels of health and greater inequalities in health, ceteris paribus, than in the first. Hence the problem of poor access will be reflected in poorer health outcomes and in lower overall goal attainment. To try to account for non-use of services because of inability to pay would be double counting in the FFC index.

4. SPRG COMMENTS AND RECOMMENDATIONS

SPRG endorses the suggestion of routinely reporting on four types of measures of the impact of household financial payments—two in the burden space, and two in the income space. This provides information that is useful to policy makers for different questions that they might wish to address. SPRG also accepts that the new mathematical formulation of the FFC index is an improvement on the original formulation. The need to obtain household survey data from many more datasets was a common and valid source of criticism of WHR 2000. SPRG emphasizes the need for WHO to reduce the estimation of 'missing data' to the minimum.

SPRG members noted that the cubing formula for the FFC index in WHR 2000 may have been responsible in large measure for the finding that horizontal inequality accounted for most of the inequality in financial burdens. Another factor responsible for the relatively small component of vertical inequality (compared with horizontal inequality) was that progressivity had already been built into the index through the definition of capacity-to-pay. SPRG members hypothesized that the greater the degree of progressivity that is built into capacity-to-pay, the smaller will be vertical inequality relative to horizontal inequality in the decomposition of the FFC index.

Some members were concerned about non-utilization of health services by the poor because it was unaffordable. This would lead to the poor making zero financial contributions compared with rich users making significant contributions, and result in an overestimate of measured progressivity (Ammar and Kasperian 2001).

Although the WHO proposal to take the cube root of the differences in the original formula (to transform it back into natural units) might yield better interval-scale properties for the FFC index, it would make decomposition into various components more difficult to undertake. The decomposition of the FFC index would no longer be additively separable into identifiable and easily interpretable components of inequality.

SPRG has the following further comments and recommendations.

(i) WHO should explore ways of controlling for differences in reference periods over which households are asked to report their expenditures. For any given pattern of health expenditures and income flows, the financial burden (or ratio) will be very sensitive to the time frame over which expenditures in the numerator and denominator are measured. An expenditure that is deemed to be catastrophic for a one-week reference period may not be considered catastrophic over a one-month (or longer) reference period. As reference periods differ among the country surveys that are used for the analysis of fairness of financial contributions, cross-country comparisons cannot be made without controlling for these differences.

(ii) Independently of the empirical problems involved in comparing the incidence of catastrophic health expenditures and inequality in FFC across countries, there is a prior conceptual question as to the appropriate time period for assessing financial burden. WHO needs to elaborate and justify the concept of burden with respect to which the fairness of financial contributions should be assessed.

(iii) SPRG supports the use of the poverty line to define capacity-to-pay, and encourages WHO to explore the use of variable poverty lines across different regions.

(iv) The burden need not be defined simply in terms of capacity-to-pay measured as the ratio of expenditure flows over the appropriate time period. An alternative definition might include stock variables in the denominator such as financial and other assets. WHO should explore ways—methodological and empirical—of introducing household assets into the calculation of capacity-to-pay.

(v) In different health insurance systems, there are differences in time-lags between incurring a health expenditure and receiving reimbursement. This can affect the comparability of FFC across different settings.

(vi) Some SPRG members noted that inequality in out-of-pocket payments has different policy implications compared to inequality in overall health financing. They also wished to see an assessment of the financial barriers to fair usage of health services.

(vii) Inequality in financial contributions is affected by utilization of health services when these are paid for out-of-pocket. In predominantly private health-care systems, the poor may not use services because they cannot afford them. WHO should explore the biases that result from comparing measured inequality of financial burdens when

there are different degrees of use and non-use of the system. The present WHO measure of FFC compares systems where financial contributions and utilization are independent with systems where they are endogenous and one depends on the other.

REFERENCES

Almeida, CM, P Braveman, MR Gold, CL Szwarcwald, JM Ribeiro, A Miglionico, JS Millar, S Porto, NR Costa, VO Rubio, M Segall, B Starfield, C Travassos, A Ugá, J Valente, and F Viacava (2001): Methodological concerns and recommendations on policy consequences of the World Health Report 2000. *Lancet*, 357(9269): 1692–1697.

Ammar, W and R Kasperian (2001): What is fair in financing fairness? *Lebanese Medical Journal*, 49(3).

Klavus, J (2000): The Measure of Fair Financing in the World Health Report 2000. In eds. U. Häkkinen and E. Ollila. The World Health Report 2000: What does it tell us about health systems? Analyses by Finnish Experts. Helsinki: National Research and Development Center for Welfare and Health (STAKES). *http://www.stakes.fi/english/publicati/Publications.htm*

Ministry of Health, Vietnam (2001): Comments and suggestions of Vietnam Ministry of Health/Health Policy Unit as regards the World Health Report 2000.

Navarro, V (2000): Assessment of the World Health Report 2000. *Lancet*, 356(9241): 1598–1601.

Nord, E (2002): Measures of goal attainment and performance: A brief, critical consumer guide. *Health Policy*, 59(3): 183–191.

Shaw, RP (2001): The conceptual basis and the scope of health systems performance assessment in the World Health Report 2000. Invited commentary: Regional consultation of the Americas on health systems performance assessment. 8-5-2001, Washington, D.C. *http://w3.whosea.org/hspa/back_cont_commentry.htm*

Szwarcwald, CL (2002): On the World Health Organisation's measurement of health inequalities. *Journal of Epidemiology and Community Health*, 56: 177–182.

Travassos, C (2001): Assessing health systems performance—a critical appraisal about the WHO World Health Report 2000 and future developments. Paper presented at Conference on Restructuring of Health Services and Corporate Public Health in the Era of Reforms. 5-7-2001, Maastricht, The Netherlands.

Ugá, AD, CL Szwarcwald, C Almeida, C Travassos, F Viacava, JM Ribeiro, NR Costa, P Buss, and S Porto (2000): Views on the WHO 2000 Report. Rio de Janeiro: FIOCRUZ.

Ugá, AD, CM Almeida, CL Szwarcwald, C Travassos, F Viacava, JM Ribeiro, NR Costa, PM Buss, and S Porto (2001): Considerations on methodology used in the World Health Organization 2000 Report. *Cadernos de Saude Publica*, 17(3):705–712.

Wagstaff, A (2001): Measuring equity in health care financing: Reflections on and alternatives to the World Health Organization's Fairness of Financing Index. Development Research Group and Human Development Network, World Bank. *http://www.healthsystemsrc.org/*

Wagstaff, A and E Van Doorslaer (2001): Paying for health care: Quantifying fairness, catastrophe, and impoverishment, with applications to Vietnam 1993–1998.

Paper presented at International Health Economics Association (iHEA) Conference. July 2001, York, United Kingdom.

Williams, A (2000): Science or marketing at WHO? A Commentary on 'World Health 2000'. *Health Economics*, 10(2): 93–100.

WHO Regional Office for the Americas (2001): Regional consultation of the Americas on Health Systems Performance Assessment: Final Report. 8-5-2001, Washington, D.C.

World Health Organization (2001): Report on WHO technical consultation on fairness in financial contribution. 4-10-2001, Geneva, Switzerland.

XI. COMPOSITE GOAL ATTAINMENT

1. WHR 2000

A composite index of goal attainment was constructed for each Member State as a weighted sum of attainment on each intrinsic goal (Gakidou et al. 2000; Murray et al. 2000). Weights were obtained from a world-wide-web key informant survey involving more than 1,600 participants from over 100 countries. Fifty per cent of the total weight was ascribed to health (25% to the average level and 25% to inequality), 25% to fairness of financial contributions, and 25% to responsiveness (12.5% to the average level and 12.5% to inequality). Uncertainty intervals were reported for the scores on the attainment index and the associated ranks.

2. MAIN COMMENTARIES AND CRITICISMS

The question of the composite indicator has perhaps received more comments and criticisms than any other issue related to WHR 2000. Some comments have been favourable: for example, the African regional consultation suggested that a composite index may be useful for comparison purposes (WHO Regional Office for Africa 2001). The Americas regional consultation indicated that the direct comparison offered by the composite index may help ministries of health secure increased political attention (WHO Regional Office for the Americas 2001). Several consultations indicated that the composite index might be useful for comparing health systems in countries with similar economic and other background characteristics. Some felt that the index could become useful in the future if the underlying science were improved (WHO Regional Office for South-East Asia 2001).

Many contrary opinions have also been expressed (for example, Ugá et al. 2001; Hurst and Jee-Hughes 2001; Almeida et al. 2001). These arguments can be considered under two broad headings: objections in principle and scientific objections. The objections in principle can be summarized as follows.

- nations have different objectives and priorities with respect to their health systems, which a single composite index cannot capture (Navarro 2000 and 2002; Ozwaldo Cruz Foundation 2000);

- nations operate in different environmental, economic and political circumstances, and comparison is either inappropriate or infeasible (Nord 2002; Häkkinen 2000);

- the composite is not helpful as it offers no policy guidance—more disaggregate data are needed (Nord 2002);

- many countries do not have the capacity to interpret the implications of the index, and so may make inappropriate policy responses;

- the rankings implicit in the composite index generate media coverage that may be unhelpful or misleading (Lancet 2001).

The scientific objections that were made about the WHR 2000 composite index can be summarized as follows:

- there was no agreement on whether the five components of the index were universally appropriate (Coyne and Hilsenrath 2002);

- the components of the index refer to different definitions of the health system (for example, health outcomes to a very broad definition, responsiveness to a narrow definition based predominantly on health care);

- the components of the index refer to different time periods (for example, health outcomes to a long period, responsiveness to the current period);

- the rescaling of the component indicators onto a 0 to 100 scale was arbitrary, and its consequences difficult to understand;

- the weights used in the composite index were derived from key informant interviews and were not representative of population preferences (Almeida et al. 2000; Williams 2000; Smith 2002);

- the methodology for deriving the weights was flawed—in particular, the questionnaire used did not elicit the required relative marginal valuation of an extra unit of performance (Smith 2002);

- the measurement of the individual components of the index was poor;

■ the treatment of 'missing data' was inadequate, and there were too many missing data to make the composite indicator credible (Nord 2002; McKee 2001; Häkkinen 2000);

■ the rankings reported in WHR 2000 are sensitive to the weights used (Oswaldo Cruz Foundation 2000);

■ the methods used were not validated or exposed to adequate scientific review.

Specific recommendations in the literature included:

■ WHO should publish the underlying data, but not aggregate it into a single index;

■ comparisons should be reported only for clusters of comparable countries;

■ different transformations (such as z-scores) should be used for the component measures (Oswaldo Cruz Foundation 2000);

■ different weights or component measures might be used for different clusters of countries, reflecting different circumstances, priorities and objectives;

■ WHO should offer more support for understanding the composite scores and translating into local action;

■ satisfaction, coverage and process measures should be incorporated into the index;

■ better methodology should be adopted for inferring weights (Appleby and Street 2001);

■ better methodology should be adopted for the analysis of uncertainty;

■ a research and development effort on the use on composites should be considered by WHO.

Many different suggestions were made about the advisability of continuing to publish a composite index. Some participants in the regional consultations felt that the Human Development Index had played a useful role in mobilizing opinion and political commitment, and that an aggregate index of health-system attainment could play a similar role. At the other extreme, critics felt that WHO should publish the underlying data on attainment of individual goals but should not aggregate the scores into a single index (Nord 2002).

Other commentators felt that WHO should make comparisons only within clusters of comparable countries (rather than among all 191 Member States taken together), and that it would be appropriate to use dif-

ferent sets of weights or goals for different clusters of countries (Nord 2002). If WHO chose to continue with a composite attainment index, it should offer more support to countries to understand its meaning and to translate the results of the exercise into better policy.

3. WHO Responses and Proposals

WHO has examined some of the above criticisms in preparing for the SPRG meetings. For example, the variability of weights was explored from representative population samples in more than 60 countries as part of the WHO Multi-Country Survey Study 2000-2001. Although the weights do vary, in no household survey was the average reported weight equal to zero for any component. SPRG was presented with scores from 53 countries for which data have been analysed ($n > 51,000$) and the average weights were 46% for health (25% for average level and 21% for inequality), 26% for fairness of financial contributions, and 28% for responsiveness (15% for average level and 13% for inequality). These weights are similar to the weights obtained from the internet survey conducted in 2000.

WHO also examined two methods of recalculating the overall attainment index reported in WHR 2000 to take account of differences in weights observed in the Multi-Country Survey Study (Lauer et al. 2002). In the first, each country's weights were allowed to vary between the minimum and maximum weights observed across all survey countries. For each country, weights were chosen from within this range so as to maximize its overall attainment score, given the country's scores on the five separate goals. This procedure resulted in the highest overall attainment score for each country (with the weights constrained to lie in the ranges observed), and was termed the 'benefit-of-the-doubt' score. The rank correlation between the WHR 2000 score and the 'benefit-of-the-doubt' score of countries was 0.997.

In the second method, weights were again constrained to lie within the ranges observed across the survey countries, but mathematical programming techniques (data envelopment analysis) used in Operations Research were applied to determine the best weights for each country. Weights calculated in this way yielded a third overall attainment score. The rank correlation between this alternative 'benefit-of-the-doubt' score for countries and the original WHR 2000 score was 0.984. The ranking of countries changed as a result of using these two alternative types of 'benefit-of-the-doubt' weights, but all ranks remained within the uncertainty intervals reported in WHR 2000.

WHO has therefore proposed to SPRG that the composite index should continue to be calculated and reported on routinely. Those who prefer to focus on the individual goals can do so because the separate scores would still be reported. To provide a basis for comparability, the average weight across countries would be used to estimate the overall attainment index. Overall attainment using 'benefit-of-the-doubt' weights would also be reported, as would an index based on the weights estimated for each country. Finally, WHO will continue to investigate whether there are systematic determinants of country weights, and will explore alternative methods of eliciting weights for the goals, including the use of survey questions involving trade-offs.

4. SPRG COMMENTS AND RECOMMENDATIONS

Smith (2002) has examined the case for developing a composite score of health-system performance. In summary, the arguments in favour of developing composite indicators of performance (as distinct from separate consideration of the component indicators) include the following.

- They place system performance at the centre of the policy arena, and draw the attention of senior policy makers to the issue.

- They can offer a rounded assessment of system performance.

- They enable subsequent judgements to be made on system efficiency.

- They facilitate communication with citizens and promote accountability.

- They indicate which systems represent the beacons of best performance.

- They indicate which systems represent a priority for improvement efforts.

- They may stimulate the search for better data and better analytic efforts across all of health care.

- Use of a composite performance measure recognizes the trade-offs that exist between different objectives, and leaves local policy makers free to decide along which indicators they have greatest scope for improvement.

Against this, the use of composite indicators (in preference to piecemeal scrutiny of individual perfor-

mance measures) can lead to dysfunctional outcomes for the following reasons.

- By aggregating individual measures of performance, composite indicators may disguise serious failings in some parts of some systems.

- As measures of performance become more aggregate, it becomes increasingly difficult to know to what to attribute poor performance, and therefore what remedial action to take.

- The individual elements used in the composite indicator can often be contentious.

- A composite that seeks to be comprehensive in its coverage may have to rely on very feeble or opaque data in some dimensions of performance.

- A composite that ignores dimensions of performance that are difficult to measure may give misleading messages and distort behaviour in undesirable ways.

- Current methodology for the calculation of weights is still inadequate.

- The weights used in composite indicators reflect a single set of preferences. Yet there may exist great diversity in preferences amongst policy makers and ordinary citizens—in short, a composite indicator does not respect alternative viewpoints.

In light of these observations, SPRG considers that the first requirement is that WHO makes a strategic decision whether it wishes to continue with publication of the composite scores and rankings. There will always be variation in the weights attached by individuals and nations to health-system objectives, and the decision to construct a composite is therefore ultimately a strategic (or policy) decision rather than a scientific judgement. However, the practical scientific difficulties of developing a satisfactory composite score may be an important element in informing this strategic decision.

If a decision is taken to continue to publish a composite attainment score, SPRG believes that WHO should indicate clearly that the science of composite indices is still in the process of development. Any results from this analysis should not be interpreted as a definitive judgement on health-system attainment. In addition, the following scientific issues arise.

(i) The fact that the different components of the composite index relate to different concepts of the 'health system' needs careful attention. For example, it is unrealistic to attribute current health outcomes to the current health system. For this reason, we recommend that the components of the composite index should be reconsidered in the light of the responses to WHR 2000. One possibility would be to examine whether some measures of process should be included.

(ii) The quality of many of the data used in constructing the WHR 2000 composite index was deficient. We welcome the subsequent efforts made by WHO to improve the quality of the measurement instruments used and the availability of data, and recommend that the process of data improvement continues to be given a high priority.

(iii) The treatment of 'missing data' in WHR 2000 was inadequately documented. We welcome signals that WHO is beginning to develop its thinking about this issue (Murray et al. 2001). SPRG recommends that WHO methodology in this area is developed further, in discussion with relevant experts, and that the technical judgements made in the treatment of 'missing data' are transparent and well-documented.

(iv) SPRG welcomes the principle of seeking to report uncertainty intervals around estimates of attainment. The WHR 2000 analysis of uncertainty included the construction of distributions (of estimates of attainment) based on sampling error and parameter estimation. However, it did not include 'second-order' sources of error, such as model specification or measurement errors. We recommend a more transparent approach to the treatment of uncertainty, which may inter alia require reconsidering the basis of the 'sampling distributions' from which uncertainty intervals are calculated.

(v) In order to construct the composite indicator, each of its constituent components is transformed onto a common scale of 0 to 100. These transformations are inextricably linked to the set of weights used in the composite, and should in principle be designed such that the chosen set of weights is valid at every level of attainment. (Alternatively the weights could be allowed to vary depending on the level of attainment.) We therefore recommend that WHO reconsiders the methods it uses to transform indicators, and ensures that they are consistent with the set of weights employed.

(vi) The derivation of the weights used in the composite index in WHR 2000 was rightly criticized for a number of reasons. It is imperative that WHO reconsiders its methodology for eliciting weights in order that the inferred weights are consistent with the scales used to measure a unit of attainment in each dimension. SPRG welcomes WHO efforts to seek a more representative basis for deriving weights (through WHS) and using more scientific methods to elicit respondents' preferences. We recommend that these efforts are pursued with vigour, in consultation with relevant experts.

(vii) SPRG believes it is imperative that policy makers and other users should be able to understand and act on any composite measure of performance. To that end, it recommends that, in parallel with technical improvements, WHO seeks vigorously to improve the capacity of users. Possible methods include:
   - offering a transparent exposition of the data sources and methods used (limitations as well as advances);
   - presenting more disaggregate data as a means of 'drilling down' in order to understand better the components of a composite score, perhaps in the form of a balanced scorecard;
   - developing local analytic capacity.

(viii) The natural starting point for performance assessment is a country's year-on-year change in attainment. SPRG views with some concern the likelihood that a country's composite index will change from year to year purely because of methodological changes. It therefore recommends that WHO should give careful consideration to how countries can be offered a useful time series of data which is not open to misinterpretation.

References

Almeida, CM, P Braveman, MR Gold, CL Szwarcwald, JM Ribeiro, A Miglionico, JS Millar, S Porto, NR Costa, VO Rubio, M Segall, B Starfield, C Travassos, A Ugá, J Valente, and F Viacava (2001): Methodological concerns and recommendations on policy consequences of the World Health Report 2000. *Lancet*, 357(9269): 1692–1697.

Appleby, J and A Street (2001): Health system goals: life, death, and...football. *Journal of Health Services Research and Policy*, 6(4): 220–225.

Coyne, JS and PH Hilsenrath (2002): The World Health Report 2000: Can health care systems be compared using a single measure of performance? *American Journal of Public Health*, 92(1): 30–33.

Gakidou, EE, CJL Murray, and J Frenk (2000): Measuring preferences on health system performance assessment. Global Programme on Evidence for Health Policy Discussion Papers, No. 20. Geneva, Switzerland: World Health Organization.

Häkkinen, U (2000): Assessment of the goal attainment and efficiency of health systems in the World Health Report 2000. In eds. U Häkkinen and E Ollila. The World Health Report 2000: What does it tell us about health systems? Analyses by Finnish Experts. Helsinki: National Research and Development Center for Welfare and Health (STAKES). *http://www.stakes.fi/english/publicati/Publications.htm*

Hurst, J and M Jee-Hughes (2001): Performance measurement and performance management in OECD health systems. Labour Market and Social Policy—Occasional Papers, No. 47. Paris, France: Organization for Economic Co-operation and Development (OECD).

Lancet (2001): Why rank countries by health performance? Editorial. *Lancet*, 357(9269): 1702–1703.

Lauer, J, D Evans, and CJL Murray (2002): Measuring health system attainment: the impact of variability in the importance of social goals. Global Programme on Evidence for Health Policy, mimeo. Geneva, Switzerland: World Health Organization.

McKee, M (2001): Measuring the efficiency of health systems. *British Medical Journal*, 323(7308): 295–296.

Murray, CJL, C Mathers, J Salomon, and A Lopez (2001): Evidence for health policy: Dealing with missing data, uncertainty and ignorance. Global Programme on Evidence for Health Policy, mimeo. Geneva, Switzerland: World Health Organization.

Murray, CJL, J Lauer, A Tandon, and J Frenk (2000): Overall health system achievement for 191 countries. Global Programme on Evidence for Health Policy Discussion Papers, No. 28. Geneva, Switzerland: World Health Organization.

Navarro, V (2000): Assessment of the World Health Report 2000. *Lancet*, 356(9241): 1598–1601.

Navarro, V (2002): The World Health Report 2000: Can health care systems be compared using a single measure of performance? *American Journal of Public Health*, 92(1): 31–34.

Nord, E (2002): Measures of goal attainment and performance: A brief, critical consumer guide. *Health Policy*, 59(3): 183–191.

Oswaldo Cruz Foundation, Brazilian Ministry of Health (2000): Report of the workshop "Health Systems Performance: The World Health Report 2000". 14-12-2000, Rio de Janeiro.

Rosén, M (2001): Can the WHO Health Report improve the performance of health systems? *Scandinavian Journal of Public Health*, 29(1): 76–80.

Smith, P (2002): Developing composite indicators for assessing overall system efficiency. In ed. P Smith. Measuring up: improving health systems performance in OECD countries. Paris, France: OECD.

Ugá, AD, CM Almeida, CL Szwarcwald, C Travassos, F Viacava, JM Ribeiro, NR Costa, PM Buss, and S Porto (2001): Considerations on methodology used in the World Health Organization 2000 Report. *Cadernos de Saude Publica*, 17(3): 705–712.

Williams, A (2000): Science or marketing at WHO? A Commentary on 'World Health 2000'. *Health Economics*, 10(2): 93-100.

Williams, A (2001): Science or marketing at WHO? Rejoinder from Alan Williams. *Health Economics*, 10(4): 283–285.

World Health Organization (2000): The World Health Report 2000. Health systems: improving performance. Geneva, Switzerland: World Health Organization.

WHO Regional Office for Africa (2001): General Report on the Regional Consultative Meeting on Health Systems Performance Assessment: Final Report. 18-5-2001, Harare, Zimbabwe.

WHO Regional Office for the Americas (2001): Regional consultation of the Americas on Health Systems Performance Assessment: Final Report. 8-5-2001, Washington, D.C.

WHO Regional Office for South-East Asia (2001): Report of the regional consultation and technical workshop on health systems performance assessment. 18-6-2001, New Delhi, India.

XII. Data Quality and Data Collection Strategies

1. WHR 2000

The following comments pertain to data quality and data collection methods that were employed in WHR 2000. Data availability and data quality are critical issues for all the health systems performance measures in the report and supporting technical documentation and background papers. This brief discussion on data will be confined to broader data quality and availability issues, and will specifically comment on the World Health Survey (WHS). In-depth data issues that pertain to 'Responsiveness' and 'Fairness in Financing' are discussed in the respective sections.

2. Main Commentaries and Criticisms

Some of the strongest and most widespread criticisms of WHR 2000 related to data quality and availability (for example, Williams 2000; Oswaldo Cruz Foundation 2000; Ugá et al. 2000). The main strands of criticism were as follows:

(i)   that estimates were based on covariates in the absence of primary data on fairness-in-financial contribution, responsiveness, health inequalities, non-fatal health outcomes, death rates and life tables;

(ii) that data were collected from key informants who may not be an appropriate source of information;

(iii) that data requirements for HSPA are too onerous and resource intensive;

(iv) that quality assurance was inadequate.

3. WHO Responses and Proposals

(i) Absence of primary data

For the most part WHO relied on datasets available within WHO, or on datasets consisting of national surveys, other surveys such as the DHS, and available household income and expenditure surveys. The only primary data collection efforts by WHO were a web-based survey to elicit information on the weighting of the different health goals, and a Key Informant Survey to obtain information on responsiveness in 33 countries. Acknowledging the limited scope of primary data collection for WHR 2000, new methods have been developed and surveys launched to improve data collection. This includes the World Health Survey (WHS), which will be conducted in more than 70 countries. The methodology for WHS is based on the Multi-Country Survey Study 2000–2001 and is documented in Üstün et al. (2000).

(ii) Inadequacy of key informants approach

The key informant strategy is an inexpensive method of obtaining information on certain domains. WHO argue that for some domains, properly selected key informants may in fact provide more valid and less biased responses than the general population, owing to key informants' specific knowledge of these areas. In this approach the choice of key informants requires close attention so as to avoid possible biases.

In order to address this question empirically, WHO has collected data on responsiveness and health-system goals from key informants, selected through a snowball sampling technique from lists of health professionals and administrators. The set of questions asked were a subset of those in the questionnaire for the Multi-Country Survey Study, which canvassed the general population. As these two surveys were carried out in the same countries, WHO is able to compare the responses of the key informants and the general population, and address issues of systematic bias. Facility studies and exit interviews are also being planned by WHO to address issues concerning validity.

(iii) Data collection

To build consensus on data collection strategies and avoid duplication of efforts, WHO will collaborate with national agencies as well as with international organizations carrying out surveys such as DHS, LSMS, EURO Barometer and MICS. In addition WHO will provide technical support to countries or agencies wishing to include the WHO Survey instrument in whole or in part in their ongoing data collection strategies. It will build capacity in countries that request support for the introduction of quality assurance and analytical survey techniques.

(iv) Quality assurance

WHO is putting in place a range of quality assurance instruments. The World Health Survey is an important tool to support the quality assurance process. Within Member States a competitive bidding process has been put in place for the execution of WHS.

4. SPRG COMMENTS AND RECOMMENDATIONS

Data required to calculate all five components of the composite index for WHR 2000 were absent for most countries. Where data were available, the quality was not always of a high standard.

Documentation of methods and treatment of missing data

Most critiques of health systems performance assessment repeated the comment that the methodologies used, data sources, and assumptions made in the analyses of WHR 2000 were not adequately documented (Williams 2000; Almeida et al. 2001; McKee 2001).

SPRG recommends that, as a means of gaining transparency and confidence, WHO should make particular efforts to explain the treatment of missing data, and should discuss explicitly the assumptions and extrapolations used in the next round of HSPA.

Data not available where needed most

Data availability and data quality are even more of a challenge in countries whose health systems are not well established, where health information systems are rudimentary, or where health systems have collapsed for reasons of war or strife. It is usually the case that these environments are hard to reach, but these may be countries which have the greatest need for HSPA as a tool for change.

SPRG recommends that HSPA clearly needs to acknowledge this dilemma as a limitation, even though it is recognized that WHO cannot always overcome this difficulty.

SPRG recommends that WHO should make a deliberate effort for early implementation of the WHS in those countries and environments that have the least developed health-information systems.

Data collection

Wherever possible WHO should rely on existing data collection efforts within Member States and coordinate collection activity with the respective data agencies.

Collection of country statistics

The processes adopted in collecting and collating the data used in WHR 2000 are not adequately documented.

SPRG recommends that WHO helps to strengthen national data collection processes, including the government agencies that release official country statistics and data. This approach would immediately take care of potential disputes concerning the acceptability of the data used, but for validation purposes other sources should also be explored.

Data quality

Where data are available, their quality needs to be examined very carefully before any conclusions are drawn. Appropriate validation techniques should continue to be applied.

SPRG welcomes the WHO commitment to improved quality assurance methods. It also recommends that countries should participate in the interpretation and validation of the data to ensure that they are acceptable locally.

Key informants

SPRG considers the 'key informant' approach susceptible to errors particularly for the HSPA exercise.

SPRG recommends that the 'key informant' approach should wherever possible be used alongside more objective sources of data. It also stresses that the choice of key informants needs careful consideration.

World Health Survey

WHS has been designed and developed on the basis of experience gained from the Multi-Country Survey Study 2000–2001, which was conducted in approximately 60 countries. WHS is designed on a modular basis with the intention of providing low-cost information that supplements data from national health-information systems to build up an evidence base for policy makers.

The commentaries all identify the need for reliable data and information as a basis for effective health-system monitoring. The African and European regional consultations emphasized the importance of WHS being closely aligned to national health-information systems (WHO Regional Office for Africa 2001; WHO Regional Office for Europe 2001). The SPRG view, based on discussion among colleagues and in country reports, is as follows.

- WHS is potentially very useful, and in broad terms SPRG welcomes its introduction.

- The WHS tool requires further refinement. The choice of modules needs to be reviewed for relevance.

- SPRG recommends that appropriate links are established with other statistical offices and data collection initiatives.

- The survey teams should work closely with countries to ensure that integration with their health-information systems occurs in a meaningful way. While WHS will provide data for HSPA that are currently 'missing', it should not become another parallel system for collecting information that is used exclusively for the HSPA exercise. Rather, WHS should be seen as a mechanism to strengthen existing health-information systems.

- WHS should be self-sustaining, and should not compete for local resources.

- If WHS is to become an important instrument for strengthening national health-information systems, further consideration must be given to its sampling frame. Does the sampling frame enable conclusions to be drawn at sub-national level and comparisons made over time? Local needs must be taken into account in designing the WHS sampling frame.

- The WHS sampling frame should enable information to be obtained on vulnerable groups, such as refugees and itinerant and institutional populations. It is also important that the population covered by the Survey is representative of the population as a whole, including children (and especially girls).

- The issue of cross-population comparability is addressed in Section XIII.

References

Almeida, CM, P Braveman, MR Gold, CL Szwarcwald, JM Ribeiro, A Miglionico, JS Millar, S Porto, NR Costa, VO Rubio, M Segall, B Starfield, C Travassos, A Ugá, J Valente, and F Viacava (2001): Methodological concerns and recommendations on policy consequences of the World Health Report 2000. *Lancet*, 357(9269): 1692–1697.

McKee, M (2001): Measuring the efficiency of health systems. *British Medical Journal*, 323(7308): 295–296.

Oswaldo Cruz Foundation, Brazilian Ministry of Health (2000): Report of the workshop "Health Systems Performance: The World Health Report 2000". 14-12-2000, Rio de Janeiro.

Ugá, AD, CL Szwarcwald, C Almeida, C Travassos, F Viacava, JM Ribeiro, NR Costa, P Buss, and S Porto (2000): Views on the WHO 2000 Report. Rio de Janeiro: FIOCRUZ.

Ustün, B, S Chatterji, M Villanueva, L Bendib, C Celik, R Sadana, N Valentine, C Mathers, JP Ortiz, A Tandon, J Salomon, Y Cao, XW Jun, and CJL Murray (2000): WHO multicountry household survey study on health and responsiveness 2000–2001. Global Programme on Evidence for Health Policy Discussion Papers, No. 37. Geneva, Switzerland: World Health Organization.

Williams, A (2000): Science or marketing at WHO? A Commentary on 'World Health 2000'. *Health Economics*, 10(2): 93–100.

Williams, A (2001): Science or marketing at WHO? Rejoinder from Alan Williams. *Health Economics*, 10(4): 283–285.

World Health Organization (2001): Background documentation: Scientific Peer Review Group meeting. Geneva, Switzerland.

WHO Regional Office for Africa (2001): General Report on the Regional Consultative Meeting on Health Systems Performance Assessment: Final Report. 18-5-2001, Harare, Zimbabwe.

WHO Regional Office for Europe (2001): Report of the Regional Consultation on Health Systems Performance Assessment. 3-9-2001, Copenhagen.

WHO Regional Office for South-East Asia (2001): Report of the regional consultation and technical workshop on health systems performance assessment. 18-6-2001, New Delhi, India.

XIII. Cross-Population Comparability

1. WHR 2000

In making the estimates for WHR 2000, corrections were made for major known biases in available measurements to improve cross-population comparability—for example, for under-reporting of mortality data in vital registration systems. The concept of internal consistency was used as a tool to improve the validity of epidemiological assessments.

2. Main Commentaries and Criticisms

Data criticisms of WHR 2000 were rather severe but this section deals only with the question of cross-country comparability. There has been little public debate and discussion on this issue beyond recognizing it as a problem with self-report data.

3. WHO Responses and Proposals

In examining self-assessed morbidity from survey data across the states of India, Murray and Chen (1992) reported the following findings: Kerala has the highest self-reported morbidity, and Bihar the lowest, across the Indian states. On the other hand, an objective measure of health—such as mortality—reveals that Kerala has a much higher life expectancy than Bihar. Next, a comparison between the US and Kerala shows that self-assessed morbidity in the US is much greater than in Kerala, despite life expectancy in the US being higher than that in Kerala.

What is going on? Are there features of the environment—educational, medical (e.g. frequency of exposure to the health system), income, etc.—that can explain these apparently inconsistent findings? Amartya Sen (1992) in an article in *Philosophy and Public Affairs* tried to understand these results in terms of what he called 'positional objectivity': the 'position' of the individual (in terms of education, income, etc.) matters in the response that is given—but all individuals in the same position will give the same response—hence 'positional objectivity'. In a more recent editorial in the British Medical Journal, he again emphasizes the fact that self-reported morbidity data have limitations that can make its use extremely misleading for policy purposes (Sen 2002).

WHO is seeking to make the responses of individuals comparable (whether they live in different states of India or in the US) by correcting for the 'positions' of the individuals in the different states of India and the US. This is obviously a very important exercise in obtaining health-status information from survey data that is comparable across countries. Moreover, self-reported data on health are still by far the most common source of such information around the world.

As a response to the paucity of representative population-based information on two key variables in the HSPA exercise in WHR 2000, the WHO launched the Multi-Country Survey Study on Health and Responsiveness. For the purposes of HSPA, these survey data are utilized to construct measures of: (i) health-adjusted life expectancy (HALE), and (ii) the level of responsiveness of the health system in a country. For example, the measurement of HALE includes estimates of non-fatal health that are, in part, derived from survey data on the different domains of health (e.g. mobility, cognition, affect, etc.). Similarly, the level of responsiveness of a country's health system is also based on such survey data. Respondents are asked to evaluate their experiences relating to different domains of responsiveness of the health system (e.g. autonomy, dignity, prompt attention, etc.).

There are two characteristics of these survey data that lead to the problem of cross-population comparability. First, the information on the domains is obtained on the basis of self-reporting. Respondents are asked to evaluate their own experience (or perception) with respect to various domains of health and of health-system responsiveness. Secondly, these self-report responses are categorical and ranked ordinally.

One example from the WHO Multi-Country Survey Study for the health domain of mobility illustrates the characteristics of the data. The main self-report question asks respondents how much difficulty they have had in moving around in the past 30 days. Respondents are asked to characterize their mobility using a 5-category ordinal response scale ranging from 1 to 5, where 1 is "Extreme/Cannot do", 2 is "Severe difficulty", 3 is "Moderate difficulty", 4 is "Mild difficulty", and 5 is "No difficulty".

This is where the issue of cross-population comparability arises. The problem with using these self-report data from the domains of health and responsiveness is that the responses are not comparable across countries, or even across different socio-demographic groups within countries. As Figure 61.2 illustrates, the categorical responses can be conceptualized as a mapping from the true level of the domain (here the line labelled "latent mobility scale") to the categorical responses for three different populations A, B, and C. As the figure shows, someone answering "No difficulty" in population A maps to a different interval on the true scale as someone answering "No difficulty" in populations B and C. Obversely, the same level of true mobility could be self-reported by a person in population A as representing "no difficulty", by a person in population B as representing "mild" difficulty, and by a person in population C as representing "moderate" difficulty. The reasons could be due to differing norms, expectations, and experiences of respondents from different populations.

This problem has been previously identified in the psychometrics literature on ability (IQ) testing and, more generally, in educational testing through standardized tests (e.g. GRE, SAT, GMAT, etc.). Certain groups, conditional on ability or knowledge, systematically do better on certain types of questions than other groups. This problem is known as "differential item functioning" in the educational testing and psychometrics literature (Holland and Wainer 1993). For instance, in the item response theory literature, the partial credit model (which is akin to the ordered probit model) specifies the probability of responding in one of two ordered (adjacent) categories as an increas-

ing function of a respondent's ability and a decreasing functioning of the category difficulty. For the same level of ability, the difficulties may be systematically different for different population groups, which will lead to a bias in measured ability. Although this problem is similar to the problem of cut-point shifts in measuring health or health-system responsiveness, the solution methods are somewhat different.

There are basically two strategies that WHO has developed to adjust survey responses for systematic differences in people's attitudes. Both strategies involve the use of a statistical model—the hierarchical ordered probit (HOPIT) model. The first strategy is to use the HOPIT model with 'vignettes'. The second strategy is to use the HOPIT model with measured tests. These are described in turn.

A vignette is a description of a level of ability on a given domain that respondents are asked to evaluate with respect to the same question and then on the same categorical response scale as the main self-report question. A vignette depicts a fixed level of ability on a given domain, so that for that vignette, differences in responses across countries or socio-demographic groups may be attributed to differences in cut-points for the response categories. The response category cut-points are estimated by use of the HOPIT model through a maximum likelihood procedure. These cut-point estimates are used to calibrate the respondent's own self-report in order to make it cross-population comparable. If, for example, respondents from a certain population group systematically give higher categorical responses to the vignettes than respondents from another group, this will show up as a lower cut-point for the first group in the HOPIT estimation.

A second strategy is to calibrate self-report responses using measured tests (instead of vignettes) in conjunction with the HOPIT model. Measured tests are tests of the level of ability of the underlying latent variable for a domain of health. Examples include the posturo-locomotion-manual (PLM) test for mobility, and the Snellen eye chart exam for the domain of vision. Such measured tests are used to estimate cut-point differences across population groups for calibration of self-report responses that are cross-population comparable. The set-up of the HOPIT model with measured tests is quite straightforward. The model assumes that the measured test is correlated with the underlying latent variable for a domain, and the cut-points for a particular categorical response are allowed to differ by population group.

For a variety of reasons including those related to measurement error, it appears that vignettes are a

Figure 61.2 Response category cut-point shift

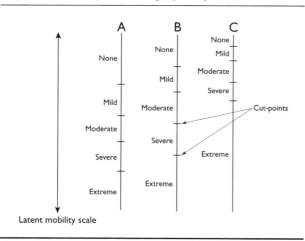

Latent mobility scale

superior mechanism than measured tests for the calibration of self-report responses. Hence, current WHO estimates of outcome measures of health and responsiveness are based primarily on the use of vignettes as a calibration strategy.

4. SPRG COMMENTS AND RECOMMENDATIONS

SPRG welcomed WHO's work in this area and recognized the importance of ensuring that the data used in the HSPA exercise are comparable across populations.

(i) The HOPIT methodology depends crucially on the assumption that the categorical responses derive from a single dimension (or attribute), which can be ordered on a unilinear scale. SPRG noted the responses should not be based on mappings by individuals that involve comparisons in two or more dimensions (of planar or higher-dimensional regions corresponding to the five categories). Application of this methodology requires that the domain of each self-report question is narrowly and unambiguously specified.

(ii) A promising avenue for future research would be to develop statistical methods that combine the information from both vignettes and measured tests in a joint estimation procedure. These methods, akin to the multiple-indicator multiple-cause models in the statistical literature, have the advantage that they take full account of all available information on a given individual, in this case the multiple sources being the individual's self-report (calibrated using vignettes) as well as his/her measured test. These types of methods can also allow for different statistical errors in information that is self-reported and information that is obtained from measured tests.

(iii) The HOPIT model depends critically on the cross-cultural reliability and consistency of the vignettes—e.g. translation problems or errors do not change the meaning of a question so that a different latent variable is being measured. SPRG recommends that the vignettes be tested further in different settings, including through back translation.

(iv) It may be possible to explore some of the problems related to (iii) above through a random coefficients version of the HOPIT model. Unlike the current version of the model, a random coefficients model allows the latent variable associated with each vignette to have its own variance (rather than the variance being the same for all vignettes). This method allows one to take account of the possibility that some vignettes may be inherently 'noisier' than others. This may be of particular relevance for vignettes referring to the middle range(s) of a domain, i.e. for vignettes that are not at either extreme of a domain.

(v) SPRG noted that the HOPIT model not only addressed the problem of cross-population comparability, but also converted the discrete (categorical) information on each domain of health and responsiveness into a continuous variable. For each individual the aggregation of these variables across the appropriate domains generates the continuous distribution from which the mean level of, and inequality in, health (or responsiveness) is estimated. Hence, the HOPIT model yields much more than cross-population comparability: it forms the basis for estimating four of the five intrinsic indicators used in HSPA.

(vi) SPRG members made several technical comments on the HOPIT methodology. Some of these are noted below.

(a) The estimates of the cut-points for a population group (e.g. country) will depend on the universe of groups included in the cut-point estimation. For example, suppose the cut-points for group A are estimated from data for groups A and B. Now, data on group C become available and the cut-points for A are re-estimated from data for all three groups A, B, and C. In general, the cut-points (and other parameter estimates) for group A will change. This could make the relative ranking between, say, groups A and B depend on the precise other groups included in the estimation (especially when considering the aggregates across domains). Hence, caution will need to be exercised in making judgements about the relative ranking between countries, which could be universe-dependent.

(b) The assumption made in the HOPIT model is that the latent variable (e.g. mobility) is unbounded (as the normal distribution is used for the error term). SPRG recommends that the WHO Secretariat check the robustness of their results to restricting the latent variable to a finite interval (e.g. through the assumption of a truncated normal distribution for the error term), as this would seem a more realistic assumption for the domains considered.

(c) SPRG members commented that it would be valuable to estimate non-linear functional forms for the latent variable equation (e.g. health production function), which might also to some extent address the problem noted in (b). A log-linear form for the health production function seems more realistic as it allows for diminishing returns to the factors that determine health (e.g. age, education, etc.), which may be more reasonable than assuming constant returns to each factor. In any case, it would be valuable to check the sensitivity of the present HOPIT results to the assumptions made about the functional form.

REFERENCES

Holland, PW and H Wainer (1993): Differential Item Functioning. Hillsdale, New Jersey: Lawrence Erlbaum Associates, Publishers.

Murray, CJL and LC Chen (1992): Understanding morbidity change. *Population and Development Review*, 18(3): 481–503.

Sen, AK (2002): Health: Perception versus observation. *British Medical Journal*, 324: 860–861.

Sen, AK (1992): Positional objectivity. *Philosophy and Public Affairs*, 22: 126–145.

XIV. Efficiency

1. WHR 2000

This section provides a commentary on the methodology used to measure health-system efficiency in the WHR 2000 statistical analysis, and on the changes proposed for the future. The methods used in WHR 2000 are outlined in World Health Organization (2000), pages 40–44, and the results given in Annex Table 10. Further details of the methods used are provided in Evans et al. (2000) and Tandon et al. (2000). The methodology was subsequently discussed at a WHO meeting of experts (World Health Organization 2001), and the analysis of efficiency with respect to healthy life expectancy has been reported in Evans et al. (2001).

To measure efficiency WHR 2000 used a frontier production function approach, an established technique employed to assess the efficiency of agricultural or industrial production, but which has been extended to the areas of education, local government, and health. This technique estimates the relationship between output and inputs to production, and the highest possible output that could have been produced for each combination of inputs. The ratio of the observed output to the maximum that could have been produced is defined as the efficiency score.

WHO modified this technique to allow for the fact that health outcomes in the absence of a functioning system would still be positive, not zero. So a minimum output level corresponding to the absence of health-system inputs was also estimated, using the relationship observed between literacy and health outcomes in the early 1900s. The inputs used to estimate efficiency in WHR 2000 were health expenditure per capita and average years of schooling of the adult population. Efficiency was estimated for the overall attainment index as well as for health attainment (HALE) separately.

The term "efficiency" is used throughout to denote the level of attainment secured by the health system in relation to spending and environmental inputs (external influences on attainment). In WHR 2000 this concept was referred to as "performance", but on the basis of the regional consultations WHO has decided to denote it as "efficiency".

2. Main commentaries and criticisms

The approach to efficiency measurement used in WHR 2000 is based on the parametric frontier estimation methods traditionally used in productivity analysis. These are analogous to usual statistical regression analyses, except that the 'error' term for any observation may be decomposed into two elements—the conventional two-sided random error, and a one-sided error attributable to inefficiency. Such productivity models have reached an advanced stage of econometric development, and have been applied in a number of different areas. The expert group assembled by WHO included some of the leading exponents of productivity modelling. It broadly endorsed the statistical approach used in WHR 2000, but it should be noted that there are those who contest the entire edifice on which modern productivity modelling is based (Newhouse 1994; Stone forthcoming).

Criticisms of the WHO methods can be considered under four headings: philosophical concerns, the theoretical production model, measurement issues, and estimation. As well as the published commentaries listed in the references below (e.g. Häkkinen 2000; Jamison and Sandbu 2001; McKee 2001; Navarro 2002; Oswaldo Cruz Foundation 2000; Gravelle et al. 2002; Grignon 2001; Richardson et al. 2002; Hollingsworth and Wildman 2002; etc.), we have also seen a number of as yet unpublished papers that we are unable to cite. We are grateful to these authors for the privileged access to their material. The concerns are listed without an attempt to judge their validity. SPRG comments and recommendations follow under heading 4 below.

Philosophical concerns

- The econometric methods used to estimate efficiency are both complex and relatively new. This makes understanding and interpretation difficult, especially for nations seeking to improve their health-system performance (Almeida et al. 2001).

- The use of the concept of efficiency may send a confused message when set alongside the objective of improving health outcomes. A country might have low absolute levels of health attainment but still be deemed technically efficient because it spends very little on its health system. The concept of efficiency makes no judgement about how much should be spent on health, but health outcomes can evidently be improved by higher expenditure.

■ The determinants of health-system performance are too complex to be reducible to a tractable statistical model, particularly in view of the poor quality of the data, the relatively small number of observations, and the lack of reliable time-series information.

■ Parametric statistical models traditionally focus on estimating the relationship between a stimulus (inputs) and a response (in this case, attainment) but not on the residual for an individual observation. In contrast, productivity models concentrate on these residuals, and therefore require much greater attention to be placed on model specification.

■ In particular, it can be argued that—in an application as complex as the WHO endeavour—it is inevitable that there is significant measurement error and that the model specification is incomplete. In these circumstances, little confidence can attach to the estimated measure of inefficiency.

■ The uncertainty analysis used by WHO is incomplete, as it does not fully consider modelling errors that are potentially important sources of uncertainty (see also Section XI).

■ Despite the progress made, there are numerous unresolved issues surrounding the methodology of productivity analysis. It may be premature to base definitive rankings of health systems on such developmental methodology.

The model of production

■ The technical consultation on 'Measurement of Efficiency of Health Systems' seemed to be comfortable with the use of a single production function (on the grounds that all countries have access to the same medical technologies). However, several commentators have argued that the health production function may not be identical between nations, suggesting that there is disagreement about whether the use of a single model is appropriate (Richardson et al. 2002; Häkkinen 2000; Nord 2002).

■ More generally, there is no consensus that the WHO approach uses an appropriate theoretical model of

the production process it seeks to capture (Pedersen 2002; Grignon 2001). For example, many of the outcome indicators in WHR 2000 are influenced strongly by factors other than the health system (e.g. war or diet), and these are inadequately captured in the WHO model of production. The treatment of income has generated particular debate. It is also argued that some of the outcome indicators—e.g. health inequality—are affected not just by the average level of inputs (e.g. education, income) but also by the distribution of inputs (inequalities in education, income) (Ammar and Awar 2001).

■ Although the proposed work on functions of the health system may help in the future, the methods used in WHR 2000 do not adequately model the 'reasons' why a given level of efficiency is observed (Grignon 2001; Pedersen 2002).

■ The chosen model does not recognize the important time lags that exist in producing health outcomes (Grignon 2001).

■ The need to calculate a "minimum" level of health attainment in the absence of a health system is contested (Gravelle et al. 2002; Häkkinen 2000).

Measurement issues

■ The description of the treatment of missing data is inadequate, as in the HSPA exercise as a whole (see Section XII). Estimates of missing data will be subject to considerable errors-in-variables, and hence will cause biases in parameter estimates and possibly in rankings (Almeida et al. 2001; Häkkinen 2000; Pedersen 2002).

■ The components of the efficiency model refer to different definitions of the health system – for example, the output measure refers to a very broad definition of the health system, whilst the input (expenditure) measure relates predominantly to expenditure on health care (Nord 2002).

■ The composite measure of output is highly contested and embraces numerous assumptions and value judgements (see Section XI), which have consequential implications for the efficiency measure.

■ Relative prices of inputs differ between nations, and estimates of total expenditure do not reflect the cost advantages in producing different outputs.

■ The measures of cost rely on PPP-adjusted estimates of expenditure, which are subject to error (in the absence of health-specific PPP factors), causing bias in parameter estimates and possibly in country ranks (Grignon 2001).

- Years of education is an inadequate proxy for external influences on health-system performance (Williams 2001; Jamison and Sandbu 2001; Häkkinen 2000; Grignon 2001).

- The methodology and data used to measure the "minimum" are contested (Williams 2001; Pedersen 2002).

Econometric methodology

- The use of the fixed-effects panel data estimator is inappropriate, given the very low degree of variation from one year to the next in most observations (Gravelle et al. 2002).

- The models used presume a fixed level of efficiency across the entire four-year period examined, which may be unrealistic (Pedersen 2002; Gravelle et al. 2002).

- The methods do not adequately treat the important contribution of income to the production of health and therefore to health system performance. The role of income needs to be properly modelled even if estimation turns out to be econometrically inconvenient (because income is highly correlated with both inputs and outputs) (Pedersen 2002).

- Formal model-selection techniques should be employed in choosing the preferred functional form for the model.

- More details are required on whether the chosen model passes the usual model misspecification statistical tests.

- There is evidence of a structural difference between developed and less-developed countries, implying the need for separate modelling (Richardson et al. 2002).

- Equally plausible alternative statistical model specifications can give rise to significantly different results (Gravelle et al. 2002; Hollingsworth and Wildman 2002; Richardson et al. 2002; Grignon 2001; Jamison and Sandbu 2001).

3. WHO RESPONSES AND PROPOSALS

The following detailed issues are highlighted in Section VI of the WHO Summary Document and in discussion documents prepared for SPRG, which include WHO proposals for further development of this work.

WHO proposes to continue developing the concept of efficiency on the grounds that health resources are scarce in all Member States. The Secretariat believes it is important to determine if those resources contribute to the greatest extent possible to the outcomes that people value. This is an important complement to the goal of finding additional resources for health.

(i) Timing
There are lags between the timing of health-system inputs and health outcomes. In WHR 2000 the assumption was made that current expenditures are highly correlated with past expenditures, but it would be preferable to use a time series of expenditures in explaining health outcomes and measuring efficiency. Data limitations prevented this in WHR 2000.

(ii) The minimum
In the absence of a health system population health (e.g. life expectancy at birth) would still be positive, so WHO argues that it is important to identify the minimum level. The minimum for WHR 2000 was estimated from limited data around 1900 when the modern health system did not exist. Only literacy was found to be correlated with health outcomes, but it would be useful to determine if there are other ways of defining the minimum.

(iii) Difficulty
Variations in the difficulty of translating inputs into outcomes were not fully captured in the production function in WHR 2000. Some, however, were subsequently analysed in the second-stage analysis.

(iv) Determinants of output
There is ongoing debate about the correct specification of the production function, but the Secretariat argues that it is critical to separate clearly the inputs to production from the factors that influence the efficiency of the production process.

(v) Determinants of efficiency
The technical consultation on this topic had suggested that the determinants of efficiency were better estimated at the same time as the estimation of efficiency rather than at a second stage, which was the approach adopted by WHO.

Because of the complexity of the issues surrounding efficiency, WHO has proposed some new analysis including: (a) estimating the traditional production function as a one-step process for efficiency simultaneously with the possible determinants; (b) a random-coefficients econometric specification of the production model. In terms of a new approach, WHO has proposed that the unobserved efficiency variable could be inferred from a multiple indicator model, which would use both the existing specification and additional models based on measures of process, such as coverage.

In light of this debate WHO proposes the following.

(i)   The questions of timing and how best to estimate the minimum are complex and the opinions of relevant outside experts will be sought. At the same time, the multiple indicator model approach is promising and should be developed further. This requires that the proposed work on coverage, discussed in Section IV of the SPRG report, should continue (with the World Health Survey providing the relevant information).

(ii) To address the question of timing, following discussion with SPRG two suggestions were made. The first was to estimate current HALE as a function of the series of past expenditures, or to use HALE at some time in the recent past, say five years ago, as a controlling variable. (The latter method has the drawback of lagged dependent variable models, while the former requires developing a historical time series of health expenditures.) The second proposal was to pursue the question of incidence-HALE—the HALE that is determined by this year's activities (Section V.A in the Summary Document). This has the advantage of being much more clearly determined by actions taken this year, but which will not produce an outcome until some time in the future. It would still be necessary to control for that part of incidence-HALE determined by actions taken in the past.

4. SPRG Comments and Recommendations

SPRG considers that there are strong arguments in favour of seeking to measure health system efficiency. Consideration of efficiency should—in principle—permit valid comparison of systems operating with different health expenditures and in different external environments. It could therefore make a vital contribution to HSPA. The WHO initiative has launched interesting technical debates and a research agenda that has the potential to advance rapidly our state of knowledge of health system performance. It has also stimulated the search for improved conceptual models

and data sources, and has made some innovative technical contributions to productivity analysis.

However, there are some important objections in principle to the method used by WHO, the most important of which are: (a) that the health system is too complex to be captured by these simple statistical models; (b) the data available are currently inadequate to support such an endeavour; and (c) the analysis is too demanding technically to be helpful to policy makers and other government officials.

In addition, it is possible to invoke numerous practical objections to the methods that have been applied, many of which are summarized above. Some of the most important are: (a) the treatment of missing data (applies to all of HSPA); (b) the treatment of influences on outcomes other than the health system; (c) the inadequate treatment of time lags; (d) the method of implementing some of the econometric techniques used; (e) the handling of uncertainty and sensitivity analysis.

We also believe that there should be complete 'transparency' of the research process relating to efficiency. As in much econometric work, the findings in WHR 2000 are the result of numerous technical judgements, and are not just the consequence of ineluctable scientific logic. Examples include the nature of the model of production, the concept of the "minimum", the treatment of missing data, and a series of econometric choices. We recognize that there may not always be consensus regarding the correct technical approach. However, it is in our view imperative that all technical judgements are capable of being understood, scrutinized and challenged by external observers. This requires preparation of a technical audit trail, publication of all methods used, and ready availability of data.

Recommendations

As the debate on WHR 2000 has demonstrated, any analysis of efficiency must be considered work-in-progress rather than a definitive judgement on health systems. On balance, we feel there is a case for continuing work in this area. However, we recommend that any continued WHO work on health-system efficiency should be presented as an ongoing research programme rather than a definitive judgement on health systems, and that progress should be reviewed at regular intervals.

The practice of publishing a league table of nations based on efficiency estimates has been highly contentious, but in the view of SPRG the decision to continue publishing league tables is a strategic and policy decision for WHO rather than a scientific one. Given the large number of technical problems that have still to be resolved, we recommend that this work should be developed further, and that any tables produced should be recognized as work-in-progress.

There are numerous possibilities for improving the data sources on which the efficiency rankings are based. These include improvement in the measurement metrics and the treatment of missing data (considered elsewhere in this report), and where possible the use of sub-national data sources. We recommend that WHO should make strenuous efforts to improve the quality and extent of data used in efficiency analysis (indeed in all of HSPA), and to adopt a transparent and careful approach to the treatment of missing data.

Particular concern has been expressed in the literature at the comparison of all health systems within a single model of production. It is possible that systems in different environmental circumstances are confronted with different production possibilities. We recommend that WHO should carefully explore the implications of incorporating environmental factors into the analysis, or developing separate models for different types of health system.

A particular conceptual weakness of methods to date has been the treatment of time. Measures of health outcome reflect years of health-system endeavour, while measures of expenditure refer to the current period. Furthermore, health-outcome measures are likely to be affected by factors other than the health system. These weaknesses suggest that contemporary measures of future (predicted) outcomes, e.g. certain process measures, may be more satisfactory measures of system performance than health-outcome measures. For this reason, we recommend that WHO should explore the scope for incorporating coverage and other measures of process into the model of efficiency.

The econometric analyses presented in WHR 2000 and subsequent variants exhibit some scientific weaknesses. We recommend that WHO engages in an ongoing consultative process with relevant experts to address the technical issues raised by outside commentators.

The treatment of uncertainty in WHR 2000 needs to be expanded as does the sensitivity analysis that was presented. We recommend that the method of modelling and presenting uncertainty should be reformulated to include a much broader scope of alternative models and assumptions.

The issues surrounding the measurement of efficiency are undoubtedly complex and require extensive data. Because of this complexity, we feel that in this area—perhaps more than in others—the input of a wide range of experts from different backgrounds is desirable. We recommend that WHO should actively consult and engage outside experts in the further development of this area, and that its analyses should be fully documented to maintain transparency.

REFERENCES

Almeida, CM, P. Braveman, MR Gold, CL Szwarcwald, JM Ribeiro, A Miglionico, JS Millar, S Porto, NR Costa, VO Rubio, M Segall, B Starfield, C Travassos, A Ugá, J Valente, and F Viacava (2001): Methodological concerns and recommendations on policy consequences of the World Health Report 2000. *Lancet,* 357(9269): 1692–1697.

Ammar, W and M Awar (2001): What does the World Health Report bring to Lebanon? *Lebanese Medical Journal,* 49(3).

Appleby, J and A Street (2001): Health system goals: life, death, and...football. *Journal of Health Services Research and Policy,* 6(4): 220–225.

Coyne, JS and PH Hilsenrath (2002): The World Health Report 2000: Can health care systems be compared using a single measure of performance? *American Journal of Public Health,* 92(1): 30–33.

Evans, D, A Tandon, CJL Murray, and J Lauer (2000): The comparative efficiency of health systems in producing health. Global Programme on Evidence for Health Policy Discussion Papers, No. 29. Geneva, Switzerland: World Health Organization.

Evans, D, A Tandon, CJL Murray, and J Lauer (2001): Comparative efficiency of national health systems: cross national econometric analysis. *British Medical Journal,* 323: 307–310.

Gravelle, H, R Jacobs, AM Jones, and A Street (2002): Comparing the efficiency of national health systems: econometric analysis should be handled with care. York: University of York. mimeo.

Grignon, M (2001): A southern European paradox: could reducing education budgets spur improvement in physicians performance? A propos World Health Report 2000. Paris: CREDES. mimeo.

Häkkinen, U (2000): Assessment of the goal attainment and efficiency of health systems in the World Health Report 2000. In eds. U Häkkinen and E Ollila. The World Health Report 2000: What does it tell us about health systems? Analyses by Finnish Experts. Helsinki: National Research and Development Center for Welfare and Health (STAKES). *http://www.stakes.fi/english/ publicati/Publications.htm*

Hollingsworth, B and J Wildman (2002): The efficiency of health production: Re-estimating the WHO panel data using parametric and non-parametric approaches to provide additional information. Melbourne: Monash University. mimeo.

Jamison, DT and ME Sandbu (2001): Global health: WHO ranking of health system performance. *Science*, 293(5535): 1595–1596.

McKee, M (2001): Measuring the efficiency of health systems. *British Medical Journal*, 323(7308): 295–296.

Navarro, V (2000): Assessment of the World Health Report 2000. *Lancet*, 356(9241): 1598–1601.

Navarro, V (2002): The World Health Report 2000: Can health care systems be compared using a single measure of performance? *American Journal of Public Health*, 92(1): 31–34.

Newhouse, M (1994): Frontier estimation: how useful a tool for health economics. *Journal of Health Economics*, 13: 317–322.

Nord, E (2002): Measures of goal attainment and performance: A brief, critical consumer guide. *Health Policy*, 59(3): 183–191.

Oswaldo Cruz Foundation, Brazilian Ministry of Health (2000): Report of the workshop "Health Systems Performance: The World Health Report 2000". 14-12-2000, Rio de Janeiro.

Pedersen, KM (2002): The World Health Report 2000: Dialog of the deaf? *Health Economics*, 11: 93–101.

Richardson, J, I Robertson, and J Wildman (2002): A Critique of the World Health Organisation's Evaluation of Health System Performance. Melbourne: Monash University. mimeo.

Rosén, M (2001): Can the WHO Health Report improve the performance of health systems? *Scandinavian Journal of Public Health*, 29(1): 76–80.

Stone, M (forthcoming): How not to measure the efficiency of public services (and how one might). *Journal of the Royal Statistical Society, Series A*.

Tandon, A, CJL Murray, J Lauer, and D Evans (2000): Measuring overall health system achievement for 191 countries. Global Programme on Evidence for Health Policy Discussion Papers, No. 30. Geneva, Switzerland: World Health Organization.

Williams, A (2000): Science or marketing at WHO? A Commentary on 'World Health 2000'. *Health Economics*, 10(2): 93–100.

World Health Organization (2000): The World Health Report 2000. Health systems: improving performance. Geneva, Switzerland: World Health Organization.

World Health Organization (2001): Report on WHO meeting of experts on the measurement of efficiency of health systems. 1-8-2001, New Orleans.

XV. Enhancing Policy Relevance

1. WHR 2000

The results of the performance assessment exercise in WHR 2000 were presented in the Statistical Annex of the Report as:

- attainment on the five intrinsic goals separately;
- attainment on the composite index;
- efficiency in terms of average health level and in terms of the composite index.

All scores were presented in rank order, with uncertainty intervals around the scores and ranks. In the overview and the first two chapters of the Report there was discussion of the potential policy uses of quantitative analysis of the health-system goals. The four chapters on functions reviewed current evidence on the relation between outcomes and provision, resource generation, stewardship, and different ways of financing. The Report did not provide country-specific interpretation of this analysis but drew general conclusions about the type of strategies which will enhance performance.

2. Main Commentaries and Criticisms

The policy uses of ranking

There was mixed feeling at the regional consultations about the value of publishing overall attainment and efficiency scores and the accompanying rankings. This topic is discussed elsewhere (see Sections XI and XIV). In relation to rankings, some participants in regional consultations argued that the overall attainment and efficiency estimates should not be reported country-by-country. An alternative suggestion was to group countries by level of attainment, e.g. high, medium and low. However, other participants saw the value of ranking as a means of focusing the attention of policy makers on the health system and its performance. Rosén (2001) welcomed the "underlying idea of generating a discussion on how well health systems function in different countries by openly reporting comparative statistics". Navarro (2001) takes a similar stance. Appleby and Street (2001) comment on how information, and ranking in particular, may be used

in different ways by policy makers and the public. In the Summary Document prepared for SPRG, WHO states that: "A tentative conclusion is that rankings are not of particular interest to the technical experts required to take the steps necessary to improve performance—although comparisons of country performance with that in a reference group of countries is useful for this purpose. However, rankings provide the means of gaining the attention of the key decision-makers who are in the position to provide more resources for health and to take the necessary actions required to demonstrate a political will to improving the performance of health systems."

Multiple goals

The fact that the WHO framework explicitly recognizes there are multiple goals for a health system has been welcomed as being useful for policy purposes (Walt and Mills 2001; McKee 2001). Appleby and Street (2001) particularly note that it is useful in thinking about trade-offs between goals.

Procedural concerns

Other comments were of a procedural nature. For example, government officials argued that countries need to be given the opportunity to comment on the estimates before they are published, that they should be given substantial advance warning before data are released to the media, and decision makers and the media need to be given more information and assistance on how to respond to performance-assessment information. The latter concern applied particularly to the uncertainty intervals around the ranks, which were either ignored or misunderstood by the media.

The need to increase confidence in and ownership of results

The perceived policy relevance of the results was partly affected by concerns about the data and the methods used (see other Sections). In addition, it was noted that confidence and ownership of results would be enhanced by more national involvement in method development, and improved capacity to apply the complex methods and tools and to interpret the results.

Summary measures of outcomes are not sufficient for policy development purposes

The measures provide information on 'how well' a health system is performing, but not on 'why' it is performing as it is. Appleby and Street (2001) observe that if countries are to respond positively to HSPA, this involves finding variables that both explain performance and are open to policy manipulation. It is argued that additional information on determinants and on intermediate goals related to health-system functions, such as access, is essential for policy development (Almeida et al. 2001; Braveman et al. 2001; Makinen et al. 2000; Nord 2002; Van der Stuyft and Unger 2000; WHO Regional Office for the Americas 2001; WHO Regional Office for Africa 2001; WHO Regional Office for the Eastern Mediterranean 2001; WHO Regional Office for Europe 2001; WHO Regional Office for South-East Asia 2001). Subnational or sub-system analyses may also be needed for policy analysis and development (Wibulpolprasert and Tangcharoensathien 2001).

The need for an explicit strategy to link assessment to policy dialogue and system development

Since the publication of WHR 2000, many have argued that the links between the measurement of performance and the development of policy requires strengthening.

A number of commentators have observed that availability of relevant information does not necessarily lead to its 'use' (Kvale 2000).

3. WHO RESPONSES AND PROPOSALS

Since the publication of WHR 2000, a number of countries have expressed interest in active collaboration with WHO to assess the performance of their own systems and to use the evidence to formulate policies to improve performance. Participants in the regional consultations also emphasized that the links between the measurement of performance and the development of policy required strengthening. To meet the country requests and suggestions of the regional consultations, the Director-General decided to group efforts under the rubric of 'Enhancing Health Systems Performance Initiative'(EHSPI). Around 30 Member States expressed interest. WHO is currently working with 20 countries from different income ranges and WHO Regions. Reasons for engaging include:

- assessment of the performance of their own health systems, or sub-systems, using the WHO framework;

- assessment of their own performance using better data than was available to WHO;

- development of national skills in the required methodologies;

- seeking support from WHO for the development of health policies and systems using the available evidence;

- contributing to the development of more practical tools for translating evidence into policy, particularly related to the four functions;

- the search for greater contact with and opportunities for learning about health systems in other countries.

EHSPI has both national and global objectives. At a national level, the aims are to:

- enable policy makers to have a better understanding of their health system's performance, and to feed this information into a national policy debate;

- link evidence to actions to improve performance;

- develop greater national capacity to monitor and improve performance.

The country level work interacts with the two global objectives:

- further development of the conceptual framework and methods;

- development of a better international evidence-base for policy advice.

Strategies to meet these objectives are discussed under the following four headings.

(i) Describing and understanding health-system performance

Outcomes. Initial work has shown that working closely with countries to carry out their own baseline assessment of attainment on the intrinsic goals is extremely useful for identifying new data sources, for undertaking new data collection where required, and for refining the indicators. For example, some countries have been interested in testing what mode of survey is the most cost-effective in obtaining the desired information, so more than one modality has been tested. Others have provided feedback which has helped to modify the indicators of the intrinsic goals or the questionnaire of the World Health Survey.

Inputs. To date, most attention has focused on improving estimates of health expenditures in countries lacking national health accounts. There are several regional initiatives supporting National Health Accounts (NHA) construction, and EHSPI has facilitated their support. A Producer's Guide to National Health Accounts for Low and Middle Income Countries,[1] jointly authored by WHO, the World Bank and USAID, will soon be published in English, French and Spanish. This interaction with NHA networks seems the most appropriate way to build evidence in this respect.

Functions. A number of countries have requested help to measure the performance of the four basic functions in their country settings. To this end, the major emphasis has been on defining an indicator of service provision that is more useful for policy than geographical access. A number of countries are testing the new WHO tool to measure effective coverage.

(ii) Implementation: linking evidence to policy

A number of participant countries have held national seminars to introduce a wider range of decision makers and researchers to the performance assessment approach, and to discuss the policy implications of findings from the baseline analysis. In addition, WHO is providing direct policy support to a small number of countries, incorporating the new information being generated from these efforts.

(iii) Sub-national performance assessment

Some have suggested that the assessment framework could be helpful in assessing and improving the performance of sub-national units. It could then become a tool for more effective stewardship and management. There will be an international meeting in 2002 to discuss the practical and methodological challenges in adapting the framework.

(iv) Building capacity in health-system performance assessment and analysis

For health systems performance assessment to be sustainable at the country level, capacity for both the diagnostic and implementation phases must be built. A variety of strategies have been piloted—ranging from straightforward briefings on using the methods, to technical support to analysts in-country or at WHO,

to formal training workshops. There have been international workshops in South Africa and Indonesia (in English), in China, and one for French speakers is scheduled in Africa in 2002.

WHO proposals for increasing policy relevance

(i) Increasing the knowledge base on health systems

- *Helping Member States monitor health-system performance*
  WHO will support the generation of better national information through the joint development of reliable, practical methods and tools, for example the World Health Survey; the CHOICE initiative (CHOosing Interventions that are Cost-Effective); tools for monitoring functions and sub-national health-system performance.

- *Policy options for health-system financing and human resources*
  WHO is building a more evidence-based understanding of policy options in health financing and human resources across the Organization.

(ii) Country support and capacity-building

- *Building national skills in the generation of information*
  Continuing the strategies mentioned above, there will also be more effort to develop local networks to provide country to country support.

- *Strengthening national health-information systems*
  Several countries wish to link baseline assessment with efforts to improve information systems. WHO proposes to take an information needs-oriented view of information system development, and review how to combine strategies such as sentinel surveillance and periodic surveys with routine facility-based reporting systems.

- *National capacity to use evidence for policy and management*
  WHO is developing a variety of strategies to build skills in policy analysis and development: national health policy reviews; the Management Effectiveness Programme; rapid health system assessments.

(iii) Expanding WHO inter-country networks on health systems
  There is a need for a more systematic approach to facilitating cross-country support in assessment and policy analysis. Existing global and regional networks include the Regional Observatories; the national health accounts partnerships; the Global

Alliance for Health Policy and Systems Research; and professional and provider networks. Where appropriate and needed, these will be more systematically strengthened. EHSPI will evolve into a network that brings together those that generate and those that use evidence.

4. SPRG COMMENTS AND RECOMMENDATIONS

SPRG noted the experience of UNICEF which presents a ranking of the performance of individual countries in its publication 'Progress of Nations'. In this publication, UNICEF reviews broad issues affecting child health and welfare but it also includes tables showing specific health achievements of individual countries in relation to their Gross National Product (GNP). From the analysis, UNICEF presents a measure called "National Performance Gap" (NPG) which is derived from the observed health indicator compared with the predicted level on the basis of the nation's GNP. This analysis has been presented for such indicators as the Under-Five Mortality Rate (U5MR), the Maternal Mortality Ratio (MMR), childhood malnutrition, etc. For example, in the case of U5MR, the national performance gap in a particular country is the difference between the actual level of U5MR and the expected level. The expected level of performance for U5MR is derived by fitting a curve to country data represented by points on a graph whose axes are GNP per capita and U5MR. The curve is fitted to match the overall shape of the country data points, using a least-squares regression method. The expected level of performance is the level predicted by the regression line for each level of GNP per capita. The NPG enables each country to assess its performance relative to its level of national income. It draws the attention of a country that is performing worse than predicted according to its GNP per capita. This gap serves to highlight problems that need special attention. Health authorities find such ranking that is based on clearly defined objective criteria easy to understand and acceptable.

Members of SPRG observed that when moving from diagnosis to policy formulation, policy makers can be faced with an overwhelming amount of information, and ways of showing the potential effects of different policy options would be useful. It was also noted in SPRG that much discussion has focused on WHO reaching top policy makers, but there are also national responsibilities in increasing the use of evidence, by orienting technocrats with managerial responsibilities.

SPRG emphasized that WHO needs to ensure that the public understands the key messages from health systems performance assessment. It will be essential for WHO to think of how to handle public relations at the global as well as national levels for the next Report on HSPA. Access to information on health systems will also be improved through the wider dissemination of country-specific analyses both in electronic and printed form.

SPRG noted that WHO will be unable to meet all demands for direct country support on health systems.

In the Summary Document WHO states that it hopes EHSPI would provide a platform to ensure the policy relevance of HSPA, and to develop national capacities for monitoring and improving performance. The initiative could also have the external benefit of contributing to the further development of the tools and methods as well as to contributing to the evidence-base for health policy advice.

SPRG recommends that WHO continue exploring this approach as a vehicle for constructive engagement with countries on health system performance and ways of improving it. It should also collaborate with countries in the development of practical methods and tools, and provide opportunities to strengthen national capacity in conducting analysis of the performance of national institutions and programmes within the health system. EHSPI will also be of value to other stakeholders in the health field. Whilst the primary focus should be on working with governments, WHO should ensure that other relevant stakeholders are informed and involved. A broad programme of technical assistance based upon the EHSPI experience should be considered.

In terms of increasing policy relevance, it is important that WHO develop indicators of the different health system functions. One can envisage a 'core' group of indicators that could be used in every country, which would facilitate comparisons of performance between health systems. Another more detailed set of function indicators could provide a menu from which Member States can select additional items. SPRG suggests that some basic principles be observed during the development of indicators of health-system functions. The indicators should:

- be policy relevant;

- be easy to use and to understand;

- be sensitive to changes in both directions;

- provide clues about the factors influencing level and change, especially those within the purview of the health system;

- be sustainable, i.e. affordable, reliably collected, and within the capacity of host countries to produce;

- be compatible with local culture and social systems.

NOTES

1 These will appear in the NHA Producer's Guide currently under preparation. It is co-funded by the World Bank, WHO and USAID, and is being jointly prepared by those agencies and a team from the Harvard School of Public Health.

REFERENCES

Almeida, CM, P Braveman, MR Gold, CL Szwarcwald, JM Ribeiro, A Miglionico, JS Millar, S Porto, NR Costa, VO Rubio, M Segall, B Starfield, C Travassos, A Ugá, J Valente, and F Viacava (2001): Methodological concerns and recommendations on policy consequences of the World Health Report 2000. *Lancet*, 357(9269): 1692–1697.

Appleby, J and A Street (2001): Health system goals: life, death, and...football. *Journal of Health Services Research and Policy*, 6(4): 220–225.

Braveman, P, B Starfield, and HJ Geiger (2001): World Health Report 2000: How it removes equity from the agenda for public health monitoring and policy. *British Medical Journal*, 323(7314): 678–681.

Kvale, G (2000): Inequalities in health. Feedback. *Bulletin of the World Health Organization*, 78(6): 856.

McKee, M (2001): Measuring the efficiency of health systems. *British Medical Journal*, 323(7308): 295–296.

Makinen, M, H Waters, M Rauch, N Almagambetova, R Bitran, L Gilson, D McIntyre, S Pannarunothai, AL Prieto, G Ubilla, and S Ram (2000): Inequalities in health care use and expenditures: empirical data from eight developing countries and countries in transition. *Bulletin of the World Health Organization*, 78(1): 55–65.

Navarro, V (2001): World Health Report 2000: Response to Murray and Frenk. *Lancet*, 357(9269): 1701–1702.

Navarro, V (2002): The World Health Report 2000: Can health care systems be compared using a single measure of performance? *American Journal of Public Health*, 92(1): 31–34.

Nord, E (2002): Measures of goal attainment and performance: A brief, critical consumer guide. *Health Policy*, 59(3): 183–191.

Rosén, M (2001): Can the WHO Health Report improve the performance of health systems? *Scandinavian Journal of Public Health*, 29(1): 76–80.

Van der Stuyft, P and JP Unger (2000): Improving the performance of health systems: The World Health Report as go-between for scientific evidence and ideological discourse. *Tropical Medicine and International Health*, 5(10): 675–677.

Walt, G and A Mills (2001): World Health Report 2000: Comments. *Lancet*, 357(9269): 1702–1703.

Wibulpolprasert, S and V Tangcharoensathien (2001): Health systems performance: What's next?. *Bulletin of the World Health Organization*, 79(6): 489.

WHO Regional Office for the Americas (2001): Regional consultation of the Americas on Health Systems Performance Assessment: Final Report. 8-5-2001, Washington, D.C.

WHO Regional Office for Africa (2001): General Report on the Regional Consultative Meeting on Health Systems Performance Assessment: Final Report. 18-5-2001, Harare, Zimbabwe.

WHO Regional Office for the Eastern Mediterranean (2001): Report on the Regional Consultation on the Conceptual Framework for Health System Performance Assessment. 9-7-2001, Ain Saadeh, Lebanon.

WHO Regional Office for Europe (2001): Report of the Regional Consultation on Health Systems Performance Assessment. 3-9-2001, Copenhagen.

WHO Regional Office for South-East Asia (2001): Report of the regional consultation and technical workshop on health systems performance assessment. 18-6-2001, New Delhi, India.

ANNEX 61.1
MEMBERS OF THE SCIENTIFIC PEER REVIEW GROUP WITH INSTITUTIONAL AFFILIATIONS

Walid Ammar
Director-General
Ministry of Public Health
Lebanon

Sudhir Anand, Chair
Professor of Economics
University of Oxford
United Kingdom

Katarzyna Kissimova-Skarbek
Krakow School of Public Health
Poland

John Eisenberg*
Director
Agency for Healthcare Research and Quality
  (AHRQ)
United States of America

Timothy Evans
Director, Health Equity
The Rockefeller Foundation
United States of America

Toshihiko Hasegawa
Director, Department of Health Care Policy
National Institute of Health Services Managements
Japan

Ana Langer
Regional Director, Latin America and the Caribbean
Population Council
Mexico

Adetokunbo O. Lucas
Adjunct Professor of International Health
Harvard School of Public Health
United States of America

Lindiwe Makubalo
Chief Director, Epidemiology Research and
  Evaluation
Department of Health
South Africa

Alireza Marandi
Chairman of the Board of Trustees
Chairman of the Board of Directors
Breastfeeding Promotion Society
Iran

Gregg Meyer**
Director, Center for Quality Measurement and
  Improvement
Agency for Healthcare Research and Quality
  (AHRQ)
United States of America

Andrew Podger***
The Secretary
Department of Health and Aged Care
Australia

Peter Smith
Professor of Economics
Centre for Health Economics (CHE)
University of York
United Kingdom

Suwit Wibulpolprasert
Ministry of Public Health
Thailand

---

*   John Eisenberg regretfully passed away on 10 March
      2002
**   Gregg Meyer joined SPRG in March 2002
***   Andrew Podger was appointed Public Services Commis-
      sioner, Commonwealth of Australia, shortly before the
      final meeting of SPRG

ANNEX 61.2
WHO MEETINGS AND CONSULTATIONS ON HEALTH SYSTEMS PERFORMANCE ASSESSMENT

1. Conference on Summary Measures of Population Health, Marrakech, Morocco, 6–9 December 1999

2. 1st Preparatory Working Group Meeting on Measuring Health Status, Geneva, Switzerland, 2–3 August 2000

3. 2nd Preparatory Working Group Meeting on Measuring Health Status, Geneva, Switzerland, 4–5 September 2000

4. Meeting of Committee of Experts on Measurement and Classification for Health, Geneva, Switzerland, 11–12 September 2000

5. Joint ECE/WHO Expert Meeting on Measuring Health Status, Ottawa, Canada, 23–25 October 2000

6. Meeting on Health Systems Performance Measurement, New Orleans, USA, 8 January 2001

7. Regional Consultation of the Americas on Health Systems Performance Assessment, WHO/AMRO, Washington, USA, 8–10 May 2001

8. Regional Consultation and Technical Workshop on Health Systems Performance Assessment, WHO/SEARO, New Delhi, India, 18–21 June 2001

9. Regional Consultation on Health System Performance, WHO/WPRO, Manila, Philippines, 3–5 July 2001

10. Regional Consultation on the Conceptual Framework for Health System Performance Assessment, WHO/EMRO, Ain Saadeh, Lebanon, 9–11 July 2001

11. Regional Consultative Meeting on Health Systems Performance Assessment, WHO/AFRO, Harare, Zimbabwe, 18–20 July 2001

12. Technical Consultation on Effective Coverage in Health Systems, Rio de Janeiro, Brazil, 27–29 August 2001

13. Regional Consultation on Health Systems Performance Assessment, WHO/EURO, Copenhagen, Denmark, 3–4 September 2001

14. Meeting on the Stewardship Function in health systems, Geneva, Switzerland, 10–11 September 2001

15. Meeting on Responsiveness Concepts and Measurement, Geneva, Switzerland, 13–14 September 2001

16. Meeting on statistical methods for enhancing the cross-population comparability of survey results, Cambridge, Massachusetts, USA, 1–2 October 2001

17. Meeting on Fairness of Financial Contribution, Geneva, Switzerland, 4–5 October 2001

18. Technical Consultation on the Measurement of Health Inequalities, Geneva, Switzerland, 7–8 November 2001

Index